# Infertility:  Male and Female

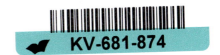

To our sons, Eytan, Yoram and Ron,
and to Danny who lives in our hearts.

*For Churchill Livingstone:*
*Publisher:* Peter Richardson
*Project Editor:* Lucy Gardner
*Copy Editor:* Pat Croucher
*Production Controller:* Neil Dickson
*Sales Promotion Executive:* Kathy Crawford

# Infertility:  Male and Female

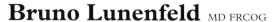

Edited

## Vaclav Insler MD FRCOG

Professor of Obstetrics and Gynaecology, Hebrew
University Hadassah Medical School, Jerusalem;
Director, Department of Obstetrics and Gynaecology,
Kaplan Hospital, Rehovot, Israel

## Bruno Lunenfeld MD FRCOG

Professor and Director, Institute of Endocrinology, The
Chaim Sheba Medical Center and Bar-Ilan University,
Israel

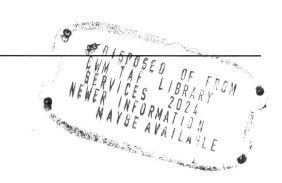
SECOND EDITION

## CHURCHILL LIVINGSTONE

EDINBURGH LONDON MADRID MELBOURNE NEW YORK AND TOKYO 1993

CHURCHILL LIVINGSTONE
Medical Division of Longman Group UK Limited

Distributed in the United States of America by Churchill
Livingstone Inc., 650 Avenue of the Americas, New York,
N.Y. 10011, and by associated companies, branches and
representatives throughout the world.

First edition 1986
Second edition 1993

ISBN 0-443-04514-3

**British Library of Cataloguing in Publication Data**
A catalogue record for this book is available from the British Library.

**Library of Congress Cataloging-in-Publication Data**
Infertility: male and female/edited by Vaclav Insler, Bruno
　　Lunenfeld. —2nd ed.
　　　　　p.　　cm
　　　　Includes bibliographical references and index.
　　　　ISBN 0-443-04514-3
　　　　I. Infertility.　I. Insler, Vaclav.　II. Lunenfeld, Bruno.
　　　　[DNLM: 1.　Infertility, Female.　2. Infertility, Male.
　　WP 570 I4375]
　　RC889.I5634　1993
　　616.692—dc20
　　DNLM/DLC
　　for Library of Congress　　　　　　　　　92–48779
　　　　　　　　　　　　　　　　　　　　　　　　CIP

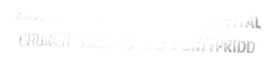

The
publisher's
policy is to use
**paper manufactured
from sustainable forests**

Printed and bound in Great Britain by
William Clowes Limited, Beccles and London

# Contents

# Contributors

**Jonathan Arbelle** MD
Lecturer, Department of Medicine,
Endocrinology Unit, Faculty of Health Sciences,
Ben Gurion University of the Negev, Soroka
Medical Center, Beer Sheva, Israel

**Benjamin Bartoov** PhD
Associate Professor, Department of Life
Sciences, Bar-Ilan University, Ramat-Gan, Israel;
Director, Male Fertility Unit, Meir Hospital,
Kfar-Saba, Israel

**Ruth Braw-Tal** PhD
A. R. O., The Volcani Center, Institute of
Animal Science, Bet Dagan, Israel

**Meinert Breckwoldt** MD
Professor and Director, Department of Obstetrics
and Gynaecology, Albert-Ludwigs-University,
Freiburg, Germany

**Cosima Brucker** MD
Scientific Assistant, Women's Hospital, Ludwig-
Maximilians, University, Munich, Germany

**Eliahu Caspi** MD
Professor of Obstetrics and Gynaecology, Asaf
Harofe Medical Center, Sackler School of
Medicine, Tel Aviv University, Tel Aviv, Israel

**Melvin R. Cohen** MD BS MS
Professor Emeritus, Northwestern University
School of Medicine, Department of Obstetrics
and Gynecology, Section of Endocrinology and
Infertility, Chicago, USA

**Alan H. De Cherney** MD
Louis E. Phaneuf Professor and Chairman,
Department of Obstetrics and Gynecology, New
England Medical Centre, Tufts University
School of Medicine, Boston, USA

**Frank D. De Leon** MD
Associate Professor, Department of Obstetrics
and Gynecology, Northwestern University,
Chicago, USA

**Emilio del Pozo** MD
Associate Professor of Medicine, University of
Basle, Switzerland

**Norbert Gleicher** MD
Professor of Obstetrics and Gynecology, and
Immunology/Microbiology/UHS/CMS;
President, The Center for Human Reproduction,
Chicago, USA

**Marek Glezerman** MD
Professor and Chairman, Departments of
Obstetrics and Gynecology, Soroka Medical
Center of Kupath Holim, Faculty of Health
Sciences, Ben Gurion University, Beer Sheba,
Israel

**Seymour M. Glick** MD
Gussie Krupp Professor of Medicine, Ben Gurion
University Health Sciences Center, Soroka
Medical Center, Beer Sheba, Israel

**Abraham Golan** MD MRCOG
Senior Lecturer, Department of Obstetrics and
Gynaecology, Assaf Harofe Medical Center, the
Sackler School of Medicine, Tel Aviv University,
Israel

**Victor Gomel** MD FRCS(C) FACOG
Professor and Head, Department of Obstetrics
and Gynecology, Faculty of Medicine, University
of British Columbia, and University and
Grace Hospitals, Vancouver, Canada

**E. S. E. Hafez** PhD (Cantab)
Executive Director, Reproductive Health Center, Kiawah Island, USA

**Gerhard Haidl** Dr med habil
Privat Dozent, Centre of Dermatology and Andrology, Justus-Liebig-University, Giessen, Germany

**Ilana Harman-Boehm** MD
Senior Lecturer, Division of Medicine, Ben Gurion University, Faculty of Health Sciences, Soroka Medical Center, Beer Sheba, Israel

**Ron Hauser** MD
Senior Physician, The Institute for the Study of Fertility, Serlin Maternity Hospital, Tel Aviv University, Israel

**Arie Herman** MD
Lecturer, Department of Obstetrics and Gynaecology, Assaf Harofe Medical Center, The Sackler School of Medicine, Tel Aviv University, Israel

**Z. T. Hommonnai** MD
Associate Professor, Tel Aviv University, Israel

**Vaclav Insler** MD FRCOG
Professor of Obstetrics and Gynecology, Hebrew University Hadassah Medical School, Jerusalem; Director, Department of Obstetrics and Gynaecology, Kaplan Hospital, Rehovot, Israel

**Elizabeth Johannisson** MD PhD
Professor, International Commitee for Research in Reproduction, Laboratory of Analytical and Quantitative Cytology (LAQC), Geneva, Switzerland

**Howard W. Jones Jr.** MD
Professor of Obstetrics and Gynecology, Eastern Virginia Medical School, Norfolk, Virginia; Chairman, Jones Institute for Reproductive Medicine, Norfolk, Virginia; Professor Emeritus, Gynecology and Obstetrics, Johns Hopkins School of Medicine, Baltimore, Maryland, USA

**J. Kremer** MD
Retired Professor in Obstetrics and Gynaecology, The Netherlands

**Herbert Kuhl** MD
Professor, Department of Gynaecology and Endocrinology, Universitats-Frauenklinik, Frankfurt am Main, Germany

**Lawrence M. Lewin** PhD
Professor and Head, Department of Chemical Pathology, Sackler School of Medicine, Tel Aviv University, Ramat Aviv, Israel

**Yair Liel** MD
Senior Lecturer, in Internal Medicine and Endocrinology, Soroka Medical Center of Kupat-Holim and the Faculty of Health Sciences, Ben Gurion University of the Negev, Beer Sheva, Israel

**Bruno Lunenfeld** MD FRCOG
Professor and Director, Institute of Endocrinology, The Chaim Sheba Medical Center and Bar-Ilan University, Israel

**Eitan Lunenfeld** MD
Fertility and IVF Unit, Department of Obstetrics and Gynaecology, Soroka Medical Center and Faculty of Health Sciences, Ben-Gurion University of the Negev, Beer Sheba, Israel

**Peter F. McComb** MB BS FRCSC FACOG
Professor, Division of Reproductive Endocrinology and Infertility, Department of Obstetrics and Gynaecology, University of British Columbia, Vancouver, Canada

**Kamran S. Moghissi** MD
Professor of Obstetrics and Gynecology and Director, Division of Reproductive Endocrinology and Infertility, Wayne State University School of Medicine, Hutzel Hospital, Detroit, USA

**H. Nachum** LPT
Medical Technical Assistant, IVF Unit, Department of Obstetrics and Gynaecology, Assaf Harofe Medical Center, The Sackler School of Medicine, Tel Aviv University, Israel

**J. Neulen** MD
Privat Dozent, Universitäts-Frauenklinik, Albert-Ludwigs University, Freiburg im Breis gau, Germany

**Gedalia F. Paz** PhD
Professor, Institute for the Study of Fertility, Serlin Maternity Hospital, Tel-Aviv, Israel

**Reuven Reich** PhD
Lecturer, Department of Pharmacology, Hebrew University of Jerusalem, Israel

**Raphael Ron-El** MD
Senior Lecturer, Department of Obstetrics and Gynaecology, Assaf Harofe Medical Center, The Sackler School of Medicine, Tel Aviv University, Israel

**Timothy Rowe** MB BS FRCSC FRCOG
Associate Professor, Department of Obstetrics and Gynaecology, University of British Columbia, Vancouver, Canada

**Kenneth J. Ryan** MD
Professor and Chairman, Obstetrics, Gynecology and Reproductive Biology, Harvard Medical School, Brigham and Women's Hospital, Boston, USA

**Wolf-Bernhard Schill** Dr med Dr med habil
Professor and Chairman, Department of Dermatology and Andrology, University of Giessen, Giessen, Germany

**Robert Schoysman** MD
Professor of Obstetrics, Vrije Universiteit, Brussels, Belgium

**Y. Soffer** MD
Senior Lecturer in Obstetrics and Gynecology, Tel Aviv University, Israel; Head, Male Infertility Clinic, Department of Obstetrics and Gynecology, Assaf Harofe Medical Center, Zenfin, Israel

**Manfred Stauber** MD
Professor, I. Universitaets-Frauenklinik, Munchen, Germany

**Patrick Taylor** MD
Professor, Department of Obstetrics and Gynaecology, University of British Columbia; Head, Department of Obstetrics and Gynaecology, St Paul's Hospital, Vancouver, Canada

**H.-D. Taubert** Dr med
Professor of Gynaecologic Endocrinology, Department of Obstetrics and Gynaecology, J.-W. Goethe-University, Frankfurt am Main, Germany

**Alex Tsafriri** PhD
Professor, Department of Hormone Research, The Weizman Institute of Science, Rehovot, Israel

**Pedro Verdugo** MD
Professor, Assistant Director, Center for Bioengineering, University of Washington, Seattle, USA

**Manuel Villalón** PhD
Assistant Professor, Unit of Reproduction and Developmental Biology, Department of Physiological Sciences, P. Catholic University of Chile, Santiago, Chile

**Haim Yavetz** MD
Senior Physician, Institute for the Study of Fertility, Serlin Maternity Hospital, Elias Sourasky Medical Center, Sackler School of Medicine, Tel Aviv University, Israel

**Leah Yogev** PhD
Senior Investigator, Soferman Institute for the Study of Fertility, Maternity Hospital, Tel Aviv, Israel

**H. P. Zahradnik** Prof Dr mcd
Leitender Oberarzt der Universitäts-Frauenklinik II, Freiburg, Germany

# Preface

During the last few years formidable progress has been made in reproductive biology and medicine. Sophisticated combination of genetic engineering with molecular biology techniques enabled identification of genes controlling the production and function of numerous hormones, growth factors and their specific receptors. Developments in organic chemistry facilitated manufacture of new artificial hormones more potent and active than their natural models. Refined blend of genetic engineering and biochemistry allowed the constitution of recombinant growth hormone, insulin, follicle stimulating hormone and luteinizing hormone. The assisted reproduction techniques have been refined and numerous new modifications were introduced. Reproductive medicine has entered a new era carrying a promise of great advancement and opening of new horizons.

In 1986, in the preface to the first edition of *Infertility: Male and Female* we stated that the amount of information generated by theoretical and clinical research in the field of reproductive physiology and infertility has been constantly increasing at a tremendous rate. Five years later, in 1991, we realized how true this statement was. Indeed, to keep abreast with the new developments the book had to be extensively updated and, to a large extent, virtually re-written. The result of those reflections is the second edition of *Infertility*. In preparing it we have tried to preserve the general philosophy applied in the first edition.

Most of the chapters have been changed and updated by the original authors. Six chapters have been written by new contributors. The general structure of the book remains essentially unchanged. Only three old chapters have been omitted and two entirely new chapters added. The amount of new data which has had to be integrated in the second edition resulted in enlargement of the volume by about 30%. We sincerely hope, however, that the readers who liked the first edition will find that the dominant principles, i.e. critical analysis of data, juxtaposition of scientific and clinical findings, unified approach to diagnosis and therapy, and consideration of male and female infertility as a joint problem of the couple, are maintained also in the new text.

We would like to express our appreciation to all the authors who willingly changed and updated their previous chapters. We are also grateful to the colleagues who wrote the new chapters, sometimes at very short notice, and did an excellent job. Thanks are also due to Ms Lucy Gardner and Ms Janice Urquhart of Churchill Livingstone, for their help and co-operation in producing this volume.

Tel-Aviv 1993
V. Insler
B. Lunenfeld

# Introduction

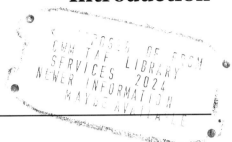

# 1. Infertility: the dimension of the problem

*Bruno Lunenfeld    Vaclav Insler*

## INFERTILITY: FUNDAMENTAL ASPECTS

Infertility is seldom, if ever, a physically debilitating disease. It may may, however, severely affect the couple's psychological harmony, sexual life and social function. Even in those societies which made family planning and birth control their official policy and social vogue, the individual couple desiring a child but unable to conceive one feels demeaned, deprived and bitter. In some cultures, childlessness may cast a heavy shadow on the physiological and social adequacy of the female and diminish the social standing of the male partner. Whatever the demographic policy of the Government and regardless of the aims proclaimed and/or pursued by the society, the individual family perceives its freedom to procreate as a most basic human right. Most cultures regard children as an extension of self, as bearers and perpetuators of the family name and tradition as well as an expansion of one's hopes, aims and strivings. The inability to procreate is thus always perceived as a denial of basic rights, an injustice and a disappointment, sometimes bordering on grief.

Most childless couples must cope with difficult psychological, family and social problems (see Chapter 28). The examination and treatment of infertility may pose additional psychological difficulties, interfere with the sexual life of the couple, and impose a financial burden on the family or on society.

Since the beginning of recorded history, the human race has placed emphasis on fertility. In the Judeo-Christian tradition, the importance of procreation is inherent in man's very creation: 'So God created man in His own image, in the image of God created He him; male and female created He them. And God blessed them, and God said unto them: Be fruitful and multiply and replenish the earth and subdue it' (Genesis 1: 27-28). Nothing more vividly demonstrates the importance of fertility to the individual than the reaction by and to those who do not have children. The grief of a woman who has failed to bear a liveborn child is no less in modern society than it was for our forefathers.

## INFERTILITY: DIMENSION OF THE PROBLEM

The estimates of prevalence and/or incidence of infertility are based on either demographic data or on health-service statistics. These sources produce diverse and inaccurate assessments. Belsey (1986) using data collected by WHO projected the prevalence of infertility among the world population. Arithmetic recalculation of those data indicated that according to demographic estimates the prevalence of infertility among the female population in the fertile age groups would be approximately 50% (including women who are fertile but perceive themselves as infertile and those of unproven fertility). As reported by health services the incidence or infertility was calculated to be approximately 16.7% (Figs 1.1, 1.2)

WHO (1991), in the framework of the Programme on Maternal and Child Health and Family Planning, Division of Family Health, collected and carefully analysed 392 publications concerning the incidence of infertility in 89 countries on five continents. Depending on geographical area, type of population, source of

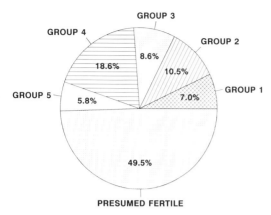

**Fig. 1.1** Prevalence of infertility in the world population calculated from demographic data. Group 1, fertile but perceiving themselves as infertile; Group 2, primary infertility; Group 3, secondary infertility; Group 4, unknown fertility; Group 5, voluntary infertility.

data and methods of their assessment, the incidence of infertility was estimated to range from 0.4% to 66.6% and that of childlessness from 0.6% to 58%. This unique study is of special interest and remarkable importance for several reasons: it reveals the impact of environmental, cultural and socioeconomic factors on infertility; it may serve as a basis for deciding in which areas and for what types of population special effort and/or additional funds should be provided to improve general health services, to combat specific endemic diseases hampering fertility and to enhance infertility treatment facilities; it also

shows that although infertility is a global problem, the methods used for its prevention and treatment must be diametrically different in various parts of the word.

The percentage of childless marriages, voluntary or involuntary, varies considerably according to society and time period. In most Western societies the figure is about 10%, although much higher percentages are found in some countries. In England and Wales, the percentage of married women with no children after 12 years of marriage fell from 13% in 1953 to 8% in 1960. In the USA, the National Fertility Survey based on personal interviews· with a multistage area probability sample of women aged 15–44 produced a reliable estimate of infertility incidence. The survey indicated that the prevalence of infertility in 1965, 1976 and 1982 did not vary significantly. There were, however, significant differences between the white and black population groups, the latter having much higher infertility rates than the former (Westhoff 1991) (Fig. 1.3). In Israel, 12.2% of women who married in 1966 remained childless after 10 years of marriage.

Acording to the United Nations Population Division the world population in 1991 was 5384 000 000. Assuming that half of the world inhabitants are women (2692 000 000), 20% of females are in the reproductive age (538 400 000) and the mean world incidence of infertility is

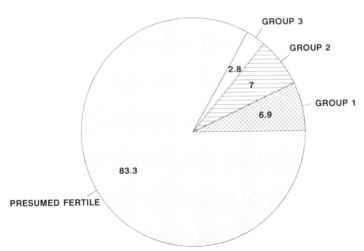

**Fig. 1.2** Incidence of infertility based on health-services data. Group 1, fertile but perceiving themselves as infertile; Group 2, primary infertility requesting treatment; Group 3, secondary infertility requesting treatment.

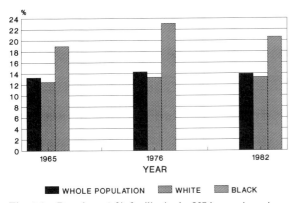

**Fig. 1.3**    Prevalence of infertility in the USA at various times and in different population groups. (Adapted with permission from Westhoff 1991).

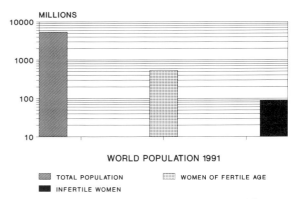

**Fig. 1.4**    The number of infertile women in the world population in 1991, based on demographic and health-services data.

16.7%, the number of infertile women throughout the globe should be approximately 90 million (Fig. 1.4). A staggering number presenting an almost unsurmountable challenge to medical services.

The population size of women between the ages 19 and 34 in the developed world in 1990 was estimated to be about 130 million. If we assume that at least 8% were infertile, than the pool of the infertile population should be above 10 million (Table 1.1), and about 700 000 new patients would enter this pool every year between the years 1990 and 1995 (Table 1.2). Although medical services in the developed countries are perfectly adequate to cope with the problem, the cost to the individual couples and the society as a whole may be difficult to bear.

The estimation of incidence of different infertility causes varies extremely between the reported series. Lunenfeld & Insler (1990) summarized the diagnostic categories established in 6549 infertile couples managed by different authors on five

**Table 1.1**    Population of women aged 19–34 years and estimated number of infertile women in developed countries in 1990

| Country | Women | Infertile women |
|---|---|---|
| Europe | 84 700 000 | 6 780 000 |
| USA | 27 700 000 | 2 220 000 |
| Canada | 2 900 000 | 230 000 |
| Japan | 12 800 000 | 1 020 000 |
| Australia | 1 900 000 | 150 000 |
| Total | 130 000 000 | 10 400 000 |

**Table 1.2**    Number of infertile women in the developed countries calculated from the number of females entering the 'fertile age pool' every year

| Country | Projected number of women | Projected number of infertile women |
|---|---|---|
| Europe | 5640 000 | 450 000 |
| USA | 1850 000 | 150 000 |
| Canada | 190 000 | 15 000 |
| Japan | 850 000 | 68 000 |
| Australia | 130 000 | 10 000 |
| Total | 8660 000 | 693 000 |

continents. The follow-up period was between 1 and 20 years, exceeding 4 years in the majority of series. The incidence of tubal factor ranged from 11.0% to 76.7%. Ovulation disturbances were detected in 10.9% of women by Nakamura (Brazil), in 42.9% by Cox (Australia) and in 49.1% by Insler (Israel). The incidence of cervical or uterine causes of infertility ranged between 3.2% and 48.0%. The cause of infertility was reported as unknown (i.e. unexplained or idiopathic) in between 3.5% and 22.1% of couples. Male infertility ranged from 26.2% to 46.6%. The incidence of multifactorial (combined) infertility is about 10% (Table 1.3). Analysis of the above data implies that the incidence of different fertility disturbances in each infertility clinic depends on the following elements:

1. The type of the population served, considering general health, endemic diseases, socioeconomic and cultural factors.

**Table 1.3**   Incidence of different infertility causes

| Author, year and country | No. of couples (years observ.) | Cause of infertility (%) | | | | | |
|---|---|---|---|---|---|---|---|
| | | Tubal | Ovulation disturbed | Cervix/uterus | Other | Unexplained | Male |
| Nakamura et al 1975 Brazil | 1000 (19) | 34.9 | 10.9 | 18.4 | 8.5 | NS | 27.9 |
| Cox 1975 Australia | 900 (9) | 11.0 | 42.9 | NS | 8.9 | 17.6 | 26.2 |
| Newton et al 1974 UK | 872 (2) | 18.0 | 27.0 | NS | 8.0 | NS | NS |
| Cocev 1972 Bulgaria | 744 (4) | 76.7 | 12.4 | 3.2 | 4.2 | 3.5 | 40.9 |
| Ratnam et al 1976 Singapore | 709 (4) | 11.7 | 22.5 | 5.8 | 14.7 | 22.1 | 23.1 |
| Dor et al 1977 Israel | 665 (15) | 16.2 | 33.4 | 5.1 | 1.2 | 16.1 | 27.9 |
| Insler et al 1981 Israel | 583 (4) | 21.4 | 49.1 | NS | 0.7 | 12.0 | 30.2 |
| Raymont 1969 Canada | 500 (10) | 32.2 | 16.9 | 25.6 | 26.2 | NS | 26.2 |
| Gunaratne 1979 Sri Lanka | 393 (1) | 15.3 | 16.2 | 16.9 | NS | NS | 41.6 |
| Anderson 1968 Denmark | 183 (3) | 36.1 | 29.5 | 48.0 | NS | 6.0 | 46.6 |

Reproduced from Lunenfeld & Insler 1990 with permission.
NS, not stated.

2. The availability and utilization of different diagnostic tests and procedures.

3. The technical knowledge and scientific interest of the medical staff.

The impact of several other factors on the incidence of different infertility causes as well as on the results of treatment must also be taken into consideration. Some types of infertility may have a genetic association (see Chapter 9), others may be connected with sexually transmitted diseases (see Chapter 27) and others may result from obesity (see Chapter 26), rapid weight loss (see

Chapter 29) or from different systemic and general diseases (see Chapters 14 and 29).

The effect of age on the incidence of infertility and on the results of therapy cannot be ignored. The classical work of Tietze et al (1950) showed that in 1727 planned pregnancies the time required for conception slightly increased with age. The American Fertility Survey indicated that the percentage of married women (excluding those surgically sterile) who were infertile increased by age from 10.6% in the 20–24-year-old to 27.4% in 40–44-year-old group (Westhoff 1991). The French Federation CECOS (1982) studied 2193 women treated by artificial insemination with donor sperm because of total sterility of the male partner. The cumulative pregnancy rates and the success rates per cycle were significantly higher in patients under 30 years of age compared to those between 30 and 35 and particularly those over 35.

There is no doubt that cigarette smoking has an adverse effect on health. The question, however, whether it results in reduced fertility of male and female subjects or of their offspring is still debatable (Rodriguez-Rigau et al 1982, Baird & Wilcox 1986).

It is obvious that the primary task of the infertility clinic is to diagnose the main cause (or causes) of infertility in each individual couple in order to be able to institute appropriate therapy within a reasonable time. Insler et al (1981) pointed out that the organization of the fertility clinic, allocation of resources, and development of diagnostic sequences and therapeutic frameworks must also be based on epidemiological studies that consider other factors such as age, socio-economic status, cultural and social habits of the population served, geographical distances, transportation means, etc.

## REFERENCES

Baird D D, Wilcox A J 1986 Future fertility after prenatal exposure to cigarette smoke. Fertil Steril 46: 368

Belsey M A, Ware H 1986 Epidemiological, social and psychosocial aspects of infertility. In: Insler V, Lunenfeld B (eds) Infertility: male and female, 1st edn. Churchill Livingstone, Edinburgh, pp 631–647.

Federation Cecos, Schwartz D, Mayaux M J 1982 Female fecundity as a function of age N Engl J Med 306: 404

Insler V, Potashnik G, Glassner M 1981 Some epidemiological aspects of fertility evaluation. In: Insler V, Bettendorf G Geissler K H (eds) Advances in diagnosis and treatment of infertility. Elsevier/North Holland, New York, pp 165–178

Lunenfeld B, Insler V 1990 Induction of ovulation: historical aspects. Bailliere's Clin Obstet Gynaecol 4: 473

Rodriguez-Rigau L J, Smith K D, Steinberger E 1982 Cigarette smoking and semen quality. Fertil Steril 38: 115

Tietze C, Guttmacher A F, Rubin S 1950 Time required for conception in 1727 planned pregnancies. Fertil Steril 1: 338

Westhoff C 1991 The epidemiology of infertility. In: Kiely M (eds) Reproductive and perinatal epidemiology. CRC Press, Boca Raton, pp 43–61

WHO 1991 Infertility: a tabulation of available data on prevalence of primary and secondary infertility. WHO, Geneva, pp 1–72

# Structural and functional basis of infertility (female)

# 2. Functional anatomy of the uterine cervix

*E. S. E. Hafez*

## GROSS ANATOMY

The cervix, cylindrical in shape, measures 3–4 cm in length. The cervix projects through the anterior wall of the vagina at the vaginal vault. The 'endocervix', lined by columnar epithelium, extends cranially from the external os to the junction of its epithelium with the endometrium. The 'ectocervix', the vaginal surface of the cervix, extends caudally from the external os to the reflection of the cervical epithelium onto the vaginal fornix (Fig. 2.1). In nulliparous women the cervical os is small and circular, whereas in parous women the os is transformed to a horizontal transverse slit bordered by a prominent anterior lip in contact with the posterior lip. This anatomical feature is altered with the introduction of a colposcope or a bivalve vaginal speculum. The two cervical lips retract, displaying a portion of the epithelium in the cervical canal. When the blades of the speculum are collapsed upon the cervix, the epithelium returns to the canal which displays its true appearance (Coppleson et al 1978).

Pregnancies cause remarkable alterations in the morphology of the cervix: increase in size due to hyperplasia and hypertrophy; and eversion of the epithelial lining of the low endocervical canal.

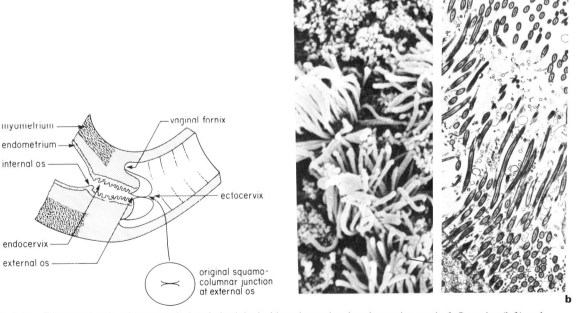

**Fig. 2.1a** Diagram showing the anatomical and physiological junctions related to the uterine cervix. **b** Scanning (left) and transmission (right) electron micrographs of ciliated cells showing cross and longitudinal sections of the kinocilia. The percentage of ciliated cells varies in different parts of the cervix.

11

Delivery may cause laceration of the cervix. After delivery, the size of the cervix decreases rapidly, due to progressive resorption of connective tissue and a decrease in the size of muscle cells. With a decline in the biosynthesis of ovarian hormones during postmenopausal life, the cervix involutes and atrophies with reduction in its weight and dimensions. The endocervical canal may be almost completely obliterated.

There are wide species differences in the gross anatomy of the uterine cervix (Hafez 1973).

The cervix and its secretions have several functions: (a) to provide receptivity to sperm penetration at or near ovulation and inhibit migration at other phases of the cycle; (b) to act as a sperm reservoir: (c) to protect spermatozoa from the hostile environment of the vagina and from being phagocytosed; (d) to provide spermatozoa with energy requirements; (e) to filter defective and immotile spermatozoa; (f) possibly to participate in the capacitation of spermatozoa (Moghissi 1973, Hafez and Thilbault 1975); and (g) to play a major physiological role during pregnancy and parturition.

## Cervical crypts and cervical canal

The cervical mucosa forms an intricate system of clefts, grooves, ridges and crypts (*plicae palmatae* or *arbor vitae uteri*) (Hafez 1980). The cervical crypts, finger-like structures separated by deep clefts, do not lie at right angles to the general plane of the epithelium, but are orientated obliquely towards the cervical canal and the external os. Colposcopically, the cervical mucosa appears in two forms: (a) rugae which are relatively coarse subdivisions appearing as two or three mounds on the cervical lip, and (b) villi separated from each other by intervillous space (Shingleton and Lawrence 1976, Coppleson et al 1978).

The human endocervical canal, fusiform in shape, ranges in length from 18 to 35 mm (an average of 27 mm). It is flattened from front to back, and measures 7 mm at its widest diameter. There are some 100 secretory units which secrete cervical mucus into the lumen of the endocervical canal (Odeblad 1966). Other authors, however, have estimated the number of cervical crypts to be much higher. Insler et al (1981) reported that, depending on the hormonal milieu, the whole length of the cervical canal contains between 9000 and 12 000 large and giant crypts. Cyclical changes occur in the diameter of the external os, dimensions of the cervical canal, tissue vascularity, and quantity and biophysical properties of cervical mucus. During the proliferative stage of the menstrual cycle, there is a progressive increase in cervical vascularity, congestion and edema, as well as secretion of cervical mucus. All these changes reach a peak just prior to or at time of ovulation, creating optimal biophysical conditions for sperm transport in the female reproductive tract. The external os reaches a diameter of 3 mm at the time of ovulation, then declines to a minimum of 1 mm.

## ANATOMICAL AND PHYSIOLOGICAL JUNCTIONS

Several anatomical and physiological junctions and structures have functional clinical significance, e.g. the squamo-columnar junction, the fibro-muscular junction, the cervico-endometrial junction, the anatomical internal os, the histological internal os, and the external os (Fig. 2.1).

## Squamo-columnar junction

Covering the vagina and ectocervix the squamous epithelium joins the columnar epithelium at the original squamo-columnar junction, a point which in 4% of women lies in the vagina itself. The cervical epithelium undergoes dramatic changes in its structure several times during the life cycle (Fig. 2.2). These alterations commence as early as fetal life and continue to the menopause. Thus this dynamic epithelium exhibits varied morphology, involving the development of a new squamous epithelium within the columnar epithelium lining the cervical canal and ectocervix (Shingleton & Lawrence 1976). The transition from the columnar epithelium is usually abrupt. The columnar epithelium, however, may extend outside the external os into the vaginal portion of the cervix. This occurs particularly in neonates and pregnant women.

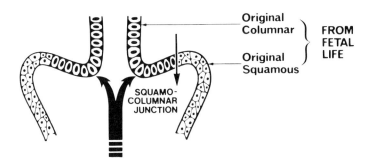

# 1. ORIGINAL EPITHELIA

a

# 2. METAPLASTIC SQUAMOUS EPITHELIUM
## –Typical transformation zone

# 3. ATYPICAL EPITHELIUM
## – Atypical transformation zone

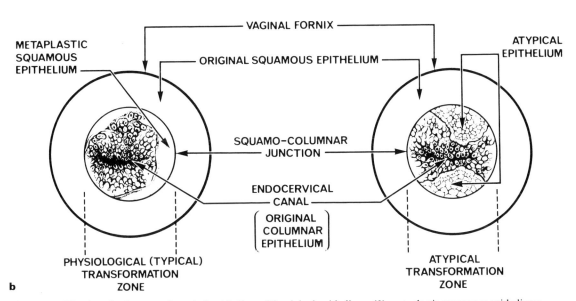

b

**Fig. 2.2a**    The three basic types of cervical epithelium: (1) original epithelium; (2) metaplastic squamous epithelium; (3) atypical epithelium which includes immature metaplastic squamous epithelium, basal cell hyperplasia, dysplasia and carcinoma in situ. **b** Distribution of epithelium within the cervix showing the basic topographical similarities within the transformation zone of the different epithelial types. (Reproduced with permission from Singer & Jordan 1976.)

The squamo-columnar junction lies within the endocervical canal during childhood, on the ectocervix in reproductive years and within the endocervical canal during menopause. The position of the junctional zone is determined by the volume of the cervical stroma which in turn depends on hormonal stimulation associated with a different electrolyte and fluid content. Depending on the age and the degree of reproductive processes the ecto-endocervical boundary varies in its topographical location; it descends during pregnancy towards the ectocervical area, but ascends in postmenopausal women. The shrinkage of the connective tissue in the cervical stroma leads to decrease in volume, and the lack of hormonal stimulation enhances this process. In young women the squamo-columnar junction is located mostly in the ectocervix and less frequently within the endocervix. In few cases, however, this junction occurs on the vaginal aspect of the portio.

The stratified squamous epithelium of the portio externa is made of several basal, parabasal, intermediate and superficial layers. The basal layer consists of a single row of cells and rests on a basement membrane. The superficial and intermediate layers contain large amounts of glycogen, which serve an important function in maintaining an acidic pH of the vaginal contents. The glycogen, released by cytolysis of desquamated cells, is metabolized by glycolytic bacterial flora of the vagina, forming lactic acid. Superficial cells are desquamated into the vaginal lumen but retain their nuclei (unlike the desquamating cells of heavily cornified epithelium such as thick skin). The rapidly regenerative nature of the basal cell is reflected in its ultrastructure, and is characterized by a high nucleus : cytoplasm ratio, prominent nucleoli, a convoluted nuclear membrane, and an abundance of ribosomes and mitochondria.

In adult women the original columnar epithelium is replaced by metaplastic epithelium at its most distal portion. The original squamo-columnar, now squamo-squamous, junction then separates the two types of squamous epithelium: original and metaplastic (Coppleson et al 1978). The 'new' squamo-columnar junction refers to the line of demarcation separating the metaplastic squamous epithelium from the original columnar epithelial junction. The epithelial lining of the low portion of the endocervical canal becomes part of the covering of the exocervix so that the original squamo-columnar junction is displaced caudally. This physiopathological process, known as 'eversion', involves no tissue destruction or replacement. The process of squamous metaplasia occurs within the area cranial to the original squamo-columnar junction and continues

sporadically during the life cycle (Coppleson et al 1978).

**Fibro-muscular junction**

The so-called 'cervical musculature', located at the junction of the muscle of the corpus uteri and the fibrous tissue of the cervix, is capable of producing a sphincter-like activity upon contraction or relaxation. The estimated muscle content in the upper segment of the cervix including this fibro-muscular junction is about 30%. There is a remarkable difference in the contractility pattern of the cervical musculature and the myometrium. The musculature of the corpus uteri is oxytocin sensitive. The musculature of the corpus uteri exhibits phasic contractions whereas that of the cervix exhibits multi-spike and tonic contractions.

**Cervico-endometrial junction**

The cervico-endometrial junction or the isthmical portion of the cervical canal has received very little attention. The anatomical and histological boundaries of this junction are still controversial. It has been defined as the part of the endometrium bounded superiorly by the 'anatomical' internal os and inferiorly by the 'histological' internal os (Fig. 2.3). There is remarkable variability in the relationship of the histological os and the anatomical os, so that they do not represent a reliable anatomical position (Danforth 1947, 1954, Danforth & Chapman 1950).

The transition from endometrial cavity to endocervix is gradual and there is no abrupt demarcation. Thus there is a gradual histological transition of the mucosa in this region from an endocervical type to an endometrial type. In the lower segments of the uterus there is a mixture of endocervical crypts and endometrial glands. Such glands are hyporesponsive: they either lag behind the functionalis glands or are totally unresponsive. The cervical stroma has a higher collagen content than the corpus endometrium, and in appearance it is more eosinophilic and less cellular.

Implantation of the blastocyst near the cervico-endometrial junction may be associated

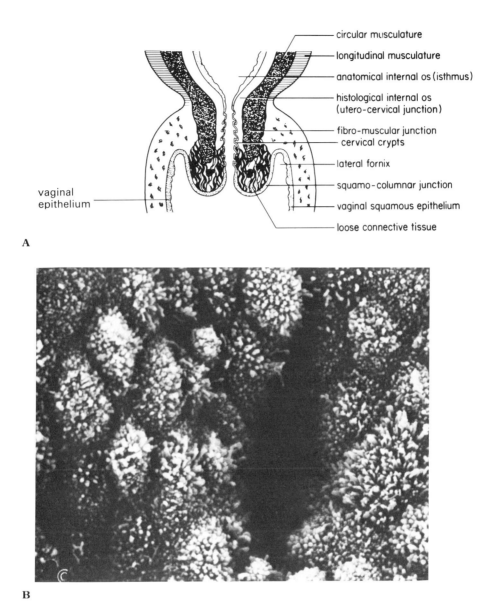

circular musculature
longitudinal musculature
anatomical internal os (isthmus)
histological internal os
(utero-cervical junction)
fibro-muscular junction
cervical crypts
lateral fornix
squamo-columnar junction
vaginal squamous epithelium
loose connective tissue

vaginal epithelium

A

B

**Fig. 2.3**   Diagrammatic illustrations of the human uterine cervix showing the cervical crypts, and various anatomical and physiological junctions. Note collagen bundles stained by Mallory's stain in cervical stroma. During nonpregnancy collagen appears as dense, tightly woven bundles of interlacing blue stain fibers whereas during term pregnancy there is loosening and the clear spaces between the collagen bundles appear due to dissociation phenomenon. The scanning electron micrographs show surface ultrastructure of endometrium, with endometrial gland; cervical epithelium with ciliated cells; and squamous epithelium showing microridge with elevated nucleus (Fig. 2.3 C, D and E overleaf). (Reproduced with permission from Hafez 1982.)

with various types of placenta previa, or result in cervical pregnancy. The management of the adenocarcinoma of the endometrium varies according to whether or not it has extended to the isthmus. Further studies on the functional anatomy of the cervico-endometrial junction may shed some light on the etiology or natural history of some of these pathologies.

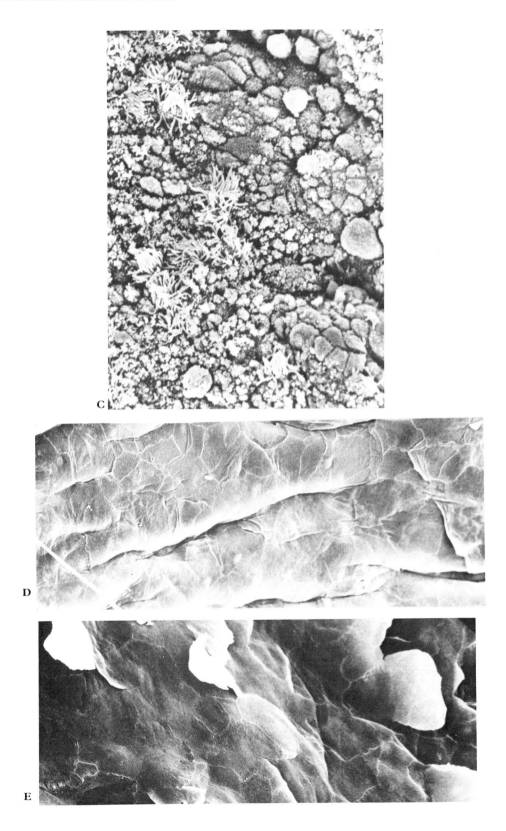

# CONGENITAL ANOMALIES OF THE CERVIX

The Mullerian ducts fuse during the 10th to 17th week of fetal life. As the fusion process is being completed, they canalize. Failure of the Mullerian ducts to fuse (resulting in uterus didelphys) and failure of the lower aspect of the right Mullerian duct to canalize (Monks 1979) result in atresia of the cervix and upper vagina.

Defects in the fusion patterns of the Mullerian duct range from incidental gross anomalies, encountered on examination of hysterectomy specimens, to severe anatomical abnormalities associated with infertility, habitual abortions, obstetrical complications or perinatal mortality. This is most frequent with uterus didelphys, uterus unicornis, and uterus duplex with a single cervix (Jones & Wheelers 1969). Thus, there is a continuous morphological spectrum of maldevelopment (Hendrickson & Kempson 1980). Congenital anomalies of the cervix are associated with atresia and aplasia of the uterus and vagina (Tables 2.1, 2.2) renal abnormalities such as unilateral renal agenesis (Wolf & Allen 1953, Wiersma et al 1976), or with endometriosis (Nunley & Kitchin 1980). Three patterns of congenital atresia of the cervix are recognized (Figs 2.4–2.6): (a) aplasia of the uterus with a nonfunctioning endometrium and amenorrhea; (b) functioning endometrium, cyclic menstruation leading to hematometra, and enlargement of the uterus; and (c) normal uterus and adnexa with or without demonstrable retrograde menstruation through the oviduct, no enlargement of the uterus, but cyclic monthly lower abdominal pain (Sherwood & Speed 1941, Zarou et al 1961, Scott et al 1971, Dillon et al 1979). Clinical characteristics vary according to the nature of the atresia and to the presence or absence of functional endometrial tissue. With normal ovaries, secondary sex characteristics develop and after menarche cyclic ovarian function occurs. With a completely functional uterus, the cervix and a portion of the upper part of the vagina are usually also present, although they may not be easily recognized (Jeffcoate 1969).

The congenital atretic cervix may be palpable as a thin fibrous cord between the vaginal apex and

**Table 2.1** Embryological classification of congenital anomalies of the uterine cervix

| Syndrome | Embryological defects and timing | Clinical presentation |
|---|---|---|
| Rudimentary or absent uterus-cervix | 8 week: failure of distal Mullerian ducts to form | First degree amenorrhea unassociated with abdominal mass or cyclic pain |
| Cervical atresia with upper vaginal atresia | 5 month: failure of canalization | Hematocolpos after menarche with periodic pain, amenorrhea |
| Double cervix (one or both functioning vaginae) | 9th–12th week | Periodic pain without complete amenorrhea associated with tense swelling of lateral vaginal wall |
| Aplastic cervix | 17th week: falure to recanalize uterus | Amenorrhea and sterility |
| Double cervix with hemiuteri and separate vaginae | 3rd week | Separate vaginal openings |
| Double cervix, externally united, uterus didelphys and separate vagina | 9th week | Asymptomatic until pregnancy, abortion, prematurity |
| Double cervix with uterus bicornuate (duplex) | 9th week | Obstetrical complications |
| Cervix with uterus septus | 12th week | Obstetrical complications |

Data from Jarcho 1946, Jones & Wheelers 1969, Benirschke 1973, Toaff 1974, Griffin et al 1976.

the uterine corpus. Such patients have neither an endocervical epithelium nor a canal. To create a functional cervical canal is quite complex. Several methods have been attempted, e.g. direct anastomosis of the vault apex to a uterine hysterotomy site, the passage of a catheter or pessary from the uterus to the vaginal vault and in the case of a rudimentary cervix, an attempt to recanalize around stents. There has been some success in creating an artificial cervical canal (Rotter 1958, Zarou et al 1961, Iversen 1966) with one case of a reported pregnancy (Zarou et al 1973). Since normal cervical mucus plays a major physiological role in sperm transport, it seems unlikely that

**Table 2.2** Clinical features of cervical anomalies in relation to infertility

| Syndrome | Associated anomalies | Clinical aspects | References |
| --- | --- | --- | --- |
| Unilateral cervical atresia | Uterus didelphys and renal agenesis on same side | Successful pregnancy occurs after surgical correction | Monks 1979 |
| Congenital atresia of cervix | Half of reported cases associated with pelvic endometriosis (probably as a result of retrograde menstruation) | Successful surgical management to preserve reproductive potential may be possible in some cases. Hysterectomy is sometimes indicated | Rotter 1958, Scott et al 1971, Geary and Weed 1973, Farber and Marchant 1975, 1976 |
| Congenital atresia of cervix and functional bicornuate uterus | Labia major and minora unremarkable. Hymen stretched to admit 2 fingers. Soft annular constriction in upper fifth of vagina | Total hysterectomy and preservation of ovaries was recommended. Reconstructrive surgery to: a. create a uterovaginal fistula to permit egress of menstrum b. establish potential of conception and pregnancy | Dillon et al 1979, Farber 1980 |
| Congenital atresia of cervix and vigina | | Surgery to preserve fertility is not recommended | Williams 1963, Jeffcoate 1969, Fritzsche and Beller 1976, Niver et al 1980 |

Uterus communicans septus, cervix septa, vagina septa

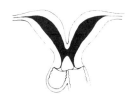

Uterus communicans bicornis, cervix duplex, vagina septa unilateralis atretica

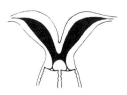

Uterus communicans bicornis, cervix duplex, vagina septa

Uterus communicans septus, cervix duplex, vagina septa

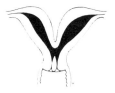

Uterus communicans bicornis, cervix septa, vagina simplex

**Fig. 2.4** Different congenital anomalies of the cervix associated with communicating uteri. (Reproduced with permission from Benson 1979, Toaff 1974.)

vaginal–uterine fistula without cervical glands would allow pregnancy. The patient who conceived (Zarou et al 1973) may have had some functioning cervical tissue. Without cervical mucus, a surgically created passage may have the eventual tendency to stenose and require further microsurgery to retain patency.

## CERVICAL EPITHELIUM

The typical cervical epithelium extends cranially from the endometrial epithelium, either to the original squamous epithelium or caudally to the metaplastic epithelium. The term 'endocervical epithelium' is erroneous, since it infers that columnar epithelium is exclusively within the cervical canal, which is not so throughout the life cycle. The original cervical epithelium is made of tall, slender, elongated columnar cells uniformly arranged in one layer and closely packed in a 'cobblestone' pattern.

The bases of the columnar cells are attached to the basement membrane by hemidesmosomes. Columnar cells consist of two types: non-ciliated secretory cells and kinociliated cells (Hafez 1972a,b, 1982) (Fig. 2.7) During pregnancy, remarkable changes occur in the cervical epithelium. Through metaplastic transformation, extensive areas of the original columnar epi-

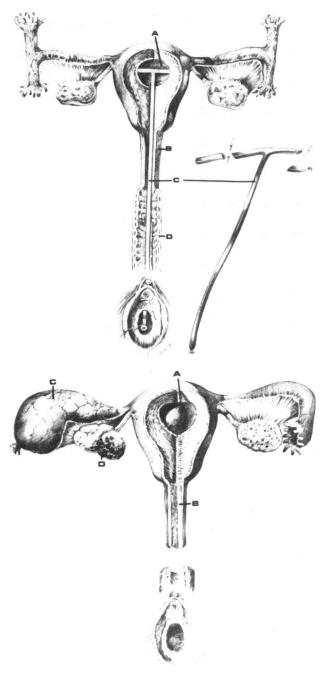

**Fig. 2.5a**  Pelvic organs showing: A endometrial cavity; B atretric cervix; C rubber T tube; D vagina. (With permission from Farber & Marchant 1975.) **b** Pelvic organs showing: A endometrial cavity; B atretric cervix; C hematosalpinx; D endometrioma. (Reproduced with permission from Farber & Marchant 1975.)

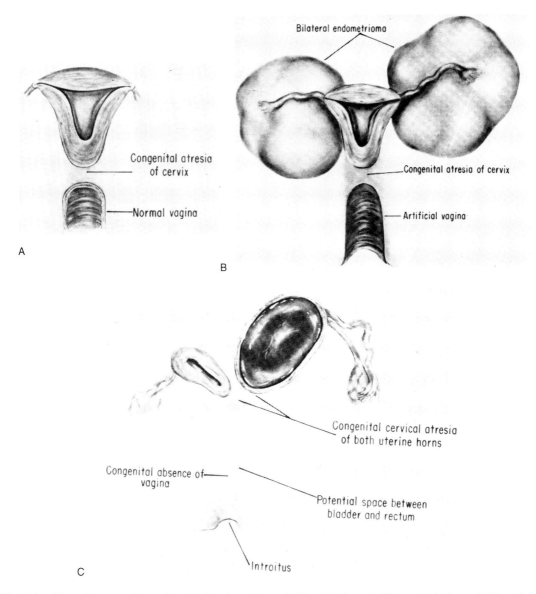

**Fig. 2.6a** Normal uterus, tubes and ovaries but the vagina ended in a blind pouch. The cervix is absent. **b** Normal uterus, tubes and ovaries but congenital atresia of the cervix and absence of the vagina. **c** The vagina is congenitally absent. A uterus didelphys is associated with rudimentary right horn and uterine tube. (Reproduced with permission from Geary & Weed 1973.)

thelium are converted into squamous epithelium. Because the cervix is a site of one of the most common forms of cancer in women, extensive investigations have been conducted on the surface ultrastructural characteristics of cervical epithelium (Komori 1965, Jordan 1976, Williams et al 1973). Cervical epithelium is also easily accessible to clinical examination and biopsy.

## Secretory cells

Secretory cells have a dome-shaped, raised surface covered with many short microvilli 2 μm long and 0.2 μm wide. Secretory cells stain deeply with periodic acid-Schiff (PAS) during the peak of the biosynthesis stage and become engorged with heterogeneous secretory granules. The subcellular

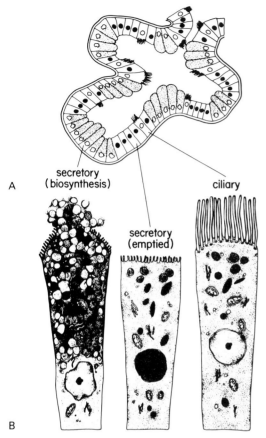

A

secretory
(biosynthesis)                              ciliary

secretory
(emptied)

B

**Fig. 2.7a** Schematic representation of secretory and ciliated cells from columnar epithelium in endocervical crypt. The secretory cells have basal, active nuclei and numerous secretory droplets during merocrine secretion. Note ciliated nonsecretory cells. A flattened basement membrane separates the epithelial cells and adjacent stroma. **b** Secretory cells (left) during biosynthesis and after storage showing heterogeneous secretory granules and cell organelles and ciliated cells (right) with kinocilia attached to basal bodies. (Reproduced with permission from Hafez 1982.)

distribution of histochemically and ultrastructurally distinguishable granules indicate the heterogeneous nature of cervical mucus (Figs 2.7, 2.8). Fibrillar bodies frequently seen in the cytoplasm of mucus-secreting endocervical cells may be a storage form of glycoprotein (Phillip 1975). The simultaneous occurrence of, and the occasional direct communication between, the light staining secretory granules and granulofibrillar bodies in endocervical cells suggest that the latter stores glycoproteins in a granulofilamentous form. The secretory activity of the cervical epitheliums involves both apocrine

and merocrine mechanisms (Nilsson & Westman 1961, Williams et al 1973).

Cyclical changes in the histochemical and ultrastructural characteristics of secretory granules correspond to cyclical changes in estrogen and progesterone levels (Moghissi 1973, Wolf et al 1978). Although cyclical morphological changes in the epithelium are inconspicuous, the viscoelastic properties of cervical mucus undergo remarkable cyclical alterations (Nilsson & Westman 1961, Williams et al 1973). The estrogen to progesterone ratio exerts an effect on the surface ultrastructural characteristics of the epithelial cells of the endocervix, e.g. cell volume, cell boundaries and morphology and pattern of microvilli.

## Ciliated cells

Ciliated cells are covered with kinocilia which beat rhythmically towards the cervical canal and the vagina. Ciliated cells are more frequent in the endocervix, particularly at the cervico-endometrial junction, and are rarely found on the ectocervix. The ciliated cells in the cervix resemble those in the endometrium and oviduct. The luminal surface of ciliated cells has surface microvilli interspersed amongst the kinocilia. The function of the ciliated cells is not clear, although it is assumed that they are involved in the mucociliary clearance of secretory macromolecules from the adjacent secretory cells.

When the growing ciliated cells reach the luminal surface, the cilia are exposed to the glandular lumen. Initially the luminal surface of the ciliated cell is concave, but as the cell develops this surface becomes convex. The cilia may also pinch off as a merocrine secretion. During this stage the cell has a characteristic fusiform-to-pear shape. Several histochemical stains are used to demonstrate the cilia, e.g. phosphotungstic acid hematoxylin (PTAH) and iron hematoxylin stains. The former demonstrates the ciliary basal bodies, whereas the latter stains the cilia themselves.

Ciliated cells have a distinctive round, smoothly contoured vesicular nucleus containing finely stippled chromatin. The cytoplasm is characterized by numerous mitochondria, free ribosomes,

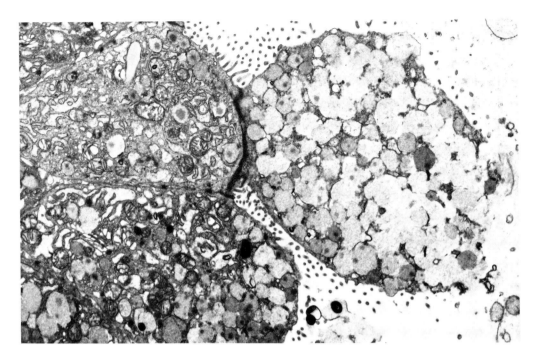

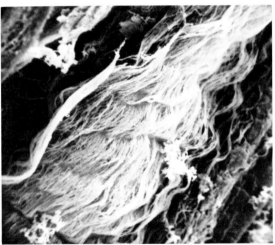

**Fig. 2.8a** Transmission electron micrograph of secretory and ciliated cells from human endocervix illustrating mechanism of cervical mucus formation. Note heterogeneity of secretory granules. **b** Microfibrillar structures of midcycle cervical mucus, showing 'parallel' arrangements. Microfibrils joined to make small macromolecules which in turn coalesce into larger macromolecules (x 12 000). (Reproduced with permission from Zaneveld et al 1975.)

occasional lysosomes, and rough and smooth surfaced endoplasmic reticulum (Shingleton & Lawrence 1976). While the nuclear features remain relatively unchanged throughout cell development, the configuration and location of the cell vary as a function of the stage of cilio-genesis. Detached ciliary tufts or clusters may be noted in cervicovaginal smears. These ciliary tufts, which are fragments of ciliated cells of the endocervical canal, are characterized by their columnar shape and by 'nippling' of the nuclei. A protruding knob of dense chromatin appears in the distal pole of the nucleus pointing toward the luminal surface. The physiological or clinical significance of this nippling is not clear but it seems to be associated with some nuclear activation such as regeneration following erosion or following estrogenic stimulation as at midcycle.

## Histochemistry of cervical epithelium

There is considerable controversy related to the histochemistry of the human cervix, primarily due to variability of cell and tissue types involved, the diversity of physiological and pathological conditions studied, and the methods used, particularly with respect to enzyme histochemistry (Blackwell & Markham 1976). Several histochemical techniques have been used to evaluate the biochemical nature of secretory granules in secretory cells (Table 2.3). For example, the Alcian blue and PAS, staining techniques have been used to distinguish acid glycoproteins localized in the mid and apical regions (Hafez 1982).

**Table 2.3**  Summary of some histochemical characteristics of the epithelium of the endocervix and ectocervix

| Histochemical parameters | Mucus-secreting columnar epithelium (endocervix) | Stratified squamous epithelium (ectocervix) |
|---|---|---|
| Mucopolysaccharides | Types of mucopolysaccharides vary throughout life cycle; in children high polymeric acid and neutral mucopolysaccharides predominate<br>Sulphomucins are more abundant than carboxymucins or neutral mucins in the adult cervix, or neutral mucins predominate<br>Quantity of mucin present varies with the stage of the menstrual cycle<br>Mucus is still abundant in postmenopausal cervix | Following diastase treatment, there is PAS-positive material in superficial layer, indicating presence of neutral mucopolysaccharides |
| Glycogen | Large amounts of mucin in the epithelium render enzyme digestion technique impossible to interpret | Glycogen present in normal squamous epithelium but absent in atypical squamous epithelium (Schiller's test)<br>Basal cells are almost devoid of glycogen but concentration increases towards the surface, with the greatest concentration being in superficial layers<br>Production of glycogen is triggered by glycogen synthesizing enzymes, with a direct correlation between sites of enzyme activity and those of glycogen accumulation |
| Enzymes | Succinic dehydrogenase, an indicator of cellular metabolism, is well defined by formazan on surface of columnar cells and in endocervical crypts<br>A wide range of alkaline phosphatase<br>β-hydroxybutyric acid dehydrogenase absent<br>α-glycerophosphate dehydrogenase present | Abundance of malic dehydrogenase in all zones except keratinized layer<br>Moderate amounts of α-glycerophosphatase dehydrogenase in deeper layers diminishing superficially<br>Glutamic dehydrogenase moderately intense in basal zone diminishing superficially<br>Phosphoamidase mostly basal diminishing superficially |
| Ultrastructure | Lateral surfaces of cells connect plasmalemma at complex interdigitating folds<br>Desmosomes connect adjacent cells with close junctions, particularly near luminal surface<br>Irregularly shaped nuclei with distributed chromatin and conspicuous nucleoli<br>Numerous rough endoplasmic reticulum; Gegi zones in close juxtaposition to secretory droplets fill supranuclear cytoplasm<br>Apocrine and merocrine secretion represented by apical bulging at luminal border | Hemidesmosomes spaced at intervals along convoluted processes of basal epithelial cells; these attachments possess focal condensations of plasma membrane parallel by a thin electron-dense line and fine filaments extending to basement membrane<br>Microvilli extend into intercellular spaces and adjacent cell membranes joined by desmosomes<br>Lobulated large nucleus with coarsely distributed chromatin and a single or double nucleoli |

Adapted from  Foraker 1962, David & Woolf 1963, Sorvari 1969, Hiersch 1970, Fand 1973, Langley & Crompton 1973, Blackwell & Markham 1976, Hafez 1982.

Secretory cells of the cervical epithelium contain uniformly electronlucent or mixed density (electronlucent with dense inner core) granules located apically. Uniformly electrondense granules, confined to the basal region of cells, correspond to the neutral glycoproteins (Chilton et al 1980a,b). In ovariectomized or postmenopausal women, intracellular neutral glycoproteins and acid glycoproteins, as well as electronlucent and mixed density granules, are depleted. The administration of exogenous estrogen to postmenopausal or ovariectomized women restores morphological and biosynthetic characteristics of the cervical epithelium.

The secretory cell undergoes dramatic cytological changes representing a cell cycle. During the *biosynthetic stage* the secretory cell becomes engorged with heterogeneous mucous granules without any apparent vacuoles (Hafez 1982). During the *secretory stage* the cell contains cytoplasmic PAS-positive spaces, vacuoles and some heterogeneous mucous granules. During the *exhaustion phase* the cells are characterized by dilated endoplasmic reticulum, empty cytoplasmic vacuoles, and the absence of mucous granules. The application of cell separation procedures to disperse endocervical cells offers a new approach to the study of hormonal modulation of endocervical cytodifferentiation and mucus secretion (Chilton et al 1980a,b).

**Squamous epithelium**

The original squamous epithelium consists of polygonal flat cells made primarily of glycogen and arranged in five to ten layers, separated from the stroma by a distinct basement membrane. The cells have a centrally raised nuclear area, with raised terminal bars between adjacent cells. Their surface shows a typical pattern of microridges which are approximately 0.15 μm wide with a space of about 0.25 μm between them (Jordan 1976). There is great variability in the length (up to 40 μm) of these microridges, which show branching and anastomosis. Microridges less than 1.0 μm long are uncommon on normal squamous cells (Jordan 1976). Microridges do not have a specific pattern, but peripherally they are arranged parallel to the cell boundaries.

The physiological significance of plasma membrane microridges is unknown. However, their unique presence in the superficial cells of squamous mucous membranes is likely to increase surface adhesiveness (Ferenczy & Richart 1974) and to provide resistance to sideways movements (Williams et al 1973). Microridges are related to the topographic configuration of mature squamous cells containing disulfide-rich keratin or keratin precursors.

Prominent terminal bars (about 0.5 μm high seem to be formed by the folding over and interdigitation of the edges of adjacent cells (Hackeman et al 1968, Shingleton et al 1968). The cell cytoplasm contains numerous mitochondria and free ribosomes, and an occasional Golgi complex and rough endoplasmic reticulum. The squamous epithelium differentiates under the influences of estrogen and progesterone, with the more mature superficial cells exfoliating into the vagina and being replaced by the metabolically active basal cell layer (Papanicolaou 1954).

The superficial cells have degenerated, pycnotic nuclei and are rich in intracytoplasmic glycogen and microfilaments, the latter providing for their rigidity (Friedrich 1973, Ferenczy & Richart 1974). The absence of desmosomes between the upper superficial cells explains their loose attachment and easy desquamation. The cells beneath the superficial cell layer, the intermediate cells, have abundant PAS — positive intracellular glycogen, which is responsible for the clear, vacuolated appearance of their cytoplasm (Williams et al 1973, Hafez et al 1975). Intermediate cells produce numerous desmosome tonofilament complexes which derive from the underlying parabasal cells. Radioautographic studies in vitro (Ferenczy & Richart 1974) have demonstrated increased nuclear DNA synthesis in this celluar region, which suggests a beginning of intracytoplasmic glycogenization (Ferenczy & Gelfand 1979).

CERVICAL STROMA

The connective tissue of the cervical stroma is made of ground substance, fibrous constituents and cellular elements. The ground substance contains proteoglycan, hyaluronic acid, chondroitin-4-6 sulfate, dermatan sulfate, heparan sulfate and keratan sulfate associated with proteins. The fibrous constituents include collagen, elastin and reticulin. Cellular elements comprise mast cells, fibroblasts and wandering cells. Collagen is made basically of chains of several amino acids such as glycine, proline, hydroxyproline, lysine or hydroxylysine. A molecule of glycine occurs in every third position throughout most of the polypeptide chains and large amounts of proline and hydroxproline are found in the other two positions (Hirakawa & Ito 1979). The structure of stroma is obstetrically important in view of the biodynamics of the cervix. The patterns of reticulin, elastin and interfibrous ground substances facilitate the dilatation of the cervix at delivery. The dissociation of the collagen fibers, which become widely separated from one another, causes the loosening of cervical tissues and increases clear spaces between collagen bundles.

Prostaglandins can interfere with the connective tissue within the cervical stroma, which is abundantly innervated by monaminergic nerves utilizing norepinephrine (NE) as transmittor. Wilhelmsson et al (1982) investigated the influence in vitro of $PGE_2$, alone and in combination with NE, on the incorporation of [3]H-labelled proline into cervical tissue proteins. Slices, 1 mm thick, of cervical tissue were incubated in buffer containing [3]H-labelled proline, fortified with $PGE_2$ and/or NE and the incorporation into total protein was measured. In the luteal phase NE decreased the incorporation of [3]H-labelled proline but this inhibition was altered into a moderate stimulation in the concomitant presence of $PGE_2$. Both clinical and experimental studies have shown that prostaglandins per se can interfere with the biophysical and biochemical properties of the cervix.

## LIGAMENTS AND SUPPORTING TISSUES

The uterosacral ligaments and lateral ligaments hold the cervix in position. The uterosacral ligaments are composed of mainly fibrous tissues which connect the supravaginal portion of the cervix and upper vagina to the 2nd, 3rd and 4th sacral vertebrae. The lateral ligaments (transverse cervical ligaments, cardinal ligament, ligament of Mackenrodt) lie at the base of the broad ligament, where fascial ligaments contain connective tissue and smooth muscle (Singer & Jordan 1976). They form an inverted U which is attached medially to the anterior, superior and posterior marginal walls of the supravaginal cervix, and laterally and below to the white line and fascia of the levator ani muscles (Fluhmann & Dickmann 1958, Fluhmann 1961).

Anteriorly, the supravaginal portion is separated from the bladder by a distinct layer of connective tissue, the parametrium, which also extends to the sides of the cervix and laterally between the layers of the broad ligament. Posteriorly, the supravaginal cervix is covered with peritoneum which continues down over the posterior vaginal wall to be reflected onto the rectum, forming the rectouterine pouch, or pouch of Douglas (Singer & Jordan 1976).

### Vascular, nerve and lymph supplies

The arterial blood supply to the cervix is arranged bilaterally and directed from three main sources: directly from the uterine artery, from its cervicovaginal branch, and from the vaginal artery (Gustafson 1976). In the squamous epithelial region of the cervix, vessels of similar size communicate with each other forming a well-regulated capillary network below the epithelium. The vessels run vertically and regularly to the superficial capillary network in the lateral view. Sekiba et al (1979) studied the fine angioarchitecture of the cervix using scanning electron microscopy. In the vascular cast of the columnar epithelial region of the cervical canal, the structure is more undulating than in the squamous epithelium and has many avascular cavities at the site of cervical crypts. The net layer is thick because of piles of capillary meshworks, a very different pattern from that of the squamous epithelium.

In typical ectopic lesions with many grape-like villi, the vascular structure is different from that of the columnar epithelium or squamous epithelium, with many chain-like vessels corresponding to the central blood vessel of the villus. Two types of vascular structures are associated with cervical dysplasia. The 'basket' structure corresponding to colposcopic mosaic is easily recognized, with network more dense than normal. In colposcopic punctuation, individual tips of hairpin-like vessels are slightly irregular compared to the inflammatory hairpin-like vessels (Sekiba et al 1979).

The cervix is innervated from three plexuses of the pelvic autonomic nervous system, the superior, middle and inferior hypogastric. Norepinephrine is the major sympathetic neurotransmitter, whereas dopamine, epinephrine, acetylcholine and prostaglandins are involved. α- and β-receptors are involved in the neural mechanisms of catecholamines. α-receptors, most responsive to epinephrine, are usually excitatory, causing uterine contractions, while inhibitory β-receptors relax the uterus.

The cervix is much more richly innervated in the region of the internal os than the external os. The sensory nerve supply of the cervix is intimately related to its automatic supply. The cervix is supplied with adrenergic (sympathetic) and cholinergic (parasympathetic) fibers. There is an extensive adrenergic network at the internal os, where smooth muscles are abundant, and throughout the cervix in relation to blood vessel walls (Rodin & Moghissi 1973).

The cervix has a rich lymphatic supply, yet it is difficult to identify the precise arrangements of its lymphatic capillary bed. A rather irregularly

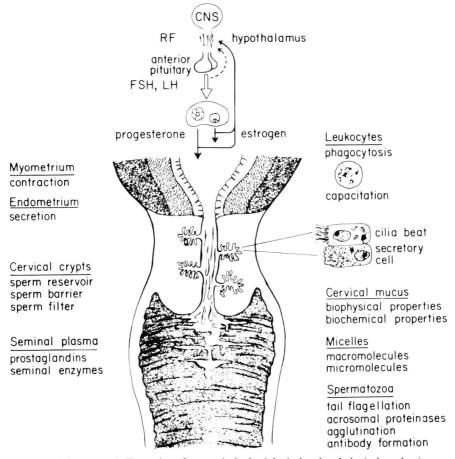

**Fig. 2.9** Diagrammatic illustration of anatomical, physiological and pathological mechanisms involved in sperm transport through the human cervix. (Reproduced with permission from Hafez 1976.)

arranged bed underlies the epithelium of the endocervical clefts and drains into the stroma where it continues outwards in a series of perforating lymphatic capillaries which pass to the outer areas of the stroma. These perforating vessels receive drainage from a second capillary bed also located in the stroma. At the periphery of the cervix the lymphatic drainage opens out into a coarse network, the serosal lymphatic plexus, which retains its designation even though the bulk of the organ is not covered by serosa (Gustafson 1976).

## SPERM TRNSPORT IN THE CERVIX

There are three recognizable stages of sperm transport within the cervix; rapid, short transport;

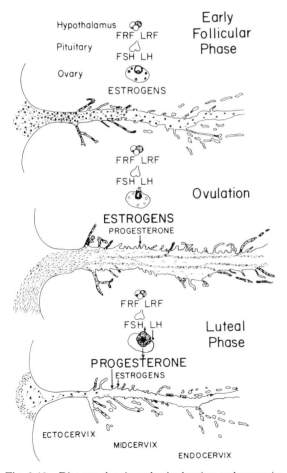

**Fig. 2.10**  Diagram showing selective barriers and reservoirs of spermatozoa in the female reproductive tract. (Reproduced with permission from Hafez 1980)

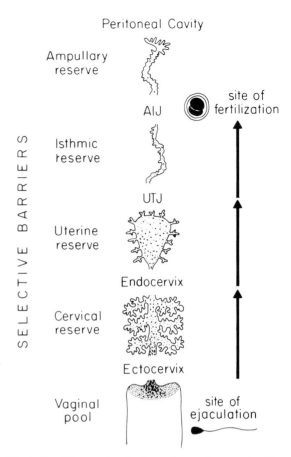

**Fig. 2.11**  Diagram showing the patterns of sperm migration from the cervix to the uterus when intercourse takes place during early follicular phase, at ovulation, and the luteal phase. Note channels of cervical mucus in which spermatozoa are aligned parallel to micelles of cervical mucus during midcycle. Sperm migration is inhibited under progesterone influence. (Reproduced with permission Hafez 1973)

colonization; and slow prolonged release (Figs 2.9–2.11) (Hafez 1980).

## Rapid transport

Immediately after deposition of semen into the vagina, spermatozoa penetrate the micelles of the cervical mucus where 'vanguard' spermtozoa are quickly transported through the cervical canal. This phase takes 10–20 min and may be facilitated by increased contractile activity of the myometrium during courtship and coitus. Some spermatozoa reach the internal os of the cervix within a few minutes after ejaculation, and may reach the site of fertilization very rapidly. Whether

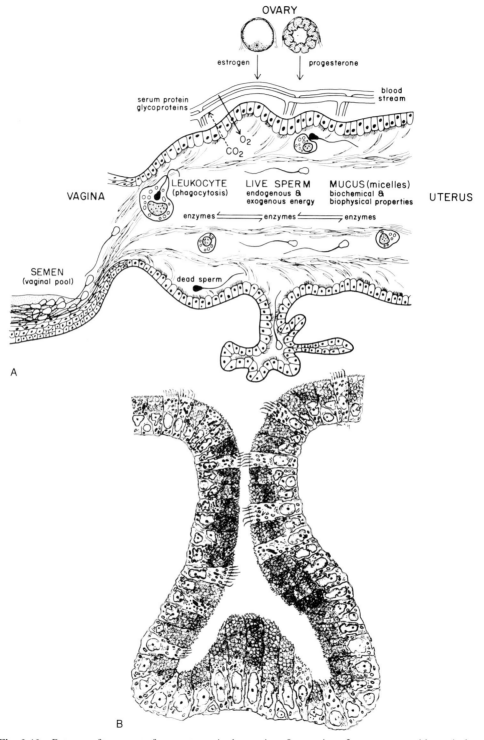

**Fig. 2.12**   Patterns of transport of spermatozoa in the cervix. **a** Interaction of spermatozoa with cervical mucus and cervical crypts **b** Diagrammatic illustration of human cervical crypt where colonization of spermatozoa takes place. (Reproduced with permission from Phillip 1972.) **c,d** Scanning electron micrographs showing interaction of sperm heads with the ciliated cells of the cervical mucosa.

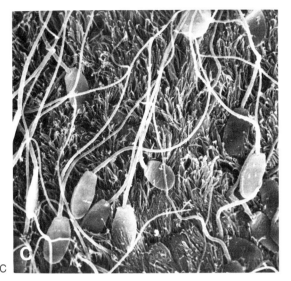

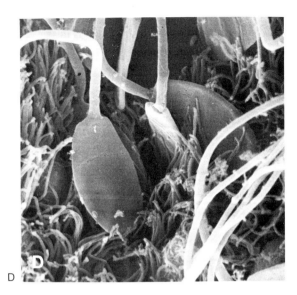

**Fig. 2.12**   C-D

the vanguard sperm entering the oviduct are those that participate in fertilization of the ovum is not known. Fertilization seems to occur only when an optimal number of spermatozoa reach the site of fertilization.

## Colonization of sperm reservoirs

Massive numbers of spermatozoa are trapped in the complex mucosal folds of the cervical crypts (Figs 2.12, 2.13). Insler et al (1981) reported that the number of spermatozoa stored in cervical crypts depends on the hormonal milieu. In women pretreated with estrogen the entire length of the cervical canal contained approximately 150 000, 180 000 and 53 000 sperm cells 2, 24 and 48 h following insemination respectively. After gestagen pretreatment the number of spermatozoa colonizing the cervical crypts was significantly lower being 47 000 at 2 h and 3000 at 24 h after insemination. This process is facilitated by the fact that the micelles of the cervical mucus help to direct spermatozoa to the cervical crypts, where the reservoirs are formed. Fewer leukocytes are found in secretion of the vagina or uterus, thus less phagocytosis of spermatozoa takes place in the cervix. Concentration gradients of spermatozoa are established in female reproductive tracts within a short time after intercourse. The more spermatozoa that enter the

cervical reservoir, the more that reach the oviduct, thus increasing the chance of fertilization. In addition, the larger the reservoir, the longer an adequate population of spermatozoa will be maintained in the oviduct. Spermatozoa may leave the cervix by their own motility or may be passively transported by cervical and uterine contractions.

## Slow release and transport

After adequate sperm reservoirs are established within the reproductive tract, the spermatozoa are released sequentially for prolonged periods. This slow release, which involves the innate motility of spermatozoa and the contractile activity of the myometrium and mesosalpinx, ensures continued availability of spermatozoa for transport into the oviduct to effect fertilization of the egg.

Because of the abundance of ciliated cells at the utero-cervical junction and at the outlets of cervical crypts, it seems that the best of kinocilia may control the alignment of mucus macromolecules in vivo. The kinetics of sperm colonization in the cervical crypts depend on the hydrodynamic, biophysical, physiological, biochemical and immunological interactions between motile and immotile spermatozoa and cervical mucus. It is not known whether the spermatozoa that initially contact the cervical mucus have any

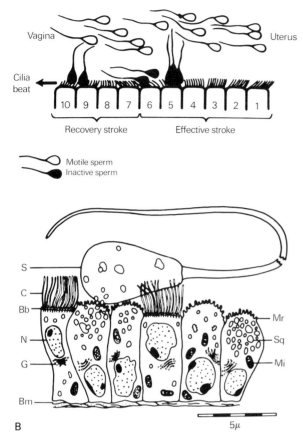

B

**Fig. 2.13 a** Diagrammatic illustration showing the effective and recovery strokes of kinocilia in relation to transport of motile and inactive spermatozoa. **b** Diagrammatic illustration showing the anatomical and physiological interactions among cervical crypt, cervical mucus and spermatozoa. Bm, basement membrane, Bb, basal body; C, cilia; G, Golgi complex; Mi, mitochondria; Mr, microvilli; N, nucleus; S, spermatozoon; Sg, secretory granules.

locomotive advantage or disadvantage over those that follow. Katz et al (1981) studied the 'vanguard' and 'following' human and bovine spermatozoa in fresh ovulatory cervical mucus of their respective species. Sperm movement characteristics in flat capillary tubes were recorded using high-speed cinemicrography. Analysis of covariance and stepwise multiple regression techniques were used to apply the data to a mathematical model of the hydrodynamics of the sperm–mucus interaction. In both species, vanguard spermatozoa swim faster than their followers, although their flagellar beat frequencies do not differ. This difference is due to an alteration of mucus properties by the vanguard sperm. Increased mucus

elasticity, resulting in decreased flagellar thrust of following sperm, may have contributed. An increase in the adhesive forces between the sperm surface and the mucus microstructure is another possible factor (Katz et al 1981).

There are remarkable variations in sperm

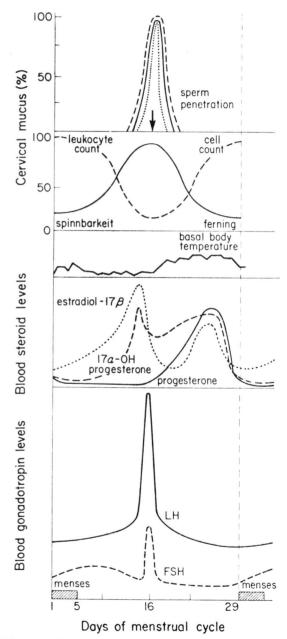

**Fig. 2.14** Cyclical changes in sperm penetrability in cervical mucus as they relate to cyclical fluctuation in endocrine profile and biophysical characteristics of cervical mucus.

penetrability in cervical mucus throughout the menstrual cycle (Fig. 2.14). This has clinical significance in evaluating postcoital tests.

## PATHOPHYSIOLOGICAL CHANGES

### Oncological transformation

The mucosa of the internal and external cervix is made of three types of epithelium: original columnar, original squamous, and metaplastic squamous. The columnar epithelia line the endo-cervical canal and are continuous with the endometrium. The squamous epithelium of the ectocervix is continuous with the vaginal epithelium. A well-defined junction between the columnar and squamous epithelium, located within the cervical canal, may undergo 'squamous metaplasia', whereby columnar epithelium that has been everted onto the ectocervix is replaced by squamous epithelium (Coppleson et al 1978). Cervical neoplasia may even be initiated during the process of metaplasia.

In some cases of adenosis, the columnar epithelium shows marked dysplastic and hyperplastic changes. The cells become crowded and acquire a malignant appearance. However, the surface projections become bleb-like in appearance rather than their usual fine microvillious configuration. In some instances, mucin seems to be extruded from these blebs. At early preinvasive stages of neoplasia, the superficial cell layer acquires a disorganized appearance and the cells become smaller (approximately 20 μm) and more rounded. Cell junctions become less prominent than normal superficial squamous cells.

The preclinical stages of squamous carcinoma have been extensively studied (Shingleton et al 1968, Shingleton & Lawrence 1976). In cervical metaplasia the columnar epithelium is transformed into squamous epithelium. Colposcopy and scanning electron microscopy (Williams et al 1973) have been used to identify the various stages of tissue transformation. Early stages of metaplasia are characterized by a shortening of the columnar cells, the presence of cuboidal-type cells, and the appearance of larger cells among the regular columnar cells. The surfaces of these cells are covered with short, closely packed microvilli without terminal bars. In advanced stages of metaplasia, the new squamous epithelium consists of mature cells with a microridge surface structure.

Carcinoma-in-situ is quite different in appearance from normal epithelium. The epithelium has a disorganized appearance with an uneven surface, in contrast to the appearance of normal squamous epithelium. The cells are rounded and of irregular shape and size, have no well-defined intercellular junction, and are covered with numerous microvilli about 0.15 μm in diameter. The presence of these microvilli in addition to the rounded shape of the cells may interfere with the interdigitation of adjacent surfaces, thus leading to increased exfoliation of these cells.

### Cervical factor/unexplained infertility

Some 5% of infertile women have cervical factor of infertility. Several factors reduce the quantity/quality of cervical mucus associated with reduced viability of sperm; previous surgery/cryosurgery of the cervix, cautery, cone biopsy, cervical stenosis, absence of functional cervical crypts, postpartum dilatation and curettage (D & C), previous abortion, and prenatal exposure to diethylstilbestrol. Chronic cervicitis may cause chronic vaginal discharge or spotting. Similar infections, such as pelvic inflammatory disease (PID), may destroy cervical crypts and contaminate cervical mucus with leukocytes.

In certain women with hypothalamic dysfunction and normal prolactin/androgen, serial determinations of the cervical mucus score and/or well-timed postcoital tests may reveal persistently poor cervical mucus with predominantly immotile sperm. Patients treated with clomiphene may exhibit poor cervical mucus in spite of elevated estrogen level as a result of multiple follicular development. If sperm penetrability in cervical mucus does not improve after clomiphene/estrogen therapy IUI (intrauterine insemination) could be recommended. Therapy with hMG-hCG may also serve as a second-line therapy in such patients as it induces ovulation without deleterious effect on the cervical mucus (Lunenfeld & Lunenfeld 1990). Little is known about the effectiveness of pulsatile GnRH to treat patients with poor cervical mucus production.

## Postmenopausal changes

The postmenopausal exocervix is flattened and protrudes into the vaginal vault. Menopause is associated with sclerosis of the cervical stroma. The columnar epithelium of the endocervix becomes flat, similar to the squamous epithelium of the ectocervix. At the squamo columnar junction, there is distinct demarcation between columnar and squamous epithelium without proliferation. The epithelial cells become flattened and hexagonal, with distinct boundaries. The cells are reduced in volume and the microvilli become slender.

## Diethylstilbestrol abnormalities

In utero diethylstilbestrol (DES) exposure is associated with vaginal adenosis, extensive ectropion, annular cervical rings, cockscomb deformity of the anterior cervical lip (Herbst et al 1972, Robboy et al 1977), incompetent cervix (Singer & Hochman 1978, Schmidt 1980), and elongated endocervical canal. The DES-related structural abnormalities in the cervix may be associated with connective tissue alterations that predispose to abnormal patterns. The smaller diameter of the endocervical canal may also contribute to the increased propensity for cervical stenosis.

The size of the area of vaginal adenosis seems to depend on the stage in the mother's pregnancy when DES was administered (Herbst et al 1975a,b). The large area of original columnar epithelium within the transformation zone undergoes metaplasia. This change is accelerated after puberty when vaginal pH falls due to the onset of estrogenic stimulation.

## Immunological parameters/postcoital test

The immune system in women is capable of local secretion of immunoglobulins. Antisperm antibodies are present in cervical mucus or solubilized cervical mucus in the absence of humoral antisperm antibodies in 3–10% of women. Hence, the need to study cervical mucus in the event of poor sperm survival despite negative serological results for antisperm antibodies (Bronson et al 1986) (See Chapters 13, 14 and 22).

In certain cases of 'unexplained infertility', the poor survival and/or penetration of sperm in cervical mucus may be associated with immunity to spermatozoa, although not invariably. The period of time when spermatozoa establish reservoirs in the cervical crypts varies among women as well as among different menstrual cycles in the same patient. The cervical mucus undergoes remarkable functional changes in viscoelasticity/ penetrability to sperm as a result of increased relative hydration by transudated water, caused by alterations in the endocervical microvasculature in response to increased levels of estrogens.

REFERENCES

Benirschke K 1973 Congenital anomalies of the uterus with emphasis on genetic causes. In: Hettig A T, Norris H J, and Abel M R (eds) The uterus. Williams and Wilkins, Baltimore, p 68

Benson R C (ed) 1979 Current obstetric/gynecologic diagnosis and treatment. Lange Medical Publisher, Los Altos, California, p 152

Blackwell P, Markham R 1976 The histochemistry of the cervical epithelium. In: Jordan J A, Singer A (eds) The cervix, Saunders, London, ch 6

Bronson R A, Cooper G W, Rosenfeld D L 1986 Factors affecting the population of the female reproductive tract by spermatozoa: Their diagnosis and treatment. Semin Reprod Endocrinol 4: 387

Chilton B S, Nicosia S V, Sowinski J M, Wolf D P 1980a Isolation and characterization of rabbit endocervical cells. J Cell Biol 86: 172

Chilton B S, Nicosia S V, Laufer M R 1980b Effect of estradiol-17 on endocervical cytodifferentiation and glycoprotein biosynthesis in the ovariectomized rabbit. Biol Reprod 23: 677

Coppleson M, Pixley E, Reid B (eds) 1978 Colposcopy, 2nd edn. Thomas, Springfield, Illinois

Danforth D N 1947 The fibrous nature of the human cervix and its relation to the isthmic segment in gravid and non gravid uteri. Am J Obstet Gynecol 53: 541

Danforth D N 1954 The distribution and functional activity of the cervical musculature. Am J Ostet Gynecol 68: 1261

Danforth D N, Chapman J C F 1950 The incorporation of the isthmus uteri. Am J Obstet Gynecol 59: 979

David J, Woolf R B 1963 Histology and fine structure of the adult human cervix uteri. Clin Obstet Gynecol 6: 265

Dillon W P, Mudaliar N A, Wingate M B 1979 Congenital atresia of the cervix. Obstet Gynecol 54: 126

Fand S B 1973 The histochemistry of human cervical epithelium. In: Blandau R J, Moghissi K S (eds) The biology of the cervix. University Chicago Press, Chicago ch 7

Farber M 1980 Cervical atresia (letter). Obstet Gynecol 55: 765

Farber M, Marchant D J 1975 Congenital absence of the uterine cervix. Am J Obstet Gynecol 121: 414

Farber M, Marchant D J 1976 Reconstructive surgery for congenital atresia of the uterine cervix. Fertil Steril 27: 1277

Ferenczy A, Gelfand M M 1979 The cytodynamics of normal and neoplastic cervical epithelium. Gynecol Surv 34: 808

Ferenczy A, Richart R M 1974 Female reproductive system: dynamics of scanning and transmission electron microscopy. John Wiley, New York

Fluhmann C F 1961 The cervix uteri and its diseases, W B Saunders, Philadelphia, p 30

Fluhmann C F, Dickmann Z 1958 The basic pattern of the glandular structures of the cervix uteri. Obstet Gynecol 11: 543

Foraker A G 1962 Histochemistry of the uterine cervix: normal exocervical metaplastic, dysplastic, intra-epithelial and invasive carcinomatous epithelium. Ann N Y Acad Sci 93: 632

Friedrich E R 1973 The normal morphology and ultrastructure of the cervix. In Blandau R J, Moghissi K (eds) The biology of the cervix. University of Chicago Press, Chicago, p 76

Fritzsche R, Beller F K 1976 Ein Fall von Zervixaplasie. Geburtschilfe Frauenheilkd 36: 524

Geary W L, Weed J D 1973 Congenital atresia of the uterine cervix. Obstet Gynecol 42: 213

Griffin J E, Edwards C, Madden J D, Harrod M J, Wilson J D 1976 Congenital absence of the vagina: the Mav Rokitansky–Kuster–Hauser syndrome. Ann Intern Med 85: 224

Gustafson R C 1976 The vascular, lymphatic and neural anatomy of the cervix. In: Jordan J A, Singer A (eds) The cervix. Saunders, London, p 79

Hackemann M, Grubb C, Hill K R 1968 The ultrastructure of normal squamous epithelium of cervix uteri. J Ultrastruct Res 22: 443

Hafez E S E 1972a Scanning electron microscopy of the female tract. J Reprod 9: 119

Hafez E S E 1972b Scanning electron microscopy of rabbit and monkey female reproductive tract. Reprod Fertil 30: 293

Hafez E S E 1973 The comparative anatomy of the mammalian cervix. In: Blandau R J, Moghissi K S (eds) The biology of the cervix. AMP: Ann Arbor, p 23

Hafez E S E (ed) 1976 Human semen and fertility regulation in men. C V Mosby, St Louis

Hafez E S E 1980 Gamete transport. In: Human reproduction: conception and contraception, 2nd edn. Harper and Row, New York

Hafez E S E 1982 Structural and ultrastructural histology of the uterine cervix. Reproduction 5: 243

Hafez E S E, Thilbault C (eds) 1975 The biology of spermatozoa. S Karger, Basel

Hafez E S E, Barnhart M I, Ludwig H et al 1975 Scanning electron microscopy of human reproductive physiology. Acta Obstet Gynecol Scand Suppl 40: 3

Hendrickson M R, Kempson R L (eds) 1980 Surgical pathology of the uterine corpus. Saunders, Philadelphia

Herbst A L, Kurman R J, Scully R E 1972 Vaginal and cervical abnormalities after exposure to stilbestrol in utero. Obstet Gynecol 40: 287

Herbst A L, Scully R E, Robboy S J 1975a Problems in the examination of the DEX exposed female. Obstet Gynecol 46: 353

Hebst A L, Poslanzer D C, Robboy S J, Friedlander L, Scully R E 1975b Prenatal exposure to stilbestrol — a prospective comparison of exposed female offspring with unexposed controls. N Engl J Med 11 292: 334

Hiersch H D 1970 Funktionell Morphologie des fetalen and kindlichen cervicalen Drusenfeldes im Uterus. Ergeb Anatom Entwicklung 43: 1

Hirakawa S, Ito A 1979 Dynamic changes of collagen in human ripening uterine cervix at term pregnancy. Scientific Exhibit 9th World Congress of Gynecology/Obstetrics, Tokyo, Japan

Insler V, Glezerman M, Bernstein D, Zeidel L, Misgav N 1981 Cervical crypts and their role in storing spermatozoa In: Insler V, Bettendorf G, Geissler K-H, (eds) Advances of Diagnosis and Treatment of Infertility. Elsevier North Holland, New York, p 195

Iversen S 1966 Congenital atresia of the cervix uteri. Nord Med 75: 41

Jarcho J 1946 Malformations of the uterus. Am J Surg 71: 106

Jaszczak S, Hafez E S E 1973 Sperm migration through the uterine cervix in the macaque during the menstrual cycle. Am J Obstet Gynecol 225: 1070

Jeffcoate T N A 1969 Advancement of the upper vagina in the treatment of haematocolpos and haematometra caused by vaginal aplasia. Pregnancy following the construction of an artificial vagina. J Obstet Gynaecol Br Commonw 76: 961

Jones H W Jr, Wheelers C R 1969 Salvage of the reproductive potential of women with anomalous development of the Mullerian ducts: 1868–1968–2068. Am J Obstet Gynecol 104: 343

Jordan J A 1976 Scanning electron microscopy of the physiology epithelium. In: Jordan J A, Singer A (eds) Saunders, London, ch 4

Katz D F, Brofeldt B T, Bloom T D, Bondurant F W, Hanson F W 1981 Vanguard spermatozoa alter the properties of cervical mucus. Biol Reprod 10: 143

Komori A 1965 Electron microscopic studies on the cyclic changes of the pseudoerosion epithelium of the human uterine portio vaginalis. J Jap Obstet Gynaecol Soc 12: 17

Langley F A, Crompton A C 1973 Epithelial abnormalities of the cervix uteri. In: Recent results in cancer research, vol 40. William Heinemann Medical Books, London, p 17

Lunenfeld B, Lunenfeld E 1990 Ovulation induction: HMG In: Seibel M M (ed) Infertility: a comprehensive test. Appleton & Lange, Connecticut, ch 23

Moghissi K S 1973 Sperm migration through the human cervix. In: Elstein M, Moghissi K S, Borth R (eds) Cervical mucus in human reproduction. Scriptor, Copenhagen, p 128

Monks P 1979 Uterus didelphys associated with unilateral cervical atresia and renal agenesia. Aust NZ J Obstet Gynaecol 19: 245

Nilsson O, Westman A 1961 The ultrastructure of the epithelial cells of the endocervix during the menstrual cycle. Acta Obstet Gynecol Scand 40: 223

Niver D H, Barrette G, Jewelewicz R 1980 Congenital atresia of the uterine cervix and vagina: three cases. Fertil Steril 33: 25

# 3. Functional anatomy of the uterus

*Elizabeth Johannisson*

## INTRODUCTION

The size and configuration of the human uterus undergo dramatic changes throughout life. In fact the human uterus is constantly manipulated by the ovarian hormones. In the premenarchal period, when ovarian secretion of steroids is negligible, the uterus is small and inactive. The shape is dominated by a large cervix, which mainly accounts for more than half of the uterine length. At menarche when the ovaries start their production of sex steroids the uterus responds by increasing in size and by cyclically altering the mucosa.

During reproductive life the uterus body (corpus) gradually expands and the cervix becomes less predominant. In adult nulliparous women the uterus measures approximately 5 cm at its broadest extent and 7–8 cm along its long axis. The cervix measures approximately 3–4 cm in length. The uterine cavity has a triangular shape with the lumina of the Fallopian tubes at two angles and the endocervical canal at the third angle. The length of the cavity is approximately 6 cm and its total volume 3–8 ml. Although the uterine cavity has almost the same configuration as the uterus, it is smaller in size as a consequence of the thick uterine muscular wall, the *myometrium*. It is covered with a mucosa, the *endometrium*, the cyclic changes of which are a prerequisite for implantation of a conceptus. During reproductive life pregnancy provokes the most important physiological deviation from the nulliparous adult uterus. The uterus enlarges greatly due to hypertrophic and hyperplastic changes in the myometrium and significant changes take place in the endomet-

rium as well as in the cervical part. After delivery the uterus decreases in size, mainly due to resorption of connective tissue in the myometrium, but it never returns to its nulliparous size.

After the menopause, with the waning of the synthesis of ovarian sex steroids, the uterus involutes and becomes atrophic. A significant decrease in weight and dimensions takes place. The muscular layer diminishes in thickness and the mucosa becomes thin and atrophic.

Among the components of the functional anatomy of the uterus described above, the changes of the mucosa or the *endometrium* may be of particular importance. Under physiological conditions the uterine mucosa is considered to closely gauge the ovarian activity. The cyclic alterations occurring in the endometrium during reproductive life are a prerequisite for the ultimate function of the uterus — to house and support the conceptus — and the morphological and biochemical changes of the uterine mucosa are likely to play an important role in the implantation of a fertilized oocyte. The molecular events that accompany embryo attachment and implantation after the blastocyst has entered the uterine cavity and hatched through its zona pellucida are still incompletely understood, and infertility problems related to defects in the implantation process are often considered as 'unexplained infertility'.

In view of the importance of the uterine mucosa for the implantation and support of the conceptus, the present review is mainly concerned with alterations of the human endometrium during the normal menstrual cycle and at the time of early pregnancy.

## MORPHOLOGICAL ALTERATIONS OF THE ENDOMETRIUM DURING THE NORMAL MENSTRUAL CYCLE

During the normal menstrual cycle the human endometrium undergoes significant morphological changes as already described in 1950 by Noyes et al. In principle the cycle can be divided into two phases—preovulatory and postovulatory. During the preovulatory phase the endometrium is mainly influenced by estrogens produced by the ovaries. Via the estrogen receptor mechanism the steroid can act on its target organ. At the time when estrogens are predominantly produced by the ovaries the proliferative activity of the endometrium is stimulated. The mucosa composed of the epithelium lining the uterine cavity, the glandular epithelium and the stroma of the functional layer of the endometrium starts to grow. During the postovulatory phase the production of progesterone following the development of the corpus luteum significantly modifies the morphology of the endometrium. These changes occur with great precision, in particular during the first 6 days after ovulation (Johannisson et al 1982, 1987, Dockery et al 1988a,b, Li et al 1988, Dockery & Rogers 1989). In studies using biopsy material timed in relation to the LH peak, basal vacuoles start to appear in the glandular epithelium between days LH−1/0 and LH+1/+2. The number of basal vacuoles then gradually increases up to day LH+4. After day LH+6 basal vacuoles are only occasionally observed in the glandular epithelium. Recent studies by Dockery et al (1990) have also revealed a dramatic increase in the packing density of the stroma between LH+2 and LH+6.

By day LH+6 the very precise day-to-day changes in the uterine mucosa are over. After LH+6 the morphological changes occurring in the endometrium during the normal menstrual cycle are mainly in the stroma. For instance, Dockery et al (1990) reported a substantial decrease (P<0.01) in the packing density of the endometrial stroma.

Days LH+6/+7 are likely to correspond to the beginning of the implantation window. The stromal oedema is reported to be maximal and the increase in volume density of the glands is significant (P<0.001) (Johannisson et al 1987).

At LH+8 to LH+10 other changes also take place in the stroma, e.g. development of predecidua around the spiral arteries as well as in the superficial part of the functional layer of the endometrium. If no implantation occurs, the endometrium undergoes regressive changes, starting approximately at days LH+11/+12 (Johannisson 1990). The volume density of the glands decreases and neutrophils start to invade the endometrial stroma.

## THE DIFFERENT MORPHOLOGICAL COMPONENTS OF THE ENDOMETRIUM

Although the whole endometrium as such must be considered as a target organ for endogeneous and exogeneous steroids, where the various structural components are likely to interact with each other, it is most likely that each structural component of the endometrium has a specific function.

There are several ways to describe the functional morphology of the human endometrium. One of these is to describe the microscopical findings of the basal layer next to the myometrium and to compare the findings with those observed in the functional layer next to the uterine cavity, the 'classical way' to deal with the description. Another approach would be to deal with the individual components of the endometrium such as the *lining epithelium, the glands, the stroma and the vessels* and to describe the morphological changes in each endometrial component in women having physiological 'normal' menstrual cycles and in women with infertility problems where the implantation has failed to occur in spite of optimal ovarian stimulation for in vitro fertilization.

A number of recent studies have reported on specific properties of endometrial glands and stroma (e.g. Maslar & Riddick 1979, Tseng et al 1987, Loke et al 1989). New methods for morphometric measurements of biopsy specimens also open new avenues to deal with the specific endometrial structures as separate components (Johannisson et al 1982, 1987, Li et al 1987, 1988, 1989). In the present review the various endometrial components will be dealt with under separate headings.

## The lining surface epithelium

Several decades ago light microscopic (Hamperl 1950) and transmission electron microscopic studies (Borell et al 1959) of the human endometrium during the normal menstrual cycle reported that cyclic changes occur in the lining epithelium of the uterine cavity and that some lining epithelial cells carried cilia. More recent studies using scanning electron microscopy confirmed the previous findings of cyclic changes occurring in the ciliated as well as in the non-ciliated epithelial cells of fertile women during the physiological menstrual cycle. (Johannisson & Nilsson 1972, Ludwig & Metzger 1976). The cilia and the microvilli were found to be well developed in the preovulatory phase, whereas clods were formed from the ciliae and the microvilli of the cell surfaces during the postovulatory phase.

Scanning electron microscopic studies from material obtained from female fetuses and postmenopausal women did not reveal any ciliated cells (Ludwig & Metzger 1976). It is therefore postulated that the development of ciliated cells might be related to the influence of estrogens. Changes similar to those described in the lining epithelium of the human endometrium have been reported to occur also in the baboons (Wilborn et al 1984). In these non-human primates, comparative scanning and transmission electron microscopic studies revealed cyclic changes in the ciliated cells. The increase in ciliated cells was likely to be related to the administration of estrogens.

Scanning electron microscopic studies of the endometrium in women with infertility problems are rare, probably due to difficulties in the definition of 'unexplained infertility'. At present there is a considerable lack of knowledge with regard to factors important for implantation, and the histological features of the uterine lining epithelium which may characterize the optimal conditions for the implantation of a human blastocyst are not completely understood.

In the studies by Johannisson & Nilsson (1972) the ciliated cells were unevenly distributed in the uterine cavity. The number of ciliated cells was scanty in the tubal corners whereas they were scattered all over the epithelial surface of the fundus area and highly increased towards the endocervix. Ciliated cells were found in higher concentration around the gland openings. The function of the ciliated cells is still not completely understood but the distribution of the ciliated cells seems to support the theory that the cilia are involved in the transport of endometrial secretory product. Studies in baboons (Wilborn et al 1984) also support this theory.

Most secretory products present in the uterine cavity are likely to originate from the glands (Enders 1967). However, secretory activity has also been demonstrated in the endometrial lining epithelium, e.g. acid mucous glycoproteins (Hester et al 1968). Acid mucous glycoproteins are likely to participate in the formation of the glycocalyx of the surface epithelial cells. Membrane glycoproteins are rich in the amino acids threonine and serine, the hydroxyl group of which carry oligosaccharide side-chains similar to those of the mucous glucoproteins. The type and amount of endometrial surface glycoproteins seem to be dependent on the ovarian steroid production. Cyclic changes have been reported to take place in the composition of the glycocalyx of the endometrial lining epithelium with a significant increase in the postovulatory phase (Thor et al 1987). Similar changes were already reported by Jansen et al (1985) who found a significant increase ($P=0.005$) in endometrial surface glycocalyx on the third day after the LH peak. In the same endometrial material accurately timed in relation to the LH-peak Jansen et al (1985) also found a decrease in electronegativity of the glycocalyx coinciding with the increase of glycoprotein cell-surface coat. In chemical terms this represents replacement of highly acid sulfated surface glycoprotein with moderately acid sialyated glycoprotein, a reaction which is likely to be a part of the influence of progesterone on the human endometrium. The decrease in electronegativity of the glycocalyx of the endometrial lining epithelium may be required for a normal implantation and it cannot be excluded that disturbances in the glycocalyx pattern may impede a successful implantation, particularly in the adhesion phase of the implantation.

Permeability factors of the surface lining epithelium with possible passage of substances between the endometrial vessels and the uterine cavity have been reported to exist (Luukainen et al 1984). However, such factors have not been sufficiently studied during the normal menstrual cycle or in relation to infertility.

## The endometrial glands

During reproductive life characteristic changes occur in the endometrial glands of the human endometrium during the normal menstrual cycle. The endometrium cannot be described as one 'organ' having the same histological structure, function and metabolic properties. For instance, the morphological changes occurring in the basal layer of the mucosa differ histologically from those of the upper functional layer. The endocervical part does not have the same steroid receptor concentration as the uterine fundus area, etc. (Tsibris et al 1981). The endometrial biopsy usually represents a part of the functional layer of the fundus area of the uterine mucosa. It was therefore felt that the present review should be limited to the description of this part of the endometrium.

The morphological changes occurring in the endometrial glands are easy to identify and can be assessed quantitatively by morphometric methods (Fig. 3.1). The number of glands per square millimeter is approximately 20 and this number has not been shown to vary significantly during the cycle (Johannisson et al 1987) (Fig. 3.2). Nor does the diameter of the glands vary significantly during the preovulatory phase (Fig. 3.2). On the other hand, a significant correlation has been found between the diameter of the glands and the mean of the daily levels of estradiol 72 h preceding the time of the biopsy (Johannisson et al 1982). Therefore it cannot be excluded that the development of the glands during the preovulatory phase is dependent on the estrogens produced by the ovarian follicles. This hypothesis is supported by immunochemical studies, which have shown that approximately 50% of the glandular cells stained positively for estrogen receptors in the early preovulatory phase, whereas only a small portion of progesterone receptors stained positively (Garcia et al 1988). Early studies have already shown that estrogens stimulate the growth of the target organ cells (Segal & Scher 1967). It is

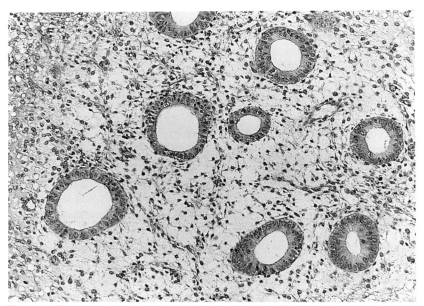

**Fig. 3.1**   Human endometrium obtained at the day of the LH surge. The mucosa is characterized by a slightly oedematous stroma and a glandular epithelium showing pseudostratification and a large number of mitoses. At the day of ovulation, represented by the LH surge, the endometrium displays a histological pattern which corresponds to 'late proliferation'. ($\times$ 163).

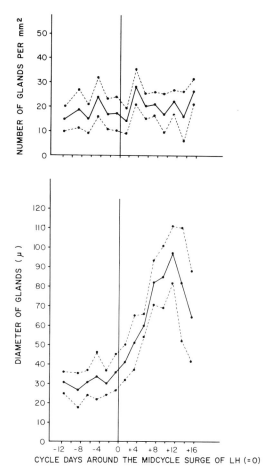

**Fig. 3.2** Number of glands per mm² and diameter of the transversally sectioned glands. The data represent mean values at 48-h periods ± SD grouped around the midcycle LH surge. A total of 90 women with timed biopsies was studied.

with their nuclei at different levels, giving rise to pseudostratification.

During the preovulatory phase, the endometrial glandular cells , when viewed electronmicroscopically, are all characterized by cytoplasmic structures compatible with high proliferative activity. A large number of ribosomes is present in the cytoplasm and a gradual increase in the development of the rough endoplasmic reticulum has been reported (Verma 1983, Cornillie et al 1985). In the late preovulatory phase glycogen particles have been described in the cytoplasm of the glandular epithelium (Themann & Schünke 1963).

The full development of the glands including the synthesis of estrogen and progesterone receptors are likely to be important factors for an adequate transformation of the uterine mucosa into a secretory endometrium with optimal conditions for implantation. The results of preliminary experiments have suggested the need for synchronization between the estrogen production of the ovarian follicles and the biochemical and morphological development of the endometrium. Premature exposure to small amounts of progesterone in the very early proliferative phase (CD(cycle day) 2–6) did not have any significant influence on the endometrial histology when compared with the control samples, whereas exposure to the same small amount of progesterone in the late preovulatory phase (CD 7–11) induced significant morphological changes such as diminished number of glandular mitoses, decrease in the height of the glandular epithelium and reduced pseudostratification (Xing Shumin et al 1983). Furthermore, the administration of antiestrogens (e.g. used for the stimulation of the follicular activity in relation to in vitro fertilization) has been reported to be followed by a decreased glandular volume in the endometrium (Bonhoff et al 1990, Rogers et al 1991).

Most morphological studies related to infertility have so far been focused on the development of the secretory activity of the endometrium in the postovulatory phase. However, the follicular development and the estrogen production during the preovulatory phase may be equally important for the achievement of a uterine environment suitable for implantation of a

therefore not surprising to find that the DNA-RNA values are significantly increased during the early preovulatory phase (LH–11 to LH–4) (Johannisson et al 1987). Unfortunately, the number of mitoses is not a very reliable index of the proliferative activity of the glands. The number of glandular mitoses varies greatly during the preovulatory phase and shows a significant decrease between days LH–3/–2 and LH–1/0 (P< 0.05).

A rapid growth of the epithelium of the glands occurs during the preovulatory period preceding LH–3/–2. The size of the glands does not keep pace with this growth and the tall columnar epithelial cells finally pile up against each other fertilized oocyte. Marchini et al (1991) recently reported that the proliferative activity in glands and stroma was higher in women undergoing controlled ovarian hyperstimulation with buserelin acetate and human gonadotrophins. Furthermore, morphometric evaluation of this material revealed early secretory changes which were unrelated to increasing circulating progesterone levels. The physiological optimal estrogen 'priming' during the normal menstrual cycle and the potential need for the synchronization between the development of the ovarian follicles and the growth and receptor synthesis of the endometrium is still incompletely understood. A better knowledge in this respect may improve the success rate of many in vitro fertilization programmes. The current success rate rarely exceeds 25% per cycle of treatment (Ethics Committee of the American Fertility Society 1990) whereas apparently healthy embryos are achieved in vitro in about 75% of the treated cycles (Jones 1984).

The production of progesterone following ovulation introduces a number of changes in the morphology of the endometrial glands during the normal menstrual cycles. Between LH-1/0 and LH+1/+2 basal vacuoles start to appear in the glandular epithelium. (Fig. 3.3). In fact there is a gradual increase in the number of vacuolated cells up to day LH+4. The basal vacuoles then remain until day LH+6. At days LH+7/+8 the basal vacuoles of the glandular cells have almost completely disappeared. Usually the presence of basal vacuoles in the glandular cells is considered as an effect of progesterone (Pincus 1965). However, it may not be the most sensitive index of progestational activity and probably not the most specific one either. Judging from its occurrence in the endometrium of ovariectomized women treated exclusively with estrogen, the specificity of the basal vacuoles of the glandular cells as a criterion of progestational action upon the endometrium may be questioned (Ferin 1971). Similar views were recently expressed by Marchini et al (1991). During the first 6 days following ovulation the glandular mitoses completely disappear and after day LH+6 no more glandular mitoses can be found. The glandular diameter as well as the volume density of the glandular lumen show a linear increase

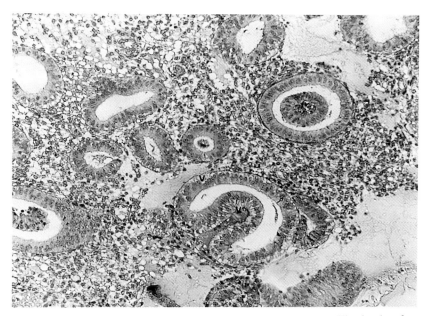

**Fig. 3.3** Endometrium obtained on the second day after the LH surge. The density of the stroma is increased. Some of the glands have started to develop regular basal vacuoles in the epithelium whereas other glands are still characterized by histological changes corresponding to 'late proliferation'. (×163).

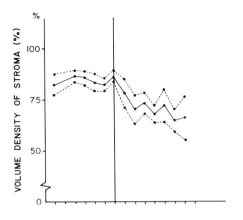

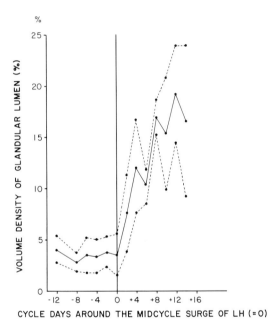

CYCLE DAYS AROUND THE MIDCYCLE SURGE OF LH (=0)

**Fig. 3.4** Volume density of the stroma and of the glandular lumen expressed as a percentage of the total endometrial volume. Mean values of 48-h periods ± SD derived from 90 women with normal menstrual cycles and grouped around the LH surge.

from day LH–1/0 to day LH+11/+12 (Fig. 3.4) and the height of the glandular epithelium significantly diminishes from day LH+3/+4 to LH+15/+16 (Johannisson et al 1987) (Fig. 3.5).

Provided that the endometrial biopsy is timed in relation to the LH surge, the cellular events in the glandular epithelium during the first 6 days after ovulation seem to be very precisely regulated and the interindividual variations are negligible. This regularity in the development of morpholog-

ically well-defined changes has been reported by Li et al (1987, 1988, 1989) and by Dockery et al (1988a) using morphometric analysis of endometrial biopsies.

Electron microscopic studies of the glandular structure during the first 6 days after ovulation revealed the development of a nuclear channel system composed of two to five tubules (Clyman 1963, Ancla et al 1965, Terzakis 1965, Wynn & Woolley 1967, Dockery et al 1988b). After day LH+6 the nuclear channel system was reported to have disappeared. The significance of this nuclear structure is still not fully understood.

Postovulatory changes of the glandular cells were also observed electron microscopically in the cytoplasm. In the early postovulatory phase glycogen particles were found to be scattered throughout the cytoplasm. Cornillie et al (1985) described these particles as accumulated close to the nucleus. This phenomenon might be related to the initiation of the secretory activity of the endometrium. On day LH+4 giant mitochondria and subnuclear 'vacuoles' were described in the glandular epithelium (Dockery et al 1988b), and in biopsies obtained at day LH+6 a smooth endoplasmic reticulum was found in the apical part of the cells. Furthermore the Golgi apparatus was well developed with a prominent vesicular structure. All these morphological events occurring in the endometrium suggest an active secretory activity (Dockery et al 1988b).

Although the morphological changes of the endometrial glands during the pre- and postovulatory phase of the menstrual cycle coincide with the changing levels of the estradiol and progesterone in plasma, there does not seem to be any simple relationship between the circulating hormone levels and the morphometric indices. The concentration and localization of estradiol and progesterone receptors have therefore been considered as an important mediating factor between the plasma steroid levels and the histological changes of the endometrium. At the time of ovulation a marked staining of progesterone receptors has been reported in the majority of the glandular cells (75%) (Garcia et al 1988, Lessey et al 1988). In this respect it is noteworthy that the estrogen receptors have been reported to be associated not only with the initiation of

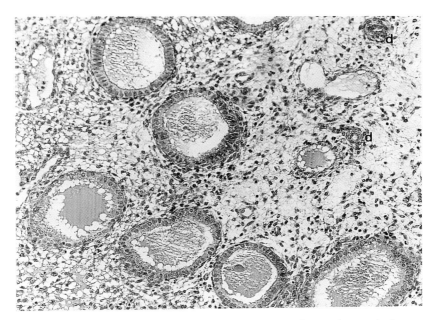

**Fig. 3.5** Endometrium obtained on day LH + 9. The stroma shows a decrease in the packing density with development of an edema. The glands are dilated with secretory products present in the lumina and low 'exhausted' epithelium. Predecidual changes (d) start to develop around the arterioles. The veins show slight dilatation. (x 163).

DNA–RNA transcription and protein synthesis of the glandular cells but also with the synthesis of the progesterone receptors (Milgrom et al 1970).

During the postovulatory phase the estradiol and progesterone receptor content either declines or disappears in the glandular epithelium (Garcia et al 1988, Lessey et al 1988). The balance of evidence therefore suggests that the estrogen and progesterone receptors both play an important role in the growth and differentiation of the glandular epithelium during the menstrual cycle. The complex interaction between ovarian steroid production, the steroid receptor synthesis and the final morphological and biochemical events taking place in the endometrium is likely to play an important role in the process of implantation. In this respect the stroma also has to be taken into consideration.

## The endometrial stroma

Whereas the histological and immunochemical changes of the endometrial glands are most prominent during the first 6 days after ovulation, the changes of the stroma are dominating from LH+7/+8 to the onset of menstruation. The endometrial stroma is a complex structure consisting of mesenchymal cells with pluripotential properties. During the preovulatory phase the stroma is mainly composed for fibroblasts which produce macromolecular precursors of collagen and elastic fibers. The fibroblasts show a slow growth reaching a maximum of mitotic figures at the time of ovulation (Johannisson et al 1987). During the preovulatory phase the cytoplasm of the stromal cells contains a large number of ribosomes but other cytoplasmic organelles such as the Golgi apparatus and the mitochondria are poorly developed (Sengel & Stoebner 1970). Estradiol and progesterone receptors are only present in a small portion of the stroma cells in the early part of the preovulatory phase. However, at the time of ovulation approximately 50% of the stroma cells are stained positively for progesterone and estradiol receptors (Garcia et al 1988).

Later during the postovulatory phase the stromal cells participate in the production of glycoproteins of the extracellular matrix as well as in the degradation of this matrix by synthesizing collagenase and other proteoglycan-degrading enzymes (Werb et al 1977). Mast cells and lymphocytes are also frequently present in the stroma of the endometrium. As revealed by the electron microscope the endoplasmic reticulum becomes more prominent and the mitochondria increase in size and number (Verma 1983). Some cytoplasmic extensions containing glycogen granules have also been described in the extracellular matrix (Cornillie et al 1985).

The major changes in the morphology of the endometrial stroma take place 8–10 days after ovulation, when the stroma becomes edematous and starts to develop predecidual changes around the spiral arteries (Fig. 3.5). Approximately 10 days after ovulation predecidual changes are also observed in the superficial part of the functional layer next to the lining epithelium. Light microscopically the predecidual cells are characterized by a vesicular nucleus and abundant clear cytoplasm. By light microscopy electron microscopy the predecidual cells display a rounding of the nucleus and an increase and dilatation of the rough endoplasmic reticulum including the Golgi apparatus (Verma 1983, Cornillie et al 1985). An accumulation of glycogen and various lysosomal enzymes has also been reported (Schmidt-Matthiesen 1963a). The importance of the predecidual reaction of the endometrium during the postovulatory phase for the nidation of a blastocyst and the early embryo development has been widely discussed. A number of proteins have been identified, e.g. PP14, a protein immunologically similar to pregnancy-associated endometrial $\alpha_1$-globulin (Seppälä et al 1988, Julkunen et al 1990) and PP12, which is likely to be identical with the low-molecular mass of insulin-like growth factor-binding protein (IGFBP) (Wahlström & Seppälä 1984, Julkunen et al 1988). Among the factors which are likely to be involved in the development of the decidualization of the human endometrium, insulin-like growth factors (IGFs) or somatomedins have been claimed to play a significant role (Koistinen et al 1986). In this respect it is noteworthy that the insulin-like growth factor-binding protein (IGFBP) has been postulated to be involved in specifying the proliferation of the endometrial fibroblasts which later differentiate into decidual cells (Bell 1989).

The decidualization of the human endo-

metrium during the postovulatory phase is not only associated with characteristic morphological patterns, but is also accompanied by prolactin secretion (Maslar & Riddick 1979). The production of this hormone has been shown to be highly correlated with the degree of histological decidualization, and more recent studies by Irwin et al (1989) have shown that the prolactin production by the stroma cells can be stimulated by progesterone in vitro in a dose-dependent manner. Other hormones such as the prostaglandins ($PGF_{2\alpha}$ and $PGE_2$) have been reported to be present in the endometrium (Abel et al 1980, Kasamo et al 1986) and prostaglandin endoperoxide synthesis have been demonstrated in the decidualized endometrial stromal cells in early pregnancy (Price et al 1989).

The development of the predecidua in the endometrium during the postovulatory phase is also followed by a significant increase in fibronectin and laminin forming the extracellular matrix (Wewer et al 1985). A pattern of pericellular distribution of laminin was found around the individual decidual cells in vitro and this reaction was found to be identical to that observed in vivo (Loke et al 1989).

The intrauterine implantation may take place only during a limited period of time ('the implantation window') and therefore the uterine environment could be indifferent, favorable or hostile to an embryo. Among the embryo-toxic substances, cholic acids have been found in high concentration in the human uterine fluid between the 22nd and 25th day of the menstrual cycle (Psychoyos et al 1989). The presence of the cholic acids in the uterine fluid coincided with the nonreceptive period of the postovulatory phase and it was suggested that this substance may be one of the factors responsible for embryo toxicity.

Retarded development of the glandular and stromal components of the endometrium has often been considered to be one possible cause of infertility. However, in the current literature, the prevalence of retarded endometrial development in women with unexplained infertility varies greatly from 8% to 65% (Jones & Pourmand 1962, Wentz 1980, Cook et al 1983, Cumming et al 1985, Huang 1986, Gerhard et al 1990). In 1989 Li et al reported that the prevalence of retarded endometrium was higher in women with infertility. However, no significant difference was found between fertile and infertile women in two other studies (Balasch et al 1985, Davis et al 1989). To some extent the varying results presented in the literature might be explained by the the lack of precise reference to the time of ovulation. Recent studies have shown important individual variations in the length of the preovulatory and postovulatory phase in normally menstruating fertile women (Johannisson et al 1987), and the traditional criteria of Noyes et al (1950) based on a hypothetic 'normal' 28-day cycle divided into a postovulatory and preovulatory phase of equal length may have to be modified using more precise reference points than the onset of the first and second menstrual bleeding. The LH surge may be a more precise reference for ovulation. Interobserver variability alone has also been found to be high, indicating false-positive diagnosis of the luteal phase defect (Li et al 1989). Finally one single plasma progesterone value is unlikely to reflect the function of the corpus luteum and, together with the lack of precision in the traditional endometrial dating, the risk of false-positive diagnosis of defective corpus luteum function should not be underestimated. During recent years the diagnosis of retarded endometrium related to corpus luteum deficiency has greatly improved. In a recent study Li & coworkers (1990) evaluated the luteal phase in a group of 49 women with unexplained infertility. The LH surge was used for precise timing of the various measurements, the histology of the endometrial biopsy was assessed by quantitative morphometric methods and the progesterone concentration was determined by integrating the daily levels from LH+1 to the end of the luteal phase. Overall 10 (20%) of the women were considered to have retarded development of the endometrium and out of these only four were associated with an integrated progesterone concentration below the normal range. Li & coworkers (1990) concluded that there was no difference 'in age, duration of infertility, follicular phase length, magnitude of estrogen surge, magnitude of LH surge, maximum follicular diameter and luteal phase length between women with a normal or defective luteal phase, defined

either by endometrial morphology or integrated progesterone concentration'. The retarded development of the endometrium may therefore be an abnormal response of the endometrium itself rather than the consequence of a deficient corpus luteum function. It cannot be excluded that the various secretory activities which are likely to be important for the normal implantation process are seriously modified in the retarded endometrium. Additional studies using the now available improved methods for the assessment of the endometrial biopsy material are required to elucidate the functional relationship between the retarded endometrium and the presence of infertility.

## Endometrial vascularization

There are a number of studies describing the uterine vessels including the vascular structure of the myometrium and that of the endometrium (for review see Schmidt-Matthiesen 1963b, Johannisson 1990).

The vessels of the myometrium and the *basal* layer of the endometrium have been reported to be little influenced by ovarian hormone production. The spiral arteries passing through the myometrium into the basal layer of the endometrium are of special interest. At the entry of these arteries into the basal uterine mucosa their vascular wall is characterized by a thick muscular layer containing an elastic lamina. No major changes have been reported to take place in this lower part of the spiral arteries during the physiological menstrual cycle.

In the *functional* layer of the endometrium extensive changes take place in vascularization, including the spiral arteries, the arterioles, the capillaries, the venous lakes and the veins. These changes are highly sensitive to the influence of ovarian hormones during the normal menstrual cycle (Peek et al 1992) and early pregnancy (Robertson 1987). During the preovulatory phase the vascular system of the functional endometrial layer is characterized by rapid growth. The most distal parts of the spiral arteries become connected to the subepithelial capillary plexus via arterioles, but they also develop small branches at irregular intervals in the functional layer (Fanger & Barker 1961, Ramsey 1977). At the time of ovulation the spiral arteries start to increase in thickness mainly due to a gradual increase in the amount of collagen, elastin and acid mucopolysaccharides in the vascular wall (Schmidt-Matthiesen 1963a,b). During the second half of the menstrual cycle the spiral arteries grow even larger and longer. This growth does not keep pace with the other components of the endometrial stroma, the fibroblasts stop their proliferative activity at days LH+3/+4. As a consequence the tortuosity of the spiral arteries becomes more developed after day LH+6. Somewhat later in the postovulatory phase — at approximately day LH+9/+10—predecidual changes start to appear around the spiral arteries.

The subepithelial capillary plexus also undergoes changes during the normal menstrual cycle. During the preovulatory phase the capillaries are all thin walled and the capillary lumen is narrow. In the early postovulatory phase the lumens of the capillaries progressively increase in diameter (Sheppard & Bonnar 1980). The dilatation reaches its maximum around LH+7 to LH+10, at the time when nidation of the blastocyst is likely to take place (Peek et al 1992). Up to day LH+7/+10 the number of capillaries is also likely to increase and at that time a complex meshwork of capillaries is present in the upper functional layer of the endometrium. The observation made in the endometrial biopsies timed in relation to the LH surge supports the results of animal experiments, indicating that the vascular dynamics and the functional properties of the endometrial capillaries are important factors for the implantation and nidation process of a blastocyst.

During the postovulatory phase there is a close connection between the thin capillaries and the arterioles as well as the venules, which are often dilated and sometimes form venous lakes. It has been postulated that these highly dilated venules and venous lakes play an important role in regulating the blood volume and the rate of the blood flow in the superficial part of the endometrium (Ramsey 1977). Arteriovenous shunts have also been suggested to be responsible for the formation of the venous lakes (Dalgaard 1945, Schlegel 1945), although there is controversy about this theory (Bartelmez 1956).

Dilatation of the superficial endometrial capillaries is likely to coincide with increased permeability of the endothelial cells (Fig. 3.6). This increased permeability has already been described at the beginning of the implantation process in rodents (Psychoyos 1971, Abrahamsohn et al 1983). An increase in capillary permeability is likely to permit complexes of serum proteins to cross the blood vessel walls and provoke a stromal edema. In the human endometrium the stromal edema reaches its maximum around LH+10/+11, immediately after maximal dilatation of the capillary lumen has been reached. (Johannisson et al 1987). The blood flow as well as the permeability of the endothelial cell membranes and the development of stromal edema may all contribute to the establishment of optimal conditions for the implantation of a blastocyst. However, more studies using precisely timed human endometrial material have to be carried out in order to better elucidate the role of these factors in infertility.

Another factor still poorly understood in the endometrial vascularization is the mechanism triggering the onset of menstruation. Fifty years ago Markee (1940) introduced a model for studying the menstrual bleeding occurring in the human endometrium. By using intraocular transplants of human endometrium in monkeys he managed to show that the menstrual bleeding in these transplants started in relation to a strong vasoconstriction in the distal segment of the spiral arteries. The bleeding seemed to take place through gaps in the cellular lining of the arterioles. Markee (1940) calculated the blood loss in endometrial transplants to be 12.5 ml through gaps in the cellular lining, whereas gaps in the capillaries accounted for 5 ml of blood loss and the rupture of the venules caused a blood loss of 6.25 ml. Diapedesis was calculated to give a minor blood loss of 1.25 ml in the transplants. Ruptures of the capillary cell walls (Fig. 3.7), and disintegration of endometrial tissue (Fig. 3.8) surrounding the vessels have also been reported in relation to the onset of menstruation (Sixma et al 1980, Kim-Björklund et al 1991).

It is generally believed that the onset of endometrial bleeding and desquamation of the uterine mucosa is a consequence of decreasing plasma levels of ovarian steroids. In normally menstruating women the onset of menstruation

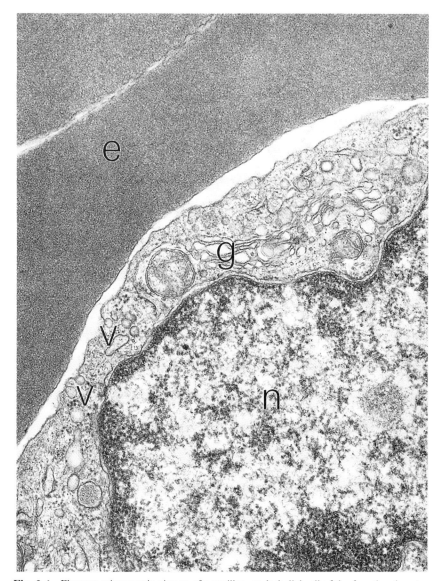

**Fig. 3.6** Electron microscopic picture of a capillary endothelial cell of the functional part of the endometrium at day LH + 2. The cytoplasm is characterized by a well-developed Golgi apparatus (g) and a system of 'plasmolemmal vesicles' (v) which are likely to be important for the permeability. n, nucleus; e, erythrocyte. ($\times$ 33 240).

is, however, not invariably associated with low circulating levels of estradiol and progesterone (Landgren et al 1980). The mechanism responsible for the onset of any endometrial bleeding episodes including irregular bleedings may therefore be more complex than previously believed.

A number of controversies exist regarding the direct effect of sex steroids on the uterine blood vessels. Perret-Applanat et al (1988) used immunochemical methods specific for steroid receptors and demonstrated a positive reaction for estrogen and progesterone receptors in the muscle cells (tunica media) of the uterine arteries. The uterine capillaries and the veins were all reported to be negative for the immunoreactivity. Press & Greene (1988) could not localize any progesterone receptors in the smooth muscle cells of the uterine vessels.

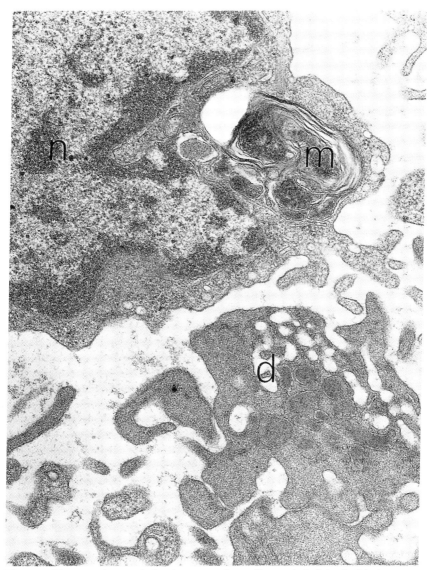

**Fig. 3.7** Electron micrograph showing a part of a capillary endothelial cell of the human endothelium at the onset of menstruation. The cytoplasm displays a number of degenerative changes such as myelin figures (m) and lysis of mitochondria and other cytoplasmic organelles. n, nucleus, d, degenerated cell. (× 33 240).

The endothelium lining the endometrial vessels has only been sporadically studied in the uterine mucosa during the normal menstrual cycle. Most immunocytochemical studies have reported a negative reaction for estrogen and progesterone receptors in the uterine endothelial cells (Perret-Applanat et al 1988, Press & Green 1988). However, this lack of immunoreactivity for estrogen and progesterone receptors in the uterine endothelial cells does not seem to exclude cyclic changes in these cells which could be related to the influence of the sex hormones. Immunocytochemical studies of Factor VIII — an important component in the process of blood coagulation — displayed a gradually increased activity during the preovulatory phase (Zhu Pengdi & Zhao Gu 1988). The same authors reported the absence of a positive reaction in the

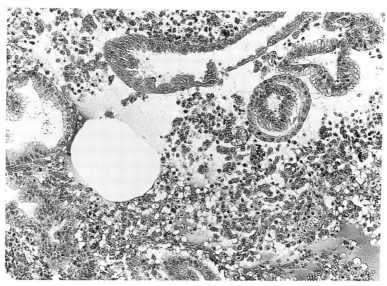

**Fig. 3.8**   Human endometrium obtained at the onset of menstruation. Strong degenerative changes are observed in the stroma and the vascular system. The infiltration of neutrophils is important. The glandular epithelium also shows degenerative changes although the basal membrane still keeps the glandular configuration together. ($\times$ 163).

uterine endothelium in the late postovulatory phase and at the time of the onset of menstruation. The findings suggest an influence of sex hormones on the synthesis of Factor VIII with a potential effect on the blood coagulation mechanism. In this respect it may be noteworthy that capillary fragility in general has been reported to be increased at the time of menstruation (Salvatore 1952).

Female infertility may be associated with various types of abnormal bleedings. Although in many cases of unexplained infertility regular menstrual cycles are common, abnormalities such as oligomenorrhea and hypermenorrhea may be present. The causes of abnormal bleedings can be different. Organic lesions like adenomyosis, endometriosis, leiomyomas or polyps may be the cause, but ovulatory dysfunctional uterine bleedings may also occur. In the latter case the infertility may be related to midcycle spotting, polymenorrhea and oligomenorrhea. The uterine vascularization including the endothelium is likely to be one of the important factors involved in the complex mechanism of implantation of a blastocyst in the human endometrium. It cannot be excluded that it also plays a role in an abnormal

response of the endometrium to circulating progesterone and a retarded development of the uterine mucosa during the postovulatory phase. In a comprehensive review of the endothelium Majno & Joris (1978) state that 'it has become more and more obvious that endothelia differ in structure, function and metabolic properties not only in different organs, but in different parts of the same organ and even in different segments of a single microcirculatory loop'. Only a limited number of studies have been done on the endometrial endothelium. The role of the ovarian steroids in modifying the membrane permeability and the protein synthesis of the endometrial endothelium needs to be further investigated.

## CONCLUSION

Unexplained infertility is a matter of concern in the treatment of infertile couples. Although there might be multiple reasons for this type of infertility, it has been repeatedly suggested that disturbances in the development of the endometrium during the postovulatory phase could be an important factor. The improved technology of in vitro fertilization and the discrepancy between the current success rate (approximately 25% per cycle of treatment) and the number of apparently healthy embryos transferred to the uterine cavity (approximately 75%, Jones 1984) has also renewed the interest in endometrial factors which may be important for implantation. The molecular events which accompany the implantation process in the human endometrium are unfortunately still poorly understood. This lack of knowledge may to some extent be explained by the fact that the process of implantation in the human species is likely to be unique. There is a great variation in the implantation process among different species and results from animal experiments cannot be unconditionally extrapolated to humans. The morphological and biochemical changes occurring in the human endometrium during the normal menstrual cycle represent a highly complex system of hormonally regulated events and it is most likely that disturbances in the synchronization of these events interfere with the optimal conditions of fertility. During the last decade more precise and accurate technology for studying the endometrium has been developed. Simple methods for the detection of ovulation have made it possible to obtain endometrial biopsies timed in relation to the LH surge. Morphometric measurements of the uterine mucosa have allowed a more objective assessment of the histological changes including statistical analyses, and highly sophisticated techniques for the detection of steroid-specific proteins in the endometrial tissue have been established. Nevertheless, endometrial factors related to infertility are still incompletely known. A multidisciplinary effort including gynecologists, biologists, biochemists, histologists and other experts in the field might contribute to a better understanding of recent gaps in the knowledge.

## REFERENCES

Abel M H, Smith S K, Baird D T 1980 Suppression of concentration of endometrial prostaglandin in early intra-uterine and ectopic pregnancy in women. J Endocrinol 85:379

Abrahamsohn P, Lundkvist O, Nilsson O 1983 Ultrastructure of the endometrial blood vessels during implantation of the rat blastocyst. Cell Tissue Res 229: 269

Ancla M, Simon P, De Brux J, Robey M 1965 Modifications endométriales aprés administration prolongée de lynestrenol. Etude au microscope optique et électronique. Gynécol Obstét 64: 231

Balasch J, Vanrell J, Creus M, Marquez M, Gonzalez-Merlo J 1985 The endometrial biopsy for diagnosis of luteal phase deficiency. Fertil Steril 44:699

Bartelmez G W 1956 Premenstrual and menstrual ischemia and the myth of endometrial arteriovenous anastomoses. Am J Anat 98: 69

Bell S C 1989 Decidualization and insulin-like growth factor (IGF) binding protein: implications for its role in stromal cell differentiation and the decidual cell in haemochorial placentation. Hum Reprod 4: 125

Bonhoff A, Johannisson E, Bohnet H G 1990 Morphometric analysis of the endometrium of infertile patients in relation to peripheral hormone levels. Fertil Steril 54: 84

Borell U, Nilsson O, Westman A 1959 The cyclic changes occurring in the epithelium lining the endometrial glands. An electron-microscopie study in the human being. Acta Obstet Gynecol Scand 38: 364

Clyman M J 1963 A new structure observed in the nucleolus of the human endometrial epithelial cells. Am J Obstet Gynecol 86: 430

Cook C L, Raoch V, Yussman M A 1983 Plasma gonadotrophin and sex steriod hormone levels during early, midfollicular and midluteal phase of women with luteal phase defects. Fertil Steril 40: 45

Cornillie F J, Lauweryns J M, Brosens I 1985 Normal human endometrium. An ultrastructural survey. Gynecol Obstet Invest 20: 113

Cumming D C, Honore L C, Scott J Z, Williams K P 1985 The late luteal phase in infertile women: comparison of simultaneous endometrial biopsy and progesterone levels. Fertil Steril 43: 715

Dalgaard J B 1945 The blood vessels of the human endometrium. Acta Obstet Gynecol Scand 26: 342

Davis O K, Berkeley A S, Naus G J, Cholst I N, Freedman K S 1989 The incidence of luteal phase defect in normal, fertile women, determined by serial endometrial biopsies. Fertil Steril 51: 582

Dockery P, Rogers A W 1989 The effects of steroids on the fine structure of the endometrium. Baillière's Clin Obstet Gynaecol 3: 248

Dockery P, Li T C, Rogers A W, Cooke I D, Lenton E A 1988a The ultrastructure of the glandular epithelium in the timed endometrial biopsy. Hum Reprod 3: 826

Dockery P, Li T C, Rogers A W, Cooke I D, Lenton E A, Warren M A 1988b An examination of the variation in timed endometrial biopsies. Hum Reprod 3: 715

Dockery P, Warren M A, Li T C, Rogers A W, Cooke I D, Mundy J 1990 A morphometric study of the human endometrial stroma during periimplantation period. Hum Reprod 5: 112

Enders A C 1967 The uterus in delayed implantation. In: Wynn R M (ed) Cellular biology of the uterus. North Holland Publishing Company, Amsterdam, p 184

Ethics Committee of the American Fertility Society 1990

Ethical considerations of the new reproductive technology. Fertil Steril 53 (suppl 2): 378

Fanger H, Barker B E 1961 Capillaries and arterioles in normal endometrium. Obstet Gynecol 17: 543

Ferin J 1971 The effects of progesterone on the human utero-vaginal tract. In: International encyclopedia of pharmacology and therapeutics, section 48, vol 1. Pergamon, Oxford, Ch 22

Garcia E, Bouchard P, De Brux J et al 1988 Use of immunocytochemistry of progesterone and estrogen receptors for endometrial dating. J Clin Endocrinol Metab 67: 80

Gerhard I, Bechthold E, Eggert-Kruse W, Heberling D, Runnenbaum B 1990 Value of endometrial biopsies and serum hormone determinations in women with infertility. Hum Reprod 5: 906

Hamperl H 1950 Ueber die 'hellen' Flimmerepithelzellen der menschlichen Uteruschleimhaut. Virchows Arch [A] 319: 265

Hester L L, Kellett W W III, Spicer S S, Williamsson H O, Pratt-Thomas H R 1968 Effects of sequential oral contraceptive on endometrial enzyme and carbohydrate histochemistry. Am J Obstet Gynecol 102: 771

Huang K E 1986 The primary treatment of luteal phase inadequacy: progesterone versus clomiphene citrate. Am J Obstet Gynecol 155: 824

Irwin J C, Kirk D, King R J, Quigley M M, Gwatkin R B 1989 Hormonal regulation of human endometrial stromal cells in culture: an in vitro model for decidualization. Fertil Steril 52: 761

Jansen R P S, Turner M, Johannisson E, Landgren B M, Diczfalusy E 1985 Cyclic changes in human endometrial surface glycoproteins: a quantitative histochemical study. Fertil Steril 44: 85

Johannisson E 1990 Endometrial morphology during the normal cycle and under the influence of contraceptive steroids. In: d'Arcangues C, Fraser 1, Newton J R & Odlind V (eds) WHO Symposium on Contraception and Endometrial Bleeding. Cambridge University Press, Cambridge, pp 53-80

Johannisson E, Nilsson L 1972 Scanning electron microscopic study of the human endometrium. Fertil Steril 23: 613

Johannisson E, Parker R A, Langren B M, Diczfalusy E 1982 Morphometric analysis of the human endometrium in relation to peripheral hormone levels. Fertil Steril 38: 564

Johannisson E, Landgren B M, Rohr H P, Diczfalusy E 1987 Endometrial morphology and peripheral hormone levels in women with regular menstrual cycles. Fertil Steril 48: 401

Jones G S 1984 Update on in vitro fertilization. Endocrine Rev 5: 62

Jones G S, Pourmand K 1962 An evaluation of etiologic factors and therapy in 555 private patients with primary infertility. Fertil Steril 13: 398

Julkunen M, Koistien R, Aalto-Setälä K et al 1988 Primary structure of human insulin-like growth factor-binding protein/placental protein 12 and tissue-specific expression of its mRNA. FEBS Lett 236:295

Julkunen M, Koistinen R, Suikkari A-M et al 1990 Identification by hybridization histochemistry of human endometrial cells expressing mRNAs encoding a uterine β-lactoglobulin homologue and insulin-like growth factor-binding protein-1. Mol Endocrinol 4: 700

Kasamo M, Ishikawa M, Yamashita K, Sengoku K, Shimizu T 1986 Possible role of prostaglandin F in blastocyst implantation. Prostaglandins 31:321

Kim-Björklund T, Landgren B M, Hamberger L, Johannisson E 1991 Comparative morphometric study of the endometrium, the fallopian tube and the corpus luteum during the post-ovulatory phase in normally menstruating women. Fertil Steril 56: 842

Koistinen R, Kalkkinen N, Huhtala M L et al 1986 Placental protein 12 is a decidual protein that binds somatomedin and has as identical N terminal amino acid sequence with somatomedin-binding protein from human amniotic fluid. Endocrinology 118: 1375

Landgren B M, Undén A L, Diczfalusy E 1980 Hormonal profile of the cycle in 68 normally menstruating women. Acta Endocrinol (Copenh) 94: 89

Lessey B A, Killiam A P, Metzger D A, Haney A F, Greene G L, McCarty K S Jr 1988 Immunohistochemical analysis of human uterine estrogen and progesterone receptors throughout the menstrual cycle. J Clin Endocrinol Metab 67: 334

Li T C, Rogers A, Lenton E, Dockery P, Cooke I 1987 A comparison between two methods of chronological dating of human endometrial biopsies during the luteal phase and their correlation with histologic dating. Fertil Steril 48: 928

Li T C, Rogers A W, Dickery P, Lenton E A, Cooke I D 1988 A new method of histologic dating of human endometrium in the luteal phase. Fertil Steril 50: 52

Li T C, Dockery P, Rogers A W, Cooke I D 1989 How precise is histologic dating of endometrium using the standard dating criteria? Fertil Steril 51: 759

Li T C, Lenton E A, Dockery P, Cooke I D 1990 A comparison of some clinical and endocrinological features between cycles with normal and defective luteal phases in women with unexplained infertility. Hum Reprod 5: 805

Loke Y W, Gardner L, Burland K, King A 1989 Laminin in human trophoblast–decidua interaction. Hum Reprod 4: 457

Ludwig H, Metzger H 1976 The human female reproductive tract. In: Ludwig H, Metzger H (eds) A scanning electron microscopic atlas New York: Springer, pp 331–441

Luukainen T, Nilsson C G, Allonen H, Haukamaa M, Toivonen J 1984 Intrauterine release of levonorgestrel. In: Zatuchni G L, Goldsmith A, Shelton J D, Sciarra J J (eds) Long-acting contraceptive delivery systems. Harper & Row, Philadelphia, pp 601–612

Majno G, Joris 1 1978 Endothelium 1977: a review. Adv Exp Med Biol 104: 169–225

Marchini M, Fedele L, Bianchi S, Losa G A, Ghisleitta M, Candiani G B 1991 Secretory changes in preovulatory endometrium during controlled ovarian hyperstimulation with buserelin acetate and human gonadotrophins. Fertil Steril 55: 717

Markee J E 1940 Menstruation in intraocular endometrial transplants in the Rhesus monkey. Contrib Embryol Carnegie Inst Wash 28: 219

Maslar I A, Riddick D M 1979 Prolactin production by human endometrium during the normal menstrual cycle. Am J Obstet Gynecol 135: 731

Milgrom E, Atger M, Baulieu E E 1970 Progesterone in uterus and plasma. IV Progesterone receptor (S) in guinea pig uterus cytosol. Steroids 16: 741

Noyes R W, Hertig A T, Rock J 1950 Dating the endometrial biopsy. Fertil Steril 1: 3

Peek M, Landgren B-M, Johannisson E 1992 The

endometrial capillaries during the normal menstrual cycle; a morphometric study. Hum Reprod (in press)

Perret-Applanat M, Groyer-Picard M T, García E, Lorenzo F, Milgrom E 1988 Immunohistochemical demonstration of estrogen and progesterone receptors in muscle cells of uterine arteries in rabbits and humans. Endocrinology 123: 1511

Pincus G 1965 The control of fertility. Academic, New York, p 162

Press M F, Greene G L 1988 Localization of progesterone receptors with monoclonal antibodies to human progestin receptor. Endocrinology 122: 1165

Price T M, Kauma S W, Curry T E, Clark M R 1989 Immunohistochemical localization of prostaglandin endoperoxidase synthase in human fetal membranes and decidua. Bio Reprod 41: 701

Pyschoyos A 1971 Methods for studying changes in capillary permeability in the rat endometrium. In: Daniel J C (ed) Methods in mammalian embryology. W H Freeman, San Francisco, pp 334–338

Psychoyos A, Roche D, Gravanis A 1989 Is cholic acid responsible for embryo-toxicity of the postreceptive uterine environment? Hum Reprod 4: 832

Ramsey E M 1977 Vascular anatomy. In: Wynn R M (ed) Biology of the uterus. Plenum, New York, pp 59–76

Robertson W G 1987 Pathology of the pregnant uterus. In Fox H (ed) Obstetrical and gynecological pathology. Churchill Livingstone, Edinburgh, pp 1149–1176

Rogers P A, Polson D, Murphy C R, Hosie M, Susil B, Leoni M 1991 Correlation of endometrial histology, morphometry and ulrasound appearance after different stimulation protocols for in vitro fertilization. Fertil Steril 55: 583

Salvatore C A 1952 Capillary fragility and menstruation. Surg Gynecol Obstet 95: 13

Schlegel J V 1945 Arteriovenous anastomes in the endometrium in man. Acta Anat 1: 284

Schmidt-Matthiesen H 1963a Histochemie. In: Schmidt-Matthiesen H (ed) Das normale menschliche Endometrium. George Thieme Verlag Stuttgart, pp 149–224

Schmidt-Matthiesen H 1963b Vaskularisierung. In: Schmidt-Matthiesen H (ed) Das normale menschliche Endometrium. George Thieme Verlag, Stuttgart, pp 149–224

Segal S J, Scher W 1967, Estrogens, nucleic acids and protein synthesis in uterine metabolism. In Wynn R M (ed) Cellular biology of the uterus. North Holland Publishing Company, Amsterdam, pp 114–150

Sengel A, Stoebner P 1970 Ultrastructure de l'endometre humain normal. 1 Le chorion cytogene. Z Zellforsch mikrosk Anat 109: 245

Seppälä M, Julkunen M, Koskimies A et al 1988 Proteins of the human endometrium. In: In vitro fertilization and other assisted reproduction. Ann N Y Acad Sci 541: 432

Sheppard B L, Bonnar J 1980 The development of vessels of the endometrium during the menstrual cycle. In: Diczfalusy E, Fraser I S, Webb, F T G (eds) Endometrial bleeding and steroidal contraception. Pitman, Bath, pp 65–77

Sixma J J, Christiaens G C M, Haspels A A 1980 The sequence of haemostatic events in the endometrium during normal menstruation. In: Diczfalusy E, Fraser I S, Webb F T G (eds) Endometrial bleeding and steroidal contraception. Pitman, Bath, pp 86–96

Terzakis J A 1965 The nucleolar channel system of human endometrium. J Cell Biol 27: 293

Themann H, Schünke W 1963 Die Feinstruktur der Drüsenepithelien des menschlichen Endometriums. Elektronen optische. Morphologie. In: Schmidt-Matthiesen (ed) Das normale menschliche Endometrium. Georg Thieme Verlag, Stuttgart, pp 111–148

Thor A, Viglione M J, Muraro R, Ohuchi N, Schlum Gorstein F 1987 Monoclonal antibody B 72.3 reactivity with human endometrium: a study of normal and malignant tissues. Int J Gynecol Pathol 6: 234

Tseng L, Mazella J, Chen G A 1987 Effect of relaxin on aromatase activity in human endometrial stroma cells. Endocrinology 120: 2220

Tsibris J C M, Fort F L, Cazenave C R et al 1981 The uneven distribution of estrogen and progesterone receptors in human endometrium. J Steroid Biochem 14: 997

Verma V 1983 Ultrastructural changes in human endometrium at different phases of the menstrual cycle and their functional significance. Gynecol Obstet Invest 15: 193

Wahlström T, Seppälä M 1984 Placental protein 12 (pp 12) is induced in the endometrium by progesterone. Fertil Steril 41: 781

Wentz A C 1980 Endometrial biopsy in the evaluation of infertility. Fertil Steril 33: 121

Werb Z, Mainardi C L, Vater C A, Harris E D 1977 Endogeneous activation of latent collagenase by rheumatoid synovial cells. Evidence for a role of plasminogen activator. New Engl J Med 296: 1017

Wewer U M, Faber M, Liotta L A, Albrechtsen R 1985 Immunochemical and ultrastructural assessment of the nature of the pericellular basement membrane of human decidual cells. Lab Invest 53: 624

Wilborn W H, Hyde B M, Pope V Z et al 1984 Comparative effects of norgestimate, northisterone and medroxyprogesterone acetate on the microanatomy of baloon endometrium. In: Zatuchni G L, Goldsmith E, Shelton J D, Sciarra J J (eds) Long acting contraceptive delivery systems. Harper & Row, Philadelphia, pp 296–315

Wynn R M, Woolley R S 1967 Ultrastructural cyclic changes in the human endometrium. II Normal postovulatory phase. Fertil Steril 18: 721

Xing Shumin, Johannisson E, Landgren B M, Diczfalusy E 1983 Pituitary, ovarian and endometrial effects of progesterone released prematurely during the proliferative phase. Contraception 27: 177

Zhu Pengdi, Zhao Gu 1988 Observation of the activity of Factor VIII in the endometrium of women with regular menstrual cycles. Hum Reprod 3: 273

# 4. Functional anatomy of the Fallopian tube

*P. Verdugo    M. Villalón*

*To Professor Richard J. Blandau, for the wealth of his contributions which will serve as inspiration to many generations to come*

## INTRODUCTION

The understanding of tubal function has widespread clinical significance for both the systematic development of new therapeutic strategies to cure iatrogenic or pathogenic tubal infertility, and for the establishment of more reliable yet less invasive contraceptive methods. However, notwithstanding more than a century of research efforts, most of the present knowledge about the oviduct is, if not empirical, at least largely phenomenological and, certainly, not sufficient to predict the function of the Fallopian tube in any single species (Blandau & Verdugo 1976). Although millions of human embryos make their journey through women's oviducts every day, the physiological mechanisms that move the gametes and the zygotes in the oviduct are still largely unknown and remain one of nature's most challenging secrets.

Despite the large volume of published material, progress in the objective understanding of the function of the Fallopian tube has been rather slow and many critical aspects of this subject are still highly speculative and controversial. This is partly because broad variations in the physiological control of tubal function among different species have virtually prevented the establishment of a reliable experimental model to predict the control of tubal function in women; and partly because the urgency to control human population has induced the establishment of research policies to support preferentially applied investigation

aimed at the short-term development of contraceptive methods, rather than to encourage fundamental research aimed at the understanding of the physiological mechanisms that control fertility. As a consequence, a high proportion of modern research in reproduction has become largely phenomenological, adding more and more to a catalogue of information that contains too many 'results', yet very few answers to even the most fundamental questions about tubal physiology. Thus, the job for a reviewer can be rather complex, especially if the assignment is not to publish a new edition of the 'Fallopian catalogue of results' but to write a comprehensive report of the progress in the understanding of tubal function.

In the present chapter, preference will be given to ideas supported by quantitative data or sound physical theory rather than to unsupported speculation or strictly descriptive results. However, when phenomenological observations are pertinent, appropriate attention will be given to them. This chapter begins with a description of the anatomy of the human oviduct. Emphasis will be given to the comparative facets in order to infer how the tube has evolved in adapting to the particular reproductive plan found in the human species. The comparative aspects are not discussed as a detailed continuum, but rather illustrated in a set of particular models in species where the reproductive plan is clearly different.

The function of the oviduct has evolved from a simple ejaculatory channel of eggs in lower species to the highly complex organ found in species with internal fertilization. In vertebrates, the tube conditions the gametes, guides the journey to their encounter, and provides a proper chemical environment for their mating. It also supplies nutriment to the zygote in its first few hours of life, and delivers the new embryo into the uterine cavity for final nidation in a timely manner.

A summary review of the functional heterogeneity of oviductal function among different species, together with a short discussion on redundancy in tubal function and the characteristic stochastic patterns of tubal transport, is the framework used here for understanding gamete transport in the oviduct. Other pieces of the puzzle that deserve consideration are the effectors of the tube. In most species, the function of the oviduct arises from a complex and poorly understood interaction of three effectors that are present in different proportions in each segment of the oviduct. A discussion of the control of these effectors, muscle, ciliated and secretory cells, is critical for the comprehension of their interaction in tubal function. The chapter closes with the formulation of a working hypothesis that is consistent with previous observations, and that can serve to guide the search for the many pieces of the puzzle that are still missing.

## ANATOMY OF THE OVIDUCT

In the early stages of the evolutionary ladder, the oviduct can be distinguished as a differentiated component of the reproductive tract connecting the ovary to the uterus. It is present in both worms and insects. It reaches a very high stage of development in fish and, especially, in birds and reptiles, where it functions not only as a transporting organ of gametes but also as an assembly line wherein the egg is provided with storage reservoirs of water and nutrients, and a hard mineral shell which supports and protects the zygote during its early development (Richardson 1935). In vertebrates, the oviducts are derived from the paramesonephric (Mullerian) ducts. In contrast to the mesonephric (Wolfian) ducts of the male, which require androgenic stimulus to complete their development, the morphogenesis of the paramesonephric ducts in the female is fairly independent of hormonal influences (Price 1974). In mammals the early development of the paramesonephric ducts is similar in both sexes and is characterized by the formation of two or

more clefts of the coelomic epithelium near the cranial region of the primitive urogenital ridge. Later on, however, these structures degenerate in the male whereas in the female they continue their development (Price & Ortiz 1965). In humans, the paramesonephric ducts develop during the 4th to 5th week of embryonic life (Foulconer 1951). From the ostial end, the paramesonephric invaginations form a duct which grows caudally in parallel with the existing Wolfian system (Gruenwald 1941b Burns 1955). In the 7- to 8-week-old human female embryo, the lower ends of the paramesonephric ducts fuse to the mesonephric bodies whereupon the mesonephric ducts initiate a regression that is complete by the 12th week of fetal life (Hunter 1930). The cranial or oviductal regions of the paramesonephric ducts undergo marked growth during the 4th and 5th month of fetal life and become clearly distinguishable from the caudal or uterine region by their characteristic coiling and smaller diameter (Hunter 1930). Differentiated muscle cells and connective tissue of the wall and ciliated cells of the mucosal lumen begin to appear in the human oviducts by the 3rd to 4th lunar months. During the 7th to 8th months, the mucosa is well developed, and, although no secretory activity is present, the characteristic differences in the mucosal folding and wall thickness between the ampullas and the isthmi can be clearly distinguished (Hunter 1930, Glenister & Hamilton 1963). At birth, the various muscle layers of the tubal wall and the tubal epithelium are fully developed and demonstrate contractile, ciliary and secretory activity (Stegner 1961). Comparative studies indicate that, although the organogenetic progression of the oviducts in different mammals follows a rather similar plan, there are slight but clear differences in the morphogenetic development of the various segments of the tube, especially of the utero-tubal junctions and the fimbriated ends. These differences are reflected later on by the characteristic anatomical and functional variations found in the oviducts of different mammalian species (Strauss 1964).

In the adult, the oviducts have a cylindrical shape and form an important segment of the reproductive tract; they anastomose to the uterus or uterine cornua by their caudal end, and, depending upon the species, their proximal (cephalic) ends may open freely to the abdominal cavity or form bursas around the ovaries. The oviducts are wrapped within two sheets of the abdominal serosa which, after encircling the tube, fuse together forming the mesosalpinx, that loosely connects the oviduct to the posterior peritoneum and also enclose a thin sheet of muscle fibres, as well as supporting ligaments, nerves, blood vessels, and lymphatics.

The smooth muscle of the tubal wall encircles a complex array of intricately folded mucosa that fills the central core of the tube leaving only a virtual lumen that varies greatly depending upon the amount of secretion and the specific segment of the tube. The length of the oviducts varies, not only among species, but also among individuals. Since oviducts are contractile organs, their length also changes with the tone of their muscle wall. In humans, the average length of the extrauterine portion of the oviducts is about 11 cm; it can vary from 6 to 15 cm (Woodruff & Pauerstein 1969).

Depending upon the anatomical localization, the amount of circular smooth muscle of the wall, the degree of folding and cellular composition of the mucosa, as well as the autonomic innervation, it is possible to distinguish four distinct segments along the oviduct. Moving from the rostral to the caudal end, these segments are: the *fimbria*, the *ampulla*, the *isthmus* and the *intramural oviduct*

(Fig. 4.1). The zone between the ampulla and the isthmus is known as the ampullary-isthmic junction (AIJ), and that between the isthmus and the entrance to the uterus as the utero-tubal junction (UTJ). A cylindrical muscle sheath known as the lamina muscularis encircles the mucosa along the entire length of the oviduct. Anatomically, the junctional zones correspond to sites that show marked changes in the thickness and the diameter of the cylindrical sheath of smooth muscle that encircles the mucosa, and in the complexity of the folding and cellular distribution of the mucosa that fills the virtual lumen of the tube. This anatomical feature should be kept in mind since, as will be shown later, it explains why the junctional zones can function as gates or sites where large gradients of mechanical energy exist, resulting in the typical discontinuities observed in tubal transport.

## THE FIMBRIA

The human fimbria is a membranous structure located at the end of the infundibular portion of the ampulla. In Italy during the early musical Rococo period, Gabriellus Fallopius compared the fimbria to the 'bell-like mouth a bronze trumpet, the trumpet of the uterus' (Fallopius 1561). However, it perhaps resembles better the shape of a semifolded umbrella that, when

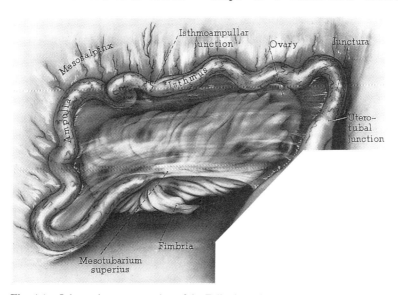

**Fig. 4.1**  Schematic representation of the Fallopian tube.

extended, can cover a rather large area, yet converge to a single central point, the ostial end of the ampulla. Underlying the serosa in close contact with the lamina propria of the mucosa is a thin layer of longitudinally oriented smooth muscle which, in humans, extends between the two serosal leaves of the fimbria ovarica forming the 'musculus atrahens tubae' (Stange 1952a,b). Like the rest of the oviduct, the outer surface of the fimbria is covered by a thin serosal layer that, depending upon the species, serves either to connect it loosely to the ovary (the fimbria ovarica in humans) or to attach it firmly to the ovary, surrounding it and forming a bursa ovarica, as in

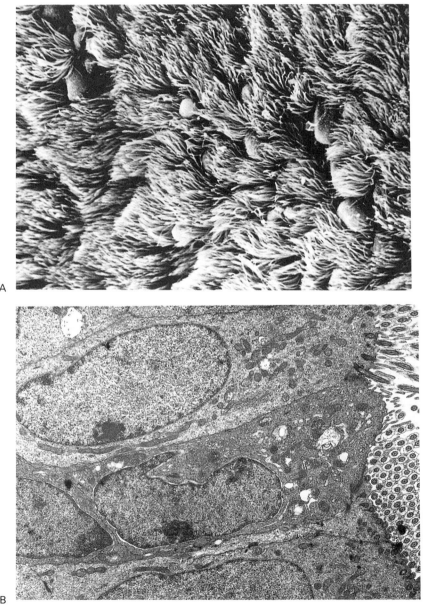

A

B

**Fig. 4.2**   Scanning electron micrograph from the mucosa of a human oviduct. Notice in **a** the presence of ciliated cells, and dome-shaped goblet mucus secretory cells. **b** A transmission electron micrograph of ciliated cells of the human tubal mucosa.

the cat. Underlying the serosa in close contact with the lamina propria of the mucosa is a thin layer of longitudinally oriented smooth muscle which, in the human, extends between the two serosal leaves of the fimbria ovarica forming the 'musculus atrahens tubae' (Stange 1952b). Like the rest of the oviduct, the innermost surface of the fimbria is covered by a highly convoluted mucosa that in this region is particularly rich in both ciliated and secretory cells that together with 'peg' and basal stem cells form a cylindrical epithelium (see Fig. 4.2). Contractile activity of the fimbriae can be observed routinely during laparotomy in several animal species, including humans. Ciliary movements of the fimbrial mucosa are oriented radially with their active stroke in a centripetal direction converging toward the ostial end of the ampulla (Rumery & Eddy 1974).

## THE OSTIUM

The ostium marks the opening of the ampullary lumen into the abdominal cavity. At this point, the smooth muscles of the walls become more peripherally located and form a ring around the mucosa-filled lumen of the tube. At the ostial end

of the oviduct, muscle fibers undergo a complicated rearrangement whereby spiral and longitudinal muscle bundles interlace and virtually form a functional sphincter (Stange 1952a).

## THE AMPULLA

The ampulla extends from the ostium to the AIJ. Its length varies in different species; in humans it is the longest section of the oviduct, reaching 5–10 cm. It is characterized by the abundance and complexity of its intricately folded mucosa, which often completely fills the tubal lumen, and is surrounded by a typically thin layer of smooth muscle (Fig. 4.3).

Histologically, the mucosa that lines the ampulla can be classified as a cylindrical monostratified epithelium, containing ciliated, secretory, 'peg' and basal cells. In the ampulla, as in the fimbria, ciliated cells are more numerous than nonciliated cells and are rich in microvilli. The intramural smooth muscle of the wall of the ampulla is organized peripherally and forms a thin ring that (compared to the isthmus) encompasses a rather large circumference around a mucosa-filled virtual lumen (Fig. 4.3). Generally, the inner smooth muscle is circular and the outer

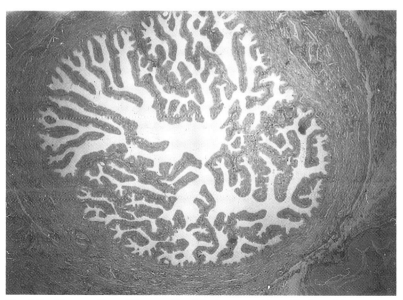

**Fig. 4.3** Cross-section of the ampulla of the human oviduct. Notice a thin muscle ring surrounding a core of highly convoluted mucosal folds. (Courtesy of Professor Croxatto)

predominantly longitudinal. However, muscle fibers are not clearly segregated according to orientation, as in the isthmus; instead they form both spiral windings and longitudinal bundles that often interweave and sometimes form a continuum with the interserosal muscle of the mesosalpinx.

## THE ISTHMUS

In most of the species, the AIJ can be better distinguished by palpation than by visual observation. The characteristic increase in the thickness of the intramural smooth muscle of the isthmus as compared to that of the ampulla marks the AIJ with a distinct change of consistency in the middle third section of the oviduct. Also, beginning at this point and extending throughout the remainder of the isthmus, the mucosa, which fills the lumen of the tube, is reduced to a few primary folds that drastically decrease the cross-sectional diameter occupied by mucosal epithelia. Conversely, the smooth muscle of the wall markedly and drastically increases to form a sheath about three times thicker in cross-section

and encircling a diameter five times smaller than those in the ampulla (Figs 4.3, 4.4). These muscle fibers are organized in bundles of similar orientation. In humans, there is a thin inner longitudinal muscle layer that runs at the foot of the mucosal folds; an intermediate muscle layer oriented circularly that occupies the largest proportion of muscle wall thickness; and a thick outer helicoidally oriented longitudinal muscle layer which forms a continuum with the interserosal muscle of the mesotubarium.

The epithelium that lines the internal surface of the isthmus is similar to the epithelium found in the mucosa of the ampulla except that the ratio of the density of ciliated cells to that of nonciliated, especially secretory cells, is lower.

## THE INTRAMURAL SEGMENT

At their caudal end, the oviducts penetrate the uterine wall to form the intramural segment. The anatomical configuration of this region varies greatly among different species and even among individuals. Reports on the trajectory of the tubal lumen inside the uterine wall, on the pattern of

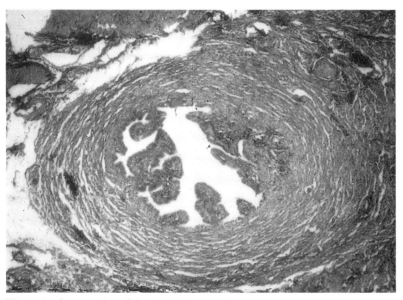

**Fig. 4. 4**  Cross-section of the middle isthmus of a human oviduct. Notice the increased thickness and decreased diameter of the smooth muscle ring of the wall. Notice also the decrease in complexity and in the number of mucosal folds that fill the lumen. (Courtesy of Professor Croxatto).

folding of the mucosa, and on the arrangement of the periluminal smooth muscle are somewhat controversial.

It is thought that a stop-flow mechanism is necessary to avoid retrograde contamination of the tube and peritoneum. Functional studies in different species seem to suggest that hormonal influences might control the resistance to flow across the intramural section. However, attempts to demonstrate the existence of a true anatomical uterotubal sphincter, especially in primates, have not been conclusive.

In humans, the length of the intramural segment of the tube varies from 1 to 2.5 cm. Its trajectory inside the uterine wall can be straight, curved, or even convoluted (Hermstein & Neustadt 1924, Sweeney 1962). As expected for a structure surrounded by contractile tissue, the luminal diameters also vary greatly, from 100 μm to 4 mm (Sweeney 1962, Rocker 1964), and probably reflect the various degrees of contracture at which the preparation was fixed.

The epithelium that lines the folded lumen of the intramural section undergoes a transition whereby, as it approaches the uterine cavity, the number of ciliated cells decreases and the typical features of the endometrial mucosa become apparent (Hermstein & Neustadt 1924). However, the most consistent morphological feature of the intramural section of the tube among different species is the drastic increase of the thickness of the smooth muscle that surrounds its lumen. This anatomical feature must be carefully considered, since contractions of the perilumenal smooth muscle, namely the myometrium, could greatly modify the flow resistance of the intramural section, especially in tubes with convoluted intraluminal trajectory (Andersen 1928), and could be responsible for the uterotubal valvular effects reported in the past (Black & Asdell 1959).

## BLOOD AND LYMPHATIC CIRCULATION

Blood is supplied to the oviduct by a mesovaric interanastomotic arterial ring fed from both the adnexal branches of the uterine artery and the tubal branch of the ovarian artery forming a rich collateral network which assures adequate perfusion of both the ovary and the oviduct (Borell & Fernstrom 1953, Watanabe 1963).

It is thought that both sympathetic and local vascular control exist in the oviduct; however, their functional significance has not been explored. The venous blood drains from interconnected capillary networks in the mucosa, the muscularis and the subserosa, which form three corresponding venous plexuses that merge in the subserosa and drain into an extrinsic circuit which follows the arterial supply (Gatsalov 1963).

In humans, the lymphatic drainage derives from three interconnected lymphatic networks in the mucosa, muscularis and subserosa forming intramural plexuses that seem to vary depending upon the segment of the oviduct and the sexual maturity of the subject (Sampson 1937). The extrinsic collecting system runs via the mesosalpinx and broad ligament and drains into the para-aortic nodes (Reiffenstuhl 1964).

## INNERVATION

The tube is innervated by both efferent autonomic nerves and afferent visceral nerves. The autonomic nervous system provides control for the tubal efferents via sympathetic and parasympathetic connections (Mitchell 1938). The efferent visceral fibers, on the other hand, are thought to be connected to Paccini receptors in the mucosa (Chiara 1959) and to transmit pain sensation via the ovarian plexus and splanchnic nerve entering the spinal cord from T11 to L2. Extrinsic preganglionic sympathetic innervation arises from T10 to L2. Synaptic relays take place via the hypogastric, ciliac or presacral plexus, further establishing their connections to the oviduct by long postganglionic fibers, or via the uterovaginal plexus, which connects to the oviduct by short postganglionic fibers (Owman & Sjöstrand 1967, Sjöberg 1967, El-Badawi & Schenk 1968). The application of new histochemical methods of fluorescence detection of catecholamines (Falck et al 1962) has revealed that in humans the intramural adrenergic terminals of the oviduct are mostly attached to the circular muscle layer and are distributed in direct proportion to the amount of circular muscle fibers, i.e. sympathetic innervation of the ampulla is sparse and reduced to vascular terminals whereas the thick circular muscle layer in the isthmic wall is supplied by a rich network of adrenergic terminals (Owman et al 1967).

Parasympathetic innervation reaches the oviduct via both vagal and sacral fibers with synaptic relays in the ovarian or the pelvic plexuses respectively. Their postganglionic connections form a network of submucosal terminals (Mitchell 1938).

## PHYSIOLOGY OF THE OVIDUCT

New life, like a chemical reaction, is born out of the encounter of two reactants. The movement of diffusing reactants is random, and chemical collisions are therefore governed by the law of probability. Likewise, in species with external fertilization gamete encounter is still very much a matter of chance, and the probability of successful collisions is increased by the production of large quantities of gametes and sometimes by some chemotactic attraction. Within this framework, the evolutionary development of internal fertilization can be interpreted as an improvement that increases the probability of successful fertilization by funnelling the gametes into a tube that guides the journey to their encounter. In more evolved species, this tube not only transports the gametes at the opportune time to their mating site but also provides safe lodging for the spermatozoa as they wait for the ova. It also preconditions the gametes for fertilization. It supports the zygote during its early hours of life and, in those species with internal development, it delivers the zygote at the proper time for final nidation into the uterine cavity. Although man has witnessed this complex and remarkably precise sequence of biological events for many years, our present understanding of the physiology of the Fallopian tube is still vastly obscure.

## PHENOMENOLOGY OF GAMETE TRANSPORT

The brief review that follows is concerned primarily with the phenomenological description of the transport of gametes from the opposite ends of the reproductive tract to the site of fertilization

and the transport of the zygote from the site of fertilization to its locus of nidation in the uterus. It describes the general features of tubal transport in mammals and discusses the effect of hormones and microsurgical interventions on tubal transport.

### Egg and zygote transport

The broad variation of gamete transport in different species has prevented both the formulation of a general hypothesis to explain this process, and the establishment of an experimental animal model that mimics gamete transport in humans. Nevertheless, there are a few functional features of tubal transport that are fairly similar among mammals and deserve further examination. These features throw some light on the underlying mechanism of tubal transport and can help in the formulation of a general hypothesis from which to predict and test our understanding of tubal function. Successful fertilization of the ovum and, in some species, the nidation and further development of the embryo require that the tubal transport of the gametes and zygote take place within relatively strict timing constraints. Ovum transport seems to be remarkably well timed to the specific reproductive plan in each species (Chang & Pickworth 1969). Observations in different mammals indicate that transport of the egg from the ostial end of the tube to the uterus can vary widely among species; yet in each species it is fairly constant (Croxatto & Ortiz 1975, Harper 1988). Features that are consistent among mammals are the different ovum transport rate in the various segments of the tube and the sometimes long stationary periods when the egg or the zygote resides in the junctional zones. In the rabbit, for instance, total tubal transport of the egg lasts for 3 days, only a few minutes of which are spent in the ampulla, the rest being spent in pausing at the UIJ and moving through the isthmus (Greenwald 1961, Harper 1966, Boling & Blandau 1971, Pauerstein et al 1974a). Ovum transport in primates also lasts 3 days. In humans ovulation takes place about 28–36 h after the LH peak (Peters & McNatty 1980). The ovum arrives at the uterus about 96–120 h after the LH peak, and thus, the actual tubal transport time is approximately 80 h (Diaz et al 1980). However, in primates there is a long ampullary transit period that is followed by a rapid isthmic transport. For instance, in the case of the baboon (*Papio anubis*), and the rhesus monkey (*Macaca mulatta*), as in humans, the ampullary transit periods last 36–46 and 72 h respectively (Rock & Hertig 1944, Noyes et al 1966, Eddy et al 1975, 1976, Croxatto et al 1978a). In many species the time profile of tubal transport shows stationary periods just before the egg enters the isthmus or at the isthmus itself and just before it enters the uterus (Black & Asdell 1958, Brundin 1964, Greenwald 1967). An issue that has not yet been well defined is the influence of fertilization on tubal transport. For instance, the human embryo arrives at the uterus at an early 7- to 12-cell stage of development, and there is no clear evidence that denudation or fertilization of the ovum can effect its transport to the uterus (Allen et al 1930, Hertig et al 1956, Croxatto 1974).

Another characteristic feature found in all the mammalian species where egg transport has been directly observed is the unique pattern of discrete pendular motions displayed by the egg inside the oviduct. This remarkable feature was among the first observations to be reported by early investigators of tubal physiology (for review see Lim & Chao 1927). However, the significance of those observations did not become apparent until recently when the quantitative assessment of egg movements in the oviduct, using computer analysis of cinematographic records, revealed that egg motions in the rabbit ampulla have the characteristic features of a random walk superimposed upon a continuous nonperiodic process (Verdugo et al 1976, Hodgson et al 1977). The same pattern of random egg movement has been more recently demonstrated in ampullary transport in primates (Villalón et al 1992). Figure 4.5 shows a typical position–time record of egg movements in the ampulla of a pig-tailed monkey (*Macaca* nemestrina) at the time of ovulation. The statistical analysis of instantaneous velocity of the egg obtained from this record is illustrated in Figure 4.6 and shows that the probability of prouterine versus proovarian motion follows the typical features of a Gaussian distribution shifted

approximately 34 μm/s in a prouterine direction. This rather simple analysis prompted the suggestion that ovum transport is probably a process where random and nonrandom components interact with each other to produce the typical pendular movement of the egg in the oviduct. These studies also strongly suggest that the random component of egg movements is probably due to muscle contractions, whereas the prouterine shift shown by the probability distribution of transport velocities (34 μm/s in the monkey, and about 100 μm/s in the rabbit) is dependent

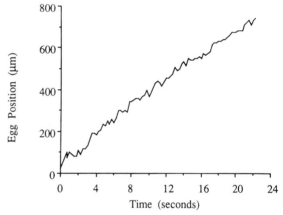

**Fig. 4.5**   Position versus time plot of ovum transport in the monkey oviduct, obtained by digitizing cinematographic records. Notice the presence of the typical random pendular motions of the egg along the lumen of the tube.

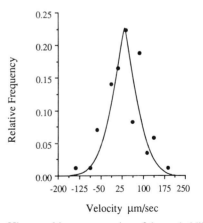

**Fig. 4.6**   Histographic representation of the probability distribution of velocities of egg motion during tubal transport in the ampulla of a pig-tailed monkey *Macaca* conchesuma at the time of ovulation. Notice that the velocities form a symmetrical Gaussian distribution balance at a bias of about 34 μm in the prouterine direction.

upon ciliary action (Verdugo et al 1976, 1980a, Verdugo 1982, Villalón et al 1991). These predictions are further supported by experiments in which the pharmacological inhibition of tubular contraction in the rabbit resulted in a pattern of unidirectional egg movement, devoid of pendular motions, at approximately 100 μm/s (Halbert et al 1976).

Results of the statistical analysis of detailed measurements of ovum transport in the rabbit ampulla prompted the formulation of a general hypothesis of stochastic oviductal gamete transport (Verdugo et al 1976, 1980a) that is now gaining widespread acceptance (Harper 1988), and that will be covered in more detail in the final section of this chapter.

## Hormonal effects on ovum transport

Although the mechanisms by which hormones modulate the tubal effectors responsible for the transport of gametes in the oviduct are still not understood, the temporal profile of variations in circulating hormones and their relation to the temporal profile of gamete transport in the oviduct have been well established for a variety of species, including humans. In a few instances, cause–effect relationships between physiological or pharmacological hormone levels and changes in tubal transport have been identified.

With the exception of the typical pulse increase of estrogen level that consistently precedes ovulation in mammals, the temporal profile of circulating ovarian steroids varies in different species. For example, changes in the level of progestins demonstrate broad variations among species. In the rabbit, progestins rise a few hours before ovulation (1.5–4 h after coitus), fall very low by the time of ovulation and initial tubal transport, and rise again 24 h after ovulation (Hilliard & Eaton 1971). In the guinea-pig, which is a cyclic ovulator having a tubal transport profile very similar to that of primates, passage is slow through the ampulla and rapid through the isthmus. Progestins are low on days 1 and 2 of the cycle, and increase by the time of isthmic transport during day 3 (Challis et al 1971, Maia et al 1977). In the rat, estradiol increases rapidly between days 3 and 4 after ovulation which is the

time eggs start to move from the oviduct into the uterus, whereas progesterone reaches a maximum level on day 3, and by day 4 has returned to low levels of concentration in plasma (Forcelledo et al 1981). In primates, including humans, tubal transport takes place while progestin levels continuously rise (Mishell et al 1971, Pauerstein et al 1978, Batra et al 1980). Although the precise effects of steroids on the human oviduct have not been identified, the concentration of steroids in tubal tissue is higher than in plasma, and receptors for these hormones are indeed present in the tube (Devoto et al 1980, Verhage et al 1980, Pino et al 1982).

Pharmacological levels of steroids show a broad variety of effects on tubal transport. Since Burdick & Pinkus (1935) first demonstrated that postcoital treatment with estrogen can arrest ovum transport and induce 'tube locking' of the egg in the mouse and the rabbit, many other investigators have shown that estrogen and progesterone as well as prostaglandins can produce drastic changes in tubal transport. However, hormonal effects on transport vary broadly in different species. The effect of estrogens and progesterone on egg transport is not only species specific, but also varies with the dose, the time of administration and the presence or absence of one or both of these hormones as well as their temporal interrelationship in the treatment (Pauerstein et al 1976). For instance, very similar estradiol treatments that produce 'tube locking' in the mouse and the rabbit can induce accelerated tubal transport in the rat, while not showing any effect in humans (Greenwald 1961, Banik & Pincus 1964, Harper 1968, Humphrey 1968, Croxatto et al 1978b).

The influence of timing of hormonal treatment upon ovum transport is well illustrated by the various effects of progestational steroids in the rabbit. Equivalent doses of these hormones given for 3 days before ovulation accelerate tubal transport; given at and after ovulation they delay the transport of eggs (Chang 1967, Kendle & Telford 1970, Pauerstein et al 1974a). Similarly, estrogen-induced delay of ovum transport in the rabbit is also time-dependent (Pauerstein et al 1974b).

Pharmacological intervention of sympathetic agonists or blockage of tubal sympathetic activity by either pharmacologic or surgical methods have failed to change the time course of ovum transport, probably the only exception being the reversal of estrogen-induced 'tube locking' by α-adrenergic blockers as observed in the rabbit (Eddy & Black 1974, Pauerstein et al 1970, 1974b). Prostaglandins $F_{2\alpha}$ and $E_1$ stimulate tubal contractions and produce marked acceleration of ovum transport in the rabbit. However, prostaglandin $E_2$, which strongly inhibits tubal contractility, does not affect tubal transport (Aref et al 1973). Some inhibitors of prostaglandin synthesis can also accelerate the time-course of ovum transport in the rabbit. Their effect seems to be associated with variations in the ratio of synthesis inhibition among different prosta-glandins, since drugs that preferentially inhibit synthesis of prostaglandin $E_2$ or prostaglandin $F_{2\alpha}$ are more effective accelerators than those that depress the synthesis of both prostaglandins (Valenzuela et al 1977).

Notwithstanding the strong stimulation of tubal contractility produced by prostaglandin $F_{2\alpha}$ in the human oviduct and its accelerating effect on tubal transport in animals, its application in humans has failed to demonstrate any effect on tubal transport (Croxatto et al 1978b).

## Tubal microsurgery

Microsurgery has become an excellent method to separate the functional roles of the different sections of the oviduct in tubal transport. It has turned out to be a most powerful and revealing experimental tool. The number of classically established speculative dogmas about tubal structure and function that has fallen victim to new direct and objective evidence obtained by micro-surgery is impressive, and it continues to grow as new evidence accumulates. The early work of Estes was a harbinger of the advances to come contributed by microsurgery. His observations that ova ovulated into the uterine cavity, bypassing the oviduct, can be fertilized and sustain normal development dismissed both the notion that in humans fertilization requires strict environmental conditions which are uniquely provided by oviductal secretions, and the notion that oviductal secretions are critical for zygote nidation into the uterus (Estes & Heitmeyer 1934, Adams 1979). We know now that the concept of structural and functional integrity of the fimbria ovarica for normal ovum pickup is probably not valid (Metz & Mastroianni 1979), that the requirement of the ampullar integrity for successful reproduction is doubtful (McComb et al 1981), and that the concept that the AIJ function is a sympathetically controlled gate that critically regulates the passage of the egg to the isthmus is clearly wrong (Eddy et al 1977). The idea that the isthmic passage of the zygote is essential for appropriate uterine nidation also seems unwarranted in view of successful pregnan-cies from eggs fertilized in vitro (Trounson et al 1982, Ahuja et al 1985). Thus, for successful fertilization and development the transtubarian passage of the egg and/or the zygote might be sufficient but are not necessary. What is left after this microsurgical cleanup is the simple idea that in both rabbits and humans decreased tubal length leads to lower pregnancy rates (McComb & Gomel 1979, Silber & Cohen 1980, McComb et al 1981).

## Sperm transport in the oviduct

Although internal fertilization clearly improves the chances of successful gamete mating, fertiliza-tion still remains a highly chancy process in that a large number of spermatozoa are required in the vagina in order that only one, or just a few, fertilize one or a few corresponding ova.

In mammals, the female genital tract actively captures and stores the ejaculated sperm. From the storage sites, the sperm is then steadily released and transported to the upper oviduct. By slow release, a slow but continuous concentration of sperm is maintained at the site of fertilization for a period that in many species can last for several days (Bishop 1969).

Therefore, sperm is not transported as a single bolus to the site of fertilization. In most mammals after sperm is deposited in the vagina, a typical initial transport is observed in which a small proportion of the spermatozoa moves rapidly from the vagina all the way up to the fimbria in just a few minutes, probably saturating one or more storage compartments along the genital tract (Warren 1938, Evans 1933, Rubinstein et al 1951, VanDermark & Moeller 1951, Adams 1952, Chang & Sheaffer 1957, Mattner 1963). However, the majority of the sperm remain in the isthmus, until the time of ovulation when they start to slowly move to the upper oviduct where fertilization occurs (Harper 1973b, Hunter 1975, Hunter et al 1982, Hunter & Wilmut 1983). Thereby, the period of potential fertilization from a single coital event, which in some species can last only a few seconds, is extended prolonging the period of potential fertilization to several hours or even several days depending upon the survival of the sperm in storage and their release and transport to the site of fertilization.

Although a postcoital rapid sperm movement along the whole female genital tract seems to be fairly consistent among many different species, the timing of the slow sperm release that follows and the arrival of the sperm to different segments of the oviduct seem to vary widely and to be closely adapted to the timing of the reproductive plan of each species. Here, as in ovum transport, there seem to be also some stationary or storage periods which vary from species to species. In the rabbit, for example, the rapid phase of sperm transport takes place in just a few minutes. There is some disagreement whether these sperm survive long enough to participate in the fertilization of the ovum that takes place several hours later (Chang & Pincus 1964, Overstreet & Cooper 1978). In any event, the bulk of the sperm that prolongs the chances of gamete mating is stored in the lower isthmus and is continuously released by the time of ovulation (Harper 1973a). In humans, during the periovulatory period, there is also a phase of rapid transport that brings the sperm up to the fimbria within a few minutes after coitus or artificial insemination (Rubinstein et at 1951, Settlage et al 1973, Ahlgren 1975, Croxatto et al 1975). In this instance, however, there is no evidence to substantiate the idea that the quickly transported sperm do not compete for fertilization of the ovum, especially since the need for sperm capacitation in humans has not been demonstrated. After the rapid initial mobilization, human sperm is steadily released from as yet not-

well-identified storage sites along the human genital tract and transported to the site of fertilization. The role of the human cervix as a sperm storage compartment is now well established (Insler et al 1980) and sperm have been shown to remain motile within the cervical mucus for up to 7 days (Perloff & Steinberger 1964). There is evidence that transport of fertilizing sperm remains active in humans for a maximum of up to 120 h after coitus (Ferin et al 1973), an indication that the viability of sperm is maintained for long periods. Thus, in natural contraception, a period of 4–5 days of sperm viability should be considered.

It is now well accepted that sperm need not be motile to be transported along the female genital tract since both dead spermatozoa and even inert material introduced in the vagina are equally well transported (Van Dermark & Moeller 1951, Akester & Inkster 1961, Egli & Newton 1961, Mattner 1963). In several species of invertebrates, sperm motility is not required for fertilization and its role even in mammals has been challenged (Chang & Thorsteinsson 1958). However, there is a good correlation between low sperm motility and male infertility, especially when sperm are challenged by the increased fluidic load offered by cervical mucus (Insler et al 1979). Whether sperm motility is essential for their survival while stored in the genital tract has not been tested. However, it is known that the genital tracts of the mouse, rat, and rabbit are invaded by leukocytes 15–20 h after coitus. These leucocytes have been shown to remove the sperm from the genital tract within 24 h after coitus (Austin 1957, Bedford 1963, Howe 1967). The role of sperm motility in avoiding this postcoital phagocytosis has not yet been evaluated, although it could explain the observed correlation between low sperm motility and male infertility.

In summary, the legacy of phenomenological research in tubal transport is a catalogue of data on particular cases, rather than a body of structured understanding. We have learned a great deal about how to manipulate empirically the transport of gametes in a large number of animal species, yet many of these studies have revealed very little about the fundamental mechanisms that control this critical process.

## MECHANISMS OF TUBAL TRANSPORT: A STANDING CHALLENGE

The goal in the previous sections of this chapter was to review briefly yet critically the phenomenology of tubal transport. This section attempts to decipher the mechanisms of gamete transport in the oviduct, establishing first the fundamental constraints that need to be considered — how tubal function is strictly conditioned to the reproductive plan of each species, and how redundancy is built in to the function of the tube. We then consider the function and control of the mechanical effectors of the oviduct, and finally move toward the formulation of a general working hypothesis of tubal transport.

### From Sir Isaac to Gabriellus: the uniqueness of the nonunique

A convenient starting point to define those constraints is to briefly consider the overall comparative aspects of the structure and function of the reproductive system. Comparative anatomy and physiology of mammalian species show that, with few exceptions, organ systems follow a well-defined single model. For instance, if the model theory of Sir Isaac Newton (1735) is applied to the circulatory system in mammals, and the specified corrections for the appropriate scale factors are considered, it becomes clear that the cardiovascular systems of the mouse and the elephant are virtually the same, both structurally and functionally (Lambert & Teissier 1927). The architecture of the various subcomponents and the general anatomical plan are indeed the same. The functional role of equivalent subcomponents and the overall strategy of operations of the whole system are identical. For example, in the case of the control of arterial pressure, the general program that governs the servo-mechanisms that modulate the function of each subcomponent and integrate the overall operation of the system are indeed very similar (Günther & Leon de la Barra 1966).

The reproductive system in mammals, on the other hand, also follows a single Newtonian model. However, in this case the similarities are limited to the anatomical design and to the equivalent functional roles of the mechanical effectors of the reproductive organs. Unlike the other systems, the programs of operations that control reproductive function, as for instance the timing of the tubal transport, are indeed very different among different species. Although superficially this deviation from the model theory observed in the reproductive system strikes us as a paradox, it is in fact not so. The basic difference between reproduction and other functions arises from their respective missions; in the one to support the life of the individual, in the other to maintain the species. For instance, circulation serves as a material, energy and information exchange system for an individual. Since, in this regard, individuals of various species differ only on a scale factor related to their total number of cells, with the appropriate scaling, the same system and same program of operation can function safely in different species. The reproductive system, on the other hand, is certainly optimized to secure the survival of the species and is remarkably well adapted to the particular reproductive plan of each species. Since reproductive plans vary widely among mammals because they are determined by different mating patterns, environmental conditions, seasonal changes, etc., it is not surprising to find striking variations in the programming of the servomechanisms that control gamete transport among different species.

The corollary of the deviation of the reproductive system from a single Newtonian model is that whereas in other organ systems physiological mechanisms documented on the basis of animal experimentation can, in general, be extrapolated to the human, in reproductive physiology, the validity of experimental evidence among different species is very limited and sometimes misleading. Therefore, any attempt to develop a general model to understand and guide further exploration in tubal function in mammals must take into consideration that, despite a similar anatomy of the tubes and the presence of the same mechanical effector in the oviduct of the various species, the physiological program that controls tubal gamete transport among the various species is strictly adapted to the particular timing constraints of the reproductive plan of each species.

## Redundancy in tubal function

Perhaps the most significant implication of the results of microsurgical research on tubal function is the strong reaffirmation that gamete transport in the tube must be a redundant system of a high order, where two, three or more functionally convergent subsystems are stacked together to virtually guarantee a high reliability of operation (Verdugo et al 1980a). A direct corollary of this principle is that different effectors, or different mechanisms of tubal transport, or in this instance, different segments of the tube, may be *sufficient* but yet not *necessary* for successful tubal function. Thus, the observation that reproduction can still exist in oviducts with paralysed cilia (Afzelius et al 1978) cannot be interpreted as evidence that cilia do not have a role in ovum transport. Conversely, the observation that in oviducts with arrested muscle contractions, ciliary action can still carry the egg across the ampulla (Halbert et al 1976), cannot be interpreted as evidence that muscle contraction has only a secondary role in ampullary transport. Even the recent observation that some segments of the oviduct can be microsurgically excised without detriment, cannot be interpreted as proof of the lack of a functional role of any particular segment in tubal physiology (Winston 1980).

Interspecies heterogeneities and redundancy in tubal transport function need to be emphasized both because they are important constraints for the formulation of a general conceptual model for the investigation of the mechanisms of tubal transport, and because ignorance of these principles has probably been the single most common source of controversy in tubal physiology. The past and present existence of 'schools of thought', built on the basis of speculations about what factors are more or less important in oviductal transport or on contradictory evidence obtained in different species, are evidence of our perilous progress in the objective understanding of the function of the oviduct.

## The mechanical effectors of the oviduct

In every segment of the tube of all mammalian species, gamete transport results from a complex and still poorly understood interaction of muscle contractions, ciliary activity and secretory function. Since hormone levels can drastically and reproducibly modify tubal transport rates, it is believed that the timing of this process must be controlled by hormonal influences on the tubal mechanical effectors that generate the forces that move the gametes and the zygote. Therefore, in attempting to understand the role of the tubal effector on the mechanisms of oviductal gamete transport, it is convenient to study how the action of the effector relates to the movement of material inside the tube. By this method we can infer what particular aspects of a intricate effector response are meaningful indicators of the role of this effector in tubal transport and then assess how responsive those indicators are to the regulatory actions of hormones.

However, one of the most salient problems in attempting to characterize the effectors of the oviduct is our ignorance of the precise mechanisms of gamete transport and the specific role of each tubal effector. For instance, when measuring the action of a hormone, say for example in tubal muscle activity, we must critically examine which features of an often complex contractile response are meaningful indicators of its role in tubal transport. Only after defining what particular aspect of the complex pattern of tubal muscle contraction determines tubal transport is it possible to meaningfully characterize the functional control of this effector.

The physiology of tubal effectors will be approached here by considering two different, although related, questions. The first concerns the cellular physiology of myosalpinx and ciliated cells, and focuses on verifying which hormones or neurotransmitters elicit response in the effector cell and what is known about the molecular mechanisms of hormonal action at the cellular level. The other question concerns the relationship between effector response and tubal transport and the specific role of each effector in gamete transport. How does muscle contraction or ciliary action move the gametes in the tube, and how is this mechanism modulated by hormonal or neurohormonal controls? Whereas direct evidence of the cellular physiology of effector response in in vitro preparations is readily available, it is often of limited significance in regard to organ function of the tube. Inferences on the role of tubal effectors in gamete transport are, with few exceptions based on indirect evidence and, in most instances, are also of uncertain significance. None the less, a short and critical examination of available evidence is warranted to gain insight into what is known of the physiology of tubal effectors.

### The myosalpinx

Although the detailed mechanism by which muscle contractions move material in the oviduct is still somewhat controversial, it is now well established that tubal contractions alone are sufficient for gamete and embryo transport since successful reproduction in humans with immotile cilia syndrome has been documented (Afzelius et al 1978). Attempts to establish a cause–effect relationship between muscle contractions and tubal transport by a variety of in vivo and in vitro techniques to measure contractile activity of the tube are still moot and have been more the subject of speculation than systematic experimental interrogation. There is, in fact, very little direct evidence to explain how muscle contractions of the tubal wall integrate their action in time and space to transport the gametes. The following sections will examine how contractions take place in the tube, the structural distribution of smooth muscle in the tubal wall, and the effects of hormones on tubal smooth muscle contractions.

**Tonic and phasic contractions** In muscle, the phosphorylation of myosin by myosin light chain kinase is the paramount mechanism in the regulation of contraction. This reaction is controlled by the concentration of cytosolic $Ca^{2+}$ ($[Ca^{2+}]i$) via Ca-calmodulin. The chain of intracellular events that links the stimulus to the mechanical response is called excitation-contraction coupling. In smooth muscle, there are two modes of excitation-contraction coupling: electromechanical coupling, and pharmacochemical coupling. Electromechanical coupling is produced by variations in membrane potential of the myocyte. Membrane depolarization results in changes of $[Ca^{2+}]i$ due to influx of $Ca^{2+}$ via voltage-gated Ca-channels. Changes in membrane potential can also increase $[Ca^{2+}]i$ by depolarization-induced release of $Ca^{2+}$ from intracellular storage sites. Conversely, hyperpolarization of the smooth muscle myocyte inhibits both $Ca^{2+}$ mobilization and contraction. Pharmacomechanical coupling is also mediated by fluctuations of $[Ca^{2+}]i$. In this case, cytosolic $Ca^{2+}$ can increase by either influx of this cation from the extracellular space by ligand-gated or second messenger-gated Ca-channels, or else by agonist-induced $Ca^{2+}$ release from intracellular storage (Proser 1974, Kamm & Stull 1989, Somlyo & Somlyo 1990).

While in the oviduct spontaneous pacemaker activity can result in depolarization-mediated contraction (Talo & Hodgson 1978), hormonal actions can induce contraction with or without changes in membrane potential. On the other hand, depolarization is not always associated with tubal contraction. For instance, oviductal smooth muscle depolarized by increased extracellular potassium can undergo both contraction or relaxation as a response to pharmacological stimulation (Sullivan & Marshall 1970, Higgs & Moawad 1974). Conversely, contraction or relaxation can take place with no apparent changes in membrane potential (Triggle 1972). This eventual divergence of association between electrical and contractile activity of the myosalpinx must be kept in mind for the interpretation of studies in which myoelectric recordings have been used as a sole index of contractile activity of the oviduct.

The smooth muscle of the oviduct demonstrates both phasic and tonic activity; i.e. does not only undergo transient twitch-like contractions but it can also vary its resting or basal tone. Detailed measurements of transport of supravitally stained eggs in cumulus inside the oviduct by cinematographic recording and computer image analysis have revealed that phasic muscle contractions of the tube are responsible for the typical random pendular motions of the egg which have been observed in the oviducts of a variety of species, including primates (Tam et al 1975, Verdugo et al 1976, Hodgson et al 1977, Villalón et al 1991). These pendular motions are produced by contractions of the circular smooth muscle of the oviductal wall (Hodgson et al 1977). Measurements of myoelectric activity, which usually precedes contraction, show that, under a broad range of hormonal influences, electrical activity in the rabbit and human oviduct takes place randomly along the tubal wall, not following any preferential pacemaker. Electrical activation propagates for short segments of random length in both prouterine and antiuterine directions with no preferential direction (Daniel et al 1975, Talo & Hodgson 1978, Talo 1992). Recordings of myoelectric activity show that along the wall of excised human oviducts there are multiple pacemaker sites, depending upon the time in the menstrual cycle and the segment of the tube. These pacemaker sites can change location, and the propagation of myoelectric activity can change from periods of short-ranged directed propagation to periods of complete randomness of propagation (Talo & Pulkkinen 1982). Directed propagation of myoelectric activity and the corresponding movement of material takes place through very short tubal length and can reach up to 1 or 2 mm/s. Contractions last for only a few seconds before reversing direction, resulting in a characteristically random pattern of intraluminal flow and very slow rates of net tubal transport (Tam et al 1975, Verdugo et al 1976, Hodgson et al 1977, Villalón et al 1992). However, there is indirect quantitative evidence that tubal motility can become partially derandomized resulting in biasing of contraction-driven egg motions in the rabbit oviduct (Verdugo 1982). The significance of bias in the propagation of oviductal contractions will be discussed in detail later in this section.

Measurements of changes of diameter of the oviduct that reflect the contractions of the circular smooth muscle agree with some of the observations of myoelectric activity in that they also fail to demonstrate long-range propagated peristalsis; instead they show that contractions take place simultaneously at different points along the oviduct and propagate only for short random length segments of the tube (Verdugo 1985). Although peristaltic activity of the oviduct has been cited in the past as the basic mechanism of tubal gamete transport, this has been based only on indirect evidence obtained by highly invasive measurements of pressure changes in the tube (Maia & Coutinho 1970) or by optical transducer

methods that have not been rigorously validated to measure tubal contractions (Halbert et al 1977). Quantitative recordings of long-range propagated peristaltic activity in the oviduct to support this contention will have to await the development of new objectively validated non-invasive transducers (Blandau et al 1975).

In summary, available evidence shows that myoelectric and contractile activity of the circular smooth muscle of the oviduct, responsible for tubal transport, seems to propagate for short random length segments and with equal probability in either pro- or antiuterine directions (Daniel et al 1975 Hodgson et al 1977, Hodgson & Talo 1978, Talo & Hodgson 1978). Accordingly, material in the lumen of the oviduct is randomly moved from contracted segments to relaxed or less contracted neighboring segments in the typical pendular pattern that has been observed in the past. Although these pendular motions of the egg show the characteristic features of a random collection, the existence of a bias in a pro- or antiuterine direction cannot be ruled out. This quantal probabilistic pattern of motion is a fundamental feature of tubal transport and needs to be considered to explain the regulation of ovum transport (Verdugo 1982).

***Laplace and the wall of the oviduct*** A critical aspect of the role of muscle in tubal transport function is the shape and distribution of smooth muscle, especially the circular muscle along the length of the oviduct. Histological sections in all mammalian species that have been studied show that smooth muscle forms a ring in the wall of the tube and that, whereas the radius encircled by the ring decreases, the wall thickness of the ring increases in a discrete mode from the ampulla to the isthmus and the intramural section of the tube (Figs 4.3, 4.4).

The law of Laplace (1821) predicts that the force exerted *against* the wall by a pressure P, inside a cylinder of radius R and wall thickness S, like the one encircled by the myosalpinx, is balanced by tension T, developed in the wall. According to the law of Laplace (Fig. 4.7) the tension (T) per unit cross-sectional area supported by the wall is equal to the ratio of the product of the cylinder's radius (R) by the pressure (P) inside the cylinder, over the thickness

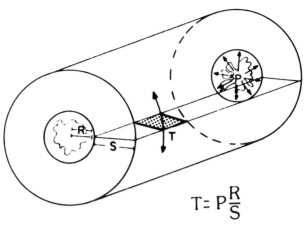

$$T = P\frac{R}{S}$$

**Fig. 4.7**  Schematic representation of the application of Laplace's law to the oviduct. S is the thickness, and R is the radius of the muscular ring that encircles the mucosa-filled lumen of the oviduct. P is the pressure *against* the tubal wall. T represents the tension per unit cross-sectional area *in* the tubal wall. Notice that for equal intraluminal pressure P, the tension T increases with R and decreases with S according to $T = P \times R/S$.

of the cylinder's wall (S). Accordingly, for equal tension per unit cross-sectional area developed by contractions in the wall, the resulting intraluminal pressure generated is inversely proportional to the radius and directly proportional to the wall thickness. Therefore, because of the increasing thickness of muscle tissue in the tubal wall and the decreasing radius it encircles, equal amounts of tension per unit of cross-sectional area generated by muscle contractions result in different luminal pressures along the various sections of the tube. These differences according to Laplace's law turn out to be proportional to the ratio of wall thickness over radius for each section:

$$P_{amp} : P_{isth} : P_{intr} = (S/R)_{amp} : (S/R)_{isth} : (S/R)_{intr}$$

From measurements of published as well as our own material the corresponding S/R ratios in ampulla, isthmus and intramural sections turn out to be approximately $1 : 5 : 50$. Thus, in order for a segment of contracting ampulla near the AIJ to inject material into the isthmus the maximum phasic pressure inside the ampullary segment should be five times the basal tonic internal pressure in the neighboring isthmic segment. Therefore, transport will probably not proceed beyond the AIJ unless the basal tone of the isthmus decreases allowing the contractile activity of the ampulla to move material into the isthmic lumen. Obviously the larger the transported egg or egg surrogate the lower should be the required isthmic basal tone for the egg to move into the isthmus. The same argument also applies to the UTJ. Thus the law of Laplace predicts that eggs would be often retained at the junctional zone simply because these are regions of the oviduct where particularly high differences of S/R exist. These gating effects in the junctional zones result from the architecture of the tube, rather than from the existence of any particular sphincter mechanism, as has been postulated in the past (Brundin 1964). The law of Laplace explains why microsurgical anastomosis of sections with very different thickness to radius ratio do not perform well in ampullouterine anastomosis. Laplace also explains why the longer the tubal amputation the lower the chance of successful tubal function, since the nearer to the uterus the higher the mechanical energetic gradient the egg will find in entering the tubal lumen. Last but not least, this law explains why the site of dilatation of the oviduct in the hydrosalpinx is the ampulla since, given equal pressure, the tension per unit cross-sectional area of the wall will be about five times higher in the ampulla than in the isthmus, i.e.

small pressures can generate very large tensions and hence more dilatation of the ampullary wall. The more the ampulla dilates, the larger is its radius and the increase in pressure required to dilate it even further is less, very much like the inflation of a rubber balloon, which is also predicted by Laplace to be difficult initially but easier as it inflates. Experimental data on pressure/volume relationships in different segments of the oviduct also confirm the predictions of the Laplace law, in that the pressure required to dilate the ampulla is much smaller than the pressure to dilate the isthmus (Talo 1975).

In summary, the movement of material in the tubal lumen is determined by the frequency and the distance that phasic contractions of the circular muscle propagate along the tubal wall. On the other hand, junctional pauses of tubal transport are probably due to the tonic activity of the myosalpinx and determined by the built-in uneven increases of smooth muscle between different segments of the tubal wall. The time–space characteristics of tubal contractions, which are the only aspects of contractions that are cause–effect related to tubal transport, cannot be reliably established from in vitro studies or from measurements of tubal intraluminal pressure in vivo. Thus, the significance of most of the available data on tubal contractility is difficult to ascertain.

***Hormonal actions on tubal muscle*** Although the detailed molecular mechanisms by which hormonal influences control the contractility of the oviductal smooth muscle cell are complex and not yet completely understood, the effects of a variety of hormones and neurotransmitters on tubal smooth muscle contractility have been well documented. Hormonal or neurohormonal influences can independently affect the phasic and/or the tonic behavior of the oviductal smooth muscle, and longitudinal and circular muscle fibers can respond differently to hormonal influences.

*The effect of ovarian steroids on the control of tubal contractility* The influence of ovarian steroids on gamete transport has been well documented (Chang 1976) and their effect on tubal contractile activity has also been extensively investigated. However, attempts to establish a cause–effect

relationship of the action of steroids on tubal motility and gamete transport are still largely speculative. Studies of tubal contractile activity in human subjects in situ at different periods of the menstrual cycle have given conflicting results whose significance in relation to either tubal transport or the mechanism of steroid action is difficult to interpret (Croxatto et al 1978b, 1979).

None the less, studies conducted in vitro of both spontaneous and simulated motor activity of longitudinal as well as circumferential tubal smooth muscle of different segments of the oviducts in a variety of experimental animals and in humans have contributed to the understanding of the effect and the mechanism of action of various steroids in tubal motility. Estradiol has been shown to potentiate tubal motility whereas progesterone inhibits it (Spilman & Harper 1974, Borda et al 1975, Gimeno et al 1976). As shown in later sections, the effect of steroids on tubal motility is thought to be mediated by the action of sympathetic transmitters and prostaglandins. However, there are indications that steroids may also directly modulate tubal contractility (Hodgson et al 1973, Nozaki & Ito 1987). Notwithstanding the direct or indirect action of steroids, the control of steroid tissue receptors in the oviduct must be taken into account when considering how tubal contractility is regulated. Steroids, like other hormones, are thought to initiate their cellular action by specifically binding to a receptor molecule which then triggers a chain of biochemical events that brings about a specific and characteristic cellular response.

Steroid receptors have been found in the tube (Batra et al 1980, Devoto et al 1980, Verhage et al 1980, Pino et al 1982). Quantitative studies of both cytosolic and nuclear steroid receptors at different times in the menstrual cycle and in different segments of the human oviduct indicate that estradiol and progesterone receptor levels rise to a maximum during the late proliferative phase and decrease after ovulation (Robertson et al 1975, Pollow et al 1981). The concentration of both receptors is two to three times higher in the ampulla than in the isthmus and infundibulum (Flickinger et al 1974, Punnonen & Lukola 1981). However, the mechanism that controls the number of receptors in the oviduct is still speculative. Increased receptor concentration in the preovulatory period could be related to an inductive effect of estradiol; the postovulatory decrease could be explained by the inhibitory effect of progesterone on receptor synthesis (Pollow et al 1981).

Regional variations in receptor concentrations between ampulla and isthmus are probably due to different distributions of receptor concentration in the mucosa rather than in the muscle tissue. However, there is no direct evidence on receptor distribution in endosalpinx and myosalpinx.

The understanding of how steroid receptors are regulated in the oviduct might turn out to be of critical clinical importance. The pathophysiology of hydrosalpinx and eventually of pelvic inflammatory disease (PID) could be the result of tubal hypoestrogenism produced by estrogen receptor depletion resulting from decreased synthesis or increased destruction of oviductal estrogen receptor sites. Although at present this mechanism is speculative, it is suggested by the muscle and epithelial atrophia observed in human hydrosalpinx and in many cases of PID as shown by recent observations of Devoto et al (1983). For this reason, the experimental hydrosalpinx produced by tubal ligation may have little significance as a model for human hydrosalpinx.

In summary, estrogen potentiates and progesterone inhibits contractility of oviductal smooth muscle. Steroid action is regulated by the turnover of steroid receptors and is probably exerted indirectly by regulating the synthesis and/or release of sympathetic agonists and prostaglandins and the turnover of their corresponding receptors. However, as shown in previous sections, the significance of studies of 'tubal contractility' in regard to tubal transport continues to be uncertain.

*Sympathetic actions on oviductal smooth muscle*
The oviducts are densely innervated by a complex network of long and short postganglionic sympathetic fibers. The circular muscle bundles of the tubal wall are innervated mainly by short fibers, and receive most of the sympathetic afferents. Hence, the sympathetic innervation is rich in the isthmus and rather sparse in the ampulla.

Sympathetic terminals have varying degrees of catecholamine content and turnover which,

especially in the short postganglionic fibers, have been shown to correlate with changes in ovarian steroids (Owman et al 1974, 1976). In humans, during the luteal, progesterone-dominated phase of the menstrual cycle, the oviducts demonstrate a net weight-independent increase in norepinephrine (NE) as compared to the secretory, estrogen-dominated phase (Owman et al 1976). Similar changes have been shown in monkeys and guinea-pigs (Thorbert et al 1978). In the rabbit oviduct, however, NE is higher in estrus than in diestrus (Bodkhe & Harper 1973). The NE content in both the rabbit and guinea-pig oviduct is reduced and this effect is reversed by estradiol (Sjöberg 1967, Kennedy & Marshall 1977). However, sympathetic nerve stimulation of tubal smooth muscles can be maintained in spite of severe reduction of norepinephrine in sympathetic terminals (Burnstock 1979). On the other hand, studies concerning modulation of spontaneous sympathetic nerve activity by steroids are somewhat contradictory (Marshall 1981).

The effect of catecholamines is mediated by the binding of these neurotransmitters to specific receptor molecules located in the membrane of the effector cell. The chain of intracellular events that takes place after the adrenergic receptor has been occupied and leads to the activation of the effector cell has now been well established and can be found in any of several excellent reviews recently published. Adrenergic receptors, depending upon their actions, their pharmacological potency and the inhibition of their effect by specific antagonist, have been classically divided into alpha ($\alpha$) and beta ($\beta$). In oviductal smooth muscle of different species, as well as in smooth muscle of other organs, $\alpha$-adrenergic receptors mediate excitation and $\beta$-receptors lead to inhibition of contraction (Nakanishi & Wood 1968, Levy & Lindner 1972, Polidoro et al 1976, Hodgson & Eddy 1975).

Although the role of adrenergic control of tubal motility and transport is still controversial, evidence obtained in animals and in humans from in vitro and in vivo studies shows that the effect of adrenergic agents seems to be modulated by steroid action (Korenaga & Kadota 1981). The effect of norepinephrine, for instance, a dual $\alpha$- and $\beta$-receptor agonist but with preferential α-receptor stimulation, varies with different tubal segments, muscle layers, and degrees of steroidal domination. Such variations may help to explain many of the past controversies.

If now seems well accepted, however, that estrogen modulates the α-receptor actions and progesterone the β-receptor actions in the oviduct (Brundin 1965, Hodgson & Pauerstein 1974, Moawad et al 1976). Also, longitudinal muscle fibers show different sensitivity to α-adrenergic agonists than do circularly oriented muscle fibers (Hodgson & Pauerstein 1974).

It has been suggested in the past that the AIJ and the isthmus may function as an adrenergically controlled sphincter that regulates the passage of the egg to the isthmus (Brundin 1965). This idea is consistent with the 'tube-locking' phenomena of egg retention in the AIJ in the rabbit, which can be reversed by α-adrenergic blockers (Pauerstein et al 1970).

However, observations that both pharmacological and surgical denervation of the oviduct and, more recently, microsurgical resection of the AJI do not affect normal fertility have severely weakened the idea of an adrenergic sphincter in the tube (Greenwald 1967, Eddy & Black 1974, Pauerstein et al 1974b). Nevertheless, from Laplacian considerations, it seems clear that a decrease of basal tone might be necessary to allow passage of the egg from the ampulla into the isthmus. This prediction is consistent with recent observations that isthmic circular myosalpinx seems to undergo reversal from α- to β-receptor response by the time to isthmic transport in both the rabbit and the human oviduct (Korenaga & Kadoka 1981). Nevertheless, in humans β-agonists as well as estradiol and prostaglandin $F_{2\alpha}$ have failed to modify the normal course of tubal egg transport, an indication that hormonal or pharmacological interventions that drastically modify contractile activity in the human oviduct do not necessarily affect ovum transport. (Croxatto et al 1978b, 1979). In the rabbit, both surgical and chemical denervation (by 6-hydroxidopamine) fail to disrupt tubal transport (Pauerstein et al 1974b). This is also the case with pharmacological manipulations to either decrease, by reserpine, or to increase endogenous catecholamine by inhibition of monoamine

oxidase, or else by α- or β-adrenergic blockade (Pauerstein et al, 1970a,b, Bodkhe & Harper 1972, Polidoro et al 1974).

In summary, the abundant adrenergic innervation of the myosalpinx does not seem to play a central part in the functional control of this effector, at least concerning the role of muscle contractions in tubal transport.

*Effect of prostaglandins on tubal smooth muscle*
Prostaglandins (PG) are one of the most widely found extracellular messengers, and in mammals they modulate a broad variety of effectors. They are short-lived products derived from arachidonic acid. They are usually synthesized near the effector site and are found in a variety of tissues, including the mammalian oviduct where they have a powerful modulating effect on the two mechanical effectors of the tube, ciliated and smooth muscle cells.

The amount, the distribution and the effect of prostaglandins varies, depending upon the different types of prostaglandins, the species, the segment of the tube, and the level of steroids. In the rabbit, for instance, estrogen potentiates both the synthesis of $PGF_{2\alpha}$ and the stimulation of tubal contraction produced by $PGF_{2\alpha}$. Conversely, progesterone inhibits both the local synthesis of and the response of tubal smooth muscle to $PGF_{2\alpha}$ and it potentiates the effect of $PGE_1$ on tubal contractility of the proximal isthmus. The observed pharmacological effects are consistent with physiological changes of contractile patterns and tubal transport during periods of estrogen and/or progesterone dominance during the rabbit estrous cycle (Spilman 1976).

In the monkey, the effect of PGs depends upon the time in the cycle. During preovulatory phases, $PGE_1$ and $PGE_2$ have no effect on spontaneous tubal contractions; during the postovulatory phase, they may sometimes inhibit contractility; however, during the luteal phase they clearly suppress spontaneous tubal contractions. On the other hand, $PGF_{2\alpha}$ has no effect on contractility during the follicular phase, but it strongly stimulates contractions immediately before and during ovulation (Spilman & Harper 1975).

Although $PGF_{2\alpha}$ exhibits α-adrenergic synergism and β-adrenergic antagonisms, and conversely $PGE_2$ demonstrates α-antagonism and β-synergism, the effector actions of catecholamines and prostaglandins are independent (Spilman & Harper 1974).

Human oviducts also contain prostaglandins (Vastik-Fernandez et al 1975), they can strongly influence tubal contractility. Studies conducted both in vivo and in vitro show that in general, $PGF_{2\alpha}$ stimulates and $PGE_2$ inhibits contractions in the different tubal segments at different times during the menstrual cycle. However, there are two exceptions: the outermost (uterine) spiral layer of the UTJ follows the pattern of response of the myometrium to PGs in that it is stimulated by $PGE_2$; during the periovulatory period, contractions of the innermost longitudinal muscle layer of the isthmus are stimulated, rather than inhibited, by $PGE_2$ (Gimeno et al 1979). In the rabbit myosalpinx the number of binding sites of $PGF_{2\alpha}$ and $PGE_2$ changes in the different segments of the tube and at different times of the cycle (Riehl & Harper 1981). However, pharmacological interventions using exogenous prostaglandins as well as efforts to interfere with PG synthesis, their release, or their metabolism have rather minor effects on oviductal transport (Hodgson 1976, Valenzuela et al 1977). These results suggest that, as in the case of catecholamines, PGs can indeed modify tubal contractility. However, their role in controlling those aspects of myosalpinx activity that are relevant to tubal transport must be rather limited.

*Action of peptides on myosalpinx contractility* The application of immunocytochemical methods as well as radioimmunoassay techniques have revealed the presence of several peptides in the oviduct of human and experimental animals. Those include: Neuropeptide Y (Stjernqvist et al 1983); the vasoactive intestinal peptide VIP (Alm et al 1980); Substance P (Huang et al 1984); and α-aminobutyric acid GABA (Martin del Rio 1981, Erdö et al 1983). Many of these substances have also been shown to affect the contractile activity of tubal smooth muscle. However, there is no evidence that peptides can produce changes in ovum transport or in fertility. For instance, VIP has been found in the isthmus in humans (Alm et al 1980). VIP can also strongly inhibit spontaneous motor activity of both the circular and

longitudinal muscle fibers of human isthmus and ampulla, and had been thought to control the tone of the isthmic region (Helm et al 1982a,b). However in ovulating rabbits, high doses of VIP failed to alter ovum transport and fertility (Fredericks et al 1983).

### Oviductal cilia

Various densities of ciliated cells have been found in the mucosa lining the convoluted internal surface of the oviduct in all vertebrate animals. It is now well established that, with a few species variations, estrogen influences the presence and density of cilia in the mucosa of the oviduct. In some species such as the rabbit, castration can lead to complete deciliation which can be reversed by exogenous estrogen (Frenko 1954). The same trophic effect of estrogen can be observed in the oviduct of immature rhesus monkeys, where it can strongly increase the density of epitheliary cilia (Allen 1928).

Although in some primates there are cyclic variations in the density of oviductal cilia in relation to the estrous cycle (Joachimovits 1935, Brenner 1967), in humans the observed changes seem to affect more the height of the ciliated epithelium than the number of cilia. The oviductal epithelium is low (10 μm) in periods of progesterone domination; its height doubles in periods of estrogen domination; and it shows signs of atrophy in the late menopausal state (Westman 1930, Andrews 1951, Fredericsson 1959, Gaddum-Rosse et al 1975).

The involvement of oviductal cilia in gamete transport was postulated very early (Lim & Chao 1927), yet it continued to be a highly speculative and controversial issue until recently when direct evidence indicated that, in the absence of muscle contractions, ciliary activity is sufficient to drive the ovum throughout the ampulla of the rabbit (Halbert et al 1976). Although ciliary action is sufficient to power tubal transport, it certainly does not seem to be necessary, since individuals suffering from Afzelius immotile cilia syndrome have been shown to undergo normal reproduction (Afzelius et al 1978). These findings have been subject to controversial interpretations owing to the idea that the roles of muscle and ciliary actions in the oviduct are mutually exclusive. This apparent paradox can be explained on the basis of redundancy in oviductal function, i.e. both muscle contractions and ciliary movement might not be necessary yet each could be sufficient to ensure the transport of gametes (Verdugo et al 1980a,b).

In primates, as in most other mammalian species, cilia beat in a prouterine direction throughout the different segments of the tube (Gaddum-Rosse & Blandau 1976). The regulation of ciliary movements in the oviduct has only recently begun to be systematically explored. The present understanding of the physiology and pharmacology of oviductal ciliated cells is meager and the significance of much of the available data is uncertain. The application of yet unvalidated methods to detect ciliary movements and the presence of mucus-secreting cells in the oviductal mucosa make it difficult to ascertain unequivocally the significance of much of the published material. For instance, hormonal actions on ciliated cells cannot be unequivocally established by measuring ciliary movements in the oviduct, since hormones can affect ciliary activity and/or secretory activity producing changes in the rheological properties of the secreted mucus and thereby indirectly changing ciliary movements due to variations of the fluidic load on the ciliated cells. For example, there are data that show that the frequencies of ciliary beat in various sections of the human and rabbit oviduct demonstrate variations during different periods of the sexual cycle (Borell et al 1957, Westrom et al 1977). The interpretation of this evidence, however, in regard to the site of hormonal action can be equivocal since hormonal effects taking place in ciliated and/or secretory cells can result in a change of ciliary activity.

The introduction of a new objective, reproducible and objectively validated method of measuring ciliary movement based on laser Doppler spectroscopy (Lee & Verdugo 1976, Verdugo & Golborne 1988) together with the development of a mucus-free tissue culture preparation of oviductal ciliated cells (Rumery et al 1971) has facilitated the study of oviductal cilia. These techniques have unequivocally demonstrated that ciliated cells of the oviduct are responsive to hormones. For instance, PGs $F_{2\alpha}$, $E_1$ and $E_2$ in concentrations equivalent to those found in vivo have been shown to stimulate oviductal ciliary activity (Verdugo 1980, Verdugo et al 1980b). β-adrenergic agonists also stimulate oviductal cilia (Villalón & Verdugo 1982) and, although there is no direct effect of ovarian steroids on ciliary activity, preliminary data obtained in our laboratory suggest that either estrogen or progesterone alone strongly potentiate β-adrenergic stimulation. However, when oviductal ciliated cells of the rabbit are simultaneously pretreated with estrogen and progesterone β-stimulation is strongly inhibited.

We now know that the cilio-stimulating effect of PGs and β-adrenergic agonists, as well as the recently discovered purinergic ($P_2$) actions on ciliated cells of the rabbit oviduct, are all mediated by changes of cytosolic $Ca^{2+}$ concentration by either release of intracellular $Ca^{2+}$, or by entry of $Ca^{2+}$ into the ciliated cell via Ca-channels (Villalón et al 1989, Villalón & Verdugo 1990).

The stimulating effect of prostaglandin $E_2$ on ciliary activity in vitro correlates very well with prostaglandin $E_2$-induced acceleration of the ciliary-driven component of tubal transport in situ, as shown by stochastic analysis of ovum transport in the rabbit oviduct (Verdugo 1982).

Whereas the function of cilia in the defense of the airways of the lung has been well established, the role of tubal cilia in the defense mechanism of the genital tract has not been objectively evaluated and remains to be explored.

**From Einstein to Fallopius: a stochastic model for tubal gamete transport**

Previous sections have given a short, phenomenological description of the available pieces of the tubal transport puzzle. In this section, an attempt will be made to sort these pieces within the conceptual framework of a general working hypothesis. The two fundamental issues that need to be considered are the identification of the mechanism that *moves* the gametes in the tube—the kinetics of tubal transport—and the mechanisms responsible for the characteristic *pauses* in tubal transport—the statics of tubal transport.

*The kinetics of tubal transport*

A convenient starting point to establish the mechanisms that move the gametes is to study the movement of the ovum inside the tube. As described in previous sections, in all species where tubal transport has been directly observed the egg is moved in the tube in discrete steps following a random pendular bidirectional pattern. The statistical analysis of the amplitude and velocity of pendular egg motions in the oviduct reveals that they form a random collection. However, the Gaussian distribution of velocities recorded while the egg undergoes pendular motion can demonstrate variable degrees of prouterine *shift* and/or *skewing* that can change, depending upon the hormonal regime.

The random characteristics of the pendular motions imply that the forces that drive them must also be random. The presence of a prouterine *skewing* as shown by an asymmetric Gaussian distribution indicates some degree of derandomization of movement that reflects an increase of the probabilities of prouterine motions of the egg over proovarian motions (Fig. 4.8). The presence of a prouterine *shift* or bias of the whole Gaussian distribution indicates the existence of a unidirectional nonrandom force acting on the egg (Verdugo et al 1976). For instance, the instantaneous velocity of pendular

motions of the egg in the monkey ampulla in estrus is a Gaussian distribution shifted about 35 μm/s in a prouterine direction (Fig. 4.6). PGE$_2$ at low concentrations produces both a marked skewing and an increase in the shift of this distribution (Verdugo 1982), showing some degree of preferential prouterine spread of contractions and also an increase in ciliary drive of the egg. Measurements of the motion of ovum surrogates in the isthmus of the rabbit demonstrate that in this section of the oviduct the eggs also undergo discrete random pendular motions, except that in between the pendular displacements, the egg surrogates can remain stationary for variable and sometimes long periods of time (Bourdage 1982).

The cause–effect relationship between random pendular motions and phasic muscle contractions of the tube and the shift of the probability distribution and ciliary action was tentatively predicted by stochastic analysis of ovum transport (Tam et al 1975, Verdugo et al 1976). This argument was later validated by direct evidence (Halbert et al 1976; Hodgson et al 1977). The statistical analysis of egg motions is also in agreement with the finding of random tubal myoelectric activity (Daniel et al 1975, Hodgson & Talo 1978, Talo & Hodgson 1978). Computer analysis of wall deformations also indicates that the phasic contractile activity of the oviduct is probably random, and determines a corresponding pattern of movement of the ovum that is bidirectional, discrete and random.

Changes in the rate of ovum transport dependent upon *derandomizing* contraction-driven pendular motions of the egg are simple to visualize. For instance, if segmental contractions become propagated for longer distances along the tube in a prouterine direction, the tubal transport is accelerated. Thus, hormones could change the rate of tubal transport by making the propagation of contractions along the tube asymmetrical (Verdugo 1980, Talo & Pulkinen 1982).

Changes in the rate of tubal transport dependent upon ciliary drive, although complex in their detailed rheology, are easy to visualize as a control mechanism since their action is undirectional. Hormones could vary the ciliary drive and cause changes in ovum transport (Verdugo et al 1980b, Verdugo 1982).

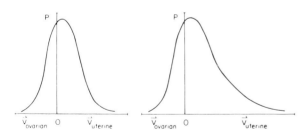

**Fig. 4.8** Schematic representation of two alternatives of regulation of ampullary ovum transport as shown by the histogram of probability distribution of ovum velocities in the oviduct. The left curve illustrates ciliary-drive-dependent accelerations as shown by an increase in the *bias* of the Gaussian distribution of random ovum velocities. The right curve displays muscle-driven-dependent acceleration as shown by *skewing* of the Gaussian distribution of random ovum velocities. Notice the asymmetry of the probability distribution indicating derandomization of ovum transport, as it results from increased probability of muscle-driven motions in a prouterine direction.

The aspect of tubal transport which is less simple to explain is how a pattern of truly *random* motions can result in net prouterine or proovarian transport and how this transport can be regulated. A convenient approach to this question is to find a physical formulation that accurately describes the nature of the movements that take place during tubal transport and thereby predicts its behavior, making explicit the implicit control mechanism that regulates it. This formulation should account for the coexistence of random and nonrandom motions and should consider the particular boundary conditions existing in the oviduct. The formulation developed by Langevin to describe how charged particles diffuse in a field of external force fulfils these requisites, since it combines the Einstein diffusion equation, to account for the random Brownian motion (which, in this case, is represented by muscle-driven motions of the egg) with a constant drag produced by the interaction of the particle charge and the electric field (which, in this case, is represented by the action of the cilia).

The application of Langevin's formulation to describe and predict ovum transport in the rabbit ampulla has been experimentally verified (Verdugo et al 1980a) and demonstrates that the movements of the egg in the ampulla can indeed be represented as a random walk in a field of continuous force. Although the mathematical derivation, which will not be presented here, might appear complex, it is conceptually very simple. The formulation predicts that variations in ampullary ovum transport can take place by changes in the ciliary drag or by changes in the random motions of the egg produced by muscle contractions. On the other hand, the long isthmic transport could result from the drive produced by a purely stochastic mechanism without the intervention of ciliary drive, i.e. if the motions of the egg in the isthmus are random, as it has been recently shown (Bourdage 1982), then isthmic transport can be simply described by the Einstein diffusion equation for Brownian motion (Einstein 1905, 1908). How can a truly random pattern of movement, as in Brownian motion, lead to net prouterine transport? The particular set of boundary conditions that can satisfactorily explain this apparent paradox is known in physics

as Einstein's 'theorem of the drunken sailor'. It states that if a drunk man is randomly walking on the sidewalk, with a wall to bounce on one side (reflecting barrier) and the edge of the street to fall on the other (absorbing barrier), it can be predicted that he will irrevocably fall to the street and that *the time* it will take him to fall is proportional to the square of the width of the sidewalk and inversely proportional to the product of *the square of the length of his random steps*, in the width axis of the sidewalk, and *the frequency of his stepping* (Fig. 4.9).

The corresponding boundary conditions for the oviduct are the ciliary drive from the ampullary side, that functions as a reflecting barrier bouncing the egg back into the isthmus, and the UTJ or the uterus, that functions as an absorbing barrier, invariably trapping the egg as it moves into its cavity. If these boundary conditions are valid then, according to Einstein, the time of isthmic transport should be directly proportional to three times the square of the length of the isthmus and inversely proportional to the product of the length of the random pendular motions (averaged) multiplied by the frequency of motion (Verdugo et al 1976, 1980a, Portnow et al 1977). Direct measurements of ovum surrogate movement in the rabbit isthmus have recently become available and show that surrogate movements in the isthmus are also pendular and random as indicated by the typical Gaussian distribution of their magnitudes. The average length of isthmic pendular movements is about 1 mm, and they occur at frequencies that vary from about 5 movements per min at 24–48h after coitus to about 10 movements per min at 60–72 h after coitus. The pendular activity in the isthmus, unlike that in the ampulla, is not continuous but is discrete, interrupted by quiescent periods of 20–45 min (Bourdage 1982). Using his own measurements and the Einstein equation for random motion in one dimension proposed by our model (Verdugo et al 1980a), Bourdage computed a predicted isthmic transport time of 2.5 h as opposed to the generally accepted 45–60 h. Taking into account this discrepancy, notwithstanding that the statistical distribution of isthmic pendular motions follow a perfectly Gaussian distribution, Bourdage argues against

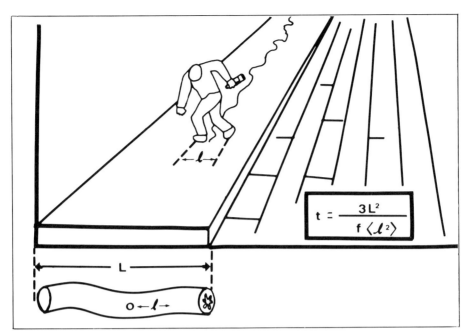

**Fig. 4.9**  Schematic representation of Einstein's theorem of the drunken sailor. t is the time it will take for the drunk to fall on the street, L is the width of the sidewalk, f is the frequency of the drunk's stepping and l is the length of the drunk's steps in the transversal coordinate of the sidewalk.

the validity of a random mechanism of ovum transport in the isthmus. There is a fallacy in this argument, however. A Gaussian distribution is indeed the mathematical signature of a random process. Secondly, Einstein's equation does not consider arrests of movement of the objects undergoing random motion like those observed in the isthmus (Einstein 1908). Unfortunately, Bourdage neither considered nor measured systematically the long stationary periods the egg undergoes in the isthmus, making invalid their conclusion. Most important, however, his data show that inside the isthmus the movements of the ovum are indeed random, although they seem to follow in the time domain a Markovian rather than a Brownian pattern of movement.

According to Einstein's equation the physiological regulation to a purely random transport mechanism can be efficiently controlled by changing the *length* and/or the *frequency* of the pendular motions. Hodgson et al (1977) have demonstrated that the length of the pendular motions depends on how far random contractions propagate along the oviductal wall. There are indications that both the frequency of contractions and their propagation are under hormonal control, since by the time of isthmic transport 48–60 h after human chorionic gonadotropin (hCG), higher frequency and longer distance of propagations of random myoelectric activity have been observed as compared to those of controls obtained 18–24 h after hCG. (Talo & Hodgson 1978). Estrogen-induced acceleration of ovum transport is accompanied by increases in the distance of propagation of myoelectric activity; progesterone-induced acceleration of egg transport is accompanied by increased frequency of myoelectric activity (Hodgson & Talo 1978). Thus, experimental evidence strongly supports the mechanisms of control of tubal transport predicted by the Einstein diffusion equation. Although not implicit in Einstein's formulation, an additional factor that could change tubal transport rate is a variation of the length of time that the ovum stays stationary as shown by Bourdage (1982).

Another interesting prediction of the stochastic hypothesis of tubal transport is that transported materials that either overcome or are not affected by ciliary drive should not suffer the effect of a 'reflecting barrier'. If, furthermore, contractions remain random along the length of the oviduct, because of Laplace's law, the tube will transport these materials in a proovarian direction. The argument is that for any given set of equally contracting segments of muscle in the tubal wall, the more caudal the position, the more pressure they will develop because their radius is smaller and their wall is thicker. Therefore, a pressure gradient should rapidly drive these materials in a proovarian direction. The involvement of a dynamic gradient in the rapid phase of sperm transport is predicted by Laplace and remains as a possible alternative to be experimentally tested.

*The statics of tubal transport*

A corollary of Laplace's law in the oviduct is that for tubal transport to move in a prouterine direction, the tonic contractile activity of the downstream oviduct should decrease. This prediction is valid regardless of the transport driven by random segmental contractions with appropriate boundary conditions (the 'drunk sailor mechanism') or by programmed contractility that propagates preferentially in a prouterine direction. The argument of this corollary states that in order for a segment (n) to propel material in a prouterine direction, the tonic tension of the neighboring segment (n + 1) in the uterine side, should be lower than the maximum phasic tension generated by segment (n). As mentioned earlier, this corollary of Laplace's law can explain the gating effects that produce the observed pauses in tubal transport. The validity of this prediction also remains to be experimentally tested in the future.

In summary, according to the stochastic model, changes in the rate of ovum transport can take place: (a) by variations of the ciliary drive; (b) by changing the periods that the egg remains stationary; (c) by changes in the frequency and/or the length of random motions, or (d) by derandomizing of the muscle contractions, such that the probability of movement in one direction becomes larger than that in the other. Some of these predicted mechanisms of control have been validated experimentally. Others remain to be verified.

## CLOSING REMARKS

The understanding of tubal transport remains a challenge. However, out of the chaos of information and misinformation, a picture is slowly beginning to emerge. The anatomy of the mammalian oviduct suggests strongly a unique biomechanical design with built-in functional implications as shown by the law of Laplace. The mechanisms by which the mechanical effectors of the oviduct transport the gametes are also becoming better defined. The control system of the effectors, although following a different program of operation in different species, contains in all cases a biphasic hormonal network of commands, a yin-yang design in which, for every effector action, there are two or more hormonal messages to either potentiate or inhibit the effector response, giving a broad and very efficient span of control. In primates, for example, the built-in program of operation that controls tubal function seems to be strongly imprinted and nonresponsive to environmental or experimental interventions. In other species, such as rodents, it seems to be highly susceptible to environmental or experimental manipulation.

Very few answers emerge from this short review. Much remains to be learned. However, a plan to search for the missing pieces of the puzzle has been outlined here in the form of a working hypothesis of high predictive power. It is not to be taken as a new dogma regarding tubal function but to be used as a conceptual framework to continue our systematic interrogation of this remarkable trumpet of Dr Fallopius.

# REFERENCES

Adams C E 1952 A study of fertilization in the rabbit: the effect of post-coital ligation of the fallopian tube or uterine horn. J Endocrinol 13: 296

Adams C E 1979 Consequences of accelerated ovum transport, including a re-evaluation of Estes' opereation. J Reprod Fertil 55: 239

Afzelius B A, Cramer P, Mossberg B 1978 On the function of cilia in the female reproductive tract. Fertil Steril 29: 72

Ahlgren M 1975 Sperm transport and survival in the human Fallopian tube. Gynecol Invest 6: 206

Ahuja K K, Smith W, Tucker M, Craft I 1985 Successful pregnancies from the transfer of pronucleate embryos in an outpatient in vitro fertilization program. Fertil Steril 44: 181

Akester A R, Inkster I J 1961 Cine-radiographic studies of the genital tract of the rabbit. J Reprod Fertil 2: 507

Allen E 1928 Reaction of immature monkey (*Macacus rhesus*) to injections of ovarian hormone. J Morphol 46: 479

Allen E, Pratt J P, Newell Q U, Bland L J 1930 Human tubal ova; related corpora lutea and uterine tubes. Contrib Embryol Carneg Inst 29: 7

Alm P, Alumets J, Håkanson R et al 1980 Origin and distribution of VIP nerves in the genito-urinary tract. Cell Tissue Res 205: 337

Andersen D H 1928 Comparative anatomy of the tubo uterine junction. Histology and physiology in the sow. Am J Anat 42: 255

Andrews M C 1951 Epithelial changes in puerperal fallopian tube. Am J Obstet Gynecol 62: 28

Aref I, Hafez E S E, Kamar G A R 1973 Postcoital prostaglandins in vivo. Oviductal motility and egg transport in rabbits. Fertil Steril 24: 671

Austin C R 1957 Fate of spermatozoa in the uterus of the mouse and rat. J Endocrinol 14: 335

Banik U K, Pincus G 1964 Estrogen and transport of ova in the rat. Proc Soc Exp Biol 116: 1032

Batra S, Helm G, Owman C, Sjöberg N O, Walles B 1980 Female sex steroid concentrations in the ampullary and isthmic regions of the human fallopian tube and their relationship to plasma concentrations during the menstrual cycle. Am J Obstet Gynecol 136: 986

Bedford J M 1963 Morphological reaction of spermatozoa in the female reproductive tract of the rabbit. J Reprod Fertil 6: 245

Bishop D W 1969 Sperm physiology in relation to the oviduct. In: Hafez E S E, Blandau R J (eds) The mammalian oviduct. University of Chicago Press, Chicago, p 231

Black D L, Asdell S A 1958 Transport through the rabbit oviduct. Am J Physiol 192: 63

Black D L, Asdell S A 1959 Mechanism controlling entry of the ova into rabbit uterus. Am J Physiol 197: 1275

Blandau R J, Verdugo P 1976 An overview of gamete transport comparative aspects. In: Harper M J K, Pauerstein C J, Adams C E, Coutinho E M, Croxatto H B, Paton D M (eds) Ovum transport and fertility regulation. Scriptor, Copenhagen, p 138

Blandau R J, Boling J L, Halbert S, Verdugo P 1975 Methods for studying oviductal physiology. Gynecol Invest 6: 123

Bodkhe R R, Harper M T K 1972 Changes in the amount of adrenergic neurotransmitter in the genital tract of untreated rabbits, and rabbits given reserpine or iproniazid during the time of egg transport. Biol Reprod 6: 288

Bodkhe R R, Harper M T K 1973 Mechanism of egg transport: changes in amount of adrenergic transmitter in the genital tract of normal and hormone-treated rabbits. In: Segal S J, Crozier P A, Corfman P G, Condliffe P G (eds) The regulation of mammalian reproduction. Thomas Press, Illinois p 364

Boling J L, Blandau R J 1971 Egg transport through the ampullae of the oviducts of rabbits under various experimental conditions. Biol Reprod 4: 174

Borda E, Sterin-Borda L, Gimeno M F, Sterin-Speziale N, Gimeno A L 1975 Motility of the rat oviductal tract isolated in different stages of the sex cycle. Int J Fertil 20: 170

Borell V, Fernstrom I 1953 The adnexal branches of the uterine artery. Acta Radiol 40: 561

Borell V, Nilsson O, Westman A 1957 Ciliary activity in the rabbit fallopian tube during oestrous and after copulation. Acta Obstet Gynecol Scand 36: 22

Bourdage R J 1982 Mechanism of control of ovum transport through the oviductal isthmus and into the cornu in rabbits. Doctoral Thesis, University of Washington. University Microfilm, p 1

Brenner R M 1967 The biology of oviductal cilia. In: Hafez E S E, Blandau R J (eds) The mammalian oviduct. University of Chicago Press, Chicago, p 203

Brundin J 1964 A functional block in the isthmus of the rabbit fallopian tube. Acta Physiol Scand 60: 295

Brundin J 1965 Distribution and function of adrenergic nerves in the rabbit fallopian tube. Acta Physiol Scand (Suppl) 66: 1

Burdick H O, Pincus G 1935 The effect of oestrin injections upon the developing ova of mice and rabbits. Am J Physiol III: 201

Burns R K 1955 Urogenital system. In: Willier B H, Weiss P A, Hannburger V (eds) Analysis of development. Saunders Philadelphia, p 462

Burnstock G 1979 Autonomic innervation and transmission. Br Med Bull 35: 255

Challis J R, Heap R B, Ilingworth D V 1971 Concentration of estrogen and progesterone in the plasma of non-pregnant and lactating guinea-pigs. J Endocrinol 51: 333

Chang M C 1967 Effect of progesterone and related compounds on fertilization, transportation, and development of rabbit eggs. Endocrinology 81: 125

Chang M C 1976 Estrogen, progesterone and egg transport. Overview and identification of problems. In: Harper M J K, Pauerstein C J, Adams C E, Coutinho E M, Croxatto H B, Paton D M (eds) Ovum transport and fertility regulation. Scriptor, Copenhagen, p 473

Chang M C, Pickworth S 1969 Egg transfer in the laboratory animal. In: Hafez E S E, Blandau R J (eds) The mammalian oviduct. University of Chicago Press, Chicago, p 389

Chang M C, Pincus G 1964 Fertilizable life of the rabbit sperm deposited into different parts of the female tract. Proceedings of the Fifth International Congress on Animal Reproduction, Trento, p 377

Chang M C, Sheaffer D C 1957 Number of spermatozoa ejaculated at copulation, transported into the female tract, and present in the male tract of the golden hamster. J Hered 48: 107

Chang M C, Thorsteinsson T 1958 Effects of urine on

motility and fertilizing capacity of rabbit spermatozoa. Fertil Steril 9: 231

Chiara F 1959 Study of the fine innervation of the female genital tube. Ann Obstet Gynecol 81: 1161

Croxatto H B 1974 The duration of egg transport and its regulation in mammals. In: Coutinho A M, Fuchs F (eds) Physiology and genetics of reproduction. Part B. Plenum, New York, p 159

Croxatto H B, Ortiz M E 1975 Egg transport in the Fallopian tube. Gynecol Invest 6: 215

Croxatto H B, Faundes A, Medel M et al 1975 Studies on sperm migration in the human female genital tract. In: Hafez E S E, Thibauld C G (eds) The biology of spermatozoa. Karger, Basel, p 56

Croxatto H B, Ortiz M E, Diaz S, Hess R, Balmaceda J, Croxatto H D 1978a Studies on the duration of egg transport by the human oviduct. II. Ovum location at various intervals following luteinizing hormone peak. A M J Obstet Gynecol 132: 629

Croxatto H B, Ortiz M E, Guiloff E et al 1978b Effect of 15($S$)-IS-methyl prostaglandin $F_{2\alpha}$, on human oviductal motility and ovum transport. Fertil Steril 30: 408

Croxatto H B, Ortiz M E, Diaz S, Hess R 1979 Attempts to modify ovum transport in women. J Reprod Fertil 55: 231

Daniel E E, Lucien P, Posey V A, Paton D M 1975 A functional analysis of the myogenic control system of the human fallopian tube. Am J Obstet Gynecol 121: 1046

Diaz S, Ortiz M E, Croxatto H B 1980 Studies on the duration of ovum transport by the human oviduct. III. Time interval between the luteinizing hormone peak and the recovery of the ova by transcervical flushing of the uterus in normal woman. Am J Obstet Gynecol 137: 116

Devoto L, Soto E, Magofke, A M, Sierralta W 1980 Unconjugated steroids in the Fallopian tube and peripheral blood during the normal menstrual cycle. Fertil Steril 33: 613

Devoto L, Pino A M, Soto E, Gutler A 1983 Estradiol and progesterone nuclear and cytosol receptors of hydrosalpinx. Fertil Steril 42: 594

Eddy C A, Black D L 1974 Ovum transport through rabbit oviducts perfused with 6-hydroxydopamine. J Reprod Fertil 38: 189

Eddy C A, Garcia R G, Kraemer D C, Pauerstein C J 1975 Detailed time course of ovum transport in the rhesus monkey (*Maccaca mulata*). Biol Reprod 13: 363

Eddy C A, Turner T T, Kraemer D C, Pauerstein C J 1976 Pattern and duration of ovum transport in the baboon (*Papio anubis*). Obstet Gynecol 47: 658

Eddy C A, Antonini R, Pauerstein C J 1977 Fertility following microsurgical removal of the ampullary-isthmic junction in rabbit. Fertil Steril 28: 1090

Egli G E, Newton M 1961 The transport of carbon particles in the human female reproductive tract. Fertil Steril 12: 151

Einsten A 1905 Uber die von der molekularkinetichen Theorie der warme geforderte bewegung von ruhenden flussingkeiten suspendierten teilchen. Ann Physik 17: 549

Einstein A 1908 Elementare theorie der brownshen bewegund. Z Elektrochem 14: 235

El-Badawi A, Schenk E A 1968 The peripheral adrenergic innervation apparatus: I. Intraganglionic and extraganglionic adrenergic ganglion cells. Z Zellforsch Abt Histochem 87: 218

Erdö S L, László A, Szporny L, Zsolnai B 1983 High density of specific GABA binding sites in human Fallopian tube. Neurosci Lett 42: 155

Estes W L Jr, Heitmeyer P L 1934 Pregnancy following ovarian implantation. Am J Surg 24: 563

Evans E I 1933 The transport of spermatozoa in the dog. Am J Physiol 105: 287

Falck B, Hillard N A, Thieme G, Torp A 1962 Fluorescence of catecholamines and related compounds condensed with formaldehyde. J Histochem Cytochem 10: 348

Fallopius G 1561 Observaciones anatomicae. Venice Ferin Thomas K, Johansson E D B 1973 Ovulation detection. In: Hafez E S E, Evans E I (eds) Human reproduction: conception and contraception. Harper and Row, New York, p 260

Ferin J, Thomas K, Johanisson E D B 1973 Ovulation detection. In: Hafez E S E, Evans T N (eds) Human reproduction—conception and contraception. Harper and Row, Maryland p 260

Flickinger D M, Muechler E K, Mikhail G 1974 Estradiol receptors in the human fallopian tube. Fertil Steril 25: 900

Forcelledo M L, Vera R, Croxatto H B 1981 Ovum transport in pregnant, pseudopregnant, and cyclic rats and its relationship to estradiol and progesterone blood levels. Biol Reprod 24: 760

Foulconer R J 1951 Observations on the Mullerian grove in human embryos. Contrib Embryol 34: 159

Fredericks C M, Lundquist L E, Mathur R S, Ashton S H, Landgrebe S C 1983 Effect of VIP upon ovarian steroids, ovum tansport and fertility in the rabbit. Biol Reprod 28: 1052

Fredericsson B 1959 Histochemical observations on the epithelium of human fallopian tubes. Acta Obstet Dynecol Scand 58: 109

Frenko B 1954 Die epithelien des eileiters und ihre hormonalen reaktionen. Z Mikrosk/Anat Forsch 61: 99

Gaddum-Rosse P, Blandau R J 1976 Comparative observations on ciliary currents in mammalian oviducts. Biol Reprod 14: 605

Gaddum-Rosse P, Rumery R E, Blandau R J, Thiersch J B 1975 Studies on the mucosa of postmenopausal oviducts: surface appearance, ciliary activity and the effect of estrogen treatment. Fertil Steril 26: 951

Gatsalov M D 1963 The intraorganic venous bed of the human fallopian tube. Arkh Anat 2: 87

Gimeno M F, Borda E S, Sterin-Borda L, Sterin-Speziale N, Gimeno A L 1976 Contractile activity of the oviduct and the mesosalpinx isolated from guinea pigs in different phases of the sex cycle. Effect of several pharmacological influences. Int J Fertil 21: 31

Gimeno A L, Sterin-Speziale N, Landa A, Zapata C, Gimeno M F 1979 Spontaneous motility of isolated mesosalpinx-free isthmic and ampullar segments from human oviducts, and the influence of indomethacin and prostacyclin(PC). Int J Fertil 24: 281

Glenister T W, Hamilton W J 1963 The embryology of sexual differentiation in relation to the possible effects of administering steroid hormones during pregnancy. J Obstet Gynecol Br Common W 70: 13

Greenwald G S 1961 A study of the transport of ova through the rabbit oviduct. Fertil Steril 12: 80

Greenwald G S 1967 Species differences in egg transport in response to exogenous estrogen. Anat Rec 157: 163

Gruenwald P 1941 The relation of the growing Mullerian

duct to the Wolffian duct and its importance for the genesis of malformations. Anat Rec 81: 1

Günther B, Leon de la Barra B 1966 Physiometry of the mammalian circulatory system. Acts Physiol Lat 16: 32

Halbert S A, Tam P Y, Blandau R J 1976 Egg transport in the rabbit oviduct: the roles of cilia and muscle. Science 191: 1052

Halbert S A, Verdugo P, Boling J L, Blandau R J 1977 In vivo studies of contraction wave propagation and its role in sperm and egg transport in the oviductal isthmus of rabbits. Biophys J 17: 266C

Harper M J K 1966 Hormonal control of transport of eggs in cumulus through the ampulla of the rabbit oviduct. Endocrinology 78: 568

Harper M J K 1968 Interference with early pregnancy in rats by estrogen. Mechanism of action of dienestrol. Anat Rec 162: 433

Harper M J K 1973a Relationship between sperm transport and penetration of eggs in the rabbit oviduct. Biol Reprod 8: 441

Harper M J K 1973b Stimulation of sperm movement from the isthmus to the site of fertilization in the rabbit oviduct. Biol Reprod 8: 369

Harper M J K 1988 Gamete and zigote transport. In: Knobil E, Neil J (eds) The physiology of reproduction. Raven Press, New York, p 103

Helm G, Håkanson R, Leander S, Owman C, Sjöberg N O, Sporrong B 1982a Neurogenic relaxation mediated by VIP in the isthmus of the human Fallopian tube. Regul Pept 3: 145

Helm G, Owman C, Sjöberg N O, Walles B 1982b Motor activity of the human fallopian tube in vitro in relation to plasma concentration of estradiol and progesterone and the influence of noradrenaline. J Reprod Fertil 64: 233

Hertig A T, Rock J, Adams E C 1956 A description of 34 ova within the first 17 days of development. Am J Anat 98: 435

Hermstein A, Neustadt B 1924 Intramural portion of the Fallopian tube. Z Geburtshilfe Gynaekol 88: 43

Higgs C, Moawad A H 1974 The effect of ovarian hormones on the contractility of the rabbit oviductal isthmus. Can J Physiol Pharmacol 52: 74

Hilliard J, Eaton L W 1971 Estradiol-l 7b, progesterone and 20α-hydroxypregn-4-en-3-one in rabbit ovarian venous plasma. II. From mating through implantation. Endocrinology 89: 522

Hodgson B J 1976 Effect of indomethasin and ICI 46474 administered during ovum transport on fertility in rabbits. Biol Reprod 14: 451

Hodgson B J, Eddy C A 1975 The autonomic nervous system and its relationship to ovum transport: a reappraisal. Gynecol Invest 6: 162

Hodgson B J, Pauerstein C J 1974 The effect of ovulation on the response of rabbit oviduct to adrenergic agonists in vitro. Biol Reprod 10: 346

Hodgson B J, Talo A 1978 Spike burst in the rabbit oviduct. II. Effect of estrogen and progesterone. Am J Physiol 234: E439

Hodgson B J, Sullivan K, Pauerstein C J 1973 The role of sympathetic nerves in the response of oviduct and uterus to field stimulation. Eur J Pharmacol 23: 107

Hodgson B J, Talo A, Pauerstein C J 1977 Oviductal ovum surrogate movement interrelation with muscular activity. Biol Reprod 16: 394

Howe G R 1967 Leucocyte response to spermatozoa in ligated segments of the rabbit vagina, uterus and oviduct. J Reprod Fertil 13: 563

Huang W M, Gu J, Blank M A, Allen J M, Bloom S R, Polak J M 1984 Peptide-immunoreactive nerves in the mammalian female genital tact. Histochem J 16: 1297

Humphrey K W 1968 The effect of oestradiol-3, 17 beta on tubal transport in the laboratory mouse. J Endocrinol 42: 17

Hunter R H 1930 Observations on the development of the human genital tract. Contrib Embryol 22: 91

Hunter R H F 1975 Physiological aspects of sperm transport in the domestic pig, Sus scrofa. II. Regulation, survival, and fate of cells. Br Vet J 131: 681

Hunter R H F, Wilmut I 1983 The rate of functional sperm transport into the oviducts of mated cows. Anim Reprod Sci 5: 167

Hunter R H F, Barwise L, King R 1982 Sperm transport, storage and release in the sheep oviduct in relation to the time of ovulation. Br Vet J 138: 225

Insler V, Bernstein D, Glezerman M, Misgav N 1979 Correlation of seminal fluid analysis with mucus penetrating ability of spermatozoa. Fertil Steril 32: 316

Insler V, Glezerman M Zeidel L, Bernstein D, Misgav N 1980 Sperm storage in the human cervix: a quantitative study. Fertil Steril 33: 288

Joachimovits R 1935 Studien zur menstruation, ovulation, aufbau und pathologie des weiblichen genitales bei mensch und affe, eileter und over. Biol Generalis 11: 281

Kamm K E, Stull J T 1989 Regulation of smooth muscle contractile elements by second messengers. Annu Rev Physiol 51: 299

Kendle K E, Telford J M 1970 Investigations into the mechanism of anti-fertility action of minimal doses of megestrol acetate in rabbits. Br J Pharmacol Chemother 40: 759

Kennedy D R, Marshall J M 1977 Effects of adrenergic nerve stimulation on the rabbit oviduct: correlation with norepinephrine content and turnover rate. Biol Reprod 16: 200

Korenaga M, Kadoka T 1981 Changes in mechanical properties of the circular muscle of the isthmus of the human fallopian tube in relation to hormonal domination and postovulatory time. Fertil Steril 36: 343

Lambert R, Teissier G 1927 Theorie de la similitude biologique. Ann Physiol Physico-chim 3: 212

Lee W I, Verdugo P 1976 Laser light scattering spectroscopy: a new application in the study of ciliary activity. Biophys J 16: 1115

Levy B, Lindner H R 1972 The effects of adrenergic drugs on the rabbit oviduct. Eur J Pharmacol 18: 15

Lim R K S, Chao C 1927 On the mechanism of the tube transportation of ova. Chin J Physiol 1: 175

Maia H S, Coutinho E M 1970 Peristalsis and antiperistalsis of the human Fallopian tube during the menstrual cycle. Biol Reprod 2: 305

Maia H J R, Salinas L A, Fernandez E, Pauerstein G J 1977 Time course of ovum transport in the guinea pig. 28: 863

Marshall J M 1981 Effects of ovarian steriods and pregnancy on adrenergic nerves of uterus and oviduct. Am J Physiol 240: C165

Martin del Rio 1981 γ-Aminobutyric acid system in rat oviduct. J Biol Chem 256: 1174

Mattner P E 1963 Spermatozoa in the genital tract of the ewe. II. Distribution after coitus. Aust J Biol Sci 16: 688

Mattner P E, Braden A W 1963 Spermatozoa in the genital

tract of the ewe: I. Rapidity of transport. Aust J Biol Sci 16: 473

McComb P, Gomel V 1979 The influence of fallopian tube length on fertility in the rabbit. Fertil Steril 31: 673

McComb P, Boer-Meisel M, Gomel V 1981 The influence of fallopian tube ampullary length on the fertility of the rabbit. Int J Fertil 26: 30

Metz K G P, Mastroianni L Jr 1979 Dispensability of fimbriae: ovum pick-up by tubal fistulas in rabbit. Fertil Steril 32: 329

Mishell D R, Nakamura R M, Crosignani P G, Stone S, Kharma K, Nagata V, Thorneycroft I H 1971 Serum gonadotropin and steroid patterns during normal menstrual cycle. Am J Obstet Gynecol 111: 60

Mitchell G A G 1938 The innervation of the ovary, uterine tube, testis and epididymis. J Anat 72: 508

Moawad A H, Hedqvist P, Kim M H 1976 Correlation of plasma estrogen and progesterone levels with in vitro adrenergic responses in the isthmus of the human oviduct. In: Harper M J K, Pauerstein C J, Adams C E, Coutinho E M, Croxatto H B, Paton D M (eds) Ovum transport and fertility regulation. Scriptor, Copenhagen, p 276

Nakanishi H, Wood C L 1968 Effects of adrenergic blocking agents on human fallopian tube motility in vitro. J Reprod Fertil 16: 21

Newton I 1735 Philosophiae naturalis principia mathematica. Lib Sec, Sec VII, Propositio 32: 294

Noyes R W, Clewe T H, Bonney W A, Burrus S B, DeFeo V J, Morgenstern L L 1966 Searches for ova in the human uterus and tubes. I. Review, clinical methodology and summary of findings. Am J Obstet Gynecol 96: 157

Nozaki M, Ito Y 1987 Changes in physiological properties of rabbit oviduct by ovarian steroids. Am J Physiol 252: R1059

Overstreet J W, Cooper G W 1978 Sperm transport in the reproductive tract of the rabbit. I. Rapid transit phase of transport. II. The sustained phase of transport. Biol Reprod 19: 101

Owman C, Sjöstrand N O 1967 Difference in rate of depletion and recovery of noradrenaline in 'short' and long sympathetic nerves after reserpine treatment. Life Sci 6: 2549

Owman C, Rosengren E, Sjöberg N O 1967 Adrenergic innervation of the human female reproductive organs: a histochemical and chemical investigation. Obstet Gynecol 30: 763

Owman C, Sjöberg N O, Sjöstrand O 1974 Short adrenergic neurons a peripheral neuroendocrine mechanism. In: Fujiwara M, Tanaka C (eds) Amine fluorescence histochemistry. Igaku-Shoin, Tokyo p 47

Owman C, Falk B, Johansson E D B et al 1976 Autonomic nerves and related amine receptors mediating motor activity in the oviduct of monkey and man: a histochemical, chemical and pharmacological study. In: Harper M J K, Pauerstein C J, Adams C E, Coutinho E M, Croxatto H B, Paton D M (eds) Ovum transport and fertility regulation. Scriptor, Copenhagen, p 256

Pauerstein C J, Fremming B D, Matin J E 1970a Influence of progesterone and alpha-adrenergic blockade upon tubal transport of ova. Gynecol Invest 1: 257

Pauerstein C J, Fremming B D, Martin J E 1970b Estrogen induced tubal arrest of ovum: antagonism by alpha-adrenergic blockade. Obstet Gynecol 35: 671

Pauerstein C J, Anderson V, Chatkoff M L, Hodgson B J

1974a Effect of estrogen and progesterone on the time course of tubal ovum transport in rabbits. Am J Obstet Gynecol 120: 299

Pauerstein C J, Hodgson B J, Fremming B D, Martin J E 1974b Effects of sympathetic denervation of the rabbit oviduct on normal ovum transport and on transport modified by estrogen and progesterone. Gynecol Invest 5: 121

Pauerstein C J, Sabry A, Hodgson B J 1976 Temporal relationships critical to estrogen-induced delay of ovum transport. Fertil Steril 27: 1308

Pauerstein C J, Eddy C A, Croxatto H D, Hess R, Siler-Khodr T M, Croxatto H B 1978 Temporal relationships of estrogen, progesterone, and luteinizing hormone levels to ovulation in women and infrahuman primates. Am J Obstet Gynecol 130: 876

Perloff W H, Steinberger E 1964 In vivo survival of spermatozoa in cervical mucus. Am J Obstet Gynecol 88: 439

Peters H, McNatty K P 1980 The ovary: a correlation between structure and function. University of California Press, Berkeley

Pino A M, Devoto L, Soto E, Castro O, Sierralta W 1982 Changes in the cytosolic and nuclear estradiol receptors of normal Fallopian tube throughout the menstrual cycle. J Steroid Biochem 16: 193

Polidoro J D, Howe G R, Black D L 1974 The effects of adrenergic drugs on ovum transport through the rabbit oviduct. J Reprod Fertil 35: 331

Pollow K, Inthraphuvasak J, Manz B, Grill H J, Pollow B 1981 A comparison of cytoplasmic and nuclear estradiol and progesterone receptors in human fallopian tube and endometrial tissue. Fertil Steril 36: 615

Portnow J, Talo A, Hodgson B J 1977 A random wall model of ovum transport. Bulletin of Mathematical Biology 39: 349

Price D 1947 An analysis of the factors influencing growth and development of the mammalian reproductive tract. Physiol Zool 20: 213

Price D, Ortiz E 1965 The role of fetal androgen in sex differentiation in mammals. In: DeHann R L, Ursprung H (eds) Organogenesis. Holt, Rinehart and Winston, New York, p 229

Proser C L 1974 Smooth muscle. Ann Rev Physiol 36: 503

Punnonen R, Lukola A 1981 Binding of estrogen and progestin in the human Fallopian tube. Fertil Steril 36: 610

Reiffenstuhl G 1964 The lymphatics of the female genital organs. Lippincott, Philadelphia

Richardson K C 1935 The secretory phenomena in the oviduct of the fowl, including the process of shell formation examined by the microin-cineration technique. Philos Trans R Soc Lond [Biol] 225: 149

Riehl R M, Harper M J K 1981 Preparation of smooth muscle cell suspensions from the rabbit oviduct and prostaglandin binding analysis. Endocrinology 109: 1011

Robertson D M, Landgren B M, Guerrero R 1975 Oestradiol receptor levels in the human fallopian tube during the menstrual cycle. Acta Endocrinol (Copenh) 80: 705

Rock J, Hertig A T 1944 Information regarding the time of human ovulation derived from a study of 3 unfertilized and 11 fertilized ova. Am J Obstet Gynecol 47: 343

Rocker I 1964 The anatomy of the utero-tubal junction area. Proc Soc Med 57: 707

Rubinstein B B, Strauss H, Lazarus M L, Hankin H 1951

Sperm survival in women: motile sperm in the fundus and tubes of surgical cases. Fertil Steril 2: 15

Rumery R E, Eddy E M 1974 Scanning electron microscopy of the limbriae and ampullae of the rabbit oviduct. Anat Rec 178: 83

Rumery R E, Phinney E, Blandau R J 1971 Culture of mammalian embryonic ovaries and oviducts. In: Daniel Jr (ed) Methods in mammalian embryology. Freeman, New York, p 472

Sampson J A 1937 The lymphatics of the mucosa of the fimbriae of the fallopian tube. Am J Obstet Gynecol 33: 91

Settlage D S F, Motoshima Tredway D R 1973 Sperm transport from the external cervical os to the fallopian tubes in women: a time and quantitation. Fertil Steril. 24: 655

Silber S J, Cohen R 1980 Microsurgical reversal of female sterilization: the role of tubal length. Fertil Steril 33: 598

Sjöberg N O 1967 The adrenergic transmitter of the female reproductive tract: distribution and functional changes. Acta Physiol Scand (Suppl) 305: 5

Somlyo A P, Somlyo A V 1990 Flash photolysis studies of excitation-contraction coupling, regulation, and contraction in smooth muscle. Ann Rev Physiol 52: 857

Spilman C H 1976 Prostaglandins, oviductal motility and egg transport. In: Harper M J K, Pauerstein C J, Adams C E, Coutinho E M, Croxatto H B, Paton D M (eds) Ovum transport and fertility regulation. Scriptor, Copenhagen, p 197

Spilman C H, Harper M J K 1974 Comparison of the effects of adrenergic drugs and prostaglandins on the rabbit oviduct motility. Biol Reprod 10: 549

Spilman C H, Harper M J K 1975 Effects of prostaglandins on oviductal motility and egg transport. Gynecol Invest 6: 186

Stange H H 1952a Functional morphology of the fimbriate end of the human oviduct and the epoophoron. Arch Gynaekol 182: 77

Stange H H 1952b Comparative morphologic studies on human fallopian tube in extreme functional states: question of existence of infundibular sphincter. Zentralse Gynakol 74: 1176

Stegner H E 1961 Das epithel der tuba uterina des neugeborenen. Elektronen mikroskopishe befunde. Z Zellforsch 55: 247

Stjernqvist M, Emson P, Owman C, Sjöberg N O, Sundler F, Tatemoto K 1983 Neuropeptide Y in the female reproductive tract of the rat. Distribution of nerve fibers and motor effects. Neurosci Lett 39: 279

Strauss F 1964 Neibliche Geschlechtsorgane (l). In: Helmcke J G, vonLengerken H, Starck D, Wermuth H (eds) Handbuch der Zoologie. Water de Gruyter, Berlin p l

Sullivan S F, Marshall J M 1970 Quantitative evaluation of effects of exogenous amines on contractility of human myometrium. Am J Obstet Gynecol 107: 139

Sweeney W J 1962 The interstitial portion of the uterine tube. Its gross anatomy course and length. Obstet Gynecol 19: 3

Talo A 1975 Amplitude variation of the pressure cycles in and between segments of the rabbit oviduct in vitro. Biol Reprod 13: 249

Talo A 1991 How the myosalpinx works in gamete and embryo transport. Arch Med Biol Exp 24: 361

Talo A, Hodgson B J 1978 Spike burst in the rabbit oviduct: I. Effect of ovulation. Am J Physiol 234: E430

Talo A, Pulkkinen M O 1982 Electrical activity in the human oviduct during the menstrual cycle. Am J Obstet Gynecol 142: 135

Tam P Y, Verdugo P, Blandau R J 1975 A quantitative approach to evaluating egg transport in the oviduct. Proc ACEMB E3: 320

Thorbert G B, Alm P, Rosengren T 1978 Cyclic- and steroid-induced changes in adrenergic neurotransmitter level of guinea pig uterus. Acta Obstet Gynecol Scand 57: 45

Triggle D L 1972 Adrenergic receptors. Ann Rev Pharmacol 12: 185

Trounson A E, Mohr L H, Wood C, Leeton J F 1982 Effect of delayed insemination on in vitro fertilization, culture and transfer of human embryos. J Reprod Fertil 64: 285

Valenzuela G, Ross H D, Harper M J K, Pauerstein C J 1977 Effect of inhibitors of prostaglandin synthesis and metabolism on ovum transport in the rabbit. Fertil Steril 28: 992

VanDermark N L, Moeller A N 1951 Speed of spermatozoa transport in reproductive tract of estrous cow. Am J Physiol 165: 674

Vastik-Fernandez, Gimeno M F, Lima F, Gimeno A L 1975 Spontaneous motility and distribution of prostaglandins in different segments of human fallopian tubes. Am J Obstet Gynecol 122: 663

Verdugo P 1980 $Ca^{2+}$-dependent hormonal stimulation of ciliary activity. Nature (Lond) 283: 764

Verdugo P 1982 Stochastic analysis of ovum transport: the effect of prostaglandin $E_2$. Cell Motility (Suppl) 1: 85

Verdugo P 1985 Functional anatomy of the Fallopian tube (1986). In: Insler V, Lunenfeld B (eds) Infertility: male and female. Churchill Livingstone, London, p 26

Verdugo P, Golborne C 1988 Remote detection of ciliary movement by fiber optic laser-Doppler spectroscopy. IEEE Trans Biomed Eng 35: 303

Verdugo P, Blandau R J, Tam P Y, Halbert S S 1976 Stochastic elements in the development of deterministic models of egg transport. In: Harper M J K, Pauerstein C J, Adams C E, Coutinho E M, Croxatto H B, Paton D M (eds) Ovum transport and fertility regulation. Scriptor, Copenhagen, p 126

Verdugo P, Lee W I, Halbert S A, Blandau R J, Tam P Y 1980a A stochastic model for oviductal egg transport. Biophys J 29: 257

Verdugo P, Rumery R, Tam P Y 1980b Hormonal control of oviductal ciliary activity: effect of prostaglandins. Fertil Steril 33: 193

Verhage H G, Akbar M, Jaffe R C 1980 Cyclic changes in cytosol progesterone receptor of human Fallopian tube. J Clin Endocrinol Metab 51: 776

Villalón M, Verdugo P 1982 Hormonal regulation of ciliary function in the oviduct: the effect of beta-adrenergic agonists. Cell Motility (Suppl) 1: 59

Villalón M, Verdugo P 1990 Stimulus-response coupling in mammalian ciliated cells: the role of $Ca^{2+}$ in prostaglandins stimulation. In: Vergara J, Jaimovich E, Bacigalupo J, Hidalgo C (eds) Transduction in biological systems. Pergamon Press, New York, p 221

Villalón M, Hinds T R, Verdugo P 1989 Stimulus-response coupling in mammalian ciliated cells: demonstration of two mechanisms of control for cytosolic $Ca^{2+}$. Biophys J 56: 1255

Villalón M, Verdugo P, Boling J L, Blandau R J 1991 The transport of cumulus egg masses through the ampullea of the oviducts in the pig-tailed, *Macaca* nemestrina. Arch Med Biol Exp 24: 351

Watanabe A 1963 Studies on the vascular system of human fallopian tube. J Jap Obstet Gynecol Soc (Abstr) 10: 199

Warren M R 1938 Observations on the uterine fluid of the rat. Am J Physiol 122: 602

Westman A E 1930 Studies of the function of the mucous membrane of the uterine tube. Acta Obstet Gynecol Scand 10: 288

Westrom K, Mardh P A, Mecklenburg C V, Hakansson C H 1977 Studies on ciliated epithelia of the human genital tract. II. The mucociliary wave pattern of fallopian tube epithelium. Fertil Steril 28: 955

Winston R M L 1980 Microsurgery of the Fallopian tube: from fantasy to reality. Fertil Steril 34: 521

Woodruff J D, Pauerstein C J (eds) 1969 The fallopian tube: anatomy. Williams and Wilkins, Baltimore, p. 22

# 5. The endocrine pattern and control of the ovulatory cycle

*K. J. Ryan*

## BRAIN–HYPOTHALAMUS–PITUITARY–OVARIAN INTERRELATIONSHIPS

### Introduction

The ovulatory cycle upon which fertility depends is regulated by an elaborate neuroendocrine system involving the brain (of which the hypothalamus is a subunit), adenohypophysis and ovaries. Internal and external environmental cues (light, smell, temperature, metabolic alterations, emotion) received by sensory input to the central nervous system (CNS) are relayed by synaptic transmission to hypothalamic neurons which process and transform the neural input into a neurosecretory endocrine outflow that regulates the pituitary production of gonadotropins and prolactin (Reichlin 1981). The pituitary endocrine products in turn regulate ovarian steroidogenesis and ovulation. The Scharrers have termed this overall process 'a neuroendocrine reflex', since a closed loop is formed by the released hormones which have feedback actions on the brain, hypothalamus and pituitary (Scharrer & Scharrer 1962).

Diagnosis and treatment of specific abnormalities of the infertile female depend to a large extent upon an understanding of the structural and functional components of this neuroendocrine reflex. The interrelationships of the ovarian cycle can best be presented in terms of a *primary neuroendocrine complex* that can operate autonomously in isolation, and a *secondary neuroendocrine control system* that is largely regulatory in nature (Fig. 5.1).

The primary neuroendocrine complex consists of: the medial basal hypothalamus, the adenohypophysis (pars distalis or anterior pituitary) and

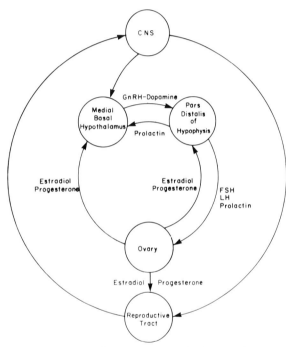

**Fig. 5.1** Diagram of primary neuroendocrine complex composed of medial basal hypothalamus, pars distalis of hypophysis and ovary (inner circle) and secondary neuroendocrine control system composed of higher CNS centers and reproductive tract (outer circle).

the ovary which, functioning as an interacting system, can drive the cyclic ovarian function necessary for fertility (Szentagothai et al 1968, Knobil 1980). Except for basic metabolic requirements, this system functions autonomously in the primate in the absence of the reproductive tract and even when separated from other CNS centers (Knobil 1980). In other mammals reproductive tract factors (luteolysins) and preoptic CNS neurons are important for cyclicity and timing.

On the other hand, the primary neuroendocrine complex in the primate cannot function normally in the absence of either the medial basal hypothalamus, adenohypophysis or ovary. Cyclic function and coordination of the three components is achieved by the absolute dependence of the endocrine activity of the adenohypophysis upon hypothalamic gonadotropin releasing hormone (GnRH), dependence of the ovary upon pituitary gonadotropins, and dependence of the adenohypophysis upon ovarian steroid 'feedback' actions. Cyclicity and synchrony are achieved by this interdependence. As the ovarian follicle grows and secretes increasing amounts of estradiol in response to pituitary gonadotropins, the rise in estradiol 'triggers' a cyclic surge release of luteinizing hormone (LH) from the pituitary at just the right time to cause ovulation of an appropriately matured egg in a follicle which is ready to rupture (Knobil 1980, DiZerega et al 1981). The cycle is ended when the resulting corpus luteum completes its finite life span as determined by 'luteolytic' mechanisms in the ovary (Behrman et al 1979) and a feedback induced drop in pituitary gonadotropins.

The *secondary neuroendocrine control system* of the ovulatory cycle is regulatory in nature and can modulate the primary system and turn it off or on by appropriate inputs from the CNS to the medial basal hypothalamus (Szentagothai et al 1968). This is achieved by inducing changes in the amount and periodicity of GnRH secretion upon which the adenohypophysis depends (Knobil 1980). Environmental changes such as light, the amount of water and food, sounds, odors and temperature all influence reproduction via this regulatory system. Seasonal breeding of animals and reproductive behavior which depends upon visual and olfactory cues operate under these mechanisms (Van Tienhoven 1968). Emotional effects on the human cycle in conditions such as pseudocyesis, anorexia nervosa and 'hypothalamic amenorrhea' are additional examples of the potential of this regulatory system (Marshall & Kelch 1979). Maturation of the primary neuroendocrine complex at the time of puberty probably involves release of the hypothalamus from inhibitory inputs from higher centers in the CNS (Knobil 1980).

While the secondary neuroendocrine control system is permissive and regulatory and not an essential factor in the ovarian cycle, its inappropriate function is probably the basis for infertility in most cases associated with anovulation and amenorrhea.

## Anatomy and reproductive function of the endocrine hypothalamus

The hypothalamus is a phylogenetically ancient part of the CNS that is involved by reciprocal connections with other parts of the nervous system in the vegetative functions of the autonomic nervous system, primitive behavior, emotion, water and electrolyte control via the neurohypophysis as well as the regulation of all adenohypophyseal endocrine secretion. The reproductive role of the hypothalamus is thus one subset of its overall complex role as an integrative way station for many bodily processes. It is in a unique position to link and influence reproductive cycles with behavioral, environmental and metabolic changes (Knigge & Silverman 1974).

The hypothalamus is derived embryologically from the floor of the diencephalon and in the adult extends from just rostral to the optic chiasm to a plane caudal to the mammillary bodies. It is bisected by the third ventricle and joins the thalamus superiorly at a lateral sulcus in the wall of the third ventricle. Parts of the lateral margins of the hypothalamus are formed by the optic tracts and its base is the floor of the third ventricle. The inferior portion of the hypothalamus (tuber cinereum or infundibulum) forms a stalk that continues into an infundibular process (posterior pituitary or neurohypophysis). The infundibulum is invaginated by a recess of the third ventricle and comes in apposition to the adenohypophysis at the median eminence of the hypothalamus which contains a confluence of neurosecretory axon terminals and the vessels of the hypophyseal portal system (Knigge & Silverman 1974; (Fig. 5.2).

The neurosecretory endocrine function of the hypothalamus was first established for the *magnocellular* neurons which produce oxytocin and vasopressin. This system is composed of the supraoptic and paraventricular nuclei, which

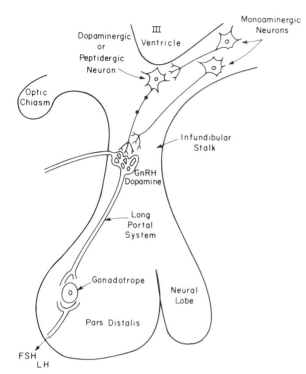

**Fig. 5.2**  Relationships of hypothalamic neurons to adenohypophysis and hypophyseal portal vascular system.

contain large, well-characterized cell bodies with axons that extend down the infundibulum stalk to terminate largely in the neurohypophysis. Oxytocin and vasopressin are packaged in a carrier protein, *neurophysin*, which makes the system visible under the microscope and helped in the establishment of the concept of axon transport of peptides and neurosecretion. This neurosecretion is largely into the peripheral circulation Knigge & Silverman 1974, Reichlin 1981).

The nerve cells concerned with reproductive neurosecretion controlling the ovary are part of the *parvicellular* system, smaller, less well-characterized (than the magnocellular system) neurons that terminate in the median eminence and secrete, among other hypophysiotropic and inhibiting substances, dopamine and GnRH for transport to the adenohypophysis.

GnRH and dopamine production occurs in the arcuate and periventricular nuclei (Fuxe & Hökfelt 1969, Ajika 1980, Palkovits 1982). The medial basal hypothalamus, containing these nuclei and the median eminence, is in apposition to the anterior pituitary, and when this area of the

hypothalamus is physically severed from the rest of the CNS caudal to the optic chiasm and anterior to the mammillary bodies, it can still maintain cyclic ovarian function. (GnRH is also synthesized in the preoptic area, which is necessary for cyclicity in the rat but not in primates.) Destruction of the arcuate nucleus of the medial basal hypothalamus obliterates pituitary release of gonadotropins, but its function can be replaced by infusion of GnRH, which is now presumed to be secreted from this nucleus (Knobil 1980). Hypothalamic amenorrhea can also be treated with pulsatile GnRH in the human (Crowley & McArthur 1980).

In the medial basal hypothalamus of the rhesus monkey, in or near the arcuate nucleus, Knobil has identified rhythmic, pulsed electrical activity that is synchronous with the pulsed release of LH (luteinizing hormone). The pulsatile pattern of LH is in turn used as an indirect measure of the pulse frequency of GnRH secretion. The area of the hypothalamus responsible for this electrical activity is the putative pulse generator that times the pulsed release of GnRH (Knobil 1989). The frequency of this electrical activity can be shown to vary during the cycle and to be influenced by estrogens and opiates. The isolated perifused medial basal hypothalamus from fetal or adult human sources also releases GnRH in a pulsed manner (Yen 1991).

There are extensive two-way neural connections between the endocrine hypothalamus and the CNS via the medial forebrain bundle from the limbic and mesencephalic-reticular circuits (Knigge & Silverman 1974, Reichlin 1981). These course through the lateral margins of the hypothalamus and provide connections to the medial hypothalamic nuclei. There are also direct connections to the medial hypothalamus, such as that of the stria terminalis from the amygdala and the medial corticohypothalamic tract.

The medial basal hypothalamus can be experimentally converted into an 'isolated hypothalamic island' by severance from these neural connections, which defines the minimal portion of the CNS needed to serve cyclic reproductive function in the primate (Szentagothai et al. 1968, Knobil 1980). The special features of this island include the dopaminergic and GnRH secreting neurons with their tuberoinfundibular tracts terminating in the median eminence of the hypothalamus. Capillary loops of the hypophyseal portal system allow vascular communication with the pituitary. In addition, specialized ependymal cells of the floor of the third ventricle extend to the perivascular space of this capillary system. There is thus access to this area of the brain by the cerebrospinal fluid as well as by the peripheral vascular system.

The essential role of the hypothalamus for pituitary function was originally established by interruption of the hypophyseal portal vascular connection by stalk section or by pituitary transplantation away from the hypothalamus. Under these circumstances the pituitary secretes prolactin, which is under chronic inhibition from hypothalamic dopamine. These studies prompted the search for the neurohormones of the hypothalamus, ending in the discovery of the hypothalamic releasing factors for thyroid stimulating hormone and gonadotropins.

GnRH, or luteinizing hormone releasing hormone (LH-RH), is a decapeptide that has been sequenced for amino acid composition and has also been synthesized (Burgus et al 1971, Matsuo et al 1971). This is the major chemical (endocrine) link between the hypothalamus and the pituitary. Administered in vivo or in vitro it can specifically cause synthesis and release of both pituitary LH and follicle stimulating hormone (FSH). Although still considered a possibility, the existence of a separate FSH releasing hormone has not been established.

## Anatomy and reproductive function of the pituitary

The anterior pituitary (adenohypophysis, pars distalis) is derived embryologically from Rathke's pouch, an out-pouching from the oral cavity. The posterior pituitary (infundibular bulb, neurohypophysis) is derived from a continuous extension of magnocellular neuronal axons that course through and make up a large part of the infundibular stem and terminate in the infundibular bulb.

The two separately derived components (Rathke's pouch and infundibular bulb) fuse together to form the *pituitary gland*, which joins the hypothalamus superiorly around the infundibular stem at a region of the ventral hypothalamus designated the *median eminence*. Some anterior pituitary cells form a collar around the infundibular stalk and are designated the *pars tuberalis*.

The adult pituitary occupies a cavity in the sphenoid bone, the *sella turcica*, which is separated from the cranial cavity by a reflection of the dura designated the *diaphragmatic sela*, through which the stalk and hypophyseal portal vessels penetrate.

The adult pituitary is 10 mm × 13 mm × 6 mm, weighs 0.5 g, of which three-quarters is the *pars distalis* (Daughaday 1981).

The pituitary contains many cell types which have been characterized by histochemical or immunological staining procedures. Specific cell types have been assigned production of growth hormone, prolactin, thyrotropin, corticotrophin and FSH and LH (Baker 1974).

The prolactin-secreting cells (lactotropes) stain red with erythrosin or carmosin, are shown to contain prolactin by cytoimmunological localization, and are distributed in the wings of the pars distalis. These cells increase in activity and mitoses in response to estrogens and pregnancy. Estrogen restricts access of dopamine to prolactin granules in the lactotropes (Gudelsky et al 1981).

The gonadotropes produce both FSH and LH (probably in a single cell), as evidenced by immunoperoxidase stains, and are located diffusely throughout the adenohypophysis.

FSH is a glycoprotein compound of two amino acid chains α and β that contain 18% carbohydrate and 5% sialic acid. The molecular weight is around 32 000.

LH is also a glycoprotein composed of two amino acid chains (α and β) of roughly the same size as FSH and with a similar molecular weight. The carbohydrate content of LH is 16% with 1% sialic acid.

The α chains of FSH and LH are identical while the β chains differ and thereby confer the immunological and biological specificity for the two hormones. The serum half-life of FSH is longer than that of LH, reflecting its higher sialic acid content, removal of which speeds metabolism by the liver (Daughaday 1981).

Prolactin is a protein of 199 amino acids,

containing no carbohydrate, with a molecular weight of 22 000, sharing many amino acid sequences with growth hormone and placental lactogen. The shared amino acid sequences have made identification and separation of human prolactin from growth hormone difficult.

FSH and LH are synthesized and secreted in response to GnRH with an important modulating effect of estrogens on the pituitary cells. Estrogen influences the number of GnRH receptors on the gonadotropes, which increases after castration (Marshall et al 1980). Prolactin release is stimulated by thyroid releasing hormone (TRH) and possibly by other releasing substances (serotoninergic), but its major control is by tonic inhibition from hypothalamic dopamine (Fang & Shian 1981, Krulich et al 1981).

*Hypophyseal portal system*

The unique feature of the hypothalamic/pituitary relationship is the privileged access of the pituitary to blood draining directly from the median eminence of the hypothalamus, which brings neurosecretory inhibiting and releasing hormones directly to the cells of the pituitary which respond to them. In addition, pituitary hormones (endorphins, gonadotropins, prolactin) can have limited access to the hypothalamus by flow in the opposite direction (a short feedback loop) (Motta et al 1969). The pituitary relies on the hypophyseal portal system for its major blood supply and if the vessels are severed necrosis of the pituitary occurs.

Arterial blood follows a path from the internal carotid to the superior hypophyseal arteries that enter the anterior median eminence, forming capillary loops and then a linear array of venous portal (long portal system) vessels lying parallel to the pituitary stalk (pars tuberalis and infundibular stem) and penetrating the diaphragma sela to distribute blood to the pars distalis (Porter et al 1974).

The trabecular and inferior hypophyseal arteries contribute to vessels that enter the posterior median eminence and form a short venous portal system from the distal infundibular stem to the pituitary.

The capillary loops of the hypophyseal portal system are located in the median eminence in close proximity to neurosecretory axon and ependymal cell terminals. The pattern of flow of blood to the pituitary was considered to be regionally specific since clamping of half the vessels of one side causes ipsilateral necrosis of that half of the pituitary. It was imagined that the releasing hormones from axon terminals specific for a given pituitary cell type drained to that cell type. Porter, however, suggests that the blood flow is variable and random (Porter et al 1974).

The dependence of the ovaries upon pituitary gonadotropins was established by hypophysectomy experiments which resulted in gonadal atrophy. Pituitary function can be replaced by exogenous administration of FSH and LH. The feedback effect of ovarian hormones in the pituitary was established by castration experiments in which pituitary gonadotropin rose markedly, indicating release from negative feedback. Exogenous ovarian hormones can then lower gonadotropins and induce a positive feedback if the dose and timing are appropriate.

## Anatomy and function of the ovaries

Mature ovaries are paired organs normally 4 cm $\times$ 3 cm $\times$ 1 cm in size, slung to the back of the broad ligament under the Fallopian tubes by a peritoneal reflection, the *mesovarium*. The medial pole of the ovary is attached by a ligament to the uterus and the lateral pole is supported by the infundibulopelvic ligament, a peritoneal reflection which carries the ovarian vessels.

The ovary has at least two major functions, production of steroid hormones and gametogenesis (Peters & McNatty 1980). These are carried out largely in organelles (follicles and corpora lutea) that cyclically develop and regress each month (Ryan & Smith 1965, Savard et al 1965). The ovary is divided into a *hilar* region through which blood supply and nerves enter from the mesovarium, an outer *cortical* region in which resting follicle-containing germ cells reside, and a central *medulla* composed largely of stromal cells. The ovary is invested during early embryonic development with a finite number of oocytes, their division having stopped and the oocytes remaining in meiotic arrest at the diplotene stage until stimulated to resume meiosis prior to ovulation or atresia. The number of oocytes in the germ cell pool at puberty is around 300 000, of which only a few hundred will actually ovulate, while the rest regress at various stages of development throughout life until depletion after the menopause (Baker 1963). The resting oocytes are first invested with a single layer of granulosa cells and constitute the primordial follicles.

The dynamics of the ovary are such that from the resting pool of primary follicles 0.05 mm in size a cohort is recruited after ovulation each month to undergo proliferation of granulosa cells and thecal cells, maturation and growth of the oocyte, and antrum formation. The follicles seem to migrate or enlarge downward from the cortex toward the medulla as they become active. At the start of menstruation a small number of the follicle pool at the 4 mm size are stimulated by gonadotropins to enlarge and develop further. To move from a 0.05-mm primary follicle during the recruitment process to a 4-mm antral follicle takes approximately 3 months. It is from the pool of 4-mm size follicles that one is selected each month for ovulation. It takes an additional 2 weeks for the selected follicle to grow from 4-mm to 25 mm and be developmentally ready for ovulation (Adashi 1991). The follicle destined to ovulate enlarges to approximately 25 mm, accumulates about 5 ml of antral fluid and increases its granulosa cell number to around 50 million. The oocyte enlarges from 25 µm to 100 µm in diameter and just before ovulation resumes meiosis and extrudes its first polar body in response to the LH surge. After ovulation the remaining ruptured follicle wall and cells are reorganized into a *corpus luteum* with follicular granulosa and thecal cells undergoing differentiation and enlargement (luteinization). Those follicles that did not ovulate undergo atresia along the way and by the end of the menstrual cycle, most follicles over 5 mm have regressed (McNatty et al 1979a, Peters & McNatty 1980).

The systemic endocrine changes of the cycle involve largely the follicle destined to ovulate, which captures FSH in its antral fluid and stimulates aromatase (estrogen production) of the granulosa cells (McNatty et al 1979b).

Meanwhile, the theca is stimulated by LH to produce the androgen precursor of granulosa cell estrogens. Both FSH and LH are thus needed for follicular development and the two cell types, theca and granulosa, must work together to produce the estrogen (Dorrington & Armstrong 1979, McNatty et al 1979a, Richards 1979). There is some confusion in the literature on the interaction of the cells of the follicle for estrogen production. Part of the problem has been the use of cells from different species and/or insufficient attention paid to the time in the cycle when a follicle was studied and whether the follicle was 'healthy' or atretic (Ryan 1979a). For all species, the theca synthesizes androgens under LH stimulation and the granulosa aromatizes androgens under FSH stimulation. When the granulosa cell has developed LH receptors, by the effects of both estrogens and FSH, it can be stimulated to aromatize with LH (Richards 1979). Thecal androgen is usually a precursor for granulosa conversion to estrogen. The species differences are seen in the absolute specificity of these reactions. In the horse and human, the theca can clearly aromatize and the granulosa can synthesize androgens. The cells from follicles early in the cycle (even in the human) probably favor thecal androgen formation and granulosa aromatization. However, cells from atretic follicles do not aromatize well at all (Fig. 5.3).

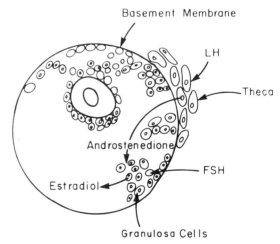

**Fig. 5.3** Relationship of granulosa and theca in steroid production by the ovary.

In any case, the need for LH for the theca and FSH for the granulosa explains the observation that both gonadotropins are necessary for follicular development. The estrogen and FSH in the follicle induce LH receptors in the granulosa cells and by the time of ovulation and subsequent corpus luteum formation the granulosa cells have the capacity to respond to LH for progesterone and estrogen production (Richards 1979). The rise in estrogen from the preovulatory follicle triggers the midcycle LH surge which causes ovulation. There is also a change in the mechanism of steroid production in the corpus luteum such that LDL-cholesterol (low-density lipoprotein bound to cholesterol) can be taken up by the cell to facilitate the conversion of cholesterol to progesterone (Tureck & Strauss 1982).

Those follicles that cannot capture FSH and produce estrogens, produce excess androgens and undergo atresia (Peters & McNatty 1980). The oocytes are influenced by the follicular microenvironment and those germ cells isolated from follicles with FSH, high granulosa cell number and high estrogen production most readily resume meiosis and undergo germinal vesicle breakdown and polar body extrusion. Oocytes from atretic follicles are less likely to survive (McNatty et al 1979b). Gonadotropins from the fetal pituitary are necessary for germ cell survival during intrauterine life. When the ovary is fully developed after 7 months of gestation, follicles remain in a quasi-resting state until gonadotropins rise at puberty. Follicles do develop to the antral stage and undergo atresia during childhood, but ovulation is absent. At puberty both FSH and LH are necessary to initiate cyclic folliculogenesis, ovulation and corpus luteum function.

The essential features of the primate cycle are:

1. Ovulation occurs randomly each month from either ovary.

2. It takes 3 months for the primary follicle to grow and develop from a size of 0.05 mm to an antral follicle of 4 mm during the recruitment process and an additional 2 weeks to reach a size of 25 mm just prior to ovulation.

3. If that follicle is destroyed, it takes another 2 weeks to recruit another follicle since all of its cohort will have become destined for atresia (DiZerega & Hodgen 1981).

4. Excess FSH and LH (such as with exogenous administration) can recruit more than one follicle and produce superovulation.

5. The rising estrogen of the preovulatory follicle triggers an LH surge to cause resumption of meiosis of the oocyte and rupture of the follicle within 24–36 h.

6. Follicular development includes induction of LH receptors in granulosa cells by estrogen and FSH. The resulting corpus luteum needs LH to function.

7. The corpus luteum cells change their mechanism of steroidogenesis by converting blood-borne cholesterol (LDL-cholesterol) to progesterone (Tureck et al 1982). The LDL-cholesterol is taken up by special cell surface receptors.

8. The primate corpus luteum once formed will regress within 12–14 days because of the local production of luteolytic agents (prostaglandins) and a reduction in gonadotropins due to negative feedback.

9. The corpus luteum is derived from the ruptured follicle and luteal deficiency probably results from poor follicular development (McNatty 1979, Sheehan et al 1982a).

## AUTOCRINE AND PARACRINE FACTORS WITHIN THE OVARY

There are regulatory and developmental aspects of ovarian function that cannot be completely explained by the traditional actions of either steroids or gonadotropins. This gap in our knowledge prompted a quest for intraovarian regulatory agents that might explain the missing links in our knowledge of how the ovary works (Channing 1979, DiZerega et al 1982). These unexplained regulatory events include: (a) the continued meiotic arrest of oocytes from fetal life until just prior to their ovulation; (b) the extensive blood vessel proliferation and then regression around the follicles and corpora lutea as they proceed through the processes of folliculogenesis and ovulation or atresia, luteinization and luteolysis; (c) massive granulosa and thecal cell proliferation, growth and differentiation during folliculogenesis not explained by direct effects of gonadotropins (Channing 1979, DiZerega et al 1982); (d) how only one follicle is ordinarily selected for ovulation; (e) the dominance over bilateral ovarian function exerted by the preovulatory follicle and the subsequent corpus luteum.

Over the past decade many peptide growth promoting, differentiating and inhibitory substances have been isolated from the ovary that can explain some of these ovarian events. For many of these peptide factors, there is now evidence for synthesis within the ovary, evidence of specific granulosa or thecal cell membrane receptors and evidence for biological action within the ovary by in vivo or in vitro studies.

### Insulin-like growth factor-I

Insulin-like growth factor-I (IGF-I) is also known as somatomedin-C, a mediator of pituitary growth hormone action found in peripheral sera. It is a straight-chain peptide of 70 amino acids with homology to proinsulin and an insulin-like growth factor-II. The IGFs are synthesized in the liver under the influence of growth hormone, and IGF-I is synthesized in granulosa cells under the influence of estrogens with enhancement by growth hormone. IGF-I acts on granulosa cells by augmenting basal and gonadotropin-stimulated endocrine functions and growth. There is an IGF binding protein in follicular fluid similar to one found in peripheral sera which can block gonadotropin-induced steroid synthesis.

IGF-I acts on the thecal cell to augment androgen production either directly or by enhancing LH activity. There is a form of polycystic ovary syndrome characterized by hirsutism, hyperandrogenism and insulin resistance (see also Chapter 26). The elevated insulin in such cases may increase androgens by stimulating thecal or stromal production of male hormone via IGF-I receptors with which insulin cross-reacts. Such cases also tend to have lower sera IGF-I binding protein which may also free up

more IGFs to stimulate ovarian androgen production (Ryan 1990, Adashi 1991).

### Inhibins, activins, transforming growth factor-β, Mullerian inhibiting substance family of ovarian proteins

Inhibin is the name given to the long elusive water soluble gonadal substance that specifically inhibits pituitary release of FSH. Although originally considered a testicular hormone, inhibin was first isolated from ovarian sources. It is a protein with a molecular weight of 32 000 composed of a heterodimer made up of an alpha subunit of 18 000 and one of two possible beta subunits (A and B) of molecular weight 14 000. There are thus two inhibins (A and B) depending on which of the two beta subunits is involved with a common alpha subunit. They are joined by disulfide bonds. Homodimers of the beta subunits of inhibin have been described and designated as activin A, B or AB depending upon which of the beta subunits are involved. Inhibin inhibits FSH release and synthesis at the pituitary level while activin fosters FSH release and synthesis and inhibits inhibin action in the pituitary cell. While inhibin sera levels and patterns of release have been described during the menstrual cycle, active secretion of activin has not yet been verified. A factor with inhibin-like properties was shown to occur in the follicle (DiZerega et al 1981, Lefevre et al 1981) and to be produced by the granulosa cell under FSH stimulation (Lee et al 1981). There is an unrelated protein, follistatin, found in follicular fluid that is a binding protein for activin and counteracts its action at the pituitary cell level. FSH stimulates the production of inhibin in the ovary and this activity is enhanced by IGF-I.

Inhibin and activin have receptors on ovarian cells and can produce biological effects in vitro. In general, inhibins inhibit, and activins augment gonadotropin actions on endocrine function. One exception is augmentation of LH-stimulated androgen production by the theca which activin inhibits. Whether these agents have specific local roles in the ovary is not yet established but inhibin has been suggested as a possible oocyte meiosis inhibitor (Ryan 1990, Yen 1991) (see also Chapter 6).

Transforming growth factor-β (TGF-β) was originally isolated from conditioned media of viral transformed cells, but it is synthesized in normal cells including in the ovary. This protein is a dimer that shares homologies with the beta chains of inhibins and activins. Like activins, TGF-β can augment FSH release and some FSH effects on ovarian cells. TGF-β has been shown to augment meiotic maturation in immature rats (Ryan 1990).

Mullerian inhibiting substance (MIS) is a glycoprotein produced by embryonic testes which causes regression of Mullerian structures as part of normal fetal male sexual development. MIS is also found in testes at later stages of life, is synthesized by granulosa cells and found in the ovary. It shares structural homologies with inhibins, activins and TGF-β. It has been suggested that MIS is an oocyte maturation inhibitor (Ryan 1990, Adashi 1991).

**Epidermal growth factor and transforming growth factor-α**

Epidermal growth factor (EGF) is a 53 amino acid peptide first isolated from rat salivary glands and shown to accelerate eruption of teeth and opening of the eyelids in newborn mice. It is a very active mitogen for many cell types including granulosa cells and it is known to act in the ovary. Transforming growth factor-α (TGF-α) is a 50 amino acid peptide isolated from viral transformed cells as well as the ovary. It shares significant homologies with EGF, uses the same membrane receptor and has the same actions. These factors inhibit FSH action on granulosa cells and augment granulosa cell proliferation and IGF-I production (Ryan 1990).

**Fibroblast growth factor**

Fibroblast growth factor (FGF) was first isolated from the pituitary and the brain but has since been shown to be produced in many tissues including the ovary. FGF is a complete angiogenic factor and cellular mitogen, and is believed to be the major factor in blood vessel proliferation in the follicle and corpus luteum. FGF also inhibits some FSH actions on the ovary (Ryan 1990).

**Relaxin**

Relaxin is a protein with a structural homology to insulin which has been known to influence the contractility of the uterus and to loosen the ligaments of the pelvic girdle. Its role in human reproduction is still speculative but it can be produced in the ovary and corpus luteum (Weiss et al 1977, Schwabe et al 1978).

FEEDBACK MECHANISMS

The ovarian cycle is a consequence of the integration of the primary neuroendocrine complex (hypothalamus–pituitary–ovary) into an interactive control system with negative and positive endocrine feedback elements as well as neural inputs of the secondary neuroendocrine system from higher CNS centers.

The timing of the primate cycle, the length of the follicular phase and day of ovulation, and the length of the luteal phase are dependent primarily on ovarian signals. It is for this reason that the 'clock' is said to reside in the ovary.

**Negative feedback**

During the phase of follicular development, LH stimulates thecal androgen production and FSH stimulates granulosa conversion of thecal androgen to estrogen. The estrogen (which is also necessary for reproductive tract development) feeds back on the gonadotropes of the pituitary to keep both FSH and LH at an appropriately low level (Kobayashi et al 1978, Goodman et al 1981, Goodman & Karsch 1980, Muldoon and Singh 1980). Estrogen also acts at the hypothalamic level. This is a closed loop negative feedback system (Reichlin 1981). If the estrogen were not present, both FSH and LH would rise as is seen after castration or the menopause. During the luteal phase of the cycle, the corpus luteum produces both estrogen and progesterone under the stimulation of LH, and both these steroids keep gonadotropins at an appropriate level by action on the pituitary and hypothalamus (Rance et al 1981). Destruction or removal of the corpus luteum triggers a subtle change in gonadotropins that can then stimulate a new follicular phase.

Estrogen and progesterone receptors have been detected on dopamine and endorphin neurons in the medial basal hypothalamus. It is believed that steroids do not act directly on GnRH neurons or the pulse generator, but instead influence them indirectly by acting on norepinephrine, dopamine or endorphin neurons which secondarily modulate the pulse generation. A major point of action of the steroids is on the pituitary itself. The way in which inhibin and activins function in feedback control remains to be established (Yen 1991).

## Positive feedback

As the follicle destined to ovulate develops, it secretes increasing amounts of estrogen which maintains negative feedback but also upon reaching a high enough serum level triggers an LH surge by direct action on the pituitary. The mechanism of this addition of a 'cyclic' positive signal over the 'tonic' negative estrogen effect has not been defined. This positive feedback estrogen signal comes from the predominant preovulatory follicle which if destroyed or removed results in a drop in estrogen and failure of an LH surge to occur (DiZerega & Hodgen 1981). Since it takes about 12–14 days to develop the follicle to the point of producing the required estrogen signal, the next ovulation is delayed by that period of time (DiZerega & Hodgen 1981). Those follicles not destined to ovulate will become atretic and cannot substitute for the predominant preovulatory follicle if it is removed. The preoptic area of the hypothalamus is important for positive feedback in the rodent but not the primate (Szentagothai et al 1968, Knobil 1980).

## Short feedback loop

Throughout the cycle, prolactin is kept low by hypothalamic dopamine reaching the pituitary lactotropes. Any rise in prolactin caused by releasing factors or neural elements reaches the hypothalamus and increases hypothalamic

dopamine which returns prolactin to basal levels. The hypothalamic dopamine induced by prolactin can also inhibit or modulate GnRH release (Evans et al 1982).

FSH and LH synthesized by the pituitary can moderate GnRH release by reaching the hypothalamus by the same short feedback loop via the hypophyseal portal system transport from pituitary back to the brain (Motta et al 1969, Mezey & Palkovits 1982).

## Neural inputs and feedback to the hypothalamus

The key to the synthesis and secretion of appropriate amounts of FSH and LH is stimulation by the hypothalamic GnRH which is itself released in pulsed amounts at hourly intervals into the hypophyseal portal system. The GnRH effect is dependent not only on the amount but on the interval of pulsed secretion. Steady infusions of GnRH inhibit pituitary secretion while alterations in the pulse rate can change FSH and LH ratios as well as limit their release (Knobil 1980).

The GnRH peptidergic neurons are in turn regulated by neurotransmitters released by other neurons at the perikarya or axon terminals (Ojeda et al 1982). Feedback effects can be either negative or positive. The neurotransmitters released include norepinephrine which is believed to be stimulating and dopamine (acting now as a neurotransmitter) which is believed to be inhibitory for GnRH release. The endogenous opioids (endorphins, enkephalins) inhibit GnRH release possibly via the intermediary of controlling norepinephrine effects (Blankstein et al 1981, Motta & Martini 1982). Opioid antagonists (naloxone) increase GnRH release suggesting a tonic inhibitory role for the opioids. Estrogens, progesterone and prolactin all regulate GnRH release presumably indirectly via effects on catecholamines.

The relationship of the pineal to the hypothalamus and reproductive function is well established in many animal species but its role in the primate is less well established. Melatonin, a specific neuroendocrine product of the pineal, is secreted under the control of light–dark cycles via inputs to it from the retinal accessory optic tracts and postganglionic sympathetic neurons. Light inhibits and dark stimulates melatonin production. Melatonin inhibits gonadotropin by inhibiting GnRH centrally and also has direct inhibitory effects on the gonads of experimental animals (Wurtman & Moskowitz 1977). The phenomena of constant-light estrus in rodents and seasonal breeding cycles of many animals are undoubtedly dependent upon this system. Although no effects of light on reproductive cycles in the human have been well established, a report suggests that the timing on the day of the LH surge is seasonal in women, occurring mostly in the afternoon in spring and early morning in other seasons. Ovulation was calculated to occur in the morning in spring and in the evening in autumn and winter (Testart et al 1982).

## Pharmacological effects on feedback mechanisms

Drugs can influence GnRH release by influencing neurotransmitter synthesis, release, metabolism or receptor binding. Catecholamine-depleting agents such as reserpine can cause a prolactin increase while dopamine receptor agonists like bromocriptine can inhibit prolactin at the pituitary level. Endorphin is also involved in prolactin control (Ragavan & Frantz 1981). Dopamine receptor blockers like metoclopramide can cause prolactin increases. Naloxone, which blocks opioid receptors, can cause an increase in LH during the luteal phase of the cycle, suggesting alterations in endogenous opioid effects throughout the cycle (Quigley & Yen 1980, Ropert et al 1981, Wilkes & Yen 1981).

## Feedback at the level of the ovary

Estrogens synthesized by the follicle can increase the sensitivity of the follicle cells to gonadotropins. In addition, it has been postulated that substances (proteins) produced by the dominant follicle and corpus luteum reduce the capacity of other follicles in either ovary to develop and hence maintain a single ovulatory event in the cycle (DiZerega et al 1982).

GnRH has been reported to bind to the receptors in ovarian tissue and inhibit response to gonadotropins. This is clearly demonstrated for the rodent ovary in both the follicle and corpus luteum, but results in the primate vary (Asch et al 1981b, Casper et al 1982, Tureck et al 1982). Applicability to primate ovaries is still in question and it is not known whether hypothalamic GnRH is the natural ligand for such a receptor.

GnRH agonists can also cause luteolysis in the human and in the rhesus monkey, and this effect can be overcome by exogenous human chorionic gonadotropin (Bergquist et al 1980, Asch et al 1982, Sheehan et al 1982a, b). The presumption is that the effect is via down regulation (see below) of receptors on the pituitary thereby decreasing FSH and LH output, since hypophysectomy negates the luteolytic effect (Asch et al 1981a). Prolactin at high serum levels can also inhibit steroid production by action on the human ovary (Demura et al 1982).

## Receptor mechanisms

The action of GnRH, gonadotropins and many of the growth factors is mediated by high affinity, cell membrane receptors, which when bound to ligand induce second messenger signals such as adenyl cyclase, protein kinases or calcium mobilization. Such cell membrane receptors have been described on gonadotropes in the pituitary for GnRH and on granulosa and thecal cells of the ovary for gonadotropins and growth factors. By mobilizing more than one second messenger, GnRH can at the same time increase pituitary cell gonadotropin release from stores by changes in calcium and new gonadotropin synthesis via a protein kinase (Yen 1991).

The action of steroids is mediated via high affinity nuclear receptors which when bound to steroid influence the transcription for new protein synthesis. It is generally recognized that hormones and growth factors can act in typical endocrine fashion via secretion into the blood stream for access to a target cell, and also act in paracrine and autocrine fashion by influencing adjacent cells or even the cell of origin. Receptors for estrogens and progestogens have been identified in the brain, hypothalamus and pituitary (McEwen 1976) as well as the reproductive tract and breast.

In the brain and hypothalamus the distribution of estrogen receptors covers areas known to be connected with control of reproductive processes, including localization on neurons producing neurotransmitters (Sar & Stumpf 1981).

One important aspect of hormone interaction with membrane receptors is that an excess of hormone may cause desensitization or down regulation which uncouples activation of adenyl cyclase. This may be followed by an actual decrease in the number of receptors, which in the rodent gonad can take up to a week to be replaced (Amsterdam et al 1979).

After the ligand (gonadotropin) is bound to the cell surface receptor the complex is internalized and processed within the cell. It is believed that the ligand is degraded and the receptor recycled (Hunzicker-Dunn et al 1979). If excess gonadotropin is present, desensitization and down regulation occur and the response is dose dependent. GnRH and its agonists inhibit rather than stimulate pituitary synthesis and release of gonadotropins if these agents are not administered in pulses at the correct dose. Continuous infusion of GnRH causes pituitary refractoriness and it is likely that the pulsatile pattern is an integral part of normal stimulating action (Knobil 1980).

## HORMONAL PATTERN OF THE OVULATORY CYCLE

It is now possible to measure many of the hormones involved in the ovulatory cycle daily or at short intervals throughout the day and night. When performed on a group of women with supposedly normal cycles, such data provide patterns of endocrine gland activity which define the interrelationships of the system (Landgren et al 1980).

### Releasing hormones

Although still controversial, an immunoassayable level of GnRH can be measured throughout the cycle. The pattern is one of roughly hourly fluctuations with a definite peak in the periovulatory period. This suggests that GnRH activity is increased around the middle of the cycle and may

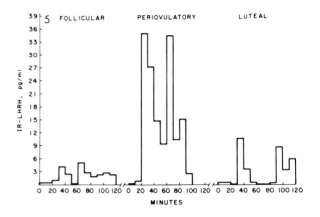

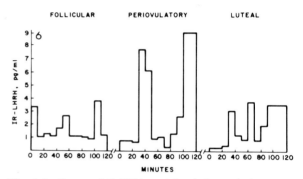

**Fig. 5.4**   Pattern of GnRH in peripheral plasma during normal ovulatory cycles of two female subjects. (Reproduced with permission from Elkind-Hirsch et al 1982.)

be a normal event (Elkind-Hirsch et al 1982; Fig. 5.4).

### Gonadotropins

LH is released in roughly hourly pulses although the pattern seems to change as the cycle progresses (Backstrom et al 1982). Pulse frequency of LH rises from the early follicular to late follicular phase. Mean LH levels gradually rise over the follicular phase, peak as a surge in response to rising estradiol about 1 day after the peak of follicular estradiol, and then decline to levels in the luteal phase which are lower than those in the follicular portion of the cycle and in less frequent pulses (Backstrom et al 1982). A standard notation is to make the day of the LH peak day 0 and count forwards or back from this event to time ovarian events. The midcycle peak level is 5–20 times higher than LH levels in the rest of the cycle. FSH seems to rise toward the

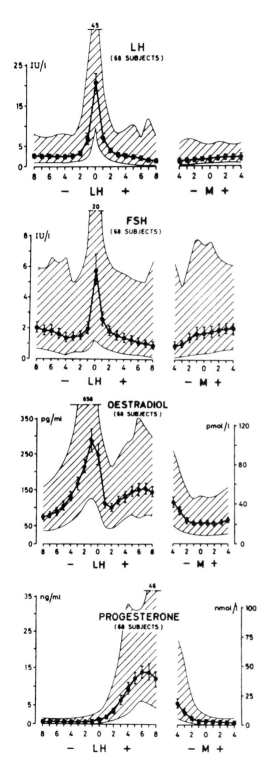

**Fig. 5.5** Pattern of gonadotropins and steroids in plasma during the cycle. (Reproduced with permission from Landgren et al 1980.)

late luteal phase and for the first few days of the follicular period, it then declines, rises concomitant with the LH peak, and drops in the first part of the luteal phase. FSH fluctuations are normally lower than for LH since both its mean serum levels are lower and its biological half-life is longer. The midcycle peak FSH level is roughly two to ten times higher than in the remainder of the cycle.

The amplitude and frequency of LH pulses are dependent upon steroid feedback. It has been suggested that estrogens have their principal negative effect on the amplitude of the LH while progesterone has a principal effect on the frequency of LH pulses. This would explain the change in pulse frequency during the cycle with a lower frequency in the luteal phase (Goodman et al 1981, Goodman & Karsch 1980; Fig. 5.5).

## Steroids

The principal steroids secreted during the follicular phase by the preovulatory follicle are estradiol, estrone and possibly 17α-hydroxy-progesterone. Both ovaries secrete smaller amounts of many other steroids presumably from other elements in the ovaries (follicles destined for atresia and stroma) (Aedo et al 1980a). The principal steroids secreted during the luteal phase by the ovary bearing the corpus luteum include progestrone, 20α-dihydroproges-terone, 17α-hydroxyprogesterone, estradiol and estrone (Aedo et al 1980b). Both ovaries contribute many other steroids to the periphery from elements other than the luteal tissue.

### Estradiol

Estradiol levels rise progressively to a peak value 1 day prior to (or on the day of) the peak level of LH. The rate of rise seems to be inversely proportional to the length of the follicular period. This estradiol comes from the major preovulatory follicle since if it is destroyed, estradiol levels drop to a basal amount. Estradiol drops precipitously after the LH surge prior to rupture of the follicle. A lower flat secondary peak of estradiol is observed over the luteal phase, due to secretion

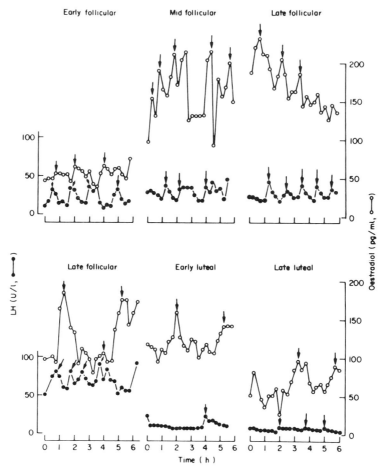

**Fig. 5.6**   Pulsatile pattern of LH and estradiol during the menstrual cycle. The lower panel is a continuation of the upper panel. (Reproduced with permission from Backstrom et al 1982.)

from the active corpus luteum. The follicular peak of serum estradiol is three to nine times higher than levels in the early part of the cycle. The luteal peak serum estradiol level is about one-third that of the preovulatory peak (Landgren et al 1980; Fig. 5.6).

*Progesterone*

Progesterone increases in the serum 1 day after the LH surge (possibly from the preovulatory follicle) and then rises steadily due to luteal secretion to a peak about 6 days after the LH release. The luteal peak serum level of progesterone is around 20 times the follicular progesterone levels (Landgren et al 1980).

## Correlations of hormonal levels and secondary effects in the cycle

The normal menstrual cycle has a mean length of 28 days with a range from 24 to 35 days. The first day of menstruation is ordinarily designated day 1 of the cycle. The follicular phase (from the first day of the menses to and including the day of the LH surge) can range from 9 to 23 days with a mean of 15. This measurement, made by careful studies from Diczfalusy's laboratory, is much more reliable than estimates based on the basal body temperature rise. The length of the follicular phase is negatively correlated with the estradiol levels, suggesting that a more rapid rise of estradiol secretion provokes an earlier

**Table 5.1** Ovarian steroids during the menstrual cycle

| | | Estradiol | Progesterone | 17-OH-progesterone | Androstenedione | Testosterone |
|---|---|---|---|---|---|---|
| Plasma level (pg/ml) | Follicular | 50–60 | 400–950 | 300–400 | 1590–1980 | 380–604 |
| | Periovulatory | 330–700 | | 1740–2000 | | |
| | Luteal | 200 | 2100–10 000 | 1740–2000 | | |
| Production rate (mg/day) | Follicular | 0.081–0.166 | 2.1–2.9 | 0.3 | 3.3 | 0.26–0.5 |
| | Periovulatory | 0.445–0.945 | | 3–4 | | |
| | Luteal | 0.204–0.270 | 22.1–25 | 3–4 | 4.2 | |
| Metabolic clearance rate (l/day) | | 0.1055–0.1350 | 2200 | 2000 | 1610–2150 | 690–890 |

ovulation (also may be seen when high levels of exogenous FSH and LH are given) (Landgren et al 1980).

The luteal phase (from the day after the LH peak to the day before onset of menses) varies from 8 to 17 days with a mean of 13. The ratio of the follicular to luteal phase lengths is about 1, but can range from 0.7 to 1.8. Recent data suggest that the cycle is more variable in a normal population than was popularly supposed. Fully one-third of cycles studied had the LH peak before day 12 or after day 18.

*'Normal' hormonal values throughout the cycle*

Since laboratories all over the world may use different standards or techniques for hormone measurement, absolute 'normal' values for the ovarian cycle are difficult to establish. Each laboratory must provide a range of normality for their experience and population.

Fortunately, secondary clinical signs can provide important information on the presence or absence of adequate amounts of many of the

hormones in question, without the need to measure them directly.

Prolactin determination has become an important guide in cases of amenorrhea and anovulation to detect microadenomas or other defects in the neuroendocrine system.

Absolute values and ratios of FSH and LH are of assistance in determining ovarian failure or in providing a clue to the etiology of anovulation as in polycystic ovary syndrome.

Estradiol levels are seldom of use except to monitor follicular development and the potential for superovulation when exogenous FSH and LH are used to induce ovulation.

Progesterone levels have been used to verify luteal presence and function with the requirement that a minimum level be reached (Hull et al 1982) and/or maintained for at least 5 days (Landgren et al 1980).

Many laboratories have reported on the production rates, metabolic clearance rates and serum levels of ovarian steroids and these data are summarized in Table 5.1. (Ryan 1979b, Sheehan et al 1982b).

REFERENCES

Adashi E Y 1991 The ovarian life cycle. In: Yen S S C, Jaffe B B (eds) Reproductive endocrinology, 3rd edn. W B Saunders, Philadelphia, pp 181–237
Aedo AR, Pedersen P H, Pedersen S C, Diczfalusy E 1980a Ovarian steroid secretion in normally menstruating women. 1. The contribution of the developing follicle. Acta Endocrinol 95: 212
Aedo A R, Pedersen P H, Pedersen S C, Diczfalusy E 1980b Ovarian steroid secretion in normally menstruating women. 2. The contribution of the corpus luteum. Acta Endocrinol 95: 222

Ajika K 1980 Relationship between catecholaminergic neurons and hypothalamic containing neurons in the hypothalamus. In: Martini L, Ganong W F (eds) Functions in neuroendocrinology, Vol 6. Raven, New York, p 1
Amsterdam A, Kohn F, Nimrod A, Lindner H R 1979 Lateral mobility and internalization of hormone receptors to human chorionic gonadotropin in cultured rat granulosa cells. In: Channing C P, Marsh J M, Sadler W (eds) Ovarian follicular and corpus luteum function. Plenum, New York, p 69
Asch R H, Eddy C A, Schally A V 1981a Lack of luteolytic

effect of D-TRP-6-LH-RH in hypophysectomized rhesus monkeys (*Macaca mulatta*). Biol Reprod 25: 936

Asch R H, Van Sickle M, Rettori V et al 1981b Absence of LH-RH binding sites in corpora lutea from rhesus monkeys. J Clin Endocrinol Metab 53: 215

Asch R H, Siler-Khodr T M, Smith C G, Schally A V 1982 Luteolytic effect of D-Trp[6]-luteinizing hormone-releasing hormone in the rhesus monkey. J Clin Endocrinol Metab 52: 565

Backstrom C T, McNeilly A S, Leask R M, Baird D T 1982 Pulsatile secretion of LH, FSH, prolactin, oestradiol and progesterone during the human menstrual cycle. Clin Endocrinol 17: 29

Baker B L 1974 Functional cytology of the hypophysial pars distalis and pars intermedia. In: Knobil E, Sawyer W H (eds) Handbook of physiology: Section 7, Endocrinology. IV. The pituitary and its neuroendocrine control part 1. American Physiological Society Washington, DC, p 45

Baker T G 1963 A quantitative and cytological study of germ cells in human ovaries. Proc R Soc (B) 158: 417

Behrman H R, Luborsky-Moore J L, Pang C Y, Wright K, Dorflinger L J 1979 Mechanisms of $PGF_2\alpha$ action in functional luteolysis. In: Channing C P, Marsh J M, Sadler W (eds) Ovarian follicular and corpus luteum function. Plenum, New York, p 557

Bergquist C, Nillius S J, Wide L 1980 Luteolysis induced by a luteinizing hormone-releasing hormone agonist is prevented by human chorionic gonadotropin. Contraception 22: 341

Blankstein J, Reyes F I, Winter J S D, Faiman C 1981 Endorphins and the regulation of the human menstrual cycle. Clin Endocrinol 14: 287

Burgus R, Butcher M, Ling N, et al 1971 Structure moleculaire du facteur hypothalamique (LRF) d'origine ovine controlant la sécrétion de l'hormone gonadotrope hypophysaire de lutéinisation (LH). Compt Rend Acad Sci 273: 161

Casper R F, Erickson G F, Rebar R W, Yen S S C 1982 The effect of luteinizing hormone-releasing factor and its agonist on cultural human granulosa cells. Fertil Steril 37: 406

Channing C P 1979 Follicular non-steroidal regulators. In: Channing C P, Marsh J M, Sadler W (eds) Ovarian follicular and corpus luteum function. Plenum, New York, p 327

Crowley W F, McArthur J W 1980 Stimulation of the normal menstrual cycle in Kallman's syndrome by pulsatile administration of luteinizing hormone-releasing hormone (LHRH). J Clin Endocrinol Metab 51: 173

Daughaday W H 1981 The adenohypophysis. In: Williams R H (ed) Textbook of endocrinology. Saunders, Philadelphia, p 73

Demura R, Ono M, Demura H, Shizume K, Oouchi H 1982 Prolactin directly inhibits basal as well as gonadotropin stimulated secretion of progesterone and 17β-estradiol in the human ovary. J Clin Endocrinol Metab 54: 1246

DiZerega G S, Hodgen G D 1981 Folliculogenesis in the primate ovarian cycle. Endocrinol Rev 2: 27

DiZerega G S, Turner C K, Stouffer R L, Anderson L D, Channing C P, Hodgen G D 1981 Suppression of follicle-stimulating hormone dependent folliculogenesis during the primate ovarian cycle. J Clin Endocrinol Metab 52: 451

DiZerega G, Gobelsmann U, Nakamura R M 1982 Identification of protein (s) secreted by the preovulatory ovary which suppresses the follicle response to gonadotropins. J Clin Endocrinol Metab 54: 1091

Dorrington J H, Armstrong D T 1979 Effects of FSH on gonadal functions. Recent Prog Horm Res 35: 301

Elkind-Hirsch K, Ravnikar V, Schiff I, Tulchinsky D, Ryan K J 1982 Determinations of endogenous immunoreactive luteinizing hormone-releasing hormone in human plasma. J Clin Endocrinol Metab 54: 602

Evans W S, Cronin M J, Thorner M O 1982 Hypogonadism in hyperprolactinemia: proposed mechanisms. In: Ganong W F, Martini L (eds) Frontiers in neuroendocrinology, vol 7. Raven, New York, p 77

Fang V S, Shian L R 1981 A serotonergic mechanism of the prolactin-stimulating action of metoclopramide. Endocrinology 108: 1622

Fuxe K, Hökfelt T 1969 Catecholamines in the hypothalamus and the pituitary gland. In: Ganong W F, Martini L (eds) Frontiers in neuroendocrinology. Oxford University Press, New York, p 47

Goodman R L, Karsch K J 1980 Pulsatile secretion of luteinizing hormones: differential suppression by ovarian steroids. Endocrinology 107: 1286

Goodman R L, Bittman E, Foster D L, Karsch F J 1981 The endocrine basis of the synergistic suppression of luteinizing hormone by estradiol and progesterone. Endocrinology 109: 1414

Gudelsky G A, Nansel D D, Porter J C 1981 Role of estrogen in the dopaminergic control of prolactin secretion. Endocrinology 108: 440

Hull M G R, Savage P E, Bromhan D R, Ismail A A A, Morris A F 1982 The value of a single serum progesterone measurement in the midluteal phase as a criterion of a potentially fertile cycle ('ovulation') derived from treated and untreated conception cycles. Fertil Steril 37: 355

Hunzicker-Dunn M, Jungmann R, Derda D, Birnbaumer L 1979 LH-induced desensitization of the adenyl cyclase system in ovarian follicles. In: Channing C P, Marsh I M Sadler W (eds) Ovarian follicular and corpus luteum function. Plenum, New York, p 27

Kobayashi R M, Lu K H, Moore R Y, Yen S S C 1978 Regional distribution of hypothalamic luteinizing hormone releasing hormone in proestrous rats: effects of ovariectomy and estrogen replacement. Endocrinology 102: 98

Knigge K M, Silverman A J 1974 Anatomy of the endocrine hypothalamus. In: Knobil E, Sawyer W H (eds) Handbook of physiology: Section 7, endocrinology IV. The pituitary and its neuroendocrine control, part 1. American Physiological Society, Washington DC, p 1

Knobil E 1980 The neuroendocrine control of the menstrual cycle. Recent Prog Horm Res 36: 53

Knobil E 1989 The electrophysiology of the GnRH pulse generator. J Steroid Biochem 33: 669

Krulich L, McCann S M, Mayfield M A 1981 On the mode of the prolactin release inhibiting action of the serotonin receptor blockers metergoline, methysergide, and cyproheptadine. Endocrinology 108: 1115

Landgren B M, Unden A L, Diczfalusy E 1980 Hormonal profile of the cycle in 68 normally menstruating women. Acta Endocrinol 94: 89

Lee V W K, McMaster J, Quigg H, Findlay J, Leversha L 1981 Ovarian and peripheral blood inhibin concentrations increase with gonadotropin treatment in immature rats. Endocrinology 108: 2403

Lefevre B, Kraiem Z, Epstein Y et al 1981 Inhibin-like

activity and steroid content in human follicular fluid during the periovulatory period. Int J Fertil 26: 295

Marshall J C, Kelch R P 1979 Low dose pulsatile gonadotropin-releasing hormone in anorexia nervosa: a model of human pubertal development. J Clin Endocrinol Metab 49: 712

Marshall J C, Bourne G A, Frager M S, Pieper D R 1980 Pituitary GnRH receptors–physiological changes and control of receptor number. In: Mahesh V B, Muldoon T G, Saxena B B, Sadler W A (eds) Functional correlates of hormone receptors in reproduction. Elsevier, New York, p 93

Matsuo H, Baba Y, Nair R M G, Arimura A, Schally A V 1971 Structure of the porcine LH and FSH releasing hormone. 1. The proposed amino acid sequence. Biochem Biophys Res Commun 43: 1334

McEwen B S 1976 Steroid receptors in neuroendocrine tissues. Topography, subcellular distribution and functional implications in subcellular mechanisms. In: Naftolin F, Ryan K J, Davies I J (eds) Reproductive neuroendocrinology. Elsevier, Amsterdam, p 277

McNatty K P 1979 Follicular determinants of corpus luteum function in the human ovary in ovarian follicle and corpus luteum function. In: Channing C P, Marsh J M, Sadler W (eds) Ovarian follicle and corpus luteum function. Plenum, New York, p 465

McNatty K P, Makris A, Degrazia C, Osathanondh R, Ryan K J 1979a The production of progesterone, androgens and estrogens by granulosa cells, thecal tissue and stromal tissue from human ovaries in vitro. J Clin Endocrinol Metab 49: 687

McNatty K P, Smith D M, Makris A, Osathanondh R, Ryan K J 1979b The microenvironment of the human antral follicle: interrelationships among the steroid levels in antral fluid, the population of granulosa cells and the status of the oocyte in vivo and vitro. J Clin Endocrinol Metab 49: 851

Mezey E, Palkovits M 1982 Two-way transport in the hypothalamo-hypophyseal system. In: Ganong W, Martini L (eds) Frontiers in neuroendocrinology, vol 7. Raven, New York, p 1

Motta M, Martini L 1982 Effect of opioid peptides on gonadotrophin secretion. Acta Endocrinol 99: 321

Motta M, Fraschini F, Martini L 1969 'Short' feedback mechanisms in the control of anterior pituitary function. In: Ganong W F, Martini L (eds) Frontiers in euroendocrinology. Oxford University Press, New York, p 211

Muldoon T G, Singh P 1980 Correlations between control of LH secretion and estrogen receptor dynamics in the anterior pituitary and hypothalamus. In: Mahesh V B, Muldoon T G, Saxena B B, Sadler W A (eds) Functional correlates of hormone receptors in reproduction. Elsevier, New York, p 65

Ojeda S R, Negro-Vilar A, McCann S M 1982 Evidence for involvement of α-adrenergic receptors in norepinephrine-induced prostaglandin $E_2$ and luteinizing hormone-releasing hormone release from the median eminence. Endocrinology 110: 409

Palkovits M 1982 Neurotransmitter distribution in the brain. In: Ruf K B, Tolis G, Karger S (eds) Frontier of hormone research, vol 10, advances in neuroendocrine physiology. S. Karger, New York, p 15

Peters H, McNatty K P 1980 The ovary. University of California Press, p 175

Porter J C, Ondo J G, Cramer O M 1974 Nervous and vascular supply of the pituitary gland. In: Knobil E, Sawyer W H (eds) Handbook of physiology: section 7 endocrinology IV. The pituitary and its neuroendocrine control part 1. American Physiological Society, Washington DC, p 33

Quigley M E, Yen S S C 1980 The role of endogenous opiates on LH secretion during the menstrual cycle. J Clin Endocrinol Metab 51: 179

Ragavan V V, Frantz A G 1981 Opioid regulation of prolactin secretion: evidence for a specific role of β-endorphin. Endocrinology 109: 1769

Rance N, Wise P M, Barraclough C A 1981 Negative feedback effects of progesterone correlated with changes in hypothalamic norepinephrine and dopamine turnover rates, median eminence luteinizing hormone-releasing hormone and peripheral plasma gonadotropins. Endocrinology 108: 2194

Reichlin S 1981 Neuroendocrinology. In: Williams R H (ed) Textbook of endocrinology. W B Saunders, Philadelphia, p 589

Ropert J F, Quigley M E, Yen S S C 1981 Endogenous opiates modulate pulsatile luteinizing hormone release in humans. J Clin Endocrinol Metab 52: 583

Richards J S 1979 Hormonal control of ovarian follicular development, a 1978 perspective. Recent Prog Horm Res 35: 343

Ryan K J, Smith O W 1965 Biogenesis of steroid hormones in the human ovary. Recent Prog Horm Res 21: 367

Ryan K J 1979a Granulosa–thecal cell interaction in ovarian steroidogenesis. J Steroid Biochem 11: 799

Ryan K J 1979b Biosynthesis and metabolism of ovarian steroids. In: Behrman S J, Kistner R W (eds) Progress in infertility, 2nd edn. Little Brown, Boston, p 281

Ryan K J 1990 The endocrinology and paracrinology of the ovary. In: Edwards BG (ed) Establishing a successful human pregnancy. Raven, New York, pp 63–76

Sar M, Stumpf W E 1981 Central noradrenergic neurones concentrate ³H-oestradiol. Nature 289: 500

Savard K, Marsh J M, Rice B F 1965 Gonadotropins and ovarian steroidogenesis. Recent Prog Horm Res 21: 285

Scharrer E, Shcharrer B 1962 Neuroendocrinology. Columbia University Press, New York

Schwabe C, Steinetz B, Weiss et al 1978 Relaxin. Recent Prog Horm Res 34: 123

Sheehan K L, Casper R F, Yen S S C 1982a Luteal phase defects induced by an agonist of luteinizing hormone-releasing factor: a model for fertility control. Science 215: 170

Sheehan K L, Casper R F, Yen S S C 1982b Induction of luteolysis by luteinizing hormone-releasing factor (LRF) agonist sensitivity, reproductibility and reversibility. Fertil Steril 37: 209

Szentagothai J, Ferko B, Mess B, Halasz B 1968 Hypothalamic control of the anterior pituitary. Akademia Kiado, Budapest, p 1

Testart J, Frydman R, Roger M 1982 Seasonal influence of diurnal rhythms in the onset of the plasma luteinizing hormone surge in women. J Clin Endocrinol Metab 55: 374

Tureck R W, Strauss J F III 1982 Progesterone synthesis by luteinized human granulosa cells in culture. The role of de novo sterol synthesis and lipoprotein-carried sterol. J Clin Endocrinol Metab 54: 367

Tureck R W, Mastroianni J L, Blasco L, Straus J F III 1982

Inhibition of human granulosa cell progesterone secretion
by a gonadotropin-releasing hormone agonist. J Clin
Endocrinol Metab 54: 1078

Van Tienhoven A 1968 Environment and reproduction. In:
Reproductive physiology of vetebrates. W B Saunders,
Philadelphia, p 388

Weiss G, O'Byrne E M, Hochman J A, Goldsmith L T,
Rifkin I, Steinetz B G 1977 Secretion of progesterone and
relaxin by the human corpus luteum at midpregnancy and
at term. Obstet Gynecol 50: 679

Wilkes M M, Yen S S C 1981 Augmentation by naloxone of
efflux of LRF from superfused medial basal hypothalamus.
Life Sci 28: 2355

Wurtman R J, Moskowitz M A 1977 The pineal organ. N Eng
J Med 296: 1329

Yen S S C 1991 The human menstrual cycle. In: Yen S S C,
Jaffe R B (eds) Reproductive endocrinology, 3rd Edn. W B
Saunders, Philadelphia, ch 8, pp 273–308

# 6. Follicular development and the mechanism of ovulation

*A. Tsafriri    Ruth H. Braw-Tal    R. Reich*

## INTRODUCTION

Ovulation, i.e. the release of a fertilizable mature ovum, is the final stage of a protracted process of folliculogenesis, follicle and oocyte growth and development. In this chapter some of the changes and regulatory mechanisms involved in follicular development and in ovulation will be reviewed. This is not intended to be an exhaustive review. The interested reader is referred to the following books covering various aspects of ovarian function: (Jones 1978, Zuckerman & Weir 1978, Peters & McNatty 1980, Guraya 1985, Knobil & Neill 1988).

## FOLLICULAR DEVELOPMENT

### Folliculogenesis

Formation of follicles is initiated in some species during embryonic life (e.g humans, monkeys, cows, pigs) and in others during the neonatal period (e.g. rats, mice) or even later during the 2nd or 3rd week of life (e.g. hamsters, cats, rabbits). In the early stage of ovarian development oocyte nuclei lie together in nests without a clear plasma membrane separating them. The oocytes within each nest ate at the same stage of meiotic prophase (leptotene, zygotene or pachytene; Fig. 6.1). The transformation of oocyte nests into separate oocytes, each surrounded by a few granulosa cells, and formation of a basement membrane around these oocytes is termed folliculogenesis. The major source of granulosa cells appears to be the rete ovarii with a varying contribution of the surface epithelium (Byskov 1975, 1986, Peters 1978). However, whereas removal of the rete ovarii before the initiation of folliculogen-

esis prevents formation of follicles, the removal of surface epithelium has no effect on follicle formation in the mouse (Byskov 1974b, Byskov et al 1977). The process of folliculogenesis starts at the innermost part of ovarian cortex and spreads to its periphery. The resulting 'primordial' or 'primary' follicles form the pool from which follicles begin to grow throughout fetal, prepubertal and pubertal life. Oocytes which do not become enclosed by granulosa cells usually degenerate (Ohno & Smith 1964).

### Classification of follicles

A classification of follicles first proposed for the mouse (Pedersen & Peters 1968) and later adapted to the human (Peters et al 1978, Gougeon 1986; Fig. 6.2) has proved most useful for analysing follicular development. Thus, four groups of follicles can be distinguished:

1. The small, nongrowing follicle (also called *primordial* or *primary follicle*) consists of a small oocyte, a few flattened granulosa cells and a basement membrane. They lie in the outer cortex of the ovary and represent the pool of resting follicles.

2. The *preantral follicle* (also called *secondary, medium* or *growing follicle)* is the one that enters the growing phase. Its oocyte begins to grow and granulosa cells enlarge and multiply to form two or three layers around the oocyte. The zona pellucida forms and cells of the ovarian stroma organize into the theca layers.

3. The *antral follicle* contains a fully grown oocyte, several layers of granulosa cells, an antrum filled with fluid and, outside the basement membrane, well-differentiated theca layers.

# OOCYTE MEIOSIS

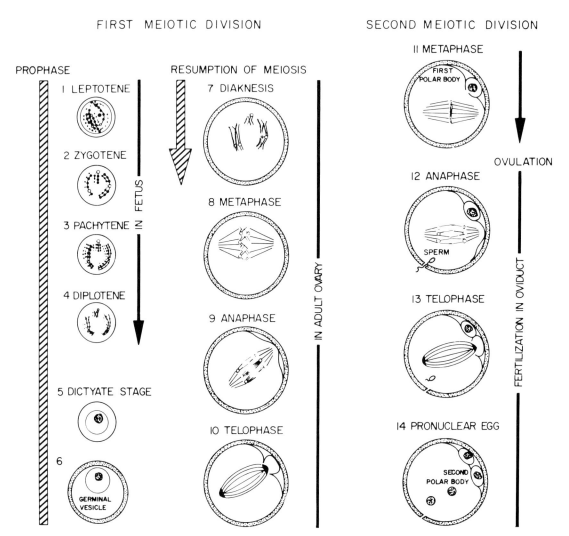

FIRST MEIOTIC DIVISION

SECOND MEIOTIC DIVISION

PROPHASE

RESUMPTION OF MEIOSIS

1 LEPTOTENE

2 ZYGOTENE

3 PACHYTENE

4 DIPLOTENE

5 DICTYATE STAGE

6

GERMINAL VESICLE

IN FETUS

7 DIAKNESIS

8 METAPHASE

9 ANAPHASE

10 TELOPHASE

IN ADULT OVARY

II METAPHASE

FIRST POLAR BODY

OVULATION

12 ANAPHASE

SPERM

13 TELOPHASE

14 PRONUCLEAR EGG

SECOND POLAR BODY

FERTILIZATION IN OVIDUCT

**Fig. 6.1**  Oocyte meiosis. For simplicity only three pairs of chromosomes are depicted. 1–4, prophase stages of the first meiotic division, which occur in most mammals during fetal life. At zygotene (2) the homologous maternal and paternal chromosomes begin to pair, and at pachytene (3), they are paired along their entire length, thus forming bivalents. During pachytene, each homologue cleaves longitudinally to form two sister chromatids, so that each bivalent forms a tetrad. During this stage, interchange of genetic material between maternal and paternal chromatids may occur by crossing over. At diplotene (4), the chromosomes begin to separate, remaining united at the chiasmata. The meiotic process is arrested at this stage ('first meiotic arrest'), and the oocyte enters the dictyate stage. When meiosis is resumed, the first maturation division is completed (7–11). Ovulation occurs usually at the metaphase II stage (11) ('second meiotic arrest'), and the second meiotic division (12–14) takes place in the oviduct following sperm penetration. (Reproduced with permission from Tsafriri 1978.)

4. The *large antral follicle* (also referred to as *Graafian follicle*) which reaches its maximum diameter and is fully responsive to the preovulatory surge of gonadotropins.

It has become evident that granulosa cells of such follicles do not constitute a homogeneous tissue, but show regional specializations. There are distinct differences between the mural granu-

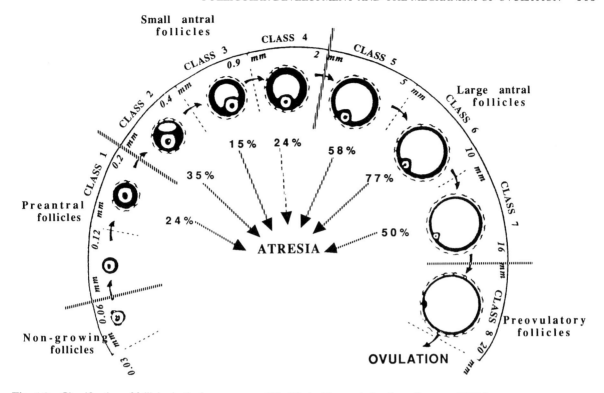

**Fig. 6.2**    Classification of follicles in the human ovary. (Modified with permission from Gougeon 1986.)

losa adjacent to the basement membrane, periantral granulosa and the cumulus cells in localization of peptide hormone receptors, steroidogenic and other enzymes and presumably other metabolic activities (Lindner et al 1977, Rao et al 1991).

## Follicular growth before puberty

### Fetal life

In humans and monkeys follicular growth starts during fetal life (van Wagenen & Simpson 1965). The first small follicles appear during the 4th month of gestation and around the 6th month many preantral follicles can be located in the innermost part of ovarian cortex. Antral follicles often develop during the last 2 months of fetal life and the ovary of the newborn is often crowded with large antral follicles (Potter 1963, Peters et al 1978). However, these follicles show signs of degeneration or atresia and of irregular growth (Peters et al 1978). During late gestation, fetal

ovaries synthesize testosterone and inhibin, a gonadal glycoprotein with selective follicle stimulating hormone (FSH) suppressing activity (Albers et al 1989a,b).

Anencephalic human fetuses have a greatly reduced pituitary gland which contains only about 2% of the normal gonadotropin content (Grumbach & Kaplan 1973). Ovaries of such fetuses at term are small and contain very few preantral and no antral follicles (Baker & Scrimgeour 1980, H. R. Braw, unpublished observations). Also, hypophysectomy in utero of rhesus monkeys resulted in impaired growth of follicles (Gulyas et al 1977). These studies suggest that gonadotropins of the fetal pituitary are involved in follicular growth and that the pituitary – ovarian feedback mechanism is already functional during fetal life.

### Prepuberty

In primates, follicular growth which has begun during fetal life continues throughout childhood (van Wagenen & Simpson 1965, Peters et al 1976). All the follicles beginning to grow before puberty are doomed to degeneration. Follicles undergo atresia at various stages of their development, but the percentage of atretic follicles increases as follicular development advances (Table 6.1; Vermande-vanEck 1956, Koering 1969, Himelstein-Braw et al 1976). Primate ovaries are active in inhibin and steroid secretion during the postnatal period (Channing et al 1984).

Follicular growth in childhood is impaired by cytotoxic drugs and abdominal irradiation. In some cases these agents even reduce the pool of the small nongrowing follicles (Miller et al 1971, Himelstein-Braw et al 1977), thus causing irreversible ovarian damage and ovarian failure at puberty (Shalet et al 1976).

In other mammalian species follicular growth begins in prepubertal life. In fact, in some species, the number of follicles starting to grow prior to puberty is much higher than their number in the mature animal. Follicles reach the antral stage and premature ovulation can be induced by exogenous gonadotropins.

It seems that follicular development in prepubertal animals is related to a rise in basal levels of gonadotropins in the blood. Blockage of the increase in serum FSH concentration, that occurs in immature rats between 7 and 21 days after birth, results in a decrease in the number of follicles beyond the primary stage of follicular development (Fagbohun et al 1990). However, administration of gonadotropin antiserum to newborn mice did not prevent the initiation of follicular growth (Eshkol & Lunenfeld 1972, Nakano et al 1975) but such treatment for 2 weeks resulted in poorly organized granulosa, ill-defined basal membrane and deficient development of the thecal layers and of follicular vasculature. Furthermore, normal follicular development could be restored by substitution with exogenous gonadotropins. While FSH restored normal preantral follicle formation, both FSH and luteinizing hormone (LH) were needed for the development of antral follicles (Eshkol et al 1970, Purandare et al 1976). These data seem to indicate that gonadotropins affect the ovary even when the number of gonadotropin receptors in granulosa cells is very low (Presl et al 1972, 1974) and before that ovarian responsiveness to LH in terms of cAMP formation is established (Lamprecht et al 1973, Kolena 1976).

## Follicular growth in sexually mature mammals

### During the estrous cycle of rodents

The dynamics of follicular growth in rodents has been examined by radiolabelling of granulosa cells or the zona pellucida (Pedersen 1970, Oakberg & Tyrrell 1975, Chiras & Greenwald 1977, Hage et al 1978). In these species approximately 10 ova are released at each estrous cycle of 4–5 days. Four to five cycles are needed for a follicle that begins to grow to reach ovulation. The preovulatory surge of LH induces ovulation (see below); it was suggested that the periovulatory secretion of FSH is necessary for the selection of follicles destined to ovulate on the next estrous cycle (Schwartz 1974, Greenwald & Siegel 1982). This suggestion was confirmed in the rat by demonstrating that abolishing the preovulatory surge

**Table 6.1** Number of oocytes lost by ovulation and atresia during the fertile period in different mammalian species

| Species | Total no. of oocytes at the onset of the fertile period | Total no. of oocytes that ovulate during the fertile period | % of follicles that disappear by atresia |
|---|---|---|---|
| Human | 390 000 | 360 | 99.9 |
| Monkey | 200 000 | 280 | 99.9 |
| Dog | 70 000 | 60 | 99.9 |
| Guinea-pig | 15 000 | 270 | 99 |
| Pig | 100 000 | 1190 | 98 |
| Mouse | 3 000 | 630 | 77 |
| Rat | 5 000 | 1260 | 75 |

With permission from Byskov 1978.

deprives the ovary of early antral follicles (390–500 µm in diameter), and that they can be restored by exogenous FSH (Welschen & Dullaart 1976, Hirshfield & Midgley 1978a,b, Hirshfield 1986). Recent studies in the hamster show that periovulatory changes in gonadotropins enhance DNA synthesis and progesterone production of small preantral follicles (Roy & Greenwald 1985, 1986). These data were corroborated by administration of an antiserum to FSH on the day of proestrus, which resulted in delay of ovulation of the next cycle without affecting ovulation the next night (Sheela Rani & Moudgal 1977). This effect is probably exerted by preventing atresia of late preantral and early antral follicles (Hirshfield 1986, Hirshfield & Midgley 1978b). Similar antiatretic effect of pregnant mare's serum gonadotropin (PMSG) was observed in mice and rats (Peters et al 1975, Braw & Tsafriri 1980a).

Both FSH and LH are needed for normal follicular development during the estrus cycle but their ratio and relative importance may vary at different stages of the cycle. Presumably, FSH is essential for the recruitment of the developing follicles and for prevention of atresia of developing follicles. This results in the selection of the dominant follicle(s), while their final maturation is dependent on LH.

*During the estrous cycle of domestic animals*

The length of the estrous cycle is about 17 days in sheep and 21 days in the cow and in the sow. It is characterized by a long luteal phase (14–17 days) and a short follicular phase (3–4 days). In the ewe, two 'waves' of follicular development occur. The first 'wave', from day 1 to 12, yields large antral follicles (> 2 mm), seen on days 7–9, which become atretic. The second 'wave' from day 12 to ovulation, recruits one or two large follicles that grow rapidly after luteolysis on day 14 and eventually ovulate (Driancourt et al 1985). Experimentally induced regression of the corpus luteum result in ovulation within 72–96 h (Baird 1983). Differentiation of the dominant follicle is associated with progressive increase of LH levels, as pituitary LH output is released from suppression by progesterone. Plasma concentration of

FSH falls progressively due to the negative feedback of estradiol and inhibin secreted by developing follicle(s) (Mann et al 1989, Campbell et al 1990, Findlay et al 1990a). Follicular development beyond 2.5 mm is dependent on adequate stimulation by both LH and FSH, and continues despite the falling plasma FSH concentrations (McNeilly et al 1986). Administration of low doses of FSH for 48 h from the initiation of luteolysis, which prevented the normal preovulatory decline in plasma FSH concentration, caused a significant increase in mean ovulation rate (Henderson et al 1988). Administration of bovine follicular fluid to anestrous ewes lowered plasma FSH concentration by 70% and reduced the number of non-atretic large antral follicles without altering the total number of follicles. Hourly injection of 50 µg FSH together with follicle fluid increased the number of nonatretic follicles and granulosa cell aromatase activity (McNatty et al 1985, McNeilly 1985). As follicle size increases, the sensitivity of sheep granulosa cells to FSH increases (Henderson et al 1987). This may be important in ensuring that final maturation of follicles occurs in spite of declining plasma FSH concentrations during the preovulatory period. The increasing sensitivity of granulosa cells to FSH in large ovulatory follicles probably protects them from undergoing atresia due to low plasma FSH concentrations, while smaller follicles, less sensitive to FSH, are likely to become atretic.

*During the menstrual cycle*

Several reviews on the development of ovarian follicles during the menstrual cycle of primates have been published (Ross & Lipsett 1978, diZerega & Hodgen 1981, McNatty 1981, Baird 1983, Gougeon 1986, Greenwald & Terranova 1988, Gougeon 1990). While in domestic animals (e.g. the ewe and the cow), large antral follicles are present at each day of the cycle, in primates, large antral follicles (class 6–8, Fig. 6.2) are present in the ovary only during the follicular stage of the menstrual cycle (Gougeon & Lefévre 1983). This difference in the pattern of follicular growth seems to be related to the difference in steroid secretion from the corpora lutea: whereas in primates the corpus luteum secretes progesterone and estradiol, that of the ewe and cow secretes progesterone, but not estradiol. The elevated level of LH and FSH allow the development of large antral follicles throughout the luteal phase of farm animals, whereas in primates FSH is elevated only during the periovulatory and the early follicular phase (Baird et al 1975, McNatty et al 1975).

Removal of the corpus luteum or the dominant follicle in the rhesus monkey or human results in ovulation only after 13–15 days (Goodman et al 1977, diZerega & Hodgen 1981, Nilsson et al 1982). Moreover, during the luteal phase in the human, only a small number of follicles are nonatretic (0–4/ovary) and the largest of these are less than 5 mm in diameter (McNatty et al 1983). It seems, therefore, that the basal levels of gonadotropins during the luteal phase of primates are insufficient to sustain the development of antral follicles to the preovulatory stages.

In primates, the dominant follicle can be identified during the early or mid-follicular phase of the menstrual cycle (monkey: diZerega &

Hodgen 1981; human McNatty 1981: Gougeon & Lefévre 1983). It is recruited from the population of healthy follicles, 2–3 mm in diameter (class 5, Figs 6.2, 6.3), present during late luteal phase (Gougeon & Lefévre 1983). In humans, during the early follicular phase, the dominant follicle can be identified by size (> 5 mm in diameter), and high mitotic index of its granulosa cells (Gougeon & Lefévre 1983). By mid-follicular phase the dominant follicle reaches 13 mm in diameter and shows an increase in its thecal vascularization, hypertrophy of theca cells and thickening of the granulosa layer. The next nonatretic follicle never exceeds 6 mm in diameter. Presumably the dominant follicle is selected among the several small antral follicles due to its responsiveness to the elevated concentration of FSH in the blood. During this phase, the dominant follicle accumulates high levels of FSH and estradiol in its fluid (McNatty et al 1975, Bomsel-Helmreich et al 1979) and establishes itself as a major source of the circulating estrogen.

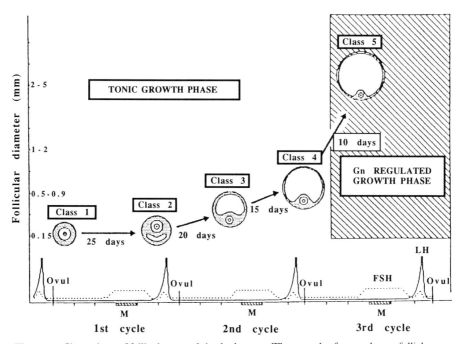

**Fig. 6.3** Chronology of follicular growth in the human. The growth of an ovulatory follicle spans during three subsequent cycles. The time estimated for follicular development through each stage is expressed in days. Ovul, ovulation; M, menstruation. (Reproduced with permission from Gougeon 1990.)

In the human in mid-follicular phase (Day 7) the largest healthy follicle has already established dominance (Baird & Fraser 1975, Baird 1983). Increasing secretion of estradiol causes a reduction of secretion of FSH but not LH (Baird & Fraser 1975, Zeleznik & Kubik 1986). Without exposure to sufficient FSH, granulosa cells of small antral follicles are incapable of aromatizing androstenedione to estradiol (see below) but retain a capacity to metabolize it to dihydrotestosterone (DHT) that inhibits aromatization and estradiol synthesis (Hillier et al 1980, McNatty 1981). As a result, these follicles lose the ability to support their own growth and consequently undergo atresia. At the same time, the dominant follicle develops a certain degree of autonomy. Its theca layer is well developed and is characterized by increased capacity to bind hCG (diZerega & Hodgen 1980, Zeleznik et al 1981). The thecal cells mainly produce androstenedione but also have the ability to secrete estrogen (Channing 1969, Channing & Coudert 1976, McNatty 1981). Granulosa cells of the dominant follicle have a well-developed aromatase activity that enables them to sustain an estrogen-enriched follicular microenvironment despite an increased output of thecal androgen. During mid to late follicular phase the granulosa cells of preovulatory follicles do not seem to require stimulation by FSH in order to metabolize androgen to estrogen (Zeleznik & Kubik 1986), and the capacity of the follicle to produce estrogen is limited only by the amount of aromatizable substrate produced by the theca. Thus the preovulatory follicle gains control of its own development by stimulating its own growth and simultaneously preventing further maturation of other follicles by reducing the levels of circulating FSH.

## Changes in follicular responsiveness to hormones

The hormonal factors involved in follicular development and the changes in follicle cell responsiveness to gonadotropins have been reviewed (Richards 1980, Richards & Hedin 1988). Here, only the major principles involved will be summarized. Initiation of follicle growth is apparently not dependent upon gonadotropic stimulation but is related to an as yet unknown signal, probably of ovarian origin. Thus, gonadotropin deprivation by hypophysectomy or administration of antisera does not prevent growth of preantral follicles, whereas it does prevent the development of antral follicles (Mauléon 1969, Eshkol et al 1970, Nakano et al 1975, Purandare et al 1976, McNeilly et al 1986).

In vitro studies with 1- or 4-day-old rat ovaries seem to indicate that the ovary acquires some degree of steroidogenic activity independently of gonadotropins (Funkenstein et al 1980, Funkenstein & Nimrod 1981). Preantral and small antral follicles are unable to synthesize estradiol. Synthesis of estradiol requires a sustained rise in serum LH and the consequent differentiation of theca cells, including stimulation of androgen synthesis. Theca androgens are then converted to estradiol by the aromatase enzyme system in the granulosa cells. Estradiol, in turn, is obligatory for the differentiation of granulosa cells (Hsueh et al 1984).

It has been shown that theca cells of preantral and antral follicles have receptors for LH and that granulosa cells of most follicles, including small preantral ones, have receptors for FSH. Only in large preovulatory follicles do the granulosa cells also have receptors for LH (Eshkol & Lunenfeld 1972, Presl et al 1972, Channing & Kammerman 1973, Zeleznik et al 1974, Kammerman & Ross 1975, Richards et al 1976, Richards 1980). Preovulatory follicles not only acquire more LH receptors but also are capable of producing more cAMP in response to gonadotropins. Both estradiol and cAMP are key regulators of granulosa cell differentiation, ovulation and luteinization. Action of LH via cAMP on theca and granulosa cells is mediated by cAMP-dependent protein kinases. The regulatory subunit of cAMP-dependent protein kinase type II, a major phosphoprotein of rat preovulatory follicles, is induced in granulosa cells by synergistic actions of estradiol and FSH (Richards et al 1984, Ratoosh et al 1987) and is decreased by LH surge and luteinization (Hedin et al 1987b). Subtle increases in LH and cAMP stimulate $P_{450}$-17$\alpha$ hydroxylase mRNA in the theca leading to an increase in biosynthesis of androstenedione, while the LH surge decreases synthesis of $P_{450}$-17$\alpha$ hydroxylase (Hedin et al 1987c).

In contrast, mRNA for $P_{450}$ side-chain cleavage increases gradually during follicle development and is markedly stimulated by the LH surge and high concentration of cAMP and then appears to be constitutively expressed in corpora lutea (Goldring et al 1986). Thus, it appears that low and high concentrations of cAMP act to turn on or turn off the expression of specific genes at specific times during follicular development.

The development of receptors to LH on granulosa cells seems to have a decisive role in follicle development. Using hypophysectomized immature rats the role of estrogen and FSH in the proliferation of granulosa cells has been demonstrated. Both of these hormones stimulated granulosa cell divisions and their action was additive suggesting action through different intracellular mechanisms (Rao et al 1977). Further, estrogen alone did not increase granulosa cell gonadotropin receptors, but estrogen priming enhanced FSH stimulation of the development of FSH and LH receptors on granulosa cells (Zeleznik et al 1974, Louvet & Vaitukaitis 1976, Richards et al 1976, Ireland & Richards 1978). As already mentioned, in addition to its effect on the increase of granulosa cell LH receptors, FSH enhances granulosa cell aromatizing activity (Armstrong et al 1979).

LH also plays an important role in early follicular development. Thus hCG enhanced the effects of FSH in estrogen-primed hypophysectomized rats (Ireland & Richards 1978). However, the mechanism(s) by which hCG promotes the action of FSH on follicular development remains obscure. Administration of testosterone or estradiol could not replace hCG in this respect (Richards 1978). In the pregnant rat, in the presence of elevated basal FSH, sustained increases in serum LH (but not FSH) support the development of preovulatory follicles (Richards 1980, Bogovich et al 1981). In the mature follicle, receptors for LH are not equally distributed among granulosa cells; mural cells contain more receptors than those close to the antrum (Zeleznik et al 1974, Amsterdam et al 1975). A summary of hormonal control of follicular development was presented by Richards (1978, 1980) and Richards & Hedin (1988).

## Atresia

The term 'atresia' is often used to describe various processes which lead to loss of germ cells from the ovary by means other than ovulation (Ingram 1962, Byskov 1978, Peters & McNatty 1980). These include degeneration of germ cells before folliculogenesis, degeneration of small nongrowing follicles and of growing follicles. It is reasonable to assume that the mechanisms involved in degeneration at these various stages of development are different. Here we will refer only to the degeneration of antral follicles as atresia (Weir & Rowlands 1977).

Only a few of the follicles which start to grow reach ovulation (Table 6.1). The proportion of atretic and healthy follicles is fairly constant during fertile life and varies among species. Thus in the rat 70% of the antral follicles are atretic (Mandl & Zuckerman 1950), in the mouse 50% (Jones 1956), in the rabbit 60% (Pincus & Enzmann 1937) and in the human 50–75% (Block 1951). In several species the percentage of atretic follicles becomes higher with increase in follicle size (Pincus & Enzmann 1937, Vermande-vanEck 1956, Himelstein-Braw et al 1976, Gougeon 1986, 1990; Fig. 6.2).

Consecutive stages of atresia of antral follicles have been described as follows:

*Early atresia (stage I)*, characterized by a small number of granulosa cells with pyknotic nuclei (<10%), usually close to the follicular antrum, while some of the granulosa cells are still in mitosis. This coincides with a reduction in $^3$H-labelled thymidine incorporation by the granulosa cells (Byskov 1974a).

*Stage II of atresia* showing many pyknotic granulosa cells (10–30%), very little if any thymidine incorporation, few cells in mitosis and the follicular antrum containing cell debris. The basement membrane loses its integrity and leukocytes infiltrate the granulosa layers. The oocyte shows meiotic-like changes. At such an advanced stage of atresia the follicle cannot be rescued by PMSG treatment and is doomed to degenerate (Hirshfield 1989).

*Stage III of atresia*, characterized by reduction in the number of granulosa cells, none of them in mitosis, and follicular collapse. The theca is hypertrophied and the cells contain lipid droplets.

Labelled rabbit and sheep atretic follicles have been shown to disappear within 7 days (Hill & White 1933, Smeaton & Robertson 1971). In the mouse it was estimated that it takes 4 days for an antral follicle to reach stage III of atresia (Byskov 1974a).

*Experimental approaches to atresia*

The major problem in studying follicular atresia is the fact that it can be recognized only in retrospect. In order to circumvent this, atresia of large preovulatory follicles was induced in several laboratories by abolishing the surge of gonadotropins either by repeated injections of Nembutal on the day of proestrus and consecutive days, by hypophysectomy on the morning of proestrus, or by administration of antibodies to gonadotropins (Braw & Tsafriri 1980b, Terranova 1980, Uilenbroek et al 1980, Bill & Greenwald 1981). It was found that blocking the preovulatory surge of gonadotropins resulted in an advanced stage of atresia within 3–4 days (Braw & Tsafriri 1980b, Uilenbroek et al 1980), but total deprivation of gonadotropins by hypophysectomy resulted in advanced atresia within 48 h (Braw et al 1981).

Surprisingly, the total steroidogenic activity of atretic follicles is even higher than that of healthy unstimulated follicles (Moor et al 1978, Braw & Tsafriri 1980b, Taya & Greenwald 1980, Terranova 1980, Braw et al 1981). However, the pattern of steroids produced is considerably different in atretic follicles: whereas in healthy preovulatory follicles estrogen is the major steroid secreted prior to and during the first hours after gonadotropic stimulation, progesterone is the major steroid secreted by atretic follicles. Furthermore, sheep, cow and human atretic follicles secrete elevated amounts of both progesterone and androgen, and small amounts of $E_2$, indicating an interference with aromatizing enzymes (Moor et al 1978, Henderson et al 1987). In the rat and in the hamster, on the other hand, 17 : 20 side-chain splitting activity, rather than aromatase, seems to be affected first and only the secretion of progesterone is enhanced, whereas both androgen and estrogen secretion is very low (Braw & Tsafriri 1980b, Uilenbroek et al 1980, Braw et al 1981). In both groups the loss of estrogen secretion by atretic follicles is a common feature.

The mechanisms initiating atresia of antral follicles are not known. Several mechanisms have been suggested: degeneration of theca and reduction of follicular capillary bed restricting the availability of nutrients to the granulosa cells (Hay et al 1976); substances from other growing and atretic follicles (Peters et al 1973); and steroid and protein hormones. Administration of androgens to experimental animals increases the number of atretic follicles (Payne & Runser 1959, Hillier & Ross 1979). Likewise, administration of dihydrotestosterone to immature rats primed with PMSG resulted in a decrease in ovulation rate accompanied with reduction in the number of granulosa cells and aromatase activity in all follicles in the size range between <200 and >400 μm (Conway et al 1990). Furthermore, precocious exposure of follicles to LH also has an atretogenic effect (Louvet et al 1975, Hillier et al 1980). Accordingly, premature induction of LH surge in women results in regression of the dominant follicle (Cargille et al 1973, Friedrich et al 1975). As mentioned above, in rodents prevention of the preovulatory surge of gonadotropins results in the degeneration of the preovulatory follicles. Administration of PMSG prevents the atresia of antral follicles (Peters et al 1975, Braw & Tsafriri 1980a). Injection of PMSG on the morning of estrus prevented atresia of large antral follicles that normally occur between estrus and metestrus (Hirshfield 1986). Similarly PMSG and FSH decrease the number of atretic follicles in bovine and ovine ovaries (Monniaux et al 1984, McNatty et al 1985). These effects of PMSG are mediated, at least in part, by estrogen (Louvet et al 1975). Thus exogenous estrogen reduces the percentage of degenerating follicles and reverses the deleterious effects of dihydrotestosterone (Conway et al 1990). In primates, suppression of gonadotropin secretion during the mid to late follicular phase by exogenous estrogen or follicular fluid results in atresia of antral follicles (diZerega & Hodgen 1981, Zeleznik & Kubik 1986).

*Paracrine hormones and atresia*

Inhibin and activin were originally identified as gonad-derived peptide hormones that modulate FSH secretion from the anterior pituitary. These are TGFβ-related dimeric protein hormones sharing a common β-subunit. Inhibin is a disulfide-linked heterodimer (Ling et al 1985, Miyamoto et al 1985, Rivier et al 1985, Robertson et al 1985) and activin is formed by the dimerization of the inhibin β chains (Ling et al 1986, Vale et al 1986). Injection of human recombinant inhibin into the ovarian bursa of immature rats resulted in an increase in the number of medium-sized antral follicles (350–500 μm in diameter). In contrast, injection of human recombinant activin caused follicular atresia. Moreover, activin prevented the stimulatory action of PMSG on follicular development (Woodruff & Mayo 1990). Inhibin production by granulosa cells is stimulated by gonadotropins in vitro (Bicsak et al 1986) and in vivo (Davis et al 1988). Thus, the effect of gonadotropins on follicular development and atresia may be mediated by the paracrine action of inhibin, activin and most likely other locally produced factors.

## FOLLICULAR FLUID

Follicular fluid (FF) accumulates between granulosa cells of growing follicles; its appearance and the formation of follicular antrum are important markers in follicular development. FF consists of plasma transudate and of follicular secretions like glycosaminoglycans and steroids. Since the blood vessels do not penetrate follicular basement membrane, FF forms the immediate milieu of the granulosa cells and the oocyte. Hence, the contents of FF influence and reflect follicular steroidogenesis, oocyte maturation, ovulation, and transformation to a corpus luteum. A brief description of follicular fluid composition follows. More details may be found in other reviews (McNatty 1978, Guraya 1985, Lipner 1988).

## Physicochemical properties

Follicular fluid is a slightly viscous straw-colored fluid. Its pH is somewhat lower than that of serum or plasma and is mostly controlled by the partial pressure of follicular carbon dioxide ($P_{CO_2}$) (Shalgi et al 1972). Its osmolality is similar or somewhat lower than that of plasma and the high content of coloidal material in the follicular fluid of some farm animals may produce a colloidal osmotic pressure of 21.5 cmH$_2$O (Zachariae 1959). Concentrations of sodium, magnesium, zinc, copper, chloride and inorganic phosphate ions are similar to those of serum (Lutwak-Mann 1954, Olds & VanDemark 1957, Shalgi et al 1972, Schuetz & Anisowicz 1974, Chang et al 1976, Knudsen et al 1978, Knudsen et al 1979), whereas the concentration of potassium ions in FF of women, cows and pigs was found to be higher than that of serum. However, this higher concentration of potassium ions may probably be attributed to release of the ion from degenerating granulosa cells due to postmortem changes during collection and handling of ovaries prior to the aspiration of FF (Knudsen et al 1978, 1979).

## Proteins

The concentration of proteins in FF is similar to or somewhat lower than that in plasma. Proteins of FF are either produced by follicle cells or transudated from the plasma. Most serum proteins have been identified in FF, but at concentrations different from those in plasma. It seems that the size of the molecule is one of the determinants of accumulation in FF. Thus the relative concentrations of serum proteins in FF were found to be inversely related to their molecular weights (Andersen et al 1976, Shalgi et al 1973). This finding led Shalgi et al (1973) to suggest that the follicular membrane functions as a molecular sieve. Apparently, in atretic and cystic follicles this sieving action is impaired; they thus contain higher concentrations of large proteins. However, some of these proteins may originate from degenerating follicle cells and leukocytes (Marion et al 1968). In healthy follicles the concentration of proteins of high molecular weight increases with the follicle's development (Andersen et al 1976).

Many enzymes have been identified in FF and most of them are common also in other tissues (Edwards 1974, Espey 1974, Lipner 1973). However, some enzymes such as collagenase, plasminogen and its activators, proteases and their inhibitors may be involved in follicular rupture (Beers et al 1975, Espey 1978b, see below).

## Proteoglycans (glycosaminoglycans)

Proteoglycans are composed of a core protein to which glycosaminoglycans (GAGs) are covalently attached to form a complex. The GAGs are composed of recurring disaccharide units, each of which contains a derivative of aminohexose, usually D-glucosamine or D-galactosamine. At least one of the two sugars contains an acid carboxylate or sulfate, which make GAGs highly charged polyanions. Holding cations and water within their domain, GAGs confer tissues their resiliency, form solutions of high elasticity and viscosity and stabilize the extracellular matrix. Proteoglycans in FF possess molecular mass estimated between $7.5 \times 10^5$ and $2.5 \times 10^6$ Daltons (Yanagishita & Hascal 1979, Grimek & Ax 1982). This size exceeds the molecular weight cut-off for the blood – follicular barrier (see above), and GAGs are retained within the follicle.

The GAGs chondroitin sulfate and heparan sulfate are the predominant isomers found in follicular fluid of mammals (Jensen & Zachariae 1958, Zachariae 1957, Zachariae & Thorsoe 1966, Ax el al 1985). It seems that the ratio between these two forms of mucopolysaccharides is reponsible for the changes in the viscosity of the fluid. In some species the viscosity of antral fluid is reduced (cow, rat and hamster, reviewed by (Zachariae & Thorsoe 1966) and in others it is increased (human, rhesus monkey; (McNatty et al 1975) as ovulation approaches. Heparin-like anticoagulants were found in the FF of women, sows, cows, bitches and rabbits (Stangroom & Weevers 1962). Anticoagulant activity of the fluid might be important to prevent clotting and entrapping of the ovulated oocyte.

## Gonadotropins and prolactin

The levels of gonadotropins in FF vary with the size of the follicle, its stage of maturation and with the estrous cycle, generally reflecting the circulating blood levels.

FSH has been found to be present in most human antral follicles. During the follicular phase, concomitantly with follicular growth there is an increase in FSH levels in some of the follicles. In the large follicles (>8 mm) FSH levels increased further even when they decreased in plasma. However, FSH levels in FF did not exceed 60% of plasma levels (McNatty et al 1975). LH could not be detected in all the follicles; a greater proportion of large follicles (>8 mm) contained LH than did small ones (<8 mm). Further, LH could be detected only in follicles also containing FSH, and LH did not exceed 30% of plasma level (McNatty et al 1975). Prolactin was always detected in FF and its levels were highly variable: much lower (8%) or higher (180%) than in plasma. Prolactin concentration was highest in small follicles and it decreased with follicular growth (McNatty et al 1975).

## Steroids

The steroidogenic activity of antral follicles is remarkably high and hence the concentration of some steroids in FF reaches levels which are 40 000–100 000-fold higher than in plasma. The follicles contain progestins, androgens and estrogens (Edwards 1974, McNatty et al 1975, 1976). Follicular steroid content, and mainly the ratio of follicular androgen to estrogen, is an important indicator of follicular activity and the prospect of its reaching ovulation (McNatty et al 1979). Thus, in women most antral follicles contain more androgen than estrogen and only the few having more estrogen than androgen continue to mature. In sheep, on the other hand, most antral follicles have more estrogen than androgens and more follicles grow and mature than in women (Peters & McNatty 1980).

## Other hormones and growth factors

In recent years our concepts of endocrine regulation have been widely broadened to include, in addition to blood-borne chemical messengers, also paracrine and autocrine (see Tsafriri et al

1988) and even intracrine (O'Malley 1989) hormones. Such local regulation plays an important, yet not fully appreciated, role in ovarian function. The FF is rich in many such hormones or factors, some of them known also from other tissues and some acting also as classical hormones. This area is the subject of very active research and cannot be exhaustively reviewed here. More details can be found in several reviews (Tsafriri et al 1988, Vale et al 1986, Ying 1988, Adashi et al 1989, Hsueh et al 1989, May & Schomberg 1989, de Jong et al 1990, Findlay et al 1990b, and proceedings of meetings Fujii & Channing 1982, Channing & Segal 1982, Sairam & Atkinson 1984, Franchimont 1986, Burger et al 1987, Hodgen et al 1988, Hirshfield 1989). Of the inhibin- or TGFβ-related proteins, inhibin, with FSH-suppressing activity and activin, with FSH-stimulating activity, were isolated from follicular fluid (Vale et al 1988, Ying 1988, Findlay et al 1990b). Another polypeptide, though structurally unrelated to the TGFβ family, follistatin—with FSH release suppressing activity—was also isolated from follicular fluid (Robertson et al 1987, Ueno et al 1987). Follistatin has recently been shown to have activin- and inhibin-binding activity and its pituitary and gonadal actions may be related to binding of activin or inhibin (Nakamura et al 1990, Kogawa et al 1991, Shimonaka et al 1991). The possible role of these factors is discussed in the section dealing with follicular development and atresia (see p 112) and oocyte maturation (see p 119).

TGFβ is secreted by the interstitial-thecal cell of rat, bovine and porcine ovaries (Bendell & Dorrington 1988, Hernandez et al 1990, Skinner et al 1987). TGFβ modifies FSH and other hormone actions on granulosa cells (reviewed by Knecht et al 1989) and inhibits interstitial-thecal cell androgen production (Magoffin et al 1989, Hernandez et al 1990). TGFβ action on oocyte maturation will be discussed below (see p 119).

Epidermal growth factor (EGF), originally identified in extracts of mouse submaxillary glands and shown to induce proliferation of skin epithelial cells (Levi-Montalcini & Cohen 1960) and tumor growth factor α(TGFα), detected through decrease in EGF binding in sarcoma virus-induced cell transformation (Todaro et al

1976), bind to the same receptor and elicit similar responses (Derynck 1986).

EGF-like activity has been detected in porcine follicular fluid (Hsu et al 1987) and TGFα and its message were expressed in theca cells (Kudlow et al 1987, Skinner & Coffey 1988). Many and diverging actions of EGF were observed, including stimulation of granulosa cell proliferation (Bendell & Dorrington 1990) and inhibition of FSH stimulation of aromatase activity and induction of LH receptors (reviewed by May & Schomberg 1989). In addition, EGF (Dekel & Sherizly 1985) and TGFα (Tsafriri & Hsueh 1989) induced the resumption of meiosis in follicle-enclosed oocytes. Thus, EGF/TGFα may play an important role in regulation of ovarian function.

Insulin-like growth factors (IGFs) can be divided into two distinct groups: basic IGF or IGF-I (identical to somatomedin C) and neutral IGFs or IGF-II (its murine equivalent formerly referred to as multiplication stimulating activity—MSA) (Adashi et al 1989). IGF-I content of porcine FF of large follicles exceeded that of serum or that of small follicles, suggesting its local production (Hammond et al 1988). Recently, evidence for granulosa cell production, reception and action of IGF-I (or II) as well as for theca-interstitial cell IGF reception and action has been presented. In general, IGF-I seems to amplify gonadotropin action on follicular development, probably via coordination of granulosa-theca cell cooperation and thus effecting follicular selection (Adashi et al 1989).

Fibroblast growth factors (FGFs) have been originally identified in pituitary and brain extracts (Esch et al 1985). Two different forms of FGF, basic and acidic, have been identified based on their isoelectric points (Gospodarowicz et al 1985, Baird & Hsueh 1986). The two forms of FGF have 55% amino acid sequence homology and share the same receptor, but basic FGF (bFGF) has higher biopotency than acidic FGF (aFGF). By reverse transcription-polymerase chain reaction ovarian expression of basic and acidic FGF was demonstrated (Koos & Olson 1989, Koos & Seidel 1989. Bovine granulosa cells in culture produce bioactive FGF and express the bFGF gene (Neufeld et al 1987).

bFGF is mitogenic for bovine and porcine granulosa cells (Gospodarowicz & Bialecki 1979, Gospodarowicz et al 1977a, 1977b). In rat granulosa cells bFGF binding sites were demonstrated (Baird et al 1989) and in vitro bFGF inhibited FSH stimulation of estrogen production, but enhanced progesterone secretion at low doses of FSH (Baird & Hsueh 1986). Furthermore, bFGF stimulated granulosa cell tissue type plasminogen activator (t-PA) expression, follicular PGE synthesis and induced the maturation of follicle-enclosed oocytes (LaPolt et al 1990). Thus FGFs may play an important role in regulation of ovarian function.

Besides the growth factors known from other organs, additional putative paracrine and autocrine factors were described in FF (reviewed by Tsafriri et al 1988). The current status of oocyte maturation inhibitor (OMI) will be described below (see p 118).

## OVULATORY CHANGES

The preovulatory surge of gonadotropins induces a series of changes in various follicular compartments culminating in the release of a fertilizable ovum and in the transformation of the follicle into a corpus luteum. The preovulatory surge of gonadotropins includes both LH and FSH and exogenous immunopurified (Tsafriri et al 1976a) or human recombinant FSH (Galway et al 1990) can induce the ovulatory response. However, since administration of an antibody directed towards the β-subunit of LH to proestrus rats prevented the ovulatory response, it was concluded that, at least in the rat, the amount of FSH normally secreted during the proestrus surge is inadequate to induce ovulation by itself (Tsafriri et al 1976a). Some of the changes occurring in the preovulatory follicle are described below.

### Luteinization

Luteinization of the preovulatory follicle is defined by morphological changes, such as cell hyperplasia and accumulation of lipid droplets, and functionally, by enhanced production of progesterone (Rondell 1974, Channing & Tsafriri

1977, Channing 1980, Hillensjö 1981, Gore-Langton & Armstrong 1988). The salient features of follicular steroidogenesis (Fig. 6.4) and of the changes associated with ovulation will be outlined.

The pioneering study of Falck (1959) suggested the interdependence of granulosa and theca cells in follicular estrogen production. However, only later studies revealed the exact role of these two cell types in follicular steroidogenesis. Thus, culturing separately hamster granulosa cells and thecal tissue established that theca cells favor androgen production and granulosa cells aromatization (Makris & Ryan 1975). This concept was supported by similar studies in the rabbit (Erickson & Ryan 1975, 1976), rat (Dorrington et al 1975, Fortune & Armstrong 1977), and sheep (Moor 1977), and led to the 'two-cell, two-gonadotropin' concept of ovarian steroidogenesis, namely that thecal tissue is stimulated by LH to produce androgen, which when transported to the granulosa cell compartment can be converted through FSH-induced aromatization, to estrogens.

In addition to interstitial – theca and granulosa cell synergism in estrogen production, evidence has been presented for similar synergism between the two cell types in thecal androgen production (Batta et al 1980, Makris & Ryan 1980, McNatty et al 1980, Armstrong et al 1981, Lischinsky & Armstrong 1983). Likewise, theca – granulosa cooperation is also involved in progesterone synthesis in the human (Batta et al 1980, McNatty et al 1980).

The changes in follicular steroidogenesis associated with the ovulatory stimulus were studied extensively in the rat and found to be mediated by enhanced follicular cAMP formation (Lindner et al 1974, Marsh 1976). It was shown that rat follicles explanted prior to the preovulatory surge of gonadotropins and cultured in a hormone-free medium produce predominantly estradiol and only low amounts of androgens and progestins. Exposure to LH in vivo or in vitro resulted in an overall stimulation of follicular steroidogenesis within 1–2 h. After 4–6 h of culture, production of androgens and estrogen levelled off, whereas secretion of progesterone remained at a higher rate (Tsafriri et al 1973, Lindner et al 1974,

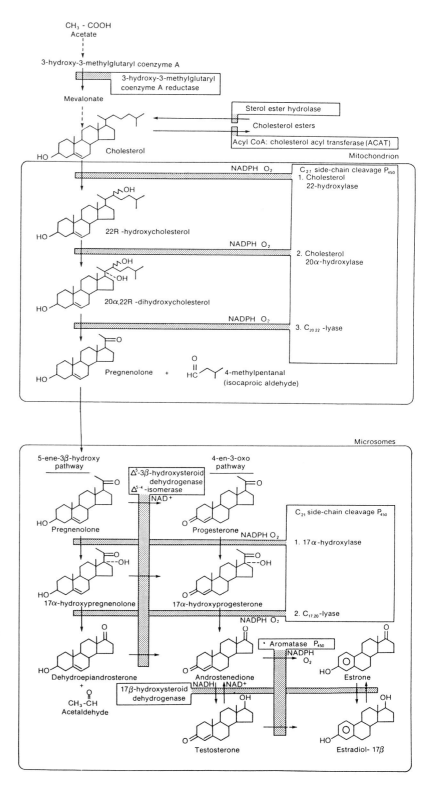

**Fig. 6.4** The principal biosynthetic pathways in the ovary for production of the progestins, androgens and estrogens. Cholesterol may be synthesized de novo from acetate or derived from preformed sources. The metabolism of cholesterol to the sex steroids is carried out sequentially by several enzyme systems, each with several catalytic functions. Thus, the conversion of cholesterol to androgens involves three enzyme systems: cholesterol ($C_{27}$-sterol) side-chain cleavage P-450, $C_{21}$-steroid side-chain cleavage P-450, and $\Delta$-3$\beta$-hydroxysteroid dehydrogenase: $\Delta^{5-4}$ isomerase. Subsequent conversion of $C_{19}$-steroids to estrogens is carried out by aromatase P-450 enzyme(s). The enzyme systems are distributed in different subcellular sites as indicated. (Reproduced with permission from Gore-Langton & Armstrong 1988.)

Hillensjö et al 1976, Hillensjö et al 1977, Goff & Henderson 1979). Addition of actinomycin D, at a dose selectively inhibiting RNA synthesis, suppresses the LH-stimulated progesterone synthesis but enhances follicular estrogen production (Tsafriri et al 1973, Lieberman et al 1975). This may indicate that the preovulatory decline in follicular estrogen production is dependent on follicular protein synthesis. Since the decline in estrogen production is accompanied by a fall in androgen, it was suggested that the LH surge suppresses the 17:20-side-chain cleavage enzymes (Lindner et al 1974). Indeed, inhibition of 17:20-side-chain cleavage enzymes has been demonstrated (Hamberger et al 1978, Suzuki & Tamaoki 1979). Similarly, addition of testosterone to rat follicles previously exposed to LH restored estradiol production, suggesting that aromatase was not affected (Hillensjö et al 1977). Similar changes in follicular steroid synthesis have been observed in the sheep (Moor 1973, Seamark et al 1974, Hay & Moor 1975a), rabbit (Mills & Savard 1973, Patwardhan & Lanthier 1976, Bahr et al 1980), hamster (Roy & Greenwald, 1987), the rhesus monkey (diZerega & Hodgen 1981) and the human (Fowler et al 1978, Mori et al 1978).

## Oocyte maturation

In the human the number of germ cells reaches its peak (approximately 7 million) during the 6th month of embryonic life (Baker 1963). Mitoses of germ cells cease at that time and due to degeneration at birth only 1 million oocytes survive and their number is further reduced during prepubertal and pubertal life (Block 1951, Baker 1963).

The meiotic process is initiated in mammals during prenatal life or shortly after birth (Fig. 6.1). The oocyte reaches the diplotene stage of prophase just before or immediately after birth. At this stage, by a mechanism yet not fully understood, the meiotic process is arrested (*first meiotic arrest*). In murid rodents, the chromosomes decondense, so that they disappear from view under light microscope and resume their transcriptive activity. The oocyte, having a prominent nucleus, referred to as *germinal vesicle (GV)*, enters the *dictyate* or *diffuse diplotene stage*, in which it may persist throughout infancy and a variable period beyond the onset of puberty. During fertile life, at each estrous cycle a number of oocytes characteristic of the species resume their meiotic process after the preovulatory surge of gonadotropins. Resumption of meiosis includes chromatin condensation, disintegration of the nuclear membrane, usually referred to as *germinal vesicle breakdown (GVB)* and the abstriction of the first polar body shortly before ovulation. At ovulation, a fertilizable secondary oocyte arrested at the metaphase of the second meiotic division (*second meiotic arrest*) is released. In most mammals, fertilization occurs at the metaphase of the second meiotic division. In these species, oocytes that did not reach this stage usually cannot be penetrated by the spermatozoa or, if penetration does occur, the sperm nucleus fails to be transformed into a sperm pronucleus (Iwamatsu & Chang 1972, Barros & Munoz 1973, Niwa & Chang 1975, Usui & Yanagimachi 1976).

Several reviews on meiotic maturation are available (Thibault 1977, Tsafriri 1978, Eppig & Downs 1984, Tsafriri & Pomerantz 1984, Schuetz 1985, Tsafriri & Pomerantz 1986, Thibault et al 1987, Dekel et al 1988, Tsafriri et al 1991a). Here some of the mechanisms involved in the control of meiotic maturation in mammals will be reviewed. For in vitro maturation of human oocytes, see Chapter 21.

Two dissimilar in vitro models have been developed for investigating meiotic maturation in mammals. The simplest is the one established by Pincus & Enzmann (1935) who demonstrated that rabbit oocytes liberated from their follicles undergo spontaneous maturation in culture without hormonal stimulation. Such spontaneous maturation of oocytes, denuded from their enveloping cumulus cells or within their cumulus complex, has been described in all mammalian species examined (reviewed by Biggers 1972, Tsafriri 1978) and is widely employed for studying certain physiological aspects of oocyte maturation. However, this model does not represent the physiological events since: (a) in vivo oocyte maturation is clearly dependent upon the preovulatory surge of gonadotropins (reviewed by Lindner et al 1974, Tsafriri 1978); (b) with the exception of murids, only a very low percentage of oocytes matured in this way are capable for normal fertilization and subsequent embryonic development (Thibault 1977, Staigmiller & Moor 1984, Mattioli et al 1988a,b).

In the second model, consisting of explanted preovulatory follicles, resumption of meiosis is dependent upon hormonal stimulation (Neal & Baker 1973, Thibault & Gerard 1973, Moor & Trounson 1977, Tsafriri et al 1972, Thibault 1977, Mattioli et al 1988a,b, Meinecke & Meinecke–Tillman 1981). Hormonal stimulation of explanted follicles was found to result in mature fertilizable oocytes, and subsequent to fertilization a high percentage of the ova transferred to foster mothers developed into normal young in the rabbit (Thibault et al 1975a,b) and in the sheep (Moor & Trounson 1977). This model permitted the analysis of some of the mechanisms involved in the hormonal induction of meiosis: the role of gonadotropins, steroids, prostaglandins, cyclic AMP, intercellular junctions, macromolecular synthesis and follicular energy metabolism. However, being a multicompartmental model it does not permit the localization of the primary site of gonadotropin action on resumption of meiosis or the analysis of the cascade of events involved in this response.

*Follicular regulation of oocyte maturation*

**Inhibition of meiosis by granulosa cells** The spontaneous maturation of isolated oocytes led Pincus & Enzmann (1935) to suggest that, within the follicle, nuclear maturation is inhibited by a follicular product. This suggestion was supported by the finding that meiosis was inhibited in porcine oocytes by coculture with segments of follicle wall, provided that they included healthy granulosa cells, or with granulosa cells. By contrast, the theca layer only (Foote & Thibault 1969, Tsafriri & Channing 1975) or ovarian bursa (Leibfried & First 1980b) failed to suppress the spontaneous maturation. Likewise, meiosis was prevented in porcine oocytes transferred to host follicles (up to 12 oocytes/follicle) and cultured in hormone-free medium (Meinecke & Meinecke-Tillman 1981, Fleming et al 1985). Furthermore, coculture of porcine oocytes with porcine granulosa cells (Tsafriri & Channing

1975, Sato & Ishibashi 1977) or extroverted follicles (Mattioli et al 1986) inhibited their spontaneous maturation, the degree of inhibition depending upon granulosa cell number. Addition of rat oocytes to rat granulosa cells previously cultured for 24 or 48 h, suppressed the resumption of meiosis. This inhibitory effect of rat granulosa cells was reversed by the addition of LH (5 μg/ml) to the cocultures (Fig. 6.5; Tsafriri et al 1977, 1979). Likewise, the spontaneous maturation of bovine oocytes was suppressed by coculture with granulosa cells (Sirard & Bilodeau 1990a,b).

Extracts of granulosa cells, as well as medium in which granulosa cells had been previously cultured, inhibited the resumption of meiosis (Tsafriri et al 1976b, Sato & Ishibashi 1977). Collectively, these results suggest that within the follicle meiosis is kept in abeyance by an oocyte maturation inhibitor (OMI) produced by the granulosa cells.

**OMI** Follicular fluid (FF) from ovaries of rabbit, ovine, bovine, porcine, hamster and human origin was found to exert an inhibitory effect upon the spontaneous maturation of isolated oocyte (Fig. 6.5; Chang 1955, Tsafriri & Channing 1975, Gwatkin & Anderson 1976, Jagiello et al 1977, Tsafriri et al 1977, Hillensjö et al 1978). This inhibitory effect is not species specific; thus human FF inhibited the maturation of porcine (Hillensjö et al 1978) and rat (Hillensjö et al 1981a) oocytes, bovine FF inhibited hamster oocytes (Gwatkin & Andersen 1976) and porcine FF inhibited the maturation of rat oocytes (Tsafriri el al 1977). The OMI activity in porcine FF appears to decline in the course of follicular growth (Stone et al 1978, Van de Wiel et al 1983).

**The chemical nature of OMI** OMI activity has been partially purified and characterized (for review see Channing et al 1982, Channing & Segal 1982). It appears to be a peptide of less than 2000 Dalton (Tsafriri et al 1976b, Stone et al 1978, Pomerantz et al 1979, Tsafriri & Pomerantz 1986, Tsafriri et al 1991a). OMI from bovine FF (Gwatkin & Anderson 1976) appears to have similar properties. However, definitive isolation and chemical characterization of OMI are still to be accomplished.

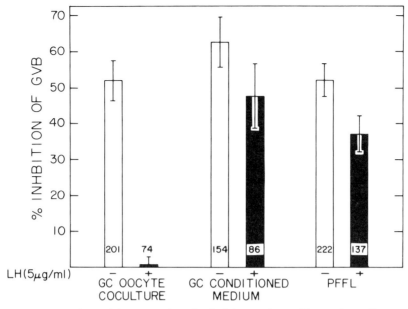

**Fig. 6.5**  Inhibition of the resumption of meiosis by coculture with granulosa cells, granulosa cell-conditioned medium and the low molecular weight fraction of porcine follicular fluid. Rat oocytes were added to dishes in which granulosa cells (GC, $10^6/0.2$ ml) had been cultured for 24 h (GC-oocyte coculture), to a medium obtained after culture of GC ($10^6$/ml) of 48 h (GC-conditioned medium) or in the presence of the low molecular weight fraction of porcine follicular fluid (PFFL). The oocytes were cultured for 6 h with (black columns) or without (white columns) added LH (5 μg/ml). Vertical brackets, s.e. (mean). The number of oocytes examined is indicated. (Modified with permisson from Tsafriri & Bar Ami 1982)

Recent studies have implicated transforming growth factor-β (TGF-β) and inhibin-related proteins, inhibin, activin and anti-Müllerian hormone (AMH; also related to as Müllerian-inhibiting factor — MIF) in the regulation of oocyte maturation. In our hands, none of the hormones tested, TGF-β, inhibin, activin and AMH, inhibited the spontaneous maturation of rat oocytes in vitro (Tsafriri & Hsueh 1989, Tsafriri et al 1988, 1991b). Thus, we could not confirm the observations that inhibin (O et al 1989) or AMH (Takahashi et al 1086, Ueno et al 1988) have OMI-like activity. It should be noted, however, that the concentrations of inhibin tested by us (due to limited supply) were lower than the $ED_{50}$ (40 nM or 120 ng/ml) reported later to be effective (O et al 1989).

A most promising clue for the identification of OMI was provided by the observations of Buscaglia and his colleagues (1989). They reported that the 35-kDa form of porcine follis-tatin (FS — an ovarian glycoprotein suppressing pituitary cell FSH secretion), but not the C-terminal truncated 32-kDa form, exerted OMI-like activity on rat and mouse oocytes. Moreover, the addition of an antibody against the C-terminal of 35-kDa FS (27 amino acid peptide) prevented the OMI-like activity of FS and of porcine follicular fluid. In our hands the 35-kDa FS, as well as the 27 amino acid peptide, had no demonstrable OMI activity. Nevertheless, we did confirm the ability of the antiserum against the C-terminal peptide of FS to abolish the inhibitory action of partially purified OMI preparations of porcine follicular fluid on maturation of rat oocytes. While we cannot say whether follicular OMI is derived from the C-terminal of FS, the cross-reaction between the antiserum towards the 27 amino acids fragment of FS and OMI from porcine follicular fluid offers a unique opportunity to purify the elusive OMI (Tsafriri et al 1991b). Furthermore, in view of the recent demonstration that FS has activin- and inhibin-binding activity (Nakamura et al 1990, Kogawa et al 1991,

Shimonaka et al 1991), it is possible that the stimulatory activity of high concentrations of activin (Itoh et al 1990) on meiotic maturation is related to its binding to FS.

On the basis of studies with mouse oocytes, hypoxanthine was found to exert OMI-like activity. Hypoxanthine and possibly other purines were, therefore, suggested to be responsible for OMI activity of porcine FF (Downs et al 1985, 1986, Eppig et al 1985). Hypoxanthine or adenosine were not detected in bovine FF, in spite of its OMI activity. Furthermore, bovine oocytes showed only limited sensitivity to purines (Sirard & First 1988, Sirard & Bilodeau 1990b).

Purine bases were demonstrated to modulate oocyte levels of cAMP, most probably by inhibiting cAMP-phosphodiesterase activity (Downs & Eppig 1987, Downs et al 1989). Furthermore, microinjection of an inhibitor of cAMP-dependent protein kinase (PKI) induced the resumption of meiosis in oocytes cultured in a medium containing hypoxanthine or guanosine (Downs et al 1989). It seems, therefore, that purines affect resumption of meiosis by raising oocytes cAMP to levels inhibitory for meiosis (see 'Role of cAMP in the regulation of meiosis', below). Such action of purine bases does not exclude the possibility of other follicular factors suppressing in parallel the resumption of meiosis. Indeed, Downs et al (1985) observed an additional inhibitory fraction in porcine FF which was not removed by charcoal extraction. The relative resistance of OMI activity to proteolysis, in some of the studies, cannot be taken as conclusive evidence that OMI is not a peptide. A small peptide may be a very poor substrate for proteases and/or the appropriate sensitive peptide bond may not be present. Hence the final identification of OMI as a purine base or a peptide must await confirmation in several mammalian test systems. Of course, the coexistence of follicular mechanisms suppressing meiosis by a peptide and by purine base(s) is a possibility which cannot be dismissed at the present.

***Physiological significance of OMI*** The inhibitory action of a porcine OMI preparation can be reversed by change of medium after 24 h incubation with the inhibitor (Stone et al 1978, Hillensjö et al 1979a,b) or by the addition of an antibody prepared against the OMI fraction (Tsafriri et al 1979). Thus, the inhibition of maturation of OMI appears not to be due to a toxic effect.

In vivo or in follicle-enclosed oocytes in vitro, resumption of meiosis is induced by LH. Hence the ability of LH to overcome the inhibition of meiosis by FF, by coculture with granulosa cells or by granulosa cell-conditioned medium, lends support to the view that OMI may have a physiological role in the regulation of meiosis (Mattioli et al 1988a,b, Gwatkin & Andersen 1976, Tsafriri et al 1977, 1979, Tsafriri & Channing 1975).

The cumulus cells appear to have an important role in the regulation of meiosis. Whereas OMI from porcine FF inhibited the resumption of meiosis of oocytes cultured within their intact cumuli, it did not interfere with the maturation of totally denuded pig (Hillensjö et al 1979b) or rat (Tsafriri & Bar-Ami 1982) oocytes. It appears, therefore, that OMI exerts its inhibitory action upon meiosis not directly on the oocyte, but through the mediation of the cumulus cells.

Some investigators were unable to demonstrate OMI activity in follicular preparations. Granulosa cells did not inhibit maturation of cow, sow or ewe oocytes, whereas FF showed such activity (Jagiello et al 1977). By contrast, Sato and coauthors (Sato & Ishibashi 1977, Sato & Koide 1984) found porcine follicular fluid to be inactive, whereas coculture with granulosa cells inhibited resumption of meiosis. Leibfried & First (1980a,b) found bovine and porcine FF as well as granulosa cells to be inactive, but coculture with follicle hemisections prevented meiosis and this was overcome by addition of LH. However in a later study from the same laboratory, bovine FF inhibited the maturation of bovine oocytes (Sirard & First 1988). These discrepant findings may be related, at least in part, to low OMI activity of follicular fluid and of granulosa cell cultures, the finding that fluid and granulosa cells from large follicles are devoid of OMI activity, instability of OMI, and differences in the methods of oocytes collection and culture.

In conclusion, there seems to be little doubt that the somatic cells of the follicle exert control over the resumption of meiosis in mammals, but the detailed mechanism is still subject to further investigation. Whereas in preantral follicles the oocytes are still incompetent to resume meiosis (Bar-Ami & Tsafriri 1981), it seems that in antral follicles, meiosis is prevented by local paracrine factors produced by granulosa and cumulus cells. Both the yet unidentified peptide OMI and hypoxanthine fulfil several of the criteria of physiological regulators of meiosis. Further studies are needed in order to determine their precise role in the regulation of oocyte maturation and these must await for full chemical identification of OMI.

***In vitro maturation of follicle-enclosed oocytes*** When preovulatory follicles are explanted from adult cycling PMSG-treated immature rats on the day of proestrus into hormone-free medium, the behavior of the oocytes depends upon the time of follicle isolation. Oocytes explanted before 1400 h, i.e before the preovulatory surge of gonadotropins, remain in the dictyate stage throughout a 24-h culture period. On the other hand, in follicles explanted later on the afternoon of the same day, following the gonadotropin surge, the oocytes resume meiosis in culture (Ayalon et al 1972, Hillensjö 1976). Explantation of follicles prior to the endogenous surge of gonadotropins allowed us to study the hormonal induction of meiosis in vitro. LH, hCG, FSH and $PGE_2$ all triggered the resumption of meiosis in such follicle-enclosed oocytes (Hillensjö 1976, Tsafriri et al 1972).

Resumption of meiosis was also induced by gonadotropins in cultured follicle-enclosed oocytes of sheep (Hay & Moor 1973, Miller & Jagiello 1973, Moor & Trounson 1977), cow (Thibault et al 1975a,b), pig (Gerard et al 1979, Meinecke & Meinecke-Tillman 1981), rabbit (Thibault & Gerard 1973) and hamster (Gwatkin & Andersen 1976).

***Role of cAMP in the regulation of meiosis*** Many of the agents inducing the resumption of meiosis in follicle-enclosed oocytes in vitro also stimulate the production of cAMP (Tsafriri et al 1972, Lindner et al 1974, Hillensjö 1976). Indeed, injection of the cAMP derivative dibutyryl cAMP (dbcAMP) into the follicular antrum (Tsafriri et al 1972) or a transient exposure of follicles to 8-bromo-cAMP (Hillensjö et al 1978), dbcAMP or isobutylmethylxanthine

(IBMX) (Dekel et al 1981) all triggered the resumption of meiosis. By contrast, the continuous presence of cAMP derivatives or inhibitors of phosphodiesterase prevented LH-triggered resumption of meiosis in follicle-enclosed oocytes (Lindner et al 1974, Hillensjö et al 1978, Dekel et al 1981). Derivatives or stimulators (forskolin) of cAMP and inhibitors of phosphodiesterase also inhibited the spontaneous maturation of isolated oocytes (Cho et al 1974, Hillensjö 1976, Hillensjö et al 1976, 1978, Dekel & Beers 1978, 1980, Dekel et al 1984, Vivarelli et al 1983, Racowsky 1984, 1985).

It seems, therefore, that whereas cAMP is probably involved in the mediation of the meiosis-inducing action of LH in the somatic cell compartment, elevated cAMP levels within the oocyte inhibit the resumption of meiosis. It was suggested, therefore, that cAMP may serve as a physiological inhibitor of meiosis in the mammalian oocyte (Lindner et al 1974, Dekel & Beers 1978, Moor et al 1980, Dekel et al 1981, Dekel & Sherizly 1983, Sherizly et al 1988). Indeed, in mouse and rat oocytes a decrease in cAMP preceded resumption of meiosis (Aberdam et al 1987, Schultz et al 1983). This decrease apparently occurred before or during the time in which follicle and cumulus cell cAMP levels was increasing (Schultz et al 1983). Likewise, incubation of rat oocytes with an invasive adenylate cyclase from bacteria of the genus *Bordatella*, elevated oocyte cAMP levels and inhibited the resumption of meiosis, while removal of the enzyme resulted in a drop of oocyte cAMP levels and resumption of meiosis (Aberdam et al 1987, Dekel et al 1985). These results support the notion that elevated levels of oocyte cAMP maintain meiotic arrest and that an intra-oocyte drop in cAMP allows the resumption of meiosis.

The dual role of cAMP in the regulation of oocyte maturation was elegantly demonstrated recently by Dekel et al (1988). Inhibition of resumption of meiosis in follicle-enclosed ova stimulated by LH or in cumulus-enclosed ova maturing spontaneously was achieved by continuous culture in the presence of IBMX ($ED_{50}$ = 0.03 mM) or dibutyryl cAMP ($ED_{50}$ = 5.0 mM). By contrast, induction of ovum maturation in follicle-enclosed oocytes was achieved by transient exposure to IBMX ($ED_{50}$ = 0.13 mM) or dibutyryl cAMP ($ED_{50}$ = 25 mM). Thus, the induction of maturation is achieved by much higher concentrations of the phosphodiesterase inhibitor or the cyclic nucleotide analogue. These findings show that basal sustained levels of follicular cAMP maintain meiotic arrest, while a LH-stimulated surge of the nucleotide is required to exert the maturation-inducing action of the hormone.

### Role of cumulus-oocyte communication
In immature oocytes the cumulus cells are closely apposed to the zona pellucida which is studded with numerous cytoplasmic projections, whereas the cumulus cells encircling mature oocytes are loosely organized and very few projections remain in the zona pellucida (Zamboni 1972, Szöllösi 1975, Szöllösi et al 1978). Also, ionic coupling and transfer of molecules are maximal before gonadotropic stimulation and decrease gradually afterwards (Gilula et al 1978, Dekel et al 1981, Sherizly et al 1988). These findings led to the hypothesis that the release of the oocyte from follicular suppression of meiosis is the result of breakdown of cumulus – oocyte communication, possibly induced by the ovulatory hormone (Lindner et al 1974, Dekel & Beers 1978, Gilula et al 1978, Dekel et al 1981). The influence of LH on resumption of meiosis may be secondary to its action on the sequestration of the oocyte. However, several of the early observations seemed incompatible with this suggestion. Thus, the disruption of oocyte – cumulus cell communication followed, rather than preceded, germinal vesicle breakdown. This was inferred from the observed reduction of the transport of choline or uridine to ovine, mouse, porcine and rat oocytes (Moor et al 1980, Eppig 1982), and from the termination of ionic coupling of the cumulus and the oocyte (Dekel et al 1981).

Later studies demonstrated that transfer of amino acids (Colonna & Mangia 1983) and uridine (Salustri & Siracusa 1983) to the oocyte is linearly dependent on their uptake by cumulus cells. Indeed when relative uptake was examined, there was a strict correlation between the resumption of meiosis and oocyte–cumulus uncoupling in mouse oocytes (Salustri & Siracusa 1983).

Furthermore, when rat follicle-enclosed oocytes were examined at various time intervals after LH/hCG stimulation, a 50% reduction in uridine uptake was observed already 1 h after the hormonal stimulus, when intact GV is still present in almost all oocytes (Sherizly et al 1988). Similarly, a reduction in oocyte – cumulus dye and metabolic coupling was observed in hamster oocytes concomitantly with GVB (Racowsky & Satterlie 1985). Also, when resumption of meiosis was triggered by EGF, oocyte – cumulus communication was reduced prior to GVB in rat follicle-enclosed oocytes (Dekel & Sherizly 1985).

Quantitative analysis of freeze-fractured rat cumulus – oocyte complexes revealed a dramatic decrease in the net area of cumulus gap junctions following the ovulatory stimulus and prior to GVB (Larsen et al 1986), thus providing a structural basis for the observed reduction in cumulus – oocyte communication. An additional consideration regarding oocyte-follicle cell communication was raised in a study by Motlik et al (1986). Examination of the changes in the association between cumulus oophorus and mural granulosa cells in follicles from PMSG, hCG-treated pigs revealed deposition of mucous matrix already 16 h after hCG stimulation, prior to GVB which occurs only 20–24 h after hCG. The importance of mural granulosa–cumulus coupling in regulation of meiosis has been suggested already by Foote & Thibault (1969). Recently, Racowsky et al (1989) observed a significant and progressive decrease in gap junction area in the membrana granulosa underlying the cumulus cell stalk with an increasing percentage of oocytes committed to mature after stimulation of ovulation by hCG in the hamster.

Collectively, these findings are compatible with the suggested communication of an inhibitory signal from the somatic cell compartment of the follicle to the oocyte. The rate of transfer of the inhibitory signal may be modulated at several points: oocyte – cumulus, cumulus – cumulus or cumulus – mural granulosa or even granulosa – granulosa cell junctions. At present, there is sufficient evidence supporting the transfer of cAMP to the oocyte (Dekel 1988). Further studies are required to determine whether other regulators of meiosis are transmitted to the ovum or their effect is exerted at the level of follicular somatic cell compartment.

### Maturation of the cumulus oophorus

The cells of the cumulus oophorus, namely the few layers of cells enclosing the oocyte, undergo characteristic changes following the preovulatory surge of gonadotropins. These include morphological changes, such as cellular dispersion (Blandau 1955), withdrawal of cumulus cell processes and transversing the zona pellucida (Zamboni 1976), which result in breakdown of cumulus cell – oocyte communication (Eppig 1980, Moor et al 1980, Dekel et al 1981, Phillips & Dekel 1991) and appearance of pseudopodia-like processes. Biochemical changes include synthesis of mucopolysaccarides (Eppig 1979a,b) and specifically hyaluronic acid (Salustri et al 1989), increased production of lactate (Billig et al 1983) and progestins (Hillensjö & Channing 1980, Hillensjö 1981, Hillensjö et al 1981b) and decrease in oxygen consumption (Dekel et al 1976, Magnusson et al 1977, Magnusson & Hillensjö 1981). FSH, but not LH, induced mucification and hyaluronic acid synthesis in mouse cumulus complexes in vitro (Eppig 1979a,b). Similarly, FSH was more effective than LH in enhancing progesterone synthesis by rat cumuli in culture (Hillensjö et al 1982). This hormone specificity is probably not physiologically important, since in vivo or in vitro LH is equally effective in inducing maturational changes in the follicle-enclosed cumuli (Hillensjö 1976, Hillensjö et al 1976, Eppig 1980).

The possible involvement of cumulus cells in the regulation of meiosis is discussed above. It should be noted that hyaluronic acid synthesis by cumulus cells is stimulated by an oocyte factor(s) (Buccione et al 1990, Salustri et al 1989, 1990). Nevertheless, since most of the carefully examined maturational changes in the cumulus follow, rather than precede, resumption of meiosis (Dekel et al 1981, Eppig 1980, Moor et al 1980, Leibfried & First 1982), it does not seem likely that any of these changes serves as a signal for the resumption of meiosis. Furthermore, the physiological role of cumulus maturation remains obscure. It is possible that the greater mass of

cumulus complex ensures its transport of the oocyte from the stigma to the site of fertilization (Mahi-Brown & Yanagimachi 1983).

## FOLLICULAR RUPTURE

The process of follicular rupture, frequently related to as 'ovulation' (Fig. 6.6), has attracted much interest recently. Numerous reviews have been published on this aspect of ovarian function (Rondell 1970, 1974, Lipner 1973, 1988, Espey 1974, 1978b, 1980, LeMaire et al 1987, Marsh & LeMaire 1974, Parr 1975, Thibault & Levasseur, 1988, Goetz et al 1991, Tsafriri et al 1991a). Two major developments in this field were the establishment of the in vitro perfused ovary model (Ahrén et al 1975, Janson 1975, Janson et al 1978, 1982, Wallach et al 1978, Löfman et al 1982, LeMaire et al 1982, Koos et al 1984b, Yoshimura & Wallach 1987) and the application of advanced biochemical and physiological approaches. Here some of the structural, biochemical, biophysical and vascular aspects of follicular rupture will be reviewed.

### Structural changes in follicular wall associated with ovulation

The mature preovulatory follicle is embedded within the connective tissue matrix of the ovary and only a small part of it protrudes from the ovarian surface. At its apex the following layers are distinguished; (a) a single layer of surface epithelium; (b) collagenous connective tissue consisting of the tunica albuginea and the theca externa, this contributes most of the tensile strength of the follicle wall (Espey 1967b); (c) theca interna, a well-vascularized layer containing differentiated fibrocytes very active in steroidogenesis; (d) granulosa cells which are separated from the theca interna by the basal lamina and enclose the follicular fluid-filled cavity.

The most important structural changes leading to ovulation are those of the connective tissue of the tunica albuginea and theca externa. As ovulation approaches there is dissolution of the extracellular matrix and dissociation of thecal collagen (Espey 1967a,b). These changes in the connective tissue are accompanied by increased permeability

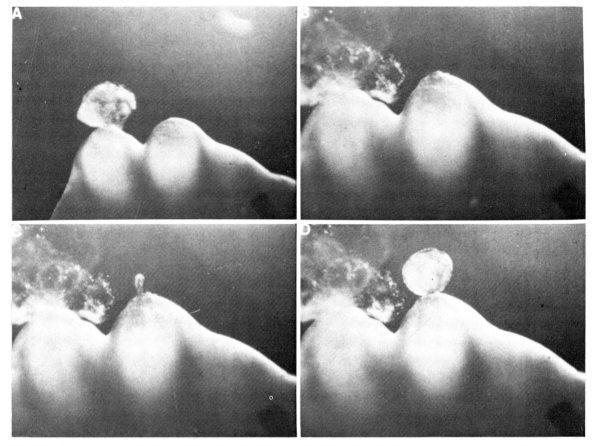

**Fig. 6.6** Sequence of events of an ovulation. In **a** the follicle on the left had ovulated just prior to photography. The cumulus cell mass containing the oocyte remained attached to the surface of the ovary. In **b** the follicle on the right shows cone formation and in **c** there is an initial spurt of cumulus cells through the ruptured follicular wall. In **d** the extrusion of cumulus mass and the oocyte is completed. (Reproduced with permission Löfman et al 1982.)

of the blood vessels resulting in leakage of erythrocytes and edema of follicular tissue (Zachariae 1958, Bjersing & Cajander 1974, Parr 1974, Abisogun et al 1988).

**Biophysical-mechanical changes**

An increase in intrafollicular pressure was for long assumed to be the cause of rupture and extrusion of the oocyte – cumulus complex. However, direct measurements of intrafollicular pressure did not demonstrate any significant increase in rat (Blandau & Rumery 1963), rabbit (Espey & Lipner 1963) and pig (Bronson et al 1979) follicles approaching ovulation. Nevertheless, an increase in follicular volume, related to the LH-

induced increase in follicular blood flow and the decrease in vascular resistance, leading to hyperemia, was demonstrated (Janson 1975). Follicular rupture occurs at constant pressure and is preceded by a marked increase in follicle volume. As ovulation approaches, an increase in follicular wall distensibility and a decrease in its tensile strength was observed (Espey 1967a, Rondell 1964).

**Vascular and related changes**

Periovulatory changes in ovarian and follicular microcirculation were described (Janson 1975, Lee & Novy 1978, Murdoch et al 1983). These studies revealed initial increase in blood flow, which in the sheep was followed by a decrease (Murdoch et al 1983). It is possible that eicosanoids are involved in ovulation by modulating follicular microcirculation. Indeed, in the rabbit, indomethacin reduced the LH-induced hyperemic response (Lee & Novy 1978) and in the ewe it prevented the second-phase reduction in follicular blood flow (Murdoch et al 1983). In the rat, inhibitors of cyclooxygenase and of lipoxygenase prevented the hCG-induced increase in uptake of labelled iodinated bovine serum albumin.

Platelet activating factor (PAF; 1-O-alkye-2-acetyl-sn-glycero-3-phosphocholine) is a potent bioactive phospholipid. In addition to triggering aggregation and degranulation of platelets, PAF induces margination and activation of neutrophils. Furthermore, PAF is released upon activation of leukocytes. We have demonstrated a preovulatory increase in ovarian and follicular neutrophils, triggered by hCG (Daphna-Iken et al 1989). In view of these changes common to ovulation and inflammation, we have examined the possible involvement of PAF in ovulation. Unilateral injection into the ovarian bursa of a specific PAF antagonist BN52021, isolated from the Chinese tree *Ginkgo biloba* (Braquet et al 1985), or its analogue BN52111 resulted in a dose-dependent inhibition of follicle rupture from the treated ovary. The inhibition was prevented when the antagonists and PAF were administered into the ovarian bursa simultaneously with hCG. By contrast, administration of PAF to rats that were not stimulated by exogenous hCG and had their endogenous surge of LH blocked by Nembutal failed to induce ovulation by itself (Abisogun et al 1989, Daphna-Iken et al 1989). A decrease in ovarian PAF was observed after stimulation of ovulation by hCG (Espey et al 1989b). While the precise mechanisms by which PAF is involved in ovulation remain to be determined, the above results support the suggested role of PAF in periovulatory changes in ovarian microcirculation and thereby also in ovulation.

Additional vasoactive substances were implicated in ovulation. During the menstrual cycle prorenin (a large molecular weight precursor of the active enzyme renin) rises following the LH surge (Sealey et al 1985, 1987) or hCG stimulation (Itskovitz et al 1987). Likewise, renin-like activity was located in FF (Fernandez et al 1985) and it is, therefore, possible that renin substrate is converted into angiotensin II in the ovary. Indeed, angiotensin binding sites were located in the ovary (Husain et al 1987, Pucell et al 1987, Daud et al 1989). Finally, the angiotensin antagonist, saralasin, blocked ovulation in immature rats (Pellicer et al 1988) and in rat perfused ovaries (Peterson et al 1989). This inhibitory effect in immature rats was reversed by simultaneous injection of angiotensin II with the antagonist (Pellicer et al 1988).

Likewise, kinins were implicated in ovulation. Thus, bradykinin induced ovulation in perfused ovaries (Brännström & Hellberg 1989) and this effect was prevented by a competitive antagonist of bradykinin (Hellberg et al 1991).

The involvement of histamine in ovulation has been suggested on the basis of its ability to mimic the hyperemic action of LH (Wurtman 1964) and the ability of antihistamines to block the hyperemic action of LH (Piacsek & Huth 1971). Nevertheless the role of histamine in ovulation remains obscure in view of the conflicting data obtained in various experimental models (see detailed reviews by Lipner 1988 and Goetz et al 1991). Finally, the role of oxygen free radicals in ovulation was shown by the use of the scavenging enzymes superoxide dismutase (SOD) and catalase. SOD and the combination of SOD and catalase reduced the number of ovulating follicles and prolonged the time interval between the gonadotropic stimulation of ovulation and follicle rupture in rabbit perfused ovaries (Miyazaki et al 1991). Similarly, SOD reduced the number of ovulated ova in immature rats (A. Tsafriri et al, unpublished observations). These results suggest a role for oxygen free radicals in follicle rupture.

The demonstration of perifollicular muscle-like cells containing myoid proteins in the rat (Amsterdam et al 1977, O'Shea 1970, Osvaldo-Decima 1970), mouse (Fumagalli et al 1971), rabbit (Fumagalli et al 1971, Bjersing & Cajander 1974), monkey (Osvaldo-Decima 1970) and human (Okamura et al 1972) led to the suggestion that ovarian contractions may be involved in follicular rupture. Ovarian contractions were demonstrated in several species, and these were enchanced by α-adrenergic (Rocerto et al 1969) and serotonergic stimulation and by various peptides such as enkephalins, substance P and VIP (Lipner 1988). Furthermore, inhibitors of smooth muscle contraction prevented ovulation in the hamster (Martin & Talbot 1981). However, the involvement of ovarian contractions in follicular rupture was questioned by others (Burden & Lawrence 1980, Didio et al 1980, Espey 1978a,). It remains to be determined whether ovarian contractility has an obligatory role in follicular rupture and the expulsion of the oocyte – cumulus complex.

## Metabolic and biochemical changes

Microscopical examination of the wall of ovulatory follicles revealed dissolution of the connective tissue matrix and of collagen fibres in the tunica albuginea and theca externa. These structural changes were correlated with an increase in distensibility of the follicular wall (see above). It was suggested early on by Schochet (1916) that proteases may play a role in ovulation. Indeed,

many enzymes have been identified in follicular tissues or fluid, including proteolytic enzymes (Reichert 1962, Espey & Rondell 1967), hyaluronidase (Zachariae 1958), acid phosphatases and esterases (Banon et al 1964), collagenase-like activity (Espey 1975, Espey & Coons 1976, Morales et al 1978, Fukumoto et al 1981, Curry et al 1985, Reich et al 1985c,d) and plasminogen activator (Beers 1975, Beers et al 1975, Strickland & Beers 1976, Canipari & Strickland 1985, Ny et al 1985, Reich et al 1985b, 1986, Milwidsky et al 1989). It was shown that injection of proteolytic enzymes into the follicular antrum resulted in follicular rupture (Espey & Lipner 1965) and application of enzyme solutions to follicular wall resulted in ovulatory changes (Espey 1967a, Espey & Rondell 1967, Rondell 1970). Here the evidence for the involvement of two proteolytic enzyme systems, interstitial collagenase and the plasmin activating system, in mammalian ovulation is reviewed. The stimulation of ovarian collagen degradation seems to be closely regulated by ovarian eicosanoids. Since steroidogenesis appears to be required for follicle rupture it will be discussed in brief. A simplified sheme depicting some of the factors implicated in

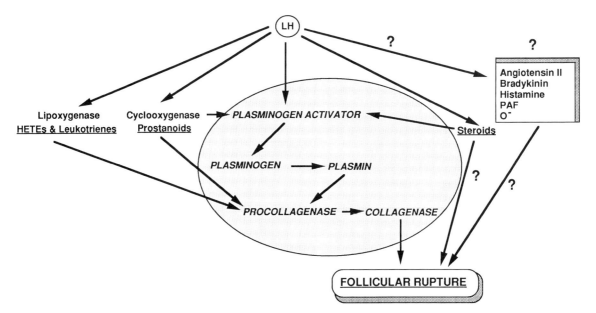

**Fig. 6.7**   A simplified scheme of some of the factors involved in follicle rupture during ovulation. The central role of the proteolytic cascade is emphasized and some of the factors involved in the modulation of proteolytic enzyme expression and activity. Further details in the text.

the regulation of ovarian proteolysis required for follicle rupture is presented in Figure 6.7

*Collagenase*

In view of the extensive changes in follicular collagen it appeared that collagenase should play a major role in follicular rupture. Nevertheless, early experiments to extract follicular collagenase and to demonstrate its ability to degrade the follicular wall were not successful (Espey & Stacy 1970), nor has a correlation between collagenase activity and ovulatory changes been demonstrated (Fukumoto et al 1981, Morales et al 1978, 1983). This failure should probably be attributed to the following characteristics of mammalian collage-nase: (a) it is secreted as an inactive zymogen (Collier et al 1988); (b) it is firmly bound to its natural substrate in the ovarian thecal collagen fibers; and (c) it is kept inactivated by serum and follicular fluid inhibitors and activated by protease activators (Grant et al 1987, He et al 1989). To circumvent these difficulties, ovarian collagen was labelled by local administration of $^{3}$H-labelled proline, and collagen metabolism and/or catab-olism was followed by assessing $^{3}$H-labelled hydroxyproline levels in acid hydrolysates of ovarian tissue. By this approach, a significant degradation of labelled ovarian and follicular collagen was detected following the gonadotropin surge (Reich et al 1985c,d). Recently, employing special extraction procedures (Reich et al 1987) and rigorous in vitro activation, Curry et al (1985) confirmed an LH/hCG-induced rise in ovarian collagenase activity. More recently, using cDNA probes for interstitial and type IV collagenases, we found a highly significant increase in the expres-sion of interstitial collagenase mRNA at 3–6 h following hCG administration to PMSG-treated immature rats. Collagenase IV, responsible for the degradation of basement membrane collagen IV, was expressed much later, at 9 h following the treatment (Reich et al 1991). The role of collage-nases in follicular rupture was corroborated also by using inhibitors of collagenase, such as cysteine (Reich et al 1985c,d), a microbial metalloprotease inhibitor (talopeptine; Ichikawa et al 1983b), and specific inhibitors of interstitial (Brännström et al 1988) collagenases.

Metalloproteinases, the enzymes including the collagenases, are locally regulated by specific serum- and tissue-borne inhibitors. Indeed, Abisogun et al (1986) have shown a significant increase in $^{125}$I-$\alpha_2$-macroglobulin uptake into rat ovaries following gonadotropin stimulation. Recently, tissue inhibitor of metalloproteinases (TIMP) has been identified in ovarian tissues (Curry et al 1989, Woessner et al 1989) and shown to be induced by gonadotropins (Curry et al 1988, Reich et al 1991).

*Plasminogen activator (PA)*

The demonstration of a preovulatory increase in plasminogen activator (Beers 1975, Beers & Strickland 1978) and the ability of plasmin to decrease the tensile strength of Graafian follicle wall (Beers 1975), led to the suggestion that PA may be involved in the ovulatory process. It was suggested that plasmin, the product of PA action on plasminogen, activates latent collagenase and thereby initiates the proteolytic processes culmi-nating in follicular rupture (Beers & Strickland 1978, Espey 1978b). In vitro studies revealed that granulosa cells contribute 80–90% of total follic-ular PA activity (Reich et al 1986). Most of granu-losa cell PA activity is secreted into the culture media, whereas intact follicles or theca tissue retain the activity within the tissue (Reich et al 1985b, 1986). These findings suggest that the theca tissue serves as a specific barrier which prevents the secretion of PA into the extrafollic-ular compartment and thereby allows localized action of PA within the follicular wall.

Two different molecular types of PA have been identified in mammalian tissues, the urokinase type (u-PA) and the tissue type (t-PA). These enzymes are products of different genes (Ny et al 1984, Riccio et al 1985, Suenson et al 1984). On the basis of electrophoretic mobility and immunoabsorption, both molecular types of PA were identified in rat, mouse and human follicles. In the rat, both PAs were present in granulosa and in theca compartments and the granulosa cells contributed 80–90% of the total follicular activity. Upon gonadotropin stimulation, a significant increase in t-PA was observed in both the granulosa and theca (Reich et al 1986). A similar increase in human granulosa cells was observed by Reinthaller et al (1990). Nevertheless, in mice u-PA, rather than t-PA, seems to be the gonadotropin stimulated type of PA (Canipari et al 1987). Inhibitors of serine proteases prevented ovulation in vivo (Akazawa et al 1983a,b, Reich et al 1985b), in hamster ovaries in vitro (Ichikawa et al 1983a) and in perfused rat ovaries (Woessner et al 1989). Furthermore, $\alpha_2$-antiplasmin and antibodies raised against t-PA suppressed ovulation rate in rats (Tsafriri & Hsueh 1989). A delayed administration of these inhibitors or antibodies (> 4 h after hCG) was ineffective in blocking ovulation (Reich et al 1985b, Tsafriri & Hsueh 1989). Collectively, these data support the hypothesis of involvement of the plasmin generating system at an early step in ovulation.

Ovarian steroids were found to synergize with LH in stimulating follicular PA secretion. Furthermore, addition of inhibitors of steroidogenesis or of aromatase inhibited the LH-stimulated PA activity. This inhibition could be restored by progesterone, testosterone and estradiol-17β, but not the nonaromatizable 5α-dihydrotestosterone (Reich & Tsafriri 1984, Reich et al 1985b).

Specific inhibitors of PA have also been described (Hekman & Loskutoff 1988). The study of Ny et al (1985) demonstrated that granulosa cells secrete PAI-1 and that FSH suppressed this activity. Human FF was also found to contain PAI-1 (Jones et al 1989), suggesting local regulation of ovarian PA activity by specific inhibitors.

*Eicosanoids*

Several studies demonstrated an increase in follicular prostaglandin synthesis after gonadotropic stimulation (Ainsworth et al 1975, 1984, LeMaire et al 1973, Armstrong & Zamecnik 1975, Bauminger & Lindner 1975). This increase is associated in the rat with a dose- and time-dependent induction of cyclooxygenase enzyme in the preovulatory follicles (Hedin et al 1987a, Huslig et al 1987, Brännström et al 1989). It was shown that the stimulation of PGE synthesis by LH is not dependent upon steroid synthesis (Bauminger & Lindner 1975), and that most follicular responses to LH, such as ovum matura-

tion, activation of adenylate cyclase, steroidogenesis and luteinization, proceed undisturbed even when prostaglandin synthesis is inhibited by drugs (reviewed by Zor & Lamprecht 1977). The exception is follicular rupture, which is prevented by administration of indomethacin (Armstrong & Grinwich 1972, Orczyk & Behrman 1972, Tsafriri et al 1972, Wallach et al 1975b), or intrafollicular injection of antiserum to $PGF_{2\alpha}$ in rabbits (Armstrong et al 1974). The inhibitory action of indomethacin was overcome by administration of $PGE_2$ to rats (Tsafriri et al 1972), $PGF_{2\alpha}$ to rhesus monkeys (Wallach et al 1975a) and both, $PGE_2$ and $PGE_{2\alpha}$ restored ovulation in the ewe (Murdoch et al 1986) and in the perfused rat ovary (Sogn et al 1987). Furthermore, in the perfused rabbit ovary $PGF_{2\alpha}$ was able to induce follicular rupture by itself, albeit somewhat earlier than LH (Holmes et al 1983). Collectively, these results suggest that prostaglandins have a physiological role in follicular rupture.

More recent studies revealed the importance of an additional group of arachidonic acid products in follicle rupture, the lipoxygenase-derived metabolites. We have shown that inhibitors of the lipoxygenase pathway block ovulation in dose-dependent manner (Reich et al 1983). In a later study, it was shown that incorporation of radio-labelled substrates into lipoxygenase products was stimulated by gonadotropins and lipoxygenase activity was located within the preovulatory follicle (Reich et al 1985a, 1987).

An increase in the levels of several lipoxygenase products was observed by radioimmunoassay following hCG stimulation of ovulation in the rat (Espey et al 1989a, Tanaka et al 1989). These included an early rise in leukotriene (LT) $B_4$ and the peptidic LTs ($LTC_4$, $D_4$ and $E_4$, measured with an antibody recognizing them as a group), the products of 5-lipoxygenase and a later rise of 15-hydroxyeicosatetraenoic acid (15-HETE). While these studies support the involvement of lipoxygenase products in ovulation, pharmacological inhibitors of lipoxygenases facilitated, rather than suppressed, the LH-stimulated ovulation in perfused rabbit ovaries (Hellberg et al 1990). Likewise, the rise in sheep follicular $LTB_4$ occurred only after follicle rupture and inhibitors of lipoxygenases did not affect ovulation in the sheep (Carvalho et al 1989). It remains to be determined whether these opposing results obtained with inhibitors of lipoxygenases are due to species differences or the methods employed.

Our recent studies indicate that eicosanoids mediate the LH/hCG-induced rise in ovarian collagenolytic activity (Reich et al 1985a, Tsafriri et al 1990). Inhibitors of eicosanoid synthesis suppressed the hCG-induced rise in ovarian interstitial collagenase mRNA expression as revealed by Northern-blot analysis, thus suggesting the involvement of eicosanoids in the regulation of collagenase synthesis. The reduced levels of collagenase mRNA may be due to reduced transcription or reduced stability of the message. However, since positive regulation of metalloproteinase gene expression seems to occur mainly at the level of transcription (Matrisian 1990), it is likely that the increase in ovarian interstitial collagenase expression is regulated similarly. By contrast, the expression of colagenase IV or of the metalloproteinase inhibitor TIMP was not altered by the inhibitors of eicosanoid synthesis (Reich et al 1991.)

Evidence has been obtained that human follicles or follicle cells can produce eicosanoids, products of both cyclooxygenase (Plunkett et al 1975, Liedtke & Seifert 1978, Patwardhan & Lanthier 1981, Feldman et al 1986), and lipoxygenase (Feldman et al 1986) pathways. Likewise, an increase in FF prostanoid levels was observed following hCG (Darling et al 1982, Lumsden et al 1986). In hCG-stimulated patients, in addition to prostanoids, $LTB_4$ and $LTC_4$, $D_4$ and $E_4$ were demonstrated (Priddy et al 1989). Finally, administration of cyclooxygenase inhibitors, azapropazone and indomethacin, to healthy cycling women markedly suppressed ovulation in response to hCG (Killick & Elstein 1987). Thus, it seems that eicosanoids play an essential role in follicle rupture also in the human.

*Steroids*

The issue whether ovarian steroidogenesis is essential for follicle rupture has been discussed at length over the last years (reviewed by Espey 1989, Tsafriri et al 1987). Early studies have shown that progesterone induces distensibility of sow follicles while neither FSH nor estrogen could do so. This effect of LH on the follicle wall could be mimicked by cAMP and prevented by an inhibitor of 3β-hydroxysteroid dehydrogenase, and the inhibition could be reversed by exogenous progesterone (Rondell 1970). Administration of aminoglutethimide and cyanoketone, drugs that block the synthetic pathway to progesterone, results in inhibition of follicle rupture (Lipner & Greep 1971, Lipner & Wendelken 1971). Hypophysectomy of rats on the afternoon of the day of proestrus resulted in blockage of follicular rupture, and this was effectively reversed by three consecutive injections of progesterone (5–10 mg each), suggesting an essential role of steroids in ovulation. This conclusion was challenged by Bullock & Kappauff (1972) who could dissociate between the effect of these inhibitors on plasma progesterone levels and on follicle rupture; thus they could induce ovulation by hCG when the rise in plasma progesterone was attenuated by aminoglutethimide, and cyanoketone prevented ovulation even when steroid plasma levels remained unaffected. Nevertheless, it is possible that plasma levels of progesterone are not a precise indicator of follicular levels of steroids, which are probably involved in follicular rupture through paracrine mechanisms. Recently, the ability of another inhibitor of 3β-hydroxysteroid dehydrogenase, epostane, to inhibit follicular rupture in the rat, was demonstrated, and this inhibition was overcome by administration of progesterone (Snyder et al 1984). Ovulation in the ewe was blocked by isoxazol, an inhibitor of progesterone synthesis (Murdoch et al 1986). Furthermore, administration of the progesterone receptor antagonist RU 38486 partially blocked ovulation in mature and immature rats in which ovulation was triggered by hCG (Tsafriri et al 1987). This supports the paracrine role of progesterone, exerted through its interaction with cellular receptors, in the mediation of LH/hCG induction of follicular rupture.

The role of ovarian steroids was closely examined in the model of perfused ovary which affords study of follicular rupture in vitro (Janson et al 1982, Lambertsen et al 1976). In perfused rabbit ovaries inhibition of cholesterol chain cleavage enzyme by aminoglutethimide or of 3β-hydroxysteroid dehydrogenase did not affect follicle rupture induced by gonadotropin (Holmes et al 1985, Yoshimura et al 1986). By contrast, an inhibitor of 3β-hydroxysteroid dehydrogenase significantly reduced the ovulation from perfused rat ovaries stimulated by a combination of LH and IBMX (Brännström & Hellberg 1989). The preovulatory decline in follicular estrogen is not required for follicular rupture in the rabbit, since addition of estrogen (10 μg/ml) to the perfusate did not inhibit ovulation, in spite of a more than two-fold increase in follicular estradiol-17β content (LeMaire et al 1982). Likewise, blockade of the early rise in estrogen by an inhibitor of aromatase did not affect follicular rupture in perfused rat ovaries (Koos et al 1984a, Morioka et al 1988). While inhibition of steroidogenesis did not affect ovulatory response of perfused ovaries in the rabbit, addition of progesterone into the perfusate modified it. Progesterone (6.7 μg/ml) somewhat enhanced follicular rupture in one study (Hamada et al 1979) and it reduced the number of ovulating ovaries in another, employing a higher dose of

progesterone (10 μg/ml) (Holmes et al 1985). Thus, a modulatory role of progesterone in follicular rupture in vitro cannot be excluded. Collectively, the data presented seem to suggest the involvement of steroids, most probably progesterone, in follicular rupture. Nevertheless, their specific role remains obscure and species differences may exist.

## ACKNOWLEDGEMENTS

We thank Mrs M. Popliker, Mrs R. Slager and Mrs A. Tsafriri for their skilful technical assistance and Mrs M. Kopelowitz for excellent secretarial help. Our studies reviewed here were supported, in part, by grants from the GIF, The German-Israel Foundation for Scientific Research and Development, Jerusalem, Israel, the Basic Research Foundation of the Israel Academy of Sciences and Humanities, Jerusalem, Israel and the Henri Beafour Institute, Le Plessis Robinson, France.

## REFERENCES

Aberdam E, Hanski E, Dekel N 1987 Maintenance of meiotic arrest in isolated rat oocytes by the invasive adenylate cyclase of *Bordetella pertussis*. Biol Reprod 36: 530

Abisogun A O, Braquet P, Tsafriri A 1989 The involvement of platelet activating factor in ovulation. Science 243: 381–383

Abisogun A O, Daphna-Iken D, Reich R, Kranzfelder D, Tsafriri A 1988 Modulatory role of eicosanoids in vascular changes during the preovulatory period in the rat. Biol Reprod 38: 756

Adashi E Y, Resnick C E, Hernandez E R, Svoboda M E, Van Wyk J J 1989 Potential relevance of insulin-like growth factor 1 to ovarian physiology: from basic science to clinical application. Semin Reprod Endocrinol 7: 94

Ahrén K, Janson P O, Selstam G 1975 A technique for perfusion of rabbit ovaries *in vitro*. Methods Enzymol 39: 1

Ainsworth L, Baker R D, Armstrong D T 1975 Preovulatory changes in follicular fluid prostaglandin F levels in swine. Prostaglandins 9: 915

Ainsworth L, Tsang B H, Marcus G J, Downey B R 1984 Prostaglandin production by dispersed granulosa and theca interna cells from porcine preovulatory follicles. Biol Reprod 31: 115

Akazawa K, Matsuo O, Kosugi T, Mihara H, Mori N 1983a The role of plasminogen activator in ovulation. Acta Physiol Lat Am 33: 105

Akazawa K, Mori N, Kosogi T, Matsuo O, Mihara H 1983b Localization of fibrinolytic activity in ovulation of the rat follicle as determined by the fibrin slide method. Jpn J Physiology 33: 1011–1018

Albers N, Bettendorf M, Hart C S, Kaplan S L, Grumbach M M 1989a Hormone ontogeny in the ovine fetus. XXIII Pulsatile administration of follicle-stimulating hormone stimulates inhibin production and decreases testosterone synthesis in the ovine fetal gonad. Endocrinology 124: 3089

Albers N, Hart C S, Kaplan S L, Grumbach M M 1989b Hormone ontogeny in the ovine fetus. XXIV Porcine follicular fluid 'inhibins' selectively suppress plasma follicle-stimulating hormone in the ovine fetus. Endocrinology 125: 675

Amsterdam A, Koch Y, Lieberman M E, Lindner H R 1975 Distribution of binding sites for human chorionic gonadotropin in the preovulatory follicle of the rat. J Cell Biol 64: 894

Amsterdam A, Lindner H R, Gröschel-Stewart V 1977 Localization of actin and myosin in the rat oocyte and follicular wall by immunofluorescence. Anatom Rec 197: 311

Andersen M M, Kroll J, Byskov A G, Faber M 1976 Protein composition in the fluid of individual bovine follicles. J Reprod Fertil 48: 109

Armstrong D T, Goff A K, Dorrington J H 1979 Regulation of follicular estrogen biosynthesis. In: Midgley A R, Sadler W A (eds) Ovarian follicular development and function. Raven, New York, pp 169–181

Armstrong D T, Grinwich D L 1972 Blockade of spontaneous and LH-induced ovulation in rats by indomethacin, an inhibitor of prostaglandin biosynthesis. Prostaglandins 1: 21

Armstrong D T, Zamecnik J 1975 Preovulatory elevation of rat ovarian prostaglandin F and its blockade by indomethacin. Mol Cell Endocrinol 2: 125

Armstrong D T, Grinwich D L, Moon Y S, Zamecnik J 1974 Inhibition of ovulation in rabbits by intrafollicular injection of indomethacin and $PGF_{2\alpha}$ antiserum. Life Sci 14: 129

Armstrong D T, Weiss T J, Selstam G, Seamark R F 1981 Hormonal and cellular interactions in follicular steroid biosynthesis by the sheep ovary. J Reprod Fert 30 (Suppl 30): 143

Ax R L, Belling M E, Grimek H J 1985 Properties and regulation of synthesis of glycosaminoglycans by the ovary. In: Toft D O, Ryan R J (eds) Proceedings of the Fifth Ovarian Workshop. Ovarian Workshops, Champaign, IL, pp 451–480

Ayalon D, Tsafriri A, Lindner H R, Cordova T, Harrel A 1972 Serum gonadotropin levels in pro-estrous rats in relation to the resumption of meiosis by the oocytes. J Reprod Fertil 31: 51

Bahr J, Gardener R, Schenck P, Shahabi N 1980 Follicular steroidogenesis: effect of reproduction condition. Biol Reprod 22: 817

Baird A, Hsueh A J W 1986 Fibroblast growth factor as an intraovarian hormone: differential regulation of steroidogenesis by an angiogenic factor. Regul Pept 16: 243

Baird A, Emoto N, Gonzalez A M, Fauser B, Hsueh A J W 1989 Fibroblast growth factors as local mediators of gonadal function. In: Hirshfield A N (eds) Growth factors and the ovary. Plenum, New York, pp 151–160

Baird D T 1983 Factors regulating the growth of the preovulatory follicle in the sheep and human. J Reprod Fertil 69: 343

Baird D T, Fraser I S 1975 Concentration of oestrone and oestradiol in follicular fluid and ovarian venous blood of women. Clin Endocrinol 4: 259

Baird D T, Baker T G, McNatty K P, Neal P 1975 Relationship between the secretion of the corpus luteum and the length of the follicular phase of the ovarian cycle. J Reprod Fertil 45: 611

Baker T G 1963 A quantitative and cytological study of germ cells in the human ovaries. Proc R Soc Lond [Biol] 158: 417

Baker T G, Scrimgeour J B 1980 Development of the gonad in normal and anencephalic human fetuses. J Reprod Fert 60: 193

Banon P, Brandes D, Frost J K 1964 Lysosomal enzymes in the rat ovary and endometrium during the estrous cycle. Acta Cytol 8: 416

Bar-Ami S, Tsafriri A 1981 Acquisition of meiotic competence in the rat: role of gonadotropin and estrogen. Gamete Res 4: 463

Barros C, Munoz G 1973 Sperm–egg interaction in immature hamster oocytes. J Exp Zool 186: 73

Batta S K, Wentz A C, Channing C P 1980 Steroidogenesis by human ovarian cell types in culture: influence of mixing of cell types and effect of added testosterone. J Clin Endocrinol Metab 50: 274

Bauminger S, Lindner H R 1975 Periovulatory changes in ovarian prostaglandin formation and their hormonal control in the rat. Prostaglandins 9: 737

Beers W H 1975 Follicular plasminogen and plasminogen activator and the effect of plasmin on ovarian follicular wall. Cell 6: 379

Beers W H, Strickland S 1978 A cell culture assay for follicle-stimulating hormone. J Biol Chem 253: 3877

Beers W H, Strickland S, Reich E 1975 Ovarian plasminogen activator: Relationship to ovulation and hormonal regulation. Cell 6: 387

Bendell J J, Dorrington J 1988 Rat thecal/interstitial cells secrete a transforming growth factor-$\beta$-like factor that promotes growth and differentiation in rat granulosa cells. Endocrinology 123: 941

Bendell J J, Dorrington J H 1990 Epidermal growth factor influences growth and differentiation of rat granulosa cells. Endocrinology 127: 533

Bicsak T A, Tucker E M, Cappel S et al 1986 Hormonal regulation of granulosa cell inhibin biosynthesis. Endocrinology 119: 2711

Biggers J D 1972 Metabolism of the oocyte. In: Biggers J D, Schuetz A W (eds) Oogenesis. University Park Press, Baltimore, pp 241–251

Biggers J D, Schuetz A W, Zamboni L 1972 Fine morphology of the follicle wall and the follicle cell–oocyte association. In: Biggers J D, Schuetz A W (eds) Oogenesis. University Park Press, Baltimore, pp 5–45

Bill II C H, Greenwald G S 1981 Acute gonadotropin deprivation. I. A model for the study of follicular atresia. Biol Reprod 24: 913

Bilig H, Hedin L, Magnusson C 1983 Gonadotrophins stimulate lactate production by rat cumulus and granulosa cells. Acta Endocrinol 103: 562

Bjersing L, Cajander S 1974 Ovulation and the mechanism of follicular rupture. VI. Ultrastructure of theca interna and the inner vascular network surrounding rabbit Graafian follicles prior to induced ovulation. Cell Tissue Res 153: 31

Blandau R J 1955 Ovulation in the living albino rat. Fertil Steril 6: 391

Blandau R J, Rumery R E 1963 Measurements of intrafollicular pressure in ovulatory and preovulatory follicles of rat. Fertil Steril 14: 330

Block E 1951 Quantitative morphological investigations of the follicular system in women. Acta Endocrinol (Copenh) 8: 33

Bogovich K, Richards J S, Reichert L E 1981 Obligatory role of luteinizing hormone (LH) in the initiation of preovulatory follicular growth in the pregnant rat: specific effects of human chorionic gonadotropin and follicle-stimulating hormone on LH receptors and steroidogenesis in theca, granulosa and luteal cells. Endocrinology 109: 860

Bomsel-Helmreich O, Gougeon A, Thebault A et al, 1979 Healthy and atretic human follicles in the preovulatory phase: differences in evolution of follicualr morphology and steroid content of follicular fluid. J Clin Endocrinol Metab 48: 686

Brännström M, Hellberg P 1989 Bradykinin potentiates LH-induced follicular rupture in the rat ovary perfused in vitro. Hum Reprod 4: 475

Brännström M, Woessner J F, Koos R D, Sear C H J, LeMaire W J 1988 Inhibitors of mammalian tissue collagenase and metaloproteinases suppress ovulation in the perfused rat ovary. Endocrinology 122: 1715

Brännström M, Larson L, Basta B, Hedin L 1989 Regulation of prostaglandin endoperoxide synthase by cyclic adenosine 3',5'-monophosphate in the in vitro-perfused rat ovary. Biol Reprod 41: 513

Braquet P, Spinnewyn B, Braquet M et al 1985 BN 52021 and related compounds: a new series of highly specific PAF-acether receptor antagonists isolated from *Ginkgo biloba*. Blood Vessels 16: 559

Braw H R, Tsafriri A 1980a Effect of PMSG on follicular atresia in the immature rat ovary. J Reprod Fertil 59: 267

Braw H R, Tsafriri A 1980b A model for atresia: follicles explanted from nembutal-treated rats. J Reprod Fertil 59: 259

Braw R H, Bar-Ami S, Tsafriri A 1981 Effect of hypophysectomy on atresia of rat preovulatory follicles. Biol Reprod 25: 989

Bronson R A, Bryant G, Balk M, Emanuele N 1979 Ultrastructural studies on the preovulatory follicle in the mouse ovary. Z Zellforsch Mikrosk Anat 100: 285

Buccione R, Vanderhyden C, Caron P J, Eppig J J 1990 FSH-induced expansion of the mouse cumulus oophorus in vitro is dependent upon a specific factor(s) secreted by the oocyte. Develop Biol 138: 16

Bullock W, Kappauf B H 1972 Dissociation of gonadotropin-induced ovulation and steroidogenesis in immature rats. Endocrinology 92: 1625

Burden H W, Lawrence I E 1980 Nerve supply of the ovary. In: Motta P M, Hafez E S E (eds) Biology of the ovary. Martinus Nijhoff, The Hague, pp 99–105

Burger H G, de Kretser D M, Findlay J K, Igarashi M (eds) 1987 Inhibin-non-steroidal regulation of follicle simulating hormone secretion, Vol 42. Serono Symposia Publications, Raven, New York

Buscaglia M, Fuller J, Mazzola T et al 1989 A new intra-ovarian function for follistatin: the inhibition of oocyte meiosis. Proceedings of the Endocrine Society USA 71: (abstr no 883)

Byskov A G 1974a Cell kinetic studies of follicular atresia in the mouse ovary. J Reprod Fertil 37: 277

Byskov A G 1974b Does the rete ovarii act as a trigger for the onset of meiosis? Nature 252: 396

Byskov A G 1975 The role of the rete ovarii in meiosis and follicle formation in the cat, mink and ferret. J Reprod Fert 45: 210

Byskov A G 1978 Follicular atresia. In: Jones R E (ed) The vertebrate ovary. Plenum New York, pp 533–562

Byskov A G 1986 Differentiation of mammalian embryonic gonad. Physiol Rev 66: 71

Byskov A G, Skakkebaek N E, Stafanger G, Peters H 1977 Influence of ovarian surface epithelium and rete ovarii on follicle formation. J Anat 123: 77

Campbell B K, Mann G E, McNeilly A S, Baird D T 1990 The pattern of ovarian inhibin, estradiol, and androstenedione secretion during the estrous cycle of the ewe. Endocrinology 127: 227

Canipari R, Strickland S 1985 Plasminogen activator in the rat ovary. Production and gonadotropin regulation of the enzyme in granulosa thecal cells. J Biol Chem 260: 5121

Canipari R, O'Connell M L, Meyer G, Strickland S 1987 Mouse ovarian granulosa cells produce urokinase-type pasminogen activator, whereas the corresponding rat cells produce tissue-type plasminogen activator. J Cell Biol 205: 977

Cargille C M, Vaitukaitis J L, Bermudez J A, Ross G T 1973 A differential effect of ethinyl estradiol on plasma F S H and L H related to time of administration in the menstrual cycle. J Clin Endocrinol Metab 36: 87

Carvalho C B, Yeik B S, Murdoch W J 1989 Significance of follicular cyclooxygenase and lipoxygenase pathways of metabolism of arachidonate in sheep. Prostaglandins 37: 553

Chang M C 1955 The maturation of rabbit oocytes in culture and their maturation, activation, fertilization and subsequent development in Fallopian tube. J Exp Zool 128: 378

Chang S C S, Jones J D, Ellefson R D, Ryan R J 1976 The porcine ovarian follicle: I. Selected chemical analysis of follicular fluid at different developmental stages. Biol Reprod 15: 321

Channing C P 1969 Steroidogenesis and morphology of human ovarian cell types in tissue culture. J Endocrinol 45: 297

Channing C P 1980 Progesterone and estrogen secretion by cultured monkey ovarian cells: influences of follicular size, serum luteinizing hormone levels, and follicular fluid estrogen levels. Endocrinology 107: 342

Channing C P, Coudert S P 1976 Contribution of granulosa cells and follicular fluid to ovarian estrogen secretion in the rhesus monkey in vivo. Endocrinology 92: 590

Channing C P, Kammerman S 1973 Characteristics of gonadotropin receptors of porcine granulosa cells during follicle maturation. Endocrinology 92: 531

Channing C P, Segal S (eds) 1982 Intraovarian control mechanisms. Advances in experimental medicine and biology, Plenum, New York

Channing C P, Tsafriri A 1977 The mechanism of action of LH and FSH upon the ovary in vitro. Metabolism 26: 413

Channing C P, Tanabe K, Hahn D, Phillips A, Charracher R 1984 Inhibin activity and steroid hormone levels in ovarian extracts and ovarian vein plasma of female monkeys during postnatal development. Fertil Steril 42: 453

Chiras D D, Greenwald G S 1977 An autoradiographic study of long-term follicular development in the cyclic hamster. Anat Rec 188: 331

Cho W K, Stern S, Biggers J D 1974 Inhibitory effect of dibutyryl cAMP on mouse oocyte maturation in vitro. J Exp Zool 187: 383

Collier I E, Smith K, Kronberg A et al 1988 The structure of human skin fibroblast collagenase gene. J Biol Chem 263: 10711

Colonna R, Mangia F 1983 Mechanisms of amino acid uptake in cumulus-enclosed mouse oocytes. Biol Reprod 28: 797

Conway B A, Mahesh V B, Mills T M 1990 Effect of dihydrotestosterone on the growth and function of ovarian follicles in intact immature female rats primed with PMSG. J Reprod Fertil 90: 267

Curry T E, Dean D D, Woessner J F, LeMaire W J 1985 The extraction of a tissue collagenase associated with ovulation in the rat. Biol Reprod 33: 981

Curry T E, Sanders S L, Pedigo N G, Ester R S, Wilson A E, Vernon M W 1988 Identification and characterization of metalloproteinase inhibitor activity in human ovarian follicular fluid. Endocrinology 123: 1611

Curry T E J, Dean D D, Sanders S L, Pedigo N G, Jones P B C 1989 The role of ovarian proteases and their inhibitors in ovulation. Steroids 54: 501

Daphna-Iken D, Chun S Y, Abisogun A O, Tsafriri A 1989 Platelet-activating factor, ginkgolides and follicle rupture during ovulation. In: Braquet P (ed) Ginkgolides—chemistry. J R Prous Science Publishers, Barcelona, pp 835–844

Darling M R N, Joyce M, Elder M G 1982 Prostaglandin $F_{2\alpha}$ levels in the human ovarian follicle. Prostaglandins 23: 551

Daud A I, Bumpus F M, Husain A 1989 Angiotensin II: does it have a direct obligate role in ovulation? Science 245: 870

Davis S R, Burger H G, Robertson D M, Farnworth P G, Carson R S, Krozowski Z 1988 Pregnant mare's serum gonadotropin stimulates inhibin subunit gene expression in the immature rat ovary: dose response characteristics and relationships to serum gonadotropins, inhibin and ovarian steroid content. Endocrinology 123: 2399

de Jong F H, Grootenhuis A J, Klaij I A, Van Beurden W M O 1990 Inhibin and related proteins: localization, regulation, and effects. In: Porter J C, Jezová D (eds) Circulating regulatory factors and neuroendocrine function. Plenum, New York, pp 271–293

Dekel N 1988 Spatial relationship of follicular cells in the control of meiosis. In: Haseltine F P (ed) Meiotic inhibition: molecular control of meiosis. Alan R Liss, New York, pp 87–101

Dekel N, Beers W H 1978 Rat oocyte maturation in vitro: relief of cyclic AMP inhibition by gonadotropins. Proc Natl Acad Sci USA 75: 3469

Dekel N, Beers W H 1980 Development of rat oocyte in vitro: inhibition and induction of maturation in the presence or absence of the cumulus oophorus. Develop Biol 75: 247

Dekel N, Sherizly I 1983 Induction of maturation in rat follicle-enclosed oocyte by forskolin. FEBS Lett 151: 153

Dekel N, Sherizly I 1985 Epidermal growth factor induces maturation of rat follicle-enclosed oocytes. Endocrinology 116: 406

Dekel N, Aberdam E, Hanski E 1985 Invasive bacterial adenylate cyclase maintains the meiotic arrest in isolated rat oocytes. In: Toft D O, Ryan R J (eds) Proceeding of the Fifth Ovarian Workshop. Ovarian Workshops, Champaign, Illinois, pp 65–69

Dekel N, Anerdam E, Sherizly I 1984 Spontaneous maturation in vitro of cumulus-enclosed rat oocytes is inhibited by forskolin. Biol Reprod 31: 244

Dekel N, Hultborn R, Hillensjö T, Hamberger L, Kraicer P 1976 Effect of luteinizing hormone on respiration of the preovulatory cumulus oophorus of the rat. Endocrinology 98: 498

Dekel N, Lawrence T S, Gilula N B, Beers W H 1981 Modulation of cell-to-cell communication in the cumulus–oocyte complex and the regulation of oocyte maturation by L H. Develop Biol 86: 356

Dekel N, Galiani D, Sherizly I 1988 Dissociation between the inhibitory and the stimulatory action of cAMP on maturation of rat oocytes. Molec Cell Endocrinol 56: 115

Derynck R 1986 Transforming growth factor-α: structure and biological activities. J Cell Biochem 32: 293

Didio L J A, Allen D J, Correr S, Motta P M 1980 Smooth muscle in the ovary. In: Motta P M, Hafez E S E (eds) Biology of the ovary. Martinus Nijhoff, The Hague, pp 107–118

diZerega G S, Hodgen G D 1980 Cessation of folliculogenesis during the primate luteal phase. J Clin Endocrinol Metab 51: 158

diZerega G S, Hodgen G D 1981 Folliculogenesis in the primate ovarian cycle. Endocrine Rev 2: 27

Dorrington J H, Moon Y S, Armstrong D T 1975 Estradiol-17β biosynthesis in cultured granulosa cells from hypophysectomized immature rats; stimulation by follicle-stimulating hormone. Endocrinology 97: 1328

Downs S M, Eppig J J 1987 Induction of mouse oocyte maturation in vivo by perturbants of purine metabolism. Biol Reprod 36: 431

Downs S M, Coleman D L, Ward-Bailey P F, Eppig J J 1985 Hypoxanthine is the principal inhibitor of murine oocyte

maturation in a low molecular weight fraction of porcine follicular fluid. Proc Nat Acad Sci USA 82: 454

Downs S M, Coleman D L, Eppig J J 1986 Maintenance of murine oocyte meiotic arrest: uptake and metabolism of hypoxanthine and adenosine by cumulus cell-enclosed and denuded oocytes. Develop Biol 117: 174

Downs S M, Daniel S A J, Bornslaeger E A, Hoppe P C, Eppig J J 1989 Maintenance of meiotic arrest in mouse oocytes by purines. Gamete Res 23: 323

Driancourt M A, Gibson W R, Cahill L P 1985 Follicular dynamics throughout the oestrus cycle in sheep. A review. Reprod Nutr Develop 25: 1

Edwards R G 1974 Follicular fluid. J Reprod Fertil 37: 189

Eppig J J 1979a FSH stimulates hyaluronic acid synthesis by oocyte–cumulus cell complexes from mouse preovulatory follicles. Nature 281: 483

Eppig J J 1979b Gonadotropin stimulation of the expansion of cumulus oophori isolated from mice: general conditions for expansion in vitro. J Exp Zool 108: 111–120

Eppig J J 1980 Regulation of cumulus oophorus expansion by gonadotropins in vivo and in vitro. Biol Reprod 23: 545

Eppig J J 1982 The relationship between cumulus cell–oocyte coupling, oocyte meiotic maturation, and cumulus expansion. Develop Biol 89: 268

Eppig J J, Downs S M 1984 Chemical signals that regulate mammalian oocyte maturation. Biol Reprod 30: 1

Eppig J J, Ward-Bailey P F, Coleman D L 1985 Hypoxanthine and adenosine in murine ovarian follicular fluid: Concentrations and activity in maintaining oocyte meiotic arrest. Biol Reprod 33: 1041

Erickson G F, Ryan K J 1975 The effect of LH/FSH, dibutyryl cyclic AMP, and prostaglandins on the production of estrogens by rabbit granulosa cells in vitro. J Exp Zool 195: 153

Erickson G F, Ryan K J 1976 Stimulation of testosterone production in isolated rabbit thecal tissue by LH/FSH, dibutyryl cyclic AMP, $PGF_{2\alpha}$ and $PGE_2$. Endocrinology 99: 452

Esch F, Ueno N, Baird A et al 1985 Primary structure of bovine brain acidic fibroblast growth factor (FGF). Biochem Biophys Res Commun 133: 554

Eshkol A, Lunenfeld B 1972 Gonadotrophic regulation of ovarian development in mice during infancy. In: Saxena B B, Berling C G, Gandy H M (eds) Gonadotrophins. Wiley Interscience, New York, pp 335–346

Eshkol A, Lunenfeld B, Peters H 1970 Ovarian development in infant mice. Dependence on gonadotropic hormones. In: Butt W R, Crooke A C, Ryle M (eds) Gonadotropins and ovarian development. E. & S. Livingstone, Edinburgh, pp 249–258

Espey L L 1967a Tenacity of porcine Graafian follicle as it approaches ovulation. Am J Physiol 212: 1397

Espey L L 1967b Ultrastructure of the apex of the rabbit Graafian follicle during the ovulatory process. Endocrinology 81: 267

Espey L L 1974 Ovarian proteolytic enzymes and ovulation. Biol Reprod 10: 216

Espey L L 1975 Evaluation of proteolytic activity in mammalian ovulation. In: Reich E, Rifkin D B, Shaw E (eds) Proteases and biological control. Cold Spring Harbor, New York, pp 767–776

Espey L 1978a Ovarian contractility and its relationship to ovulation: a review. Biol Reprod 19: 540

Espey L 1978b Ovulation. In: Jones R E (ed) The vertebrate ovary. Plenum, New York, pp 503–532

Espey L L 1980 Ovulation as an inflammatory reaction: a hypothesis. Biol Reprod 22: 73

Espey L L 1989 The role of steroids in mammalian ovulation. In: Tsafriri A, Dekel N (eds) Follicular development and the ovulatory response, vol 23, Ares-Serono Symposia, Rome, pp 189–198

Espey L L, Coons P J 1976 Factors which influence ovulatory degradation of rabbit ovarian follicles. Biol Reprod 14: 233

Espey L L, Lipner H 1963 Measurements of intrafollicular pressures in the rabbit ovary. Am J Physiol 205: 1067

Espey L L, Lipner H 1965 Enzyme-induced rupture of rabbit Graafian follicle. Am J Physiol 208: 208

Espey L L, Rondell P 1967 Estimation of mammalian collagenolytic activity with a synthetic substrate. J Appl Physiol 23: 757

Espey L L, Stacy S 1970 Failure of an ovarian collagenolytic extract to decompose the connective tissue in the mature sow graafian follicle. Fed Proc 29: 833

Espey L L, Tanaka N, Okamura H 1989a Increase in ovarian leukotrienes during hormonally induced ovulation in the rat. Am J Physiol 256: E753

Espey L L, Tanaka N, Woodard D S, Harper M J K, Okamura H 1989b Decrease in ovarian platelet-activating factor during ovulation in the gonadotropin-primed immature rat. Biol Reprod 41: 104

Fagbohun C F, Dads M D, Metcalf J P, Ashiru O A, Blake C A 1990 Blockage of the selective increase in serum follicle-stimulating hormone concentration in immature female rats and its effects on ovarian follicular population. Biol Reprod 42: 625

Falck B 1959 Site of production of oestrogen in rat ovary as studied in microtransplants. Acta Physiol Scand Suppl 163 47: 1

Feldman E, Haberman S, Abisogun A O et al 1986 Arachidonic acid metabolism in human granulosa cells: evidence for cyclooxygenase and lipoxygenase activity in vitro. Hum Reprod 1: 353

Fernandez C A, Tarlatzis B C, Rzasa P J et al 1985 Renin-like activity in ovarian follicular fluid. Fertil Steril 44: 219

Findlay J K, Clarke I J, Robertson D M 1990a Inhibin concentrations in ovarian and jugular venous plasma and the relationship of inhibin with follicle-stimulating hormone and luteinizing hormone during the ovine estrus cycle. Endocrinology 126: 528

Findlay J K, Sai X, Shukovski L 1990b Role of inhibin-related peptides as intragonadal regulators. Reprod Fertil Develop 2: 205

Fleming A D, Kuehl T J, Armstrong D T 1985 Maturation of pig and rat oocytes transplanted into surrogate pig follicles in vitro. Gamete Res 11: 107

Foote W D, Thibault C 1969 Recherches experimentales sur la maturation in vitro des ovocytes de turie et de veau. Ann Biol Anim Biochem Biophys 9: 329

Fortune J E, Armstrong D T 1977 Androgen production by theca and granulosa isolated from proestrous rat follicles. Endocrinology 100: 1341

Fowler R E, Fox N L, Edwards R G, Walters D E, Steptoe P C 1978 Steroidogenesis by cultured granulosa cells aspirated from human follicles using pregnenolone and androgens as precursors. J Endocrinol 77: 171

Franchimont P (ed) 1986 Paracrine control. Clinics in endocrinology and metabolism, W.B. Saunders, London

Friedrich F, Kemeter P, Salzer H, Breitenecker G 1975 Ovulation inhibition with human chorionic gonadotrophin. Acta Endocrinol 78: 332

Fujii T, Channing C P (eds) 1982 Non-steroidal regulators in reproductive biology and medicine, In: Advances in the biosciences, Pergamon, Oxford

Fukumoto M, Yajima Y, Okamura H, Midorikawa O 1981 Collagenolytic enzyme activity in human ovary: An ovulatory enzyme system. Fertil Steril 36: 746

Fumagalli Z, Motta P, Calvieri S 1971 The presence of smooth muscular cells in the ovary of several mammals as seen under the electron microscope. Experientia 27: 682

Funkenstein B, Nimrod A 1981 Control of developmental processes in cultured neonatal ovaries. In: Byskov A G, Peters H (eds) Development and function of reproductive organs. Excerpta Medica, Amsterdam, pp 307–318

Funkenstein B, Nimrod A, Lindner H R 1980 The development of steroidogenic capability and responsiveness to gonadotropins in cultured neonatal rat ovaries. Endocrinology 106: 98

Galway A B, LaPolt P S, Tsafriri A, Dargan C M, Boime I, Hsueh A J W 1990 Recombinant follicle-stimulating hormone induces ovulation and tissue plasminogen activator expression in hypophysectomized rats. Endocrinology 127: 3023

Gerard M, Menezo Y, Rombauts P, Szöllösi D, Thibault C 1979 In vitro studies of oocyte maturation and follicular metabolism in the pig. Ann Biol Anim Biochem Biophys 18: 1521

Gilula N B, Epstein M L, Beers W H 1978 Cell-to-cell communication and ovulation: a study of the cumulus–oocyte complex. J Cell Biol 78: 58

Goetz F W, Berndtson A K, Ranjan M 1991 Ovulation: mediators at the ovarian level. Vertebrate endocrinology: fundamentals and biomedical implications. 4, part A. Academic, New York, pp 127–203

Goff A R, Henderson K M 1979 Changes in follicular fluid and serum concentrations of steroids in PMS treated immature rats following LH administration. Biol Reprod 20: 1153

Goldring N B, Farkash Y, Goldschmit T, Orly J 1986 Immunofluorescent probing of the mitochondrial cholesterol side-chain cleavage cytochrome P-450 expressed in differentiating granulosa cells in culture. Endocrinology 119: 2821

Goodman A L, Nixon W E, Johnson D K, Hodgen D 1977 Regulation of folliculogenesis in the cycling rhesus monkey: selection of the dominant follicle. Endocrinology 100: 155

Gore-Langton R E, Armstrong D T 1988 Follicular steroidogenesis and its control. In: Knobil E, Neill J (eds) The physiology of reproduction, 1. Raven, New York, pp 331–385

Gospodarowicz D 1988 Molecular characterization of fibroblast growth factor and possible role in early and late embryonic development. In: Hirshfield A N (eds) Growth factors and the ovary. Plenum Press, New York, pp 75–92

Gospodarowicz D, Bialecki I I 1979 Fibroblast and epidermal growth factors are mitogenic agents for cultured granulosa cells of rodent, porcine and human origin. Endocrinology 104: 757

Gospodarowicz D, Cheng J, Lui G M, Bohlen P 1985 Corpus luteum angiogenic factor is related to fibroblast growth factor. Endocrinology 117: 301

Gospodarowicz D, Ill C R, Birdwell C R 1977a Effect of fibroblast and epidermal growth factors on ovarian cell proliferation in vitro. I. Characterization of the response of granulosa cells for FGF and EGF. Endocrinology 100: 1108

Gospodarowicz D, Birdwell C R 1977b Effect of fibroblast and epidermal growth factors on ovarian cell proliferation in vitro. II. Proliferative response of luteal cells to FGF but not EGF. Endocrinology 100: 1121

Gougeon A 1986 Dynamics of follicular growth in the human: a model from preliminary results. Human Reproduction 1: 81

Gougeon A 1990 Follicular growth to ovulation. In: Edwards R G (eds) Establishing a successful human pregnancy, 66. Raven, New York, pp 49–62

Gougeon A, Lefévre B 1983 Evolution of the diameters of the largest healthy and atretic follicles during the human menstrual cycle. J Reprod Fertil 69: 497

Grant G A, Eisen A Z, Marmer B C, Roswil W T, Goldberg G I 1987 The activation of human skin fibroblast procollagenase. J Biol Chem 262: 5886

Greenwald G S, Siegel H I 1982 Is the first or second periovulatory surge of FSH responsible for follicular recruitment in the hamster? Proc Soc Exp Biol Med 170: 225

Greenwald G S, Terranova P F 1988 Follicular selection and its control. In: Knobil E, Neill J, Ewing L L, Greenwald G S, Markert C L, Pfaff D W (eds) The physiology of reproduction, 1. Raven, New York, pp 387–445

Grimek H J, Ax R L 1982 Chromatographic comparisons of chondroitin-containing proteoglycans from small and large bovine ovarian follicles. Biochem Biophys Res Commun 104: 1401

Grumbach M M, Kaplan S L 1973 Ontogenesis of growth hormone, insulin, prolactin and gonadotrophin secretion in the human foetus. In: Cross K W, Nathanielz P (eds) Fetal and neonatal physiology. Cambridge University Press, Cambridge, p 362

Gulyas B J, Hodgen G D, Tullner W W, Ross G T 1977 Effects of fetal and maternal hypophysectomy on endocrine organs and body weight in infant Rhesus monkeys (*Macaca mulatta*): with particular emphasis on oogenesis. Biol Reprod 16: 216

Guraya S S 1985 Biology of ovarian follicles in mammals. Springer, Berlin

Gwatkin R B L, Andersen O F 1976 Hamster oocyte maturation in vitro inhibition by follicular components. Life Sci 19: 527

Hage A J, Groen-Klevant A C, Welschen R 1978 Follicle growth in immature rat ovary. Acta Endocrinol 88: 375

Hamada Y, Wright K H, Wallach E E 1979 The effect of progesterone and human chorionic gonadotrophin on ovulation in the in vitro perfused ovary. Fertil Steril 32: 335

Hamberger L, Hillensjö T, Ahrén K 1978 Steroidogenesis in isolated cells of preovulatory follicles. Endocrinol 103: 771

Hammond J M, Hsu C, Klindt J, Tsand B K, Downey B R 1988 Gonadotropins increase concentrations of immunoreactive insulin-like growth factor-I in porcine follicular fluid in vivio. Biol Reprod 38: 304

Harman S M, Louvet J, Ross G T 1975 Interaction of estrogen and gonadotropins on follicular atresia. Endocrinology 96: 1145

Hay M F, Moor R M 1973 The Graafian follicle of the sheep: relationship between gonadotropins, steroid production morphology and oocyte maturation. Ann Biologie Anim Biochim Biophys 13: 241

Hay M F, Moor R M 1975a Distribution of $\Delta^5$-3-hydroxysteroid dehydrogenase activity in the Graafian follicle of the sheep. J Reprod Fert 43: 313

Hay M F, Moor R M 1975b Functional and structural relationships in the Graafian follicle population of the sheep ovary. J Reprod Fertil 45: 583

Hay M F, Cran D G, Moor R M 1976 Structural changes occurring during atresia in sheep ovarian follicles. Cell Tissue Res 169: 515

He C, Wilhelm S M, Pentland A P et al 1989 Tissue cooperation in proteolytic cascade activity human interstitial collagenase. Proc Natl Acad Sci 86: 2632

Hedin L Gaddy-Kurten D, Kurten R, DeWitt D L, Smith W, Richards J S 1987a Prostaglandin endoperoxide synthetase in rat ovarian follicles: content, cellular distribution, and evidence for hormonal induction preceding ovulation. Endocrinology 121: 722

Hedin L, McKnight G S, Lifka J, Durica J, Richards J S 1987b Tissue distribution and hormonal regulation of messenger ribonucleic acid for regulatory and catalytic subunits of adenosine 3',5'-monophosphate-dependent protein kinases during ovarian follicular development and luteinization in the rat. Endocrinology 120: 1928

Hedin L, Rodgers R J, Simpson E R, Richards J S 1987c Changes in content of cytochrome $P450_{17\alpha}$, cytochrome $P450_{scc}$, and 3-hydroxy-3-methylglutaryl CoA reductase in developing rat ovarian follicles and corpora lutea: correlation with theca cell steroidogenesis. Biol Reprod 37: 211

Hekman C M, Loskutoff D J 1988 Bovine plasminogen activator inhibitor 1: specificity determinations and comparison of the active, latent, and guanidine-activated forms. Biochemistry 27: 2911

Hellberg P, Holmes P V, Brännström M, Olofsson J, Janson P O 1990 Inhibitors of lipoxygenase increase the ovulation rate in the in vitro perfused luteinizing hormone-stimulated rabbit ovary. Acta Physiol Scand 138: 557

Hellberg P, Larson L, Olofsson J, Hedin L, Brännström M 1991 Stimulatory effects of bradykinin on the ovulatory process in the in vitro-perfused rat ovary. Biol Reprod 44: 269

Henderson K M, McNatty K P, Smith P et al 1987 Influence of follicular health on the steroidogenic and morphological characteristics of bovine granulosa cells in vitro. J Reprod Fertil 79: 185

Henderson K M, Savage L C, Ellen R L, Ball K, McNatty K P 1988 Consequences of increasing or decreasing plasma FSH concentrations during the preovulatory period in Romney ewes. J Reprod Fertil 84: 187

Hernandez E R, Hurwitz A, Payne D W, Dharmarajan A M, Purchio A F, Adashi E Y 1990 Transforming growth factor-β 1 inhibits ovarian androgen production: gene expression, cellular localization, mechanisms(s), and site(s) of action. Endocrinology 127: 2804

Hill M, White W E 1933 The growth and regression of follicles in the oestrous rabbit. J Physiol 80: 174

Hillensjö T 1976 Oocyte maturation and glycolysis in isolated pre-ovulatory follicles of PMS-injected immature rats. Acta Endocrinol Copenh 82: 809

Hillensjö T 1981 Steroid biosynthesis by granulosa, thecal and stromal cells: their interaction. In: Franchimont P, Channing C P (eds) Intragonadal regulation of reproduction. Academic London, pp 33–60

Hillensjö T, Channing C P 1980 Gonadotropin stimulation of

steroidogenesis and cellular dispersion in cultured porcine cumuli oophori. Gamete Res 3: 233

Hillensjö T, Batta S K, Schwartz-Kripner A, Wentz A C, Sulewski J, Channing C P 1978 Inhibitory effect of human follicular fluid upon the maturation of porcine oocytes in culture. J Clin Endocrinol Metab 47: 1332

Hillensjö T, Bauminger S, Ahrén K 1976 Effect of luteinizing hormone on the pattern of steroid production by preovulatory follicles of Pregnant Mare's Serum Gonadotropin-injected immature rats. Endocrinology 99: 996

Hillensjö T, Hamberger L, Ahrén K 1977 Effect of androgens on the biosynthesis of estradiol 17 β by isolated preovulatory rat follicles. Molec Cell Endocrinol 9: 183

Hillensjö T, Ekholm C, Ahrén K 1978 Role of cyclic AMP in oocyte maturation and glycolysis in the pre-ovulatory rat follicle. Acta Endocrinol Copenh 87: 377

Hillensjö T, Channing C P, Pomerantz S H, Schwartz-Kripner A 1979a Intrafollicular control of oocyte maturation in the pig. In Vitro 15: 32

Hillensjö T, Kripner A S, Pomerantz S H, Channing C P 1979b Action of porcine follicular fluid oocyte maturation in vitro: possible role of cumulus cells. In: Channing C P, Marsh J M, Sadler W A (eds) Ovarian follicular and corpus luteum function. Plenum, New York, pp 283–291

Hillensjö T, Chari S, Magnusson C, Daume E, Sturm G 1981a Inhibitory effects of low molecular weight fractions of human follicular fluid upon rat granulosa cells and oocyte in vitro. In: Semm K, Mettler K (eds) International Congress Series No. 551 (Proceedings II World Congress of Human Reproduction). Excerpta Medica, Berlin

Hillensjö T, Magnusson C, Svensson U, Thelander H 1981b Effect of LH and FSH on progesterone synthesis in cultured rat cumulus cells. Endocrinology 108: 1920

Hillensjö T, Magnusson C, Ekholm C, Billig H, Hedin L 1982 Role of cumulus cells in oocyte maturation. In: Segal S J, Channing C P (eds) Intraovarian control mechanisms. Plenum, New York, pp 175–188

Hillier G S, Ross G T 1979 Effects of exogenous testosterone on ovarian weight, follicular morphology an intraovarian progesterone concentration in estrogen-primed hypophysectomized immature female rats. Biol Reprod 20: 261

Hillier S G, van den Boogaard A M Y, Reichert A M J, Reichert L E J, van Hall E V 1980 Alterations in granulosa cell aromatase activity accompanying preovulatory follicular development in the rat ovary with evidence that 5a-reduced C19 steroids inhibit the aromatase reaction in vitro. J Endocrinol 84: 409

Himelstein-Braw R, Byskov A G, Peters H, Faber M 1976 Follicular atresia in the infant human ovary. J Reprod Fertil 46: 55

Himelstein-Braw R, Peters H, Faber M 1977 Influence of irradiation and chemotherapy on the ovaries of children with abdominal tumours. Br J Cancer 36: 269

Hirshfield A N 1986 Patterns of [$^3$H] thymidine incorporation differ in immature rats and mature, cycling rats. Biol Reprod 34: 229

Hirshfield A N, (ed) 1989 Growth factors and the ovary. Plenum, New York

Hirshfield A N, Midgley A R Jr. 1978a Morphometric analysis of follicular development in the rat. Biol Reprod 19: 597

Hirshfield A N, Midgley A R J 1978b The role of FSH in the selection of large ovarian follicles in the rat. Biol Reprod 19: 606

Hodgen G D, Rosenwaks Z, Spieler J M (eds) 1988 Nonsteroidal gonadal factors: physiological roles and possibilities in contraceptive development. Conrad International Workshop, The Jones Institute Press, Norfolk

Holmes P V, Janson P O, Sogn J et al 1983 Effects of P G F$_{2\alpha}$ and indomethacin on ovulation and steroid production in the isolated perfused rabbit ovary. Acta Endocrinol 104: 233

Holmes P V, Sogn J, Schillinger E, Janson P O 1985 Effects of high and low preovulatory concentrations of progesterone on ovulation from the isolated perfused rabbit ovary. J Reprod Fertil 76: 393

Hsu C J, Holmes S D, Hammond J M 1987 Ovarian epidermal growth factor-like activity. Concentrations in porcine follicular fluid during follicular enlargement. Biochem Biophys Res Commun 147: 242

Hsueh A J W, Adashi E Y, Jones P B C, Welsh J T H 1984 Hormonal regulation of the differentiation of cultured ovarian granulosa cells. Endocrine Rev 5: 76

Hsueh A J, Bicsak T A, Jia X C et al 1989 Follicle-stimulating hormone: structure and function of a glycoprotein hormone. In: Clark J H (eds) Recent progress in hormone research, 45. Academic, San Diego, C A, pp 209–277

Husain A, Bumpus F M, De Silva P, Speth R C 1987 Localization of angiotensin II receptors in ovarian follicles and the identification of angiotensin in rat ovaries. Proc Nat Acad Sci USA 84: 2489

Huslig R L, Malik A, Clark M R 1987 Human chorionic gonadotropin stimulation of immunoreactive prostaglandin synthase in rat ovary. Molec Cell Endocrinol 50: 237

Ichikawa S, Morioka H, Oda M, Oda K, Murao S 1983a Effects of various proteinase inhibitors on ovulation of explanted hamster ovaries. J Reprod Fertil 68: 407

Ichikawa S, Ohta M, Morioka H, Murao S 1983b Blockage of ovulation in the explanted hamster ovary by a collagenase inhibitor. J Reprod Fertil 68: 17

Ingram D L 1962 Atresia. In: Zuckerman S (ed) The ovary, 1. Academic, New York, pp 247–273

Ireland J J, Richards J S 1978 A previously undescribed role for luteinizing hormone (LH: hCG) on follicular cell differentiation. Endocrinology 102: 1458

Itoh M, Igarashi M, Yamada K et al 1990 Activin A stimulated meiotic maturation of the rat oocyte in vitro. Biochem Biophys Res Commun 166: 1479–1484

Itskovitz J, Sealey J E, Glorioso N, Rosenwaks Z 1987 Plasma prorenin response to human chorionic gonadotropin in ovarian-hyperstimulated women: correlation with the number of ovarian follicles and steroid hormone concentrations. Proc Nat Acad Sci USA 84: 7285

Iwamatsu T, Chang M C 1972 Sperm penetration in vitro of mouse oocytes at various times during maturation. J Reprod Fertil 31: 237

Jagiello G, Graffeo J, Ducayen M, Prosser R 1977 Further studies of inhibitors of in vitro mammalian oocyte maturation. Fertil Steril 28: 476

Janson P O 1975 Effects of luteinizing hormone on blood in the follicular rabbit ovary as measured by radioactive microspheres. Acta Endocrinol 79: 122

Janson P O, Amato F, Weiss T, Ralph M, Seamark R F 1978 On the isolated perfused sheep ovary as a model for the study of ovarian function. Fertil Steril 30: 230

Janson P O, LeMaire W J, Källfelt B 1982 The study of ovulation in the isolated perfused rabbit ovary. I. Methodology and pattern of steroidogenesis. Biol Reprod 26: 456

Jensen E V, Zachariae F 1958 Studies on the mechanism of ovulation: Isolation and analysis of acid mucopolysaccharides in bovine follicular fluid. Acta Endocrinol (Copenh) 27: 356

Jones E C 1956 The aging ovary. Thesis, University of Birmingham

Jones P B C, Vernon M W, Muse K N, Curry J T E 1989 Plasminogen activator and plasminogen activator inhibitor in human preovulatory follicular fluid. J Clin Endocrinol 68: 1039

Jones R E (ed) 1978 The vertebrate ovary. Plenum, New York

Kammerman S, Ross J 1975 Increase in numbers of gonadotropin receptors on granulosa cells during follicle maturation. J Clin Endocrinol Metab 41: 546

Killick S, Elstein M 1987 Pharmacologic production of luteinized unruptured follicles by prostaglandin synthetase inhibitors. Fertil Steril 47: 773

Knecht M, Feng P, Catt K J 1989 Transforming growth factor-beta: autocrine, paracrine, and endocrine effects in ovarian cells. Semin Reprod Endocrinol 7: 12

Knobil E, Neill J 1988 In: Ewing L L, Greenwald G S, Markert C L, Pfaff D W (eds) The physiology of reproduction. Raven, New York

Knudsen J F, Litkowski L J, Wilson T L, Guthrie H D, Batta S K 1978 Concentrations of hydrogen ions, oxygen, carbon dioxide and bicarbonate in porcine follicular fluid. J Endocrinol 79: 249

Knudsen J F, Litkowski L J, Wilson T L, Guthrie H D, Batta S K 1979 Follicular fluid electrolytes and osmolality in cyclic pigs. J Reprod Fertil 57: 419

Koering M J 1969 Cyclic changes in ovarian morphology during the menstrual cycle in *Macaca mulatta*. Am J Anat 126: 73

Kogawa K, Nakamura T, Sugino K, Takio K, Titani K, Sugino H 1991 Activin-binding protein is present in pituitary. Endocrinology 128: 1434

Kolena J 1976 Ontogenic development of the responsiveness in cAMP synthesis to L H and $PGE_1$ and gonadotropin receptors in the rat ovary. Biol Neonate 29: 96

Koos R D, Feiertag M A, Brodie A M H, LeMaire W J 1984a Inhibition of estrogen synthesis does not inhibit luteinizing hormone-induced ovulation. Am J Obstet Gynecol 148: 939

Koos R D, Jaccarino F J, Magaril R A, LeMaire W J 1984b Perfusion of the rat ovary in vitro methodology, induction of ovulation and pattern of steroidogenesis. Biol Reprod 30: 715

Koos R D, Olson C E 1989 Expression of basic fibroblast growth factor in the rat ovary: detection of mRNA using reverse transcription-polymerase chain reaction amplification. Molec Endocrinol 3: 2041

Koos R D, Seidel R H 1989 Detection of acidic fibroblast growth factor mRNA in the rat ovary using reverse transcription-polymerase chain reaction amplification. Biochem Biophys Res Commun 165: 882

Kudlow J E, Kobrin M S, Purchio A F et al 1987 Ovarian transforming growth factor-a gene expression: immunohistochemical localization to the theca-interstitial cells. Endocrinology 121: 1577

Lambertsen C J, Greenbaum D F, Wright K H, Wallach E E 1967 In vitro studies of ovulation in the perfused rabbit ovary. Fertil Steril 27: 178

Lamprecht S A, Zor U, Tsafriri A, Lindner H R 1973 Action of $PGE_2$ and LH on ovarian adenylate cyclase, protein kinase and ornithine decarboxylase activity during postnatal development and maturity in the rat. J Endocrinol 57: 217

LaPolt P S, Yamoto M, Veljkovic M et al 1990 Basic fibroblast factor induction of granulosa cell tissue-type plasminogen activator expression and oocyte maturation: potential role as a paracrine ovarian hormone. Endocrinology 127: 2357

Larsen W J, Wert S E, Brunner G D 1986 A dramatic loss of cumulus cell gap junctions is correlated with germinal vesicle breakdown in rat oocytes. Develop Biol 113: 517

Lee W, Novy M J 1978 Effects of luteinizing hormone and indomethacin on blood flow and steroidogenesis in the rabbit ovary. Biol Reprod 18: 799

Leibfried L, First N L 1980a Effect of bovine and porcine follicular fluid and granulosa cells on maturation of oocyte in vitro. Biol Reprod 23: 699

Leibfried L, First N L 1980b Follicular control of meiosis in the porcine oocyte. Biol Reprod 23: 705

Leibfried L, First N L 1982 Preovulatory changes in cumulus – oocyte complex of the hamster. Anat Rec 202: 339

LeMaire W J, Yang N S T, Behrman H H, Marsh J M 1973 Preovulatory changes in the concentration of prostaglandins in rabbit Graafian follicles. Prostaglandins 3: 367

LeMaire W J, Curry T E, Morioka N et al 1987 Regulation of ovulatory processes. In: Stouffer R L (ed) The primate ovary. Plenum New York, pp 91–111

LeMaire W J, Janson IO, Källfelt B J et al 1982 The preovulatory decline in follicular estradiol is not required for ovulation in the rabbit. Acta Endocrinol Copenh 101: 452

Levi-Montalcini R, Cohen S 1960 Effects of the extract of the mouse submaxillary salivary glands on the sympathetic system of mammals. Ann N Y Acad Sci 85: 324

Lieberman M E, Barnea A, Bauminger S, Tsafriri A, Collins W P, Linder H R 1975 LH-effect on the pattern of steroidogenesis in cultured Graafian follicles of the rat: dependence on macromolecular synthesis. Endocrinology 96: 1533

Liedtke M P, Seifert B 1978 Biosynthesis of prostaglandins in human ovarian tissues. Prostaglandins 16: 825

Lindner H R, Tsafriri A, Lieberman M E et al 1974 Gonadotropin action on cultured Graafian follicles: mechanism of induction of maturation of the mammalian oocyte. Recent Prog Horm Res 30: 79

Lindner H R, Amsterdam A, Salomon Y et al 1977 Intraovarian factors in ovulation: determinants of follicular response to gonadotrophins. J Pieprod Fertil 51: 215

Ling N, Ying S, Ueno N, Esch F, Denoroy L, Guillemin R 1985 Isolation and partial characterization of a Mw 32,000 protein with inhibin activity from porcine follicular fluid. Proc Nat Acad Sci USA 82: 7217

Ling N, Ying S Y, Ueno N et al 1986 Pituitary FSH is released by a heterodimer of the β-subunits from the two forms of inhibin. Nature (Lond) 321: 779

Lipner H 1973 Mechanism of mammalian ovulation. In: Greep R (ed) Handbook of physiology, endocrinology. II, part 1. American Physiological Society, Washington, DC, pp 409–437

Lipner H 1988 Mechanism of mammalian ovulation. In: Knobil E, Neill J (eds) The physiology of reproduction. Raven, New York, pp 447–488

Lipner H, Greep R O 1971 Inhibition of steroidogenesis at various sites in the biosynthetic pathway in relation to induced ovulation. Endocrinology 88: 602

Lipner H, Wendelken L 1971 Inhibition of ovulation by inhibition of steroidogenesis in immature rats. Proc Soc Exp Biol Med 136: 1141

Lischinsky A, Armstrong D 1983 Granulosa cell stimulation of thecal androgen synthesis. Canad J Physiol Pharmacol 61: 472

Löfman C O, Janson P O , Källfelt B J, Ahrén K, LeMaire W J 1982 The study of ovulation in the isolated perfused rabbit ovary. II. Photographic and cinematographic observations. Biol Reprod 26: 467

Louvet J P, Vaitukaitis J L 1976 Induction of FSH receptor in rat ovaries by estrogen priming. Endocrinology 97: 366

Louvet J P, Harman S M, Schreiber J R, Ross G T 1975 Evidence for a role of androgens in follicle maturation. Endocrinology 97: 366

Lumsden M A, Kelly R W, Templeton A A, van Look P F A, Swanston I A, Baird D T 1986 Changes in the concentration of prostaglandins in preovulatory human follicles after administration of hCG. J Reprod Fertil 77: 119

Lutwak-Mann C 1954 Note on the chemical composition of bovine follicular fluid. J Agric Sci 44: 477

Magnusson C, Hillensjö T 1981 Further studies on the gonadotrophin-induced inhibition of respiration in the preovulatory rat cumulus oophorus. Acta Physiol Scanda 113: 17

Magnusson C, Hillensjö T, Tsafriri A, Hultborn R, Ahrén K 1977 Oxygen consumption of maturing rat oocytes. Biol Reprod 17: 9

Magoffin D A, Gancedo B, Erickson G F 1989 Transforming growth factor-β promotes differentiation of ovarian thecal-interstitial cells but inhibits androgen production. Endocrinology 125: 1951

Mahi-Brown C A, Yanagimachi R 1983 Parameters influencing ovum pickup by oviductal fimbria in the golden hamster. Gamete Res 8: 1

Makris A, Ryan K J 1975 Progesterone, androstenedione, testosterone, estrone and estradiol synthesis in hamster ovarian follicle cells. Endocrinology 96: 694

Makris A, Ryan K J 1980 The source of follicular androgens in the hamster follicle. Steroids 35: 53

Mandl A M, Zuckerman S 1950 The number of normal and atretic ova in the mature rat. J Endocrinol 6: 426

Mann G E, Campbell B K, McNeilly A S, Baird D T 1989 Passively immunizing ewes against inhibin during the luteal phase of the oestrus cycle raises the plasma concentration of FSH. J Endocrinol 123: 383

Marion G B, Gier H T, Choudary J B 1968 Micromorphology of the bovine ovarian follicular system. J Anim Sci 27: 452

Marsh J M 1976 The role of cyclic AMP in gonadal steroidogenesis. Biol Reprod 14: 30

Marsh I M, LeMaire W J 1974 The role of cyclic AMP and prostaglandins in the actions of luteinizing hormone. In: Moudgal N R (ed) Gonadotropins and gonadal function. Academic, New York, pp 376–390

Martin G G, Talbot P 1981 The role of follicular smooth muscle cells in hamster ovulation. J Exp Zool 216: 469

Matrisian L M 1990 Metalloproteinases and their inhibitors in matrix remodeling. TIG 6: 121

Mattioli M, Galeati G, Seren E 1986 Pig oocyte maturation in vitro and evaluation of their developmental capability by IVF. Atti Soc It Sci Vet 40: 200

Mattioli M, Galeati G, Bacci M L, Seren E 1988a Follicular factors influence oocyte fertilizability by modulating the intercellular cooperation between cumulus cells and oocyte. Gamete Res 21: 223

Mattioli M, Galeati G, Seren E 1988b Effect of follicle somatic cells during pig oocyte maturation on egg penetrability and male pronucleus formation. Gamete Res 20: 177

Mauléon P 1969 Oogenesis and folliculogenesis. In: Cole H H, Cupps P (eds) Reproduction in domestic animals. Academic, New York, pp187–215

May J V, Schomberg D W 1989 The potential relevance of epidermal growth factor and transforming growth factor-alpha to ovarian physiology. Sem Reprod Endocrinol 7: 1

McNatty K P 1978 Follicular fluid. In: Jones R E (eds) the vertebrate ovary. Plenum, New York, pp 215–259

McNatty K P 1981 Hormonal correlates of follicular development in the human ovary. Australian J Biol Sci 34: 249

McNatty K P, Hunter W M, NcNeilly A S, Sawers R S 1975 Changes in the concentration of pituitary and steroid hormones in the follicular fluid of human Graafian follicles throughout the menstrual cycle. J Endocrinol 64: 555

McNatty K P, Baird D T, Bolton A, Chambers P, Corker C S, McLean H 1976 Concentration of oestrogens and androgens in human ovarian venous plasma and follicular fluid throughout the menstrual cycle. J Endocrinol 71: 77

McNatty K P, Makris A, De Grazia C, Osathanondh R, Ryan K J 1979 The production of progesterone, androgens and oestrogens by human granulosa cells in vitro and in vivo. J Steroid Biochem 11: 775

McNatty K P, Makris A, De Grazia C, Osathanondh R, Ryan K J 1980 Steroidogenesis by recombined follicular cells from the human ovary in vitro. J Clin Endocrinol Metab 51: 1286

McNatty K P, Hillier S G, Van den Boogard A M J, Trimbos-Kemper T C M, Reichert J L E, Van Hall E V 1983 Follicular development during the luteal phase of the human menstrual cycle. J Clin Endocrinol Metab 56: 1022

McNatty K P, Hudson N, Gibb M et al 1985 FSH influences follicle viability, oestradiol biosynthesis and ovulation rate in Romney ewes. J Reprod Fert 75: 121

McNeilly A S 1985 Effect of changes in FSH induced by bovine follicular fluid and FSH infusion in the preovulatory phase on subsequent ovulation rate and corpus luteum function in the ewe. J Reprod Fertil 74: 661

McNeilly A S, Jonassen J A, Fraser H M 1986 Suppression of follicular development after chronic LHRH immunoneutralization in the ewe. J Reprod Fertil 76: 481

Meinecke B, Meinecke-Tillman S 1981 Induction and inhibition of meiotic maturation of follicle-enclosed porcine oocytes in vivo. Theriogenology 216: 205

Miller W A, Jagiello G 1973 Gonadotropin dependency of isolated ovine ovarian follicles cultured in vitro. Fertil Steril 24: 609

Miller J J I, Williams G F, Leissring J C 1971 Multiple late complications of therapy with cyclophosphamide, including ovarian destruction. Am J Med 50: 530

Mills T M, Savard K 1973 Steriodogenesis in ovarian follicles isolated from rabbit before and after mating. Endocrinology 92: 788

Milwidsky A, Kaneti H, Pinci Z, Laufer N, Tsafriri A, Mayer M 1989 Human follicular fluid protease and antiprotease activities: a suggested correlation with ability of oocytes to undergo in vitro fertilization. Fertil Steril 52: 274

Miyamoto K, Hasegawa Y, Fukuda M et al 1985 Isolation of porcine follicular fluid inhibin of 32K daltons. Biochem Biophys Res Commun 129: 396

Miyazaki T, Sueoka K, Dharmarajan A M, Atlas S J, Bulkley G B, Wallach E E 1991 Effect of inhibition of oxygen free radical on ovulation and progesterone production by the in vitro perfused rabbit ovary. Reprod Fertil 91: 207

Monniaux D, Mariana Y C, Gibson W R 1984 Action of PMSG on follicular population in the heifers. J Reprod Fertil 70: 243

Moor R M 1973 Oestrogen production by individual follicles explanted from ovaries of sheep. J Reprod Fertil 32: 545

Moor R M 1977 Sites of steroid production in ovine Graafian follicles in culture. J Endocrinol 73: 143

Moor R M, Trounson A O 1977 Hormonal and follicular factors affecting maturation of sheep oocytes in vitro and their subsequent developmental capacity. J Reprod Fertil 49: 101

Moor R M, Hay M F, Dott H M, Cran D G 1978 Macroscopic identification and steroidogenic function of atretic follicles in sheep. J Endocrinol 77: 309

Moor R M, Smith M W, Dawson R M C 1980 Measurement of intercellular coupling between oocytes and cumulus cells using intracellular markers. Exp Cell Res 126: 15

Morales T I, Woessner J F, Howell D S, Marsh J M, LeMaire W J 1978 A microassay for the direct demonstration of collagenolytic activity in Graafian follicles of the rat. Biochim Biophys Acta 524: 428

Morales T I, Woessner J F J, Marsh J M, LeMaire W J 1983 Collagen, collagenase and collagenolytic activity in rat Graafian follicles during follicular growth and ovulation. Biochim Biophys Acta 756: 119

Mori T, Fujita Y, Suzuki A, Kinoshta Y, Nishimura T, Kanbegawa A 1978 Functional and structural relationships in steroidogenesis in vitro by human ovarian follicles during maturation and ovulation. J Clin Endocrinol Metab 47: 955

Morioka N, Brännström M, Koos R D, LeMaire W J 1988 Ovulation in the perfused ovary in vitro: Further evidence that estrogen is not required. Steroids 51: 173

Motlik J, Fulka J, Flèchon J E 1986 Changes in intercellular coupling between pig oocytes and cumulus cells during maturation in vivo and in vitro. J Reprod Fertil 76: 31

Murdoch W J, Nix K J, Dunn T G 1983 Dynamics of ovarian blood supply to periovulatory follicles of the ewe. Biol Reprod 28: 1001

Murdoch W J, Peterson T A, Van Kirk E A, Vincent D L, Inskeep E K 1986 Interactive roles of progesterone, prostaglandin, and collagenase in the ovulatory mechanism of the ewe. Biol Reprod 35: 1187

Nakamura T, Takio K, Eto Y, Shibai H, Titani K, Sugino H 1990 Activin-binding protein from rat ovary is follistatin. Science 247: 836

Nakano R, Mixumo T, Katayama K, Tojo S 1975 Growth of ovarian follicles in the absence of gonadotrophins. J Reprod Fertil 45: 545

Neal P, Baker T G 1973 Response of mouse ovaries in vivo and in organ culture to pregnant mare's serum gonadotrophin and human chorionic gonadotrophin. I. Examination of critical time intervals. J Reprod Fertil 33: 399

Neufeld G, Ferrara N, Mitchell R, Schweigerer L, Gospodarowicz D 1987 Granulosa cells produce basic fibroblast growth factor. Endocrinology 121: 597

Nilsson L, Wikland M, Hamberger L 1982 Recruitment of an ovulatory follicle in the human following follicle-ectomy and luteectomy. Fertil Steril 37: 30

Niwa K, Chang M C 1975 Fertilization of rat eggs in vitro at various times before and after ovulation with special reference to fertilization of ovarian oocytes matured in culture. J Reprod Fertil 43: 435

Ny T, Elgh F, Lund B 1984 The structure of the human tissue type plasminogen activator gene. Correlation of intron and exon structures to functional and structural domains. Proc Nat Acad Sci USA 81: 5355

Ny T, Bjersing L, Hsueh A J W, Loskutoff D J 1985 Cultured granulosa cells produce two plasminogen activators and an antiactivator, each regulated differently by gonadotropins. Endocrinology 116: 1666

O W, Robertson D M, de Kretser D M 1989 Inhibin as an oocyte meiotic inhibitor. Molec Cell Endocrinol 62: 307

Oakberg E F, Tyrrell P D 1975 Labeling the zona pellucida of the mouse oocyte. Biol Reprod 12: 477

Ohno S, Smith J B 1964 Role of fetal follicular cells in meiosis of mammalian oocytes. Cytogenetics 3: 324

Okamura H, Virutamasen P, Wright K H, Wallach E E 1972 Ovarian smooth muscle in the human being, rabbit, and cat. Am J Obstet Gynecol 112: 183

Olds D, VanDemark N L 1957 Composition of luminal fluid in bovine female genitalia. Fertil Steril 8: 345

O'Malley B W 1989 Editorial: did eucaryotic steroid receptors evolve from intracrine gene regulators? Endocrinology 125: 1119

Orczyk G P, Behrman H R 1972 Ovulation blockade by aspirin or indomethacin: In vivo evidence for a role of prostaglandin in gonadotrophin secretion. Prostaglandins 1: 3

O'Shea J D 1970 An ultrastructural study of smooth muscle-like cells in the theca externa of ovarian follicles in the rat. Anat Rec 167: 127

Osvaldo-Decima L 1970 Smooth muscle in the ovary of the rat and monkey. J Ultrastruc Res 29: 218

Parr E L 1974 Histological examination of the rat ovarian follicle wall prior to ovulation. Biol Reprod 11: 483

Parr E L 1975 Rupture of ovarian follicles at ovulation. J Reprod Fertil (Suppl) 22: 1

Patwardhan V V, Lanthier A 1976 Effect of ovulatory dose of LH on the concentration of oestrone, oestradiol and progesterone in the rabbit ovarian follicles. Acta Endocrinol 82: 792

Patwardhan V V, Lanthier A 1981 Prostaglandins PGE and PGF in human ovarian follicles: endogenous contents and in vitro formation by theca and granulosa cells. Acta Endocrinol 97: 543

Payne R W, Runser R H 1959 Quantitative response of the rat ovary to pituitary gonadotrophin as modified by estrogen. Endocrinology 65: 383

Pedersen T 1970 Follicle kinetics in the ovary of the cyclic mouse. Acta Endocrinol 64: 304

Pedersen T, Peters H 1968 Proposal for a classification of

oocytes and follicles in the mouse ovary. J Reprod Fertil 17: 555

Pellicer A, Palumbo A, DeCherney A H, Naftolin F 1988 Blockage of ovulation by an angiotensin antagonist. Science 240: 1660

Peters H 1978 Folliculogenesis in mammals. In: Jones R E (ed) The vertebrate ovary. Plenum, New York, pp 121–144

Peters H, McNatty K P 1980 The ovary. Granada Publishing, London

Peters H, Byskov A G, Faber M 1973 Intraovrian regulation of follicle growth in the immature mouse. In: Peters H (ed) The development and maturation of the ovary and its function. Excerpta Medica, Amsterdam, pp 20–23

Peters H, Himelstein-Braw R, Faber M 1976 The normal development of the ovary in childhood. Acta Endocrinol 82: 617

Peters H, Byskov A G, Grinsted J 1978 Follicular growth in fetal and prepubertal ovaries of human and other primates. In: Ross G T, Lipsett M B (eds) Gynecological endocrinology. W.B. Saunders, London, p 469

Peters H, Byskov A G, Himelstein-Braw R, Faber M 1975 Follicular growth: the basic event in the mouse and human ovary. J Reprod Fertil 45: 559

Peterson C M, Zhu C, Mukaida T, LeMaire W J 1989 The angiotensin II antagonist, saralasin, inhibits ovulation in the perfused rat ovary. Biol Reprod 40: 56

Phillips D M, Dekel N 1991 Maturation of the rat cumulus – oocyte complex: structure and function. Molec Reprod Develop 28: 297

Pacsek B E, Huth J F 1971 Changes in ovarian venous blood flow following cannulation: effect of luteinizing hormone (LH) and antihistamine. Proc Soc Exp Biol Med 138: 1022

Pincus G, Enzmann E V 1935 The comparative behaviour of mammalian eggs in vivo and in vitro. J Exp Med 62: 655

Pincus G, Enzmann E V 1937 The growth, maturation and atresia of ovarian eggs in the rabbit. Journal of Morphology 61: 351–383

Plunkett E R, Moon Y S, Zamecnik J, Armstrong D T 1975 Preliminary evidence of a role for prostaglandin F in human follicular function. Am J Obstet Gynecol 123: 392

Pomerantz S, Tsafriri A, Channing C P 1979 Studies on purification and actions of an oocyte maturation inhibitor isolated from porcine follicular fluid. In: Gross E, Meienhofer J (eds) Peptides, structure and biological function. Pierre Chemical Company, Rockford, IL pp 765–774

Potter G 1963 The ovary in infancy and childhood. In: Grady H G, Smith D E (eds) The ovary. Williams and Wilkins, Baltimore, pp 11: 23

Presl J, Pospisil J, Figarova V, Wagner V 1972 Developmental changes in uptake of radioactivity by the ovaries, pituitary and uterus after $^{125}$I-labeled human chorionic gonadotrophin administration in rats. J Endocrinol 52: 585

Presl J, Pospisil J, Figarova V, Krabec Z 1974 Stage-dependent changes in binding of iodinated FSH during ovarian follicle maturation in rats. Endocrinol Exp (Bratisl) 8: 291

Priddy A R, Killick S R, Elstein M et al 1989 Ovarian follicular fluid eicosanoid concentrations during the pre-ovulatory period in humans. Prostaglandins 38: 197

Pucell A G, Bumpus F M, Husain A 1987 Rat ovarian angiotensin II receptors. J Biol Chem 262: 7076

Purandare T V, Munshi S R, Rao S S 1976 Effect of antisera to gonadotropins on follicular development and fertility of mice. Biol Reprod 15: 311

Racowsky C 1984 Effect of forskolin on the spontaneous maturation and cyclic AMP content of rat oocyte cumulus complexes. J Reprod Fertil 72: 107

Racowsky C 1985 Effect of forskolin on maintenance of meiotic arrest and stimulation of cumulus expansion, progesterone and cyclic AMP production by pig oocyte-cumulus complexes. J Reprod Fertil 74: 9

Racowsky C, Satterlie R A 1985 Metabolic, fluorescent dye and electrical coupling between hamster oocytes and cumulus cells during meiotic maturation in vivo and in vitro. Devel Biol 60: 318

Racowsky C, Baldwin K V, Larabell C A, DeMarais A A, Kazilek C J 1989 Down-regulation of membrana granulosa gap junctions is correlated with irreversible commitment to resume meiosis in golden Syrian hamster oocytes. Eur J Cell Biol 49: 244

Rao M C, Richards J S, Midgley J A R, Reichert J L E 1977 Regulation of gonadotropin receptors by luteinizing hormone in granulosa cells. Endocrinology 101: 512

Rao I M, Mills T M, Anderson E, Mahesh V B 1991 Heterogeneity in granulosa cells of developing rat follicles. Anat Rec 229: 177

Ratoosh S L, Hedin L, Lifka J, Jahnsen T, Richards J S 1987 Hormonal regulation of the synthesis and mRNA content of the regulatory subunit of cyclic AMP-dependent protein kinase type II in cultured rat ovarian granulosa cells. J Biol Chem 262: 7306

Reich R, Tsafriri A 1984 Mechanisms involved in follicular rupture in the rat. In: McKerns K, Naor Z (eds) Hormonal control of the hypothalamo – pituitary – gonadal axis. Plenum, New York, pp 337–353

Reich R, Kohen F, Naor Z, Tsafriri A 1983 Possible involvement of lipoxygenase products of arachidonic acid pathway in ovulation. Prostaglandins 26: 1011

Reich R, Kohen F, Slager R, Tsafriri A 1985a Ovarian lipoxygenase activity and its regulation by gonadotropin in the rat. Prostaglandins 30: 581

Reich R, Miskin R, Tsafriri A 1985b Follicular plasminogen activator: involvement in ovulation. Endocrinology 116: 516

Reich R, Tsafriri A, Mechanic G L 1985c The involvement of collagenolysis in ovulation in the rat. Endocrinology 116: 521

Reich R, Tsafriri A, Mechanic G L 1985d Role of collagenolysis in ovulation in the rat. In: Toft D O, Ryan R J (eds) Proceedings of the 5th Ovarian Workshop, pp 167–173

Reich R, Miskin R, Tsafriri A 1986 Intrafollicular distribution of plasminogen activators and their hormonal regulation in vitro. Endocrinology 119: 1588

Reich R, Daphna-Iken D, Chun S Y et al 1991 Preovulatory changes in ovarian expression of collagenases and tissue metalloproteinase inhibitor mRNA: Role of eicosanoids. Endocrinology 129: 1869

Reich R, Haberman S, Abisogun A O et al 1987 Follicular rupture at ovulation: collagenase activity and metabolism of archidonic acid. In: Naftolin F, deCherney A H (eds) The control of follicle development, ovarian and luteal function: lessons from in vitro fertilization. Raven, New York, pp 317–329

Reichert J E 1962 Endocrine Influences on rat ovarian proteinase activity. Endocrinology 70: 697

Reinthaller A, Bieglmayer C, Kirchheimer J C, Christ G, Deutinger J, Binder B R 1990 Plasminogen activators, plasminogen activator inhibitor, and fibronectin in human granulosa cells and follicular fluid related to oocyte maturation and intrafollicular gonadotropin levels. Fertil Steril 54: 1045

Riccio A, Grimaldi G, Verde P, Gebastio G, Boast S, Blasi F 1985 The human urokinase plasminogen activator gene and its promotor. Nucl Acid Res 13: 2759

Richards J S 1978 Hormonal control of follicular growth and maturation in mammals. In: Jones R E (ed) The vertebrate ovary. Plenum, New York, pp 331–360

Richards J S 1980 Maturation of ovarian follicles: actions and interactions of pituitary and ovarian hormones on follicular cell differentiation. Physiol Rev 60: 51

Richards J S, Hedin L 1988 Molecular aspects of hormone action in ovarian follicular development, ovulation, and luteinization. Annual Review of Physiology 50: 441–463

Richards J S, Ireland J J, Rao M C, Bernath G A, Midgley A R J, Reichert L E J 1976 Ovarian follicular development in the rat: hormone receptor regulation by estradiol, follicle stimulating hormone and luteinizing hormone. Endocrinology 99: 1562

Richards J S, Haddox M, Tash Y S, Walter U, Lohmarin S M 1984 Adenoside 3', 5'-monophosphate-dependent protein kinase and granulosa cell responsiveness to gonadotropins. Endocrinology 114: 2190

Rivier C, Rivier J, Vale W 1985 Inhibin-mediated feedback control of follicle-stimulating hormone secretion in the female rat. Science 234: 205

Robertson D M, Foulds L M, Leversha L et al 1985 Isolation of inhibin from bovine follicular fluid. Biochem Biophys Res Commun 126: 220

Robertson D M, Klein R, de Vos F L et al 1987 The isolation of polypeptides with FSH suppressing activity from bovine follicular fluid which are structurally different to inhibin. Biochem Biophys Res Commun 149: 744

Rocerto T, Jacobowitz D, Wallach E 1969 Observations of spontaneous contractions of the cat ovary in vitro. Endocrinology 84: 1336

Rondell P 1964 Follicular perssure and distensibility. Am J Physiol 207: 590

Rondell P 1970 Biophysical aspects of ovulation. Biol Reprod 2 (suppl): 64

Rondell P 1974 Role of steroid synthesis in the process of ovulation. Biol Reprod 10: 199

Ross G T, Lipsett M B 1978 Hormonal correlates of normal and abnormal follicle growth after puberty in humans and other primates. Clin Endocrinol Metab 7: 561

Roy S K, Greenwald G S 1985 An enzymatic method for dissociation of intact follicles from the hamster ovary: histological and quantitative aspects. Biol Reprod 32: 203

Roy S K, Greenwald G S 1986 Effect of FSH and LH on incorporation of [3H] thymidine into follicular DNA. J Reprod Fertil 78: 201

Roy S K, Greenwald G S 1987 In vitro steroidogenesis by primary to antral follicles in the hamster during the periovulatory period: effects of follicle-stimulating hormone, luteinizing hormone and prolactin. Biol Reprod 37: 39

Sairam M R, Atkinson L E (eds) 1984 Gonadal proteins and peptides and their biological significance. World Scientific Publishing, Singapore

Salustri A, Siracusa G 1983 Metabolic coupling, cumulus expansion and meiotic resumption in mouse cumuli oophori cultured in vitro in the presence of FSH or dcAMP, or stimulated in vivo by hCG. J Reprod Fertil 68: 335

Salustri A, Yanagishita M, Hascall V C 1989 Synthesis and accumulation of hyaluronic acid and proteoglycans in the mouse cumulus cell-oocyte complex during FSH-induced mucification. J Biol Chem 264: 13840

Salustri A, Yanagishita M, Hascall V C 1990 Mouse oocytes regulate hyaluronic acid synthesis and mucification by FSH-stimulated cumulus cells. Develop Biol 138: 26

Sato E, Ishibashi T 1977 Meiotic arresting action of the substance obtained from cell surface to porcine ovarian granulosa cells. Jpn J Zootechnol Sci 48: 22

Sato E, Koide S S 1984 A factor from bovine granulosa cells preventing oocyte maturation. Differentiation 26: 59

Schochet S S 1916 A suggestion as to the process of ovulation and ovarian cyst formation. Anat Rec 10: 447

Schuetz A W 1985 Local control mechanisms during oogenesis and folliculogenesis. In: Browder L W (eds) Developmental biology. A comprehensive synthesis, 1. Plenum Press, New York, pp 3–83

Schuetz A W, Anisowicz A 1974 Cation and protein composition of ovarian follicular fluid of the pig: relation to follicle size. Biol Reprod 11: 64

Schuetz A W, Dubin N H 1981 Progesterone and prostaglandin secretion by ovulated rat cumulus cell-oocyte complexes. Endocrinology 108: 457

Schultz R M, Montgomery R R, Belanoff J R 1983 Regulation of mouse oocyte meiotic maturation: implication of a decrease in oocyte cAMP and protein dephosphorylation in commitment to resume meiosis. Develop Biol 97: 264

Schwartz N B 1974 The role of FSH and LH and of their antibodies on follicular growth and on ovulation. Biol Reprod 10: 236

Sealey J E, Atlas S A, Glorioso N, Manapat H, Laragh J H 1985 Cyclical secretion of prorenin during the menstrual cycle: synchronization with luteinizing hormone and progesterone. Proc Nat Acad Sci USA 82: 8705

Sealey J E, Cholst I, Glorioso N et al 1987 Sequential changes in plasma luteinizing hormone and plasma prorenin during the menstrual cycle. J Clin Endocrinol Metab 6: 1

Seamark R F, Moor R M, McIntosh J E W 1974 Steroid hormone production by sheep ovarian follicles in culture in vitro. J Reprod Fertil 41: 143

Shalet S M, Beardwell C G, Morris Jones P H, Pearson D, Orrell D H 1976 Ovarian failure following abdominal irradiation in childhood. Br J Cancer 33: 655

Shalgi R, Kraicer P F, Soferman N 1972 Gases and electrolytes of human follicular fluid. J Reprod Fertil 28: 335

Shalgi R, Kraicer P F, Rimon A, Pinto M, Soferman N 1973 Proteins of human follicular fluid: The blood-follicle barrier. Fertil Steril 24: 429

Sheela Rani C S, Moudgal N R 1977 Role of proestrus surge of gonadotropins in the initiation of follicular maturation in the cyclic hamster: a study using antisera to follicle stimulating hormone and luteinizing hormone. Endocrinology 101: 1484

Sherizly I, Galiani D, Dekel N 1988 Regulation of oocyte maturation: communication in the rat cumulus-oocyte complex. Human Reprod 3: 761

Shimonaka M, Inouye S, Shimasaki S, Ling N 1991

Follistatin binds to both activin and inhibin through the common beta-subunit. Endocrinology 128: 3313

Sirard M A, Bilodeau S 1990a Effects of granulosa cell co-culture on in-vitro meiotic resumption of bovine oocytes. J Reprod Fertil 89: 459

Sirard M A, Bilodeau S 1990b Granulosa cells inhibit the resumption of meiosis in bovine oocytes in vitro. Biol Reprod 43: 777

Sirard M A, First N L 1988 In vitro inhibition of oocyte nuclear maturation in the bovine. Biol Reprod 39: 229

Skinner M K, Coffey R J 1988 Regulation of ovarian cell growth through the local production of transforming growth factor-a by theca cells. Endocrinology 123: 2632

Skinner M K, Keski-oja J, Osteen K G, Moses H L 1987 Ovarian thecal cells produce transforming growth factor-β which can regulate granulosa cell growth. Endocrinology 121: 786

Smeaton T C, Robertson H A 1971 Studies on the growth and atresia of Graafian follicles in the ovary of the sheep. J Reprod Fertil 25: 243

Snyder B W, Beecham G D, Schane H P 1984 Inhibition of ovulation in rats with epostane, an inhibitor of 3β-hydroxysteroid dehydrogenase (41865). Proc Soc Exp Biol Med 176: 238

Sogn J H, Curry T E, Brannstrom M et al 1987 Inhibition of follicle-stimulating hormone induced ovulation by indomethacin in the perfused rat ovary. Biol Reprod 36: 536

Staigmiller R B, Moor R M 1984 Effect of follicle cells on the maturation and developmental competence of ovine oocytes matured outside the follicle. Gamete Res 9: 221

Stangroom J E, Weevers R de G 1962 Anticoagulant activity of equine follicular fluid. J Reprod Fertil 3: 269

Stone S L, Pomerantz S H, Schwartz-Kripner A, Channing C P 1978 Inhibitor of oocyte maturation from porcine follicular fluid: further purification and evidence for reversible action. Biol Reprod 19: 585

Strickland S, Beers W H 1976 Studies on the role of plasminogen activator in ovulation. In vitro response of granulosa cells to gonadotropins, cyclic nucleotides and prostaglandins. J Biol Chem 251: 5694

Suenson E, Lötzen O, Thorsen S 1984 Initial plasmin degradation of fibrin as the basis of a positive feed-back mechanism in fibrinolysis. Eur J Biochem 140: 513

Suzuki K, Tamaoki B I 1979 Enzymological studies of rat luteinized ovaries in relation to acute reduction of aromatizable androgen formation and stimulated production of progestin. Endocrinology 104: 1317

Szöllösi D 1975 Ultrastructural aspects of oocyte maturation and fertilization in mammals. In: Thibault C (ed) La Fécondation. Masson, Paris, pp 13–35

Szöllösi D, Gérard M, Ménézo Y, Thibault C 1978 Permeability of ovarian follicle; corona cell – oocyte relationship in mammals. Ann Biol Anim Biochem Biophys 18: 511

Takahashi M, Koide S S, Donahue P K 1986 Müllerian inhibiting substance as oocyte meiosis inhibitor. Molec Cell Endocrinol 47: 255

Tanaka N, Espey L, Okamura H 1989 Increase in ovarian 15-hydroxyeicosatetraenoic acid during ovulation in the gonadotropin-primed immature rat. Endocrinology 125: 1373

Taya K, Greenwald G S 1980 In vitro and in vivo ovarian steroidogenesis in the long term hypophysectomized hamster. Endocrinology 106: 1093

Terranova P F 1980 Effect of phenobarbital-induced ovulatory delay on the follicular population and serum levels of steroids and gonadotropins in the hamster: a model for atresia. Biol Reprod 23: 92

Thibault C 1977 Are follicular maturation and oocyte maturation independent processes? J Reprod Fertil 51: 1

Thibault C, Gerard M 1973 Cytoplasmic and nuclear maturation of rabbit oocytes in vitro. Ann Biologie Anim Biochem Biophys 13: 145

Thibault C, Levasseur M C 1988 Ovulation. Human Reprod 3: 513

Thibault C, Gerard M, Menezo Y 1975a Acquisition par l'ovocyte de Lapine et de Veau du facteur de decondensation du noyau du spermatozoide fecondant (MPGF). Ann Biol Anim Biochen Biophys 15: 705

Thibault C, Gerard M, Menezo Y 1975b Preovulatory and ovulatory mechanisms in oocyte maturation. J Reprod Fertil 45: 605

Thibault C, Szöllösi D, Gerard M 1987 Mammalian oocyte maturation. Reprod Nutr Develop 27: 865

Todaro G J, De Larco J E, Cohen S 1976 Transformation by murine and feline sarcoma viruses specifically blocks binding of epidermal growth factor to cells. Nature 264: 26

Tsafriri A 1978 Oocyte maturation in mammals. In: Jones RE (eds) The vertebrate ovary. Plenum, New York, pp 409–442

Tsafriri A, Bar-Ami S 1982 Oocyte maturation inhibitor: a 1981 perspective. In: Channing C P, Segal S J (eds) Intra-ovarian control mechanisms, advances in experimental medicine and biology Vol 147. Plenum, New York, pp 145–160

Tsafriri A, Channing C P 1975 An inhibitory influence of granulosa cells and follicular fluid upon porcine oocyte meiosis in vitro. Endocrinology 96: 922

Tsafriri A, Hsueh A J W 1989 Transforming growth factor-β inhibits LH-induced maturation of rat oocytes. In: Hirshfield A N (ed) Growth factors and the ovary. Plenum, New York, pp 209: 212

Tsafriri A, Pomerantz S H 1984 The control of ovum maturation in mammals: comparative aspects. In: Sairam S H, Atkinson L E (eds) Gonadal peptides and proteins. World Scientific Publishing Co., Singapore, pp 191–206

Tsafriri A, Pomerantz S H 1986 Oocyte maturation inhibitor. In: Franchimont P (ed) Clinics in endocrinology and metabolism, 15/1, WB Saunders, London, pp 157–170

Tsafriri A, Lindner H R, Zor U, Lamprecht S A 1972 Induction in vitro of meiotic division in follicle-enclosed rat oocytes by LH, cyclic AMP and prostaglandin $E_2$. J Reprod Fertil 31: 39

Tsafriri A, Lieberman M E, Barnea A, Bauminger S, Lindner H R 1973 Induction by LH of ovum maturation and of steroidogenesis in isolated Graafian follicles of the rat: role of RNA and protein synthesis. Endocrinology 93: 1378

Tsafriri A, Lieberman M E, Koch Y et al 1976a Capacity of immunologically purified FSH to stimulate cyclic AMP accumulation and steroidogenesis in Graafian follicles and to induce ovum maturation and ovulation in the rat. Endocrinology 98: 655

Tsafriri A, Pomerantz S H, Channing C P 1976b Porcine follicular fluid inhibitor of oocyte meiosis: Partial characterization of the inhibitor. Biol Reprod 14: 511

Tsafriri A, Channing C P, Pomerantz S H, Lindner H R 1977 Inhibition of maturation of isolated rat oocytes by porcine follicular fluid. J Endocrinol 75: 285

Tsafriri A, Weinstein Y, Bar-Ami S, Channing C P,

Pomerantz S H, Lindner H R 1979 The control of meiotic maturation of the rat oocyte. In: Conti E (ed) Research on steroids. Academic New York, pp 193–798

Tsafriri A, Abisogun A O, Reich R 1987 Steroids and follicular rupture at ovulation. J Steroid Biochem 27: 359

Tsafriri A, Picard Y, Josso N 1988 Immunopurified anti-Müllerian hormone does not inhibit spontaneous maturation in vitro of rat oocytes. Biol Reprod 38: 481

Tsafriri A, Daphna-Iken D, Abisogun A O, Reich R 1990 Follicular rupture during ovulation: Activation of collagenolysis. In: Mashiach S, Ben-Rafael Z, Laufer N, Schenker J G (eds) Advances in asssisted reproductive technologies. Plenum, New York, pp 103–112

Tsafriri A, Reich R, Abisogun A O 1991a The ovarian egg and ovulation. In: Lamming G E (ed) Marshall's physiology of reproduction. III. Churchill Livingstone, London, in press

Tsafriri A, Veljkovic M V, Pomerantz S H, Ling N 1991b The action of transforming growth factors and inhibin-related proteins on oocyte maturation. Bull Assoc Anat 75: 109

Ueno N, Ling N, Ying S, Esch F, Shimasaki S, Guillemin R 1987 Isolation and partial characterization of follistatin. A novel $M_r$ 35,000 monomeric protein that inhibits the release of follicle stimulating hormone. Proc Nat Acad Science USA 84: 8282

Ueno S, Manganaro T F, Donahoe P K 1988 Human recombinant Müllerian inhibiting substance inhibition of rat oocyte meiosis is reversed by epidermal growth factor in vitro. Endocrinology 123: 1652

Uilenbroek J T J, Woutersen P J A, van der Schoot P 1980 Atresia of preovulatory follicles: gonadotropin binding and steroidogenic activity. Biol Reprod 23: 219

Usui N, Yanagimachi R 1976 Behaviour of hamster sperm nuclei incorporated into eggs at various stages of maturation, fertilization and early development. J Ultrastruc Res 57: 276

Vale W, Rivier J, Vaughan J et al 1986 Purification and characterization of an FSH-releasing protein from porcine ovarian follicular fluid. Nature (Lond) 321: 776

Vale W, Rivier C, Hsueh A et al 1988 Chemical and biological characterization of the inhibin family of protein hormones. Recent Prog Horm Res 44: 1

Van de Wiel D F M, Bar-Ami S, Tsafriri A, de Jong F H 1983 Oocyte maturation inhibitor, inhibin and steroid concentrations in porcine follicular fluid at various stages of the oestrous cycle. J Reprod Fertil 68: 247

van Wagenen G, Simpson M E 1965 Embryology of the ovary and testis in *Homo sapiens* and *Macaca mulatta*. Yale University Presss, New Haven

Vermande-vanEck G J 1956 Neo-ovogenesis in adult monkey. Anat Rec 125: 207

Vivarelli E, Conti M, DeFelici M, Siracusa G 1983 Meiotic resumption and intracellular cAMP levels in mouse oocytes treated with compounds which act on cAMP metabolism. Cell Differ 12: 271

Wallach E E, Bronson R, Hamada Y, Wright K H, Stevens V C 1975a Effectiveness of prostaglandin $F_{2\alpha}$ in restoration of HMG-HCG induced ovulation in indomethacin-treated rhesus monkeys. Prostaglandins 10: 129

Wallach E E, de la Cruz A, Hunt J, Wright K H, Stevens V C 1975b The effect of indomethacin on HMG-HCG induced ovulation in the rhesus monkey. Prostaglandins 9: 645

Wallach E E, Wright K H, Hamada Y 1978 Investigation of mammalian ovulation with an in vitro perfused rabbit ovary preparation. Am J Obstet Gynecol 132: 728

Weir B J, Rowlands J W 1977 Ovulation and atresia. In: Zuckerman S, Weir B J (eds) The ovary, 1. Academic, New York, pp 265–301

Welschen R, Dullaart J 1976 Administration of antiserum against ovine follicle-stimulating hormone or ovine luteinizing hormone at pro-oestrus in the rat: effects of follicular development during the oncoming cycle. J Endocrinol 70: 301

Woessner J J F, Butler W J, LeMaire W J, Morioka N, Mukaida T, Zhu C 1989 The role of collagenase in ovulation in the rat. In: Tsafriri A, Dekel N (eds) Follicular development and the ovulatory response, 23. Ares-Serono Symposia, Rome, pp 167–178

Woodruff T K, Mayo K E 1990 Regulation of inhibin synthesis in the rat ovary. Annu Rev Physiol 52: 807

Wurtman R J 1964 An effect of luteinizing hormone on the fractional perfusion of the rat ovary. Endocrinology 75: 927

Yanagishita M, Hascal V C 1979 Biosynthesis of proteoglycans by rat granulosa cells cultured in vitro. J Biol Chem 254: 12355

Ying S 1988 Inhibins, activins, and follistatins: gonadal proteins modulating the secretion of follicle-stimulating hormone. Endocrine Rev 9: 267

Yoshimura Y, Wallach E E 1987 Studies of the mechanism(s) of mammalian ovulation. Fertil Steril 47: 22

Yoshimura Y, Hosoi Y, Atlas S J, Bongiovanni A M, Santulli R, Wallach E E 1986 The effect of ovarian steroidogenesis on ovulation and fertilizability in the in vitro perfused rabbit ovary. Biol Reprod 35: 943

Yoshimura Y, Espey L, Hosoi Y et al 1988 The effects of bradykinin on ovulation and prostaglandin production by the perfused rabbit ovary. Endocrinology 122: 2540

Zachariae F 1957 Studies on the mechanism of ovulation: autoradiographic investigations on the uptake of radioactive sulphate into the ovarian mucopolysaccharides. Acta Endocrinol (Copenh) 26: 215

Zachariae F 1958 Studies on the mechanism of ovulation. Permeability of the blood – liquor barrier. Acta Endocrinol 27: 339

Zachariae F 1959 Acid mucopolysaccharides in the female genital system and their role in the mechanism of ovulation. Acta Endocrinol Copenh 33 (suppl 47):11

Zachariae F, Thorsoe H 1966 Hormonal control of acid mucopolysaccharides in the female genital tract. In: Asboe Hansen G (ed) Hormones and connective tissue. Munksgaard, Denmark, pp 257–281

Zamboni L 1972 Comparative studies on the structure of mammalian oocytes. In: Biggers J D, Schuetz A W (eds) Oogenesis. University Park Press, Baltimore, M D pp 5–45

Zamboni L 1976 Modulation of follicle cell oocyte association in sequential stages of mammalian follicle development and maturation. In: Crosignani P G, Michell D R (eds) Ovulation in the Human. 1–30, Academic Press, London and New York

Zelezink A J, Kubik C J 1986 Ovarian responses in macaques to pulsatile infusion of follicle-stimulating hormone (FSH) and luteinizing hormone: increased sensitivity of the maturing follicle to FSH. Endocrinology 119: 2025

Zeleznik A J, Midgley J A R, Reichert J L E 1974 Granulosa cell maturation in the rat: increased binding of human chorionic gonadotropin following treatment with follicle-stimulating hormone in vivo. Endocrinology 95: 818

Zeleznik A J, Schuler H M, Reichert L E J 1981
Gonadotropin-binding sites in the Rhesus monkey ovary:
role of the vasculature in the selective distribution of human
chorionic gonadotropin to the preovulatory follicle.
Endocrinology 109: 356

Zor U, Lamprecht S A 1977 Mechanism of prostaglandin
action in endocrine glands. In: Litwack G (ed) Biochemical
actions of hormones, 4. Academic, New York, pp 85–133
Zuckerman S, Weir B J (eds) 1978 In: Zuckerman S, Weir B J
(eds) The ovary. Academic, New York

# Structural and functional basis of infertility (male)

# 7. Functional anatomy of the male accessory sex organs (physiology and mechanism of regulation)

*Gedalia F. Paz   Haim Yavetz   Leah Yogev   Zwi T. Homonnai*

## INTRODUCTION

This chapter presents the most common and recent information concerning the anatomy, innervation, and blood and lymph supplies of the male accessory sex organs of man. A detailed description of the physiology of each organ and the regulation of its various compartments by the endocrine and neural systems follows. Attention is devoted to the cellular and subcellular regulatory mechanisms, in order to elucidate the possible role of different materials and products in regulating male reproduction. Due to the paucity of information concerning the human male reproductive organs, we discuss data obtained from animal studies in order to present a complete picture. This is true especially for areas dealing with regulatory mechanisms.

Pathological changes in the accessory sex organs may lead to subfertility of the male. The understanding of the processes that lead to the malformation of the various organs is a crucial part of the search for treatment methods for these patients. The same information can be used for the treatment of infertility on the one hand, and for the development of male contraceptive devices through interruption of accessory sex organ function, on the other.

The understanding of the physiology of erection and ejaculation is an important issue in seeking a solution in cases of impotence. The use of a pharmacological approach in addition to new methods of diagnosis, is an interesting avenue in the treatment of disorders in this field.

The ejaculate is composed of spermatozoa and seminal plasma. Since each of these two components is known to influence the chemical composition of the other, it is important to study the composition of the seminal plasma and the secretions from the different accessory glands. Thus, the assessment of the secretory function of each of the accessory sex glands could be of value in dealing with fertility problems, urological complaints and sexual dysfunction.

In this chapter the accessory sex organs, except for the testis itself, are discussed from the standpoint of the correlation between their structure and function.

## DEVELOPMENT OF THE MALE ACCESSORY SEX ORGANS AND THEIR CONTROL

The primary development of a male rather than a female gonad in mammals is determined by the presence of a Y chromosome. The other property unique to the Y chromosome is the occurrence of a cell-surface antigen (designated H-Y), which distinguishes male from female (McLaren 1987).

The notion that H-Y was a single molecular species responsible for triggering the indifferent gonad to differentiate into the testis, became a widely accepted hypothesis. Data are presented which suggest that although H-Y is a male-specific factor and may play a role in male sex determination, it is unlikely that it is the primary inducer of testis differentiation (Goldberg 1988).

The initial diversion of germ cells to the male pathway in the fetal life of the mouse, that is the formation of amitotic TI-prospermatogonia, is an indirect effect of the Y: the Y-chromosomal testis-determining gene (Tdy) acts to create a testis and the testicular environment causes the germ cells to follow the male pathway. The first direct effect of the Y in the germ line occurs at the initiation of the spermatogenic cycles (approximately 1 week after birth) when a Y-chromosomal gene (Spy) is needed for normal spermatogonial survival and progression to meiosis. The capacity to produce H-Y antigen also has the Spy function, raising the possibility that H-Y antigen is the mediator of Spy activity. The Y is next required in the male germ line during meiotic prophase, when it provides a pairing partner for the X chromosome (Burgoyne 1987). Since antibodies to the H-Y antigen are available, it is possible to detect and separate sperm cells bearing the Y chromosome and H-Y antigen. This method has been introduced recently in bovine semen (Ali et al 1990).

In the 8th week, the first typical Leydig cells appear; these will fill the space between the sex cords and make up more than half the volume of the fetal testis by the 14th to 18th week of

gestation. The main events in the development of the male accessory sex organs, as well as in the appearance and disappearance of organs and factors as a function of fetal age, are depicted in Figure 7.1.

An immunocytochemical method, based on the use of a polyclonal antibody raised against purified bovine anti-Müllerian hormone (AMH) (Josso & Picard 1986), was used to detect AMH in Sertoli cell cytoplasm of various mammalian species, including human. In human testicular tissues, AMH is detectable up to 6 years of age. In rats, AMH production is initiated at 13 days postcoitum, peaks between 15 and 17 days, and is no longer detectable 1 week after birth. Preliminary results indicate that there may be a relationship between the amount of immunoreactive AMH present in testicular biopsies of intersex patients and the degree of regression of the Müllerian ducts on the ipsilateral side. This may help to elucidate whether persistence of Müllerian ducts results from lack of testicular production of AMH, or from peripheral resistance of the Müllerian primordia to the hormone (Tran et al 1987). AMH, also called Müllerian-inhibiting substance or factor, was measured by an interspecific enzyme-linked immunoassay (Elisa) in the serum of normal children and adults of both sexes and in boys with various developmental disorders. AMH levels were high in normal males under 2 years of age, fell progressively in older boys and decreased sharply at puberty. Serum AMH was not detectable in adults or in females at any age, with very rare exceptions. AMH serum concentrations were significantly decreased in infants with disorders of sex differentiation, particularly testicular dysgenesis, and increased in patients with delayed puberty. AMH shows promise as a marker of testicular function in infancy (Josso et al 1990). Findings indicate that adult mammalian granulosa cells are capable of producing immunoreactive and bioactive AMH at a rate apparently similar to that already demonstrated for mature Sertoli cells and add yet another item to the homologies reported between male and female somatic gonadal cells (Vigier et al 1984). Ultimately AMH causes the Müllerian duct to regress, thus preventing the development of the uterus and Fallopian tubes in the male,

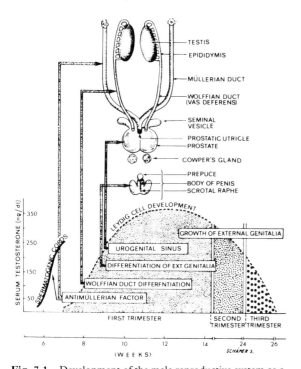

**Fig. 7.1** Development of the male reproductive system as a function of age of the fetus throughout development and the concentration of testosterone in serum. The organs in the upper area of the figure schematically represent the organs under control. The different shaded areas under the curve of testosterone concentration represent the three different trimesters of pregnancy

leaving a small residual portion of the prostatic utricle (Glenister 1962).

Studies have shown that Leydig cells between the cords of the testis extensively produce testosterone. Both in vitro and in vivo studies have shown synthesis of testosterone by Leydig cells from acetate or from precursor steroid sulfates. The temporal pattern of this synthesis coincides closely with that of the differentiation of the male urogenital tract. Differentiation of the urogenital duct system takes place after the 8th week of fetal life when testosterone is first synthesized. Testosterone is the principal steroid in extracts of human fetal testes. It stimulates the development of epididymis, vas deferens, seminal vesicles and ejaculator ducts from the Wolffian ducts. In addition, testosterone promotes virilization of the urogenital sinus and urogenital tubercle leading to the formation of the prostate, male urethra, penis and scrotum. The virilizing effect of testosterone is local rather than systemic.

The differentiation of the urogenital sinus and external genitalia begins at 9 and 10 weeks. By the 10th week, male fetuses can be recognized by the appearance of external genitalia. Coincidental with the peak in serum testosterone levels (14–16 weeks), seminal vesicles become recognizable and the urethra reaches the meatus. The glans is covered by the prepuce. The prostate acquires its definitive form by about the 20th week. During the 2nd and 3rd trimesters of gestation, all the sex organs are formed and their further development is dependent on the continued presence of testosterone. Leydig cell numbers and steroidogenic activity decrease during the 3rd trimester, increase for a short period at about term, and thereafter decline sharply until prepubertal age. Two major androgens that control accessory sex organ differentiation and development are recognized: (a) testosterone, which virilizes the Wolffian ducts, promoting the differentiation of cells that form the epididymis, vas deferens and seminal vesicles; and (b) dihydrotestosterone (DHT), formed in the anlagen of the prostate and external genitalia prior to the onset of phenotypic development due to the appearance of the enzyme 5-α-reductase. DHT controls the virilization of the tubercule sinus (prostate,

Cowper's glands) and urogenital sinus (external genitalia).

According to the results of tissue recognition experiments by Cunha et al (1980, 1981), androgens exert their effect via the mesenchymal cells of the undifferentiated urogenital tract, influencing the epithelial cells to develop and proliferate by the classical mode of action. Androgen receptor activity in the developing mouse urogenital tract is confined to the mesenchymal cells (Shannon et al 1981). Even in the adult organism, androgen-dependent organs such as the prostate require continuous interaction with the associated mesenchymal cells for continued epithelial expression.

Several genetic defects in male development have been described. Various gene mutations affecting an enzyme in the pathway of cholesterol to testosterone conversion have been identified, all resulting in incomplete virilization of the male urogenital tract. The phenotypic appearance is dependant on the extent of enzyme deficiency (Wilson 1978). A second class of human genetic defects involves the lack of DHT formation due to the partial or total deficiency of 5-α-reductase activity or the presence of 5-α-reductase inhibitors (synthetic progestins). The mutant males have female external genitalia but normal male Wolffian structures that end in a vagina (Peterson et al 1977). A third class of defects has been described in embryos lacking androgen receptors, leading to abnormal male phenotypic development, i.e. testicular feminization. This X-linked disorder was first studied in the mouse and rat (Lyon & Howkes 1970). A similar form of human testicular feminization has been described in males, in which external genitalia are characteristically female and internal genitalia absent, except for undescended testes. Cultures of genital skin fibroblasts were used to study this defect (Keenan et al 1974). The fourth class of mutations to be considered manifests a phenotype similar to that in Tm mice. These aberrant males have normal levels of 5-α-reductase activity and normal levels of androgens. Changes in the affinity of the hormone –receptor complex to chromosomal acceptor sites and related changes in the events taking place thereafter, prevent physiological expression of the mutation. As described above, there is extensive genetic heterogenicity in androgen resistance in man (Wilson et al 1981a,b).

In conclusion, the female pattern of development is the basic pattern in mammalian sexual differentiation. It proceeds, unless androgens are produced by the developing fetal testis, in response to genetic signals (Y-chromosome, H-Y antigen). Masculinization, virilization and accessory sex organ development take place only if the androgens are present and their enzymatic pathways active, and if the receptors in the target organs are of adequate concentration and appropriate activity. A deficiency in any of the above will lead to sex malformation and defects in the male embryo (Faiman et al 1981).

## THE EPIDIDYMIS AND EFFERENT DUCTS

### Embryology

The human epididymis originates from the mesonephros. During regression of the mesonephros at the 3rd to 4th month of embryonic development, 8–12 mesonephric tubules in the mesonephric ridge connect to the neighbouring gonadal ridge and form the efferent ducts (MacCallum 1902), while the remaining longitudinal section of the mesonephric duct (Wolffian duct) becomes the epididymis. Both the efferent ducts and epididymis increase in length and volume, becoming coiled after full development.

### Anatomy of the epididymis

The epididymis is covered by the tunica albuginea and rests close to the testis. It extends as an elongated structure from the cranial to the caudal pole of the testis. The epididymis begins from the efferent ducts and continues into the vas deferens. Coiled efferent ducts emerge from the rete testis and constitute most of the caput epididymis. The efferent ducts join the coiled epididymis tube and then form the corpus and cauda portions thereof. The length of the epididymis and associated ducts has been measured to be 5–6 m (Lanz & Neuhauser 1964).

Based on morphological criteria (diameter of the lumen, height and cytological characterization of the epithelial cells, cell organelles and cell surfaces) (Holstein 1969), eight sections have been distinguished in the epididymis. There is a proximal decrease in the width of the lumen, the narrowest area being located at the transition between the corpus and the cauda. The remaining cauda sections have a wide lumen.

The epithelium of the epididymis consists of two types of cells: principal and basal cells. The principal cells are high and columnar, but their morphological characteristics vary along the different sections of the epididymis, especially in the cauda, where they are often small and contain few organelles and small stereocilia. The infranuclear compartment of the principal cells is rich in rough endoplasmic reticulum (RER). The supranuclear compartment has numerous mitochondria and Golgi complexes. The apical portion of the cytoplasm has many membrane-bound vesicles with an electron-dense granular material, multivescular bodies and lysosomes. Stereocilia emanate from the apex of the cell. The micropinocytotic vesicles present near the cell surface indicate that resorption occurs. Occasionally cytoplasmic protrusions extend into the lumen or may be found sequestered from the cells as vesicles among the luminar contents. These protrusions are considered as evidence of secretory activity of the epididymal epithelium.

The basal cells are spherical and are interspersed between the more numerous principal cells. They do not extend toward the luminal surface of the epithelium and are characterized by lipofuscin-like cytoplasmic inclusions. Their morphology remains constant throughout the epididymis.

Varying numbers of spermatozoa, immature germ cells, and fragments of cells (nuclei, organelles, membranes) are found in the lumen of the epididymis. Large phagocytes containing spermatozoa or fragments of cells are also found (Holstein 1969).

The subepithelial layer consists of thin, smooth muscle cells; it gradually increases in thickness proximodistally. Most of the muscle cell bundles are oriented circularly. At the junction of the corpus and cauda a layer of thick smooth muscle cells is superimposed on the subepithelially located bundles of thin smooth muscle cells (Baumgarten et al 1971). At the beginning of the vas deferens, which has three distinct layers of smooth musculature (Pabst 1969), the thin smooth muscle cells are replaced by layers of ordinary thick, smooth muscle cells. Ultra-structural studies reveal that these smooth muscle cells resemble myofibroblasts that may represent poorly differentiated smooth muscle elements.

## Anatomy of the efferent ducts

Four different sections have been described, based on the width of the lumen of the duct and on the typical appearance of the epithelial cells (height and structure). The proximal end has a wide lumen, while the distal part has a narrow lumen. The lumen is lined with epithelial cells possessing microvilli; some of them also have cilia. This structure hints at the secretory and resorptive activities of the lumen, predominantly in the proximal sections, and at its absorptive activities in the distal sections. Both sections have many nonciliated cells (Holstein 1976), possessing protruding apices and suggesting secretory activity. These cells are often present in shallow areas of the epithelium forming intra-epithelial glands (Vendrely 1981).

## Physiology of the epididymis

The epididymis is a convoluted canal in which the final steps of sperm maturation and development take place.

For a long time the epididymis has been considered to be a simple duct in which spermatozoa are stored and through which they pass upon ejaculation. Studies performed mainly on animals and a few studies in humans, established the concept that beyond serving as a conduit and storage for spermatozoa, the epididymis sustains a maturation process that results in the acquisition of progressive motility and fertilizing ability by spermatozoa (Shilon et al 1978). However, recent reports have doubted the need for spermatozoa to travel or to accumulate in the epididymis as a prerequisite to display fertilizing ability, since isolated spermatozoa from the epididymis were able to fertilize human oocytes (Silber 1980, 1988).

The literature so far points to the cooperative phenomena taking place in the epididymis, which include the interaction of sperm, luminal fluid, epididymal epithelium and the blood and lymph vascular compartments in the control of the maturation process that the sperm undergo during transit within the epididymis. The epididymal epithelium has all the attributes of being very active metabolically. Two major functions have been described: *absorption* and *secretion*. The net result of these functions determines the composition of the luminal milieu. Merocrine secretion has been demonstrated in the cell apex of the principal secretory cells of the epididymis (Nicander & Malmquist 1977). Other authors have also shown apocrine and holocrine types of secretion.

The epididymis synthesizes certain compounds that are secreted into the lumen of the canal. These include protein, carnitine, lipids, glycerylphosphorylcholine (GPC), carbohydrates, steroids and other small molecules (Hamilton 1977). Several of these are of great importance in the determination of the fate of spermatozoa suspended in the luminal fluid.

### Proteins

Particular interest has been paid to the biosynthesis of glycoproteins. The principal cells that line the duct of the epididymis and vas deferens synthesize and secrete a number of specific proteins. The sequence of protein biosynthesis in the epididymal cells is similar to the classic one: amino acids are taken up from the blood into the RER and built up as polypeptide and glycoproteins which migrate to the Golgi complex where final glycosylation occurs. They are concentrated in secretion vacuoles which are released into the lumen (Kanka & Kopecny 1977, Flickinger 1979).

A polyacrylamide gradient slab gel electrophoretogram of samples of rat fluid from various portions of the epididymis and vas deferens revealed the following:

1. Many blood proteins appear in the epididymal fluid as a result of ultrafiltration.

2. The relative amounts of some proteins vary along the epididymis, which indicates secretion, absorption or proteolytic activities.

3. Epididymal fluid contains many low molecular weight proteins.

4. A number of epididymal proteins disappear in the vas deferens (Wong et al 1981).

Two specific proteins were found in the epididymis: galactosyltransferase (Hamilton 1980) and α-lactalbumin (Hamilton 1981). Both play a role in glycosylation of spermatozoal surfaces as spermatozoa progress through the epididymis. Kohane et al (1979) used [125]I-labelled specific protein (SEP) in order to establish a radioimmunoassay for this protein, which is produced by the epididymis and is androgen dependent. Specific protein has been shown to be attached to the spermatozoa obtained from the cauda epididymis. Thus, SEP may play a role in sperm maturation since Orgebin-Crist & Jahad (1978) showed that DHT controls the induction of sperm maturation in cultured rabbit epididymal tubules, the process being blocked by the simultaneous addition of RNA or protein synthesis inhibitors.

A progressive motility-sustaining factor (PMSF) was isolated from human epididymal fluid and was found to stimulate the motility of oligoasthenozoospermic specimens (Sheth et al 1981). It was shown in cattle and monkeys that the PMSF is a glycoprotein of epididymal origin which plays a physiological role in the acquisition of sperm motility (Brandt et al 1978). Other proteins are secreted into specific regions of the epididymis and subsequently become associated with spermatozoa (Kohane et al 1980, Orgebin-Crist 1981).

The free amino acids in the epididymis consist of high concentrations of glycine, glutamic acid, alanine and serine in the epididymal plasma of mice, rats, rabbits and rams. The significance of the presence of free amino acids in the epididymal fluid is not clear; it is supposed that they play a role in the sperm maturation mechanism (Huang & Johnson 1975).

The composition of proteins and amino acid

changes along the epididymal canal, implying that different mechanisms may be involved in their secretion and absorption, and also that spermatozoa may have a direct effect on protein composition (Crabo & Hunter 1975).

*Carnitine*

Carnitine and acetylcarnitine have been found in extremely high concentrations in the epididymal fluid (Marquis & Fritz 1965). Carnitine is not synthesized in the epididymis but is accumulated in the epididymal cells following its absorption from the blood; afterwards it is secreted into the lumen of the epididymis.

Carnitine is involved in fatty acid metabolism. Casillas (1972) used isolated mitochondria from bull epididymal sperm to show that the addition of carnitine stimulated the oxidation of palmitic acid up to 40-fold. Since spermatozoa are dependent on fatty acid metabolism, carnitine may play a crucial role in preserving sperm viability in the epididymis. It may also play a role in the determination of osmotic pressure and may, after ejaculation, stimulate motility (Hinton et al 1981).

Carnitine can be used as an epididymal marker for the detection of luminal obstructions. Soffer et al (1981) subjected semen samples obtained from 399 patients to the auxanographic procedure. Thirty samples were scored low in total carnitine content (7.5%); 14 of these were azoospermic and 16 were severely oligozoospermic. These results, and those of other studies of this group and of other investigators (Frenkel et al 1974), imply that low carnitine levels can be attributed either to epididymal dysfunction or to obstruction of the reproductive tract.

The semen ejaculated after vasectomy does not contain secretions from the testis or the epididymis, but mainly consists of secretions from the seminal vesicles, the prostate gland and of a small contribution from the vas deferens. Since prostatic fluid obtained by prostatic massage contains only traces of carnitine and its acetyl derivates, carnitine in man originates mainly from the epididymis (Frenkel et al 1974) and the seminal vesicle. Postvasectomy specimens contain only 40% of the free carnitine and 52% of the total carnitine found in the prevasectomy semen. These findings can contribute to the evaluation of the epididymal function and help in the diagnosis of obstructions in the epididymis and/or vas deferens (Wetterauer & Heite 1980, Fahimi et al 1981).

The possible role of carnitine in human semen was studied by correlating its levels in the ejaculate with sperm quality (concentration, motility and morphology); however, no correlation could be established (Paz et al 1977). Thus, although carnitine and its derivatives are secreted and metabolized by the epididymis and may play an important role in situ by directly affecting spermatozoa (which accumulate carnitine), its importance in the ejaculate is still not established.

## Lipids

Lipids constitute an important part of the substrates used by the epididymal spermatozoa during their transit period. Total lipids represent 1.25% of the total wet weight of the epididymal tissue. Phospholipids form 64%, cholesterol 12% and glycerides 24% of the total lipids. This information is useful in following the changes in the function of the epididymis as reflected in semen evaluation (Sheriff 1980).

## Glycerylphosphorylcholine

Glycerylphosphorylcholine (GPC) is synthesized by the epithelial cells of the epididymis and is secreted and accumulated in high concentrations (up to 1 g%) in various animals, including man. The physiological role of GPC is not clear, but it may help to maintain the osmotic pressure balance in the lumen. Sperm are not able to metabolize exogenous GPC; thus it does not serve as an endogenous substrate (Mann & Lutwak-Mann 1981). Glycerylphosphorylcholine is secreted by the holocrine type of secretion, apparently under androgen control. Frenkel et al (1974) have shown that over 70% of the GPC is secreted by human epididymis, so it can serve as an indicator-maker of epididymal function. None the less, the level of GPC in the ejaculate was not found to be correlated with sperm quality (Paz et

al 1977) and thus its physiological importance and its involvement in reproduction remain obscure.

## Carbohydrates

Small carbohydrate molecules (fructose, glucose and citric acid) have been reported to be virtually absent from epididymal plasma (Mann & Lutwak-Mann 1981). In contrast, studies using [$^3$H]-labelled galactose have shown direct involvement of the epididymal epithelium in the synthesis of complex carbohydrates, involving the acitivity of the Golgi complex (Fleischer et al 1969). The epididymal secretion is rich in sialic acids, which are incorporated into sialomucoproteins and effect the acrosome of the maturing spermatozoon (Prasad et al 1973).

## Steroids

There are some indications that the epididymis can synthesize steroids in vitro in addition to metabolizing testosterone (Gloyna & Wilson 1969). Enzymes involved in steroidogenesis have been identified in the epididymal tissue resulting in the production of testosterone and dihydroepiandrosterone. Thus, in addition to the steroids supplied by testicular fluid reaching the epididymis via the blood supply, the tissue itself may supply small amounts of androgens, which are essential for the maintenance of epididymal activity.

## Absorption

The absorptive activity of the epithelial cells of the epididymis is an important part of the canal function, since it determines the concentration of materials in the luminal fluid, thus affecting the composition of the epididymal fluid. In vivo, samples of epididymal fluid can be obtained using micropuncture techniques. Microsamples from four areas of the rat epididymis were analysed for $Na^+$ and $K^+$ concentrations and for sperm density. Natrium values declined while $K^+$ and sperm concentrations increased from the caput toward the corpus epididymis. This was explained by the substantial loss of reabsorbed water as well as of both cations. This may play a role in regulation of sperm maturation (Turner et al 1977). Studies of rabbit epididymal fluid showed that the epididymis actively absorbs $Na^+$ and $Cl^-$ and actively secretes GPC, protein, carnitine, alkaline phosphatase, $\beta$-$N$-acetylglucosaminidase and mannosidase and acid deoxyribonuclease. Potassium accumulates due to the degeneration of spermatozoa (Jones 1974). Direct measurement of pH values in different segments of the epididymis of the rat, compared with the seminiferous tubules, revealed acidification of the fluid leaving the testis (pH = 6.64, compared to 7.30 in the testis) (Levine & Kelly 1978).

Rat epididymal caput epithelium was shown to have the capacity of reabsorbing inhibin from the drained rete testis fluid. This function is very important in the regulation of follicle stimulating hormone (FSH) release, since inhibin plays a role in the negative feedback of FSH (Le Lannous et al 1979). Electron microscopic evidence of the absorptive functions of the epididymis has also been reported in man, rabbits, hamsters and rats (Friend 1969).

Reabsorption activity has been documented for the efferent ducts before the meatus enters the proximal epididymis (Crabo & Gustafsson 1964). The structural details of this activity do not differ significantly from similar processes in other cell types. Crabo (1965) eatimated that more than 90% of the fluid that leaves the testis in the bull and in the boar is reabsorbed in the efferent ducts and in the first part of the epididymis. The initial stages of fluid movement probably involve micropinocytosis at the luminal plasmalemma. In contrast to water resorption, which takes place only in the proximal lumen, the particulate absorption occurs all along the canal. Under some experimental conditions, epithelial cells in various parts of the epididymis are also capable of absorbing portions of spermatozoa (phagocytosis) (Nicander 1965).

Thus, all along the epididymal canal processes of secretion and absorption take place, resulting in the formation of epididymal fluids that differ in their composition depending on their location in the canal. The biochemical composition of human epididymis and vas deferens was studied by Riar et al (1972). Their results showed changes in protein, alkaline phosphatase, acid phosphatase, glycogen, lactic acid, GPC and lipid along the canal. It is likely that these differences are important for the establishment of the milieu appropriate for the specific subcellular changes associated with the sperm's acquisition of fertilizability.

## Sperm maturation

Most studies have been performed on animals and have been concentrated on changes occurring in the spermatozoa during their transport through the epididymis. Spermatozoa isolated from different segments of the guinea-pig epididymis differ with respect to metabolism (Frenkel et al 1973a), morphology (Fawcett & Phillips 1969) and nucleotide pattern (Frenkel et al 1973b). Changes in enzymes activity have been observed in the sperm of the bull during transit within the epididymis (Waldschmidt & Karg 1972). Cytoplasmic droplets located at the midpiece continuously migrate during the passage of sperm through the epididymis. Migration was found to be greatest in the region from the proximal to distal caput epididymis.

Alteration in animal sperm membrane lactin-binding properties (Olson & Danzo 1981), as well as glycoprotein composition (Brown et al 1983) and iodination characteristics (Olson & Danzo 1981) associated with sperm epididymal transport, have been described. Other studies indicate that during epididymal transit, spermatozoa undergo metabolic changes such as acquisition of increased capacity for glycolysis (Hoskins et al 1975), modification of adenylcyclase activity (Casillas et al 1980), and alternation in cellular phospholipid fatty acid content (Voglmayr 1975).

It has been proposed that metabolism of sperm in situ probably occurs at a very slow rate, in view of the absence of appreciable quantities of utilizable carbohydrate, and since the diffusion of oxygen into the densely packed cells of the epididymal duct is probably also restricted. Paz (unpublished data) used a Beckman oxygen microelectrode in order to measure the partial tension of oxygen ($PO_2$) in the cauda epididymis and vas deferens of guinea-pigs and compared the results with values in the vena cava posterior of

Nembutal-anesthetized animals. Results showed $PO_2$ values of 9.5 ± 2.0, 7.6 ± 2.2 and 38.4 ± 1.2 mmHg (mean ± s.e.) in the lumen of the vas deferens, cauda epididymis and vena cava posterior, respectively. Thus, the spermatozoa in the cauda epididymis and vas deferens exist in semianaerobic conditions, which may be reflected in the low metabolic rate and the unique metabolic patterns of the spermatozoa.

Nevertheless, several indirect studies have shown that some of the changes known to occur in the animal epididymis occur in the human organ as well. An increased formation of disulphide (S–S), bonds was recorded (Bedford et al 1973), as well as changes in the ability to bind positively charged colloidal ferric oxide to the surface of spermatozoa from different segments of the epididymis in man. The formation of S–S bonds is important in the stabilization of the spermatozoa (Reyer et el 1976). Morton et al (1978) showed that in humans the first area where motile sperm was found was the corpus epididymis. There was a correlation between the amount of free calcium surrounding the sperm within the cauda epididymis and sperm motility.

Apart from these chemical changes which occur along with sperm transport in the epididymis, there is a great deal of evidence in animals that the transport is associated with increasing ability to: (a) move in a progressive manner; (b) bind to the zona pellucida; (c) bind and fuse with the zone-free vitellus; (d) fertilize eggs in vitro, and (e) fertilize eggs after in vivo insemination (Shilon et al 1978, Cooper 1986, Amann 1987, Blaquier et al 1988).

In vitro studies, inducing metabolic maturation of epididymal isolated spermatozoa by treatment with caffeine, revealed the linkage between sperm maturation and their fertilizing capacity (Shilon et al 1978). This finding has been used clinically, in treating asthenozoospermic specimens derived from subfertile men (Homonnai et al 1976) and in artificial insemination (Barkay et al 1977a). It was believed that in human epididymis the fertilizing capacity of spermatozoa is acquired in the distal portions of the canal.

Qualitative changes in sperm motility were observed along the human epididymis (Bedford

et al 1973, Dacheux et al 1987). Sperm retrieved from the distal portion of the duct displayed a better motility rate and degree than those obtained from the proximal portions. Studies performed with spermatozoa collected at the time of vasectomy or during epididymovasostomy in the distal region of the epididymis, demonstrated an increased ability to bind, fuse with and penetrate the vitellin membrane compared to sperm from proximal parts (Hinrichsen & Blaquier 1980, Moore et al 1983). There are reports of in vitro fertilization (IVF) successes achieved with sperm isolated from the vas deferens (Pryor et al 1984) and from the corpus epididymis (Jequier et al 1990) of men with obstructive azoospermia but not with sperm from the caput epididymis (Pryor 1987). These studies suggest that the more epididymis the sperm passes through, the greater the motility rate and the chance of their fertilizing ability. In contrast, however, motile spermatozoa have been recovered in the ejaculate after end-to-end anastomosis of the vas deferens to the efferent duct (Silber 1988). A few reports of pregnancies achieved by sperm removed from sperm reservoirs (Brindley et al 1986) or spermatocele (Jimenez Cruz 1980) have been reported. Even pregnancy following IVF with sperm obtained from the efferent duct of men with vas deferens agenesis was reported (Silber et al 1987, Silber 1988). These contradictory results were evaluated and summarized recently (Cooper 1990), stating that under certain circumstance, human epididymal and testicular spermatozoa may have the ability to fertilize eggs both in vivo and in vitro. However, since the 'fertility profile' of the human epididymis cannot be explored, a fair assumption would be that fertilizing capacity develops fully in the distal part of the epididymis. Motility and fertilizing capacity observed in sperm obtained from pathological tissue, although of great clinical interest, preclude definitive statements about the function of the normal epididymis.

**Control of epididymal function**

The functional integrity of the epididymis is clearly dependent upon testicular hormones. Testosterone and DHT are the major androgens controlling epididymal function. It is interesting that the minimal dose of androgen required to maintain the epididymis at control values after castration is four times the dose required to maintain other male accessory sex organs (Prasad et al 1973).

Within the epididymis there appear to exist regional differences in response to androgens (higher in cauda than in caput) and also in the different cell types. In order to maintain their structural integrity, stereocilia require much lower levels of androgens than those required for the maintenance of the secretory activity of the epithelium. The threshold of androgens required to maintain the fertilizing ability to sperm is higher that that needed for retention of sperm motility (Dysson & Orgebin-Crist 1973).

The hormonal dependence of fluid absorption has been studied in isolated rat cauda epididymis with intact blood supply. It was found that fluid reabsorption in rat cauda epididymis is dependent on the presence of androgens in the circulation. Aldosterone did not effect fluid reabsorption, but luteinizing hormone (LH), FSH and vasopressin produced a significant increase in its rate. Epinephrine, but not norepinephrine, was very stimulating. Both $\alpha$- and $\beta$-receptors may be present in the epididymal epithelium and may play a phyiological role in the regulation of fluid reabsorption in the cauda epididymis (Wong & Yeung 1977).

The function of the epididymis is mainly controlled by DHT, as has been demonstrated in studies in vitro on perfused proximal epididymal segments of the rabbit (Orgebin–Crist & Jahad 1978). The results of their studies indicate that the development of the sperm fertilizing ability was dependent on the effect of DHT on the epididymal epithelium. This was evident from the observation of binding and consequently the synthesis of new RNA and protein molecules.

An active $5$-$\alpha$-reductase-NADPH has been shown to exist in the human epididymis. The properties of $5$-$\alpha$-reductase in the microsomal fraction are similar to those in the nuclear fraction (Kinoshita et al 1980). This enzyme has a considerable affinity for testosterone.

The epididymal cells have specific intracellular receptors. A cytoplasmic receptor for testosterone was isolated and characterized in the cytosol of epididymal cell of rhesus monkeys. This receptor had a higher affinity for DHT than for testosterone, and was different from androgen-binding protein (ABP) of testicular origin, or sex hormone-binding globulin (SHBG) of blood origin (Blaquier 1974). A specific ABP of Sertoli cell origin has been shown to have a high affinity for both $5$-$\alpha$-DHT and testosterone. A preponderance of published evidence suggests that ABP is either lost or deactivated as it moves along the epididymis (Purvis & Hansson 1978). This means that testosterone and DHT from the seminiferous tubules are released into the epididymal fluid after degradation of ABP. These findings may explain the data showing higher levels of androgens in the epididymal fluid than in the circulation (Hansson et al 1975). ABP has been identified in the rat epididymis (Musto et al 1978). Its presence in human epididymis has been confirmed and it was shown to be a separate entity from SHBG (Lipschultz et al 1977). Thus, high levels of androgens are found in the epididymal fluid due to two sources: tubular fluid and the circulation.

In addition to androgens, prolactin has been found to be active in the epididymis in stimulating epididymal growth synergistically with DHT (Kreider et al 1977). Specific prolactin receptors were identified in the epididymal tissue and found to be time and temperature dependent (Orgebin-Crist & Djiane 1979). Prolactin increased the uptake of testosterone by the caput epididymis of the rat (Baker et al 1977). Thus, as in other accessory glands, androgens and prolactin act together in controlling the glandular function.

Attention has been given to the possible role of temperature in the control of epididymal function, since the rate of sperm transport in the epididymis may be a factor effecting the quality of ejaculated spermatozoa. Thus, in the presence of normal spermatogenesis, accelerated transport of the spermatozoa in the epididymis may cause the appearance of defective spermatozoa. This was the picture in the ejaculates of rabbits. The biology of the scrotum and temperature regulation together played a crucial role in the determination of the fate of spermatozoa in the male tract. Studies on experimental surgical deflection of the epididymis into the abdomen showed that high temperature accelerated sperm transport without affecting its quality (Bedford 1978).

Of particular interest is the function of the epididymis in testicondid animals such as the hyrax (Bedford & Millar 1978), where the epididymal maturation process is similar to that of scrotal mammals. The prolonged storage of spermatozoa in these animals, in addition to the preservation of fertilizing capacity, can be explained by inherent differences in the character of the spermatozoa themselves, rather than by the activity of the epithelial environment (Bedford & Millar 1978).

The epididymis is a target organ for male contraception. In view of its dynamic role in the development and maintenance of the functional integrity of spermatozoa, it constitutes an ideal extragonadal site for control of fertility in the male by selective alteration of its function. A few drugs have been shown to act through the epididymis. α-Chlorohydrin (Paz & Homonnai 1982) and 6-chlorodeoxyglucose (Ford & Waites 1978) cause a decrease in sperm metabolism and motility and hence a fall in spermatozoal fertilizing capacity (Paz & Homonnai 1982).

## THE VAS DEFERENS

### Anatomy

The vas deferens is a tube, 35–45 cm long, with a diameter of $0.85 \pm 0.07$ mm (Brueschke et al 1974). It extends from the tail of the epididymis, runs along its medial site, through the inguinal canal, to the neck of the seminal vesicle, it then fuses with the seminal vesicle, forming the ejaculatory duct, which passes through the prostate and opens into the floor of the prostatic urethra at the level of the verumontanum. Within the scrotum and inguinal canal runs the spermatic cord, which is surrounded by the tunica vaginalis, and includes the vas deferens, spermatic artery, veins of the pampiniform plexus surrounding the artery, lymphatic vessels and nerves of the testis and epididymis, and the cremasteric muscle. At the internal inguinal ring, the vas deferens leaves the spermatic cord, curves and enters the pelvis.

The vas deferens is divided into five portions: epididymal, scrotal, inguinal, pelvic and ampullar. Histologically, the vas is composed of adventitial, muscular, and mucosal layers. The adventitial layer is composed of a sheath of connective tissue that is rich in blood vessels and small nerve branches. The thick muscular layer consists of an inner and outer longitudinal and an interposed circular smooth muscular layer (Pabst 1970). Along the vas deferens and linked to it, run the vessels and nerves leading to and coming from the testicle. The mucosal layer of the vas is composed of pseudostratified epithelium which contains basal cells and three types of tall and thin columnar cells: principal cells, pencil cells and mitochondria-rich cells. All these show stereocilia and irregular convulated nuclei. The principal cell is much more frequent in the proximal part of the vas and the proportion of the two other cells increases towards the distal portion of the vas (Paniagua et al 1981). Among the vas deferens, some additional changes take place. The epithelial height decreases towards the distal end, the longitudinal folds of the epithel are simple proximally and become complexed distally, and the entire thickness of the muscle layer gradually decreases. All these changes suggest that the ductus is more than a passive channel for sperm transport from the epididymis to the ampulla.

Before it penetrates the prostate, the vas deferens dilates with a glandular enlargement, forming the ampulla (Fig. 7.2). In this area the epithelium becomes thicker. At the final portion of the ampulla, the seminal vesicles join; from there on, the vas deferens enters the prostate opening into the prostatic urethra. The segment that runs in the prostate is called the ejaculatory duct and presents a mucous layer similiar to that of the ampulla, but without a muscular layer.

### Physiology and control of the vas deferens

The vas deferens of many animal species has for years served as a model for the study of neuromuscular anatomy and physiology on the one hand, and of the possible use of its obstruction (vasectomy, devices, occlusions, etc.) as male contraception, on the other hand. The vas deferens acts as a canal transporting spermatozoa

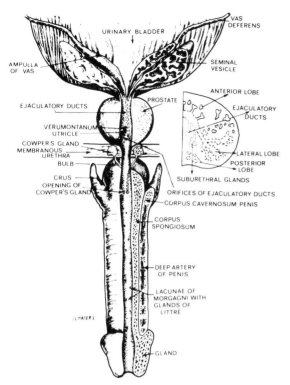

**Fig. 7.2** Shematic presentation of the male accessory sex organs depicted from a posterior view. On the left are the closed organs, on the right, the open organs. The insert on the right is a schematic drawing of the glandular appearance of the different prostatic lobes

from the cauda epididymis to the ampulla where most of the spermatozoa are stored prior to ejaculation. Thus, in the study of the physiology of the vas deferens, two aspects were most attractive: the control of sperm transport and the study of the possible role of its epithelial lining in controlling the final steps of sperm maturation, as well as in regulating the number of spermatozoa available for emission.

Martins et al (1940) reported that while only six of 11 epididymides showed spontaneous motility, 29 of 42 human vasa exhibited tonic-rhythmic contraction upon administration of epinephrine. Pitocin produced no definite response. Acetylcholine elicited a less constant response. It is generally agreed that acetylcholine activity is of minimal importance (McLeod et al 1973).

Histamine, 5-hydroxytryptamine and isoproterenol have also been found not to affect in

vitro human vas deferens preparations significantly (McLeod et al 1973). Ventura et al (1973) extended these studies and demonstrated the existence of spontaneous motility of the human vas deferens in an organ bath with perfusion. Rhythmic contractions were recorded. Norepinephrine infusion markedly increased the force and frequency of the spontaneously active vas. The authors proposed that the intrinsic rhythmicity of the human vas deferens is dependent upon the local concentration of norepinephrine, while the powerful contractions that propel the sperm from the epididymis to the urethra during ejaculation are controlled by the sympathetic nervous system through the α-adrenergic nerves. The structure and function of the vas deferens are under androgen regulation, since the human duct converts testosterone to DHT (Dupuy et al 1979). Castration in monkeys caused atrophy of the duct and testosterone administration resulted in restoration of the vas (Dinakar et al 1977).

Microscopic studies showed that the mucosal layer of the vas contains a basal layer of cuboidal cells and a luminal layer of columnar cells that may possess microvilli or cilia. The composition of the mucosal layer may help to explain its possible role in the regulation of the number and quality of transported spermatozoa. Activities of deoxyribonuclease and proteolytic enzymes have been demonstrated in this layer.

The ampulla is a glandular enlargement of the terminal portion of the vas deferens. It is considered to be the last storage space for spermatozoa before ejaculation. The physiological function of the ampulla and the biochemical properties of the ampullar spermatozoa are largely unknown. Evidence in the bull, however, has shown that the number of spermatozoa in the ampulla is normally sufficient for one ejaculate. In the human, estimates of the percentage of the total ejaculate that originates in the proximal vas and epididymis range from 10% (Batra 1974) to 60–70% (Freund & Davis 1969).

Studies on spermatozoa isolated from the vas deferens have shown that these spermatozoa differ metabolically (Frenkel et al 1973a,b) and microscopically (Fawcett & Phillips 1969) from those of the epididymis. Thus, the fluids secreted by the cells of the duct, as well as the cells themselves, may affect the quality of the transported sperm, indicating a continuous maturation process of spermatozoa, starting in the epididymis.

Long sexual rest in the bull results in a low quality of the first ejaculate, implying destructive action of the ampullary secretions. Similar data have been recorded in men after long periods of abstinence (Martin–Delson et al 1973). The ejaculate, although being hyperzoospermic, contains a large percentage of abnormal forms. Thus, disintegration of ageing spermatozoa in the vas is a method for controlling the number of spermatozoa produced in the ejaculate. This supports the concept that the vas deferens is not an inert canal but rather a very active one, controlling two important factors: sperm quality and sperm transport for emission.


## THE PROSTATE

### Embryology

The fetal prostate develops around the opening of the Wolffian ducts as a series of solid outgrowths from the endodermal prostatic urethra. The prostate eventually encloses the ejaculatory ducts and the prostatic utricle. It completely surrounds the area of the urogenital sinus that will develop into the prostatic urethra (Tuchman-Duplessis et al 1972). By the 4th month of gestation the prostate is well differentiated.

The embryonic prostate develops into the five lobes of the mature prostate. Most of the stroma, which build the urogenital sinus, originate from mesenchyme, while the muscle cells originate from the paramesonephric mesenchyme. All the development is under strict DHT control (Bruchovsky & Wilson 1968).

The prostatic utricle is the residue of the united Müllerian ducts in the male, and is situated within the colliculus seminalis (verumontanum). The utricle is usually present as a small sac that opens in the center of the verumontanum through a small, slit-like opening. The two ejaculatory ducts lie at its sides. The length of the utricle ranges between 1 and 5 mm, but in a few instances has been recorded to be as long as 11 mm (Zondek & Zondek 1974).

In the fetus, the utricle and the glands in its vicinity are the first structures to be affected by continuous and intense estrogenic stimulation. A gradual regression of metaplastic changes takes place after birth, leading to a diminution in utricle volume. Thus, prostatic lobes develop under androgenic control, and the prostatic utricle (Müllerian duct origin) under estrogenic stimulation.


### Anatomy

The prostate, which lies behind the pubic symphysis, is the largest accessory sex gland. In young and middle-aged adults, the gland is 3–4 cm in diameter and approximately 20 g in weight. It is divided into an anterior lobe, two lateral lobes connected by a median or posterior commissural lobe, and a posterior lobe. The posterior lobe lies behind the place of the ejaculatory ducts. The lateral and anterior lobes of the prostate are bound to the pubic symphysis by the puboprostatic ligaments. The broad, flattened, triangular posterior surface, which lies anterior to the rectum, contains a longitudinal midline depression called the median sulcus. Denonviellier's fascia separates the gland from the outer surface of the rectal wall, while the space of Retzius intervenes between the anterior surface of the prostate, the bladder and the symphysis. The base of the gland surrounds the neck of the bladder and the urethra as it leaves the bladder. The apex of the prostate lies at the level of the urogenital diaphragm. The cut surface is quite homogeneous in texture and gray-white in color. It is composed of branching, tubuloalveolar or tubulosaccular glands, excretory ducts, a moderate fibroelastic capsule, blood vessels, lymphatics, nerves, ganglia and sensory corpuscles.

Some investigators suggest that on the basis of morphological, functional and pathological significance, the prostate can be divided into five distinct zones (McNeal 1981, 1990).

Each zone makes contact with a specific portion of the prostatic urethra which can be taken as an anatomical landmark:

1. The anterior fibromuscular stroma which

covers the entire anterior surface of the prostate and is entirely lacking in glandular elements.

2. The peripheral zone which contains 75% of the total glandular tissue in which almost all carcinomas develop.

3. The central zone located behind the upper part of the verumontanum.

4. The preprostatic tissue which has a sphincteric function at the time of ejaculation to prevent retrograde ejaculation.

5. The transition zone which contains a small group of ducts near the junction of the proximal and distal urethral segments, where the majority of the benign prostatic hyperplasia originates.

The two ejaculatory ducts, one on each side, are formed where the ampulla of the vas deferens fuses with the neck of the seminal vesicle. The ejaculatory ducts pierce the prostate obliquely and pass into the interior of the gland. Within the prostate they converge, decrease in diameter and terminate in the floor of the prostatic urethra, in the region known as verumontanum.

Although the prostate proper is quite easily recognized, prostatic or prostatic type tissue is present in other areas as well. Prostatic tissue, different from that of the sex organ, has been found as a periurethral mass in the anterior, lateral and posterior walls of the urethra at the level of the verumontanum. The subcervical glands of Albarran and the subtrigonal glands of Homes and Jores also contain prostatic-type tissue.

## Histology

### Stroma

The gland is capsulated by regularly arranged rows of collagen, fibroblasts and elastic fibers. At intervals, the capsule forms septa that extend into the interior of the prostate, subdividing it into lobes and embedding the glands in stroma. In humans, the innermost layers of the capsule often contain many smooth muscle cells. The capsule and stroma account for 25–30% of the volume of the normal gland. Thin branches of the stroma support the epithelium and form a central core within the epithelial folds and papillae projecting

into the lumen of the gland. Small blood and lymphatic vessels accompany the stroma.

The stroma cells comprise fibroblasts, smooth muscle cells, macrophages, and mast cells. Pathophysiological conditions cause changes in the content of the different types of cells, which can be reflected during rectal examination of the prostate by changes in volume and consistency of the gland.

The smooth muscle surrounding each gland is probably involved in the expulsion of the gland's secretions. The stroma's blood vessels and nerves directly and indirectly influence the formation of the prostatic secretion and the exchange of substances between the gland and the blood.

### Parenchyma

The prostate is an aggregate structure formed from 30–50 tubuloalveolar or tubulosaccular glands of different sizes and shapes. Its 16–32 excretory ducts open into the floor and lateral surfaces of the urethra. The ducts are lined by a simple or pseudostratified columnar epithelium that becomes a transitional epithelium near its entrance into the urethra. The ducts have an irregular branching pattern as well as numerous cystic outgrowths from their tubular portions. No secretory functions have been observed in the ducts of the prostatic glands.

Two types of epithelial cells exist in the glandular structures of the prostate: secretory or glandular cells and basal nonsecretory cells. The glandular cells are the most abundant. They are usually columnar in shape; however, in many regions their shape is distorted by crowding. The basal nuclei of the glandular cells vary in shape from spherical to oval, the long axis of the nucleus coinciding with the long axis of the cell. Nucleoli are not conspicuous, and the nucleoplasm contains fine punctate areas of heterochromatin. The basal cytoplasm contains a moderate number of short mitochondria, profiles of RER and free ribosomes. Above the nucleus it is possible to find a well-developed Golgi complex, several profiles of RER, an occasional lipid droplet and single membrane-bound secretory granules and vacuoles. In addition, lipopigments have been located in either the basal or supranuclear regions of prostate glands obtained from elderly men (Aumuller et al 1979). The apical cytoplasm also contains numerous active lysosomes and dense bodies, and the plasma membrane in this area possesses a microvilli formation. The cells are joined to each other by apical functional complexes and by desmosomes (Brandes 1974, Aumuller 1983).

The basal cells are polygonal in shape, do not reach the lumen of the gland, and show little evidence of organelle polarization. They lack secretory vesicles and contain few mitochondria, little RER and poorly developed Golgi complexes. Spaces or lacunae often appear between the plasma membranes of basal and glandular cells. A moderate number of filaments and pinocytotic vesicles are present in the cytoplasm of the basal cells. The filaments probably serve a contractile function, whereas the pinocytotic vesicles are likely to be involved in the exchange of materials between the glandular epithelium and the stroma.

In the human prostate, basal cells serve primarily as stem cells which give rise to secretory epithelial cells (Merk et al 1982). They proliferate in response to a number of normal and abnormal stimuli. Repair following infection and infarction, as well as the development of benign hyperplasia, probably result from the proliferation of basal cells (Kastendieck & Altenahr 1979). The presence of a bilayered epithelium (i.e. complete, incomplete or pseudostratified) composed of both glandular and basal cells is a critical feature for distinguishing normal or benign glands from malignant glands, which contain only a single layer of modified glandular epithelial cells.

## Physiology and regulation of prostatic function

The prostate has two main functions: it serves as a sphincter, and it secretes fluid into the ejaculate.

### Sphincter

The prostate lies at the base of the bladder neck between the two sphincters of the urethra. The circularly oriented smooth muscle at the neck of the bladder and the preprostatic sphincter are involved in the release of the prostatic secretion and may also be involved in urinary continence; the smooth and striated muscle of the anterior and anterolateral portions of the prostate which fuses with the external sphincter is involved in urinary continence, and is probably only indirectly involved in the emission of semen (Blacklock 1976).

### Secretion

The prostate secretes 0.5–1.5 ml of a thin milky fluid (15–30% of the ejaculate volume) which is usually regarded as slightly alkaline (pH = 7.2), although it has also been reported to be slightly acidic (pH = 6.8) (Pfau et al 1978). The variation in pH is probably due to the level of citric acid in the fluid.

Human prostatic fluid contains a number of constituents (Table 7.1). The most well known are acid phosphatase, citric acid, polyamines and bivalent cations ($Ca^{2+}$, $Zn^{2+}$ and $Mg^{2+}$). In addition, lamellated acidophilic bodies called *Corpora amulacea* can be found in the fluid.

The secretions of the prostate are predominantly merocrine, for which membrane-linked secretory granules fuse with the cell membrane to release their contents. Apocrine secretion occasionally occurs, in which part of the cell apex becomes distended in the form of a large bleb or saccule. In this case, secretory granules and fragments of the cell components including cytoplasm, small organelles and endoplasmic reticulum are also secreted (Brandes 1974).

### Acid phosphatase

Human prostatic acid phosphatase is a dimeric protein that catalyses the hydrolysis of phosphomonoesters. It has a pH optimum in the range 4.0–6.0, which depends upon the nature of the substrate and buffer composition when tested in vitro. A standard for the enzymatic activity of prostatic acid phosphatase is that the pure enzyme catalyses the hydrolysis of 240–250 μmol *p*-nitrophenyl phosphate/mg protein per min at 25°C and pH 5.0. The enzyme also splits creatine phosphate, phosphoproteins and oligonucleotides and effects the transfer of phosphoryl groups from

**Table 7.1**  Selected components of human prostatic secretions

| Component | Possible functions |
| --- | --- |
| Acid phosphatase | Hydrolysis of phosphocholine in seminal plasma; can be used as a prostatic marker |
| Prostate-specific antigen | Specific prostatic marker |
| γ-Glutamyl transferase | Transfers γ-glutamyl group from peptides to amino acids or peptides |
| α-Amylase | Active enzyme in the ejaculate |
| Diamine oxidase | Oxidizes diamines |
| Polyamines (spermine, spermidine, putrescine) | Basic aliphatic polyamine; may be involved in growth regulating; is bacteriostatic; when oxidized, produces 'musk' odor of semen |
| Plasminogen activator | Seminal clot lysis |
| Seminin (chymotrypsin-like enzyme) | A protease, also called fibrinolysin |
| Inositol | Maintains osmotic equilibrium of seminal plasma |
| Cholesterol | Helps to stabilize sperm against thermal and environmental shock |
| Citric acid | Binds metal bivalent cations |
| Bivalent cations ($Zn^{2+}$, $Mg^{2+}$, $Ca^{2+}$) | Cofactors in enzymatic actions |

different substrates to acceptors other than solvents. Aliphatic alcohols are good acceptors of phosphoryl groups in transphosphorylation reactions. Specific inhibitors of acid phosphatase are fluoride, phosphate, arsenate, molybdate, tungstate, oxalate and L-tartrate.

Acid phosphatase activity in the prostate gland is localized in the glandular and basal epithelia (Gyorkey 1964). In the rat, the enzyme exists in secretory vacuoles localized in the perinuclear and apical areas of the epithelial cells and the activity takes place in the Golgi complex and cisternae. Synthesis, transport, packaging and exocytosis in prostatic epithelial cells take place as in other exocrine organs. The secretion is by merocrine or by reverse exocytosis. The secretory granules enter the ducts from which the enzyme can be partly reabsorbed into the blood vessels, probably via the lymphatics (Serrano et al 1977). A dual localization of this enzyme in secretory granules or vacuoles and in lysosomes has been shown cytochemically by electron microscopy in various species. The lysosomal acid phosphatase is responsible for the increase of this enzyme in patients with prostatic carcinoma.

Acid phosphatases are secreted into the semen by other tissues, such as erythrocytes, platelets, liver, kidney, bones and bone marrow. The isoenzyme (defined by chromatography or isoelectric focusing) produced by the prostate can be distinguished using the inhibitory capacity of L-tartrate and formaldehyde. A highly specific and sensitive radioimmunoassay has also been developed. The method is capable of detecting 1.5–6.5 ng/mL serum, with a 5% error. A counter immunoelectrophoretic method which measures both enzymatic activity and antigenicity at the same time has also been developed (MacDonald et al 1978).

The synthesis and secretion of the enzyme are hormone dependent and increase under androgen stimulation. The secretion of the enzyme can also be affected by age, disease, emotional excitement and pharmacological treatment. Castration, hypophysectomy and treatment with estrogens all suppress acid phosphatase secretion. Inflammatory conditions also diminish its secretion (Eliasson et al 1970, Girgis et al 1981, Comhaire et al 1989).

The activity of the enzyme can be associated with the metabolic activity of spermatozoa by their catalysing transfer of phosphates following splitting of glycerolphosphate. Normal human semen contains several acid phosphatases of different origin. The enzyme derived from the gland accounts for only about 10–25% of the total activity in the serum (Ostrowski 1980).

Neoplastic prostatic tissue (carcinoma) contains less acid phosphatase on a gram to gram basis than does either a normal or hyperplastic prostate. Serum acid phosphatase has served for half a century as a biochemical marker for the development of the disease and for follow-up of its regression following treatment, e.g. with estrogens or antiestrogens. However, it appears that recently the measurement of prostatic-specific antigen is about to replace acid phosphatase.

Prostatic specific antigen (PSA) is a glycoprotein specific for prostate epithelial cells, formed by a single polypeptide chain of 240 amino acid residues that were isolated and purified in 1979. It has been shown that prostatic tissue, whether benign or malignant, as well as prostatic secretion, contain PSA (Chu & Murphy 1986, Lilja & Abrahamsson 1988). PSA has been suggested as a specific marker for monitoring patients with prostate carcinoma (de Vere White 1989).

## Bivalent metals

It is well established that three bivalent metals, zinc, magnesium and calcium, are accumulated and secreted in the prostatic fluid (Homonnai et al 1978a). Zinc is the most common, with its concentration in human seminal plasma ranging from 2.5 to 25.7 mg/dl (Skandhan 1981). The anatomical localization of administered $Zn^{2+}$ in the human prostate, as demonstrated by autoradiography, is in the epithelium of the glands.

The role of zinc in reproduction is still obscure, although it has been shown that spermatozoa accumulate zinc from the prostatic fluid (Kvist et al 1985) and that zinc can modulate the acrosome reaction (Delgado et al 1985), sperm motility (Arver & Eliasson 1982) and sperm chromatin decondensation (Huret 1986). Zinc was also found to be involved in the control of several enzymes. A number of zinc metalloenzymes are known, including carbonic anhydrase, carboxypeptidase, alcohol dehydrogenase, glutamic dehydrogenase, lactate dehydrogenase and alkaline phosphatase. Zinc is also known to inhibit DNAase activity, which may indicate that it contributes to the control of the destruction of spermatozoa.

Wallace & Grant (1975) hypothesized that DHT may initiate the synthesis of zinc binding protein required for the accumulation of zinc within the prostatic cells and lumen. As the epithelial cells become saturated with zinc, this cation may switch off testosterone reduction by binding to thiol groups at or near the cofactor binding site of the 5-α-reductase. Following ejaculation, 5-α-reductase activity may be restored, thus allowing the renewed accumulation of zinc within the gland.

## Citrate

Citrate is the major anion in human seminal plasma (mean 376 mg/dl). Its secretion is important in maintaining the osmotic equilibrium of the prostate and is a potent binder of metal ions (Mann & Lutwak-Mann 1981). Its secretion in the seminal plasma was suggested as a discriminative factor between semen of infected and noninfected infertile men (Comhaire et al 1989).

Citrate is produced via the tricarboxylic acid cycle and accumulates upon secretion if not utilized. Thus, the $CO_2$ production of the active prostatic cells is very low. Secretion of citrate takes place by means of the sodium pump and is under androgen control.

## Polyamines

The high concentration of aliphatic polyamines (spermine, spermidine, putrescine) in prostatic tissue and in seminal plasma is well documented (Williams-Ashman et al 1975). Human seminal plasma contains spermine (60 mg/100 ml) and about one-tenth as much spermidine and putrescine. Spermine comes mostly from the prostate, as has been shown in prostatic fluid obtained by rectal massage (Barkan et al 1978). Polyamines are synthesized in the body mainly from arginine via ornithine, catalysed by ornithine decarboxylase, which is a key enzyme controlled by testosterone in the sex organs. Other steps give rise to putrescine, spermidine and spermine.

The role of polyamines in the male reproductive tissues has been studied and a few mechanisms of control have been suggested. All three polyamines are recognized promoters of cellular growth. Putrescine was shown to serve as a growth factor produced by human fibroblasts in culture (Pohjanpelto & Raina 1972). Spermine and spermidine were able to stimulate the DNA-primed RNA polymerase. Polyamines are also involved in the phosphorylation of nonhistone chromosomal proteins (Ahmed et al 1978). The polyamines in rats are attached covalently to certain proteins involved in the formation of the ejaculated semen coagulum (Williams-Ashman & Canellakis 1979).

Direct effects of polyamines on spermatozoa

have been shown. Polyamines were found to enhance human sperm motility (Fair et al 1972), and may increase the rate of fructolysis in rat epididymal spermatozoa (Pulkkinen et al 1978).

Polyamines may also have negative effects on spermatozoa. Inhibition of the conversion of proacrosin to its active form acrosin has been shown by Parrish et al (1979). The oxidation of polyamines by diamine oxidase, especially putrescine, yields toxic aldehydes and peroxide which may affect the sperm. Pulkkinen et al (1978) showed that the oxidized spermine inhibited sperm fructolysis.

Spermine was shown to possess bacteriostatic properties that prevent the microbial growth in the seminal plasma (Grossowicz et al 1955). This may explain the difficulties in culturing semen for detection of bacteria.

The importance of polyamine biosynthesis and accumulation in cell growth processes studies makes them likely candidates for follow-up in cases of normal and abnormal tissue growth. This is valuable, especially for detecting and following carcinoma. Humans carrying tumors of the breast or colon were shown to secrete abnormal amounts of polyamines in urine (Russell 1978). It is interesting to evaluate cases of carcinoma in the sex organs and its correlation with polyamines. No definite answer is found in the literature (Russell 1978).

The development of new methods for determining polyamines using radioimmunoassay (Chaisiri et al 1979) instead of routine chemical methods (Gould et al 1975) has created a new momentum in monitoring prostatic gland activity. The most sensitive polyamine, with respect to prostatic function, was found to be spermine (Williams-Ashman et al 1975). Polyamines are known to be involved in certain events that occur in the prostatic cells. The activities of two pyridoxal phosphate decarboxylating enzymes that yield putrescine and spermidine were markedly decreased following gonadectomy and were restored by administration of testosterone. In the prostate and seminal vesicle, a coupling between RNA and polyamine synthesis probably takes place during the early phases of androgen-induced growth. Since the concentration of polyamines in the prostate of castrated controls increased only after a long period of androgen treatment, it has been suggested that these compounds do not perform a second messenger-like function relating to the biosynthesis of RNA and proteins in androgen-dependent tissues (Williams-Ashman & Reddi 1972).

## Prostatic control by androgens

It is now well established that the secretory activity of the epithelial cells of the male accessory sex glands are primarily under the control of testicular androgens. The prostate gland and other androgen target tissues accumulate androgen in significantly higher concentrations than do other somatic and nontarget tissues. Moreover, selective accumulation and retention have been demonstrated in the human organ, including the normal hyperplastic prostate and the neoplastic prostate (Attramadal et al 1975).

Testosterone in the prostate is converted rapidly to 5-α-DHT by the enzyme 5-α-reductase. The human prostate, especially in its periurethral region, will also rapidly and extensively convert testosterone to DHT. The high and prolonged uptake of androgen in the prostate is due to the presence of specific androgen receptor proteins located in the cytoplasm and nuclei of the prostatic epithelium (Liao & Fang 1969, Sufrin & Coffey 1973). A review on the receptors of male accessory sex organs has been presented by Rennie & Bruchovsky (1980). Steroid receptors are intracellular proteins that carry sites for the specific, high affinity, noncovalent binding of steroid hormones. The receptors are located in the cytoplasmic and nuclear compartments. Androgens initiate and maintain the growth and functional differentiation of the epithelial cells of male accessory sex tissues by controlling the utilization and DNA-directed synthesis of both rRNA and mRNA. The description of the mode of action of androgens and the involvement of other hormones in the regulation of prostatic function are given on page 181.

## Prostatic control by the nervous system

In all species studied, the glands are innervated by a dual sympathetic and parasympathetic efferent system, supplied by the hypogastric and pelvic nerves respectively. The influence of autonomic nerves on prostatic secretion has been studied extensively in the dog (Bruschini et al 1978). The canine prostate secretes most actively and copiously in response to electric stimulation of intact or decentralized hypogastric nerves or in response to pilocarpine, a powerful cholino-mimetic secretagogue. In contrast, pelvic nerve stimulation and cholinesterase inhibitors induce very little or no secretion. Other studies involving the administrating of stimulatory or inhibitory agents have established that secretions: (a) are effected exclusively via sympathetic pathways; (b) do not involve adrenomedullary or sympathetic adrenergic neuroterminal influence; (c) are influenced by acetylcholine released at epithelial affector sites by cholinergic postganglionic sympathetic neurons, and (d) are regulated by preganglionic cholinergic fibers of the hypogastric nerve.

The accessory glands of the dog continuously secrete at a very low rate. This persists after decentralization of the hypogastric nerve and is not affected by atropine or adrenergic blocking agents. Thus, the basal secretion is autonomous and independent of the direct and indirect autonomic neural influence and may be related to the epithelial blood supply (Smith 1975).

## Human prostatic growth and pathogenesis

Man and dog are virtually alone in the animal kingdom in their susceptibility to prostatic hyperplasia. There are a few reports on the mitotic activity of the human prostate. The human hyperplastic prostate exhibits an average labelling index of 0.36% using [$^3$H]-labelled thymidine, while a normal prostate has a lebelling index of 0.1%. This mitotic index is not located at the stromal compartment of the prostate, but rather at the epithelial cells. Thus, in the human prostate, the epithelial tissue of the peripheral zone appears to be the predominant site of the origin of carcinoma. Other studies showed a positive index between the weight of the prostate and the epithelial labelling index. A high labelling index may therefore justify prostatectomy. A method for studying the in vitro labelling index was devel-

oped using small pieces of prostatic biopsies. Good correlations were found between this and in vivo results (Senius et al 1974).

As the prostate ages it becomes more sensitive to androgens. Prostatic tissue is rich in growth factors and dehydrotestosterone receptors in the nucleus, yet mitotic cells are rare. Thus, the abnormal size of the aged prostate is not maintained by an enhancement of cell replication but rather by a decrease in the rate of cell death. These changes are likely to be mediated by estrogen and 5-α-reduced androgens (Trachtenberg et al 1980). Neonatal and prepubertal steroid imprinting may be of great importance in determining the prostatic growth (Naslund & Coffey 1986).

### Benign prostatic hypertrophy

Benign prostatic hypertrophy (BPH) takes place in the transition zone of the prostate. In this condition, the tissue concentrations of steroids are higher than normal, and the 5-α-reductase activity is also elevated. A good correlation was found between estradiol levels and BPH, especially in the development of nodules by certain actions on the stroma. Prolactin probably takes no part in BPH formation. The ratio DHT/testosterone is increased significantly in patients with BPH, which may imply stimulation of the incompletely developed glandular tissue. The androgen dependency of the prostate provides the rationale for using 5-α-reductase inhibitors for the treatment of BPH (Shapiro 1990). Benign prostatic hypertrophy is usually found in men over 40 years of age (Wilson 1980).

### Carcinoma

Carcinoma develops in the peripheral zone. This tissue binds more testosterone than does normal tissue, in spite of decreased testosterone in the circulation. Prolactin is higher in the semen of carcinoma patients. Thus, suppression of prolactin by bromocriptine may have some beneficial effects on prostatic carcinoma development.

Prostatic cancer tissue contains less DHT than

does normal tissue. The capacity to metabolize testosterone to DHT is significantly lower in carcinomatous tissue than in either normal or hyperplastic tissue (Djoseland et al 1977), indicating that malignant transformation of the prostatic epithelium is associated with diminished 5-α-reductase activity.

One might speculate whether the weak effect of cyproterone acetate on prostatic cancer as demonstrated clinically may be related to such fundamental alterations of androgen metabolism in malignant prostatic disease. It is less probable that compounds acting mainly by displacing DHT from the receptor sites will have a significant effect on prostatic cancer tissue, which contains relatively low amounts of this androgen (Djoseland et al 1977, Tveter 1981).

Since the analysis of the estradiol receptor protein content of breast tumor tissue is successfully used to predict the response to endocrine therapy of patients with advanced cancer, it has been suggested that DHT receptor levels in prostatic carcinoma may also be of value in determining the most appropriate form of therapy.

Treatment of BPH and carcinoma of the prostate includes surgery and/or hormonal antiandrogen drugs, or a combination of these treatments (Tveter 1981, Garnick 1988, Paulson 1988). Studies with implanted luteinizing hormone-releasing hormone (LHRH) analogue d-tryp-6-LHRH-ethylamide (LHRH-T) were made on geriatric male dogs with palpable prostatic hyperplasia. The treatment lasted 71 days. Testosterone levels rose for about 7 days after LHRH-T implantation and then declined. A marked decrease in the dimensions of the prostates was found in the radiographs. After testosterone levels rose, prostate dimensions increased slowly, again lagging behind the changes in testosterone. A decline in the ejaculate volume paralleled the decline in testosterone, although the sperm count remained normal for three weeks. The data suggest that LHRH analogues may be useful in the treatment of hormone responsive prostatic syndromes in man (Vickery et al 1981).

DeVoogt et al 1991, summarized the current status of GnRH analogues in the treatment of prostatic cancer:

1. All GnRH agonists provide medical castration equally well with minimal side-effects.

2. Combination with antiandrogens is important in the first 2–6 weeks of treatment with GnRH agonist to prevent flare-up.

3. GnRH agonists combined with antiandrogens cause earlier and better response.

*Chronic prostatitis*

During youth, the prostate surrounds the urethra. It is made up of many tube-like glands, each surrounded by a muscular sleeve that is believed to expel its contents during ejaculation. By the mid forties, it is common to find hypertrophy of the glandular acini. Gradual enlargement and coalescence of these nodules cause the gland to swell, pushing up the base of the bladder and pinching the urethra from both sides.

Rectal examination of the prostate may disclose a slight bagginess of the gland which, when gently massaged, releases a flow of prostatic fluid from the urethral meatus. Leukocytes in this fluid may signify inflammation diagnosed as prostatitis. Patients with prostatitis most often complain of urinary frequency and urgency, often with nocturia and terminal dysuria. Perhaps 25% of the patients are asymptomatic. Less frequent complaints include lower abdominal pain, backache, testicular aching or perineal pain. Urethral discharge occurs frequently and seems to be especially common upon arising in the morning. Prostatic tenderness, nodularity or edema occur occasionally, but absence of these signs does not exclude diagnosis of prostatitis. An acutely inflamed prostate is extremely tender and one that contains an abscess may be both tender and asymmetrical.

**The prostate and fertility**

Bacteria and other microorganisms often reach the prostate through the urethra, either by retrograde entry via the urethral meatus or by antegrade entry via contaminated urine. Most infectious processes of the male reproductive tract are neither common nor easily diagnosed. The vast majority of men with symptoms of prostatic inflammation have no clearly identifiable infecting organisms and nonbacterial, nonchlamydial epididymitis accounts for approximately 25% of the epididymal infections in young men (Berger et al 1979).

Flower (1981), in a selected review, described the various bacterial flora and inflammations of the male urogenital tract with special focus on its effect on fertility. There is insufficient data available to correlate the inflammation status with the fertility of men. Nevertheless, the evaluation of all infertile men should include urinalysis and urine culture and a thorough history and physical examination in order to uncover symptoms and signs of ongoing infection or evidence suggestive of past infection.

The possible mechanism which causes infertility in cases of chronic prostatitis may be due to secretory dysfunction of the prostate which is accompanied by chronic bacterial prostatitis. It was suggested that chronic prostatitis leads to an environment that adversely affects spermatozoa and results in subfertility. Inverse correlation between semen quality and prostatic concentration of calcium, magnesium and zinc was observed (Homonnai et al 1978a, Caldmone et al 1979). Furthermore, following therapy and intraprostatic injection of zinc, prostatic leukocytes decreased in association with a significant increase in sperm motility and normal morphology (Fahim et al 1985). Another possible mechanism for fertility impairment might be sperm agglutination as was shown by in vitro studies (Peleg & Ianconescu 1966, Teague et al 1971, Busolo et al 1984). The agglutination may result in functional abnormalities affecting sperm motility, sperm – mucus or sperm – oocyte interaction. These may be affected as well by antisperm antibodies which were shown to be excreted in chronic prostatitis. Both immunoglobulin-G (IgG) and immunoglobulin-A (IgA) have been implicated as factors of immunologically mediated infertility (Bronson et al 1984). Furthermore, chronic prostatitis is characterized by the appearance of inflammatory cells in the prostatic secretion. It was shown that infertile men had an increased number of leukocytes in prostatic secretion compared to normal men (Schaeffer 1981), and that the concentration of leukocytes in the semen correlates negatively with

sperm penetration test (Berger et al 1982, Colpi et al 1988).

The involvement of the accessory sex glands in male fertility is currently under extensive study. Since the composition of the seminal plasma affects sperm quality, it is important to determine its components (Homonnai et al 1978a). Dynamic tests evaluating the prostatic secretory function have been introduced. Ethanol, sulfamethoxazole and cephalexin have been used as external markers for monitoring prostatic secretions. These compounds were administered orally at a loading dose and their concentrations in semen and serum were estimated. Ethanol and sulfamethoxazole were secreted into the semen while cephalexin was not. No correlation was found between the rate of secretion of the above materials and the pathophysiology of the prostate or semen quality (Asher et al 1978, Paz et al 1979).

Treatment of chronic prostatitis should be specifically directed when possible. Recently, a new method of treatment using an ultra-high-frequency electric field was introduced with satisfactory results (Bogolyabov et al 1986). In cases when specific organisms are not identified but inflammation of the gland is suggested by microscopic evaluation of the semen, or by physical examination anti-inflammatory drugs in addition to wide-spectrum antibiotics are recommended.

## THE SEMINAL VESICLES

### Embryology

Primordia of the seminal vesicles become distinct at the end of the 3rd fetal month. They form longitudinal folds or evaginations in the walls of the mesonephric ducts before entering into the urethra (Pallim 1901). Sacculation of the glands is conspicuous during the 6th and 7th months (Fig 7.1). At the 6th month and later, the epithelium is simple or pseudostratified, showing some apocrine secretion. The musculature of the vesicular glands is derived from the musculature of the vas deferens. By the 6th fetal month, the seminal vesicle and the vas deferens show the same relationship to each other as in the adult. By the 7th month, the seminal vesicles attain their adult form. The seminal vesicles grow slowly until puberty (Arey 1965, Brewster 1985).

## Anatomy

The seminal vesicles of men are paired, highly convoluted pyriform glands (Fig. 7.2). Each vesicle is 5–6 cm long and 1–2 cm wide. They lie, one on each side of the midline, lateral to the ampulla of the vas deferens, posterior to the urinary bladder and superior to the prostate. Each gland is closed at its apex, open at its lower extremity and coiled. The convolutions of each vesicle, the saccules and diverticules are often so numerous that a single histological section may pass through several different regions.

The number and size of diverticules between the ridges and folds vary with the individual and from region to region in each seminal vesicle. They are thinner at their base than they are at their apex. Commonly, the recesses of the glands are filled with secretory material, but it is possible to find empty collapsed cavities. Just above the base of the prostate, each seminal vesicle ends in a narrow, duct-like structure that obliquely joins the termination of the vas deferens (ampulla) to form an ejaculatory duct.

## Histology

The gland is divided into two major compartments: *stroma* and *parenchyma*. Each has typical histological and ultrastructural appearances.

### Stroma

The lamina propria, which supports the mucosal folds and separates the epithelium from the underlying muscle layer, contains a few fibroblasts plus a moderate number of collagen and reticular fibers. In most species, this region is fairly well vascularized and rich in elastic fibers. The structural integrity of the stroma and its elastic elements, together with the volume of secretory material, determine the size of the gland.

Muscle is the prominent tissue, although the organization and orientation of its layers are often not discrete. The inner layer is composed of inter-

lacing circular and oblique smooth muscles and the outer layer predominantly contains longitudinally arranged smooth muscles. The adventitia covering the seminal vesicles is very thin. It is composed primarily of blood vessels, collagen and elastic fibers.

Hormones, especially testosterone, affect the growth, multiplication and innervation of the smooth muscle cells. During ejaculation, contraction of these muscles aids in the expulsion of the secretion from the seminal vesicles into the ejaculatory ducts.

### Parenchyma

Human seminal vesicles presumably contain two types of epithelial cells, principal or glandular cells and basal cells. Principal cells within active glands are usually columnar. Their apical surfaces are either smooth or covered with short microvilli. The nucleus is elongated and changes in size with advanced age. The basal plasmalemmae cover interdigitating cytoplasmic processes that interlock these cells at the base; comparable processes also exist on neighboring cells (Riva 1967). The arrangement of the mucosal cells varies from one area of the gland to another, and changes with advancing age or due to disturbances in hormonal status. Mucosal ridges and folds vary considerably even within the same cross-section. Through electron microscopy, developed organelles related to the secretory function, i.e. developed mitochondria, RER and Golgi complexes, have been identified (Brandes 1974).

Malformations of the male genital tract have been linked in some cases with the kidney. The absence of one testis or of one vas deferens or seminal vesicle, or of one-half of the prostate gland, or the bilateral absence of the vasa deferentia and seminal vesicles, have been demonstrated concomitantly with malformations or abnormalities of the kidney (Graham 1961, Homonnai et al 1978b).

In men, tumors of the seminal vesicle are very rare, but have been reported (Boreau 1977).

## Physiology of the seminal vesicles

The secretion of the seminal vesicles is viscid,

slightly yellowish in color and alkaline in pH. About 70% of the human ejaculate originates in the seminal vesicle. An average of 0.8–1.3 ml can be collected following digital massage. The last fraction of the ejaculate contains primarily secretions from the seminal vesicles. During sexual excitement, the seminal vesicles become tense and the smooth muscle contracts. Seminal vesicles undergo peristaltic contractions, discharging the secretion into the ejaculatory ducts and urethra.

Although the seminal plasma may not contain factors that are absolutely essential for fertilization, the secretions may nevertheless optimize conditions for sperm motility, survival and transport in both the semen and the female reproductive tract.

Fructose is the primary sugar secreted into the semen, averaging 315 mg/dl. This level of fructose is under androgenic regulation, but many factors such as storage, frequency of ejaculation, blood glucose levels and nutritional status can also affect the seminal plasma fructose concentration (Mann & Lutwak-Mann 1981). Fructose is formed via three possible enzymatic pathways, each starting with blood glucose, which undergoes isomerization and dephosphorylation to produce fructose. The employment of other enzymes such as hexokinase or sorbitol dehydrogenase will produce sorbitol from glucose (Paz et al 1980, Mann & Lutwak-Mann 1981).

Ascorbic acid, inorganic phosphorus and acid-soluble phosphorus are also present. Sorbitol, citrate inositol, prostaglandins (PG), cholinesterase and several soluble proteins are synthesized.

Proteins in the seminal vesicle fluid are few in number, may be insoluble at a certain pH, and frequently form large macromolecular aggregates (Curry & Atherton 1990). Human seminal proteins have strict species-dependent expression with some similarities in primates (Aumuller et al 1990). A specific protein, MHS-5, which was shown to be a unique marker for human semen, is a secretory product of the human seminal vesicle epithelium (Evans & Herr 1986).

A recent publication mentioned that an anti-inflammatory protein secreted from the rat seminal vesicle epithelium inhibits the synthesis

of plate-activating factor and the release of arachidonic acid and prostacyclin (Camussi et al 1990). An inhibitory effect of SV-IV, a major protein secreted from the rat seminal vesicle epithelium, on phagocytosis and chemotaxis of human polymorphonuclear leukocytes was also documented (Metafora et al 1989).

A proteinase inhibitor secreted by the seminal vesicles stabilizes the sperm's acrosomal membranes (Reddy et al 1979). In addition, uric acid, a source of reducing substances, is very highly concentrated in seminal plasma (Mann & Lutwak-Mann 1981).

Sodium and potassium are the predominant cations in seminal vesicle secretion. The usual alkaline pH of vesicular secretion may indicate that bicarbonate is an important anion, and undoubtedly citrate, too, fulfills a role as a major anion.

The protein profile of human semen contained specific proteins of both prostatic fluid and seminal vesicle fluid. One major group of proteins in seminal vesicle fluid (MW 28 000–68 000 daltons), designated as seminal vesicle-specific antigen, was observed in freshly ejaculated human semen, but disappeared when the ejaculate was allowed to stand at room temperature for 30 min. It was found that this seminal vesicle-specific antigen is the structural component of seminal coagulum (McGee & Herr 1988, Lee et al 1989).

The use of seminal vesicle-specific protein for the diagnosis of agenesis of the vas deferens and seminal vesicle in azoospermic men has been suggested by Calderon et al (1991). The absence of seminal vesicle-specific protein in seminal fluid was found to be a reliable proof of agenesis of seminal vesicle and vas deferens.

Prostaglandins were thought to originate in the prostate, but are now known to be secreted by the seminal vesicles. There are at least 15 prostaglandins in human seminal plasma (Bergstrom et al 1968), the majority of which are of the following types; $PGE_1$ (25 µg/ml), $PGE_2$ (23 µg/ml), $PGE_3$ (5.5 µg/ml), $PGF_{1\alpha}$ (3.6 µg/ml) and $PGE_{2\alpha}$ (4.4 µg/ml) (Eliasson 1963, Srivastava 1977, Templeton et al 1978, Kelly et al 1979). Prostaglandins probably account for most of the smooth muscle stimulants in human seminal plasma. They may also play some role in sperm transport in the female tract (Mandle 1972).

Since the seminal vesicles are of the same embryonic origin as the vas deferens, the congenital absence of the vas is associated with the absence of the seminal vesicle. This can be used to differentiate azoospermia due to testicular abnormalities from that of bilateral congenital absence of the vasa deferentia. In the latter case, the semen contains no fructose (Homonnai et al 1978b).

## Control of seminal vesicle function

The synthesis, production and release of constituents from the seminal vesicle have been studied to a limited extent in the rat, but not in the human. Flickinger (1974a,b) described the conventional pattern in the rat. Protein synthesis starts in the RER, with the product being transported to the Golgi complex where it is concentrated and packed into secretory vacuoles, which migrate to the apex of the cell, and are discharged in the lumen by exocytosis, as in the prostate.

The role of androgens in maintaining the accessory sex organs is well established. Testosterone production is required for the differentiation of the seminal vesicle at puberty and thereafter for proper sexual functioning. Thus, control of the seminal vesicles is similar to that of the prostate.

The epithelia of seminal vesicles are able to metabolize androgens through the steroid dehydrogenases-17β, 3-β, and 3-α (Sirigu et al 1981). Testosterone is important as a precursor of 5-α-DHT and DHT is the major androgen in the postnatal development (Shima et al 1990).

Male castration is followed by atrophy of the principal cells and cessation of secretory activity. The RER and Golgi complex becomes distrupted, the nucleus becomes pyknotic, secretory granules disappear and lysosomes increase in number, size and activity. Administration of testosterone usually reverses these changes, although this takes a few days to occur. Prolactin appears to act synergistically with testosterone; however, in some instances, it seems to function as a testosterone antagonist. As a result of tests on rats using the ergot alkaloid lisuride hydrogen maleate, an inhibitor of prolactin secretion, Aumuller et al

(1979) proposed that prolactin is an important hormone for maintaining seminal vesicle function.

The finding of a high affinity estrogen receptor in cytosol and nuclear extract suggests that estrogen, in addition to androgen, may act in the physiological regulation of this organ (Murphy et al 1980).

Recently a homogeneous class of vasopressin binding sites has been found in both seminal vesicles and renal medulla. However, the vasopressin receptors present in these tissues are different in terms of ligand specificity and adenylate cyclase activation. The density of the vasopressin receptors present in human seminal vesicles is inversely correlated with patient age, consistent with a physiological role for vasopressin in the regulation of accessory sex gland activity (Maggi et al 1989).

## THE COWPER'S AND URETHRAL GLANDS

### Embryology

The Cowper's glands (bulbourethral glands) originate from two endodermal epithelial buds growing from the pelvic part of the urogenital sinus (Chwalle 1927; Fig. 7.1). The openings of these glands are located between the membranous urethra and cavernous portions of the male urethra, one on each side. The secretory portion is derived by differentiation of mucin-producing secretory cells, which appear at the beginning of the 4th fetal month. The interstitium of the glands differentiates from the mesenchyme in situ.

The urethral glands (of Littre) develop in the second half of pregnancy from endodermal epithelial buds growing from the cavernous urethra (Fig. 7.1). The primordia of the preputial glands appear at the same time as small buds growing from the ectodermal glandopreputial lamella.

### Anatomy

The Cowper's glands are paired bodies 3–5 mm in diameter, which are homologous to Bartholin's glands in the female (Fig. 7.2). There is one gland on each side of the membranous urethra dorsal to the bulb of the penis, partially embedded in the skeletal muscle fibers of the urogenital diaphragma. The glands are divided into lobes and lobules by connective tissue. Each lobule is drained by a ductule. The ductules anastomose to form ducts, and the ducts within each gland unite to form a solitary excretory duct. Usually the ducts are surrounded by one or two layers of circular smooth muscle. The smaller ducts are lined by a simple columnar secretory epithelium, which occasionally gives rise to diverticules. The large ducts contain nonsecretory, pseudostratified or stratified columnar epithelium, and occasional mucous-producing intraepithelial glands. The excretory ducts are 3–4 cm long. They are lined by stratified columnar epithelium. The excretory ducts pierce the urogenital membrane, pass into the corpus spongiosum of the penis, and travel for 2–3 cm in the poorly defined submucosa of the bulbous urethra. They open into the floor of the urethra by two very small openings, one on each side of the midline.

**Histology**

These glands exhibit the typical arrangement of stroma and parenchyma of all the male accessory sex glands.

*Stroma*

The tubules and alveoli are surrounded by connective tissues rich in elastic fibers. Smooth muscles as well as stratified muscles are abundant.

*Parenchyma*

The squamous epithelial cells are dominant in the tubules and alveoli of the gland. Other forms such as cuboidal- or columnar-shaped cells are also present, depending upon the functional phase, age, hormonal status, and sexual activity of the man.

**Physiology and control**

The clear, visicid, mucus-like secretions of the gland are discharged during erection and possibly also during ejaculation. The glandular epithelium of the alveoli secretes droplets of mucin, which presumably aids in urethral lubrication. The secretion of the mucus, rich in sialoprotein, occurs by exocytosis and is usually associated with the appearance of large intercellular secretory canaliculi.

The Cowper's gland of the boar has been shown to posseess a mucin that inhibits corona radiata penetrating enzyme in vitro and decreases the fertilizing ability of capacitated spermatozoa in vivo (Srivastava & Gould 1973).

Scattered accessory glands can be found throughout the male reproductive tract. Common are the urethral (Littre's) and preputial (Tyson's) glands. Their secretions are discharged close to their location. No information is available on the nature and physiology of the secretion in men.

All of the glands are under strict androgen control for proliferation and secretion. They are involuted following castration or estrogen administration. Very few diseases are known in these glands (Price & Williams-Ashman 1961).

PENIS

The external genitalia in man originate in the urogenital sinus and genital tubercle (Fig. 7.1). The genital tubercle develops into the penis. The genital folds are the origin of the central raphe, displacing the urethral opening to the tip of the penis.

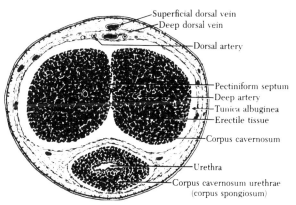

**Fig. 7.3** Drawing of a transverse section of the penis. (Redrawn and reproduced with permission from Leeson and Leeson 1970)

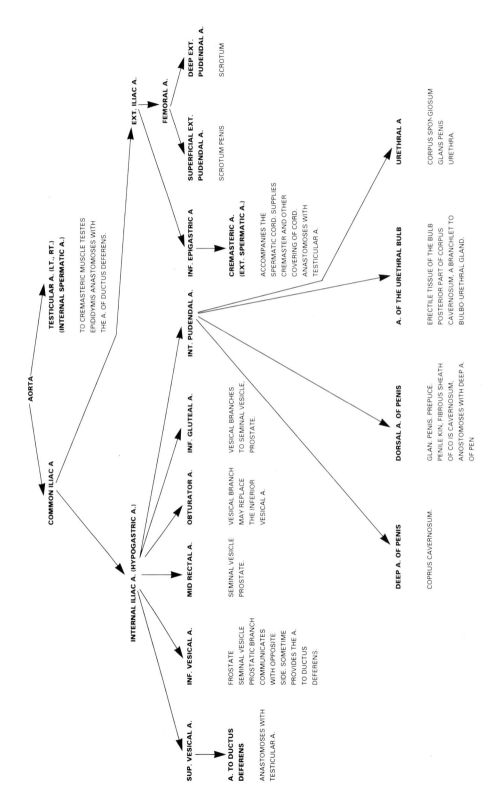

**Fig. 7.4**   Schematic presentation of the arterial blood supply to the male genital organs, based mainly on *Gray's Anatomy* (Warwick & Williams 1989).

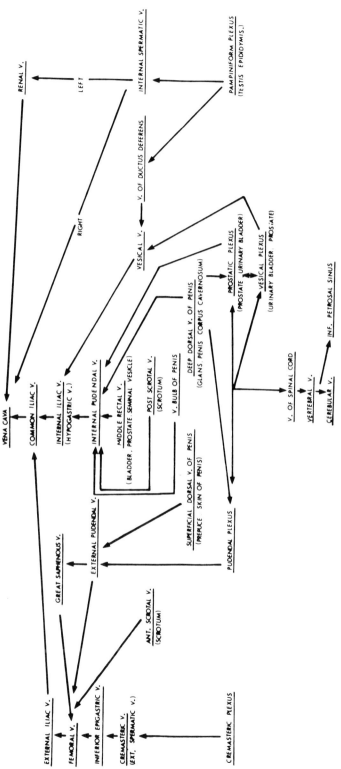

**Fig. 7.5**  Schematic presentation of the venous blood system of the male genital organs, based mainly on *Gray's Anatomy* (Warwick & Williams 1989).

The penis is attached to the front and sides of the pubic arch and is composed of three cylindrical masses of erectile cavernous tissues, blood vessels, lymph and nerves (Fig. 7.2). All of these are bound together by fibrous tissue and covered with skin. The cavernous bodies are two lateral corpora cavernosa and one median corpus spongiosum (Fig. 7.3). The corpus spongiosum (corpus cavernosum of the urethra) runs through the penis, builds the glans penis by dilatation at its distal end, and covers the ends of the two corpora cavernosa. At the proximal end (towards the prostate) the corpus forms the bulb. The three corpora are each covered by tunica albuginea, with that covering the spongiosum being much thinner than that surrounding the cavernosa.

The erectile tissue within the penis is a labyrinth of irregular blood sinuses or spaces. The sinuses are supplied by capillaries and the afferent arterioles are drained by venules. The trabeculae of the erectile tissue form the partitions between adjacent sinuses. They are composed of collagen, elastic and smooth muscle fibers, and numerous fibroblasts. The prepuce is a retractile fold of skin containing connective tissue, with smooth muscle in its interior. Sebaceous glands are present in the internal folds and in the skin that covers the glans.

The penis is supplied with blood by the deep and dorsal arteries (Figs 7.3–7.5). The deep arteries pass into the corpora cavernosa, while the dorsal arteries travel between them and the dorsal surface of the penis, supplying the skin and the fibrous sheath of the corpora cavernosa. The dorsal and deep arteries anastomose in the sheath.

Both superficial and deep veins exist in the penis. The superficial veins drain the foreskin and skin of the penis, although most of the blood is drained by the deep veins, which enter the pudendal plexus. In addition, drainage from the skin through the deep inguinal nodes has also been described. Veins from the glans penis and corpora cavernosa empty into the deep inguinal and external iliac nodes. The blood from the corpus spongiosum is drained via the superficial and deep dorsal veins. A rich lymphatic network is also found in the penis.

The nerve supply of the penis comes from the pudendal nerve and the pelvic plexus. The smooth muscles of the corpora cavernosa and the arterioles within the trabeculae of the penis receive the innervation from the pelvic plexus via the hypogastric and prostatic plexus.

## SCROTUM

Midline fusion of the genital folds forms the scrotum. The scrotum is a thin pouch of skin outside the testis, composed of muscle, elastic and collagenous tissue (Fig. 7.1). Beneath the skin is the tunica dartos, which is built up from smooth muscle fibers and connective tissue. The two tunics that surround each testis fuse to form an internal scrotal partition, the septum scroti. Under the dartos lies a layer of striated muscle and connective tissue, the cremaster fascia, which is a continuation of the internal oblique muscle and forms a sheath around the spermatic cord. The scrotum is internally lined with a layer of the tunica vaginalis, derived from the saccus vaginalis of the peritoneum, after descent of the testis. The mesothelial cells and the macrophages lying within the tunica both have phagocytic properties.

The blood supply of the scrotum is schematically represented in Figures 7.4 and 7.5. The physiology of the scrotum will be described in another chapter dealing with thermoregulation and spermatogenesis. Generally, scrotal activity is under strict androgen control.

## BLOOD SUPPLY TO THE MALE GENITAL ORGANS

### Arteries

Three arteries arising from the aorta supply the male genital tract (Fig. 7.4). The left and right testicular arteries, also called internal spermatic arteries, supply the testes, epididymides and cremasteric muscles and also anastomose with the artery of the vas deferens. In addition, the common iliac artery gives rise to the internal and external iliac arteries which supply all the other compartments of the genital organs.

### Veins

Blood drainage is based on the creation of five branches of veins that are built up by the veins of the different organs: cremasteric, pudendal, prostatic, vesical, and the pampiniform plexus (Fig. 7.5). The cremasteric and pampiniform plexuses are characterized by anastomoses between the right and left twins of plexuses and also between the cremasteric and pampiniform plexuses of the same side.

Thus, this complex system of blood drainage leads to the major vessels by different avenues. The following peculiarities characterize this venous system:

1. Connections between different venal vessels exist at each level of the system, which means that blood drained from the testes can reach the veins coming from the accessory glands. If a major vein is blocked, the blood can be collected by several alternative pathways.

2. The left and right spermatic veins reach the vena cava in different ways. The right one usually drains directly into the vena cava, while the left drains via the left renal vein.

3. An alternative route for blood coming from the prostatic, vesical and pudendal plexuses is connected to the vein of the spinal cord leading to the brain. This explains the appearance of metastases in the vertebrae and skull in many cases where the primary tumor is located in one of the accessory sex glands (Batson 1942). Generally, the blood coming from the various glands and organs can be drained directly into the vena cava (spermatic veins) or through the external and internal iliac veins which form the common iliac vein on each side.

## LYMPHATIC DRAINAGE

Parallel and close to the venal drainage is a well-developed lymphatic system. The testicular lymphatic drainage is both superficial and deep. The superficial system commences on the surface of the tunica vaginalis, and the deep system is in the epididymis and body of the testis. They form from four to eight collecting trunks which ascend with the spermatic veins in the spermatic cord and along the front of the psoas major muscle to the level where the spermatic vessels cross the aorta, and end in the lateral and preaortic groups of lumbar nodes.

Light and electron microscopic investigations have indicated that lymphatic capillaries of the testis are in close association with the vas deferens and are grouped like alveoles from where collecting vessels emerge. Collecting vessels are located at the periphery of the plexus pampiniformis, decreasing in number towards the inguinal canal. Single smooth muscle cells line the wall of the initial segments of the collecting ducts. In the proximal part of the spermatic cord, most of the lymphatic walls are lined by several layers of muscle cells. However, where collecting vessels are equipped with valves, the muscular coat is almost completely interrupted (Moller 1980).

The lymphatic vessels of the vas deferens pass to the external iliac nodes; those of the seminal vesicles are drained partly into the hypogastric and partly into the external iliac nodes. The drainage of the prostate terminates chiefly in the hypogastric and sacral nodes, but one trunk from the posterior surface ends in the external iliac nodes, and another from the anterior surface joins the vessels that drain the membranous part of the urethra.

Lymphatics from the skin of the penis drain into the superficial and deep inguinal nodes. The lymphatics of the cavernous portion of the urethra accompany those of the glans penis, and terminate with them in the deep subinguinal and external iliac nodes. Those of the membranous and prostatic portion pass to the hypogastric nodes.

## INNERVATION OF THE MALE GENITAL ORGANS

The glands receive a dual sympathetic and parasympathetic efferent innervation supplied by the hypogastric and pelvic nerves respectively. They are also connected with specific ganglia that are located on both sides of the vertebrae (sympathetic) or close to the genital organs (parasympathetic).

The hypogastric nerve is derived from the lumbar spinal cord gray matter and is connected to the upper or upper and middle lumbar sympathetic ganglia. This nerve forms most of the efferent sympathetic innervation of the male genital organs. In man, a lumbosacral plexiform nerve forms the right and left hypogastric nerves.

The pelvic nerve, usually with three or four trunks, is based on nerves derived from the upper or midsacral spinal cord gray matter.

Branches of the hypogastric nerves and the pelvic nerves build the pelvic plexus which innervates all of the genital compartments that are part of the pelvic viscera. There are also several secondary plexuses related to the genital organs; the visceral plexus, prostatic plexus, greater cavenous nerve, and lesser cavernous nerves. Organ innervation is mostly ipsilateral, but crossing over the midline leads to contralateral organ innervation as well.

Ganglia are located along neural pathways of genital organs and are composed of central and peripheral groups. The central ganglia include the inferior mesenteric ganglion and the ganglia that lie along the branches of the hypogastric and pelvic nerves. The peripheral ganglia include the hypogastric ganglion and the pelvic plexus ganglia. Elbadawi & Goodman (1980) have described the innervation of the male genital tract in great detail.

The neuromuscular transmission in the male accessory sex organs, including the vas deferens, is similar to, and based on, dual innervation by the sympathetic and parasympathetic nerves. The muscular innervation is derived from the same short neuron group that supplies the vas deferens. The predominant muscular action of the sympathetic innervation in these organs is excitatory and belongs to the α-adrenergic group. The parasympathetic innervation plays a minor role in the active muscular contraction, but is more involved in the basal muscular activity of organs during the erection phase preceding ejaculation (Elbadawi & Goodman 1980).

## ERECTION AND EJACULATION

The male sexual response consists of the same four distinct phases known in females: excitement, plateau, orgasm and resolution. In men, this response is coordinated by higher centers in the hypothalamus, limbic system and cerebral cortex and is influenced to various degrees by sex hormone levels. The basic sexual cycle is controlled by reflex mechanisms organized within the lumbosacral segments of the spinal cord. A summary of the events during erection and ejaculation is presented in Table 7.2 and Figure 7.6.

The initial event of the sexual response during the excitement phase is penile erection, which is followed by glandular emission and ejaculation.

### Erection

Erections are due to psychogenic and reflexogenic responses. The mechanism of erection involves the following steps (Fig. 7.6):

1. closure of arteriovenous anastomoses between

**Table 7.2**   Control of erection and ejaculation by the nervous system of man

| Physiological parameter | Afferent | Efferent | Central pathway | Changes in the affected organ |
|---|---|---|---|---|
| Erection | | | | |
| Reflexogenic | Pudendal nerve | Sacral parasympathetic | Sacral spinal reflex | Dilatation of arterial supply to corpus cavernosum and corpus spongiosum |
| Psychogenic | Visual, auditory, tactile, olfactory | Lumbar sympathetic, sacral parasympathetic | Supraspinal origin | |
| Glandular secretion | Pudendal nerve | Sacral parasympathetic | Sacral spinal reflex | Seminal vesicles and prostate |
| Seminal emission | Pudendal nerve | Lumbar sympathetic | Intersegmental spinal reflex (sacrolumbar) | Contraction of vas deferens, ampulla, seminal vesicles, prostate, closure of bladder neck |
| Ejaculation | Pudendal nerve | Somatic efferents in pudendal nerve | Sacral spine reflex | Rhythmic contractions of bulbocavernosus and ischiocavernosus muscles |

Reproduced from deGroat & Booth (1980) with permission of the authors and Editor of *Annals of Internal Medicine*.

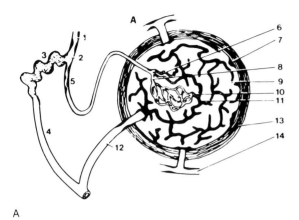

A

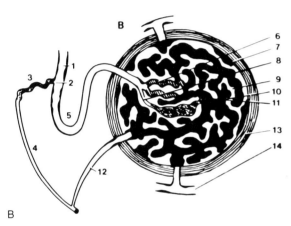

B

**Fig. 7.6** Vascular relationships of the human penis. **a** In the flaccid state, blood flows toward the corpora cavernosa in the deep artery of the penis (5). This vessel possesses intimal cushions, which tend to regulate blood flow. Almost all the blood passes directly (6) into an arteriovenous anastomosis (8), which is usually dilated in this state and connects with efferent veins (9). Minimal amounts of blood pass to the corpora cavernosa. At a point inside the corpora this artery (7) divides into branches, the helicine artery (1), which empties almost immediately into the blood spaces of erectile tissue and, after breaking up into a capillary network, it reforms into a small vein (2) and empties into a cavernous space. Cavernous spaces are drained by veins that have internal cushions (4). These pierce the tunica albuginea and constitute efferent venous return. **b** During erection, blood flow in the deep artery of the penis (5) increases. Opening (6) of arteriovenous anastomosis (8) is reduced by active vasoconstriction, resulting in a slightly dilated artery (7) passing through the tunica albuginea (3) into the cavernous body. Helicine arteries (1) dilate, and cavernous spaces fill with blood while the nutritive vessel and its venous junction (2) with cavernous space become compressed. Blood flow leaving the cavernous body (4) is not reduced despite the internal structure of these emergent veins. (Adapted and modified with permission from Conti 1952)

the deep artery of the penis and the peripheral venous return

2. constriction of penile arterioles, which facilitates the entry of blood into the three corpora covernosa
3. blocking of blood drainage by constriction of efferent penile veins.

There is contradictory evidence relating to this last step, since studies by Shirai & Ishii (1981) using two techniques, infusion of $^{133}$Xe into corpora cavernosa and cavernosography, demonstrated the existence of erections without closure of the efferent vein from the corpora cavernosa.

Intensive investigations in animal models and human volunteers have clarified the mechanism of erection. The data is reviewed by Lue & Tanagho (1987). Measurement of blood flow during erection has revealed an increase in arterial flow, sinusoidal relaxation and increased venous resistance, resulting in turgidity of the corpora cavernosa and corpus spongiosum. In the full erection phase the pressure is approximately 90–100 mmHG. In the rigid erection phase the pressure can reach values of more than 350 mmHg.

The human penis not only has unique arteriovenous shunts, but also has a specific structure of muscle fibers (pads, also called posters) that freely modify the vascular lumen. When the penis is in the flaccid state, the longitudinal and circular muscles of the afferent artery pads are contracted, reducing the volume of their lumen. Blood therefore does not enter the lumen of the corpora cavernosa. During erection both the circular and longitudinal fibers relax, causing 20–50 ml of blood to enter and fill the corpora. Due to their fibrous capsule cover, the corpora cavernosa become rigid upon filling. During erection, blood continues to pass through the penis but at a slower rate, helping to maintain erection (Weiss 1972).

The typical venous drainage of blood from the penis is due to the existence of special funnel-shaped valves located in the deep dorsal veins, which cause the delayed venous return from the corpora cavernosa (Fitzpatrick & Cooper 1975).

The two components of the autonomic nervous system are responsible for erection. The parasympathetic system is responsible for closing the arteriovenous complexes and for increasing the flow of blood into the sinuses; the sympathetic activity accounts for arteriole constriction in the other parts of the penis, which leads to increased blood pressure and flow. Penile erection is primarily an involuntary or reflex phenomenon that can be elicited by a variety of stimuli and by at least two distinct control mechanisms. For example, psychogenic erections are initiated by supraspinal centers in response to auditory, visual, olfactory, tactile and imaginative stimuli (Weiss 1972). The efferent limb of the reflex pathway can be in either the thoracolumbar (T12–L3) or the sacral autonomic outflow (S2–S4). In patients with lesions in the sacral area, reflexogenic erections are abolished, but psychogenic erection may still take place via the sympathetic innervation of the penis; in contrast, spinal lesions above T12 abolish psychogenic erections, but do not affect reflexogenic erections.

The neurotransmitters controlling penile erection may involve the following transmitters or drugs: vasoactive intestinal polypeptide, α-adrenergic blockade, acetylcholine. Based on this data it was found that intracavernous injection of vasoactive agents such as papaverine, phenoxybenzamine or a combination of papaverine and pentolamine can be used in order to induce penile erection. This is applied in the clinic as a dynamic test for evaluation of arterial, venous and sinusoidal mechanisms in order to differentiate organic from psychogenic impotence (Virag et al 1984). In addition, once it was proved to be effective, it was used routinely under careful medical supervision.

## Detumescence

Following ejaculation, blood flows out of the highly congested cavernous spaces of the penis, with consequent loss of erection. This action is clearly due to arterial constriction by the sympathetic system. In the cat, electrical stimulation of the abdominal sympathetic nerves and their pathway via the hypogastric and presacral nerves produces rapid detumescence. This effect is even more rapid than that produced by complete occlusion of the aorta.

## Ejaculation

During the second (plateau) and third (orgasm) phases of the male sexual response, the glandular secretions, emission and ejaculation take place. Emission results from the accumulation of semen in the prostatic urethra, and the propulsion of semen out of the urethra during orgasm which is concomitant with closure of the bladder neck.

During emission, reflex activity in the thoracolumbar sympathetic outflow elicits rhythmic contractions of the smooth muscle of the seminal vesicles, prostate and vas deferens, and glandular secretions into the urethra, with simultaneous closure of the urinary bladder neck, to prevent the backflow of semen into the bladder. Surgical interruption of sympathetic nerves or the administration of drugs that either block α-adrenergic receptors, deplete norepinephrine stores, or block its release (e.g. guanethidine) result in a disturbed emission.

After the emission of semen into the proximal urethra, rhythmic contractions of the bulbocavernosus and ischiocavernosus muscles and the external urethral sphincter result in ejaculation.

The autonomic nervous system controls ejaculation. Afferent stimuli from the penis gland are transmitted by the pudendal nerve into the spinal cord and the cerebral cortex. Efferent fibers, in turn, run into the throracolumbar sympathetic outflow at the spinal sympathetic ganglia T12–L3. This stimulates peristaltic contractions of the smooth muscles within the epididymis and vas deferens, which move sperm to the ampulla of the vas. Thereafter, contraction of the ampulla, seminal vesicles and prostate glands leads to emission simultaneous with the contraction of the bladder neck. The parasympathetic system from the sacral area is responsible for the emission of the material accumulated in the posterior urethra, and the delivery of the ejaculate.

The seminal plasma serves as a transport medium for spermatozoa between the male and female reproductive tracts. Human seminal plasma is composed of secretions derived from the testes, rete testes, efferent duct, epididymis, vas deferens, ampullae, seminal vesicles, prostate and the combined secretions of the Cowper's and urethral glands (Mitsuya et al 1960).

The delivery of semen in humans is usually in splits (fractions) in a well-defined fashion that involves the emission of spermatozoa from the vas and ampulla with the secretions of the Cowper's, urethral and prostatic glands in the first fractions (rich in sperm of good quality, suspended in about 30% of the whole ejaculated volume). The following splits (70% of the ejaculate) mostly include the secretions of the seminal vesicles, which rinse the remaining spermatozoa liberated from the cauda epididymis, vas deferens and ampulla. This entire process can be followed with biochemical markers for glandular function (Eliasson & Lindholmer 1976). The sensations accompanying ejaculation constitute the orgasm. Orgasm is not neccessarily affected by sympathectomy, provided that the pudendal nerves remain intact. Damage of the spinal cord in paraplegics, where the site of injury was in the thoracolumbar area, inhibits ejaculation. Only about 10% are able to achieve intromission and ejaculation following cord lesion.

*Effect of phenoxybenzamine*

Studies on the effect of phenoxybenzamine-hydrochloride (PBZ-HCl) in small doses on the fertility of male rats and men and the function of the reproductive tract have been published (Paz et al 1984). The main conclusions of the above studies and other studies performed in men were that PBZ-HCl causes a block of the sympathetic nervous system of the male sexual tract leading to aspermia (dry ejaculation) due to block of sperm transport and semen emission (Homonnai et al 1984). No changes were reported in the hormonal balance and blood pressure. The block of semen emission is the main side-effect reported in men treated with low doses (up to 20 mg/day) of PBZ–HCl. On the other hand, most men who complained of premature ejaculation reported excellent improvement in sexual response during treatment (Shilon et al 1984). Since the drug causes dry ejaculation, it was suggested as a male contraceptive (Homonnai et al 1984).

**Pathophysiology**

Sexual dysfunction includes impotence, prema-

ture ejaculation, ejaculatory failure and reduced or absent libido. The reasons for sexual dysfunction may include psychological causes, age, hormonal imbalance, vascular changes, medication and neuropathy.

Organic deficiency of erection is not common. However, any condition that interrupts the blood or nerve supply to the penis will disturb erection. Examples are carcinoma and diabetes. A study of the autonomic nervous system in the corpora cavernosa of impotent diabetics lends strong support to the idea that their sexual impotence is due to a neurological lesion of the nerve fibers that control erection (Faerman et al 1974).

Several drugs, many used for treating hypertension, block the parasympathetic nerves and interfere with erection. Drugs increasing serum prolactin (tranquilizers) are known to cause impotence through the higher centers of the brain. In addition, psychotropic drugs may influence the ejaculatory process.

Priapism is a pathological prolonged erection of the penis and is a result of impaired venous outflow. The etiology of this syndrome is attributed to psychological and neurological deviations (i.e. encephalitis, multiple sclerosis, compression of spinal medulla, etc.). Priapism is very painful and may lead to thrombotic changes of the cavernous bodies.

Retrograde ejaculation may occur if the internal sphincter fails to contract during ejaculation. The internal sphincter is stimulated through the sympathetic nerves, which may be injured during operations to replace an aneurism of the aorta, when excising pelvic cancer or performing radical pelvic surgery, or which may be blocked by drugs administered for hypertension. In some patients, the failure of bladder neck contraction is followed by the failure of seminal vesicles and vas deferens contraction. Diabetes, in some cases, may be followed by retrograde ejaculation.

SPERM TRANSPORT

Spermatogenesis ends in the release of immotile spermatozoa into the lumen of seminiferous tubuli, from which they are transported to the ampulla of the vas deferens by various methods including contractions of the myoid cells of the seminiferous tubuli, capillary forces and reabsorption of testicular fluids in the caput epididymis, and peristaltic contractions of the smooth muscles of the epididymis and vas deferens.

From the seminiferous tubule, the spermatozoa travel into the rete testis by the release of fluid and contraction of myoid cells. Rhythmic contractions of the seminiferous tubuli facilitate the release of spermatozoa and lead to their transport out of the testis into the rete testis, which is composed of 12–20 ducts in man. The rate of fluid flow through the rete testis can be measured by catheterization of the duct. Setchell et al (1969) recorded a fluid flow of 2 ml/h in the ram. In rabbits, the muscles of the tunica albuginea contract, hinting at its possible contribution to fluid and sperm transport.

Transport of spermatozoa through the epididymis, a single 6-m (20-ft) convoluted duct, takes 10–15 days in various species (Amann et al 1976). Spermatozoan transport results from the following factors; (a) fluid flow from the testis and resorption of this fluid by the caput epididymis with the movement of cilia in the efferent ducts; (b) a hydrostatic pressure gradient from the testis through the caput epididymis towards the vas deferens; and (c) muscular contractions. The epididymis is surrounded by three layers of smooth muscle (inner longitudinal, middle circular and outer longitudinal layers). These three layers of smooth muscle are also present and extend to the ampulla in the vas deferens.

The electrical activity of the smooth muscle of the rat epididymis has been studied. The highest activity was recorded in the caput and decreased towards the cauda and vas deferens. Electrical activity spreads over long distances in the distal part and caudal epididymis and in the vas. Peristaltic contractions of the caudal epididymis have also been recorded in vivo (Talo et al 1979). Contraction of the smooth muscles of the epididymis is stimulated by intraluminal pressure, action of catecholamines and neurohypophyseal hormones. The flow of sperm and fluid from the testis and the peristaltic movement of parts of the epididymal tract, have also been implicated in transport of spermatozoa (Knight 1974).

Mitsuya et al (1960), using an X-ray technique similar to angiography, injected the vas deferens

with contrast media, and were thus able to fill and visualize the ampullae and seminal vesicles. They describe the ampullae and seminal vesicles as inclined at an angle of 30° from the horizontal plane, prior to the induction of sexual excitement by masturbation. During sexual excitement and the accompanying erection, these structures assume the horizontal plane. In the pre-ejaculatory stage the seminal vesicles become tense and begin to show peristaltic movements. However, the ampulla at this stage is seen to undergo active contraction, expelling its contents into the posterior urethra via the ejaculatory duct and bypassing the seminal vesicles. This action is soon followed by seven or eight active contractions of the seminal vesicles at intervals of about 0.20 s each for the first three, and 0.04 s for the terminal contractions, the latter being stronger as well as longer. These authors conclude that the actual contractions of the seminal vesicles overlap the emissive and ejaculatory processes and emission itself, in terms of time, is largely a function of the ampullae.

In men, the vas deferens contains large amounts of catecholamines, especially norepinephrine. Although the sympathetic system is dominant (Ventura et al 1973), the vas is richly innervated with adrenergic fibers, yet has poor cholinergic innervation. It has been estimated that 10–60% of the total ejaculate originates in the proximal vas and epididymis (Freund & Davis 1969). During ejaculation, semen is released by powerful, short, adrenergically mediated contractions of the distal cauda epididymis and vas deferens; spermatozoa are then mixed with the secretions of the ampullary glands, the seminal vesicles, the prostate, and the urethral and Cowper's glands.

## REGULATION OF MALE ACCESSORY SEX ORGAN FUNCTION

Regulation of the male accessory sex organs is carried out by endocrine and neural factors. Most of the studies of regulation were performed on the prostate, particularly in rodents. The responses elicited by androgens in this tissue include the induction of glycolytic enzymes and the synthesis of RNA and DNA and the onset of cell division. Testosterone has been shown to play a regulatory role in a number of carbohydrate-metabolizing enzymes in androgen-dependent tissues. Castration of the rat is usually followed by a marked decrease in the activities of hexokinase, phosphofructokinase, pyruvate kinase, glucose-6-phosphate, 6-phosphogluconate dehydrogenase and α-glycero-phosphate dehydrogenase in the prostate and seminal vesicles. This is effectively reversed by the administration of testosterone in a dose-dependent and time-dependent manner (Singhal & Sutherland 1975). A decrease in the metabolism (oxygen consumption) of slices of the rat ventral prostate following orchidectomy was reported to be accompanied by a decrease in the activities of a number of mitochondrial enzymes and in the number of mitochondria (Edelman 1963).

The sequence and order of synthesis of materials, and their production, packing in vacuoles, and secretion are well known (Flickinger 1974a,b). The precise mechanism of the mode of action is unclear; however, there is general agreement about two basic assumptions: the site of action of androgens is at the level of the nucleus, and DHT is the androgen that mediates hormonal responses in the prostate. Thus,

although testosterone is the primary plasma androgen that induces growth of the prostate gland and other sex accessory tissues, it appears to function as a prohormone in that the active form of the androgen in the prostate is not testosterone but a metabolite, DHT (Bruchovsky & Wilson 1968). This conversion can take place directly in the prostate and seminal vesicles or in peripheral tissues. Over 90% of the testosterone is irreversibly converted to DHT through the action of NADPH and the enzyme 5-α-reductase. Although DHT is a potent androgen (1.5 to 2.5 times as potent as testosterone in most bioassay systems), its low plasma concentration and tight binding to plasma proteins diminish its direct importance as a circulating androgen affecting prostate and seminal vesicle growth.

The mode of action of testosterone on prostatic cells and on other male accessory sex organs is depicted in Figure 7.7, and is as follows:

1. Free testosterone on entering the cell by diffusion is reduced by 5-α-reductase to DHT.
2. DHT binds to a cytoplasm receptor, resulting in a receptor – DHT complex which thereafter moves to the nucleus.

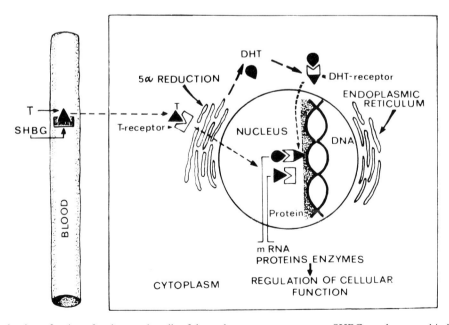

**Fig. 7.7**   Mechanism of action of androgens in cells of the male accessory sex organs. SHBG, sex hormone binding globulin; T, testosterone; DHT, dihydrotestosterone.

3. Receptor – DHT binds to the nuclear matrix and specific sequences of DNA.

4. Changes in DNA topology and chromatin. Increased transcription expression and regulation of specific genes.

5. Trimming and processing of the mRNA as it is transported through the nucleus to the nuclear pore complex.

6. Stability and transportation of mRNA into the cytoplasmic compartment to be translated into protein.

7. Transportation of the protein to specific cellular sites and its subsequent post-translational modification.

The binding of DHT to the receptor may stimulate adenylcyclase, resulting in increased production of nuclear cyclic adenosine monophosphate (cAMP). The resulting increase in nuclear cAMP may activate a specific protein kinase (histone kinase) and result in the phosphorylation of prostatic histone with a subsequent change in the DNA – histone interaction. The exposed genome would then be subject to transcription by RNA polymerase and eventual translation into an altered metabolic profile (Wilson 1972).

Two cells can have the same androgen receptors present in their nuclei, but one will respond by making one type of androgen-induced protein, while the other will produce a second type of androgen-induced protein. How androgens specify gene response remains a mystery.

Cloning of the complete coding sequence of the human androgen receptor was reported by Lubahn et al (1988). Rabbit polyclonal antibodies were raised against a synthetic peptide from the N-terminal region of the human androgen receptor. Immunocytochemical analysis of human prostate tissue demonstrated that androgen receptor is localized predominantly in the nuclei of glandular epithelial cells.

The amount of receptor in the cytoplasm and nucleus of the prostatic cell is determined by the hormonal status of the animal. In the normal prostate, most of the receptor–hormone complex is located in the nucleus while in castrated rats it is found mostly in the cytoplasm.

It is well established that part of the mechanism of androgen activity in accessory glands is through the adenylcyclase system. The ability of theophylline to potentiate the effects of a submaximal dose of testosterone on prostatic and vesicular carbohydrate metabolism has also been investigated. This is generally based on the ability of methylxanthine to inhibit the biodegradation of endogenous cAMP to $5^1$AMP by phosphodiesterase and thereby increase the intracellular pool of cAMP. When a low dose of testosterone was administered in conjunction with theophylline, the increases were of a much greater magnitude and were similar to those produced with a larger dose of testosterone. The ability of theophylline to mimic and to potentiate the influence of submaximal doses of sex steroids on accessory sex organ responses supports the concept that cAMP is involved in the sequence of events taking place in the target tissue in response to the appropriate hormone.

The direct involvement of adenylcyclase in the activity of the prostate and seminal vesicle has been demonstrated by measurement of cAMP in the accessory sex organs. It was also found that a single injection of testosterone partially reversed the decrease in cAMP concentration in the glands of castrated rats. $^3$H-labelled ATP added to glands incubated in vitro was a model to study the effect of testosterone and theophylline on the conversion of ATP to cAMP under various physiological conditions.

Another model for studying the involvement of the adenylcyclase system in the activity of the accessory sex glands was the preparation of homogenates. The addition of DHT, testosterone-proprionate or testosterone to the homogenates of broken cell preparations failed to cause any increase in the levels of adenylcyclase activity. Since the hormones are usually bound to the cytosol receptor and afterwards to the nucleus, the absence of an intact system prevented the physiological manifestation (Singhal & Sutherland 1975) thus rendering the model inappropriate.

Less than 2% of the total testosterone in human plasma is free or unbound, and the remaining 98% is bound to several different types of plasma proteins. The plasma proteins that bind steroids include human serum albumin and testosterone-estrogen-binding globulin, also denoted as SHBG. The majority of testosterone bound to plasma protein is associated with SHBG (Vermeulen 1973).

SHBG is a plasma glycoprotein that binds certain steroids. It, in turn, binds to a specific receptor on cell membranes.

The regulation of the amount of androgen that is free is an important physiological variable. This nonprotein-bound 'free testosterone' is available to diffuse into the sex accessory tissue and into liver cells for metabolism. The total plasma level of SHBG can be altered by hormone therapy.

Receptors in target organs can serve as markers for the degree of response to androgen stimulation, since they play a vital role in mediating the action of androgens and therefore can be used for determining the type of hormonal treatment of carcinomatous tissue. There is a paucity of clinical data comparing the androgen-receptor concentration in prostatic carcinoma with the response of this tissue to endocrine therapy (antiandrogens).

DHT is the most potent androgen affecting accessory gland function. It is the most potent mitogenic agent for the prostate in organ culture. However, DHT concentration in the tissue has no correlation with the mitotic rate.

Androgen stimulation affects proliferation and secretion, controlling cell proliferation by action at the gene level. The growth of the organ is due to cell proliferation, cellular hypertrophy, and the size and function of the cells. Most of the studies in this field have been carried out on castrated animals, which, after stabilization, were injected with different doses of androgens and other hormones or drugs. In the rat, the ventral prostate shrinks to its minimum size, as do the amounts of its secretions, after 10 days. The same has been found for the seminal vesicles. In most of the accessory glands, there is weight decrease concomitant with the cessation of cell renewal. This can be explained on the basis that some androgen activity, originating from the adrenal glands, is still present. It is well known that after castration the prostate undergoes atrophy. In addition, it has been shown (in the rat) that large clusters of lysosomes appear which degrade cellular material, indicating autophagia. The

administration of androgens to castrated animals promotes a dramatic increase in weight and intracellular and extracellular secretions after a delay or latent period of 2 or 3 days. The renewal process can be followed by [3]H-labelled thymidine and autoradiography which proves that DNA replication and cell proliferation are occurring. Maximal effects were found with DHT. Thus, the initial pulse in mitotic activity after androgenic stimulation is dependent on the dose and potency of androgen administered, whereas the latter stages of stimulation are independent.

Several hormones are synergistic or antagonistic to androgens in target sex organs. Some hormones may even stimulate proliferation.

*Prolactin*

Specific prolactin binding sites have been found in the rat prostate and afterwards also in other species, including man (Aragona & Friesen 1975). Castration also decreases the number of prolactin receptors in prostate membranes by 90% in the rat 4 days after orchidectomy. The effect can be reversed by testosterone administration. Estrogen may decrease a number of prolactin receptors (Barkay et al 1977b).

Golder et al (1972) first showed that relatively low doses of prolactin enhanced adenylcyclase activity in rat prostatic tissue. Larger doses had no effect or even decreased cAMP levels in the tissue. Thus, the stimulatory effect of prolactin is only in the physiological dose ranges. In the rat, it has been shown that prolactin may act independently to stimulate growth of the accessory sex organs. Prolactin can increase prostate and seminal vesicle growth both in castrated and in adrenalectomized rats. The citric acid content of the prostate of a castrated, hypophysectomized rat treated with prolactin was increased significantly. Hyperprolactin levels caused a decrease in the DHT levels in the lateral prostate in addition to increasing growth. Thus it has been suggested that prolactin may enhance rat lateral prostate growth by an androgen-independent pathway (Lee et al 1985).

Prolactin administration, combined with small doses of testosterone, stimulates the growth of the ventral and dorsal prostate as well as the seminal vesicles (Farnsworth et al 1979). The activity of prolactin on the accessory glands is also promoted by glucocorticoids, since adrenocorticotropic hormone (ACTH) in combination with prolactin increases accessory sex organ weights.

Three mechanisms of action of prolactin have been proposed: (a) direct effect of prolactin at the organ level; (b) synergizing with circulating androgens; and (c) increasing the output of androgens from the testis and adrenal glands (Negro-Vilar 1980).

When measuring prolactin levels of elderly patients or those suffering from benign prostatic hyperplasia, no clear correlation of the cause of prostate pathology and the prolactin effect is apparent (Birkoff et al 1974).

## Gonadotropins

The amount of testosterone produced by Leydig cells in the testes is controlled in part by the plasma levels of the LH released from the anterior pituitary gland. In turn, testosterone is involved in a negative feedback regulation of the pituitary by acting on the pituitary gland as well as the basal medial hypothalamus region. Testosterone treatment of both intact and castrated adult males results in a marked suppression of pituitary LH synthesis and release. An increase in the dose of testosterone will also cause the depression of FSH levels. At least part of the negative feedback by steroids on the function of the pituitary is mediated by inhibiting the secretion of the LHRH which is in the hypothalamus and is carried to the anterior pituitary via the hypophyseal portal blood supply. Gonadotropin-releasing hormone analogs or antagonists are in use for chemical castration in cases of prostatic cancer (Conn & Crowley 1991).

## Opiates

Recently, the proopiomelanocortin (POMC)-derived peptides have been identified in testicular interstitial fluid (TIF) which surrounds rat Leydig cells at concentrations several-fold higher than those of the peripheral blood. When hypophysec-tomized rats were treated with human chorionic gonadotropin (hCG), both testosterone and β-endorphin levels increased in the TIF (Valenca & Negro-Vilar 1986). These observations, together with the presence of POMC in Leydig cells, suggest synthesis and secretion of opioids in the testes. It was suggested that β-endorphin inhibits Sertoli cell division and androgen-binding protein secretion (Morris et al 1987). Endogenous opiates may also participate in the suppressive effect of testosterone on LH secretion (Veldhuis et al 1984).

## Insulin

Insulin directly promotes growth and activity of the accessory sex glands (Johansson 1976). Extensive studies have been carried out on the experimental streptozotocin diabetic rats. It has been shown that insulin insufficiency is followed by testicular atrophy, decreased testosterone production, atrophy of accessory sex glands, and sterility (Paz et al 1978a). Treatment with insulin or hCG alone was not sufficient for recovery. None the less, treatment by combining both drugs reversed the above symptoms (Paz et al 1978b). Clinical findings regarding changes in accessory sex glands of diabetic patients can be explained on the basis of these results (Schoffling 1965).

## Antiandrogens

These are substances that block the effects of androgen at the target tissue level, acting mainly by competition with androgens. Thus, antiandrogens in appropriate concentrations can cause chemical castration. Compounds that will lower androgen uptake, block androgen binding, or inhibit the formation of DHT will thus have antiandrogenic properties. Three groups of antiandrogens are known: pure antiandrogens, antiandrogens with progestational effects, and progestins.

Cyproterone acetate is a strong antiandrogen at the target tissue level, reducing the binding of DHT to intratesticular receptors (Coffey 1974), Mainwaring 1977). It had been shown to inhibit androgen-induced cell proliferation in target tissues and is thus used in anticarcinogenic treatments.

Gestagens in high concentrations (are potent inhibitors of gonadotropin secretion, with suppression of LH leading to decreased testosterone production. They can also reduce testosterone biosynthesis in the testes. Progestins (P) are the most potent inhibitors of 5-α-reductase, which may indirectly cause the antiandrogenic effects (Orestano et al 1974).

Some other antiandrogens are flutamide or spironolactone which generally demonstrate high receptor affinity such as cyproterone acetate and P. Spironolactone interacts with aldosterone and other receptors while flutamide, a nonsteroidal androgen antagonist, has an effect on its own (Neri 1977).

*Melatonin*

Melatonin has been shown to inhibit the testosterone induced growth of the prostate in castrated rats (Debeljuk et al 1970).

*Corticoids*

Corticoids affect the secretion of the male accessory sex glands and have protective, proliferative and secretory actions on the glands (Tisell 1971).

Hyperstimulation of the adrenal cortex causes the production of adrenal steroids that stimulate the growth of the prostate gland. Such stimulation of prostatic growth has been observed in both castrated, and castrated-hypophysectomized, animals, but does not occur in animals that are adrenalectomized (Tisell 1970). Nevertheless, the effect of normal levels of adrenal androgens on the prostate in noncastrated humans and adult male rats may not be significant because adrenalectomy has very little effect on prostate size, DNA, or morphology of the sex accessory tissue (Oesterling et al 1986). In castrated rats, the DHT level in the prostatic tissue is approximately 20% of that in normal intact animals. Adrenalectomy lowers the DHT to nondetectable levels without further diminution in prostate growth. This indicates that a threshold level of DHT is required in the prostate to stimulate growth and that the castrate level is below this threshold (Kyprianou & Isaacs 1987).

*Estrogens*

Only small amounts of estrogen are produced directly by the testes. This is mostly derived from the peripheral conversion of androstenedione and testosterone to estrone and estradiol via the aromatase reaction (Siiteri & MacDonald 1973).

Estrogens directly or indirectly inhibit the development and growth of the prostate gland when given in high doses, but in low doses they potentiate the proliferative effects of testosterone (Tisell 1971). This is because estrogen stimulates SHBG levels, and also competes with testosterone for binding to SHBG. However, estrogen has only one-third the binding affinity of testosterone. Therefore administration of small amounts of estrogen increases the total concentration of SHBG and this effectively increases the binding of testosterone and thus lowers the free testosterone plasma concentration.

Some estrogens like diethyl stilbestrol directly inhibit androgen-dependent DNA polymerase in human hyperplastic and neoplastic prostates, whereas the natural estrogen, estradiol, is ineffective.

The human prostate has been shown to produce and metabolize PG, and is affected by PGF, while the seminal vesicles predominantly produce $PGE_1$ and $PGE_2$. Prolactin and androgens increase $PGF_{2\alpha}$, synthesis in the prostate.

The above data demonstrate the multifactorial control of male accessory sex gland activity. Androgens (testosterone and DHT) are the dominant factors promoting this activity, sometimes in combination with prolactin, insulin and corticoids. Antiandrogens (cyproterone, progestins, estrogens in high doses) and melatonin are inhibitory. The net effect depends on the doses and duration of action.

## CLOSING REMARKS

The analysis of the fluids obtained from the male accessory sex glands, together with the properly performed evaluation of the anatomical and functional characteristics of these glands, help the clinician to diagnose and treat many andrological dysfunctions. The understanding of the regulation of organ activity, particularly of the cellular and subcellular events involved, leads to the formulation of appropriate methodology for pinpointing the defects that cause certain diseases and the malformation of organs. As a result, solutions may emerge, giving rise to great prospects for therapy.

Once these mechanisms are fully described, the possibility of developing a male contraceptive device involving the accessory sex organs is likely to become a reality. It has been proposed than an, 'ideal contraceptive drug is one that will not inhibit masculine behaviour and male libido, but will reversibly inhibit spermatozoal quality' (Homonnai & Paz 1980).

The epididymis is one of the target organs currently under investigation with respect to inhibition of its activity, leading to decreased sperm quality. The use of epididymal markers for following its activity was recommended. Other target organs for male contraception are the prostate gland and seminal vesicles which, by inhibition of secretion or production of hostile fluid, may prevent healthy sperm from reaching the female tract. The vas deferens and ampulla are also potential organs for contraceptive intervention. The inhibition of sperm transport and/or increase of phagocytosis would be effective by decreasing sperm quality in the ejaculate.

The ideas described here, and others that are mentioned in the literature, are worth investigating as part of the general effort to solve infertility and contraception problems through basic and applied science research.

## ACKNOWLEDGEMENTS

The authors wish to thank Mr S. Schafer and Mrs Renée Berman for their artistic work, and Mrs Shaina Henigman for editorial assistance.

## REFERENCES

Ahmed K, Wilson M J, Goueli S A, Williams-Ashman H B 1978 Effects of polymines on prostatic chromatin and nonhistone-protein associated protein kinase reactions. *Biochem* J 176: 739

Ali J I, Eldridge F E, Koo G C, Schanbacher B D 1990 Enrichment of bovine X- and Y-chromosome-bearing sperm with monoclonal H-Y antibody-fluorescence-activated cell sorter. Arch Androl 24: 235

Amann R P 1987 Function of the epididymis in bulls and rams. J Reprod Fertil Suppl 34: 115

Amann R P, Johnson L, Thompson D L, Pickett B W 1976 Daily spermatozoal production, epididymal spermatozoa reserves and transit time of spermatozoa through the epididymis of the rhesus monkey. Biol Reprod 15: 586

Aragona C, Friesen H G 1975 Specific prolactin binding sites in the prostate and testis of rats. Endocrinology 97: 677

Arey L B 1965 Developmental anatomy, 7th edn. W B Saunders, Philadelphia, p 313

Arver S, Eliasson R 1982 Zinc and zinc ligands in human seminal plasma: II. Contribution by ligands of different origin to the zinc binding properties of human seminal plasma. Acta Physiol Scand 115: 217

Asher I, Kraicer P F, Paz (Frenkel) G, Fainman N, Homonnai Z T 1978 The use of ethanol and sulfamethoxazol in functional evaluation of male accessory glands. Arch Androl 2: 31

Attramadal A, Tveter K J, Weddington S C et al 1975 Androgen binding and metabolism in human prostate. Vitam Horm 33: 247

Aumuller G 1983 Morphology and endocrine aspects of prostatic function. Prostate 4: 195

Aumuller G, Volki A, Seitz J 1978 Fine structure and function of the rat seminal vesicle after treatment with ergot alkaloids. Arch Androl 2 (Suppl): 56

Aumuller G, Seitz J, Lilja H, Abrahamsson P A, Von der Kammer H, Scheit K H 1990 Species and organ specificity of secretory proteins derived from human prostate and seminal vesicles. Prostate 17: 31

Baker H W G, Worgul T J, Santen R J, Jefferson L S, Bardin C W 1977 Effect of prolactin on nuclear androgens in perfused male sex accessory organs. In: Troen P, Nankin H R (eds) The testis in normal and infertile men. Raven, New York, p 379

Barkan T, Paz G, Homonnai Z T, Chayen R, Kraicer P F 1978 Spermine and citric acid in human prostatic fluid. Int J Androl 1: 393

Barkay J, Zuckerman J, Gordon S 1977a Improved quick-freezing method for human sperm with caffeine stimulation. Fertil Steril 28: 312 (Abstr)

Barkay R J, Shani J, Amit J T, Barzilai D 1977b Specific binding of prolactin to seminal vesicle, prostate and testicular homogenates of immature, mature and aged rats. J Endocrinol 74: 163

Batra S K 1974 Sperm transport through vas deferens. Review of hypothesis and suggestions for quantitative model. Fertil Steril 25: 186

Batson O V 1942 The role of the vertebral veins in metastatic processes. Ann Intern Med 16: 38

Baumgarten H G, Holstein A F, Rosengren E 1971 Arrangement, ultra-structure, and adrenergic innervation of smooth musculature of the ductuli efferentes, ductus epididymidis and ductus deferens of man. Z Zellforsch Mikrosk Anat 120: 37

Bedford J M 1978 Influence of abdominal temperature on epididymal function in the rat and rabbit. Am J Anat 152: 509

Bedford J M , Millar R P 1978 The character of sperm maturation in the epididymis of the acrotal hyrax, *Procavia capensis* and armadillo, *Dasypus novemcinctus*. Biol Reprod 19: 396

Bedford J M, Calvin H, Cooper G W 1973 The maturation of spermatozoa in the human epididymis. J Reprod Fertil Suppl 18: 199

Berger R E, Alexander E R, Harnisch J P et al 1979 Etiology, manifestations and therapy of acute epididymitis. Prospective study of 50 cases. J Urol 121: 750

Berger R E, Karp L E, Williamson R A, Koehler J, Moore D E, Holmes K K 1982 The relationship of pyospermia and seminal fluid bacteriology to sperm function as reflected in the sperm penetration assay. Fertil Steril 37: 557

Bergstrom S, Carlson L A, Weeks L R 1968 The prostaglandins: a family of biologically active lipids. Pharmacol Rev 20: 1

Birkoff J D, Lattimer J K, Frantz A G 1974 Role of prolactin in benign prostatic hypertrophy. Urology 4: 557

Blacklock N J 1976 Surgical anatomy of the prostate. In: Williams D I, Chisholm G D (eds) Scientific foundations of urology. William Heinemann Medical, Chicago, p 113

Blaquier J 1974 Androgen receptors from the epididymis of the rhesus monkey. End Ocrinol Res Commun 1: 155

Blaquier J A, Cameo M S, Cuasnicu P S et al 1988 On the role of epididymal factors in sperm fertility. Reprod Nutr Dev 28: 1209

Bogolyubov V M, Karpukhin I V, Bobkova A S, Razuvayev A V, Kozhinova E V 1986 Dynamics of spermatogenesis, hormonal and immune response of patients suffering from chronic prostatitis and sterility under bitemporal treatment with an ultra-high frequency electric field. Int Urol Nephrol 18: 89

Boreau J 1977 Diagnosis and treatment of primary malignant tumors of the seminal vesicles. In: Grindmann E, Vahlensieck W (eds) Tumors of the male genital system. Recent results in cancer research, vol 60. Springer Verlag, New York, p 157

Brandes D (ed) 1974 Male accessory sex organs: structure and function in mammals. Academic, New York

Brandt H, Acott T S, Johnson D J, Hoskins D D 1978 Evidence for an epididymal origin of bovine forward motility protein. Biol Reprod 19: 830

Brewster S F 1985 The development and differentiation of human seminal vesicles. J Anat 143: 45

Brindley G S, Scott G I, Hendry W F 1986 Vas cannulation with implanted sperm reservoirs for obstructive azoospermia or ejaculatory failure. Br J Urol 58: 721

Bronson R, Cooper G, Rosenfield D 1984 Sperm antibodies: their role in infertility. Fertil Steril 42: 171

Brown C R, von Glos K I, Jones R 1983 Changes in plasma membrane glycoproteins of rat spermatozoa during maturation in the epididymis. J Cell Biol 96: 256

Bruchovsky M, Wilson J D 1968 The conversion of testosterone and 5-α-androstane-17β-ol-3-one by rat prostate in vivo and in vitro. J Biol Chem 243: 2012

Brueschke E E, Burus M, Mannes J H, Wingfeld J R, Mayerhofer K, Zaneveld J L D 1974 Development of a reversible vas deferens occlusive device. I. Anatomical size of the human and dog vas deferens. Fertil Steril 25: 659

Bruschini H, Schmidt R A, Taragho E A 1978 Neurologic control of prostatic secretion in the dog. Invest Urol 15: 288

Burgoyne P S 1987 The role of the mammalian Y chromosome in spermatogenesis. Development 101 (suppl): 133

Busolo F, Zanchetta R, Bertoloni G 1984 Mycoplasma localization patterns on spermatozoa from infertile men. Fertil Steril 42: 412

Caldamone A A, Freytag M K, Cockett A T 1979 Seminal zinc and male infertility. Urology 13: 280

Calderon I, Abramovici H, Barak M et al 1991 The use of seminal vesicle specific protein (SVSP) for the diagnosis of agenesis of the vas deferens and seminal vesicles in azoospermic men. (in press)

Camussi G, Tetta C, Bussolino F et al 1990 An anti-inflammatory protein secreted from the rat seminal vesicle epithelium inhibits the synthesis of platelet-activating factor and the release of arachidonic acid and prostacyclin. Eur J Biochem 192: 481

Casillas E R 1972 The distribution of carnitine in male reproductive tissues and its effect on palmitate oxidation by spermatozoal particles. Biochim Biophys Acta 280: 545

Casillas E R, Elder C M, Hoskins D D 1980 Adenylate cyclase activity of bovine spermatozoa during maturation in the epididymis and the activation of sperm particulate adenylate cyclase by GTP and polyamines. J Reprod Fertil 59: 297

Chaisiri P, Harper M E, Griffiths K 1979 Plasma spermine concentration of patients with benign and malignant tumors of breast or prostate. Clin Chim Acta 92: 273

Chu T M, Murphy G P 1986 What's new in tumor markers for prostate cancer? Urology 27: 487

Chwalle R 1927 Ueber die Entwicklung der Harnblase und der primaren Harnrohre den Menschen mit besonderer Berucksichtigung der Art und Weise, in der sich die Ureteren von der urniereingangen trennen, nebst Bemerkungen uber die Entwicklung der Mullerschen Gange und des Mast. Z Anat Entwickl Gesch 83: 615

Coffey D S 1974 Effects of androgens on DNA and RNA synthesis in sex accessory tissue. In: Brandes D (ed) Male accessory organs. Structure and function in mammals. Academic, New York, p 307

Colpi G M, Roveda M L, Tognetti A, Balerna M 1988 Seminal tract inflammation and male infertility. Correlations between leukospermia and clinical history, prostatic cytology, conventional semen parameters, sperm viability and seminal plasma protein composition. Acta Eur Fertil 19: 69

Comhaire F H, Vermeulen L, Pieters O 1989 Study of the accuracy of physical and biochemical markers in semen to detect infectious dysfunction of the accessory sex glands. J Androl 10: 50

Conn P M, Crowley W F 1991 Gonadotropin-releasing hormone and its analogues. N Engl J Med 34: 93

Conti G 1952 L'erection du penis human et ses bases morphologique-vasculaires. Acta Anat 14: 217

Cooper T G 1986 The epididymis, sperm maturation and fertilisation. Springer Verlag, Heidelberg

Cooper T G 1990 In defense of a function for the human epididymis. Fertil Steril 54: 965

Crabo B 1965 Studies on the composition of epididymal content in bulls and boars. Acta Vet Scand 6 (suppl 5):1

Crabo B, Gustafsson B 1964 Distribution of sodium and potassium and its relation to sperm concentration in the epididymal plasma of the bull. J Reprod Fertil 7: 337

Crabo B, Hunter A 1975 Sperm maturation and epididymal function, In: Sciarra J, Markland C, Spiedel J (eds) Control of male fertility. Harper and Row, New York, p 2

Cunha G R, Chung L W H, Shannon J M, Reese B A 1980 Stromal epithelial interactions in sex differentiation. Biol Reprod 22: 19

Cunha G R, Shannon J M, Neubauer B L et al 1981 Mesenchymal – epithelial interactions in cell differentiation. Hum Genet 58: 68

Curry P T, Atherton R W 1990 Seminal vesicles: development, secretory products, and fertility. Arch Androl 25: 107

Dacheux J L, Chevrier C, Lanson Y 1987 Motility and surface transformations of human spermatozoa during epididymal transit. Proc Natl Acad Sci USA 513: 560

Debeljuk L, Feder V M, Panlucci D A 1970 Effects of melatonin on changes induced by castration and testosterone in sexual structure of male rats. Endocrinology 87: 1358

deGroat W C, Booth A M 1980 In: Bradley W E (ed) Aspects of diabetic autonomic neuropathy. Ann Intern Med 92: 330

Delgado N M, Carranco A, Merchant H, Reyes R 1985 Effect of bivalent cations in acrosome reaction induced by glycosaminoglycans in porcine spermatozoa. Arch Androl 14: 193

de Vere White R 1988 Prostate cancer – diagnostic dilemmas. In: Paulson D (ed) Prostatic disorders. Lea and Febiger, Philadelphia, p 261

de Voogt H J, Adensuer H, Widdra W C 1991 The use of the LHRH analogue Buserlin in the treatment of prostate cancer. A 10 years review on 1522 patients treated in 119 centers on 4 continents. Scand J. Urol Nephrol Suppl 138: 131

Dinakar R A, Dinakar N, Prasad M R N 1977 Response of the epididymis, ductus deferens and accessory glands of the castrated prepubertal rhesus monkey to exogenous administration of testosterone or 5α-dihydrotestostesterone. Indian J Exp Biol 15: 829

Djoseland O, Tveter K H, Attramadal A, Hansson V, Haugen H N, Mathiesen W 1977 Metabolism of testosterone in the human prostate and the seminal vesicles. Scand J Urol Nephrol 11: 1

Dupuy G M, Boulanger K D, Roberts K D, Blesau G, Chaspdelaine A 1979 Metabolism of sex steroids in the human and canine vas deferens. Endocrinology 104: 1553

Dysson A L M B, Orgebin-Crist M C 1973 Effect of hypophysectomy, castration and androgen replacement upon fertilizing ability of rat epididymal spermatozoa. Endocrinology 93: 391

Edelman P M 1963 Effects of castration on mitochondria of rat ventral prostate. Endocrinology 72: 853

Elbadawai A, Goodman D C 1980 Autonomic innervation of accessory male genital glands. In: Spring-Mills E, Hafez E S E (eds) Male accessory sex glands. Elsevier North Holland Biomedical Press, Amsterdam, p 101

Eliasson R 1963 Prostaglandin properties, actions and significance. Biochem Pharmacol 12: 405

Eliasson R, Lindholmer C 1976 Functions of male accessory genital organs. In Hafez E S E (ed) Human semen and fertility regulation in men. C V Mosby, St Louis, p 44

Eliasson R, Molin L, Rajka G 1970 Involvement of prostate and seminal vesicle in urethritis with special reference to semen analysis. Andrologia 2: 179

Evans R J, Herr J C 1986 Immunohistochemical localization of the MHS-5 antigen in principal cells of human seminal vesicle epithelium. Anat Rec 214: 372

Faerman I, Glocer L, Fox D, Jadrinsky M N, Rapaport M 1974 Impotence and diabetes, histological studies of the autonomic nervous fibers of the corpora cavernosa in impotent diabetic males. Diabetes 23: 971

Fahim M S, Ibrahim H H, Girgis S M, Essa H A, Hanafi S 1985 Value of intraprostatic injection of zinc and vitamin C and of ultrasound application in infertile men with chronic prostatitis. Arch Androl 14: 81

Fahimi F, Bieber L, Lewin L M 1981 The sources of carnitine in human semen. J Androl 2: 339

Faiman C, Winter J S D, Reyes F I 1981 Endocrinology of the fetal testis. In: Burger H, de Kretser D (eds) The testis. Raven, New York, p 81

Fair W R, Clark R B, Webner N 1972 A correlation of seminal polyamine levels and semen analysis in the human. Fertil Steril 23: 38

Farnsworth W E, Slaunwhite W R Jr, Sharma M et al 1979 Interaction of prolactin and testosterone in the human prostate. Urol Res 2: 49

Fawcett D W, Phillips D M 1969 Observations on the release of spermatozoa and on changes in the head during passage through the epididymis. J Reprod Fertil 6 (suppl): 405

Fitzpatrick T J, Cooper J F 1975 A cavernosogram study on the valvular competence of the human deep dorsal vein. J Urol 113: 497

Fleischer B, Fleischer S, Ozawa H 1969 Isolation and characterization of Golgi membranes from bovine liver. J Cell Biol 43: 59

Flickinger C J 1974a Synthesis, intracellular transport and release of secretory protein in the seminal vesicle of the rat as studied by electron microscpe radioautography. Anat Rec 180: 407

Flickinger C J 1974b Protein secretion in the rat ventral prostate and the relation of Golgi vesicles, cisternae and vacuoles as studied by electron microscope radioautography. Anat Rec 180: 427

Flickinger C J 1979 Synthesis, transport and secretion of protein in the initial segment of the mouse epididymis as studied by electron microscope radioautography. Biol Reprod 20: 1015

Flower J E 1981 Infections of the male reproductive tract and infertility. A selected review. J Androl 2: 121

Ford W C L, Waites G M H 1978 Chlorinated sugars: a biochemical approach to the control of male infertility. Int J Androl 2 (suppl): 541

Frenkel G, Peterson R N, Freund M 1973a Changes in the metabolism of guinea pig sperm from different segments of the epididymis. Proc Soc Exp Biol Med 143: 1231

Frenkel G, Peterson R N, Freund M 1973b The role of nucleotides and the effect of caffeine and dibutyryl cyclic AMP on the metabolism of guinea pig epididymal spermatozoa. Proc Soc Exp Biol Med 144: 420

Frenkel G, Peterson R N, Davis J E, Freund M 1974 Glycerylphosphorylcholine and carnitine in normal human semen and in postvasectomy semen: differences in concentrations. Fertil Steril 25: 84

Freund M, Davis J 1969 Disappearance of spermatozoa from the ejaculate following vasectomy. Fertil Steril 20: 163

Friend D S 1969 Cytochemical staining of multivesicular body and Golgi vesicles. J Cell Biol 41: 269

Garnick M B 1988 Management of metastatic carcinoma of the prostate—treatment options and controversies. In: Paulson D (ed) Prostatic disorders. Lea and Febiger, Philadelphia, p 369

Girgis S M, Ceinasury M K, El-Kodary M et al 1981 Diagnostic value of determination of acid and alkaline phosphatase levels of the seminal plasma of infertile males. Andrologia 16: 330

Glenister T W 1962 The development of the utricle and of

the so-called middle or median lobe of the human prostate.
J Anat 96: 443

Gloyna R E, Wilson J D 1969 A comparative study of the
conversion of testosterone to 17β hydroxy 5α
androstandione (dihydrotestosterone) by prostate and
epididymis. J Clin Endocrinol Metab 29: 970

Goldberg E H 1988 H-Y antigen and sex determination.
Philos Trans R Soc Lond Biol 322: 73

Golder M P, Boyns A R, Harper M E, Griffiths K 1972 An
effect of prolactin on prostatic adenylate cyclase activity.
Biochem J 128: 725

Gould S, Chayen R, Harell A, Toaf M E, Toaf R 1975 Gas
chromatography of urinary 17KS in female infertility
due to endocrine hyperactivity. Isr J Med Sci 11: 1219
(abstr)

Graham W H 1961 Congenital abnormalities of the kidney.
In Winsbury-White H P E, Livingstone S (eds) Textbook of
genitourinary surgery, 2nd edn. Edinburgh

Grossowics N, Rozin S, Rozansky R 1955 Factors influencing
the antibacterial action of spermine and spermidine on
*Staphylococcus aureus*. J Gen Microbiol 13: 436

Gyorkey F 1964 The appearance of acid phosphatase in
human prostate gland. Lab Invest 13: 105

Hamilton D W 1977 The epididymis. In: Greep R O,
Koblinsky M A (eds) Frontiers in reproduction and fertility
control. MIT Press, Cambridge, p 411

Hamilton D 1980 UDP-galactose, *N*-acetylglucsamine
galactosyltransferase in fluids from rat rete testis and
epididymis. Biol Reprod 23: 377

Hamilton D 1981 Evidence for alpha lactalbumin-like activity
in reproductive tract fluids of the male rat. Biol Reprod
25: 385

Hansson V, Ritzen E M, French F S, Nayfeh S 1975
Androgen transport receptor mechanisms in testis and
epididymis. In: Hamilton D W, Greep R O (eds)
Handbook of physiology, section 7—endocrinology, vol 5.
Williams and Wilkins, Baltimore, p 173

Hinrichsen M J, Blaquier J A 1980 Evidence supporting the
existence of sperm maturation in the human epididymis.
J Reprod Fertil 60: 291

Hinton B T, Brooks E D, Dott H M, Setchell B P 1981
Effects of carnitine and some related compounds on the
motility of rat spermatozoa from the caput epididymis.
J Reprod Fertil 61: 59

Holstein A F 1969 Morphologisch Studien zu Nebenhoden
des Menschen. In: Baemann W, Doerr W (eds) Zwanglose
Abhandlungen aus dem Gebiet der Normalen und
Pathologischen Anatomie, vol 20. Georg Thieme, Stuttgart,
p 91

Holstein A F 1976 Structure of the human epididymis. In:
Hafez E S E (ed) Human semen and fertility regulation in
men. C V Mosby, St Louis, p 23

Homonnai Z T, Paz G F 1980 Methods for evaluating
contraceptive techniques. In: Cunningham G R,
Schill W B, Hafez E S E (eds) Regulation of male fertility.
Martinus Nijhoff, The Hague, p 41

Homonnai Z T, Paz G, Soffer A, Kraicer P F, Harell A 1976
Effect of caffeine on the motility, viability, oxygen
consumption and glycolytic rate of ejaculate human
normokinetic and hypokinetic spermatozoa. Int J Fertil
21: 163

Homonnai Z T, Matzkin H, Fainman N, Paz G, Kraicer P F
1978a The cation composition of the seminal plasma and
prostatic fluid and its correlation to sperm quality. Fertil
Steril 29: 539

Homonnai Z T, Paz G, Kraicer P F 1978b A retrospective
diagnostic study on fifty cases of vas deferens agenesis.
Andrologia 10: 410

Homonnai Z T, Shilon M, Paz G F 1984 Phenoxybenzamine
—an effective male contraceptive pill. Contraception
29: 479

Hoskins D D, Musterman D, Hall M L 1975 The control of
bovine sperm glycolysis during epididymal transit. Biol
Reprod 12: 566

Huang H F S, Johnson A D 1975 Amino acid composition of
the epididymal plasma of mouse, rat, rabbit and sheep.
Comp Biochem Physiol 50B: 359

Huret J L 1986 Nuclear chromatin decondensation of human
sperm: a review. Arch Androl 16: 97

Jequier A M, Cummins J M, Gearon C, Apted S L,
Yovich J M, Yovich J L 1990 A pregnancy achieved using
sperm from the epididymal caput in idiopathic obstructive
azoospermia. Fertil Steril 53: 1104

Jimenez Cruz J F 1980 Artificial spermatocoele. J Urol 123:
885

Johansson R 1976 RNA, protein and DNA synthesis
stimulated by testosterone, insulin and prolactin in the rat
ventral prostate cultured in chemically defined medium.
Acta Endocrinol (Copenh) 80: 761

Jones R 1974 Absorption and secretion in the cauda
epididymis of the rabbit and the effects of degenerating
spermatozoa of epididymal plasma after castration.
J Endocrinol 63: 157

Josso N, Picard J Y 1986 Anti-Müllerian hormone. Physiol
Rev 66: 1038

Josso N, Legeai L, Forest M G, Chaussain J L, Brauner R
1990 An enzyme linked immunoassay for anti-Müllerian
hormone: a new tool for the evaluation of testicular
function in infants and children. J Clin Endocrinol Metab
70: 23

Kanka J, Kopecny V 1977 An autoradiographic study of
macromolecular synthesis in the epithelium of the ductus
epididymis in the mouse I; DNA, RNA and protein. Biol
Reprod 16: 421

Kastandieck H, Altenahr E 1979 Role of basal cells in
nonmalignant lesions of the prostate. Arch Androl 2
(suppl 1):64

Keenan B S, Meyers W S, Hadiyan A J, Jones H W, Migeon
C G 1974 Syndrome of androgen resistance in man:
Absence of 5-α-dihydrotestosterone binding protein in skin
fibroblasts. J Clin Endocrin Metab 38: 1143

Kelly R W, Cooper I, Templeton A A 1979 Reduced
prostaglandin levels in the semen of men with very high
sperm concentrations. J Reprod Fertil 56: 195

Kinoshita Y, Hosuku M, Nishimura R, Takai S 1980 Partial
characterization of 5-α-reductase in the human epididymis.
Endocrinol Japan 27: 277

Knight T W 1974 A qualitative study of factors affecting the
contractions of the epididymis and ductus deferens of the
ram. J Reprod Fertil 40: 19

Kohane A C, Carberi J C, Cameo M S, Blaquier J A 1979
Quantitative determination of specific proteins in rat
epididymis. J Steroid Biochem 11: 671

Kohane A C, Echeverria, F M C G, Pineira L, Blaquier J A
1980 Interaction of proteins of epididymal origin with
spermatozoa. Biol Reprod 23: 737

Kreider D L, Cole T C, Stallcup O T 1977 Influence of
prolactin with dihydrotestosterone on young rabbit and
bovine male reproductive organs. IRCS Libr Compend
45: 467

Kvist U, Bjorndahl L, Roomans G M, Lindholmer C 1985 Nuclear zinc in human epididymal and ejaculated spermatozoa. Acta Physiol Scand 125: 297

Kyprianou N, Isaacs T 1987 Biological significance of measurable androgen levels in the rat ventral prostate following castration. Prostate 10: 313

Lanz T von, Neuhauser G 1964 Morphometische Analyse des menschlichen Nebenhodens. Z Anat Entwicklungsgesch 124: 126

Lee C, Hopkins D, Holland J M 1985 Reduction in prostatic concentration of endogenous dihydrotestosterone in rats by hyperprolactinemia. Prostate 6: 361

Lee C, Keefer M, Zhao Z W, Kroes R, Berg L, Liu X X, Sensibar J 1989 Demonstration of the role of prostate-specific antigen in semen liquefaction by two-dimensional electrophoresis. J Androl 10: 432

Le Lannous D, Chambon Y, Le Calve M 1979 Role of the epididymis in reabsorption of inhibin in the rat. J Reprod Fertil 26(suppl): 117

Levine N, Kelly H 1978 Measurement of pH in the rat epididymis in vivo. J Reprod Fertil 52: 333

Liao S, Fang S 1969 Receptor-proteins for androgens in the mode of action of androgens on gene transcription in ventral prostate. Vitam Horm 27: 17

Lilja H, Abrahamsson P A 1988 Three predominant proteins secreted by the human prostate gland. Prostate 12: 29

Lipschultz L I, Tsai Y H, Sanborn B M, Steinberger E 1977 Androgen-binding activity in the human testis and epididymis. Fertil Steril 28: 947

Lubahn D B, Joseph D R, Sar M et al 1988 The human androgen receptor: complementary deoxyribonucleic acid cloning sequence analysis and gene expression in prostate. Molec Endocrinol 2: 1265

Lue T F, Tanagho E A 1987 Physiology of erection and pharmacological management of impotence. J Urol 137: 829

Lyon M F, Howkes S L 1970 X-linked gene for testicular feminization in the mouse. Nature (Lond) 227: 1217

MacCallum J B 1902 Notes on the Wolffian body of higher animals. Am J Anat 1: 245

McDonald I, Rose N R, Pontes E J, Choe B K 1978 Human prostatic acid phosphatase: III Counter immunoelectrophoresis for rapid identification. Arch Androl 1: 235

McGee R S, Herr J C 1988 Human seminal vesicle-specific antigen is a substrate for prostate-specific antigen (or P-30). Biol Reprod 39: 499

McLaren A 1987 Testis determination and the H-Y hypothesis. Curr Top Dev Biol 23: 163

McLeod D G, Reynolds D G, DeMaree G D 1973 Some pharmacologic characteristics of the human vas deferens. Invest Urol 10: 338

McNeal J E 1981 The zonal anatomy of the prostate. Prostate 1: 35

McNeal J 1990 Pathology of benign prostatic hyperplasia. Insight into etiology. Urol Clin North Am 17: 477

Maggi M, Baldi E, Genazzani A D et al 1989 Vasopressin receptors in human seminal vesicles: identification, pharmacologic characterization, and comparison with the vasopressin receptors present in the human kidney. J Androl 10: 393

Mainwaring W I P 1977 The mechanism of action of androgens. Monographs on endocrinology. Springer Verlag, Heidelberg

Mandle J P 1972 The effect of prostaglandin $E_1$ on rabbit sperm transport in vivo. J Reprod Fertil 31: 263

Mann T, Lutwak-Mann C L 1981 Male reproductive function and semen. Themes and trends in physiology, biochemistry and investigative andrology. Springer Verlag, Berlin

Marquis N R, Fritz I B 1965 The distribution of carnitine, acetylcarnitine and carnitine acetyltransferase in rat tissues. J Biol Chem 240: 2193

Martin-Delson P A, Shaver E, Gammal E B 1973 Chromosome abnormalities in rabbit blastocytes resulting from spermatozoa aged in the male tract. Fertil Steril 24: 212

Martins T, Valle J R, Porto A 1940 Pharmacology of the human vas deferens and epididymis. The question of the endocrine control of the in vitro motility accessory genitals. J Urol 44: 682

Merk F B, Ofner P, Qwann P W L, Leav I, Vena R L 1982 Ultrastructural and biochemical expression of divergent differentiation in prostates of castrated dogs treated with estrogens and androgens. Lab Invest 47: 437

Metafora S, Porta R, Revagnan G et al 1989 Inhibitory effect of SV-IV, a major protein secreted from the rat seminal vesicle epithelium, on phagocytosis and chemotaxis of human polymorphonuclear leukocytes. J Leukoc Biol 46: 409

Mitsuya H, Asai J, Suyama K, Ushida T, Hoseo K 1960 Application of X-ray cinematography in urology. 1. Mechanism of ejaculation. J Urol 83: 86

Moller R 1980 Arrangement and fine structure of lymph vessels in the human spermatic cord. Androloga 12: 564

Moore H D M, Hartmann T D, Pryor J P 1983 Development of the oocyte-penetrating capacity of spermatozoa in the human epididymis. Int J Androl 6: 310

Morris P L, Vale W W, Bardin C W 1987 β-Endorphin regulation of FSH-stimulated inhibin production is a component of a short loop system in testis. Biochem Biophys Res Commun 148: 1513

Morton B E G, Sagadraca R, Fraser C 1978 Sperm motility within the mammalian epididymis: species variation and correlation with free $Ca^{++}$ levels in epididymal plasma. Fertil Steril 29: 695

Murphy J B, Emmott R C, Hick L L, Walsh P C 1980 Estrogen receptors in the human prostate, seminal vesicle, epididymis, testis, and genital skin: a marker for estrogen-responsive tissues? J Clin Endocrinol Metab 50: 938

Musto N A, Gunsalus G L, Bardin C W 1978 Further characterization of androgen binding protein in epididymis and blood. Int J Androl 2 (suppl): 424

Naslund M J, Coffey D S 1986 The differential effects of neonatal androgen, estrogen and progesterone on adult rat prostate growth. J Urol 136: 1136

Negro-Vilar A 1980 Prolactin and the growth of prostate and seminal vesicles. In: Spring-Mills E, Hafez E S E (eds) Human reproductive medicine. Male accessory sex glands. Elsevier/North Holland Biomedical Press, Amsterdam, p 223

Neri R 1977 Studies on the biology and mechanisms of action of nonsteroidal androgens. In: Martini L, Motta M (eds) Androgens and antiandrogens. Raven, New York p 179

Nicander L 1965 An electron microscopical study of absorbing cells in the posterior caput epididymis of rabbits. Z Zellforsch 66: 829

Nicander L, Malmquist M 1977 Ultrastructural observations

suggesting merocrine secretion in the initial segment of the mammalian epididymis. Cell Tissue Res 184: 487

Oesterling J E, Epstein J I, Walsh P C 1986 The inability of adrenal androgens to stimulate the adult prostate—an autopsy evaluation of men with hypogonadotropic hypogonadism and panhypopituitarism. J Urol 136: 103

Olson G E, Danzo B J 1981 Surface changes in rat spermatozoa during epididymal transit. Biol Reprod 24: 431

Orestano F, Klose K, Rubin A, Knapstein P, Altwein J E 1974 Testosterone metabolism in benign prostatic hypertrophy. Invest Urol 12: 15

Orgebin-Crist M C 1981 Epididymal physiology and sperm maturation. In: Bollack C, Clavert A (eds) Progress in reproductive biology, vol 8. Epididymis and fertility: biology and pathology. Karger, Basel, p 80

Orgebin-Crist M C, Jahad N 1978 The maturation of rabbit epididymal spermatozoa in organ culture: inhibition by antiandrogens and inhibitors of ribonucleic acid and protein synthesis. Endocrinology 103: 46

Orgebin-Crist M C, Djiane J 1979 Properties of a prolactin receptor from the rabbit epididymis. Biol Reprod 21: 135

Ostrowski W 1980 Human prostatic acid phosphatase: physicochemical and catalytic properties. In: Spring-Mills E, Hafez E S E (eds) Human reproductive medicine. Male accessory sex glands. Elsevier/North-Holland Biomedical Press, Amsterdam, p 197

Pabst R 1969 Untersuchungen uber Bau und Funktion des menschlichen. Samenleeiters A Quat Entwicklungsgesch 129: 154

Pabst R 1970 Studies on the human ductus deferens. In: Holstein A F, Horstman E (eds) Advances in andrology. Grosse Verlag, Berlin, p 135

Pallim G 1901 Anatomie und Entwicklung der Prostate and Semenblase. Arch Anat Physiol 135

Paniagua R, Regardera J, Nistal M, Abaurrea M A 1981 Histological, histochemical and ultrastructural variations along the length of the human vas deferens before and after puberty. Acta Anat 111: 190

Parrish R F, Goodpasture J C, Zaneveld L J D, Polakoski K L 1979 Polyamine inhibition of the conversion of human proacrosin to acrosin. J Reprod Fertil 57: 239

Paulson D F 1988 Treatment selection in patients with prostatic carcinoma. In: Paulson D (ed) Prostatic disorders. Lea and Febiger, Philadelphia, p 287

Paz G F, Homonnai Z T 1982 A direct effect of α-chlorohydrin on rat epididymal spermatozoa. Int J Androl 5: 308

Paz G, Sofer A, Homonnai Z T, Kraicer P F 1977 Human semen analysis: seminal plasma and prostatic fluid compositions and their interrelations with sperm quality. Int J Fertil 22: 140

Paz (Frenkel) G, Kaplan R, Yedwab G, Homonnai Z T, Kraicer P F 1978a The effect of caffeine on rat epididymal spermatozoa: motility, metabolism and fertilizing capacity. Int J Androl 1: 145

Paz G, Homonnai Z T, Draznin N, Sofer A, Kaplan R, Kraicer P F 1978b Fertility of the streptozotocin diabetic male rat. Andrologia 10: 127

Paz (Frenkel) G, Ser N, Homonnai Z T, Campus A, Eylan E 1979 Absence of cephalexin in the male ejaculate following oral administration. Int J Androl 2: 308

Paz G F, Drasnin N, Homonnai Z T 1980 Sorbitol in the accessory glands of the diabetic male rat. Acta Diabetol Lat 17: 229

Paz G F, Shilon M, Homonnai Z T 1984 The possible use of phenoxybenzamine as a male contraceptive drug: studies on male rats. Contraception 29: 189

Peleg B A, Ianconescu M 1966 Spermagglutination and spermabsorption due to mycoviruses. Nature (Lond) 211: 1211

Peterson R E, Imperato-McCinley J, Gautier T, Sturla E 1977 Male pseudohermaphroditism due to steroid 5-α-reductase deficiency. Am J Med 62: 170

Pfau A, Perlberg S, Shapira A 1978 The pH of the prostatic fluid in health and disease: implications of treatment in chronic bacterial prostatitis. J Urol 119: 384

Pohjanpelto P, Raina A 1972 Identification of a growth factor produced by human fibroblasts in vitro as putrescine. Nature New Biol 235: 247

Prasad M R N, Rajalakshmi M, Gupta G, Karkun T 1973 Control of epididymal function. J Reprod Fertil Suppl 18: 215

Price O, Williams-Ashman H G 1961 The accessory reproductive glands of the mammals. In: Young W C (ed) Sex and internal secretions, part 7. Williams and Wilkins, Baltimore, p 234

Pryor J, Parsons J, Goswami R et al 1984 In vitro fertilization for men with obstructive azoospermia. Lancet ii: 762

Pryor J P 1987 Surgical retrieval of epididymal spermatozoa. Lancet ii: 1341

Pulkkinen P, Sineroiste R, Janne J 1978 Mechanisms of action of oxidized polyamines on the metabolism of human spermatozoa. J Reprod Fertil 51: 399

Purvis K, Hansson V 1978 Androgens and androgen binding in the rat epididymis. J Reprod Fertil 52: 59

Reddy J M, Stark R A, Zaneveld L J D 1979 A high molecular weight antifertility factor from human seminal plasma. J Reprod Fertil 57: 437

Rennie P S, Bruchovsky N 1980 Measurement of androgen receptors. In: Spring-Mills E, Hafez E S E (eds) Human reproductive medicine. Male accessory sex glands, vol 4. Elsevier/North Holland Biomedical Press, Amsterdam, p 265

Reyes A, Mercado E, Goicokchen B, Rasado A 1976 Participation of membrane sulfhydryl group in the epididymal maturation of human and rabbit spermatozoa. Fertil Steril 27: 1452

Riar S S, Setty B S, Kar A B 1972 Biochemical composition of primate epididymis. Curr Sci 41: 453

Riva A A 1967 Fine structure of human seminal vesicle epithelium. J Anat 102: 71

Russell D H 1978 Polyamines as markers of tumour kinetics. In: Griffiths K, Pierrepont C G, Neville A M (eds) Tumour markers, determination and clinical role. Alpha Omega Alpho, Cardiff, p 68

Schaeffer A J 1981 Prevalence and significance of prostatic inflammation. J Urol 125: 215

Schoffling K 1965 Hypogonadism in male diabetic subjects. In: Lcibcl B S, Wrenshall G A (eds) On the nature and treatment of diabetics, Excerpta Medical, Amsterdam p 505

Senius K E O, Pietile J, Arvola I, Tuohima P 1974 A simple method for the clinical determination of the mitotic activity of human prostate in vitro. J Clin Pathol 27: 880

Serrano J A, Wasserkrug H L, Serrano A A, Pand Paul B D 1977 The histochemical demonstration of human prostatic acid phosphatase with phosphorylcholine. Invest Urol 15: 123

Setchell B P, Voglmayer J K, Waites G M H 1969 A blood –

testes barrier restricting passage from blood into rete testis fluid but not into lymph. J Physiol 200: 73

Shannon J M, Cunha G R, Vanderslice H O 1981 Autoradiographic localization of androgen receptors in the developing mouse urogenital tract and mammary gland. Anat Rec 199: 232

Shapiro E 1990 Embryologic development of the prostate. Insights into the etiology and treatment to benign prostatic hyperplasia. Urol Clin North Am 17: 487

Sheriff D S 1980 The lipid composition of human epididymis. Int J Androl 3: 282

Sheth A R, Gunjukar A N, Shah G V 1981 The presence of progressive motility sustaining factor (PMSF) in human epididymis. Andrologia 13: 142

Shilon M, Paz G F, Homonnai Z T, Schoenbaum M 1978 The effect of caffeine on guinea pig epididymal spermatozoa: motility and fertilizing capacity. Int J Androl 1: 416

Shilon M, Paz G F, Homonnai Z T 1984 The use of phenoxybenzamine treatment in premature ejaculation. Fertil Steril 42: 659

Shima H, Tsuji M, Young P, Cunha G R 1990 Postnatal growth of mouse seminal vesicle is dependent on 5-alpha-dihydrotestosterone. Endocrinology 127: 3222

Shirai M, Ishii N 1981 Hemodynamics of erection in man. Arch Androl 6: 27

Siiteri P K, MacDonald P C 1973 Handbook of physiology, section 7, endocrinology, vol 11. Williams & Wilkins, Baltimore, p 615

Silber S J 1980 Vasoepididymostomy to the head of the epididymis: recovery of normal spermatozoal motility. Fertil Steril 34: 149

Silber S J 1988 Pregnancy caused by sperm from vasa efferentia. Fertil Steril 49: 373

Silber S J, Ord T, Borrerro C, Balmaceda J, Asch R 1987 New treatment of infertility due to congenital absence of vas deferens? Lancet ii: 850

Singhal R L, Sutherland D J B 1975 Cyclic 3'-5' adenosine monophosphate and accessory sex organ responses. In: Thomas J A, Singhal R L (eds) Molecular mechanisms of gonadal hormone action. University Park Press, Baltimore, p 225

Sirigu P, Cusso M, Scarpa R, Pinna A 1981 Histochemistry of some steroid-dehydrogenases in epithelia of human seminal vesicle, deferential ampulla, and prostate gland. Arch Androl 1981 7: 9

Skandhan K P 1981 Zinc in normal human seminal plasma. Andrologia 13: 346

Smith E R 1975 The canine prostate and its secretion. In: Thomas J A, Singhal R L (eds) Molecular mechanisms of gonadal hormone actions. Advances in sex hormones research, Vol 1. University Park Press, Baltimore, p 167

Soffer Y, Pace-Shalev D, Weissenberg R, Orenstein H, Nebel L, Lewin L M 1981 Survey of carnitine content of human semen using a semiquantitative auxanographic method: decreased semen total carnitine concentration in patients with azoospermia or severe oligozoospermia. Andrologia 13: 440

Srivastava K C 1977 Extraction of prostaglandins $F_{1\alpha}$ and $F_{2\alpha}$ from human seminal plasma. Z Anal Chem 285: 35

Srivastava P N, Gould K G 1973 Inhibition of the fertilizing capacity of rabbit spermatozoa by sialoproteins. Contraception 7: 65

Sufrin G, Coffey D S 1973 A new model for studying the effect of drugs on prostatic growth. In Antiandrogens and DNA synthesis. Invest Urol 11: 45

Talo A, Ulla-Marijut J, Merja-Makkula V 1979 Spontaneous electrical activity of the rat epididymis in vitro. J Reprod Fertil 57: 423

Teague N S, Boyarsky S, Glenn J F 1971 Interference of human spermatozoa motility by Escherichia coli. Fertil Steril 22: 281

Templeton A A, Cooper I, Kell R W 1978 Prostaglandin concentrations in the semen of fertile men. J Reprod Fert 52: 147

Tisell L E 1970 Effect of cortisone on the growth of the ventral prostate, the dorsolateral prostate, the coagulating gland and the seminal vesicles in castrated adrenalectomized and in castrated non-adrenalectomized rats. Acta Endocrinol 64: 637

Tisell L E 1971 The growth of the ventral prostate, the dorsolateral prostate, the coagulating glands and the seminal vesicles in castrated adrenalectomized rats, injected with estradiol and/or cortisone. Acta Endocrinol (Copenh) 68: 485

Trachtenberg J, Hicks L L, Walsh P C 1980 Androgen and estrogen receptor content in spontaneous and experimentally induced canine prostatic hyperplasia. J Clin Invest 65: 1051

Tran D, Picard J Y, Campargue J, Josso N 1987 Immunocytochemical detection of anti-Müllerian hormone in Sertoli cells of various mammalian species including human. J Histochem Cytochem 35: 733

Tuchmann-Duplessis H, David G, Haegel P 1972 Organogenesis. In: illustrated embryology, vol 2. Chapman and Hall, London, p 82

Turner T T, Hartman P K, Howards S S 1977 In vitro sodium potassium and sperm concentrations in the rat epididymis. Fertil Steril 28: 191

Tveter K 1981 The effect of antiandrogens on the prostate gland with special reference to the human prostate. Int J Androl 97 (suppl 5): 108

Valenca M M, Negro-Vilar A 1986 Proopiomelanocortin-derived peptides in testicular interstitial fluid: characterization and changes in secretion after human chorionic gonadotropin or luteinizing hormone-releasing hormone analog treatment. Endocrinology 118: 32

Veldhuis J D, Rogol A D, Samojlik E, Ertel N H 1984 Role of endogenous opiates in the expression of negative feedback actions of androgen and estrogen on pulsatile properties of luteinizing hormone secretion in man. J Clin Invest 74: 47

Vendrely E 1981 Histology of the epididymis in the human adult. In: Bollack C, Clavert A (eds) Progress in reproductive biology, vol 8. Epididymis and fertility: biology and pathology. S Karger, Basel, p 21

Ventura W P, Freund M, David J, Pannuti C 1973 Influence of norepinephrine on the motility of the human vas deferens: a new hypothesis of sperm transport by the vas deferens. Fertil Steril 24: 68

Vermeulen A 1973 The physical state of testosterone in plasma. In: Johannes VHT (ed) The endocrine function of the human testis, vol I. Academic, New York, p 157

Vickery B H, McRae G I, Borasch H 1981 Effect of prolonged systemic administration of an LHRH agonist of prostatic size and function in geriatric dogs. ASA Meeting, New Orleans. J Androl 2.31 (abstr)

Vigier B, Picard J Y, Tran D, Legeai L, Josso N 1984 Production of anti-Müllerian hormone: another homology between Sertoli and granulosa cells. Endocrinology 114: 1315

Virag R, Frydman D, Legman M, Virag H 1984 Intracavernous injection of papaverine as a diagnostic and therapeutic method in erectile failure. Andrology 35: 79

Voglmayr J K 1975 Metabolic changes in spermatozoa during epididymal transit. In: Greep R O, Astman E B (eds) Handbook of physiology, section 7. Endocrinology. Williams & Wilkins, Baltimore, p 437

Waldschmidt M, Karg H 1972 Review on metabolic and enzyme studies of spermatozoa from the ampulla ductus deferentis of bulls. Braunschweig Schering Workshop in Contraception: the masculine gender. Advances in the biosciences, vol 10. Pergamon Oxford, p 169

Wallace A M, Grant J K 1975 Effect of zinc on androgen metabolism in the human hyperplastic prostate. Biochemical Society Transactions 56th Meeting, London, p 540

Warwick R, Williams P L (eds) 1989 Gray's anatomy, 37th edn. Longman, Harlow, Essex

Weiss H D 1972 The physiology of human penile erection. Ann Intern Med 76: 793

Wetterauer U, Heite J J 1980 Carnitine in seminal plasma: its significance in diagnostic andrology. Arch Androl 4: 137

Williams-Ashman G H, Reddi A H 1972 Androgenic regulation of tissue growth and function. In: Litwack G (ed) Biochemical actions of hormones, vol 2, Academic, New York, p 257

Williams-Ashman H G, Corti A, Sheth A R 1975 Formation and functions of aliphatic polyamines in the prostate gland and in secretions. In: Goland M (ed) Normal and abnormal growth of the prostate. Thomas, Springfield, p 222

Williams-Ashman H G, Canellakis A N 1979 Polyamines in mammalian biology and medicine. Perspect Biol Med 22: 421

Wilson J D 1972 Recent studies on the mechanism of action of testosterone. N Engl J Med 287: 1284

Wilson J D 1978 Sexual differentiation. Ann Rev Physiol 40: 279

Wilson J D 1980 The pathogenesis of benign prostate hyperplasia. Am J Med 68: 745

Wilson J D, George F W, Griffin J E 1981a The hormonal control of sexual development. Science 211: 1278

Wilson J D, Griffin J E, Leshin M, George F W 1981b Role of gonadal hormones in development of the sexual phenotypes. Hum Genet 58: 78

Wong P Y D, Yeung D H 1977 Hormonal regulation of fluid reabsorption in isolated rat cauda epididymis. Endocrinology 101: 1391

Wong P Y D, Tsang A Y F, Lea W M 1981 Origin of the luminal fluid of the rat epididymis. Int J Androl 4: 331

Zondek L H, Zondek T 1964 The prostatic vesicle in the fetus and infant. Urol Invest Basel, 29, 458

# 8. Pathophysiology of the human testis

*Gedalia F. Paz    Haim Yavetz    Ron Hauser    Leah Yogev*
*Lawrence M. Lewin    Zwi T. Homonnai*

## INTRODUCTION

The functions of the testis are limited to steroido-genesis and spermatogenesis. Both are under endocrine and paracrine control. Endocrine control is mainly carried out by the gonadotropins, which in turn are regulated via the pulsatile gonadotropin releasing hormone (GnRH) secreted from the hypothalamic nuclei into the pituitary portal system (Fig. 8.1). More details appear in other chapters. Paracrine control is the fine regulation by the tissue growth factors. This is a cell-to-cell interaction which modulates the activities of the variety of cells which build up the testicular tissue. Spermatogenesis depends on special arrangements which are unique to the testis. The structure of the seminiferous tubuli, which is characterized by its blood – testis barrier, is controlled by genetic, hormonal, biochemical and environmental factors.

In this chapter, details of the structure, function and control of the events dealing with steroido-genesis and spermatogenesis will be provided. This will be followed by a description of the disorders which may occur leading to infertility or sterility. Most of the data will be focused on the human testis, but since basic research and major data are accumulated from research in animals, some of it will also be given only as a background to a better understanding of the events taking place in the human testis.

## FUNCTIONAL ANATOMY OF THE HUMAN TESTIS

### Gross anatomy

The human testis is ovoid in shape and is located within the scrotum. The length and weight are approximately 4.5 cm and 34–45 g, respectively.

### Scrotum

The scrotum is composed of six distinct layers of tissue, four of which are acquired as a result of the descent of the male gonads from their original position in the retroperitoneal area into the scrotum. The testis is attached to the caudal part of the scrotum by a fibromuscular tissue, probably a remnant of the embryonal gubernaculum. The skin is characterized by a rugate pattern, and abundance of sebaceous follicles and sweat glands. There is no subcutaneous adipose tissue. Under the skin lies a thin fibrous layer (tunica dartos) extending inwardly to form the septum, which divides the two scrotal cavities. The external spermatic, cremasteric and internal spermatic fasciae are a continuation of the layers of the abdominal wall. The innermost tunica vaginalis originates from the peritoneum. The cremasteric fascia contains a layer of striated muscle that produces retraction of the testicle due to various stimuli. When exposed to cold, the cremasteric muscle contracts, bringing the testis closer to the warmer environment of the body. A similar response takes place as a result of tactile stimulus (the cremasteric reflex) aimed at protecting the testis. The importance of the position of the testis inside the scrotum has been shown to depend upon its role in the control of testicular hypothermia.

The testicular parenchyma is composed of seminiferous tubules surrounded by interstitial tissue (Fig. 8.2). This parenchyma is covered by a capsule composed of three layers: the tunica

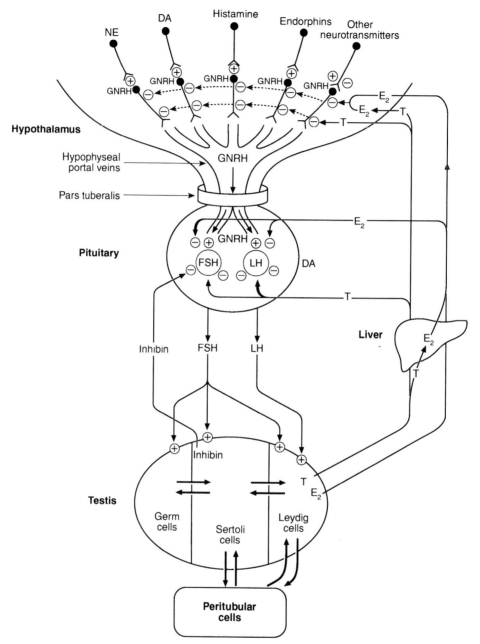

**Fig. 8.1** Feedbacks in the hypothalamus-hypophyseal-testes compartments. (Reproduced and revised with permission from Glass & Vigersky 1991)

vaginalis, tunica albuginea, and the innermost tunica vasculosa. The tunica vaginalis also has a parietal layer that lines the scrotum. Between these two layers is a space containing a small amount of serous fluid, allowing free motion of the testis within the scrotum. The tunica albug-

inea, the stronger layer of the capsule, is composed of collagen fibers, and some smooth muscle fibers (Holstein 1967). The innermost layer, the tunica vasculosa, is composed of a thin connective tissue, rich in blood vessels. Both the tunica vasculosa and albuginea penetrate the testis

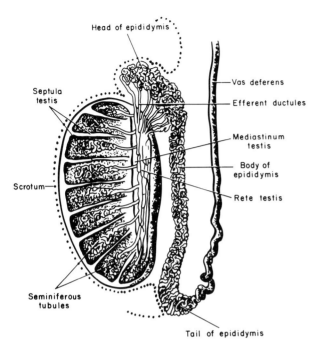

**Fig. 8.2**   Vertical section through the scrotum, testis and epididymis. Arrangement of the seminiferous tubules, rete testis and epididymis.

parenchyma, forming septa and dividing the testis into lobules. Incision through the tunica vasculosa during testicular biopsy causes bleeding, and may lead to hematoma formation, the most common complication of this procedure.

## Innervation

The innervation of the testis is primarily through the superior, the intermediate and inferior spermatic nerves. This is an adrenergic innervation to the small blood vessels of the interstitium. The origin of nerves from the intermesenteric and renal plexus may explain the nausea associated with testicular trauma, and the referred testicular pain associated with renal disease (Steinberger 1989).

## Blood supply

This is composed of three sources: the internal spermatic artery, the deferential artery, and the external spermatic or cremasteric artery. The spermatic artery arises from the aorta, and enters the posterior border of the testis directly, or after branching, and then divides into smaller branches directed toward the rete testis. Other branches form a superficial vascular network within the tunica vasculosa that gives off numerous terminal branches into the interstitium of the testis. The capillary network surrounding the seminiferous tubules and which is in close relation to Leydig cells, plays a role in the transport of hormones and nutrients from the circulation to Leydig cells, and to the seminiferous tubules (Suzuki & Nagano 1986).

Changes in the terminal pattern of the small blood vessels inside the testis may account for the distinctive, patchy degenerative events in the seminiferous tubules in cases of pathology in the arterioles related to disease and ageing.

There are two sets of veins inside the testes. One set drains the peripheral part and the vessels course centrifugally, and drain into larger veins on the surface of the testis. The other set drains a greater part of the testis. These veins course centripetally to the area of the rete testis. Both sets join the cremasteric and differential veins, to form the pampiniform plexus (Kormano & Suoranta 1971). The venous blood then drains into the spermatic vein. The right spermatic vein collects vessels from the right testis and joins the inferior vena cava, while the left spermatic vein drains blood from the left testis into the left renal vein. This difference, together with the histological structural features of veins characterized by a thin wall with little musculature, and lack of valves, are some of the implicated etiologies of vasodilatation of blood vessels in the left venous system, and may be a factor favoring formation of varicoceles (Ishigami et al 1970).

It is considered that the complex arrangement of blood vessels plays a role in a cooling process of the testis.

## Lymphatic drainage

Lymph vessels are located in the interstitial tissue of the testis, and drain into lymphatic ducts in the spermatic cord. The fluid secreted by the tubules drains through the rete testis. Obstruction of the lymphatic ducts in the spermatic cord is followed by dilatation of the interstitium only, and also causes the formation of hydrocele.

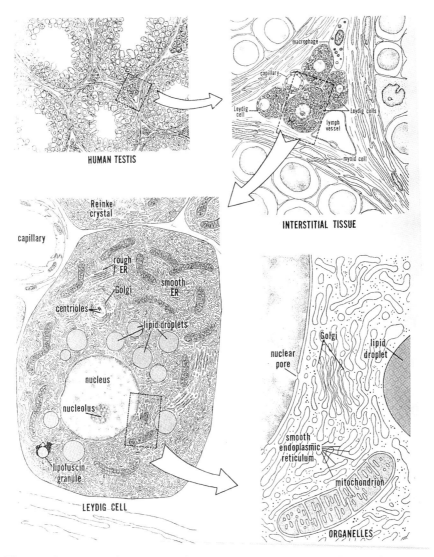

**Fig. 8.3**    Location and fine structure of human Leydig cells. (Reproduced and revised with permission from Christensen 1975)

## Histology of the testis

### Interstitium

The interstitial tissue is located in spaces among the seminiferous tubules. It contains blood and lymph vessels, fibroblastic supporting cells, macrophages, mast cells and Leydig cells. The interstitium occupies about 34% of testis volume.

***Leydig cells.*** These cells are the major source of testosterone in the male. In 1850, Franz Leydig was the first to describe these cells in several mammals, but it was about 100 years later that the evidence of testosterone secretion from these cells was proven.

Leydig cells are presented in clusters, and account for about 5–15% of the total volume of the testes in man and rats (Christensen 1975). The cells are rounded or polygonal in shape. They stain with the periodic acid-Schiff reaction, and enzymatically for 3β-hydroxy-steroid-dehydrogenase. Each cell contains a round nucleus with a nucleolus (Fig. 8.3). The ultrastructure of the human Leydig cell is characterized by prominent mitochondria, abundant smooth endoplasmic reticulum (SER), scattered patches of rough endoplasmic reticulum (RER), and lipid droplets (Christensen 1975). Leydig cells possess crystals of Reinke characterized by a lattice-like substructure. These crystals are seen only in human adult Leydig cells. Their function is not completely understood.

The number of Leydig cells in both testes of a 20-year-old male is up to 700 million, and diminishes by one-half by the age of 60. No division of Leydig cells has been observed in the testes of adult men (Kerr 1989).

*Seminiferous tubules*

The seminiferous tubules are the site of spermatogenesis. They are long, loop-like, convulated ducts with both ends terminating in the rete testis. The number of the seminiferous tubules is 600–1200, with an estimated total length of 250 m (Lennox & Ahmad 1970). Spermatozoa and fluid originating in the tubules are transported to the rete testis, and then to the epididymis. It has been suggested that the rete testes act as a valve that controls this flow (Roosen-Runge & Holstein 1978).

The seminiferous tubule is composed of wall, Sertoli and germ cells. The germ cells are described in detail in the section dealing with spermatogenesis.

***The wall*** of the tubule is composed of three concentric layers (Fig. 8.4):

1. An inner acellular basement membrane composed of a thin basal lamina, and a thicker filamentous area containing collagen and some elastic fibrils.

2. An intermediate myoid layer constituting a number of discontinuous layers of myoepithelial cells coated with a basal, lamina-like material containing actin filaments. These cells possess contractile properties. Adjacent myoid cells generally have overlapping cytoplasmic processes that decrease the intercellular space, and partially restrict movement of material to and from the tubule (Dym & Fawcett 1970).

3. An outer adventitial layer which contains fibroblasts and fibrils.

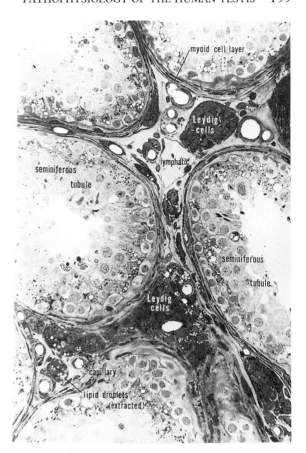

**Fig. 8.4** Light micrograph of human testis. (Reproduced and revised with permission from Christensen 1975)

***Sertoli cells.*** These are epithelial cells of mesodermal embryonic origin. They are arranged in a continuous, single layer, lining the inner aspect of the seminiferous tubule. Sertoli cells are found in a constant number after sexual maturation.

The cells are characterized by several unique, morphological features (Fig. 8.5). They have an irregular outline, with cytoplasmic projections surrounding adjacent germ cells, and an irregularly shaped nucleus, containing a prominent nucleolus. Adjacent Sertoli-cell membranes have unique tight junctional complexes. An abundance of RER and SER, dense vacuoles, and inclusion bodies are located in the cytoplasm (Kerr 1989, Ritzen et al 1989).

The Sertoli cells rest on the basement membrane of the seminiferous tubule, and each cell extends to the inner tubular lumen. Germinal

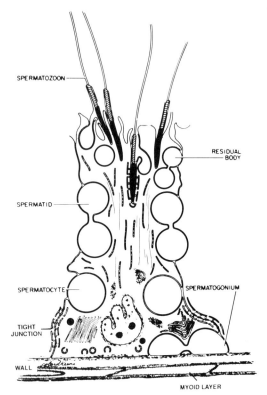

SPERMATOZOON

RESIDUAL BODY

SPERMATID

SPERMATOCYTE

SPERMATOGONIUM

TIGHT JUNCTION

WALL

MYOID LAYER

**Fig. 8.5** The Setoli cell and its surroundings: the germinal cells and the wall of the seminiferous tubule. Localization of the blood – testis barrier and the compartmentalization of the germinal epithelium by tight junctions between adjacent Sertoli cells is illustrated. (Reproduced and revised with permission from Huckins & Meacham 1991)

cells are arranged between the Sertoli cells, engulfed by their cytoplasmic projections. The undifferentiated spermatogonia are located near the basement membrane, and the more advanced forms are arranged at successively higher levels near the tubular lumen.

Sertoli cells are more than 'nursing' cells to the adjacent germinal cells. They play a crucial role in regulation of spermatogenesis.

Two types of inter-Sertoli junctions have been identified: 'tight', and less intimate junctions (Dym & Fawcett 1970). The 'tight' junction fuses with outer membranes of neighboring Sertoli cells (Fawcett 1975). Intramembranous granules, bundles of actin-like microfilaments, and cisternae of endoplasmic reticulum are present at the junction sites (Ritzen et al 1989).

Numerous studies have shown that certain substances present in the blood diffuse to the lymphatic vessels of the testes, but do not appear in fluid of the seminiferous tubules (Setchell & Waites 1975, Fawcett 1979). The specialized junctional complexes between adjacent Sertoli cells are believed to be the principal site of this blood–testis barrier. Sertoli cell 'tight' junctions subdivide the seminiferous tubule into basal and adluminal compartments. This was identified in man (de Kretser & Burger 1972, Chemes et al 1977), as well as in many other species (Dym & Fawcett 1970).

## SPERMATOGENESIS

### General considerations

The process of proliferation and differentiation of germ cells has been termed spermatogenesis, and takes place within the seminiferous tubules. The seminiferous tubules occupy approximately 70% of the testis (Johnson 1986).

The basic understanding of spermatogenesis is derived from studies in rats, and is detailed in excellent reviews (Steinberger 1971, Clermont 1972). In this section most of the data provided are on spermatogenesis in the human testis.

The long seminiferous tubules of the human testis are lined with a single continuous layer of Sertoli cells that are epithelial elements of mesodermal origin, organized in a complex helical plan (Schulze et al 1986). The germinal cells pack the spaces between Sertoli cells. In the adult testis, Sertoli cells do not divide spontaneously (Steinberger & Steinberger 1971). Adjacent Sertoli cells are joined by extensive tight junctions along their lateral borders, thereby forming an impermeable blood–testis barrier (Dym & Cavicchia 1978). Sertoli tight junctions divide the tubule into basal and adluminal compartments (Koskimies et al 1973). Germ cells develop up to the stage of leptotene primary spermatocytes within the basal compartment, which has relatively free access to the extratubular environment. Secondary spermatocytes continue their development into spermatozoa in the adluminal compartment. Because of the blood–testis barrier, any factor influencing the latter stages of spermatogenesis must be mediated through the Sertoli cells.

Within the adult testis, the rate at which germ cells mature is constant. In humans, production of spermatozoa takes 74 days (Heller & Clermont 1963). Spermatocyte maturation requires 25.3 days, with spermiogenesis extending over 21.6 days. Each primitive spermatogonium may ultimately give rise to 64 mature spermatozoa. Studies have provided evidence of a wave-form of spermatogenesis in the human testis in a helical arrangement (Schulze et al 1986).

The spermatogonial stem cells continuously supply cells for spermatogenesis in a cyclic pattern, and at the same time renew themselves to maintain a constant reservoir. Syncytial clusters of germ cells, which are progeny of the same original germ cells division, develop in synchrony. Such clones in humans contain few cells, therefore cross-sections of human tubules often display different cell associations.

No significant degeneration of human germ cells occurs between type B spermatogonia and secondary spermatocytes (Johnson et al 1987), or during spermiogenesis (Johnson et al 1981).

A 30–40% loss of germ cells occurs mainly late in meiosis during the second meiotic division (Barr et al 1971, Johnson et al 1984a).

## Spermatogenesis process

Spermatogenesis can be subdivided into four successive processes:

1. Undifferentiated spermatogonia – proliferation process
2. Spermatogonial differentiation
3. Spermatocyte development – meiosis
4. Spermatid development – spermiogenesis and spermiation.

### Proliferation

In the human testis, four spermatogonial types have been recognized ($A_{long}$, $A_{dark}$, $A_{pale}$, and B), and the possibility of additional types of A cells has recently been raised (Fig. 8.6). All type A spermatogonia have been considered for a stem cell role. The $A_{dark}$ and $A_{pale}$ spermatogonia are numerous, while the $A_{long}$ spermatogonia occur infrequently. $A_{dark}$ spermatogonia are reserve stem cells that do not normally contribute to spermatogenesis, and it has been suggested that they represent a phase of cell cycle rather than specific cell type, whereas the $A_{pale}$ are active stem cells. Type B spermatogonia, which are produced by the $A_{pale}$ spermatogonia, are differentiated cells that ultimately produce preleptotene spermatocytes (Clermont & Antar 1973) (Fig. 8.6).

### Meiosis

The final spermatogonial division generates preleptotene spermatocytes which enter a resting phase of 2.6 days, which consists of about 16% of the cycle duration. Towards the end of this period, the preleptotene spermatocytes begin to synthesize DNA for meiosis, and subsequently enter the long meiotic prophase. This process occurs in the basal compartment of the tubule, but as the cells transform into leptotene spermatocytes, syncytial clusters pass across the tight junction to enter the adluminal compartment (Dym & Cavicchia 1978). This process is passive on the part of the germ cells, and involves the interposition of slips of Sertoli-cell cytoplasm between the spermatocytes and the tubular wall. When the cytoplasmic extensions meet, new tight junctions are formed, and the existing junctions 'unzip' to provide the leptotene spermatocytes immediate access to the luminal environment. The tight junction does not depend on the presence of germ cells. Only in long-term cryptorchidism is the barrier disassembled. Thus its existence depends on hypothermia. Once the spermatocytes have traversed the tight junction, a unique morphological relationship develops between pachytene spermatocytes and Sertoli cells, which persists until spermiation. Midway through the pachytene step of meiotic prophase, the secondary spermatocytes begin to develop a number of new surface antigens. As these cells are on the luminal side of the tight junction barrier, newly formed antigens are detected which are foreign to the immunological system. Unique surface antigens foreign to the body continue to be produced throughout spermiogenesis (Means et al 1976). Although some of these antigens disappear prior to the end of the

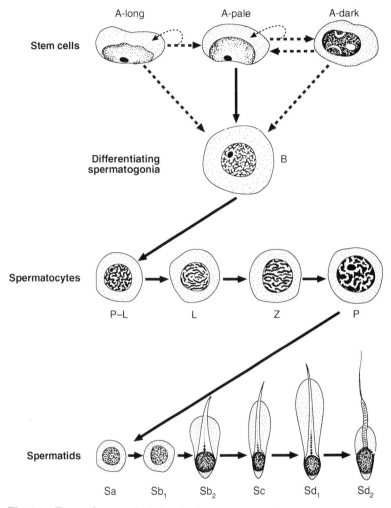

Stem cells — A-long — A-pale — A-dark

Differentiating spermatogonia — B

Spermatocytes — P–L — L — Z — P

Spermatids — Sa — Sb₁ — Sb₂ — Sc — Sd₁ — Sd₂

**Fig. 8.6**   Types of germ cells during the three processes of human spermatogenesis. Relationships between stages are indicated by arrows. Uncertain relationships are indicated by broken lines. (Reproduced with permission from Huckins & Meacham 1991 )

process, others are retained in the plasma membrane of testicular spermatozoa that have been shed.

Just prior to the first meiotic division, primary spermatocytes replicate their DNA and contain twice the normal amount (4N) (Fig. 8.7). After the first meiotic division, each secondary spermatocyte contains an haploid number of chromosomes, but the total amount of DNA in each daughter spermatocyte is equal to that of a normal somatic cell (2N), since each chromosome is in a double structure. During the second meiotic division, each double-structured chromosome divides, so that each daughter cell (spermatid) contains 23 chromosomes.

*Spermiogenesis and spermiation*

During the maturation of spermatids into spermatozoa several events occur, including formation of the acrosome, changes in nuclear morphology, and formation of the flagellum.

**Development of the acrosome**

In the initial phase of the process, the Golgi

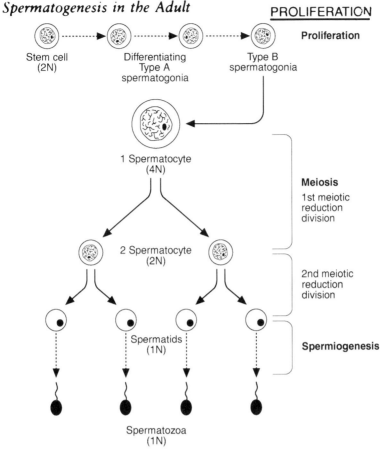

**Fig. 8.7** Description of the three processes: proliferation, meiosis and spermiogenesis. During spermatogenesis, the DNA of the primary spermatocyte is replicated, creating the first spermatocyte with twice the normal complement of DNA (4N). Two subsequent meiotic reduction divisions produce the spermatids (1N). (Reproduced and revised with permission from Huckins & Meacham 1991)

apparatus donates material for the acrosome, which is actually a modified lysosomal bag containing glycoprotein enzymes. The acrosome development can be used to determine the chronological progression of the spermatid itself. On the basis of acrosomal cap development during spermiogenesis, six stages ($Sa$, $Sb_1$, $Sb_2$, $Sc$, $Sd_1$ and $Sd_2$) have been described for the human spermatid (Clermont 1963).

Early in spermiogenesis, the spermatid nucleus remains a metabolically active spherical body. The nucleus migrates to the periphery of the cell when the acrosome is fully formed, and becomes intimately invested by the overlying plasma membrane. The end of this migration signals the gradual cessation of nuclear metabolic activity, the onset of chromatin condensation, and the beginning of nuclear elongation. At the completion of spermiogenesis, the nucleus is transformed into a dense, flattened shape, containing greatly compacted chromatin. While acrosome growth occurs at one nuclear pole, centrioles move to the opposite pole, and initiate formation of the tail. Mitochondria, originally dispersed at the periphery of the spermatid, migrate to the region of the forming tail. There they line up in an end-to-end spiral around the tail to serve eventually as the energy formation source for cell metabolism.

As spermatids begin to elongate, extensive ectoplasmic specializations appear between spermatids and Sertoli cells over the region of the acrosomal cap (Russell & Clermont 1977). This has a role in the orderly migration of the spermatids towards the lumen, and in the maintenance of contact with Sertoli cells. At spermiation, these specializations disassemble, thus releasing the individual spermatozoon into the tubular lumen. The released spermatozoa are immotile and infertile.

Recently, antigen SP-10 was detected. By following this new antigen localization, its existence was demonstrated in spermatids at each of the six-stage cycles of the seminiferous epithelium. Immunohistochemical localization of SP-10 was proven to be similar to that of the developing acrosome. The presence of SP-10 was detected within the developing acrosomal vesicle in the early steps of spermiogenesis. At the end of spermiogenesis, this antigen became associated with the inner and outer acrosomal membranes of the most mature spermatids (Kurth et al 1991).

At the conclusion of spermiogenesis, most of the cytoplasm, including the intracellular bridges and remaining organelles, is shed as a 'residual body' which is immediately phagocytosed by Sertoli cells. Phagocytosis can also be followed by monitoring lipid inclusions areas, occupied by the Sertoli cell cytoplasm (Paniagua et al 1987).

## Effect of age on spermatogenesis

Testicular weight does not increase after 20–30 years of age. Human testicular parenchyma is significantly reduced in aged men (Johnson et al 1986). Other age-related changes include decreased volume of seminiferous epithelium, increased thickness of the tubular wall, and decreased length of the tubuli.

Lower seminiferous epithelial volume in older men is associated with lower daily sperm production per man (Johnson et al 1984c, Johnson 1986).

Age-related reduction in daily sperm production in humans is significantly correlated with loss of Sertoli cells (Johnson et al 1984b). Furthermore, old men have additional germ-cell degeneration during the prophase of meiosis, in addition to the physiological germ-cell loss at the end of meiosis in the normal cycle (Johnson 1986).

*Hormonal control*

Sperm production requires the stimulatory actions of the anterior pituitary gonadotropins, luteinizing hormone (LH) (via testosterone) and follicle-stimulating hormone (FSH). Thus, initiation of sperm production does not occur in boys with prepubertal hypothalamic, hypogonadotropic hypogonadism (e.g. Kallman's syndrome). Spermatogenesis cannot be maintained in adult men who acquire gonadotropin deficiency. While it is clear that gonadotropins are necessary for spermatogenesis, the specific role of LH and FSH in the control of spermatogenesis are unclear. Studies on selective gonadotropin replacement in normal men with experimentally induced hypogonadotropic hypogonadism demonstrate that qualitatively normal sperm production can be achieved by replacement of either LH (or human chorionic gonadotropin (hCG)) or FSH alone. However, both LH and FSH are necessary to maintain quantitatively normal spermatogenesis in man.

Studies of gonadotropin replacement therapy of men with spontaneously occurring hypogonadotropic hypogonadism suggest that the requirement for FSH activity to stimulate sperm production is greatest during the initiation of spermatogenesis at the time of puberty. The re-initiation and maintenance of sperm production in men who acquire hypogonadotropic hypogonadism as adults can often be achieved with LH activity alone (Matsumoto et al 1983, Matsumoto & Bremner 1987).

Other pituitary hormones, e.g. prolactin, can also affect spermatogenesis, but their role appears to be secondary to the gonadotropins. Prolactin receptors have been located on the Leydig cells and prolactin enhances the LH-stimulated testosterone secretion (Zipf et al 1978).

LH binds to Leydig cells, and stimulates steroid hormone synthesis resulting in increased production of testosterone. Presence of high local concentrations of testosterone within the seminiferous tubules is thought to play an important role in both the initiation and maintenance of sperm

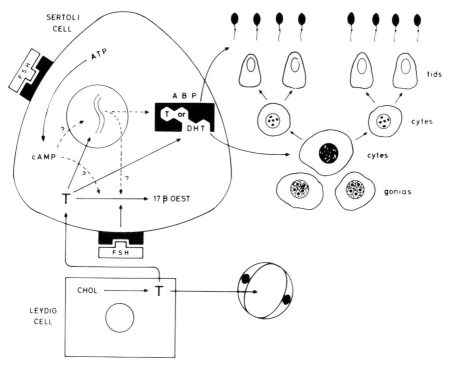

**Fig. 8.8** Effect of FSH and testosterone on Sertoli cell functions and regulation of spermatogenesis. (Reproduced with permission from Franchimont 1980)

production (di Zerega & Sherins 1980, Matsumoto & Bremner 1987). The mechanism by which testosterone regulates spermatogenesis, and the concentration of testosterone within the seminiferous tubule required for normal sperm production, are not well defined. However, the intratesticular testosterone concentration in normal human testes is 50- to 100-fold that of circulating levels (Steinberger 1975). It is still unclear whether the active androgen in the testes is testosterone or dihydrotestosterone (DHT).

FSH is delivered to the interstitial area of the testis via the arterial system (Fig. 8.8). It passes through the basement membrane of the seminiferous tubule, and binds to specific plasma membrane receptors on the Sertoli cells. It then activates adenyl cyclase, thus stimulating the production of cyclic adenosine monophosphate (cAMP). This nucleotide regulates production of new proteins, and activates protein kinases for the control of the physiology of Sertoli cells (Means et al 1976, Matsumoto & Bremner 1987).

The major protein to be demonstrated in the Sertoli cells is androgen-binding protein (ABP). Androgens produced by the Leydig cells under the stimulatory action of LH diffuse from the interstitial area into the seminiferous tubule, where they are bound by the ABP. ABP has a high affinity for androgens, and thus creates a high-androgen concentration in the vicinity of certain meiotic germ cells (controls meiosis).

It is now clearly established that in addition to ABP, the Sertoli cells secrete transferrin, inhibin, plasminogen activator, ceruloplasmin and many other compounds. Sertoli-cell products are believed to be of importance in spermatogenesis by either serving as transport proteins, sources of energy or substrates for germ cells metabolism. Recent studies demonstrated transferrin and ABP binding to germ cells during specific stages of differentiation (Sharpe 1992).

Sertoli cells surround developing sperm with their cytoplasmic processes, and are thought to nurture and coordinate the completion of sperm maturation in the seminiferous tubule.

While leucine aminotransferase (LAT) and ABP are used as Sertoli-cell markers, lactate dehydrogenase isozyme (LDH-C$_4$) is a testis-specific isozyme which is used as a germ-cell marker. LDH-C$_4$ is the predominant LDH isozyme in mammalian spermatozoa. When immunological localization of LDH-C$_4$ on human capacitated sperm was observed by indirect immunofluorescent assay, using monoclonal antibodies, a marked binding could be demonstrated to the postacrosome and some to the neck and midpiece of the sperm cell (Wang et al 1990, Reader et al 1991).

In addition, studies on the correlation between LDH-C$_4$ activity in semen sperm concentration and fertility were carried out (Eliasson & Virji 1985, Casano et al 1991).

## Seminiferous contractility

Testosterone and DHT have a biphasic effect on tubular contractility. High doses of both induce contractions of the seminiferous tubules, whereas lower doses of these hormones induce relaxation. Estradiol induces relaxation of the seminiferous tubules in a dose-dependent manner. Thus, it is suggested that steroids may be involved in the control of contraction of the human seminiferous tubule, and may regulate the movement of spermatozoa from the testes (Yamamoto et al 1989).

The isolated human seminiferous tubule is capable of undergoing contraction after exposure to noradrenaline and acetylcholine. Isoproterenol produces relaxation of the seminiferous tubule. It is indicated that these are the adrenergic alpha and beta receptors and muscarinic receptors in the myoid cells of human seminiferous tubules (Miyake et al 1986).

## STEROIDOGENESIS AND ITS CONTROL

## Steroidogenesis throughout life

De novo steroidogenesis has been demonstrated in the human testis starting from week 7 of gestation (Griffin & Wilson 1983). Plasma testosterone levels of the male embryo then rise until late in pregnancy, and fall to concentrations similar to those of females. During the first 3 months after birth testosterone levels rise, then fall by 1 year and remain low (but are slightly higher in boys than girls) until the onset of puberty. At about 11 or 12 years of age, the pituitary gland starts to secrete gonadotropins, thus stimulating testosterone production.

Normally, plasma testosterone concentrations reach adult levels at approximately 17 years of age. The adult level is maintained until late middle age, and then decreases slowly. After age 70, plasma testosterone levels decline, while sex hormone-binding globulin (SHBG) concentration increases. This results in a larger drop in free testosterone concentrations. Peripheral production of estrogen increases, resulting in a decreased androgen/estrogen ratio. This is believed to be involved in the development of benign prostatic hypertrophy, and gynecomastia in elderly men (Griffin & Wilson 1983).

## Testosterone synthesis and physiology

Testosterone is synthesized from cholesterol. The Leydig cells of the testis have been shown capable of synthesizing cholesterol de novo from acetate. In some species (e.g. pig) Leydig cells contain receptors for low density lipoprotein (LDL), and are therefore able to obtain cholesterol from circulating LDL. It is unclear what proportion of the cholesterol in human Leydig cells is obtained in this manner (Odell 1989).

The limiting step in testosterone synthesis is the cleavage of the side chain of cholesterol to yield pregnenolone. This occurs in the mitochondrial membrane, and is catalysed by an enzyme system containing cytochrome P-450, a flavoprotein, and a non-heme iron protein. The rate-limiting step in testicular steroid production, regulated by LH, occurs at this step (Rommerts & van der Molen 1989). Pregnenolone can then be converted to testosterone in the endoplasmic reticulum by a series of five enzymatically catalysed steps involving Δ-4 or Δ-5 intermediates (Fig. 8.9).

The intermediates in these pathways can be interconverted by the action of 3β-hydroxysteroid dehydrogenase (3β-HSD), and Δ-5-4 isomerase.

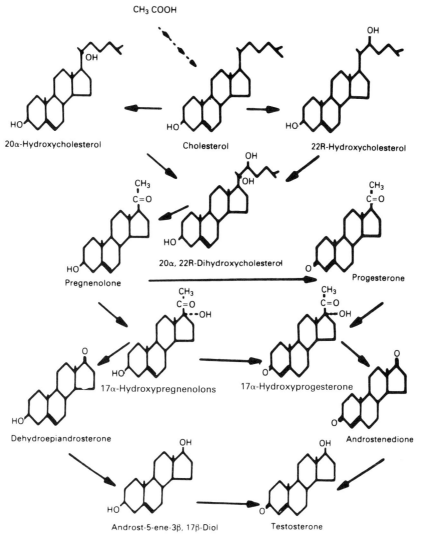

**Fig. 8.9** Pathway of testicular androgen biosynthesis. The conversion of pregnenolone to testosterone via progesterone is known as the $\Delta^4$ pathway and the conversion of pregnenolone to testosterone via dehydroepiandrosterone is known as the $\Delta^5$ pathway.

The rate of testosterone production by the $\Delta$-4 and $\Delta$-5 pathways differs in different organisms, and probably the physiologically occurring reactions include both $\Delta$-4 and $\Delta$-5 intermediates. The $\Delta$-5 pathway is predominant in the adrenals. Further details on testicular steroidogenesis may be found in an excellent review by Rommerts & van der Molen (1989).

The Sertoli cells of the seminiferous tubules are able to convert testosterone to estradiol or DHT, which may play a role in seminiferous tubule physiology. They are unable to synthesize testosterone, but have been shown to produce ABP which apparently transports testosterone or DHT into the luminal fluid of the seminiferous tubules (Granner 1988).

The peripheral effects of androgens include specific effects producing male secondary sexual characteristics, and more general anabolic effects resulting in increased weight and muscular development. The important physiological effects of testosterone are given in Table 8.1.

**Table 8.1**  Physiological effects of testosterone

Sexual differentiation during embryogenesis
Effects on gonadotropins, spermatogenesis and sexual
    functions
Effects on metabolism and various organ systems:
• Anabolic effects (effects on nitrogen balance, muscle
    development, etc.)
• Effect on lipid metabolism
• Effect on carbohydrate metabolism
• Effect on hematopoiesis and thrombus formation
• Retention of water and salt
• Effects on skin and appendages
• Other metabolic effects (including effects on the kidney,
    ventilation and hypoxic drive, and on bone metabolism)
• Effects in children (growth hormone secretion, epiphysial
    closure)
Virilizing effects/effects on genitalia
Stimulation of beard, axillary and pubic hair
Enlargement of larynx and thickening of vocal cords
Effects due to peripheral conversion to estrogen
Influence on the central nervous system, including
    development and behavior
Interactions with other drugs
Effects on the liver and hypersensitivity due to chemical
    alterations of the testosterone molecule
Teratogenic effects

## Control of steroidogenesis

Testosterone production in the Leydig cells is under feedback control involving the hypothalamic-pituitary-testis axis (Figs 8.1, 8.10). GnRH is released in a pulsatile manner from the hypothalamus into the hypothalamic-hypophyseal portal system, and stimulates the hypophysis (pituitary) to release LH and FSH. Increased unpulsatile secretion of LH can cause down-regulation of LH receptors, and desensitization of steroid responses in the target cell. This event is estradiol-mediated enzyme inhibition. Prolactin, growth hormone (GH) and insulin-like growth factor (IGF-I) are also involved in regulation of LH receptors. FSH regulates LH receptors by paracrine modulation of tubular function (Dufau 1988).

Testosterone, either directly or through its metabolites, estradiol or DHT, decreases secretion of LH from the pituitary gland. Evidence has been presented to show that estradiol decreases the amplitude of each LH discharge (achieved, in part, by decreasing the sensitivity of the pituitary to GnRH). In contrast, testosterone decreases the mean LH level by reducing the frequency of discharge, mediated by the hypothalamus (Bardin 1986) (Fig. 8.1).

The rate-limiting step in testicular steroid production depends upon the amount and activity of the cytochrome P-450 enzyme. The mechanism of LH in stimulating testicular testosterone production involves enzyme induction or activation. Leydig cells maintain, on their surfaces, high-affinity LH receptors. These receptors were identified as glycoproteins which are composed of two identical subunits associated by monocovalent interactions. The receptor-LH complex can be internalized and afterwards recycled (Dufau 1988). The binding of LH to these membrane receptors results in increased adenylcyclase activity, thus elevating the concentration of cAMP, a 'second messenger' that activates protein kinase, which in turn activates numerous

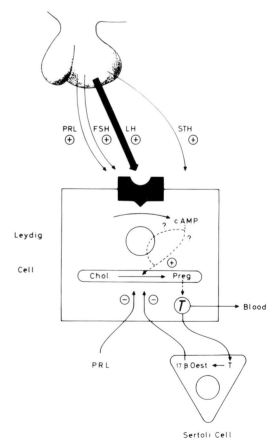

**Fig. 8.10**  Regulation of Leydig cell functions by endocrine and paracrine pathways. (Reproduced with permission from Franchimont 1980)

cellular metabolic reactions. Maximal stimulation of testosterone biosynthesis occurs, however, at LH concentrations which are not sufficient to elicit an increase in intracellular cAMP concentration. This suggests that other second messengers such as $Ca^{2+}$, inositol trisphosphate, or diacylglycerol might also be involved in regulating testosterone biosynthesis (Odell 1989).

## Steroid metabolism

Testosterone concentration is highest in the testis compartment, and this elevated concentration is necessary for supporting spermatogenesis. A portion of this testosterone is transported into the seminiferous tubules, where it is taken up by Sertoli cells (by ABP) which can metabolize it further. Sertoli cells can also produce DHT and estradiol, which may play an important physiological role there. Steroids produced by Sertoli-cell modification of testosterone may be bound to ABP, and transported in the seminiferous tubule fluid to the epididymis, where they are taken up by the epididymal epithelial cells.

Approximately 6 mg/d of testosterone is produced by the Leydig cells of a healthy young man (Fig. 8.11). It is secreted in a pulsatile manner, and binds to a specific protein, SHBG, which is synthesized in the liver, or to human serum albumin (HSA). Testosterone levels in the blood, measured by radioimmunoassay, vary from 0.3 to 1.2 µg/dl. Because of the pulsatile

nature of testosterone secretion, it is advisable to perform these measurements on samples of plasma/serum which have been collected in several portions over a 2–3 hour period (Horton 1989).

Only a small amount of free testosterone (unbound to proteins) is available for entry into the peripheral tissues. Certain organs of the male reproductive tract, such as prostate and seminal vesicle, convert testosterone to DHT, which binds to a nuclear receptor in those cells, and functions as a more active androgen than does testosterone itself. Other organs, notably adipose tissue, are capable of aromatizing testosterone to estradiol. This is the major source of the estrogen found in the blood plasma of men (Griffin & Wilson 1983). Only approximately 20% of estradiol secreted by the male (10–15 µg/d) is produced by the aromatase activity of the Leydig cell itself (Horton 1989).

The liver plays a major role in metabolizing testosterone and other steroids by oxidizing them to form 17-ketosteroids. Liver enzymes catalyse the oxidation, and a variety of conjugating enzymes convert the androgens into water-soluble glucuronides and sulfates which are excreted (primarily in urine, and to a smaller degree in bile). Some portion of the urinary metabolites (e.g. steroid sulfates) may be produced in the Leydig cell itself. Measurement of urinary 17-hydroxy steroids, once suggested as an assay for androgen excretion, is not suitable for that

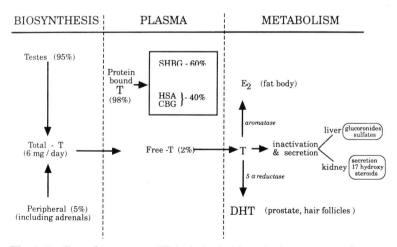

**Fig. 8.11**   Fate of testosterone (T) in the body: biosynthesis, transport and metabolism.

purpose because a large proportion of these metabolites are of adrenal rather than testicular origin (Horton 1989).

## Pathology of steroidogenesis

It is almost axiomatic that among the 5 billion humans alive today, there will be mutants in almost every gene that can be altered without causing lethality. It is therefore not surprising that mutants have been found with defective functioning of the following steps of testicular steroidogenesis: side-chain cleavage enzyme, 17α–hydroxylase, conversion of C21 to C19, reduction of 17-ketone, oxidation to Δ-4-3 ketos-teroid, and 5α-reductase. The lack of testosterone synthesis is called hypoandrogenism, and it results in the absence of male secondary sex characteristics (Table 8.1). Persons who completely lack a biosynthetic enzyme or receptor protein display a female phenotype although they have an XY genotype. Partial deficits may result in milder abnormalities. In addition to primary hypogonadism, caused by testicular defects, secondary hypogonadism is caused by decreased or defective LH secretion (Granner 1988).

In addition to the enzyme defects, there are cases where testosterone production is normal, but the receptor for testosterone is defective. In these cases, 46 XY genotypes may exhibit female phenotypes because target tissues are unable to respond to testosterone in order to induce developmental changes necessary for maleness. This syndrome is termed 'testicular feminization'.

The feminizing effects of the small amount of estradiol in the blood of normal males are counteracted by the much higher testosterone concentrations. In certain pathological situations, the estrogen may cause gynecomastia or contribute to enlargement of the prostate in benign prostatic hypertrophy (Griffin & Wilson 1983).

During sexual development of the adolescent boy, precocious puberty may occur as a result of pathological processes such as androgen production by a tumor or by tumors, causing increased gonadotropin production. Absent puberty may be caused by testicular defects, hereditary androgen resistance, or defects in the hypothalamic-hypophysial-gonadal axis. (For details see 'Pathology of testicular function').

## THERMOREGULATION

A close correlation exists between spermatogenesis and temperature. Local application of heat to the mammalian testis damages spermatogenesis, and epididymal function. Cryptochidism results in identical damage, and it is now generally agreed that its adverse effects are exerted by the higher temperature of the abdominal cavity. Spermatogenesis is therefore extremely sensitive to very small elevations of temperature in men, and some other mammals.

It has been demonstrated that experimentally induced cryptorchidism in adult rats causes damage to the germinal epithelium, and decrease in Sertoli-cell functions as reflected in low levels of inhibin and ABP.

Leydig-cell morphology and steroidogenesis in the scrotal testes of rats, compared to abdominal testes, were studied. Leydig cells in the cryptorchid testis were characterized by reduction in number, increased lipid content, changes in endoplasmic reticulum, and changes in steroid metabolites which cause decreased testosterone synthesis. In addition, relatively increased estradiol concentration was found, which may have affected cryptorchid testicular function via the paracrine mode, or by changes in the microcirculation of the testis (Bergh et al 1984).

Thermoregulation of the testis is controlled by the scrotum via a countercurrent heat-exchange system in the vessels of the spermatic cord (Waites 1970). In men, the testicular artery is usually free of convolutions, and the abdominoscrotal temperature difference averages only 2.2°C. In contrast, the ram testicular artery is extremely tortuous, and is related to an abdominoscrotal temperature gradient of 13°C.

The close relation of the veins of the pampiniform plexus to the artery is well adapted to the control of preheating or precooling of arterial blood flow to the testis.

The human scrotal skin has a very thin epidermis, and is well supplied with blood vessels. Fat is absent from the superficial fasciae, and variations in its surface area can be achieved by

PATHOPHYSIOLOGY OF THE HUMAN TESTIS   211

contractions of the dartos muscle. The sweat glands of the scrotum are critically involved in local thermoregulation. Scrotal sweat glands can discharge up to a maximum frequency of 10 times/h. This is dependent on environmental conditions (clothes, temperature, etc.)

Elevated temperature of the testis may cause a relatively low number of sperm to be produced/g of testis, poor-quality spermatozoa to be released therefrom, a rapid epididymal transport, and a minimally developed sperm storage system in the cauda epididymis (Amann 1981).

Nakamura et al (1988) showed that pachytene spermatocytes and round spermatids, cells that readily degenerate at higher temperatures, are not actively involved in DNA synthesis. Thus, inpairment of DNA synthesis in preleptotene germ cells may not be the underlying direct cause of temperature-induced spermatogenic damage, but heat may interfere with the normal mitotic process. It appears that different metabolic parameters could be affected by elevated temperatures at various stages of germ-cell development.

Present knowledge concerning the relationship between temperature and male reproductive functions comes mainly from animal studies of in vitro experiments, and from clinical observations. In animals such as the rat, rabbit, dog, sheep, ram and bull, procedures such as experimental cryptorchidism, scrotal insulation, acute febrile illness, increased ambient temperature and experimental varicocele, all alter the spermatogenic functions and inhibit spermatogenesis. Clinical studies using testicular hypothermia devices showed improvement in sperm production and quality following weeks of treatment. This may provide a new tool for treatment of infertile men once it has been proved that thermoregulation of their testes is disturbed (Zorgniotti et al 1986).

## PARACRINE REGULATION

In addition to the well-defined endocrine control, there has been increasing awareness as to the existence of a vigorous and essential paracrine activity in the testicular tissue. Studies are based on in vivo and in vitro experiments including organ culture. Purified cells such as Leydig, Sertoli, peritubular and germinal cells at various stages of development were used in the studies. Histochemical and immunocytochemical procedures have been developed to assess the purity of the cells. The combination of in vitro analysis to investigate molecular parameters, and in vivo experiments to support physiological significance were useful to elucidate cell–cell interactions (Saez et al 1991, Skinner 1991) (Fig. 8.12). Cellular interactions are based on three elements: environmental (extracellular matrix and adhesion), nutritional (nutrients, metabolites and energy), and regulatory (via paracrine/autocrine, growth factors).

In the mammalian testis, very active paracrine and autocrine regulatory processes take place between cells of the interstitial tissue (macrophages and Leydig cells), and the seminiferous tubules (Sertoli, germinal, and peritubular myoid cells). The direct effect of the factors and materials secreted and acting on each of the cells was studied and reviewed mainly in animals.

Insulin-like growth factor-I (IGF-I) is an important permissive factor involved in the maintenance and activity of most cells in the testis (Cailleau et al 1990). All major cells of the testicular tissue produce and secrete IGF-I.

Insulin-like growth factor-I has an important role in the facilitation of deoxyribonucleic acid (DNA) synthesis followed by proliferation of the cell. Most of the testicular cell types require cell proliferation (except for Sertoli cells that terminate their proliferation prior to puberty). The local production and action of growth factors are therefore required to regulate testicular cell differentiation and growth.

The production of IGF-I by a coculture system of Leydig and Sertoli cells was found to be synergistic in nature, suggesting that cell-to-cell interactions may play a role in the control of testicular IGF-I production. Jacobs et al (1991) proposed the involvement of GH and IGF-I in the human reproductive process. In women, it was clearly proven to be involved in folliculogenesis. In men, the authors were successful in inducing increased testosterone secretion and sperm production in the testes of hypogonadotropic, hypogonadal men following treatment with GH and gonadotropins. GH treatment of normogonadotropic, infertile men failed to increase sperm production although serum and seminal plasma IGF-I were found to be significantly elevated (Yavetz et al 1992a).

Vascular and lymphatic systems are well developed in the interstitium of the testis. The tissue contains macrophages and lymphocytes. Local factors are involved in stimulation of macrophages and lymphocyte cells which, in turn, produce factors that affect adjacent Leydig-cell activity (Lombard-Vignon et al 1991). Macrophages serve as a major source for interleukin-1β (IL-1β). This peptide, at maximal effective doses, stimulates steroidogenesis in vitro in isolated rat Leydig cells, and implicates these cells in paracrine control of testicular function (Verhoeven et al 1988). Thus, stimulated rat macrophages could be important in the control of Leydig-cell steroidogenesis.

## Sertoli–germ cell interactions

Sertoli cells appear to be the primary somatic cell to interact directly with the developing germinal cells, and indirectly via paracrine factors with other cells previously mentioned. An individual Sertoli cell can be in contact with five adjacent Sertoli cells at the basal surface of the cell, and 47 adjacent germinal cells at various stages of development. A rapid rate of remodelling between the cell populations in the seminiferous tubule is necessary in order to maintain spermatogenesis at a daily production rate of millions of sperm cells.

Sertoli cells also support germ-cell syncytium that connects the cells derived from an initial clone of cells. Several cell-to-cell specializations were defined in the seminiferous tubuli: the tight desmosome-gap function, the ectoplasmic specialization, and the tubulobulbar complex (Russell 1977).

Sertoli cells have been shown to metabolize glucose to lactate and pyruvate which supply energy to the cells. In addition, different transport proteins, capable of transferring nutritional components from the interstitial space into the tubule and germinal cells, a process which is critical for germ-cell survival, were identified. Sertoli cells are known for their capacity to synthesize transferrin, which in turn delivers iron to the cells in the tubule through a receptor-mediated process. Transferrin and the receptor

complex are endocytosed, and the iron is released. This function of Sertoli cells is essential in order to enable spermatogenesis to continue in a rapid, synchronized, well-controlled order. High concentrations of transferrin receptors have been localized on pachytene spermatocytes. A good correlation was established between transferrin concentration in seminal plasma, and sperm concentration in the ejaculate (Paz et al 1992). A similar transport mechanism was shown for copper by ceruloplasmin (copper transfer) and lipid metabolism by a sulfated glycoprotein-1 mechanism. Vitamins (especially vitamin A) and cofactors are also transported into the germinal cell line during spermatogenesis.

The physiological role of the regulatory interactions between Sertoli cells and germinal cells requires multichannel paracrine factors, which regulate and synchronize the processes taking place during the three phases of spermatogenesis: proliferation, meiosis and spermiogenesis. Since germinal cells are isolated from external influence and agents, the major regulation is via Sertoli-cell paracrine effects. For this reason, · cell-to-cell interaction is essential for bidirectional synchronization of the complicated process of spermatogenesis. A detailed description of the interaction between Sertoli and germinal cells is given in the reviews of Saez et al (1991) and Skinner (1991), and are depicted in Table 8.2 and Fig. 8.12.

Spermatogenesis is under the control of FSH and testosterone (via LH), which also regulate Sertoli-cell function. On the other hand, germ cells can regulate Sertoli-cell activity via structural and paracrine avenues. Regulation of Sertoli-cell function by germ cells has been suggested by in vivo and in vitro studies. Sertoli-cell morphology, as well as its function, varies along the length of the seminiferous tubules in conjunction with the stage of the spermatogenic cycle (Parvinen et al 1986). The nature of the germ-cell factors involved in these regulations is unknown. Some studies point to the importance of nerve growth factor (NGF), since it is produced by spermatids and affects Sertoli cells.

Inhibin is a glycoprotein secreted by Sertoli and Leydig cells. This is a dimer of α- and β-subunits that act to preferentially suppress pituitary FSH secretion both in vivo and in vitro (de Kretser &

**Table 8.2** Secretory products of the cells in the testis.

| Cell products | Propsed function |
|---|---|
| Leydig cells | |
| Androgens | Endocrine, paracrine, autocrine control |
| Proopiomelanocortin | Opioids, α-MSH, ACTH |
| Inhibin | Endocrine, paracrine activity |
| IGF-I | Growth, differentiation |
| IL-1β (macrophages) | Kinin activity |
| Sertoli cells | |
| ABP | Binding of androgens |
| Transferrin | Iron transport |
| Ceruloplasmin | Copper transport |
| Estrogen/aromatase | Endocrine paracrine regulation |
| Laminin, collagen | Extracellular matrix |
| Proteoglycans | Extracellular matrix |
| TGF-α, TGF-β, IGF-I, IL-1, | Growth factors which inhibit or stimulate cell physiology and proliferation |
| SC-EGF | |
| Inhibin, activin | Endocrine, paracrine |
| Mullerian inhibitory factor | Fetal Sertoli cell development |
| LHRH-like substance | Binds to Leydig cells in rats |
| Lactate/pyruvate | Metabolites, nutrients for germ cells |
| Peritubular cells | |
| P-Mod-S | Paracrine regulation of Sertoli cells |
| Fibronectin | Extracellular matrix |
| Proteoglycans | Extracellular matrix |
| TGF-α, TGF-β, IGF-1 | Growth factors |

Revised with permission from Skinner 1991. MSH, melanocyte stimulating hormone; ACTH, adrenocorticotropic hormone. ·

Robertson 1989, Robertson et al 1989). The β-subunits may also form dimers ($\beta_A\beta_A$ or $\beta_A\beta_B$) termed activin, which, in contrast to inhibin, stimulates FSH secretion in vitro (Vale et al 1986). Activin formed in gonads of animals (rat, porcine) is carried by a binding protein which is structurally similar to follistatin (Nakamura et al 1990). It is suggested that this binding protein has an autocrine or paracrine function in the gonad.

Coculturing of Sertoli cells, together with germ cells in the presence of activin, resulted in the formation of tubular elements, and after specific binding, some spermatogonal proliferation was noticed (Mather et al 1990).

Transforming growth factor-β (TGF-β) also belongs to the family with structural homology to activin, and it shows some of the paracrine activites of inhibin in the ovary.

Studies in men have shown that serum inhibin is regulated and maintained by the combination of both LH and FSH. Human chorionic gonadotropin treatment of hypogonadotropic, hypogonadal men was enough to stimulate inhibin secretion. Clinical studies of testicular disorders failed to show a firm correlation between serum FSH and inhibin (Robertson et al 1988). The levels of bioactive inhibin in human testicular extract were not significantly correlated to FSH or daily sperm production (Simpson et al 1987). Inhibin is produced by Sertoli and Leydig cells in rats (Risbridger et al 1989). This fact may explain the lack of a clear correlation between spermatogenesis and serum inhibin.

## Leydig–Sertoli cell interactions

Leydig cells are the major source of androgens in the testis, and are under strict control of LH. The androgens produced regulate male behavior and accessory sex-gland function in the usual endocrine manner, and support peritubular-myoid and Sertoli cell functions and spermatogenesis by way of paracrine activity. In addition to androgens, Leydig cells can potentially influence Sertoli cells through nonsteroidal factors. These are given in Table 8.3 and Figure 8.12.

Sertoli-cell function is also known to be regulated by β-endorphin synthesized by Leydig cells under LH control. These observations suggest that β-endorphin regulates inhibin secretion by inhibiting FSH receptors coupled to adenyl cyclase (Morris et al 1987). Leydig cells also secrete an oxytocin-like immunoreactive material which influences the contractibility of the seminiferous tubule by acting on the peritubular-myoid cells.

Testicular interstitial fluid (TIF) contains factors capable of stimulating testosterone secretion. In the rat it was found that these factors are produced within the testis, are derived from the various cell populations, and presumably are involved in the local regulation of the intratesticular testosterone levels (Sharpe & Cooper 1984).

Melsert et al (1988) recently reported that albumin present in the TIF is evidently an important regulator of testosterone production.

The direct effect of GnRH on gonadal function was shown by its inhibition of steroidogenesis in the ovary and testis when administered to

**Table 8.3**   Sertoli cell–Leydig cell regulatory interactions

| Potential paracrine factor | Site production | Site action | Actions/proposed function |
|---|---|---|---|
| Androgen | Leydig | Sertoli | Regulate/maintain function and differentiation |
| POMC peptides | Leydig | Sertoli | |
| β-Endorphin | | | Decrease FSH actions |
| MSH, ACTH | | | Increase FSH actions/cAMP |
| Stimulatory factor (FSH dependent or independent) | Sertoli | Leydig | Increase steroidogenesis |
| Inhibitory factor | Sertoli | Leydig | Decrease steroidogenesis |
| LHRH-like factor | Sertoli | Leydig | Decrease steroidogenesis |
| Estrogen | Sertoli | Leydig | Decrease steroidogenesis |
| IGF-I | Sertoli | Leydig | Increase steroidogenesis |
| TGFα | Sertoli | Leydig | Decrease steroidogenesis/increase growth |
| TGFβ | Sertoli | Leydig | Increase steroidogenesis |
| IL-1 | Sertoli | Leydig | Decrease steroidogenesis |
| Inhibin | Sertoli | Leydig | Increase steroidogenesis |

Reproduced with permission from Skinner 1991. POMC, proopiomelanocortin

hypophysectomized rats. Because the concentration of GnRH in blood is too low to directly regulate the gonads, it has been postulated that there is a GnRH-like paracrine control of gonadal steroidogenesis. Direct inhibition of gonadal steroidogenesis is mediated through specific high-affinity GnRH receptors. A biologically active GnRH-like peptide has been isolated from a rat testis, which can serve as a local modulator of steroidogenesis. Nevertheless, it has been shown that such activity does not take place in the human testis (Clayton & Huhtaniemi 1982).

Schaison et al (1984) studied the possible involvement of GnRH in regulation of testicular steroidogenesis. They used hypogonadotropic men treated by hCG with or without GnRH analog (GnRHa) and have shown that the antigonadal effect of GnRHa in men appears to be mediated exclusively through the pituitary.

The ability of Sertoli cells and seminiferous tubules to affect Leydig-cell function was initially observed by morphological studies on Leydig cells in damaged testes. Damage to seminiferous tubules caused by irradiation, increased temperature in cryptorchid testes, vitamin A deficiency, chemotherapy drugs, and diseases causing malfunction of the tubules, revealed changes in Leydig-cell function. In studies in vitro utilizing conditioned culture medium, factors secreted by Sertoli cells were identified and characterized as stimulators of Leydig-cell steroidogenesis (Table 8.3). Many of the stimulatory and inhibitory effects were observed with materials isolated from

Sertoli cell-conditioned medium, and may be attributed to the known regulatory agents investigated, i.e. IGF-1, TGF-α or TGF-β.

Sertoli cells in culture, derived mainly from immature rats, were found to produce factors that can stimulate (Sharpe & Cooper 1984, Verhoeven & Cailleau 1990) or inhibit (Vihko & Huhtaniemi 1989) steroidogenesis by Leydig cells.

Studies have shown that FSH treatment caused an increase in testosterone production by the testis. This is done indirectly by stimulating Sertoli cells, which in turn produce factors that modulate Leydig-cell function, especially in some stages of seminiferous tubules (stage VII and VIII in the rat). The spent solution obtained from stages IX to V of spermatogenesis in the rat tubuli was found to have the highest inhibitory activity on cAMP and testosterone productions. Since these stages are not dependent on androgens, all the data points to a possible short loop feedback control between Sertoli-germinal and Leydig-cell functions (Bergh 1983, Parvinen et al 1986).

Tubular fragments, taken from human testicular tissue when cultured in vitro, produced a factor that stimulated the production of testosterone by human interstitial cells, and by Percoll-purified Leydig cells from rat and mouse origin. The factor is a thermolabile and trypsin-sensitive protein, with a molecular weight > 10 000. Its activity is cAMP independent. The protein is similar in its behavior to the factor secreted by rat Sertoli cells in culture. The factor's production is stimulated by FSH and dibutylryl cAMP. Thus, a

Leydig cell-stimulating factor of tubular origin acts as a paracrine regulatory molecule responsible for the effects of FSH on Leydig-cell function (Verhoeven & Cailleau 1987).

It can be concluded that a bidirectional paracrine short-loop feedback exists in the testis, which regulates the activities of Leydig-, Sertoli- and germ-cell populations.

**Peritubular–Leydig–Sertoli cell interactions**

Peritubular cells are stromal cells that surround the seminiferous tubule, and are in contact with the basal surface of the Sertoli cells. These cells provide the structural integrity for the tubule, and also appear to be involved in contraction of the tubule. Both the peritubular and Sertoli cells are responsible for the secretion of the extracellular matrix, which plays a crucial role in maintenance of the integrity of the tubule and the efficiency of the blood–testis barrier (Table 8.2).

In several elegant studies using a dual chamber culture system, the presence of extracellular matrix was found to facilitate polarized secretion of specific Sertoli-cell markers: androgen binding protein (ABP), transferrin, inhibin and plasminogen activators (Dym et al 1987). Human Sertoli cells cultured in vitro in the presence of peritubular cells were stimulated, and produced increased amounts of transferrin (Holmes et al 1984).

Peritubular cells also influence Leydig-cell function by secreting paracrine factors which include IGF-1, EGF-like substances, TGF-α and TGF-β.

The functional, bidirectional interrelationship between peritubular and Sertoli cells indicates the presence of regulatory interactions between the two cells. The factors that may be involved in the mechanisms are given in Figure 8.12 and Table 8.2.

Sertoli cells are derived from epithelial cells which, during embryogenesis, come in close contact with the peritubular cells of mesenchymal origin. The mesenchymal-epithelial interaction plays an essential role in the development of a unique collaborative relationship leading to activation of Sertoli cells and production of trans-

ferrin, ABP and inhibition of FSH-inducible aromatase activity (Swinnen et al 1989, 1990).

Leydig and peritubular-myoid cell populations are derived from similar precursor mesenchymal embryonic origin. In the adult, several populations of Leydig cells can be defined (Bergh 1983). The endocrine cells, which are located around blood vessels, and paracrine cells which are attached to the seminiferous tubuli close to the peritubular cells. Peritubular cells are modulated by androgens produced by the Leydig cells. Specific androgen receptors are found in the peritubular cells. The cells respond to androgen stimulation by secretion of a protein named P-Mod-S, which is important for the maintenance of proper Sertoli-cell activity and spermatogenesis (Skinner et al 1988).

Recently, Skinner et al (1988) succeeded in the purification of two related paracrine factors, P-Mod-S (A) and P-Mod-S (B), with molecular weights of 56 000 and 59 000 respectively, both being thermolabile and trypsin-sensitive, and their production is enhanced by androgens.

The relevance of the paracrine regulation in idiopathic male infertility can be explained on the grounds that in these men most measurable testicular parameters are in the normal range, including reproductive hormones (except for elevated serum FSH, in some cases). Nevertheless, sperm production is abnormal. It is possible that in these cases some elements of the nature of paracrine regulation are not physiologically effective, causing an imbalance in the fine regulation of spermatogenesis, which leads to infertility. Thus, in the future, apart from the routine laboratory workup, paracrine factors will also be measured as a cascade of agents. Fertility evaluation will therefore be far more complicated and accurate.

## PATHOLOGY OF TESTICULAR FUNCTION

Normal testicular function is the final result of several harmonious factors. Genetic, hormonal, biochemical, anatomical and environmental variables have been shown to be the underlying causes of testicular dysfunction, leading to disturbed sperm production, and/or androgen secretion. This impairment is usually termed 'hypogo-

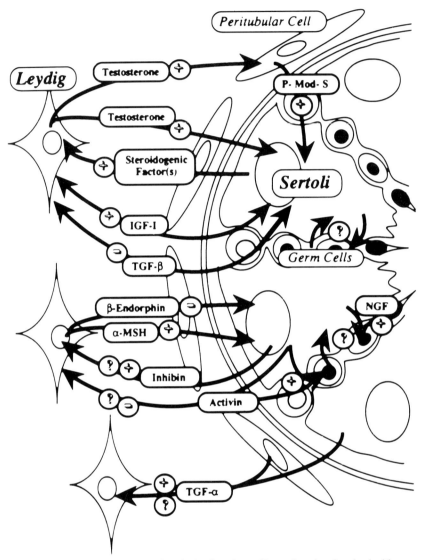

**Fig. 8.12**   Paracrine regulation of testicular functions. (Reproduced and revised with permission from Saez et al 1991)

nadism', regardless of the exact etiology. However, since the entire process in the testes is under gonadotropin control, it is common to classify the hypogonadic state into several categories: normo-gonadotropic, hypogonadotropic and hyperg-onadotropic. This classification is very practical from a clinical point of view (Table 8.4).

### Normogonadotropic hypogonadism

Some of the syndromes classified as hyper-

gonadotropic or hypogonadotropic hypogona-dism may occasionally be associated with normogonadotropin levels. However, the vast majority of these patients belong to the oligo-teratoasthenozoospermic syndrome (OTA-syndrome). This syndrome is generally characterized by poor-quality semen (low concen-tration with reduced motility and abnormal morphology) (see Ch. 12). Idiopathic OTA-syndrome is a diagnosis made by exclusion of all other etiologies which might cause the syndrome.

**Table 8.4**   Disorders leading to hypogonadism

**A. Normogonadotropic-hypogonadism**
Oligoteratoasthenozoospermia (OTA)
Disorders of different types

**B. Hypogonadotropic hypogonadism**

| *Congenital* | *Acquired* |
| --- | --- |
| Kalman's syndrome | Disorders in GnRH or gonadotropin secretion |
| Fertile eunuch syndrome | Suprasellar tumors |
| Prader–Willi syndrome | Prolactinomas |
| Laurence–Moon–Biedle syndrome | Chronic diseases |
| Mobius syndrome | |
| Multiple Lentigenes syndrome | |

**C. Hypergonadotropic hypogonadism**

| *Congenital* | *Genetic disorders* | *Enzymatic and receptor deficiency* | *Acquired* |
| --- | --- | --- | --- |
| Anorchia-testicular agenesis | Klinefelter's syndrome | 5α-reductase deficiency | Drugs |
| Testicular malposition-cryptorchidism | Chromosomal abnormalities | Testicular feminization | Chemotherapy and irradiation |
| Sertoli cell-only syndrome | XYY syndrome | Reifenstein's syndrome | Systemic diseases |
| Germinal cell arrest and hypoplasia | Ullrich–Turner's syndrome | | Heat and febrile illness |
| | Mixed gonadal dysgenesis | | |

Since sperm cells are present in the ejaculate, different empirical methods to improve its quality are employed. These include medical (drugs and hormones), surgical (high ligation of spermatic vein), and assisted reproductive technologies.

## Hypogonadotropic hypogonadism

Hypogonadotropic hypogonadism may result from developmental or acquired pituitary disease, or from failure of the hypothalamus to secrete GnRH.

### Clinical appearance

At puberty, hypogonadotropic hypogonadism results in the persistence of infantile sexual appearance resembling that of delayed puberty. The testes remain prepubertal in size, without spermatogenic activity, and the penis is small. The prostate gland is rarely palpable. The pubic and axillary hair growth is scant or absent, there is a lack of the bitemporal scalp hair recession and the voice is high-pitched. The entire body habitus is eunuchoid due to delayed epiphyseal closure in combination with diminished muscular development caused by the absence of the anabolic effect of testosterone.

However, the clinical feature of eunuchoidism is rarely encountered these days among infertile patients, since boys are usually diagnosed and treated by androgen replacement therapy at puberty. At the postpubertal age, the most common clinical symptoms are loss of potency, reduced libido, regression of secondary sex characteristics, and muscle weakness.

### Congenital syndromes

***Kallmann's syndrome*** (Kallmann et al 1944) is a familial disorder characterized by hypogonadotropic hypogonadism, partial or complete anosmia, and absence of hypothalamic GnRH secretion. This disorder is one of the most common forms of hypogonadism (Paulsen 1974).

Other developmental anomalies, i.e. craniofacial distortion, hare lip, cleft palate and cryptorchidism, are frequently associated with it. The disorder appears to be inherited as an autosomal recessive trait or an autosomal dominant trait with incomplete expressivity (Lieblich et al 1982), or by an X-linked inheritance associated with partial deletion of the short arm of the X-chromosome (Meitinger et al 1990).

In this disease, administration of GnRH will activate the pituitary gonadotropins, after some priming, to secrete LH and FSH (Yeh et al 1989).

***Fertile eunuch syndrome.*** This syndrome is characterized by spermatogenesis which coexists with variable dysfunction of Leydig cells.

Androgen function improves after treatment with hCG (Pasqualini & Bur 1950). The syndrome is a variant of hypogonadotropic eunuchoidism with variable habitus, dependent upon the extent of androgen deficiency. In the most extreme variant, the patient has an eunuchoid appearance, low plasma testosterone, and low ejaculate volume which contains apparently normal spermatozoa. In mild cases, testosterone secretion is sufficient to bring about epiphyseal closure, but insufficient to establish complete virilization. Plasma LH concentrations are at the low to normal levels, and FSH concentration is within the normal range.

It is believed that in some cases the intratesticular concentration of testosterone is high enough to maintain spermatogenesis, but in most patients the plasma concentration is too low to induce and maintain normal masculine characteristics.

*Prader – Willi syndrome.* This rare syndrome is associated with massive obesity, mental retardation, short stature, small hands and feet, cryptorchidism and diabetes mellitus. It occurs in 1/30 000 births. Chromosomal analysis reveals a high frequency of deletion and translocation involving chromosome 15q (Pauli et al 1983). The hypogonadism appears to be of hypothalamic origin, since the response to GnRH stimulation is normal (Bray et al 1983).

*Laurence – Moon – Biedle syndrome.* This rare syndrome is characterized by retarded growth, obesity, retinitis pigmentosa, syndactyly, polydactyly and mental retardation. The pathophysiology is not clear, except for the fact that there is a high rate of consanguinity among the parents. The inheritance is autosomal recessive, and the degree of gonadotropin deficiency is variable (Toledo et al 1977).

Additional syndrome complexes associated with hypogonadotropic hypogonadism include 'Mobius syndrome' (Bardin 1971), and the *multiple lentigenes syndrome* (Gorlin et al 1969), which are very rare.

### Acquired syndromes

In addition to the syndromes cited above in which there is an isolated absence of GnRH, there are several other disorders which disturb the normal function of the hypothalamus or hypophysis, and result in hypogonadotropic hypogonadism. A long list of disturbances such as neoplasms, inflammatory lesions, degenerative disorders, pituitary stalk section, vascular lesions and head trauma can cause absence of GnRH or gonadotropin secretion.

*Suprasellar tumors.* Craniopharyngioma, metastasis, or downward extension of pinealoma, and upward extension of pituitary lesions, may cause hypogonadotropic hypogonadism. The impairment in the gonadotrope's function may be partial or complete, and is caused by injury or destruction of the cells by the tumor, surgery, or as a result of the empty sella syndrome. Lesions arising below the hypothalamus may present with anterior pituitary insufficiency, growth deficit, diabetes insipidus, and impotence, while lesions arising in the hypothalamus are more likely to display a variety of symptoms, including altered food intake, and abnormal temperature control (Christy & Warren 1989).

In the absence of functional gonadotropic cells, the basal FSH and LH secretion is low, and does not respond to GnRH stimulation. Apart from the neurological manifestation associated with the tumor, the hypogonadic clinical symptoms are associated with infrequent need to shave, loss of libido or potency, and loss of body hair.

*Prolactinomas* of the pituitary are characterized by elevated serum prolactin levels and may lead to hypogonadism without any direct impairment of the gonadotrophs. Blockade of the portal veins by the adenoma may prevent the hypothalamic prolactin-inhibiting factor from reaching the hypophysis, and cause elevation of the plasma prolactin level. Hyperprolactinemia may be associated with decreased testosterone secretion, and impaired spermatogenesis (Carter et al 1978).

*Chronic diseases.* Diseases such as renal failure, cirrhosis, and infections may be followed by hypothalamic hypogonadism.

## Hypergonadotropic hypogonadism

Infertility due to primary seminiferous tubule

dysfunction and hypergonadotropic hypogonadism without other endocrine manifestations occurs frequently. The most common in this category is Klinefelter's syndrome. The next most frequent types are hypogonadism due to developmental disorders such as cryptorchidism and anorchia, and cases caused by trauma, irradiation and medical manipulation.

### Congenital syndromes

***Anorchia-testicular agenesis.*** In this syndrome patients have 46 XY chromosomes. The testes fail to develop or undergo atrophy during intrauterine life. Atrophy most likely occurs between gestational weeks 7 and 14, as a result of mechanical trauma (Huff et al 1991). The clinical findings are those of complete prepubertal castrate. The patients are born with normal external genitalia. However, no testes are present in the scrotum, and none can be detected in the inguinal canal, peritoneal cavity or the retroperitoneal space. The scrotum may contain small masses – remnants of the Wolffian duct. The patients fail to develop secondary sex characteristics, and eventually have typical eunuchoid phenotype.

The diagnosis is relatively simple. This syndrome is associated with very high serum gonadotropin levels due to the negative feedback, and very low testosterone levels. The patients will fail to respond to exogenous hCG stimulation. It is important to differentiate this condition from bilateral cryptorchidism.

***Testicular malposition (cryptorchidism).*** This category includes inguinal, abdominal or retroperitoneal testes, and in rare instances suprapubic or perineal testes. Failure of testes to descend during embryonal life or after birth will result in impairment of the spermatogenic process and androgen production. Incidence of testicular malposition is 0.8% at birth, and declines to 0.3% at puberty. The etiology of testicular malposition is not clear and may involve several factors such as hormonal, genetic, anatomical abnormalities of the descending pathway, and intrinsic defects in the testes (Yavetz et al 1992b).

Based upon their own experience as well as that of others, Hadziselimovic et al (1987) suggested treatment with GnRH as the drug of choice during the first year of life, or hCG treatment in cases where the former treatment failed to induce testicular descent. Orchidopexy should be performed after failed medical treatment and before 3 years of age. This approach is recommended in order to reduce the histopathological changes in the cryptorchid testes, which worsen with the duration of the malposition (Hezmall & Lipshultz 1982). These changes give rise to reduced sperm, generally ranging from variable degrees of oligoteratoasthenozoospermia up to azoospermia in extreme cases (Yavetz et al 1992b).

Besides the hypogonadism associated with malposition of the testes, there is a 35-fold increase in the incidence of neoplasia in the persistent cryptorchid testes (Witherington 1984).

***Sertoli-cell-only syndrome.*** This syndrome described by del Castillo et al (1947) is characterized by azoospermia associated with small seminiferous tubules and lack of germinal epithelium. An incidence of 3.4% among infertile patients was reported (Dubin & Amelar 1971).

Except for azoospermia, phenotypically the patients with this syndrome are normal males. All the other seminal characteristics seem to be normal. Thus the syndrome can be verified only by testicular biopsy. The microscopic examination reveals seminiferous tubules devoid of germ cells, lined by Sertoli cells which appear to be normal in shape. The FSH levels are normal or elevated, and the testosterone and LH levels are within the normal range. The etiology of this syndrome is not known.

***Germinal cell arrest and hypoplasia.*** These conditions are usually associated with oligozoospermia or azoospermia. In cases of germinal cells arrest, spermatogenesis is normal up to a certain stage. Thus no matured sperm are present (azoospermia). In hypoplasia, all stages of development are present but in reduced numbers. Active Leydig cells are found with normal steroidogenesis. Serum FSH is usually elevated, and LH and testosterone are in the normal range (Paulsen 1974).

*Genetic disorders*

Included in this category are some chromosomal impaired arrangements other than Klinefelter's syndrome, defects in hormone synthesis, and hormone receptor failure.

***Chromosomal abnormalities.*** The incidence of chromosomal abnormalities among patients with impaired spermatogenesis has been reported to be between 2% to 21%, being low among patients with low sperm count, and high among azoospermic men (de Kretser et al 1972, Matsuda et al 1989). The most common abnormalities are: D-D translocations, ring chromosomal abnormalities, reciprocal translocations, and Robertsonian aberrations. A 3.5% incidence of somatic chromosomal abnormalities in the infertile population and 10.5% incidence of abnormalities in the Y chromosome were also reported (Hendry et al 1976).

***Klinefelter's syndrome.*** This syndrome is the most common chromosomal abnormality associated with testicular dysfunction (up to 1/500 newborn males). Although hypogonadism was not initially regarded as part of the picture in its original description (Klinefelter et al 1942), it is now apparent that the clinical symptoms range from nearly normal external genitalia with feminine-like body hair, and diminished beard growth, gynecomastia and poor muscular development, up to the full-blown eunuchoid characteristics (Hsueh et al 1978).

The syndrome is characterized by a 47XXY karyotype pattern in 90% of patients. Other patterns include an array of extra X chromosomes, 48XXYY, 48XXXY, 49XXXXY, and a varying degree of mosaicism (46XY/47XXY). It was suggested that any phenotypic male who demonstrates two or more X chromosomes plus at least one Y chromosome in all or part of the cells in the body should be included in this syndrome (Leonard et al 1975). The mosaics account for the high proportion with unusual clinical variant. However, in the classic form of the disorder, small, firm testes with defective spermatogenesis or azoospermia are present in virtually all patients. The testicular histology consists of hyalinization and fibrosis of the seminiferous tubules (Paulsen 1974). In cases of mosaicism, areas of spermatogenesis have been described as being associated with poor sperm production (Gomez-Acebo et al 1968).

The Leydig cells are concentrated in prominent clumps and exhibit anisochromia, absence of Reinke crystals, abnormal mitochondria and endoplasmatic reticulum (Ahmad et al 1971).

The abnormalities seen in the Leydig cell correlate with the relatively low testosterone plasma concentration of most of the Klinefelter syndrome patients. The characteristically elevated plasma LH (as well as FSH) provides additional evidence of Leydig-cell impairment.

***The XYY syndrome.*** This syndrome affects approximately 0.2% of the male population. Some studies have shown that these patients have antisocial behavior because the incidence of this karyotype in the prison population is about 10-fold higher than in newborn males (Wiener et al 1968).

The phenotypic expression of this disorder is variable. Characteristically these patients are tall and have pustular acne. Occasionally spermatogenesis and steroidogenesis may be normal.

***Ullrich–Turner's syndrome.*** These are 46XY individuals who resemble phenotypic characteristics of Turner's syndrome. They are characterized by short stature, low-set ears, webbed neck and cardiovascular abnormalities. The affected patients have male external genitalia, with undescended testes being common. Spermatogenesis is rarely normal, and usually germinal aplasia occurs. The Leydig-cell function is impaired. The inheritance is autosomal, dominant and incomplete penetrance is common. (Grumbach & Conte 1985).

***Mixed gonadal dysgenesis 45X0/46XY.*** Patients with this syndrome are diagnosed at birth, however this disorder in its mildest form may not be detected until adulthood. Phenotypically the patients lack complete virilization and up to 60% have been reared as females. However, in the mildest form, normal virilization, including a complete phallic urethra has been reported. The most common karyotype is 45X0/46XY. After puberty, despite the fact that the patients develop masculine features, the seminiferous tubules lack the germinal elements and contain only Sertoli cells (Davidoff & Federman 1973).

*Enzymatic and receptor deficiency*

Five enzymatic conversions are required to synthesize testosterone from cholesterol: 20,22-desmolase, 3β-hydroxysteroid dehydrogenase, 17α-hydroxylase, 17,20-desmolase and 17β-hydroxysteroid dehydroxygenase. Impaired testosterone synthesis has been reported as a result of a defect in each of these enzymes. From a clinical point of view, such defects result in male pseudohermaphroditism. The Wollffian duct derivatives are rudimentary or absent, depending on the severity of the block. The external genitalia are female or ambiguous, with an enlarged clitoris, and blind-ended vagina.

Mullerian duct derivatives are absent because of the secretion of Mullerian duct inhibitory substances by the fetal Sertoli cells. The testes in these patients may be intra-abdominal, in the inguinal canal or in the labioscrotal folds. Plasma testosterone concentration is low, and challenging its secretion by hCG may result in a rise in the steroid precursor proximal to the enzyme block. Gonadotropin levels tend to be elevated. (New 1970, Schneider et al 1975, Zachmann et al 1982, Rosler & Kohn 1983, Hauffa et al 1985).

**5α-reductase deficiency.** Autosomal recessive inheritance deficiency of the enzyme 5α-reductase blocks the conversion of testosterone to DHT. In 46XY patients, this deficiency leads to male pseudohermaphroditism (Peterson et al 1977). Among these patients Wolffian duct derivatives are present because testosterone production is normal. The male external genitalia, however, which normally develop under the control of DHT, cannot be produced and these patients present with enlarged clitoris, urogenital sinus, labial testes and labial-like scrotum. At puberty striking virilization occurs (Imperato-McGinley et al 1991). Histological examination of adult testes shows Leydig-cell hyperplasia. Adult subjects in whom descent of testes occurs at puberty have normal spermatogenesis, while those with undescended testes have typical findings of cryptorchid testes.

The virilization at puberty is due either to the effect of the large increase in testosterone acting directly, or to the conversion of small amounts of testosterone to DHT.

**Testicular feminization (androgen-resistance syndrome).** This disorder, transmitted by an X-linked recessive gene in 46XY males, is characterized by total resistance to the virilizing and metabolic influences of testosterone. It is now apparent that the problems lie in a wide range of quantitative and qualitative defects in the intracellular receptor to DHT (Marcelli et al 1991). Thus, the androgens fail to bind to the cell nucleus receptor to exert its biological effect (Kaufman et al 1976).

In its complete form the syndrome occurs in 1/60 000 males (Meyer et al 1975). Phenotypically the patient has a female appearance. The breasts are fully developed, although the areola and nipples are rather small. Pubic and axillary hair is sparse or totally absent. The external genitalia develop to a vagina which terminates blindly and is shorter than usual. The mullerian derivatives are absent. Testes are usually found in the inguinal canal, but they may be abdominal.

These individuals have normal, or slightly elevated plasma testosterone and estrogen concentrations, elevated LH levels, and normal to slightly elevated FSH levels (Imperato-McGinley et al 1982). Histologically the testes resemble those of cryptorchid patients, with a reduced number of germ cells in the tubuli, combined with Leydig-cell hyperplasia (Ferenczy & Richart 1972). Feminization of these individuals is believed to be caused as a result of relatively high concentrations of estrogens of both testicular and peripheral conversion, acting unopposed along with androgen resistance.

In the incomplete form of testicular feminization, the appearance of the patients is similar to the complete form, except that the genitalia are ambiguous, with some pubic hair, enlarged clitoris, and partial fusion of the labioscrotal folds.

**Reifenstein's syndrome.** This rare syndrome is now regarded as a less severe variant of the androgen-resistant, genetically determined syndrome (Griffin et al 1982). The individuals are phenotypically males. However, due to the androgen deficiency during development and maturation, there is deficient virilization, gynecomastia, cryptorchid testes and severe hypospadias. Pubic hair growth is almost normal, but beard growth is scant. The Wolffian duct derivatives may be present, rudimentary or absent. Men are either azoospermic or oligozoospermic (Aiman et al 1979).

### Acquired

Different factors may impair or alter the normal process of spermatogenesis, and cause infertility. The most sensitive cell in the spermatogenic line seems to be the spermatid, while spermatogonia were found to be the least sensitive, except for *irradiation* and *chemotherapeutic drug* damage (Meistreich 1986). The Sertoli cells are also vulnerable to injury, while the Leydig cells are less affected.

Systemic diseases and *drugs* which affect one of the intratesticular cells and alter its normal function may cause hypogonadism. These factors include: environmental hazards (*heat* and irradiation); systemic diseases (diabetes mellitus, renal failure, cystic fibrosis); infectious diseases (mumps, orchitis); therapeutic drugs (dopamine blockers, sulfasalazine and furadantin); drug abuse (opioids), and vascular disturbances (varicocele). However, since these factors are discussed in detail in other chapters of this book, they will not be elaborated further here.

## CLOSING REMARKS

The endocrine regulation of testicular functions is well established. Both long- and short-loop feedbacks control the two major axes (Fig. 8.1). The GnRH–gonadotrope–LH–Leydig cell–testosterone axis and the GnRH–gonadotrope–FSH–Sertoli cell–spermatogenesis. While disturbances of the first axis are easy to diagnose and treat, according to the cause of the problem, disorders of the second axis are possible to diagnose, but if the disease is of testicular origin,

no available medical methods for monitoring and treatment are available.

Most of the cases with failure of Sertoli cell–cell interaction lead to the OTA-syndrome; hence the intensive research carried out on the paracrine regulation of testicular function. No reliable marker is available to monitor Sertoli-cell-germ–cell interaction in semen or blood. The use of inhibin and transferrin as possible intratubular markers has been proven to be unrelated to any particular step of spermatogenesis, and their intratesticular measurement is most difficult. Sharpe (1992) suggested a search for a specific marker of meiosis which is possibly secreted by Sertoli cells. This hypothetical marker, once found, can be used for monitoring sperm production, and hence provide some clue for the fine paracrine regulation of spermatogenesis. In regard to this approach, the sulfated glycoprotein-2 (SGP-2), also called 'clusterin', is a major protein product of the Sertoli cell. This protein covers the surface of the sperm cell and is endocytosed in the rete testis, but a smaller form of SGP-2 is secreted by the caput epididymis and attaches to the sperm surface. Clinical studies of this molecule have found certain value in measuring SGP-2 in seminal plasma for predicting in vitro fertilization outcome (O'Bryan et al 1990).

Thus, it is possible that in the near future new markers will be available in order to monitor spermatogenesis and the activity of the cells involved in this process. Today, it is obvious that inhibin cannot serve as a reliable marker, since it is secreted by both Sertoli and Leydig cells.

Andrologists are seeking new developments in this field in order to focus the treatment of the problem diagnosed and to obtain tools for monitoring seminiferous tubular activity.

## ACKNOWLEDGEMENT

The authors are grateful to Mrs Renée Berman for the illustrations, and Mrs Carmela Perl for the photography workup.

# REFERENCES

Ahmad K N, Dykes J R, Ferguson-Smith MA et al 1971
Leydig cell volume in chromatin-positive Klinefelter's
syndrome. J Clin Endocrinol Metab 33: 517

Aiman J, Griffin J E, Gazah J M et al 1979 Androgen
insensitivity as a cause of infertility in otherwise normal
men. Engl J Med 300: 223

Amann R P 1981 A critical review of methods for evaluation
of spermatozoa from seminal characteristics. J Androl 2: 37

Bardin C W 1971 Hypogonadotropic hypogonadism in
patients with multiple congenital defects. In: Bergsma D
(ed) Birth defects, vol 7, part 10. Williams & Wilkins,
Baltimore, pp 175–178

Bardin C W 1986 Pituitary–testicular axis, In: Yen S S C,
Jaffe R B (eds) Endocrine regulation of the reproductive
system, 2nd edn. Saunders, Philadelphia, pp 177–199

Barr A B, Moore D J, Paulsen C A 1971 Germinal cell loss
during human spermatogenesis. J Reprod Fertil 25: 75

Bergh A 1983 Paracrine regulation of Leydig cells by the
seminiferous tubules. Int J Androl 6: 57

Bergh A, Ason-Berg A, Damber J E, Hammar M, Selstam G
1984 Steroid biosynthesis and Leydig cell morphology in
adult unilaterally cryptorchid rats. Acta Endocrinol 107:
556

Bray G A, Dahms W T, Swerdloff R S, Fiser R H,
Atkinson R L, Carrel R E 1983 The Prader–Willi
syndrome. A study of 40 patients and a review of the
literature. Medicine 62: 59

Cailleau J, Vermeire S, Verhoeven C 1990 Independent
control of the production of insulin-like growth factor 1 and
its binding protein by cultured testicular cells. Molec Cell
Endocrinol 69: 79

Cater J N, Tyson J E, Tolis G, Van Vilet S, Faiman C,
Friesen H G 1978 Prolactin-screening tumors and
hypogonadism in 22 men. N Engl J Med 299: 847

Casano R, Orlando C, Serio M, Forti G 1991 LDH and
LDH-X activity in sperm from normospermic and
oligozoospermic men. Int J Androl 14: 257

Chemes H, Dym M, Fawcett D W, Jaradpour N, Sherins R J
1977 Pathophysiological observations of Sertoli cells in
patients with germinal aplasia or severe germ cell depletion.
Ultrastructural findings and hormone levels. Biol Reprod
17: 108

Christensen A K 1975 Leydig cells. In: Greep R O, Astwood
E B (eds) Handbook of physiology, section 7, vol 5.
American Physiological Society, Washington DC,
pp 57–94

Christy N P, Warren M P 1989 Other clinical syndromes of
the hypothalamus and anterior pituitary, including tumor
mass effects. In: DeGroot L J (ed) Endocrinology, vol 3.
Saunders, Philadelphia, pp 419–454

Clayton R N, Huhtaniemi I 1982 Absence of gonadotropin-
releasing hormone receptors in human gonadal tissue.
Nature 299: 56

Clermont Y 1963 The cycle of the seminiferous epithelium in
man. Am J Anat 112: 35

Clermont Y 1972 Kinetics of spermatogenesis in mammals:
seminiferous epithelium cycle and spermatogonial renewal.
Physiol Rev 52: 198

Clermont Y, Antar M 1973 Duration of the cycle of the
seminiferous epithelium and the spermatogonial renewal in
the monkey Macaca arctoides. Am J Anat 136: 153

Davidoff F, Federman D D 1973 Mixed gonadal dysgenesis.
Pediatrics 52: 725

de Kretser D M, Burger H G 1972 Ultrastructural studies of
the human Sertoli cell in normal men and males with
hypogonadotropic hypogonadism before and after
gonadotropic treatment. In: Saxena B B, Beling C G,
Gandy H M (eds) Gonadotropins. Wiley Interscience, New
York, p 640

de Kretser D M, Robertson D M 1989 The isolation and
physiology of inhibin and related proteins. Biol Reprod 40:
33

de Kretser D M, Burger H G, Fortune D, Hudson B,
Long A R, Paulsen C A, Taft H P 1972 Hormonal,
histological and chromosomal studies in adult males with
testicular disorders. J Clin Endocrinol Metab 35: 392

del Castillo E, Trabucco A, de La Balze F 1947 Syndrome
produced by absence of germinal epithelium without
impairment of the Sertoli cells. J Clin Endocrinol Matab 7:
493

di Zerega G S, Sherins R J 1980 Endocrine control of adult
testicular function. In: Burger H, de Kretser D (eds) The
testis. Raven, New York, pp 127–140

Dubin L, Amelar R D 1971 Etiologic factors in 1294
consecutive cases of male infertility. Fertil Steril 22: 469

Dufau M L 1988 Endocrine regulation and communicating
functions of the Leydig cell. Ann Rev Physiol 50: 483

Dym M, Fawcett D W 1970 The blood–testis barrier in the
rat and the physiological compartmentation of the
seminiferous epithelium. Biol Reprod 3: 308

Dym M, Cavicchia J C 1978 Functional morphology of the
testis. Biol Reprod 18: 1

Dym M, Hadley M A, Djakiew D, Byers S W 1987
Differentiation and polarized function of Sertoli cells in
vitro. Adv Exp Med Biol 219: 515

Eliasson R, Virji N 1985 LDH-C$_4$ in human seminal plasma
and its relationship to testicular function. II. Clinical
aspects. International J Androl 8: 201

Fawcett D W 1975 Observations on the organization of the
interstitial tissue of the testis and on the occluding cell
functions in the seminiferous epithelium. In: Raspe G,
Bernhard S (eds) Advances in the biosciences, Schering
Symposium on Contraception, vol 10. Pergamon, New
York, pp 83–99

Fawcett D W 1979 The cell biology of gametogenesis in the
male. Perspect Biol Med Winter: 556

Ferenczy A, Richart R M 1972 The fine structure of the
gonads in the complete form of testicular feminization
syndrome. Am J Obstet Gynecol 113: 399

Franchimont P 1980 Hormonal regulation of testicular
function. In: Cunningham G R, Schill W B, Hafez E S E
(eds) Regulation of male fertility. Martinus Nijhoff, The
Netherlands, pp 5–14

Glass A R, Vigersky R A 1991 Pituitary–testicular axis. In:
Lipshulz L I, Howards S S (eds) Infertility in the male, 2nd
edn. Mosby Year Book, St Louis, pp 21–36

Gomez-Acebo J, Parrilla R, Abrisqueta J A, Pozuelo V 1988
Fine structure of spermatogenesis in Klinefelter's
syndrome. J Clin Endocrinol Metab 28: 1287

Gorlin R J, Anderson R C, Blaw N 1969 Multiple lentigenes
syndrome. Am J Dis Child 117: 652

Granner D K 1988 Hormones of the gonads, In: Murray R K,
Granner D K, Mayes P A, Rodwell J W (eds) Harper's
biochemistry, 21st edn. Appleton and Lange, Norwalk,
pp 530–536

Griffin J E, Wilson J D 1983 Disorders of the testis. In:

Petersdorf R G, Adams R D, Braunwald E, Isselbacher K J, Martin J B, Wilson J D (eds) Harrison's principles of internal medicine, 10th edn. McGraw Hill International, Auckland, pp 689–700

Griffin J E, Leshin M, Wilson J D 1982 Androgen resistance syndromes. Am J Physiol 243: E81

Grumbach M M, Conte F A 1985 Disorders of sexual differentiation. In: Wilson J D, Foster D W (eds) Williams' textbook of endocrinology, 7th edn. Saunders, Philadelphia, pp 312–401

Hadziselimovic F, Herzog B, Bauer H 1987 Development of cryptorchid testes. Eur J Pediatr 146 (suppl 2):S8

Hauffa B P, Miller W L, Grumbach M M, Conte F A, Kaplan S L 1985 Congenital adrenal hyperplasia due to deficient cholesterol side-chain cleavage activity (20,22 desmolase) in a patient treated for 18 years. Clin Endocrinol 23: 481

Heller C G, Clermont Y 1963 Spermatogenesis in man and estimate of its duration. Science 140: 184

Hendry W F, Polani P E, Pugh R C B, Sommerville I F, Wallace D M 1976 200 infertile males: correlation of chromosome, histological, endocrine, and clinical studies. Br J Urol 47: 899

Hezmall H P, Lipshultz L 1982 Cryptorchidism and infertility. Urol Clin North Am 9: 361

Holmes S D, Lipshultz L I, Smith R G 1984 Regulation of transferrin secretion by *human* Sertoli cells cultured in the presence or absence of *human* peritubular cells. J Clin Endocrinol Metab 59: 1058

Holstein A G 1967 Die glatte muskulatur in der tunica albuginea des hodens und ihr einflus auf den spermatozoentransport in den nebenhoden. Ergebnisse Anat Anz 121: 103

Horton R 1989 Testicular steroid secretion, metabolism and mode of action, In: DeGroot L J (ed) Endocrinology, vol 3, 2nd edn. Saunders Philadelphia, pp 2146–2151

Hsueh W A, Hsu T H, Federman D D 1978 Endocrine features of Klinefelter's syndrome. Medicine 57: 447

Huckins C, Meacham R B 1991 Spermatogenesis in the adult: characteristics, kinetics and control. In: Lipshultz L I, Howards S S (eds) Infertility in the male. Mosby Year Book, St Louis, p 84

Huff D S, Wu H Y, Snyder H M 3rd, Hadziselimovic F, Blythe B, Duckett J W 1991 Evidence in favor of the mechanical (intrauterine torsion) theory over the endocrinopathy (cryptorchidism) theory in the pathogenesis of gesticular agenesis. J Urol 146: 630

Imperato-McGinley J, Peterson R E, Gautier T et al 1982 Hormonal evaluation of a large kindred with complete androgen insensitivty: evidence for secondary 5α-reductase. J Clin Endocrinol Metab 54: 931

Imperato-McGinley J, Miller M, Wilson J D, Peterson R E, Shackleton C, Gajdusek D C 1991 A cluster of male pseudohermaphrodites with 5 alpha-reductase deficiency in Papua New Guinea. Clin Endocrinol (Oxf) 34: 293

Ishigami K, Yoshida Y, Hirooka M, Mohri K 1970 A new operation for varicocele: use of microvascular anastomosis. Surgery 67: 620

Jacobs H S, Bouchard P, Conway C S et al 1991 Role of growth hormone in infertility. Horm Res 36 (suppl 1): 61

Johnson L 1986 Review article: spermatogenesis and aging in the human. J Androl 7: 331

Johnson L, Petty C S, Neaves W B 1981 A new approach to quantification of spermatogenesis and its application to germinal cell attrition during human spermiogenesis. Biol Reprod 25: 217

Johnson L, Petty C S, Porter Z C, Neaves W B 1984a Germ cell degeneration during postprophase of meiosis and serum concentrations of gonadotropins in young adult and older adult men. Biol Reprod 31: 779

Johnson L, Zane R S, Petty C S, Neaves W B 1984b Quantification of the human Sertoli cell population: its distribution, relation to germ cell numbers, and age-related decline. Biol Reprod 31: 785

Johnson L, Petty C S, Neaves W B 1984c Influence of age on sperm production and testicular weights in men. J Reprod Fertil 70: 211

Johnson L, Petty C S, Neaves W B 1986 Age-related variation in seminiferous tubules in men: a stereologic evaluation. J Androl 7: 316

Johnson L, Nguyen H B, Petty C S, Neaves W B 1987 Quantification of human spermatogenesis: germ cell degeneration during spermatocytogenesis and meiosis in testes from younger and older adult men. Biol Reprod 37: 739

Kallman F, Schonfeld W A, Barrera S E 1944 The genetic primary eunuchoidism. Am J Ment Deficiency 48: 203

Kaufman M, Straidfeld C, Pinsky L 1976 Male pseudohermaphrodism presumably due to target organ unresponsiveness to androgens: deficient 5α-dihydrotestosterone binding in cultured skin fibroblasts. J Clin Invest 58: 345–350

Kerr J B 1989 The cytology of the human testis. In: Burger H, de Kretser D (eds) The testis. Raven, New York, pp 197–229

Klinefelter H F, Reifenstein E C, Albright F 1942 Syndrome characterized by gynecomastia, spermatogenesis, without A-Leydigism and increased excretion of follicle stimulating hormone. J Clin Endocrinol 2: 615

Kormano M, Suoranta H 1971 Microvascular organization of the adult human testis. Anat Rec 170: 31

Koskimies A I, Kormano M, Alfthan O 1973 Proteins of the seminiferous tubule fluid in man: evidence for a blood testis barrier. J Reprod Fertil 32: 79

Kurth B E, Klotz K, Flickinger C J, Herr J C 1991 Localization of sperm antigen SP–10 during the six stages of the cycle of the seminiferous epithelium in man. Biol Reprod 44: 814

Lennox B, Ahmad K N 1970 The total length of tubules in the human testis. J Anat 107: 191

Leonard J M, Bremner W J, Capell P T, Paulsen C A 1975 Male Hypogonadism: Klinefelter and Reifenstein syndromes, In: Bergsma D (ed) National foundation. Birth defects original article series, genetic forms of hypogonadism, pp 17–22

Lieblich J M, Rogol A D, White B J, Rosen S W 1982 Syndrome of anosmia with hypogonadotropin hypogonadism (Kallman syndrome): clinical and laboratory studies in 23 cases. Am J Med 73: 50

Lombard-Vignon N, Grizard G, Boucher D 1991 Influence of rat testicular macrophages on Leydig cell function in vitro. Int J Androl 15: 144

Marcelli M, Zoppi S, Grino P B, Griffin J E, Wilson J D, McPaul M J 1991 A mutation in the DNA-binding domain of the androgen receptor gene causes complete testicular feminization in a patient with receptor-positive androgen resistance. J Clin Invest 87: 1123

Mather J P, Attie K M, Woodruff T K 1990 Activin stimulates spermatogonial proliferation in germ-Sertoli cell cocultures from immature rat testis. Endocrinology 127: 3206

Matsuda T, Nonomura M, Okada K, Hayashi K, Yoshida O 1989 Cytogenetic survey of subfertile males in Japan. Urologia Internationalis 44: 194–197

Matsumoto A M, Bremner W J 1987 Endocrinology of the hypothalamic–pituitary–testicular axis with particular reference to the hormonal control of spermatogenesis. Bailliere's Clin Endocrinol Metab 1: 71

Matsumoto A M, Karpas A E, Paulsen C A, Bremner W J 1983 Reinitiation of sperm production in gonadotropin-suppressed normal men by administration of follicle-stimulating hormone. J Clin Invest 72: 1005

Means A R, Fakunding J L, Hackins C, Tindall D J, Vitale R 1976 Follicle-stimulating hormone, the Sertoli cell and spermatogenesis. Recent Prog Horm Res 32: 477

Meistrich M L 1986 Critical components of testicular function and sensitivity to disruption. Biol Reprod 34: 17

Meitinger T, Heye B, Petit C et al 1990 Definitive localization of X-linked Kallman syndrome (hypogonadotropic hypogonadism and anosmia) to Xp22.3: close linkage to the hypervariable repeat sequence CRI-S232. Am J Hum Genet 47: 664

Melsert R, Hoogerbrugge J W, Rommerts F F C 1988 The albumin fraction of rat testicular fluid stimulates steroid production by isolated Leydig cells. Molec Cell Endocrinol 59: 221

Meyer W J III, Migeon B R, Migeon C J 1975 Focus on human X chromosome for dihydrotesterone receptor and androgen insensitivity. Proc Natl Acad Sci USA 72: 1469

Miyake K, Yamamoto M, Narita H, Hashimoto S, Mitsuya H 1986 Evidence for contractility of the human seminiferous tubule confirmed by its response to noradrenaline and acetylcholine. Fertil Steril 46: 734

Morris P L, Vale W W, Bardin C W 1987 Beta-endorphin regulation of FSH-stimulated inhibin production is a component of a short loop system in testis. Biochem Biophys Res Commun 148: 1513

Nakamura M, Namiki M, Oknayama A et al 1988 Optimal temperature for synthesis of DNA, RNA and protein by human testis in vitro. Arch Androl 20: 41

Nakamura T, Takio K, Eto Y, Shibai H, Titani K, Sugino H 1990 Activin-binding protein from rat ovary is follistatin. Science 247: 836

New M I 1970 Male pseudohermaphrodism due to 17α-hydroxylase deficiency. J Clin Invest 49: 1930

O'Bryan M K, Baker H W G, Saunders J R et al 1990 Human seminal clusterin (SP-40, 40) isolation and characterization. J Clin Invest 85: 1477

Odell W D 1989 The Leydig cell, In: DeGroot L J (ed) Endocrinology, vol 3, 2nd edn. Saunders, Philadelphia, pp 2137–2145

Paniagua R, Rodriguez M C, Nistal M, Fraile B, Amat P 1987 Changes in the lipid inclusion/Sertoli cell cytoplasm area ratio during the cycle of the human seminiferous epithelium. J Reprod Fertil 80: 335

Parvinen M, Vihko K K, Toppari J 1986 Cell interactions during the seminiferous epithelial cycle. Int Rev Cytol 104: 115

Pasqualini R Q, Bur G E 1950 Sindrome hipandrogenico con gametogenesis conservada: clarification de la insufficiencia testicular. Rev Assoc Med Argent 64: 6

Pauli R M, Meisner L F, Szmanda R J 1983 'Expanded' Prader–Willi syndrome in a boy with an unusual 15q chromosome deletion. Am J Dis Child 137: 1087

Paulsen C A 1974 The testes. In: Williams R H (eds) Textbook of endocrinology, 5th edn. Saunders, Philadelphia, pp 323–367

Paz G, Lewin L M, Yavetz H, Yogev L, Gamzu R, Jaffo A, Homonnal Z T 1992 Seminal plasma transferrin and male fertility. Assisted Reprod Technol/Androl (in press)

Peterson R E, Imperato-McGinley J, Gautier T, Sturla E 1977 Male pseudohermaphroditism due to steroid 5α-reductase deficiency. Am J Med 62: 170

Reader S C, Shingles C, Stonard M D 1991 Acute testicular toxicity of 13-dinitrobenzene and ethylene glycol monomethyl ether in the rat: evaluation of biochemical effect markers and hormonal responses. Fundam Appl Toxicol 16: 61

Risbridger G P, Clements J, Robertson D M, Drummond A E, Muir J, Burger H G, de Kretser D M 1989 Immuno and bioactive inhibin α-subunit expression in rat Leydig cell cultures. Molec Cell Endocrinol 67: 438

Ritzen E M, Hansson V, French F S 1989 The Sertoli cell. In: Burger H, de Kretser D (eds) The testis. Raven, New York, pp 269–301

Robertson D M, Tsonis C G, McLachlan R I et al 1988 Comparison of inhibin immunological and in vitro biological activities in human serum. J Clin Endocrinol Metab 67: 438

Robertson D M, McLachlan R I, Burger H C, de Kretser D M 1989 Inhibin and inhibin-related proteins in the male, In: Burger H, de Kretser D (eds) The testis. Raven, New York, pp 231–253

Rommerts F F G, van der Molen H J 1989 Testicular steroidogenesis, In: Burger H, de Kretser D (eds) The testis, 2nd edn. Raven, New York, pp 303–328

Roosen-Runge E C, Holstein A F 1987 The human rete testis. Cell Tissue Res 189: 409

Rosler A, Kohn G 1983 Male pseudohermaphrodism due to 17β-hydroxysteroid dehydrogenase deficiency: studies on the natural history of the defect and effect of androgens on gender role. J Steroid Biochem 39: 663

Russell L D 1977 Desmosome-like functions between Sertoli cells and germ cells in rat testis. Am J Anat 148: 301

Russell L D, Clermont Y 1977 Degeneration of germ cells in normal, hypophysectomized and hormone-treated hypophysectomized rats. Anat Rec 187: 347

Saez J M, Avallet O, Lejeune H, Chatelain P C 1991 Cell–cell communication in the testis. Horm Res 36: 104

Schaison G, Brailly S, Vuagnat P, Bouchard P, Milgrom E 1984 Absence of a direct inhibitory effect of the gonadotropin releasing hormone (GnRH) agonist D-Ser (TBU)[6], des-Gly-NH$_2$[10] GnRH ethylamine (buserelin) on testicular steroidogenesis in men. J Clin Endocrinol Metab 58: 885

Schneider G, Genel M, Bongiovanni A M et al 1975 Persistent testicular Δ5-3β-HSD deficiency in the Δ5-3β-HSD form of congenital adrenal hyperplasia. J Clin Invest 55: 681

Schulze W, Riemar M, Rehder U, Hohne K H 1986 Computer-aided three-dimensional reconstructions of the arrangement of primary spermatocytes in human seminiferous tubules. Cell Tissue Res 244: 1

Setchell B P, Waites G M H 1975 The blood–testis barrier. In: Greep R O, Astwood E B (eds) Handbook of physiology, section 7. Endocrinology, Williams and Wilkins, Baltimore, p 143

Sharpe R M 1992 Monitoring of spermatogenesis in man. Measurement of Sertoli cell-or germ cell-secreted proteins in semen or blood. Int J Androl 15: 201

Sharpe R M, Cooper I 1984 Intratesticular secretion of a factor(s) with major stimulating effects on Leydig cell testosterone secretion in vitro. Molec Cell Endocrinol 37: 159

Simpson B J B, Tsonis C G, Wu F C W 1987 Inhibin bioactivity in human testicular extracts. J Endocrinol 115: R9

Skinner M K 1991 Cell–cell interaction in the testis. Endocr Rev 12: 45

Skinner M K, Fetterolf P M, Anthony C T 1988 Purification of a paracrine factor, P-Mod-s, produced by testicular peritubular cells that modulate Sertoli cell function. J Biol Chem 263: 2884

Steinberger A, Steinberger E 1971 Replication pattern of Sertoli cells in maturing rat testis in vivo and in organ culture. Biol Reprod 4: 84

Steinberger E 1971 Hormonal control of mammalian spermatogenesis. Physiol Rev 51: 1

Steinberger E 1975 Hormonal regulation of the seminiferous tubule function. In: French F S, Hansson V, Ritzen E M, Nayfeh S N (eds) Hormonal regulation of spermatogenesis. Plenum, New York, p 337

Steinberger E 1989 Structural consideration of the male reproductive system. In: De Groot L J, Besser G M, Cahill Jr G F et al (eds) Endocrinology. Saunders, Philadelphia, pp 2123–2131

Suzuki F, Nagano T 1986 Microvasculature of the human testis and excurrent duct system. Cell Tissue Res 243: 79

Swinnen K, Cailleau J, Heyns W, Verhoeven G 1989 Stromal cells from the rat prostate secrete regulated factors which modulate Sertoli cell function. Molec Cell Endocrinol 62: 147

Swinnen K, Cailleau J, Heyns W, Verhoeven G 1990 Prostatic stromal cells and testicular peritubular cells produce similar paracrine mediators of androgen action. Endocrinology 126: 142

Toledo S P, Medeiros-Neto G A, Knobel M, Mattar E 1977 Evaluation of the hypothalamic-pituitary-gonadal function in the Bardet–Biedl syndrome. Metabolism 26: 1277

Vale W, Rivier J, Vaughan J et al 1986 Purification and characterization of an FSH releasing protein from porcine ovarian follicular fluid. Nature 321: 776

Verhoeven G, Cailleau J 1987 A Leydig cell stimulatory factor produced by human testicular tubules. Molec Cell Endocrinol 49: 137

Verhoeven G, Cailleau J 1990 Influence of coculture with Sertoli cells on steroidogenesis in immature rat Leydig cells. Molec Cell Endocrinol 71: 239

Verhoeven G, Cailleau J, Van Damme J, Billiau A 1988 Interleukin-1 stimulates steroidogenesis in cultured rat Leydig cells. Molec Cell Endocrinol 57: 51

Vihko K K, Huhtaniemi I 1989 A rat seminiferous epithelial factor that inhibits Leydig cell cAMP and testosterone production: mechanism of action, stage-specific secretion, and partial characterization. Molec Cell Endocrinol 65: 119

Waites G M H 1970 Temperature regulation and the testis. In: Johnson A D, Gomes W R, Van Demark N L (eds) The testis. Academic, New York, pp 241–279

Wang S X, Luo A M, Liang Z G, Song J F, Wang H A, Chen Y X 1990 Preparation and characterization of monoclonal antibodies against sperm specific lactate dehydrogenase $C_4$. J Androl 11: 319

Wiener S, Sutherland G, Bartholomew A A, Hudson B 1968 XYY males in a Melbourne prison. Lancet i: 150

Witherington R 1984 Cryptorchidism and approaches to its surgical management. Surg Clin North Am 64: 367

Yamamoto M, Nagai T, Takaba H, Hashimoto J, Miyake K 1989 In vitro contractility of human seminiferous tubules in response to testosterone, dihydrotestosterone and estradiol. Urol Res 17: 265

Yeh J, Rebar R W, Liu J H, Yen S S 1989 Pituitary function in isolated gonadotrophin deficiency. Clin Endocrinol 31: 375

Yavetz H, Zadik Z, Yogev L et al 1992a Effect of growth hormone on sperm quality serum hormones and IGF-1 in serum/seminal plasma. Assisted Reprod Technol/Adrol (in press)

Yavetz H, Harash B, Paz G et al 1992b Cryptorchidism: incidence and sperm quality in infertile men. Andrologia (in press)

Zachmann M, Werder E A, Prader A 1982 Two types of male pseudohermaphroditism due to 17,20-desmolase deficiency. J Clin Endocrinol Metab 55: 487

Zipf W B, Payne A H, Kelch R P 1978 Prolactin, growth hormone, and luteinizing hormone receptors. Endocrinology 103: 595

Zorgniotti A W, Cohen M S, Sealfon A I 1986 Chronic scrotal hypothermia: results in 90 infertile couples. J Urol 135: 944

# Diagnosis of infertility (female)

# 9. Classification and diagnosis of ovarian insufficiency

*M. Breckwoldt    H.P. Zahradnik    J. Neulen*

## INTRODUCTION

Normal ovarian function involves follicular maturation, selection of a dominant follicle, ovulation and corpus luteum formation. These morphological processes are associated with characteristic endocrine functions affecting the specific target organs for sexual steroids. Ovarian function is reflected by a characteristic pattern of estrogens and progesterone in peripheral blood. Proper steroid secretion of the ovary is essential in controlling hypothalamic and pituitary function. Peripheral serum levels of FSH and LH are indicative for hypothalamic-pituitary interaction. Central nervous system, hypothalamus, pituitary and ovary have to be regarded as a dynamic functional unit. Any disruption of these well-coordinated and synchronized interactions will result in ovarian dysfunction. During a physiological ovarian cycle a single mature ovum, ready for fertilization, will be released into the genital tract. In abnormal cycles, however, ovulation is either missing or markedly impaired. Thus any degree of ovarian insufficiency is incompatible with reproduction. Approximately 30–40% of female infertility patients present with ovarian dysfunction. A meaningful therapeutic approach to female infertility due to ovarian insufficiency is highly depending on diagnostic evaluation.

The most important step in the diagnostic

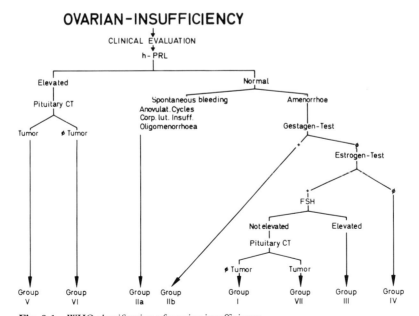

**Fig. 9.1**  WHO classification of ovarian insufficiency.

evaluation of ovarian dysfunction is a careful medical history with emphasis on menstrual bleeding patterns, use of drugs and general diseases. In addition, physical and gynecological examination including inspection and palpation of the breast, documentation of sexual hair distribution, body length and body weight can be helpful in finding the correct diagnosis. Gynecological examination should record uterine and ovarian size, vaginal cytology and cervical factors. Good spinnbarkeit and positive ferning of the cervical mucus indicate adequate estrogen production. Absent cervical secretion and atrophic vaginal epithelium are indicative of low estrogen production. A detailed medical history and a meticulous physical examination with special attention to the target organs for sexual steroids frequently provide better information than a battery of uncoordinated laboratory tests. During recent years progress has been made in understanding ovarian physiology and pathophysiology. Neuroendocrinology, psychoneuroendocrinology, molecular genetics and immunology have provided a great deal of new information regarding ovarian function and dysfunction. However, therapeutic approaches have remained largely unchanged during the last decade.

In 1976 the WHO Scientific Group on 'Agents Stimulating Gonadal Function in the Human' has proposed a widely used classification of ovarian disturbances which is helpful in the diagnostic work-up of female infertility patients. This classification as outlined in Figure 9.1 is not only of diagnostic relevance, but it meets also particular therapeutic aspects. The objective of this chapter is to describe the various groups of ovarian insufficiency in detail, to discuss the pathophysiological mechanisms and the diagnostic requirements for a meaningful classification.

## GROUP I—HYPOTHALAMIC PITUITARY FAILURE

### Definition

These patients present clinically with a history of primary or secondary amenorrhea due to reduced or absent pituitary gonadotropin release. Serum levels of FSH and LH are low and, consequently, appropriate endogenous estrogen production is missing. Exposure to progestagens will not result in withdrawal bleeding. Serum prolactin levels are within the normal range. Basal levels of cortisol can be elevated (Biller et al 1990).

### Pathophysiology

Since Knobil (1980) described the permissive role of ganadotropin releasing hormone (GnRH) for the control of the pituitary function in the Rhesus monkey, a better understanding of the interaction between hypothalamus and pituitary was provided. This concept of the permissive role of GnRH applies obviously also to the human as shown by Leyendecker et al (1981). Wildt et al (1980) have demonstrated that pulsatile exogenous administration of GnRH resulted in normal ovarian function in immature Rhesus monkeys. After discontinuation of the GnRH supplementation, cessation of gonadal function was noted. From these data and clinical findings it was concluded that the shift from a normal ovarian cycle through corpus luteum insufficiency, anovulatory cycles, oligomenorrhea to amenorrhea could be interpreted as a consequence of gradually decreasing GnRH production by the hypothalamus. The function of the GnRH-producing neurons is modulated by various catecholamines, neuropeptides and sex steroids as shown by Fuxe et al (1978). There is also evidence that enkephalins and endorphins are involved in the regulation of GnRH production. The administration of naloxone, an opioid antagonist, can result in gonadotropin increase. Ellingboe et al (1982) noted an increase of basal LH levels, peak values and frequency of LH spiking during blockade of endogenous opioid receptors by naloxone. Chronic administration of naltrexone can induce ovulatory cycles in patients with hypothalamic amenorrhea (Wildt & Leyendecker 1987). Blockade of opioid receptors, however, is obviously effective in patients with measurable endogenous estrogen levels. The effect of naloxone treatment on LH pulsatility is illustrated in Figures 9.2 and 9.3. It is well accepted that emotional stress and psychological factors can influence the hypothalamo-pituitary-

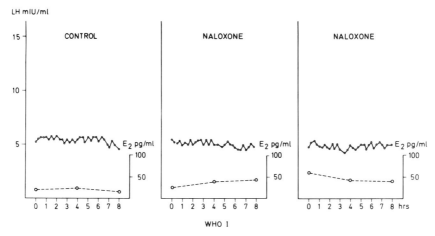

**Fig. 9.2**  LH pulsatility of a patient with hypothalamic amennorhea WHO 1: control and during nalaxone treatment.

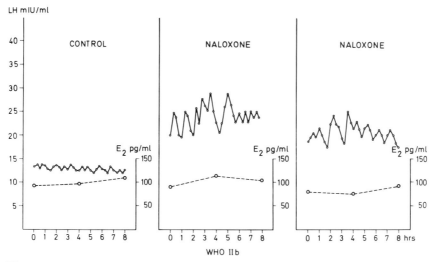

**Fig. 9.3**  Effect of nalaxone on LH pulsatility in a patient with normogonadotropic ammenorrhoea WHO 11b.

ovarian axis resulting in ovarian dysfunction. For example, anorexia nervosa, a classical psychosomatic disease, is always associated with amenorrhea, reflecting a severe impairment of the ovarian function. Patients with stress-induced amenorrhea exhibit elevated cortisol levels due to increased CRH activity (Rivier et al 1986). Neuroendocrine dysfunction in women with hypothalamic amenorrhea can be interpreted as a consequence of increased hypothalamic dopaminergic tone, increased opioid levels and decreased LH pulsatility (Berga et al 1989, Biller et al

1990, van Binsbergen et al 1990). Interactions between psychosomatic conflicts and gonadotropin secretion in amenorrheic patients have been described by Peters et al (1982). The study evaluates the pituitary responsiveness to GnRH in correlation with psychoanalytical data in 30 patients with secondary amenorrhea. According to the pituitary response to GnRH and the psychosomatic symptomatology the patients could be separated into two groups. Patients with severe psychosomatic disease complained predominantly about somatic discomfort and had a poor or absent response to GnRH. Patients presenting mainly with mental symptoms were found to be less affected by this psychosomatic disease. The LH responses to GnRH were only moderately impaired in these patients. Progress in psychotherapy was reflected by gradually increasing LH output. This study provides evidence that secondary amenorrhea may be regarded as a symptom of psychosomatic disease. This symptom is frequently found in patients with psychiatric disorders (Gregory 1957). In the normal population the rate of amenorrhea is in the range of 1–4%. Pettersson et al (1973) found an incidence of 3.3%.

Secondary amenorrhea in patients with anorexia nervosa seems to be a function of the duration and the severity of this syndrome. In these patients FSH response to GnRH was found by most investigators to exceed that of LH (Nillius & Wide 1972, Keller et al 1976, Travaglini et al 1976). During successful therapy of anorexia nervosa gonadotropin responses to GnRH can be monitored by a characteristic shift of the pituitary responsiveness to GnRH. The FSH response decreases while LH levels increase (Keller et al 1976). Improvement of LH response to GnRH after weight gain is a common finding (van Binsbergen et al 1990). The increased FSH response in anorectic patients has been interpreted as the expression of sexual immaturity. In these patients gonadotropin levels are normally low; endogeneus estrogen levels may also be below the proliferation threshold. These patients will not respond to a progesterone challenge test and should be consequently classified as belonging to group I. However, group I cannot be regarded as a pathophysiological entity. Gonadotropin, estrogen and prolactin determinations are not sensitive enough to clarify the underlying pathophysiology. Therefore it can be helpful to study the pituitary response to exogenous GnRH or to follow the plasma levels of LH and FSH at short-term intervals for spontaneous pulsatility. Leyendecker et al (1981) have studied amenorrheic patients, classified as group I according to the above-mentioned criteria. None of the patients exhibited normal spontaneous pulsatility. LH and FSH levels were constantly low, however, the pituitary response to 100 µg

GnRH was different. Some patients responded with an increase in LH only (adult response, 3a) others showed a moderate rise in both FSH and LH (prepubertal response, 3b), and a final group of patients did not respond at all indicating absent endogenous GnRH secretion (3c). The different pituitary response patterns are interpreted as consequence of different degrees of GnRH deficiency. Body weight and composition are of significant importance for the regulation of ovarian function as shown by Frisch (1988). Reduction of fat tissue below 15% of body weight is associated with ovarian dysfunction.

Isolated gonadotropin deficiency associated with anosmia is referred to as 'Kallmann's syndrome' or olfacto-genital syndrome. These patients are obviously unable to produce sufficient GnRH to achieve proper pituitary function. Consequently these patients present with primary amenorrhea. Clinical symptoms indicating ovarian activity such as breast development and growth of axillary or pubic hair are scanty or missing. The symptomatology of anosmia and hypothalamic dysfunction implies interactions between these two systems. Ellendorf et al (1979) have provided experimental evidence that stimulation of the olfactory bulb by pheromones increases its electrophysiological activity in the pig. In addition the pig is able to transmit information originating in the olfactory bulb to lower brain structures such as the nucleus amygdalae and the mediobasal hypothalamus. Immunohistochemical studies on mouse embryos provide evidence that GnRH-producing neurons and neurons of the olphactory tract are of the same origin (Schwanzel-Fukuda & Pfaff 1989). Based on these findings, Kallmanns's syndrome can be interpreted as an early degeneration of GnRH-producing neurons. Rjosk & Goebel (1978) studied the pituitary response to GnRH in two patients with Kallmann's syndrome. In both cases FSH increase was significant while the LH levels remained unchanged. This pattern is consistent with that seen in the prepubertal phase and also in patients with anorexia nervosa (Keller et al 1976, Travaglini et al 1976). The incidence of Kallmann's syndrome in the female population is estimated to be 1 : 50 000.

Postpartum pituitary necrosis (Sheehan's syndrome) as a consequence of hypovolemic shock can result in hypogonadotropic hypogonadism. Pituitary hemorrhage or ischemic infarction, however, are very rare conditions due to improved medical care during delivery. Also inflammatory diseases of pituitary tissue leading to massive destruction of the gland are rarely seen. Individual case reports of chronic lymphocystic hypophysitis have been published (McDermott et al 1988).

Hypophysectomized patients should obviously also be classified as WHO group I.

## Diagnostic approach

Amenorrheic patients with low FSH and LH levels and normal human prolactin (hPRL) in combination with a negative progesterone challenge test can be classified as group I. In addition, the pituitary response to GnRH can provide further information on the actual endocrine status. Estrogen levels in these patients are consistently low, estrogen determinations are therefore not necessarily required. The essential diagnostic tools in addition to medical history and physical examination are therefore h-PRL, FSH and LH determinations and exposure to gestagenic compounds. Space-occupying lesions in the hypothalamo-pituitary region should be excluded. Hypoplasia or aplasia of the rhinencephalon can be visualized by magnetic resonance imaging (Klingmüller et al 1987).

## GROUP II—HYPOTHALAMIC PITUITARY DYSFUNCTION

### Definition

According to the proposal of WHO this group describes patients with a variety of menstrual cycle disturbances including luteal phase insufficiency, anovulatory cycles or amenorrhea. There is evidence for endogenous estrogen production sufficient to stimulate endometrial proliferation. Consequently gonadotropin levels are within the normal range, exposure to progestagens results in withdrawal bleeding, prolactin levels are usually normal.

### Pathophysiology

For therapeutic consideration this group can be regarded as homogeneous since clomiphene or human menopausal ganadotrophin(hMG) therapy in clomiphene-non-responders are the most meaningful therapeutic regimens. However, from the pathophysiological point of view this group of patients, representing the majority of infertility patients, requires a more detailed description. Patients of group II may present with:

1. luteal phase insufficiency
2. anovulatory cycles
3. secondary amenorrhea.

For practical reasons it seems appropriate to separate these patients into two groups:

11a. patients with spontaneous menstrual bleedings
11b. amenorrheic patients.

Patients of both groups may present virilizing symptoms which may be due to hyperandrogenemia. These patients require androgen determinations for further diagnostic evaluation. The most meaningful diagnostic parameters are plasma testosterone and dehydroepiandrosterone sulfate (DHEA–S) (Schwartz et al 1981).

### Luteal insufficiency

Luteal insufficiency is incompatible with fertility. The diagnosis of a luteal defect is normally based on the basal body temperature (BBT) curve, on progesterone determinations and/or on endometrial biopsies. However, even by these parameters it is difficult to discriminate luteal insufficiency from anovulatory cycles with luteinization of the unruptured follicle. Lehmann (1978) has studied the endocrine profiles of 62 normal cycles and compared them to the data of 18 cycles with luteal defects. The main features of the insufficient cycles are described as retarded and/or reduced increase of the plasma estrogen levels followed by a continuous decrease without a second peak during the luteal phase. The progesterone levels did not exceed 5 ng/ml on average. The peak progesterone value in the apparently normal cycles were found to be of the order of 15 ng/ml. Similar concentrations in normal cycles were reported by Landgren et al (1980). Based on the data given by Strott et al (1970), Sherman & Korenman (1974) and Lehmann (1978), corpus luteum insufficiency can be interpreted as a consequence of inappropriate follicular maturation. The rise in FSH levels, beginning in the previous cycle and continuing during the menstrual period into the first part of the follicular phase, is obviously essential for normal follicular development as pointed out by Ross et al (1970). In addition, it has been discussed that corpus luteum insufficiency might be due to an inadequate LH surge (Jones & Madrigal-Castro 1970). The importance of LH secretion in determining the lifespan of the corpus luteum has been demonstrated by van de Wiele et al (1970). From these studies it was concluded that corpus luteum function requires LH stimulation. Inadequate residual LH secretion may account for a short luteal phase. It must be admitted, however, that the factors, controlling the normal lifespan of the corpus luteum are largerly unknown. In normal ovarian cycles LH pulsatility is reduced during the luteal phase to 6–9 pulses/24 h. A further reduction may result in luteal insufficiency. The role of prolactin in controlling luteal function is unclear, moderate hyperprolactinemia may also cause a luteal defect.

The physiological role of prostaglandins in the process of luteolysis is still controversial and the luteolytic effect in women has not been convincingly substantiated (Embrey 1981). In many other species such as sheep, cow, pig and guinea-pig, a uterine luteolytic factor being responsible for the normal regression of the corpus luteum has been demonstrated. In the sheep the uterine factor has been identified as $PGF_{2\alpha}$ (Horton & Poyser 1976). Direct measurements of tissue concentrations of $PGF_{2\alpha}$ and $PGE_2$ in human corpora lutea at various stages of the luteal phase provide some evidence for the physiological role of prostaglandins in the process of luteal regression (Patwardhan & Lantheir 1980).

### Anovulatory cycles

Anovulatory cycles are characterized as menstrual bleedings without preceding ovulation and corpus luteum formation. A cohort of follicles reaches a certain stage of maturation associated with measurable estrogen secretion sufficient to stimulate the endometrium. However, the dominant follicle does not reach a preovulatory stage, ovulation does not occur, the maturing follicles become atretic and estrogen secretion decreases. Since anovulatory cycles are frequently observed during adolescence it seems feasible to assume that in these cases anovulation is due to insufficient hypothalamic stimulation of the anterior pituitary (Kulin & Reiter 1973, Lehmann 1978, Leyendecker et al 1981). Lehmann (1978) has studied estrogen and progesterone patterns in patients with anovulatory cycles. The estrogen peaks were observed on average on day 20, being significantly lower than those found in normal cycles. Estrogen levels were continuously falling after the LH peak, progesterone levels were slightly elevated with maximum values of 2–3 ng/ml, reflecting luteinization of unruptured follicles. The hormone profiles explain the endometrial morphology of insufficient secretory transformation. According to the data of Lehmann it can be assumed that there is a floating shift from luteal insufficiency to anovulation. This notion is compatible with the concept proposed by Leyendecker et al (1981).

Ultrasonographic and endocrinological studies in normal and insufficient ovarian cycles provide further evidence of the difficulty in clearly separating anovulatory cycles from cycles with a luteal defect (Breckwoldt & Geisthövel 1984).

### Amenorrhea

Patients of group IIb with amenorrhea will experience withdrawal bleedings after exposure to gestagenic compounds indicating the presence of endogenous estrogens. Plasma levels of FSH and LH are found in the normal range. Ovarian insufficiency associated with secondary amenorrhea is a frequent finding during adolescence in combination with a transitory moderate weight loss. This 'weight-loss amenorrhea' has a high rate of spontaneous remission. In most cases normal ovarian function will resume without specific treatment. In these cases GnRH administration may be of prognostic value. Poor or absent pituitary response to GnRH reflects severe impairment of the hypothalamo-pituitary unit. Patients who respond well to GnRH with significant increase of LH levels and a slight rise in FSH do not require special therapy, they can be guided by a psychologically oriented gynecologist (Peters et al 1982). LH pulsatility in these patients is characterized by a high frequency but low amplitude (Genazzani et al 1990). Infertility patients with secondary amenorrhea and poor or absent pituitary response to GnRH should be referred to hMG-hCG treatment, since they normally fail to respond to clomiphene.

Group II—ovarian insufficiency—includes also polycystic ovarian disease (PCOD), a functional disturbance being associated with the clinical features of virilization and infertility. Since the description of Stein & Leventhal (1935), numerous clinical and experimental studies have been devoted to this particular subject. The pathophysiology of PCOD, however, has not been clarified (see also Chapter 26).

Yen (1980) has proposed a working hypothesis assuming that chronically elevated plasma androgens have to be considered as initiating a process that ultimately leads to anovulation. Androgens suppress the production of SHBG, thus potentiating the biological activity of androgenic steroids (Anderson 1974, Duignan 1976). Elevated levels of testosterone in PCOD patients are probably derived from ovarian secretion (De Vane et al 1975, Yen 1980), and also from extraglandular conversion of androstenedione (Kirschner & Jacobs 1971, Siiteri & McDonald 1973, Kopelman et al 1980). Serum estrone levels are higher than estradiol concentrations. This finding is consistent with the concept that in PCOD chronic acyclic estrogen production is derived largely from peripheral aromatization of androstenedione to estrone. Exogenous administration of estrone-benzoate sufficient to achieve levels two- or three-fold above normal resulted in PCOD patients in a further dissociation of FSH and LH levels. FSH decreased to levels below normal while LH remained unaffected (Chang et al 1982). In normally cycling women, however, exogenous administration of estrone-benzoate failed to alter the pattern of daily LH and FSH secretion. With regard to the lack of estrone-benzoate to induce a positive feedback on LH release, it can be assumed that estrone is responsible for the tonic secretion of LH and FSH (Baird 1976, Rebar et al 1976). Tonic secretion of LH and FSH is incompatible with ovulation. A steady state of tonic gonadotropin secretion with constantly elevated LH and low or normal FSH values is a characteristic feature of PCOD. FSH deficiency and increased intraovarian androgen concentrations inhibit obviously normal follicular maturation (Louvet et al 1975). Androgen formation by the hyperplastic theca cell layers is increased (Yen 1980), causing a reduction of follicular LH receptors (Rajaniemi et al 1980). The aromatizing capacity of C-19 steroids in granulosa cell layers in polycystic ovaries is reduced due to insufficient FSH stimulation (Erickson et al 1979).

Schwartz et al (1981) have proposed to consider PCOD as a gradually developing pathophysiological process. A typical example of a 24-h hormonal profile of a patient with PCOD is shown in Figure 9.4. LH levels are constantly elevated, episodic spiking is maintained, FSH levels are low, pulsatility is reduced. Testosterone levels are above the normal range. Endocrinologically the PCOD can be regarded as a self-sustaining system resulting in chronic anovulation. Follicles undergoing atresia are immediately replaced by a new cohort of follicles of similar limited growth potentials due to insufficient FSH stimulation. In response to permanently elevated LH levels theca and stroma cells become hyperplastic and secrete increased amounts of androstenedione and testosterone (Fig. 9.5).

The various theories of the pathogenesis of PCOD have been reviewed by McKenna (1988). Characteristic endocrine parameters are elevation of LH, LH/FSH ratio, testosterone, estrone and prolactin associated with increased peripheral insulin resistance. Patients with PCOD and hyperandrogenemia tend to be insulin resistant as evidenced by elevated peripheral insulin levels (Dunaif et al 1990, Kazer et al 1990). Association of familial virilization due to hyperandrogenemia, insulin resistance and acanthosis nigricans has been frequently described. Normalization of androgen levels, however, did not improve insulin

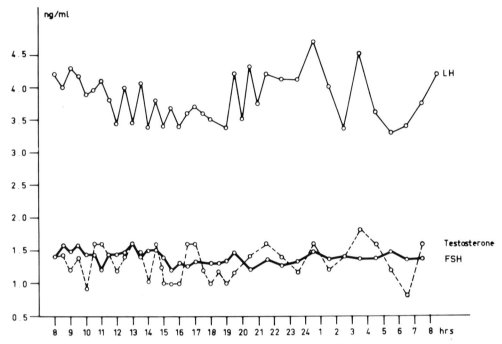

**Fig. 9.4**   Plasma levels of LH, FSH and testosterone in a patient with PCOD associated with severe hirsutism.

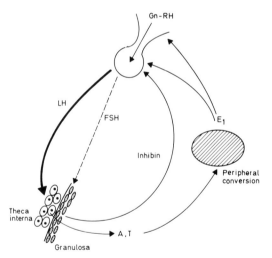

**Fig. 9.5**   Schematic representation of the pathophysiology of polycystic ovary syndrome.

resistance (Corenblum and Baylis 1990, Dunaif et al 1990). Insulin and insulin-like growth factor-I (IGF-I) are obviously involved in the production of estradiol by granulosa cells. FSH and IGF-I stimulate dose dependently and synergistically the aromatizing capacity of granulosa cells of polycystic ovaries (Erickson et al 1990). Inherited ovarian 17-ketoreductase deficiency has been discussed as a possible cause of PCOD (Toscano et al 1990). The etiology of PCOD is still a matter of debate. It has been proposed by Axelrod & Goldzieher (1976), and by Abraham & Buster (1976), that inherited enzyme defects of the 3β-ol-dyhydrogenase, the Δ 4,5-isomerase and the aromatizing system could be considered as causative. Primary ovarian enzyme deficiencies, however, do not provide satisfactory explanation since FSH supplementation can lead to normalization of follicular development, ovulation, corpus luteum function and subsequent pregnancy. Also clomiphene treatment causing elevation of the endogenous FSH levels can be effective in inducing ovulation in PCOD. The role of inhibin in the pathogenesis of PCOD is controversial. Some reports describe elevated inhibin levels in PCOD patients (Tanabe et al 1983), others were unable to confirm these findings (Buchler et al 1988).

Ovarian hyperthecosis is morphologically characterized by multiple islands of luteinized hyperplastic theca cells distributed throughout the ovarian stroma. There is evidence that this type of ovarian dysfunction is a consequence of decreased desmolase activity (Abraham & Buster 1976), resulting in increased secretion of progesterone, 17α OH-progesterone, testosterone and 5α DHT. Consequently these patients develop severe virilizing symptoms associated with menstrual irregularities and infertility. In contrast to patients with PCOD no tonic elevation of LH is observed, FSH and LH levels are rather low (Nagamani et al 1981). Patients with ovarian hyperthecosis will not respond to clomid, the pituitary response to GnRH is normal. The production rate of testosterone is eight times normal (Aiman et al 1978). Peripheral androgen levels are elevated, increasing significantly after hCG administration, and cannot be suppressed by dexamethasone (Abraham & Buster 1976). According to a study of Givens et al (1971) ovarian hyperthecosis can be inherited through an autosomal dominant pattern and should be regarded as a type of gonadal dysgenesis.

Androgen excess of adrenal origin can result in ovarian dysfunction by suppressing gonadotropin release. Congenital adrenal hyperplasia is associated with increased androgen production resulting in severe virilization with acceleration of bone age, enlargement of the clitoris, fused labia and hirsutism. Because of its striking symptomatology the diagnosis is easily established. In 95% of cases congenital adrenal hyperplasia is due to an inherited 21-hydroxylase deficiency. The gene regulating 21-hydroxylase is located on chromosome 6 closely linked to HLA genes (New 1986). Cushing's syndrome and androgen-secreting tumors can also cause hyperandrogenemia.

The observation of Steinberger et al (1979) that elevated testosterone levels in infertile patients were associated with significant prolongation of the follicular phase and increased incidence of amenorrhea and anovulation indicates that elevated androgens can result in ovarian dysfunction. Since treatment with glucocorticoids was quite effective in androgen suppression and in normalizing ovarian function resulting in subsequent pregnancy, it can be assumed that the excessive testosterone levels were of adrenal origin. Late-onset or acquired adrenal hyperplasia

can be regarded as a mild form of a congenital enzyme defect (Bouchard et al 1981). Clinical features are hirsutism, acne and menstrual irregularities.

### Diagnostic approach

For the diagnostic work-up of this rather heterogeneous group of patients it is recommended for practical reasons to separate spontaneously menstruating women (IIa) from amenorrheic patients (IIb). For patients with spontaneous menstrual bleedings the BBT curve should be used as an essential diagnostic guideline. In addition repeated progesterone determinations during the phase of elevated BBT can be used as quantitative parameters of the luteal function. Endometrial biopsies with adequate morphological staging can also be recommended. FSH and LH levels are in the normal range. Patients with virilizing symptoms and menstrual irregularities need testosterone and DHEA-S determinations. Definitely elevated androgen levels require further detailed evaluation. In patients with PCOD the FSH/LH ratio is shifted in favor of LH, testosterone may be slightly above normal. h-PRL levels are in the normal range. Patients with hyperandrogenemia of adrenal origin exhibit elevated DHEA-S levels. These patients present in general clinical evidence of virilization such as acne, hirsutism, male sexual hair distribution and alopecia. The minimum diagnostic requirements for infertility patients presenting with amenorrhea should involve progesterone challenge test, h-PRL, FSH and LH determinations. Patients with virilizing symptoms need androgen determinations. GnRH stimulation is of prognostic value and helpful in guiding the management of patients.

### GROUP III—OVARIAN FAILURE

### Definition

According to the recommendation of WHO, patients classified as group III are characterized as amenorrheic women with no evidence of ovarian estrogen production and with elevated FSH levels.

## Pathophysiology

For therapeutic considerations these patients represent a homogeneous group. However, the underlying pathomechanisms and etiologies that lead to the final status of ovarian failure are different and should be discussed in detail. As a common diagnostic feature elevated FSH levels associated with hardly detectable estrogens are indicative of primary ovarian insufficiency. Increased pituitary FSH secretion is a consequence of an absent negative feedback, the ovary is unable to produce sufficient amounts of sex steroids and inhibin, a glycoprotein which is considered important in the regulation of pituitary FSH secretion (McLachlan et al 1988). The frequency of ovarian failure is of the order of 10–15% of all cases presenting with amenorrhea (Bergh et al 1977).

## Genetic factors

In almost 30% of hypergonadotropic hypogonadism ovarian failure is genetically determined. Turner's syndrome is observed with a frequency of one per 3000 among the female population. This syndrome was originally described by Morgangi in 1768. A detailed description of this syndrome was given by Ullrich (1930) and Turner (1938). Turner assumed that the somatic symptomatology and sexual immaturity were due to pituitary dysfunction. Polani et al (1954) described X-chromatin-negative cells in patients with Turner's syndrome. The complete karyotype of 45X0 was almost simultaneously reported in the same journal in 1959 by Ford et al and by Fraccaro et al. The clinical symptomatology is characterized by two obligatory symptoms: sexual infantilism and short stature. Numerous other clinical symptoms such as webbed neck, shield chest, pigment naevi, and cubitus valgus may or may not be present. During early childhood the clinical symptoms are frequently discrete and become more and more prominent as childhood advances. The external and internal genitalia are hypoplastic, the ovaries are transformed to streak gonads composed exclusively of connective tissue without any follicular structures. Histological studies of ovarian morphology of newborn children with Turner's syndrome revealed all stages from normal structure to complete degeneration (Carr et al 1968). These findings led to the conclusion that gonadal dysgenesis is caused by rapid regression of the follicular apparatus rather than by congenital absence of oocytes. Short stature and retarded bone maturation due to the absence of endogenous sexual steroids are common during childhood and adolescence. Since puberty is not initiated the typical growth spurt during normal pubertal development is absent. The expected final height is variable, in the range of 135–152 cm. Growth hormone levels are normal (Donaldson et al 1968), IGF-I levels are normal or slightly elevated (Saenger et al 1976). The intellectual capability of patients with Turner's syndrome is normal as compared to the average population (Nielsen et al 1977). Money & Mittenthal (1970) found in 73 patients with gonadal dysgenesis a remarkable emotional stability. Sexual orientation was definitely female.

Turner's syndrome is based on a complete or partial loss of one X chromosome. The presence of both X chromosomes is essential for normal development and function of the ovaries and also for normal growth. Genes encoding for ovarian function are mainly located at the long arm (Xq). From mosaic compositions it is known that genes responsible for normal growth are localized at the short arm (Xp). Deletions of the short arm are always associated with short statute. Ninety-eight per cent of conceptuses with a karyotype of 45X0 are eliminated by spontaneous abortion, only 2% will survive. The survival rate of mosaicism with two or more cell lines of various chromosome compositions is obviously greater (Hecht & MacFarlane 1969). Gonadal dysgenesis can be associated with various cytogenetic abnormalities such as 46X,i (Xq) or 45X0/46XX, ring formation and loss of a long or short arm of one X chromosome. The impact of mosaicisms is significant with regard to ovarian differentiation. In patients with the karyotype 46XX/45X0 functional ovarian cortical tissue can be present in individual patients sufficient to include pubertal development and in some instances even fertility is maintained.

Pure gonadal dysgenesis is associated with a

karyotype of 46XX or 46XY. The phenotype of these patients is always female. As a consequence of the primary ovarian failure internal and external genital organs are hypoplastic. Growth is normal, bone age definitely retarded since the gonad is unable to produce sex steroids. Sexual and axillary hair are scanty or missing. The presence of a Y chromosome (46XY, Swyer's syndrome) indicates that the Y chromosome in these individuals is defective as it does not express the testis-determining factor. Female patients carrying a Y chromosome require gonadectomy to avoid malignant development. Malignant gonadal tumors have been observed in 30% of patients with gonadal dysgenesis based on the karyotype 46XY or 46XY/45X0 (Barr et al 1976, Helpap et al 1980).

In rare instances premature regression of ovarian tissue can be induced by autoimmune disease analagous to idiopathic Addison's disease (Irvine 1980, Luborsky et al 1990). The presence of antibodies against corticosteroid-producing cells was detected in 70% of Addison patients. A similar pathogenetic mechanism could become operative in patients with premature menopause. McNatty et al (1975) studied the sera of 23 patients with idiopathic adrenal insufficiency with proven antibodies against corticosteroid-producing cells. These antibodies reacted positive with freshly obtained human corpus luteum tissue and induced cytolysis of human granulosa cells. Studies supporting this pathogenetic concept have been published by Golonka & Goodman (1968), Ayala et al (1979) and Collen et al (1979).

Luborsky et al (1990) described 45 patients with premature ovarian failure. The sera of these patients were screened for ovarian and oocyte antibodies by ELISA. In total 69% of the reactions were positive either for ovarian tissue or for oocytes. Two patients became pregnant after glucocorticoid treatment. However, it can be assumed that this mechanism applies only to a very limited number of patients with premature menopause.

Exogenous factors such as irradiation or cytotoxic agents can cause premature ovarian failure (Himmelstein-Braw et al 1977). Chapman et al (1976) studied 41 patients with advanced Hodgkin's disease. During chemotherapy 20 patients developed hypergonadotropic ovarian insufficiency and 14 patients exhibited menstrual irregularities. In seven patients only normal ovarian cyclicity was maintained. Adjuvant chemotherapy of normally cycling women with breast cancer caused in a large proportion regression of steroid-producing ovarian tissue as reflected by increasing FSH levels (Schulz et al 1979). Since radiotherapy of Hodgin's disease has been established as the treatment of choice it has been proposed to preserve ovarian function by oophoropexy. Positive results with resumption of ovarian function are obtained in 50% (Trueblood et al 1970). It should be pointed out, however, that this is a rather optimistic figure.

Premature menopause defines follicular regression before the age of 35 years. The aetiology of this process is unknown (Zarate et al 1970) and may be related to genetic or autoimmunological factors (Moraes-Ruehsen et al 1972).

## Resistant ovary syndrome

A rare syndrome of amenorrhea in association with definitely elevated FSH levels and apparently normal ovarian follicular apparatus was first described by Jones & de Moraes-Ruehsen (1969). They reported on three patients with primary amenorrhea, elevated gonadotropins and low estrogens. Ovarian histology was absolutely normal showing follicular tissue of all developmental stages. Similar observations have been published by Starup et al (1971).

Gonadotropin resistance is a characteristic feature in patients with Rothmund–Thomson syndrome (Wieacker et al 1988). Other reports on patients with elevated FSH levels yet normal estrogen values are worth mentioning (Falk 1977). Various reports on patients with increased FSH levels being substituted with estrogens and gestagens and subsequent normalization of the ovarian function have been published (Shapiro & Rubin 1977, Johnson & Peterson 1979, Schreiber et al 1979, Wright & Jacobs 1979, Breckwoldt et al 1981). According to Schreiber et al (1979), this particular form of ovarian disturbance could be defined as intermittant ovarian failure. Rebar & Conolly (1990) reported on clinical features of 115 young women with hypergonadotropic amenorrhea. Eight of these women became pregnant after being diagnosed as hypergonadotropic. In general, hypergonadotropic ovarian insufficiency is incompatible with reproduction. However, there are some rare exceptions. Several case reports have been published. Bahner et al (1960) described a patient with a karyotype 45X0 who gave birth to a healthy child. Nielsen et al (1979) have collected data on pregnancies observed in patients with Turner's syndrome. Nine pregnancies in seven women with the karyotype 45X0 have been described. In addition data on 56 pregnancies of 23 patients with mosaicism (45X0/46XX or 47XXX) are documented. Fifteen spontaneous abortions were noted and four cases of stillbirth, in 12 cases somatic defects and malformations were evident. Three children with Down's syndrome were born and five children were identified as 45X0. The remaining 26 children were apparently normal. This high incidence of genetic abnormalities and somatic malformations requires careful monitoring of such rare pregnancies including ultrasonography and prenatal chromosome analysis. Among our patients with mosaicism we have followed two patients during pregnancy; in both cases healthy babies were delivered.

### Diagnostic approach

Careful medical history, clinical and gynecological examination are of great importance in the evaluation of patients with ovarian failure. The most relevant endocrine parameters are FSH and estrogen levels in serum. Clinical suspicion of genetically caused ovarian failure requires cytogenetic analysis. The presence of a Y chromosome needs further clarification and removal of the dysgenetic gonads. Laparoscopy and gonadal biopsy can be helpful in establishing the correct diagnosis.

## GROUP IV—CONGENITAL OR ACQUIRED GENITAL TRACT DISORDERS

### Definition

These patients present with amenorrhea due to congenital or acquired anatomical disorders of the genital tract.

### Pathophysiology

The most frequent anatomical cause of primary amenorrhea is the Rokitansky–Küster–Mayer syndrome. This syndrome is characterized by congenital absence of the vagina and failure of fusion of the two Müllerian ducts. Both separated uterine horns are solid, the endometrium is normally absent, and the ovaries appear perfectly normal in size, location and function. The failure of the Müllerian ducts to fuse completely obviously prevents the upgrowth of the epithelium of the urogenital sinus to form the vagina. This malformation is frequently associated with developmental abnormalities of the urinary tract. Lischke et al (1973) described identical twins being discordant for Rokitansky–Küster–Mayer syndrome, indicating that this type of malformation is not related to genetical disorders. The leading symptom in these patients is primary amenorrhea with normal somatic and sexual development. Gynecological examination reveals total absence of the vagina and normal breast development. Sexual and pubic hair are normal. Laparoscopy may be helpful in clarifying the anatomical situation.

Imperforate hymen with hematocolpos is easy to diagnose. The patients present with primary amenorrhea, normal sexual development, pelvic pain and hematocolpos.

The transverse vaginal septum as a consequence of canalization failure of the distal third of the vagina can be the cause of primary amenorrhea in very rare instances. Familial occurrence of this malformation suggests a genetic etiology (McDonough 1979).

Uterine amenorrhea caused by a partially or completely obliterated uterine cavity due to intrauterine adhesions are referred to as Asherman's syndrome (Asherman 1948). These adhesions ought to be considered as complications of intensive postpartum or postabortum curretings removing almost completely the basal layer of the endometrium. This syndrome, however, seems a rare complication. For diagnostic evaluation hysterosalpingography or hysteroscopy (Lindemann 1977) can be employed. In rare cases tuberculosis of the endometrium may also cause anatomical amenorrhea.

## Testicular feminization

Testicular feminization can be considered as the most common form of familial male pseudohermaphroditism. The clinical symptomatology of these phenotypic female patients is primary amenorrhea associated with scanty or absent axilliary and pubic hair. Breast development in these patients is normal. Gynecological examination reveals normal external genitalia, the clitoris is rather small. In some instances the patients present with inguinal hernia containing the gonads. In most cases, however, the gonads are intra-abdominally located. The vagina is in general short and blind ending, uterus and Fallopian tubes are absent as a consequence of the regression of the Müllerian ducts. Due to androgen insensitivity the Wolffian ducts are not stabilized and have disappeared. These patients can be easily diagnosed by general physical and gynecological examination. Medical history frequently uncovers other affected members of the family. We have seen a patient with complete testicular feminization, her family history revealed 14 additional cases.

The gonads present histologically the characteristic features of undescended testes with normal or hyperplastic Leydig cells and seminiferous tubules without spermatogenesis. For further diagnostic evaluation chromosomal analysis is required. The karyotype is 46XY, the inheritance is obviously X-linked (Meyer et al 1975).

Levels of plasma testosterone and testosterone production rates are elevated (MacDonald et al 1979), probably a consequence of increased LH secretion. Enhanced LH secretion, in turn, is obviously due to resistance of negative feedback regulation to circulating androgens. Androgen insensitivity applies to all target organs including the breast and the liver. Despite elevated testosterone levels the lipoprotein pattern is beneficial with an improved HDL/LDL cholesterol ratio (Breckwoldt et al 1989).

## Diagnostic approach

Congenital genital tract disorders causing anatomical amenorrhea can be easily diagnosed by gynecological examination. For detailed classification laparoscopy can be useful. Abnormalities of the urinary tract should be identified. Karyotyping is required when pseudohermaphroditism is suspected. Hysteroscopy may be helpful in cases of acquired anatomical uterine disorders.

## Hyperprolactinemia (see also Chapter 17)

In 1928 Stricker & Grueter provided experimental evidence for the presence of a mammotropic hormone originating in the anterior pituitary. Riddle & Braucher (1931) proposed the term 'prolactin'. In 1971 human prolactin (hPRL) was isolated and separated from human growth hormone (hGH) (Hwang et al 1971, Lewis et al 1971), consequently homologous radioimmunoassays for the quantification of hPRL were developed. Specific and sensitive detection of hPRL in biological fluids provided the basis for studying its physiological and pathophysiological significance in the human reproductive process. The regulation of hPRL synthesis and secretion is rather complex and still incompletely understood. Prolactin secretion from the anterior pituitary is mainly under tonic inhibitory control of hypothalamic dopamine. In addition, a fragment of the precursor molecule for GnRH has been shown to have potent prolactin-inhibiting properties (Nikolics et al 1985).

Several hypothalamic neuropeptides such as thyroid releasing hormone (TRH) vosoactive intestinal polypeptide (VIP), cholecystokinin (CCK) and serotonin have been shown to stimulate PRL release. Estrogens enhance PRL production as evidenced by rising peripheral PRL levels during pregnancy. Any abnormality in dopamine metabolism or in the interaction of dopamine with its receptor will result in diminished inhibition of the lactotrope causing hyperprolactinemia. Pathological hyperprolactinemia was originally suspected in various clinical syndromes presenting with galactorrhea and amenorrhea

(Chiari et al 1855, Frommel 1882, Argonz & del Castillo 1953, Forbes et al 1954). Increased secretion of hPRL is generally associated with ovarian dysfunction including luteal phase defects, anovulatory cycles, oligomenorrhea or amenorrhea. Since hyperprolactinemia is incompatible with reproduction the terms hyperprolactinemia-infertility syndrome (Crosignani & Robyn, 1977) or hyperprolactinemia-anovulatory syndrome (Bohnet et al 1976) have been proposed. Hyperprolactinemia obviously affects the GnRH pulse generator leading to impaired LH and FSH pulsatility causing reproductive dysfunction. Elevated hPRL levels are found in 15–20% of infertility patients presenting with menstrual irregularities, galactorrhea may or may not be present. These findings indicate that hPRL determinations have become an important diagnostic tool in the work-up of infertility patients.

## GROUP V—HYPERPROLACTINEMIC INFERTILE WOMEN WITH A SPACE-OCCUPYING LESION IN THE HYPOTHALAMIC-PITUITARY REGION

### Definition

Women with a variety of menstrual cycle disturbances (e.g. luteal phase insufficiency, anovulatory cycles, or amenorrhea) with elevated prolactin levels and evidence of a apace-occupying lesion in the hypothalamic-pituitary region comprise group V.

### Pathogenesis

Prolactinomas are the most frequent hormone-producing pituitary tumors (Franks et al 1975, Giannattasio & Bassetti 1990). Conventional staining of the anterior pituitary with hematoxylin and eosin demonstrates that prolactinomas contain acidophilic and chromophobe cells (Landolt 1978). Specific immunohistochemical techniques provide a more precise classification indicating that frequently pituitary adenomas produce more than one hormone. In 30–50% of patients with hyperprolactinemic amenorrhea a pituitary tumor is suggested by computed scanning X-ray of the sella turcica (Franks et al 1975, Rjosk et al 1976, Bergh et al 1977, Kleinberg et al 1977).

Macroprolactinomas of more than 10 mm in diameter normally result in enlargement of the sella. Microprolactinomas are characterized by normal size of the sella turcica with asymmetry of the sella floor (Vezina & Sutton 1974). High resolution of coronal computerized tomography allows detection of microadenomas of 2 mm in diameter (Taylor 1981). However, negative results of sella tomography do not exclude the presence of microadenomas (Tolis et al 1974, Franks et al 1975). Hardy et al (1978) detected very small microadenomas by microsurgical exploration of radiographically normal sella. It is an unsolved question whether hyperprolactinemia not depending on other endocrinopathies is generally caused by pituitary adenomas, even if a tumor is not detectable by computer tomography.

It is known that estrogens have mitogenic properties on prolactin-producing cells (Hunt 1947). This fact is well documented by the pituitary enlargement during pregnancy. In 1909, Erdheim & Stumme originally described hypertrophy and hyperplasia of the pituitary 'pregnancy cells' which were later identified as prolactin-producing cells (Goluboff & Ezrin 1969). The estrogen hypothesis is supported by the fact that prolactinomas are found more frequently in females than in males (Werder et al 1980). However, serum prolactin levels in response to estrogen exposure in patients with prolactinomas revealed variable results (White et al 1981). Prolactin levels correlate well with the size of the adenoma (Malarkey & Johnson 1976). In general patients with microprolactinomas have lower serum prolactin levels than those with macroprolactinomas. Prolactin levels above 250 ng/ml (MRC 71/222) are almost indicative of a prolactin-secreting adenoma (Kleinberg et al 1977). Moderately elevated PRL levels do not exclude the presence of microprolactinomas.

In a number of endocrinopathies hyperprolactinemia can be found as a concomitant symptom, e.g. acromegaly (Franks et al 1976), Cushing's syndrome (Berlinger et al 1977, Kleinberg et al 1977), or hyperthyrodism due to a TSH-producing tumor (Benoit et al 1980). A small proportion of prolactin-producing tumors are mixed tumors secreting additionally growth hormone (GH), adrenocortico tropin (ACTH) or TSH (Guyda et al 1973, Horn et al 1979, Kleinberg et al 1977). According to recent findings using immunohistochemical techniques the proportion of mixed tumors is much higher than previously assumed (Giannattasio & Bassetti 1990). Increased prolactin levels may also be caused by a local suppression of prolactin-inhibiting factor (PIF) input by suprasellar extension of the tumor or compression of the pituitary stalk (Franks et al 1976). A prolactinoma was described to occur concommittantly in the syndrome of multiple endocrine neoplasia (Doumith et al 1982).

## Diagnostic evaluation

The diagnostic procedure in patients with hPRL-producing pituitary tumors is guided by the peripheral hPRL levels. Patients presenting with plasma hPRL concentrations above 20–30 ng/ml (MRC 71/222) require radiological examination by X-ray of the sella turcica using computerized tomography. In addition, neurological and ophthalmological examination are obligatory. Plasma levels of hPRL can be used as a marker reflecting the tumor size.

## GROUP VI—HYPERPROLACTINEMIC INFERTILE WOMEN WITH NO DETECTABLE SPACE-OCCUPYING LESION IN THE HYPOTHALAMO-PITUITARY REGION

### Definition

As for group V women except that there is no evidence of a space-occupying lesion.

### Pathophysiology

Physiological hyperprolactinemia occurs during pregnancy. The increase in prolactin is accepted to be induced by rising estrogen levels originating from the feto-placental unit (Rigg et al 1977). It is well known that the pituitary gland increases in size throughout pregnancy to almost double its

weight at term. Erdheim & Stumme demonstrated in 1909 that this increase in weight is almost exclusively due to hyperplasia of the lactotropes. In the postpartum period hPRL remains elevated for a longer period in fully lactating women than in those who do not lactate at all. In nonlactating women hPRL decreases to normal values within 3 weeks after delivery. Puerperal infertility depends on two mechanisms:

1. Ovaries and pituitary gonadotrophs are resistant to physiological stimuli for a limited period of time of 3–4 weeks postpartum.
2. Elevated hPRL levels interfere with physiological gonadotropin release resulting in tonic acyclic FSH and LH output.

In fully lactating women hyperprolactinemia is a common finding. The number of suckling episodes determines the range of hPRL levels (Delvoye et al 1978). The more frequently the baby is nursed the higher are hPRL levels causing physiological infertility. During this phase FSH levels are normal or elevated, while LH levels remain low (Rolland & Corbey 1977). No significant changes in serum estradiol and progesterone can be detected. Suckling-induced hyperprolactinemia reduces LH pulsatility causing ovarian quiescence. Treatment with dopamine agonists results in rapid resumption of pulsatile LH and FSH secretion, and consequently restoration of ovarian function (Rolland & Corbey 1977). The most common menstrual disturbance related to hyperprolactinemia is amenorrhea. The incidence of hyperprolactinemia among amenorrheic women ranges in larger series between 13% and 20% (Franks et al 1975, Bohnet et al 1976, Rjosk et al 1976, Bergh et al 1977).

A variable proportion of hyperprolactinemia is associated with galactorrhea (Franks et al 1975, 37%; Bohnet et al 1976, 51%; Rjosk et al 1976, 89%). In some cases galactorrhea becomes apparent several years after the onset of amenorrhea (Rjosk et al 1976). Prolactin levels in galactorrhea patients are widely spread permitting no correlation (Friesen & Tolis 1977). Thus, galactorrhea has to be regarded as a facultative symptom of hyperprolactinemia without predictive value for the range of the hPRL level. Inappropriate lactation may also be associated with normal hPRL levels and normal ovarian function.

Serum hPRL levels being responsible for amenorrhea are found to be above 50 ng/ml (MRC 71/222). Prolactin levels between 30 and 50 ng/ml may be associated with minor alterations of the menstrual cycle (e.g. luteal insufficiency, anovulatory cycles). The upper limit of the normal range is considered at 15 ng/ml. The significance of hPRL levels between 15 and 30 ng/ml is difficult to define. Pathophysiological evidence of these levels should be re-evaluated by repeated determinations and/or by treatment with dopamine agonists.

In a group of 617 unselected patients with secondary amenorrhea in our department, 12% had hyperprolactinemia presenting hPRL levels above 50 ng/ml. In 3% of the patients hPRL levels were between 20 and 35 ng/ml. These values were obviously not responsible for amenorrhea because bromocriptine treatment failed to induce menstrual bleeding.

Hyperprolactinemia can also be induced by drugs being involved in dopamine-mediated processes, such as dopamine receptor blocking agents or dopamine depleting agents (Sulman 1970, Laakmann & Benkert 1977). The compounds are listed in Table 9.1.

In most cases the etiology of hyperprolactinemia remains obscure. The incidence of pituitary adenomas can be calculated to be approximately in the order of 35% (see group V).

The functional relationship between TSH and hPRL is demonstrated by stimulation of both hormones by TRH (Bowers et al 1971, Snyder et al 1973). In primary hypothyroidism TSH and h-PRL secretion are increased. Amenorrhea and galactorrhea may be found as concomitant symptoms. Thyroid hormone replacement restores the normal endocrine status (Bowers et al 1971, Snyder et al 1973).

Some studies have demonstrated a relatively high coincidence of hyperprolactinemia and PCOD (Duignan 1976, Falaschi et al 1980). It is assumed that constantly increased circulating estrogens are responsible for the enhanced hPRL secretion. These patients exhibit normal hPRL responses to TRH and dopaminergic blockade by bromocriptine (Falaschi et al 1980). Hyperprolactinemia in these patients is only moderate. A rather rare concomitant symptom of hyperprolactinemia is hirsutism (Besser et al 1977). However, these cases were not clearly separated from PCOD. Bassi et al (1977) described patients with amenorrhea and hyper-prolactinemia associated with elevated plasma levels of DHEA-S. Testosterone levels were normal in those patients and remained unaffected by bromocriptine treatment, while DHEA-S returned to normal (Seppälä et al 1976).

More detailed information on androgen metabolism in hyperprolactinemic women was given by Glickman et al (1982) and Vermeulen et al (1982). Both groups described increased free testosterone levels in hyperprolactinemia, whereas total testosterone was normal. Testosterone-

**Table 9.1**   Causes of hyperprolactinaemia

| | |
|---|---|
| 1. Physiological | — pregnancy |
| | — puerperium |
| 2. Idiopathic | — dysfunctional hyperprolactinemia |
| 3. Pituitary tumors | — macroadenomas |
| | — microadenomas |
| 4. Drugs | — dopamine receptor blocking agents: phenothiazines, e.g. chlorpromazine; butyrophenones, e.g. haloperidol; metoclopramide, sulpiride, pimozide |
| | — dopamine depleting agents: reserpine methyldopa |
| | — other: oestrogens (including high-dose oral contraceptives) |
| 5. Hypothyroidism | — reversible with thyroxine treatment |
| 6. Hypothalamic diseases | — hypothalamic and pituitary stalk lesions |
| 7. Chronic renal failure | — including hemodialysis |

binding globulin was found to be one-third lower that in healthy controls. Increased free testosterone and DHEA-S levels are suggested to be ACTH dependent since androgen production was suppressible by dexamethasone (Glickman et al 1982).

In fibrocystic breast disease with symptoms such as lumpy breast, mastodynia and galactorrea a large proportion of the patients exhibits elevated basal hPRL levels (Bischoff et al 1980, Fraioli et al 1981, Watt-Boolsen et al 1981, Peters et al 1982). In addition, increased responsiveness of the lactotropes to TRH could be demonstrated (Peters et al 1981, 1982). Watt-Boolsen et al (1981) found a significant positive relation between increased estradiol and hPRL levels in patients with mastodynia. This disease was described to be associated with luteal insufficiency (Sitruk-Ware et al 1979). However, it is difficult to clearly assess the cause–effect relationship. In these patients hyperprolactinemia is moderate and amenorrhea is uncommon (Peters et al 1982). Chronic hypersecretion of the alveolar epithelium is accepted to be a pathogenetic factor of fibrocystic breast disease (Bässler 1978). Penetration of the secretory product into the adjacent connective tissue results in peridural inflammation and fibrosis.

Fibroadenomas of the breast and macromastia have been found to coincide with elevated hPRL levels (Martin et al 1978, Peters et al 1981). Also patients with breast cancer may exhibit moderate hyperprolactinemia (Kwa et al 1974). However, the biological significance of this alteration is not clarified.

Prolactin has been found to be moderately elevated in patients with uremia (Ramirez et al 1977, Lim et al 1979). Kidney transplantation normalized hPRL levels, indicating that the kidneys are involved in hPRL metabolism and excretion (Lim et al 1979).

Mild hyperprolactinemia has been described in severe liver disease (Wernze & Burghardt 1979). In this condition inadequate metabolism of hPRL and/or decreased estrogen metabolism by the liver resulting in chronic stimulation of the lactotropes may be the pathophysiological background of hyperprolactinemia. Bauer et al (1980) found that hepatic elimination of hPRL was not markedly affected by severe liver diseases, concluding that the kidney is the main site of hPRL clearance.

Certain clinical conditions affecting thoracic nerves such as thoracotomy, herpetic infections, and breast surgery may induce hyperprolactinemia (Boyd et al 1978).

## Effect of hyperprolactinemia on pituitary and ovarian function

The role of hPRL in regulating follicular development, steroid hormone synthesis and corpus luteum formation and function in primates is at present not fully understood. The available evidence is consistent with pathophysiological effects at the hypothalamo-pituitary unit as well as at the ovarian level. For details see Chapter 17.

In hyperprolactinemic amenorrhea LH and FSH levels are within the range found during the early follicular phase. GnRH administration reveals normal or low responses of FSH and normal responses of LH. In some cases exaggerated LH responses are observed being related to elevated estradiol levels (Boyar et al 1974, Corbey et al 1977).

In hyperprolactinemic women the prolactin response to TRH is blunted or completely abolished whereas the TSH response is preserved. The lack of control of prolactin secretion by TRH suggests autonomous production by the pituitary gland and is different from what is found in physiological hyperprolactinemia. During puerperium both TRH- and suckling-induced responses are maintained intact (Jeppson et al 1976). Müller et al (1978) have proposed a pharmacological approach using nomifensine to discriminate between dysfunctional hyperprolactinemia and hPRL secreting tumors. Nomifensine, an antidepressant drug activating dopamine neurotransmission, failed to lower hPRL levels in patients with hPRL secreting pituitary tumors. In patients with dysfunctional hyperprolactinemia, however, nomifensine was quite effective in suppressing peripheral hPRL levels. These findings are not supported by the results obtained by Crosigniani et al (1980).

In summary it can be stated that none of the tests using dopamine agonists or antagonists can clearly distinguish between tumorous and nontumorous hyperprolactinemia (Kleinberg et al 1977, Crosigniani et al 1980). These findings suggest a common defect of dopaminergic control in hyperprolactinemia.

## Diagnostic approach

Medical history with particular emphasis on the use of drugs, clinical examination, BBT and repeated hPRL determinations are the most meaningful diagnostic requirements. In addition, monitoring of the menstrual cycle by progesterone determinations during the phase of elevated BBT before and while taking bromocriptine can be helpful in evaluating the underlying pathophysiology.

## GROUP VII—AMENORRHEIC WOMEN WITH SPACE-OCCUPYING LESIONS IN THE HYPOTHALAMIC-PITUITARY REGION WITH NORMAL OR LOW H-PRL LEVELS

### Definition

This group describes patients with primary or secondary amenorrhea due to anatomical lesions that interfere with the hypothalamo-pituitary interaction resulting in decreased gonadotropin secretion. Prolactin secretion is generally normal.

### Pathophysiology

In most cases craniopharyngeomas originating from Rathke's pouch are responsible for the symptomatology. Craniopharyngeoma is the most common tumor found in the pituitary region during childhood and adolescence. These tumors do not secrete any hormones but produce symptoms by damaging the adjacent structures. The clinical picture depends therefore on tumor size and location. Suprasellar extension of the tumor may cause various neurological symptoms including headache, nausea and visual field defects. A variety of endocrine disorders such as diabetes insipidus and in rare instances precocious puberty may be related to craniopharyngeomas. Intrasellar development can be associated

with general pituitary insufficiency resulting in retarded growth, hypothyroidism, adrenal insufficiency and delayed puberty. In such cases patients present with primary amenorrhea, poor or absent breast development and scanty or missing sexual hair. The bone age is retarded. FSH and LH levels in plasma are low, estrogens are low or undetectable. Craniopharyngeomas vary greatly in their morphological picture and may present as simple cystic structures containing dark oily fluid or as solid tumors composed of columnar cells.

Depending on the symptomatology, location and size of the tumor neurosurgery may be required.

## Diagnostic approach

For the diagnostic evaluation of these patients neurological and ophthalmological examinations are required including X-ray of the skull and computerized tomography. Radiologically craniopharyngeomas present characteristic features with cystic structures and calcification, FSH and LH levels are low, hPRL is found in the normal range.

## EPILOGUE

Various proposals for classification and diagnostic evaluation of ovarian dysfunctions have been made. None of these proposals, however, seems ideal since it is obviously difficult to cover all pathophysiological aspects in a relatively simple system. The main objective of any classification is of course to simplify the complexity and heterogeneity of the various forms of ovarian insufficiency. Therefore any form of classification will come up with a sort of compromise. This chapter follows largely the proposal of WHO (1976), since it seems simple enough to be easily applied to all infertility patients presenting with ovarian dysfunctions. On the other hand this classification is not only of diagnostic relevance, it is in particular aimed at therapeutic aspects and is of prognostic value. Applying this diagnostic approach in a systematic manner helps to find the correct diagnosis within a short period of time with the minimum of expenses. It should be emphasized that the most important steps in the diagnostic work-up are a complete medical history including drug consumption, a careful clinical and gynecological examination, supplemented by a few endocrine parameters: hPRL, hFSH, hLH, testosterone and DHEA-S. Diagnostic evaluation of hyperprolactinemia fairly above normal includes computer tomography of the sella turcica. GnRH stimulation is a further diagnostic tool providing additional information on the functional status of the hypothalamic-pituitary interaction. Androgen determinations are required if clinical symptoms of androgenization or virilization are present. In these cases determination of FSH/LH ratio and testosterone levels should be performed. Ultrasonography provides additional information on ovarian

morphology. Suspicion of genetic disorders needs chromosome analysis. The presence of a Y chromosome can be used as an indication for gonadectomy. Anatomical disorders of the genital tract should be clarified by laparoscopy or in rare cases by hysteroscopy.

The clinical symptomatology of space-occupying lesions in the hypothalamo-pituitary region depends on location and size of the tumor. For diagnostic evaluation detailed neurological and ophthalmological examination is required. The WHO classification of ovarian dysfunction can be simplified by combining groups V and VI, since the primary therapeutic approach using dopamine agonists is identical (vonWerder 1991).

## REFERENCES

Abraham G E, Buster J E 1976 Peripheral and ovarian steroids in ovarian hyperthecosis. Obstet Gynecol 47: 581

Aiman J, Edman C D, Worley R J, Vellios F, MacDonald P C 1978 Androgen and estrogen formation in women with ovarian hyperthecosis. Obstet Gynecol 51: 1

Anderson D C 1974 Sex-hormone-binding globulin. Clin Endocrinol 3: 69

Argonz J, del Castillo E B 1953 Syndrome characterized by estrogenic insufficiency galactorrhoea and decreased urinary gonadotropin. J Clin Endocrinol Metab 13: 79

Asherman J G 1948 Amenorrhoea traumatica (atretica) J Obstet Gynaecol Br Emp 55: 23

Axelrod L R, Goldzieher J W 1967 The polycystic ovary Acta Endocrinol 56: 255

Ayala A, Canales E S, Karchmer S, Alarc'on D, Zarate A 1979 Premature ovarian failure and hypothyroidism associated with sicca syndrome Obstet Gynecol 53: 985

Bahner F, Schwarz G, Hienz H A, Walter K 1960 A fertile female with XO sex chromosome constitution. Case report. Acta Endocrinol 35: 397

Baird D T 1976 Pituitary–ovarian relationship in disorders of menstruation. In: James V H T, Serio M, Giusti G (eds) The endocrine function of the human ovary. Academic, London p 125–133

Barr M L, Carr D H, Plunkett E R, Soltan H C, Wiens R C 1967 Male pseudohermaphroditism and pure gonadal dysgenesis in sisters. Am J Obstet Gynecol 99: 1047

Bassi F, Giusti L, Borsi G et al 1977 Plasma androgens in women with hyperprolactinaemic amenorrhoea Clin Endocrinol 6: 5

Bässler R 1978 Pathologie der Brustdrüse Spezielle Pathologische Anatomie ed Doerr E, Seifert G, Uehlinger E Springer Verlag, Berlin, ch 11

Bauer A G C, Wilson J H P, Lamberts S W J 1980 The kidney is the main site of prolactin elimination in patients with liver disease. J Clin Endocrinol Metab 51: 70

Benoit J, Tsoukas G, Gardiner R J 1980 Hyperthyroidism due to a pituitary TSH secreting tumor with amenorrhoea galactorrhoea. Clin Endocrinol 12: 11

Berga S L, Mortola J F, Suh G B, Laughlin G, Pham P, Yen S S C 1989 Neuroendocrine aberrations in women with functional hypothalamic amenorrhoea. J Clin Endocr Metab 68: 301

Bergh T, Nillius S J, Wide L 1979 Hyperprolactinaemia in amenorrhoea-incidence and clinical significance Acta Endocrinol 86: 683

Berlinger E G, Ruder H J, Wilber J F 1977 Cushing's syndrome associated with galactorrhoea, amenorrhoea and hypothyroidism a primary hypothalamic disorder. J Clin Endocrinol Metab 45: 1205

Besser G M, Thorner O M, Wass J A H 1977 Hyperprolactinaemia-hypogonadism syndrome—medical treatment. In: James V H T (ed) Endocrinology. Excerpta Medica, Amsterdam p 81–87

Biller B M K, Federoff H J, Koenig J I et al 1990 Abnormal cortisol secretion and responses to corticotropin-releasing hormone in women with hypothalamic amenorrhoea. JCEM 70: 311

Bischoff I, Rebham E M, Prestele H, Becker H 1980 Serum Prolaktin und Anamnesevergleich bei Mammazysten und zystischer Mastopathie. Geburtshilfe Frauenheilkd 40: 65

Bohnet H G, Dahlen H G, Wuttke W, Schneider H P G 1976 Hyperprolactinaemic anovulatory syndrome. J Clin Endocrinol Metab 42: 132

Bouchard P, Kuttenn F, Mowszowics J, Schlaison G, Raox-Euren M C, Mauvais-Jarvis P 1981 Congenital adrenal hyperplasia due to partial 21-hydroxylase-deficiency. Study of 5 cases. Acta endocrinol 96: 107

Bowers C Y, Friesen H G, Hwang P H, Guyda H J, Folkers K 1971 Prolactin and thyreotropin release in man by synthetic pyroglutamyl-histidyl-prolinamide. Biochem Biophys Res Commun 45: 1033

Boyar R M, Kapen S, Finkelstein J W et al 1974 Hypothalamic-pituitary function in diverse hyperprolactinemic states. J Clin Invest 53: 1588

Boyd A E III, Spare S, Bower B, Reichlin S 1978 Neurogenic galactorrhoea-amenorrhoea. J Clin Endocrinol Metab 47: 1374

Breckwoldt M, Geisthövel F 1984 Endocrinological and sonographic data in normal and insufficient cycles. In: Taubert H D, Kuhl H (eds) The inadaequate luteal phase. MTP, Lancaster, pp 103–109

Breckwoldt M, Siebers J W, Müller K 1981 Die primäre Ovarialinsuffizienz. Gynäkologe 14: 131

Breckwoldt M, Neulen J, Geyer H, Wieacker P 1989 Wirkung von Sexualsteroiden auf das Lipoproteinprofil Dtsch Med Wochenschr 113: 218–220

Buchler H M, McLachlan R I, Mac Lachlan V B, Healy D L, Burger H G 1988 Serum inhibin levels in PCO-syndrome basal levels and response to LH-RH-agonist and exogenous gonadotropin administration JCEM 66: 798

Carr D H, Haggar R A, Hart A G 1968 Germ cells in the ovaries of Xo female infants. Am J Clin Pathol 49: 521

Chang R J, Mandel F P, Lu J K H, Judd H L 1982 Enhanced disparity of gonadotropin secretion by estrone in women with polycystic ovarian disease. J Clin Endocrinol Metab 54: 490

Chapman R M, Sutcliffe S B, Malpas J S 1976 Cytotoxic-induced ovarian failure in women with Hodgkin's disease. JAMA 242: 1877

Chiari J, Braun K, Späth J 1855 Klinik der Geburtshilfe und Gynäkologie. Enke Verlag, Erlangen

Collen R J, Lippe B M, Kaplan S A 1979 Primary ovarian failure, juvenile rheumatoid arthritis and vitiligo. Am J Dis Child 133: 598

Corbey R S, Lequin R M, Rolland R 1977 Hyperprolactinaemia and secondary amenorrhoea. In Crosigniani P G, Robyn C (eds) Prolactin and human-reproduction Academic, London, p 203

Corenblum B, Baylis B W 1990 Medical therapy for the syndrome of familial virilization insulin resistance and aconthosis nigricans. Fertil Steril 53: 421

Crosigniani P G, Robyn C 1977 Prolactin and human reproduction. Academic Press, New York, London p 305

Crosigniani P G, Ferrari C, Malinverni A et al 1980 Effect of central nervous system dopaminergic activation on prolactin secretion in man: evidence for a common central defect in hyperprolactinemic patients with and without radiological signs of pituitary tumors. J Clin Endocrinol Metal 51: 1068

Delvoye P, Badawi M, Demaegd M, Robyn C 1978 Long lasting lactation is associated with hyperprolactinemia and amenorrhoea. In: Bobyn C, Harter M (eds) Progress in prolactin physiology and pathology. Elsevier North Holland, Amsterdam, p 213

De Vane G W, Czekala N M, Judd H L, Yen S S C 1975 Circulating gonadotropins estrogens and androgens in polycystic ovarian disease. Am J Obstet Gynecol 121: 496

Donaldson C L, Wegienka L C, Miller D, Forskam P H 1968 Growth hormone studies in Turner's syndrome. J Clin Endocrinol 28: 383

Doumith R, de Gennes J L, Cabane J P, Zygelman N 1982 Pituitary prolactinomas adrenal aldosterone producing adenomas gastric schwannoma and colonic polyadenomas: a possible variant of multiple endocrine neoplasica (MEN) type I. Acta Endocrinol 100: 189

Duignam N M 1976 Polycystic ovarian disease. Br J Obstet Gynaecol 83: 593

Dunaif A, Green G, Futterweit W, Dobrjansky 1990 Suppression of hyperandrogenism does not improve peripheral or hepatic insulin resistance in the polycystic ovary syndrome. JCE M 70: 669

Ellendorf E, Kouda N, MacLeod N, Reinhardt W 1979 Olfactory perception in brain unit responses to pheromones Acta Endocrinol Suppl (Copenh) 225: 421

Ellingboe J, Veldhuis J D, Mendelson J H, Kuehnle J C, Mello N K 1982 Effect of endogenous opioid blockade on the amplitude and frequency of pulsatile luteinizing hormone secretion in normal men. J Clin Endocrinol Metab 54: 854

Embrey M P 1981 Prostaglandins in human reproduction Br Med J 283: 1568

Erdheim J, Stumme E 1909 Über die Schwangerschafts-veränderung de Hypophyse. Beitr Pathol 46: 1

Erickson G F, Hsuch A W J, Quigley M E, Rebar R W, Yen S S C 1979 Functional studies of aromatase activity in human granulosa cells from normal and polycystic ovaries. J Clin Endocrinol Metab 46: 514

Erickson G F, Magoffin D A, Cragun J R, Chang R J 1990. The effects of insulin and insulin like growth factors I and II on estradiol production by granulosa cells of polycystic ovaries. J C E M 70: 894

Falaschi P, del Pozo E, Rocco A, et al 1980. Prolactin release in polycystic ovary. Obstet Gynecol 55: 579

Falk R J 1977 Euestrogenic ovarian failure. Fertil Steril 28: 502

Forbes A P, Hennemann P H, Griswold G C, Albright F 1954 Syndrome characterized by galactorrhea amenorrhea and low urinary FSH comparison with acromegaly and normal lactation. J Clin Endocrinol Metab 14: 256

Fraioli G, La Veccia V, Vita F, Santoro F, Orzi C, Marcellino L R 1981. Relationship between hormonal status and clinical response in human fibrocystic disease. In: Adlercreutz H, Bulbrook R D, van der Molen H Jm Vermeulen A, Sciarra F (eds) Endocrinological cancer, ovarian function and disease Excerpta Medica, Amsterdam p 323

Franks S, Murray M A F, Jequier A M, Steele S J, Nabarro J D N, Jacobs H S 1975 Incidence and significance of hyperprolactinemia in women with amenorrhoea. Clin Endocrinol 4: 597

Franks S, Jacobs H S, Nabarro J D N 1976 Prolactin concentrations in patients with acromegaly: clinical significance and response to surgery. Clin Endocrinol 5: 63

Frisch R E 1988 Fatness and fertility. Sci Am 258: 70

Friesen H G, Tolis G 1977 The use of bromocriptin in the galactorrhea-amenorrhea syndromes: the Canadian cooperative study. Clin Endocrinol 6 (suppl 1): 91

Frommel R 1882 Über puerperale Atrophie des Uterus Z Geburtsh Gynaekol 7: 305

Fuxe K, Löfström A, Hökfelt T, Ferland L, Anderson K et al 1978 Influence of central catecholamines on LH-RH-containing pathways. Clin Obstet Gynecol 5: 251

Genazzani A D, Petraglia F, Fabbri G, Monzani A, Monatanini V, Genazzani A R 1990 Evidence of luteinizing hormone secretion in hypothalamic amenorrhea associated with weight loss. Fertil Steril 54: 222

Giannattasio G, Bassetti M 1990 Human pituitary adenomas. Recent advances in morphological studies. J Endocrinol Invest 13: 435

Givens J R, Wiser W L, Coleman S A, Wilroy R S, Anderson R N, Fisch S A 1971 Familial ovarian hyperthecosis: a study of two families. Am J Obstet Gynecol 110: 959

Glickman S P, Rosenfield R L, Bergenstal R M, Helke J 1982 Multiple androgenic abnormalities, including elevated free testosterone, in hyperprolactinemic women. J Clin Endocrinol Metab 55: 251

Golonka J E, Goodman A D 1968 Coexistence of primary ovarian insufficiency primary adrenocortical insufficiency and idiopathic hyperparathyroidism. J Clin Endocrinol Metab 28: 79

Goluboff L G, Ezrin C 1969 Effect of pregnancy on the somatotroph and the prolactin cell of the human adenohypophysis. J Clin Endocrinol Metab 29: 1553

Gregory A J L 1957 The menstrual cycle and its disorders in psychiatric patients. J Psychosom Res 2: 199

Guyda H, Robert F, Colle E, Hardy J 1973 Histologic ultrastructural and hormonal characterization of a pituitary tumor secreting both hCG and prolactin. J Clin Endocrinol Metab 36: 531

Hardy J, Beauregard H, Robert F 1978 Prolactin-secreting pituitary adenomas: transphenoidal microsurgical treatment. In: Robyn C, Harter M (eds) Progress in prolactin, physiology and pathology. Elsevier/North Holland, Amsterdam, p 361

Hecht F, MacFarlane J P 1969 Mosaicism in Turner's syndrome reflects the lethality of XO. Lancet ii: 1197

Helpap B, Schwinger E, Spiertz K 1980 Dysgerminom bei reiner XY-gonadodysgenesie. Geburtshilfe Frauenheilkd 40: 381

Himelstein-Braw R, Peters H, Faber M 1977 Influence of irradiation and chemotherapy on the ovaries of children with abdominal tumours. Br J Cancer 36: 269

Horn K, Erhardt F, Fahlbusch R, Pickardt R, v.Werder K, Scriba P C 1979 Recurrent goiter hyperthyroidism galactorrhea and amenorrhea due to a thyrotropin and prolactin producing pituitary tumor. J Clin Endocrinol Metab 43: 137

Horton E W, Poyser N L 1976 Uterine luteolytic hormone. A physiological role for prostaglandin $F_{2\alpha}$. Physiol Rev 56: 595

Hunt T E 1947, Mitotic activity in the anterior hypophysis of ovariectomized rats after injection of estrogens. Anat Rec 97: 127

Hwang P, Guyda A, Friesen H 1971 A radioimmunoassay for human prolactin. Proc Natl Acad Sci USA 68: 1902

Irvine W J 1980 Autoimmunity in endocrine disease. Recent Progr Horm Res 36: 509

Jeppson S, Nilsson K O, Rannevik G, Wide L 1976 Influence of suckling and of suckling followed by TRH or LH-RH on plasma prolactin, TSH, GH and FSH. Acta Endocrinol 82: 246

Johnson T R Jr, Peterson E P 1979 Gonadotropin induced pregnancy following premature ovarian failute. Fertil Steril 31: 351

Jones G S, de Morcas-Ruehsen M 1969 A new syndrome of amenorrhea in association with hypergonadotropism and apparently normal ovarian follicular apparatus. Am J Obstet Gynecol 104: 597

Jones G S, Madrigal-Castro V 1970 Hormonal findings in association with abnormal corpus luteum function in the human: the luteal phase defect. Fertil Steril 21: 1

Kazer R R, Unterman T G, Glick R P 1990 An abnormality of the growth hormone/insulin like growth factor I axis in women with polycystic ovary syndrome. J C E M 71: 958

Keller E, Frick V, Schier U et al 1976 Hormonprofil bei Patientinnen mit psychogener Amenorrhoe. Fortsch der Fertilitätsforschung III. Grosse Verlag, Berlin, p 122

Kirschner M A, Jacobs J B 1971 Combined ovarian and adrenal vein catheterization to determine the site(s) of androgen overproduction in hirsute women. J Clin Endocrinol Metab 33: 199

Kleinberg D L, Noel G D, Frantz A C 1977 Galactorrhea: a study of 235 cases including 48 with pituitary tumors. N Engl J Med 296: 589

Klingmüller D, Dewes W, Krahe Th, Brecht G, Schweikert H U 1987 Magnetic resonance imaging of the brain in patients with anosmia and hypothalamic hypogonadism (Kallmann's Syndrome). J Clin Endocrinol Metab 65: 581

Knobil E 1980 The neuroendocrine control of the menstrual cycle. Recent Prog Horm Res 36: 53

Kopelman P G, Pilkington T R W, White N, Jeffcoate S L 1980 Abnormal sex steroid secretion and binding in massively obese women. Clin Endocrinol 12: 363

Kulin H E, Reiter E O 1973 Gonadotropins during childhood and adolescence: a review. Paediatrics 51: 260

Kwa H G, de Jong-Bakker M, Engelsman E, Cleton F J 1974 Plasma proclatin in human breast cancer. Lancet i: 433

Laakman G, Benkert O 1977 Effects of antidepressants on pituitary hormones. In: Laakmann G, Benkert O (eds) Depressive disorders. Schattaucer Verlag, Stuttgart, p 325

Landgren B M, Undén A L, Diczfalusy E 1980 Hormonal profile of the cycle in 68 normally menstruating women. Acta Endocrinol (Copenh) 94: 89

Landolt A M 1978 Progress in pituitary adenomas biology. Adv Tech Stand Neurosurg 5: 3

Lehmann F 1978 Untersuchungen zur menshclichen Corpus luteum Funktion. Forschritte der Fertilitätsforschung. Grosse Verlag, Berlin, ch 4

Lewis, U J, Singh R N P, Seavy B K 1971 Human prolactin isolation and some properties. Biochem Biophys Res Commun 44: 1169

Leyendecker G, Wildt L, Plotz E J 1981 Die hypothalamische Ovarialsinuffizienz. Gynäkologe 14: 84

Lim V S, Kathpalia S C, Frohman L A 1979 Hyperprolactinaemia and impaired pituitaty response to suppression and stimulation in chronic renal failure: reversal after transplantation. J Clin Endocrinol Metab 48: 101

Lindemann H J 1977 Hysteroskopie. In: Frangenheim H (ed) Die Laparoskopie in Gynäkologie, Chirugie und Pädiatrie. Thieme Verlag, Stuttgart p 162–169

Lischke J D, Curtis C H, Lamb E J 1973 Discordance of vaginal agenesis in monozygotic twins. Obstet Gynecol 41: 920

Louvet J P, Harman S M, Schreiber J R, Ross G T 1975 Evidence for a role of androgens in follicular maturation. Endocrinology 97: 366

Luborsky J L, Visintin I, Boyers S, Asari T et al 1990 Ovarian antibodies detected by immobilized antigen immunoassay in patients with premature ovarian failure. J C E M 70: 69

McDermott M W, Griesdale D E, Berry K, Wilckins G E 1988. Lymphatic adenohypophysitis. Can J Neurol Sci 15: 38

Mac Donald P C, Madden J D, Brenner P F, Wilson J D, Siiteri P K 1979 Origin of estrogen in normal men and in women with testicular feminization. J Clin Endocrinol Metab 49: 905

McDonough P G 1979 Amenorrhea: etiology approach to diagnosis. In: Wallach E E, Kempers R D (eds) Modern trends in infertility and conception control. William and Wilkins, Baltimore p 143–147

McKenna T J 1988 Pathogenesis and treatment of polycystic ovary syndrome. N Engl J Med 318: 558

MacLachlan R I, Matsumoto A M, Burger H G, de Kretser D M, Bremner W J 1988 Follicle-stimulating hormone is required for quantitatively normal inhibin secretion in men. J Clin Endocrinol Metab 67: 1305

McNatty K P, Short R V, Barnes E W, Irvine W J 1975 The cytotoxic effect of serum from patients with Addison's disease and autoimmune ovarian failure on human granulosa cells in culture. Clin Exp. Immunol 22: 378

Malarkey W B, Johnson J C 1976 Pituitary tumors and hyperprolactinemia. Arch Intern Med 136: 40

Martin P M, Kuttenn F, Serment H, Mauvais-Jarvis P 1978 Studies on clinical hormonal and pathological correlations in breast fibroadenomas. J Steroid Biochem 9: 1251

Meyer W J, Migeon B R, Migeon C J 1975 Locus on human X chromosome for dihydrotestosterone receptor and androgen insensitivity. Proc Natl Acad Sci USA 72: 1469

Money J, Mittenthal S 1970 Lack of personality pathology in Turner's syndrome: relation to cytogenetics hormones and physique. Behav Genet 1: 43

Moraes-Ruehsen M, Blizzard R M, Garcia-Bunuel R, Jones G S 1972 Autoimmunity and ovarian failure. Am J Obstet Gynecol 112: 693

Müller E E, Genazzani A R, Murru S 1978 Nomifensine: diagnostic test in hyperprolactinemic states. J Clin Endocrinol Metab 47: 1352

Nagamani M, Lingold J C, Gomez L G, Garza J R 1981 Clinical and hormonal studies in hyperthecosis of the ovaries. Fertil Steril 36: 326

New M J 1986 Erkranckung der Nebennierenrinde 11β- und 21-Hydroxylase-Mangel. In: Gupta D (Hrsg) Endokrinologie der Kindheit und Adoleszens. Thieme Verlag, Stuttgart, pp 182–228

Nielsen J, Nyborg H, Dahl G 1977 Turner's syndrome. Acta Jutlandica XLV: 1

Nielsen, J, Sillesem I, Hansen K B 1979 Fertility in women with Turner's syndrome case report and review of literature. Br J Obstet Gynaecol 86: 833

Nikolics K, Mason A J, Szouyi E 1985 A prolactin-inhibiting factor within the precursor for human gonadotropin releasing hormone. Nature 316: 511

Nillius S J, Wide L 1972 The LH-releasing hormone test in 31 women with secondary amenorrhea. Br J Obstet Gynaecol 79: 874

Patwardhan V V, Lantheir A 1980 Concentrations of prostaglandins PGE and PGF, estrone, estradiol and progesterone in human corpora lutea. Prostaglandins 20: 963

Peters F, Pickard C R, Zimmermann G, Breckwoldt M 1981 PRL, TSH and thyroid hormones in benign breast diseases. Clin Wschr 59: 403

Peters F, Richter D, Breckwoldt M 1982 Interactions between psychosomatic conflicts and gonadotrophin secretion. Acta Obstet Gynecol Scand 61: 439

Pettersson F, Fries H, Nillius S J 1973 Epidemiology of secondary amenorrhea. I. Incidence and prevalence rates. Am J Obstet Gynecol 117: 80

Polani P E, Hunter W F, Lennox B 1954 Chromosomal sex in Turner's syndrome with coarctation of the aorta. Lancet ii: 120

Rajaniemi H J, Rönnberg L, Lauppila L, Ylöstalo P, Vikko R 1980 Luteinizing hormone receptors in ovarian follicles of patients with polycystic ovarian disease. J Clin Endocrinol Metab 51: 1054

Ramirez G, O'Neill W M, Bloomer H A, Jubiz W 1977 Abnormalities in the regulation of prolactin in patients with chronic renal failure. J Clin Endocrinol Metab 45: 658

Rebar R, Judd H L, Yen S S C, Rakoff J, Vandenberg G, Naftolin F 1976 Characterization of the inappropriate gonadotropin secretion in polycystic ovary syndrome. J Clin Invest 57: 1320

Rebar R W, Connolly H V 1990 Clinical features of young women with hypergonadotropic amenorrhea. Fertil Steril 53: 804

Riddle O, Braucher P F 1931 Studies on the physiology of reproduction in birds. XXX control of the special secretion of the crop-gland in pigeons by an anterior pituitary hormone. Am J Physiol 97: 617

Rigg L A, Lein A, Yen S S C 1977 Pattern of increase in circulating prolactin levels during human gestation. Am J Obstet Gynecol 129: 454

Rivier C, River J, Vale W 1986 Stress induced inhibition of reproductive functions: role of endogenous corticotropin releasing factor. Science 231: 607

Rjosk H K, v Werder K, Fahlbusch R 1976 Hyperprolactinämische Amenorrhoe. Geburtshilfe Frauenheilkd 36: 575

Rjosk H K, Goebel R 1978 Das olfacto-genitale Syndrom. Geburtshilfe Frauenheilkd 38: 25

Rolland R, Corbey R S 1977 Hyperprolactinemia and hypogonadism in the human female. Eur J Obstet Gynecol Reprod Biol 7/5: 337

Ross G T, Cargille C M, Lipsett M B, Rayford P L et al 1970 Pituitary and gonadal hormones in women during spontaneous and induced ovulatory cycles. Recent Prog Horm Res 26: 1

Saenger P, Schwartz E, Eiedemann E, Levin L S et al 1976 The interaction of growth hormone, somatomedin and oestrogen in patients with Turner's syndrome. Acta Endocr (Copenh) 81: 9

Schreiber J R, Davajan V, Kletzky O A 1979 A case of intermittent ovarian failure. Am J Obstet Gynecol 132: 698

Schulz K D, Schmidt, Rhode O, Weymar P, Künzig, H J, Geiger W 1979 The effect of combination chemotherapy on ovarian hypothalamic and pituitary function in patients with breast cancer. Arch Gynecol 227: 293

Schwanzel-Fukuda M, Pfaff D 1989 Origin of luteinizing hormone-releasing hormone neurons. Nature 328: 161

Schwartz U, Moltz L, Hammerstein J 1981 Die hyperandrogenämische Ovarialinsuffizienz. Gynäkologe 14: 119

Seppälä M, Hirvonen E, Rante R 1976 Hyperprolactinaemia and luteal insufficiency. Lancet i: 229

Shapiro A G, Rubin A 1977 Spontaneous pregnancy in association with hypergonadrotropic ovarian failure. Fertil Steril 28: 500

Sherman B M, Korenman S G 1974 Measurement of plasma LH, FSH, estradiol and progesterone in disorder of the human menstrual cycle: the short luteal phase. J Clin Endocrinol Metab 38: 89

Siiteri P K, MacDonald P C 1973 Role of extraglandular estrogen in human endocrinology. In: Greep R O, Estwood E B (eds) Handbook of physiology, vol 2. American Physiological Society, Washington

Sitruk-Ware R, Sterkers N, Mauvais-Jarvis P 1979 Benign breast disease I: hormonal investigation. Obstet Gynecol 53: 457

Snyder P J, Jacobs L S, Utiger R D, Daughaday W H 1973 Thyroid hormone inhibition and the prolactin response to thyrotropin-releasing hormone. J Clin Invest 52: 2374

Starup J, Philip J, Sele V 1978 Oestrogen treatment and subsequent pregnancy in two patients with severe hypergonadotrophic ovarian failure. Acta Endocr (Copenh) 89: 149

Steinberger E, Smith K D, Tcholakian R K, Rodriguez-Rigau L J 1979 Testosterone levels in female partners of infertile couples. Am J Obstet Gynecol 133: 133

Strott C A, Cargille C M, Ross G T, Lipselt M 1970 The short luteal phase. J Clin Endocrinol Metab 30: 246

Sulman F G 1970 Hypothalamic control of lactation. Berlin, Springer Verlag

Tanabe K, Gagliano P, Channing C P et al 1983 Levels of inhibin F activity and steroids in human follicular fluid from normal women and women with polycystic ovary disease. J Clin Endocrinol Metab 57: 24

Taylor S 1981 High resolution of direct coronal CT of the sella: diagnosis of prolactinomas. Neuroendocrinol Left 3: 325

Tolis G, Somma M, van Capenhout J, Friesen H 1974 Prolactin secretion in sixty-five patients with galactorrhea. Am J Obstet Gynecol 118: 91

Toscano V, Balducci R, Bianchi P et al 1990 Ovarian 17-ketosteroid reductase deficiency as a possible cause of polycystic ovarian disease J C E M 71: 288

Travaglini P, Beck-Peccoz P, Ferrari C et al 1976 Hypothalamic-pituitary function in patients with anorexia nervosa. Acta Endocrinol (Copenh) 81: 252

Trueblood H W, Enright L P, Ray G R, Kaplan H S, Nelsen T S 1970 Preservation of ovarian function in pelvic radiation for Hodgkin's disease. Arch Surg 100: 236

Turner H H 1938 A syndrome of infantilism congenital webbed neck and cubitus valgus. Endocrinology 23: 256

Ullrich O 1930 Über typische Kombinationsbilder multipler Abartungen. Z Kinderheilk 49: 271

van Binsbergen C J M, Bennink H J T C, Odink J et al 1990 A comparative and longitudinal study on endocrine changes related to ovarian function in patients with anorexia nervosa. J C E M 71: 705

van de Wiele R L, Bogumil J, Dyrenfurth I, et al 1970 Mechanisms regulating the menstrual cycle in women. Recent Prog Horm Res 26: 63

Vermeulen A, Ando S, Verdonck L 1982 Prolactinomas

testosterone-binding globulin and androgen metabolism. J Clin Endocrinol Metab 54: 409

Vezina J L, Sutton T J 1974 Prolactin secreting microadenomas. A J R 120: 46

vonWerder K 1991 Therapic von Mikro und Makroprolactinomen. Dtsch med Wschr 116: 25–27 Georg Thieme Verlag Stuttgart, New York

Watt-Boolsen S, Andersen A N, Blichert-Toft M 1981 Serum prolactin and oestradiol levels in women with cyclical mastalgia. Horm Metab Res 13: 700

Werder v, K, Brendal C, Eversmann T, Fahlbusch R, Müller O A, Rjosk H K 1980 Medical therapy of hyperprolactinemia and Cushing's disease associated with pituitaty adenomas. In: Fraglia G, Giovanelli M A, Mac Leod R (eds) Pituitary microadenomas. Academic, London, p 383

Wernze H, Burghardt W 1979 Hyperprolaktinämie bei Lebererkrankungen. Med Klin 74: 1615

White M C, Rosenstock J, Anapliotou M, Maskiter K, Joplin G F 1981 Heterogenity of prolactin responses to oestradiol benzoate in women with prolactinomas. Lancet i: 1394

WHO Classification 1976 WHO consultation on the diagnosis and treatment of endocrine causes of infertility. WHO, Hamburg

Wieacker P, Peters P, Breckwoldt M 1988 Gonadotropin-resistenz beim Rothmund-Thomsen-Syndrom. Geburtshilfe. Frauenheilkd 48: 443

Wildt L, Leyendecker G 1987 Induction of ovulation by the chronic administration of naltrexone in hypothalamic amenorrhea. J Clin Endocrinol Metab 64: 1334

Wildt L, Marshall G, Knobil E 1980 Experimental induction of puberty in the infantile female rhesus monkey. Science 207: 1373

Wright C S, Jacobs H S 1979 Spontaneous pregnancy in a patient with hypergonadotrophic ovarian failure Br J Obstet Gynaecol 86: 389

Yen S S C 1980 The polycystic ovarian syndrome. Clin Endocrinol 12: 177

Zàrate A, Karchmer S, Gomez E, Castelazo-Ayala L 1970 Premature menopause. Am J Obstet Gynecol 106: 110

# 10. Investigations of tuboperitoneal causes of female infertility

*Timothy C. Rowe    Victor Gomel    Peter McComb*

## INTRODUCTION

Infertility associated with tuboperitoneal damage must be evaluated in concert with a broader investigation of all factors that may also be contributing to infertility. Indeed, a detailed investigation of all fertility parameters is necessary even if a specific abnormal tuboperitoneal factor has already been demonstrated.

The results of management of couples with infertility due to tuboperitoneal factors have improved significantly in the past two decades. The evolution of microsurgical techniques and operative laparoscopy were a major factor in the 1970s and early 1980s; subsequently, the development of in vitro fertilization and embryo transfer (IVF-ET) offered the possibility of pregnancy to women in whom a surgical approach was contraindicated or associated with minimal chance of pregnancy. One of the major requirements of assessment of tuboperitoneal factors is to help the couple decide whether the better management for them is a surgical approach, or whether it is IVF-ET. The reliability of investigations therefore becomes critical. It is true, however, that the infertility surgeon is presented with the *fait accompli* of the limitations of the current methods of investigation of the tubal and peritoneal factors, especially oviductal function.

The investigation follows the initial visit, which includes a full history, a review of the available records and prior investigations, a complete physical examination, and appropriate counselling of the patient about the investigative procedures that are to be carried out. We recommend that both partners attend this initial visit; it must be carried out in a relaxed manner and

sufficient time must be allowed. The subsequent investigation of the fertility parameters must follow a rational approach; this should include semen analysis, assessment of ovulation by endometrial biopsy or serum progesterone assay and, when deemed necessary, assay of the reproductive hormones. Other analyses, such as sperm–mucus penetration tests and assays of antisperm antibodies in the sera of the couple, semen and cervical mucus, are performed when indicated.

The major cause of infertility associated with tubal and peritoneal factors is prior pelvic inflammatory disease(PID). Although endometriosis may cause adhesions and tubal occlusion, infertility may be associated with milder forms of this disease where neither of these findings is apparent. Other, less well-understood conditions, such as salpingitis isthmica nodosa, cause an occlusion in the cornual region of the oviduct. Although cornual polyps by themselves rarely occlude the oviduct, they are much more prevalent among patients who present with infertility. Patients who have had a previous ectopic pregnancy treated by segmental excision or another mode of conservative surgery may need to be reinvestigated. A detailed history is usually helpful in pointing to the principal cause of infertility in the couple. Tubal and/or peritoneal factors must be suspected in women who acknowledge episodes of diagnosed salpingitis, postpartum sepsis, or who have used an intrauterine device for contraception. Instances of vague lower abdominal pain that may or may not have required hospitalization may represent unrecognized PID. It is interesting to note that in approximately 60% of the patients who present with terminal occlusion of the oviducts we are unable to elicit a history resembling previous PID (Gomel 1983a). This suggests that the disease process may be silent or subacute, leading to diagnostic misinterpretation or to the patient seeing no need for medical consultation.

There is a specific group of patients, the number of which has markedly increased during the past two decades, that seek a sterilization reversal. With these women, before commencing the general infertility investigation, it is essential to obtain the operative and pathology reports pertaining to the sterilization procedure, in order to assess the potential for reversal. This approach will avoid the unnecessary investigation of those who were subjected to a very damaging form of sterilization precluding reversal (such as a fimbriectomy that takes the form of a subtotal salpingectomy with removal of almost all of the ampullary segment).

Occlusive tubal disease in the absence of prior sterilization involves either the most proximal or the most distal portions of the oviduct, or both. Occlusions at other tubal sites are rare and are usually secondary to tuberculosis, endometriosis, previous ectopic pregnancy or adenomatoid tumor of the oviduct; not infrequently, it is an artefact related to a poor hysterosalpingographic technique.

Proximal tubal occlusion is mostly due to an inflammatory phenomenon, secondary to an ascending sexually transmitted disease, puerperal infection, or septic abortion. It may also be associated with salpingitis isthmic nodosa, endometriosis, tubal polyposis, or other rare causes of endosalpingitis. Distal tubal occlusion is most frequently the sequela of salpingitis. Gonorrhea and infections by bowel organisms and vaginal flora are linked strongly with this kind of pathology. More recently, chlamydia has been implicated, especially by Scandinavian authors (Westrom & Mardh 1982) in 50% of cases of salpingitis. Inflammation due to peritonitis, particularly in younger children, is frequently seen. Periadnexal adhesions and terminal occlusion of the oviduct may be secondary to peritonitis, usually following a suppurative appendicitis; this is more common in children. Conditions such as adenomatoid tumors and developmental anomalies are rarely encountered.

The techniques that are currently employed for the evaluation of tubal and peritoneal factors causing infertility include hysterosalpingography, (and selective salpingography and tubal cannulation), laparoscopy, and hysteroscopy when indicated. Hysterosalpingography was first used soon after the invention of the X-ray, and it has remained the primary procedure for the assessment of tubal patency and architecture. In the past few years the availability of 'steerable' fine cannulae has allowed cannulation of the proximal portion of the intramural segment of the oviduct for the introduction of contrast medium into the oviduct itself (selective salpingography). This allows discrimination between artefactual failure of dye to enter the intramural segment of the tube, and genuine proximal tubal obstruction. In the event of proximal obstruction, the tube can be cannulated further by the use of a finer 'steerable' cannula introduced through the initial cannula placed at the uterine tubal ostium (tubal cannulation) (Novy et al 1988).

In the last 25 years, laparoscopy has been increasingly used for infertility investigation. Hysteroscopy is a relative newcomer that has a limited role in this regard, confined especially to investigation of uterine causes of infertility. Review of the literature shows a dedication among authors to show that either hysterosalpingography or laparoscopy is a better investigative procedure. There are those who use laparoscopy early on in the investigation (before a hysterosalpingography), others that have altogether abandoned hysterosalpingography, and some who prefer the combined use of hysteroscopy and laparoscopy (Taylor 1977, Valle 1980).

It is our practice to perform hysterosalpingography first, before proceeding to a laparoscopy, unless the former procedure is contraindicated. The hysterosalpingographic findings, combined with the history of the patient, determine whether a hysteroscopy is required. Although hysteroscopy may be performed as an office procedure, it is generally done in conjunction with laparoscopy.

Although both hysterosalpingography and laparoscopy may yield essentially the same information, generally these procedures prove to be complementary. It is essential, therefore, to synthesize the information obtained from both investigations and that provided by hysteroscopy when this procedure has also been employed.

## HYSTEROSALPINGOGRAPHY

### Introduction

We consider hysterosalpingography as the initial step in the assessment of tubal and peritoneal factors leading to infertility, and an essential part of the investigation of all infertile women. Hysterosalpingography precedes laparoscopy with very few exceptions; examples of the latter would be an infertile patient found on initial assessment to have a pelvic mass, or the presence of pelvic pain sufficient to warrant an early laparoscopy. A hysterosalpingogram film on display in the operating room at the time of laparoscopy enhances greatly the surgeon's appreciation of the 'external' view of the oviduct. Hysterosalpingographic evidence of tubal patency will encourage laparoscopic salpingo-ovariolysis in the presence of periadnexal adhesions. In addition, the occasional therapeutic value of hysterosalpingography is well known; pregnancies have been reported after this procedure, even in patients with longstanding infertility (Gomel & McComb 1981).

### Contraindications

Hysterosalpingography is contraindicated in the presence of active pelvic infection and is inadvisable in a patient with a recent episode of PID. Hysterosalpingography in women with repeated infections in the past or any suggestion of recent exacerbation should be approached with caution; these patients should be treated prophylactically with antibiotics effective against both aerobic and anaerobic organisms, beginning 24 h before the procedure. A history of allergy to any contrast medium or to iodine constitutes a contraindication to the procedure.

### Medium

We routinely use a water-soluble contrast medium, Hypaque M60% (Winthrop). This avoids the inflammatory reactions associated with the use of oil-soluble contrast media, especially the granulomatous inflammation reported in the Fallopian tube and peritoneal cavity. Water-soluble media appear to be better tolerated by the patient, since the pain experienced during the procedure is usually less. They also disperse more rapidly and avoid the possibility of oil embolism. The purported advantages of oil-soluble media are two-fold: a better resolution for diagnosis and also a greater therapeutic value, with some claims that the pregnancy rate following use of oil-soluble media is higher than after use of water-soluble medium. These claims are not necessarily tenable when oil-soluble media are compared with water-soluble media unsuited for salpingography, such as Renografin (DeCherney et al 1980); this medium, high in sodium content, may cause inflammation of the tubal mucosa. In our experience, the specific water-soluble medium (Hypaque M60%) is superior. It provides excellent resolution; in particular, its lower viscosity provides greater visual detail of the lesions and the internal architecture of the oviducts (Fig. 10.1) than would be possible with oil-soluble media.

### Method

The method of performing hysterosalpingography is standardized in our unit. The procedure is carried out between the 8th and 10th days of the patient's cycle. It is important that the patient's menstrual flow has been completed for 2 or 3 days, so that menstrual tissue or fluid is not carried either into the oviduct or the peritoneal cavity. It is important also to carry out the procedure before the oocyte has resumed meiosis, which occurs at about day 12 of a normal cycle. The oocyte undergoing meiosis is radiosensitive, and thus exposure to radiation during this time should be avoided.

The patient lies on the radiographic table with the hips flexed and the vulva exposed. A plastic bivalve speculum is inserted into the vagina, and the cervix and upper vagina are washed with an antiseptic solution. Visible cervical mucus is removed. A modified Kahn cannula with a teflon acorn tip is attached to a syringe containing contrast medium and the medium is injected

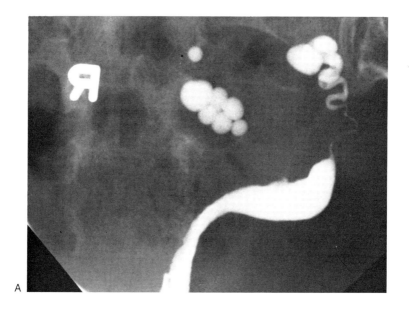

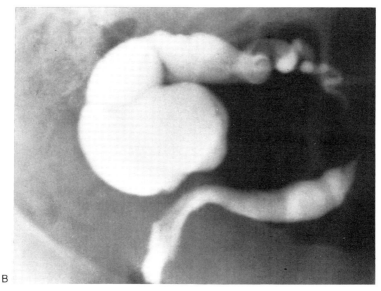

**Fig. 10.1**  Hysterosalpingography. **a** Oil-based contrast medium failing to outline a right hydrosalpinx. A unicornuate uterus is present. **b** Water-based contrast medium that depicts a right hydrosalpinx in detail. Same patient as **a**.

through the cannula to ensure removal of air bubbles. The length of the acorn tip should be no more than 1 cm. The cervix is grasped with a tenaculum and traction is applied. The cannula is inserted into the cervical canal under direct vision and counter traction applied an the tenaculum to ensure a tight seal. The bivalve speculum is then removed and the patient's legs are extended. Under fluoroscopic control, 2 ml of contrast medium (Hypaque M60%) are injected to outline the uterine cavity.

Continuous pressure is then maintained to inject contrast medium gently and slowly, governed by the patient's tolerance, until the oviducts have been outlined and free intraperitoneal spill of the dye is confirmed. Lateral rotation of the patient's hips may be necessary to allow adequate visualization of the oviducts and to confirm intraperitoneal spread. We do not find it necessary to use local anesthetic admixed with the medium, or to perform paracervical block. Similarly, we have only rarely found it necessary to administer glucagon or β-mimetic agents to overcome cornual spasm. An unhurried explanation of the procedure before beginning, and a relaxed, reassuring, performance of the procedure itself have resulted in total patient acceptance and freedom from significant discomfort. Very occasionally, a patient may become syncopal through too rapid injection of the contrast medium; administration of atropine parenterally, if required, will relieve the vasovagal symptoms. No manometry is used during instillation of the contrast medium and the pressure exerted is determined by the patient's discomfort.

Radiographs are taken when a permanent record of an abnormal feature is desired, and we follow no fixed pattern. A preliminary plain film is essential; in infertile women we have found forgotten intrauterine devices on the initial plain film, previous hysterosalpingographs having missed this diagnosis because contrast was introduced into the cavity before films were taken (Rowe & McComb 1987). It is also important to obtain films early during the procedure, in order to record properly any intrauterine lesions and the intratubal architecture. Detail of such lesions is obscured by larger amounts of contrast material in the uterus, tubes, and/or the peritoneal cavity. Manipulation of the uterus with the cannula may be necessary for better visualization of specific tubal segments. If obstruction to the flow of contrast medium is observed in the course of introduction, a film is taken at that point with sustained pressure applied to the syringe. Films are also taken at the point of dispersal of the medium into the peritoneal cavity, with anteroposterior and oblique views being recorded if the dispersal is abnormal. If one or both oviducts are distended, or if there is loculation of the dye at the fimbrial end, a follow-up film is taken at 5 min to observe dye retention. Syringe intensification (increasing pressure on the plunger of the syringe containing contrast medium to distend any enclosed space) facilitates the procedure and enchances the information obtained.

## Abnormalities

Abnormalities of hysterosalpingography are not limited to those of the oviduct. The use of a foreshortened acorn tip and the early film as soon as the contrast medium is injected allows assessment of the cervix and the endometrial cavity. If widening or funneling of the internal os is a notable feature, then cervical incompetence may be present. Furthermore, scrutiny of the uterine cavity may reveal a T-shape associated with intrauterine diethylstilbestrol therapy (Fig. 10.2), endometrial polyps (Fig. 10.3), submucous fibroids or synechiae (Figs 10.4, 10.5).

Abnormalities of the oviducts themselves may be divided into five categories: (a) abnormalities of the tubocornual region; (b) isthmic abnormalities; (c) ampullary and infundibular abnormalities; (d) abnormalities of the fimbriae; and (e) abnormalities of peritoneal spread.

The general configuration of the oviduct may provide a clue as to the specific disease entity. For example, exposure to diethylstilbestrol at the time of development of the genital tract may lead to a shorter, hypoplastic oviduct with a narrow abdominal ostium. Extremely tortuous oviducts that present no resistance to passage of the contrast medium have also been associated with infertility in the absence of specific anatomical abnormalities (Leeton & Salwood 1978). Furthermore, a general impression that the oviduct is rather fixed within the pelvis—lacking the usual mobility so characteristic of this structure—is an indication of periadnexal adhesions. Sequelae of genital tuberculosis are usually associated with typical hysterosalpingographic images.

### Abnormalities of the tubocornual region

Failure of contrast medium to enter the oviduct may be seen unilaterally or bilaterally. As mentioned previously, in our hands this is very rarely due to myometrial spasm, but where there is unilateral failure of the medium to enter the tube, this may be artifactual (Fig. 10.6). A fluid

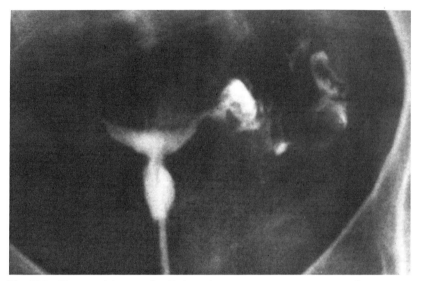

**Fig. 10.2**   Hysterosalpingography. T-shaped uterus associated with intrauterine diethylstilbestrol therapy.

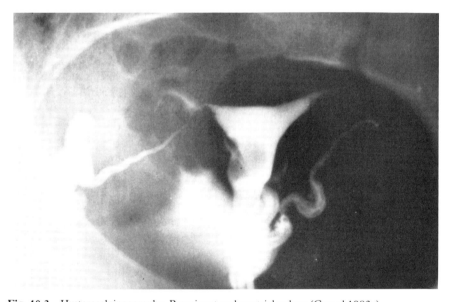

**Fig. 10.3**   Hysterosalpingography. Prominent endometrial polyps (Gomel 1983a).

column under pressure seeks the path of least resistance, and if the caliber of one tubal lumen is greater than the other, the medium may not enter the narrower lumen at all. The question of whether there is true unilateral proximal obstruction or cornual spasm can be resolved at subsequent laparoscopy, when higher intrauterine pressure can be applied under general anesthesia; or alternatively, the patent oviduct can be occluded with the probe.

In the presence of a true cornual occlusion, hysterosalpingography permits the assessment of the intramural segment. This is important, since a patent and normal intramural segment

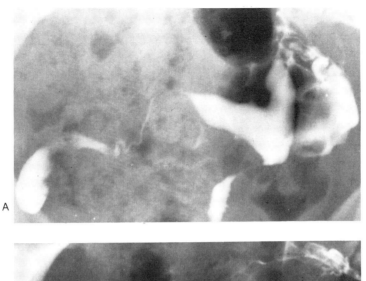

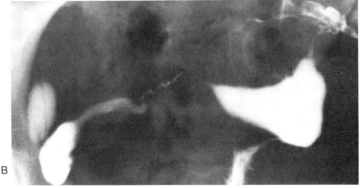

**Fig. 10.4**    Hysterosalpingography. **a** Intrauterine synechiae at the uterine fundus. **b** Postoperative film after division of the synechiae seen in **a** (Gomel 1983a).

permits a juxtauterine tubocornual anastomosis (Fig. 10.7). Selective salpingography and/or tubal cannulation may provide further information about the nature of proximal tubal obstruction.

Salpingitis isthmica nodosa may produce a radiographic picture of simple obstruction to the passage of contrast medium, usually with a tapering of the leading edge of the contrast, or there may be some evidence of interstitial spread of the contrast with small spicules of contrast apparently emanating from the intraluminal dye, giving a bushy or berry-like appearance (Fig. 10.8). In the earlier stages of the condition, this latter appearance will be associated with distal passage of dye. As the condition progresses, obstruction in the isthmus or intramural oviduct develops (McComb & Rowe 1989). Endometriosis may also provide a similiar image;

frequently in this case the punctate pattern is more pronounced and larger.

Cornual polyps are not an uncommon finding in the intramural segment of the tube or proximal isthmus. They appear as small globular or elongated images (vacuoles) surrounded by contrast medium, and they may occupy the center of the lumen or may be clearly seen at the superior or inferior margin of the oviduct (Fig. 10.9). When seen in this fashion, they obviously do not completely obstruct the passage of contrast medium. Infrequently, they may cause frank occlusion.

Where sterilization has been performed by electrocautery of the proximal isthmus, the endo-salpingeal damage may extend to the distal part of the intramural tube. In these cases, therefore, the intramural portion of the oviduct is seen to fill

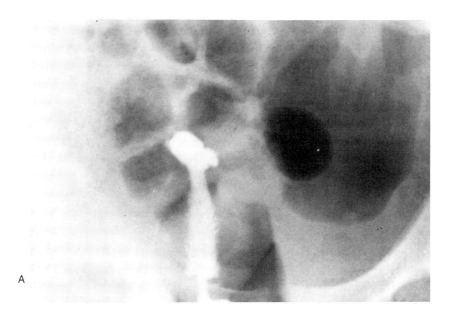

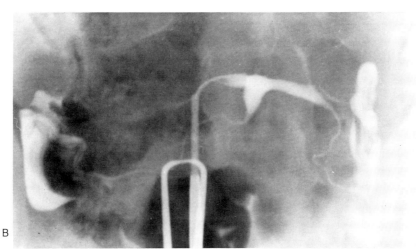

**Fig. 10.5**    Hysterosalpingography. **a** Dense intrauterine synechiae obliterating the uterine fundus. **b** Restoration of uterine cavity shown by postoperative film Same patient as **a**; pregnancy ensued.

with contrast medium reaching a tapered or blunt conclusion distally.

*Abnormalities of the isthmus*

Obstruction to the passage of dye in the isthmus is most commonly seen after surgical sterilization. Less commonly, isthmic occlusion is associated with salpingitis isthmica nodosa; rarely, it may be due to pathological entities such as tuberculosis or endometriosis. Even a previously unrecognized ectopic pregnancy may result in isthmic obstruction, although such occlusions are more frequent in the proximal ampulla near the ampullary-isthmic junction.

*Abnormalities of the ampulla and infundibulum*

Ampullary obstructions tend to have the same etiology as isthmic obstructions (Fig. 10.10). In

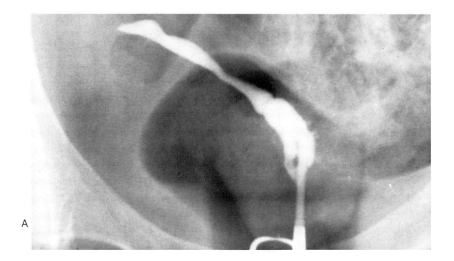

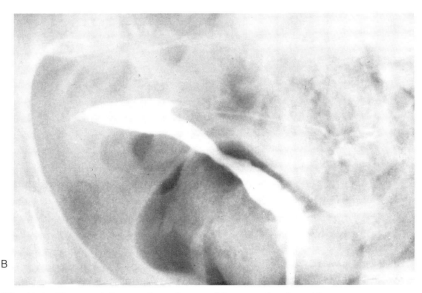

**Fig. 10.6**   Hysterosalpingography. **a** Spasm of the cornual regions. No contrast enters the oviducts. **b** Spasm resolves: contrast is seen in the interstitial oviduct, and in the isthmus of the contralateral oviduct (Gomel 1983a)

addition, endosalpingeal infections may produce intraluminal adhesions (Fig. 10.11). Careful observation of the mode of advance of the column of contrast and the observation of patchy filling defects (leopardskin appearance) indicate the presence of intraluminal adhesions.

Tubal pregnancies may infrequently arrest and may even calcify and cause an obstruction, usually in the proximal ampulla. If not absorbed, they may be associated with a round 'tumor-like' image located immediately before the obstruction.

The most frequent site for occlusion associated with tuberculous salpingitis is the proximal ampulla.

*Abnormalities of the fimbria*

Obstruction of the oviduct is seen most commonly at its terminal end. Most forms of

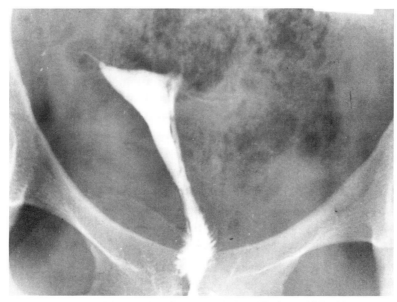

**Fig. 10.7**   Hysterosalpingography. Cornual occlusion. The interstitial oviduct is seen; tubocornual anastomosis is possible.

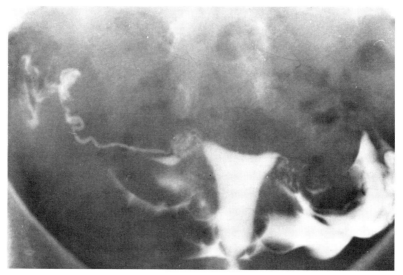

**Fig. 10.8**   Hysterosalpingography. Salpingitis isthmica nodosa. Contrast spicules are seen in the extraluminal tissues.

PID, including those caused by gonorrhea and chlamydia, as well as pelvic sepsis resulting from extragenital infections, primarily obstruct the terminal end of the oviduct (Fig. 10.12). Such obstructions are usually bilateral but may be unilateral. It is important in the first instance to inject a small amount of constrast material to demonstrate the endotubal architecture. Only thereafter is the tube distended maximally in order to define the diameter of the damaged oviduct, and to determine as far as possible the condition of the tubal musculature. The presence of longitudinal epithelial folds is associated with a good postoperative prognosis, whereas intratubal

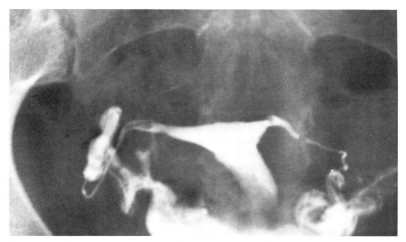

**Fig. 10.9**   Hysterosalpingography. Cornual polyps. In this case the Fallopian tubes are patent (1983a).

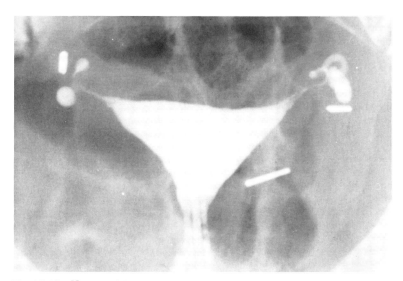

**Fig. 10.10**   Hysterosalpingography. Week clip sterilization. Note that two clips have been placed on one of the oviducts.

adhesions produce constrictions of the oviduct or, where extensive, a leopardskin pattern that has come to be associated with a poor prognosis. Such information is essential when salpingoneostomy is planned subsequently. When the tubal wall has been greatly damaged and thinned out, leakage of contrast medium into the peritoneal cavity occurs, frequently from tears in the oviductal wall resulting from increased intratubal pressure. Lateral rotation of the pelvis under fluoroscopic vision is required to detect this leakage, especially if it has occurred posteriorly. Phimosis of the distal tubal ostium is accompanied by intraluminal retention of contrast medium with slow intraperitoneal spill from the stenosed ostium. The greater the degree of phimosis, the slower will be the spill of constrast and the greater the degree of retention and intraluminal distension. In such cases, intratubal retention is frequently present in the delayed film taken 5–10 min later.

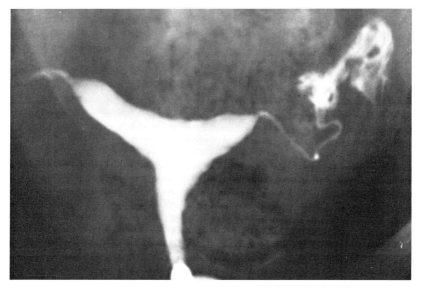

**Fig. 10.11**   Hysterosalpingography. Intraluminal adhesions within the ampulla of the oviduct — the leopard-skin appearance.

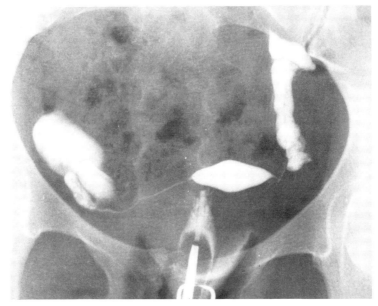

**Fig. 10.12**   Hysterosalpingography. Terminal occlusions of the Fallopian tubes. The absence of rugae carries with it a poor prognosis after reconstructive surgery.

*Abnormalities of intraperitoneal spread*

The manner in which the contrast medium passes from the distal end of the oviduct into the peritoneal cavity must be closely observed.

Manipulation with the uterine cannula, to move the uterus both vertically and laterally, is used to better assess the intraperitoneal distribution of the contrast medium. The nature of such leakage — its source, its volume and the mode of spread —

must be carefully ascertained. Typically, the presence of perifimbrial and peritubal adhesions results in localized pooling and loculation of the contrast medium around the distal ends of the oviducts, with limited intraperitoneal spread or perhaps pooling in the pouch of Douglas. The presence of distal tubal phimosis will result in slow dispersal of the contrast medium. Occasionally, ovarian cysts will be outlined by the contrast medium coursing around them, and their outlines will be seen most clearly in follow-up films. Again, lateral radiographic views will help to delineate the size and position of such lesions. At times the contrast medium is seen to pass back along the external surface of the oviduct, producing a double contour image which enables the thickness of the tubal wall to be assessed.

It is also important to observe the direction of the tubal images. Healthy oviducts are usually seen as symmetrical, horizontal trails, whereas previous pelvic suppuration will tend to have drawn the tubes towards it. Women with anomalies of Müllerian duct fusion tend to have tubal images which are more vertical, terminating at or below the pelvic brim.

*Radiographic images of pelvic tuberculosis*

Sequelae of genital tuberculosis are usually associated with typical radiographic images (Rozin 1975, Musset 1979):

1. Most frequently that of a golf-club appearance; usually only the isthmus and proximal ampulla is visualized and the isthmic segment has a rigid stovepipe appearance (Fig. 10.13).

2. Beaded appearance: the tube shows alternating segments of stenosis and dilatation (Fig. 10.14).

3. The Maltese cross appearance: in this case the tube is almost completely filled (Fig. 10.15). The tube appears rigid, often irregular, and terminates in the form of a Maltese cross, which is frequently surrounded by a halo.

4. A rosette type of image at the distal extremity of the portion of oviduct that is filled by contrast material.

5. A tube which has not completely filled and demonstrates the presence of numerous diverticula in the isthmus or proximal ampulla.

6. A tube which is not uniformly filled, where the ampulla has a leopardskin-like speckled appearance.

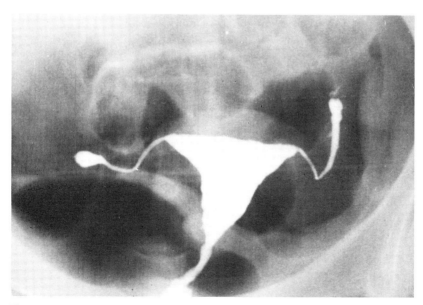

**Fig. 10.13**  Hysterosalpingography. Tuberculosis. Occlusion of the proximal ampulla — the isthmus has a rigid stovepipe appearance (Gomel 1978).

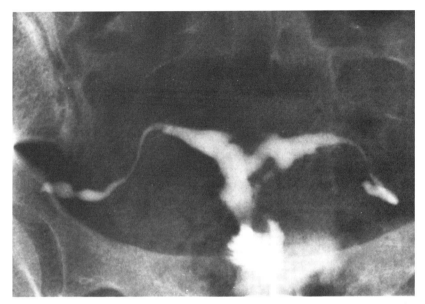

**Fig. 10.14** Hysterosalpingography. Tuberculosis. Segments of alternating stenosis and dilatation of the oviduct. Note the intrauterine synechiae (Gomel 1983a).

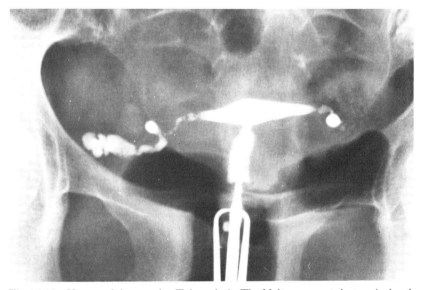

**Fig. 10.15** Hysterosalpingography. Tuberculosis. The Maltese cross at the terminal end of a rigid, irregular-shaped oviduct (Gomel 1983a).

Frequently, uterine synechiae are also present, and in addition, intravasation of the contrast material may be noted (Fig. 10.16). The presence of calcified pelvic lymph nodes or calcified inclusions in the tubal lumen with any of the above enhances the diagnosis.

The findings at the initial hysterosalping-ography may necessitate selective salpingography and tubal cannulation. Hysterosalpingography and, where indicated, selective salpingography, may provide sufficient information to reach a diagnosis regarding tuboperitoneal pathology in cases of infertility. However, in most instances a laparoscopy will be necessary since the informa-

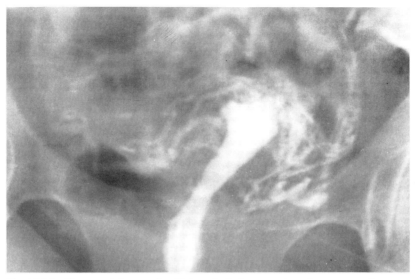

**Fig. 10.16**   Hysterosalpingography. Tuberculosis. Intravasation of contrast medium (Gomel 1983a).

tion yielded by laparoscopy is complementary to that obtained by hysterosalpingraphy.

## LAPAROSCOPY

### Investigative laparoscopy

The technique we use for laparoscopy is standard (Gomel 1977a, Gomel et al 1986). General anesthesia is induced and maintained by inhalation through an endotracheal tube. On occasions, we have used regional and even local anesthesia, but this does not afford the same degree of control as does general anesthesia. The bladder is catheterized, the pelvis examined and a tenaculum placed on the anterior lip of the cervix. A uterine cannula is secured in place by attaching it to the tenaculum. The cannula bears an acorn tip that is either a narrow-based cone or a broad-based cone, depending upon the parity of the patient. It is important to ensure a watertight seal when testing later for tubal patency. Rarely, when a satisfactory cervical seal cannot be obtained with the uterine cannula and especially in cases of apparent proximal tubal occlusion, a pediatric Foley catheter (no.8 or no.10) is fed through the cervix without prior dilatation. The balloon is then inflated with 2–3 ml of normal saline and

traction is placed on the catheter to seal the balloon against the internal os.

With laparoscopy, we prefer to use a multiple puncture technique (Gomel et al 1986). The separation of the operative axis from the visual axis permits easier manipulation of the pelvic structures with the probe and affords greater safety with operative laparoscopic procedures (Fig. 10.17). After proper abdominal palpation, we place the initial incision vertically within the umbilicus over an existing natural cleft. This renders the subsequent scar invisible. Carbon dioxide is used for insufflation and the apparatus is tested first by attaching the tubing to the insufflation apparatus and the Verres' needle to the tubing. The pressure inherent in the passage of $CO_2$ from the machine through the tubing and through the tip of the Verres' needle is measured first. With our apparatus, it varies between 4 and 6 mm Hg. This precautionary maneuver allowed a meaningful interpretation of intra-abdominal pressures later recorded. The abdominal wall is elevated, the needle is inserted slowly and deliberately, with the surgeon watching the staccato movement of the inner obturator as it proceeds through each layer of the abdominal wall. The direction of the needle is towards the hollow of the sacrum. Inserting the needle slightly to the left

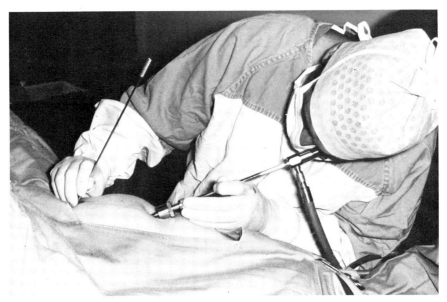

**Fig. 10.17**　Laparoscopy. The multiple puncture technique allows separation of the visual axis from the operative asix (Gomel 1983a).

of the midline allows avoidance of midline adhesions when the patient has had a previous laparotomy. Once the needle is thought to be in the peritoneal cavity, the various tests for safe positioning of the needle are carried out meticulously. If the ear is placed next to the orifice of the inserted Verres' needle and the abdominal wall is elevated briskly, then abdominal inspiration of air can be readily heard (Lacey 1976). Injection and withdrawal of normal saline tends to ascertain that lack of return of saline or of abnormal content such as blood or bowel provides indirect evidence of safe placement within the peritoneal cavity. The loss of a drop of saline, placed in the hub of the Verres' needle upon elevation of the abdominal wall, although consistent with safe placement, may also occur when the tip of the needle is in the preperitoneal space. Finally, after insufflation of $CO_2$ has been initiated, if the level of the needle is brought up against the peritoneal surface, then the pressure in the delivery system rises rapidly, whereas if the bevel is directed away from the peritoneum and the needle is applied to peritoneum once more, then the pressure does not rise if placement is correct. If there is doubt about placement, then the needle is withdrawn and reinserted through the same incision, and the

same safety checks are repeated. Should difficulty be encountered on subsequent trials then an alternative site of insertion of the needle is used. The Verres' needle may be introduced at a point two fingerbreadths below the left costal margin and immediately lateral to the rectus muscle. This site is preferable in the patient who has had numerous other abdominal surgical interventions and when adhesions are suspected. Alternatively, a point is selected in the midline approximately halfway between the umbilicus and the symphysis pubis, and the Verres' needle is inserted directly towards the fundus of the uterus. The same safety checks are then performed. It is also possible to create the pneumoperitoneum by introducing the Verres' needle into the pouch of Douglas transvaginally, through the posterior fornix (Mintz & Cognat 1973), provided that there are no contraindications (fixed retroverted uterus, pelvic mass, etc.) to the use of this approach. The degree of $CO_2$ pneumoperitoneum induced depends on the stature of the patient and the diameter of the laparoscope in use. Once appropriate pneumoperitoneum (12–14 mmHg) is achieved, the Verres' needle is removed and the laparoscopic trochar is inserted through the umbilical incision. The $CO_2$ line is attached to the cannula and the gas insufflation system is then placed on automatic delivery.

The laparoscope itself is inserted and the upper abdomen is examined. It is our experience that the majority of women who demonstrate evidence of prior PID within the pelvis proper also have relatively avascular string-like (violin string) or broader adhesions between the anterior surface of the liver and the abdominal wall. These follow perihepatitis. Delay of therapy of PID and specific gonococcal or chlamydial infections have been associated with these adhesions. Perihepatic adhesions, so characteristic of PID, are rarely found in women requesting reversal of sterilization. The laparoscope is then used to inspect the right paracolic gutter. The oblique insertion of bowel mesentery with the peritoneal cavity dictates that fluid from the pelvis will tend to track towards the liver along this route. Accordingly, it is common to find adhesions affecting the cecum (in the presence of a normal appendix) that may have originated from an inflammatory process in the pelvis.

Following this general upper abdominal inspection, the patient is placed in the Trendelenburg position and a probe is inserted suprapubically, two fingerbreadths above the symphysis pubis (Fig. 10.17). To displace the bowel from the pelvis into the abdomen, the uterus is manipulated upwards with the uterine cannula. The probe is useful in retracting bowel loops and the pelvic organs. These are inspected systematically. The degree of successful examination depends upon the normality of the pelvis. For example, when pelvic adhesions are sparse it is easy to properly visualize each structure (Fig. 10.18). However, in some cases of prior PID, ruptured appendicitis, tuberculosis or severe endometriosis, the pelvic organs and loops of bowel may be agglutinated one to another giving rise to a status that resembles a frozen pelvis (Fig. 10.19). In other instances, despite the presence of extensive adhesions, the structures themselves are not intimately adherent one to another. Here it is often possible to visualize the pelvic organs by creating windows within adhesions by using the probe or a pair of laparoscopic scissors and then by introducing the end of the laparoscope to delve into cavities within the pelvis that did not appear

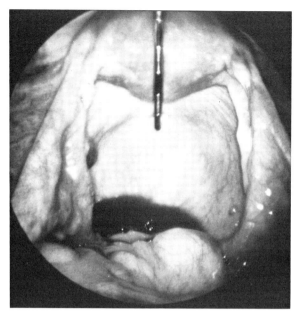

**Fig. 10.18** Laparoscopy. Fallope ring sterilization. An excellent view of the pelvis is obtained (Gomel 1983a).

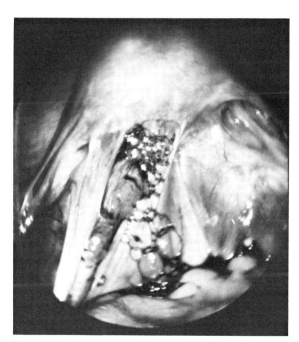

**Fig. 10.19** Laparoscopy. A frozen pelvis. The organs are confluent (Gomel 1978).

to be present at first inspection. The suprapubic probe is used as a measuring stick, a manipulator of organs and an extension of the surgeon's fingers to allow assessment of the consistency of the tissues. It is important to differentiate between extensive omental adhesions that extend to the circumference of the pelvic brim and that shield the pelvis from view, and dense pelvic adhesions bordering on a frozen pelvis where the pelvic organs are intimately glued one to another. With the omental type of adhesions, windows can be created with the use of the suprapubic probe to allow visualization of the pelvis. The probe itself may be used to break down some loose omental adhesions; but when necessary, these are best divided by direct cutting of the scar tissues at their thinnest portion with laparoscopic scissors. Broad periadnexal adhesions may shield the ovary or the distal portion of the oviduct. Proper visualization of these structures requires division of some of these periadnexal adhesions; this is best accomplished by using laparoscopic scissors. The laparoscopic scissors are inserted through a third abdominal puncture, usually in the right lower quadrant at about McBurney's point or as necessary through an entry point slightly more cranial. Care is taken to avoid the inferior epigastric vessels by direct visualization and transillumination of the abdominal wall with the tip of the laparoscope.

The pelvis is inspected in a systematic manner (Gomel et al 1986) commencing with the vesicouterine pouch and followed by the uterus. Manipulation with the uterine cannula and probe allows optimal exposure of the uterus and adnexa. Such features of the uterus as its mobility, appearance, shape, consistency and abnormal findings are noted. To inspect the cul-de-sac the uterus is anteverted by pulling downwards with the uterine cannula and manipulation with the probe. The cul-de-sac is inspected and any abnormal findings such as adhesions (their extent and density) and endometriosis (nature and extent) are noted.

The uterine ligaments are next examined for evidence of abnormalities, such as scarring and endometriosis (see also Chapter 20).

The ovaries are studied individually. Lateral movement of the uterus with the uterine cannula aids in exposure. It is important to flip the ovary around with the aid of the probe to inspect its posterior surface as well as the fossa

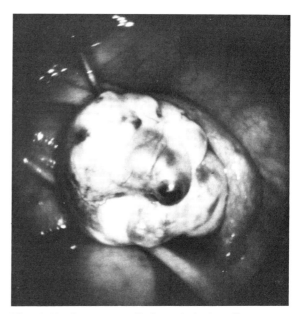

**Fig. 10.20** Laparoscopy. Endometriosis. A small endometriotic cyst is seen on the ovary (Gomel 1978).

ovarica. Furthermore, examination of the posterior surface of the ovary is essential whenever possible, since this is not infrequently the site of endometriosis (Fig. 10.20). Abnormalities such as endometriosis, cystic or solid tumors are noted.

The functional appearance of the ovary is judged according to the time of the menstrual cycle. Our infertility laparoscopies are undertaken, for the most part, during the secretory phase of the menstrual cycle to allow a concomitant endometrial sampling to be obtained for histological dating. Furthermore, it permits observation of the corpus luteum and the presence of a stigma indicating the occurrence of ovulation.

The extent of and type of periadnexal adhesions influence greatly the prognosis subsequent to reconstructive surgery (Gomel 1978). Laparoscopy is the only efficient means by which these can be assessed. When adhesions are encountered, it is important to determine the extent, density and vascularity. Pelvic and periadnexal adhesions may be filmy and avascular (Fig. 10.21), they may be thick and vascular (Fig. 10.22), the adhesive process may be cohesive and the ovaries may be intimately adherent to the pelvic side wall. This assessment

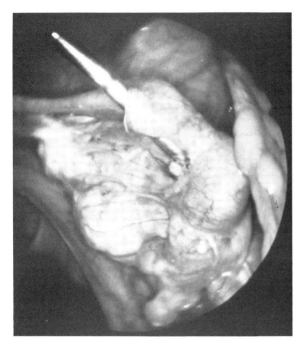

**Fig. 10.21**   Laparoscopy. Filmy, avascular periadnexal adhesions suitable for lysis at laparoscopy (Gomel 1978).

is critical, since an ovary intimately adherent to the broad ligament or pelvic side wall will demand careful dissection during reconstructive surgery,

also necessitating reconstruction of the peritoneal surface to which it is adherent. A useful exercise is to palpate the ovarian tissue (often camouflaged behind adhesions) with the suprapubic probe. Lack of mobility is a warning for the surgeon. In general, the adhesions involving ovarian tissue are of two types. The ovary may simply be held against the side wall of the pelvis by covering adhesions (associated with a better prognosis), or densely adherent to the ovarian fossa (a worse prognosis). Assessment of the tubo-ovarian relationship may be difficult in women with extensive periadnexal adhesions. However, every effort should be made to study the terminal end of the oviduct and the ovary to determine whether the tissues have 'melted' together (cohesion adhesions), for this finding makes dissection technically more difficult.

The proximal portion of the oviduct, including the cornu of the uterus, is assessed next. The uterus is deviated to allow optimal inspection. Occlusive tubal disease of the cornual region is frequently associated with fibrosis and a fusiform enlargement of the cornua. This can be gauged visually and by palpation; the swelling may be associated with polyposis or with cornual salpingitis isthmica nodosa. However, it should be

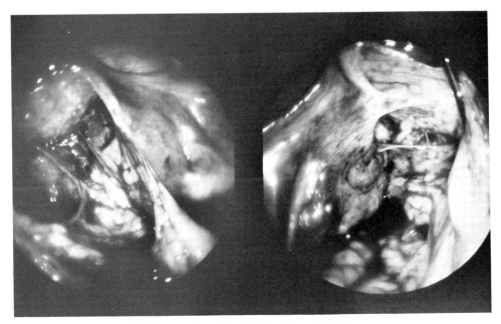

**Fig. 10.22**   Laparoscopy. Thick, vascular pelvic adhesions (Gomel 1978).

stated that occlusion of intramural oviduct proper may lead to absolutely no visible or palpable change.

The midportion of the oviduct is inspected next by noting any adhesion formation, tortuosity, tumefaction, rigidity or other abnormal appearance. The distal oviduct is subsequently assessed. The fimbriae are studied for size (are they hypoplastic?), agglutination and evidence of scarring. It is essential to position the fimbriae *en face* to ensure that fimbrial phimosis, intrafimbrial adhesions, and the covering of the fimbriae by filmy adhesions are not missed (Fig. 10.23). If there is an apparent tubal occlusion, then it is important that the surgeon visualizes the terminal end of the oviduct and its relationship to the ovary. The terminal tube may be intimately adherent to the ovary and actually covering part of the ovarian surface. The terminal portion of the oviduct may be surrounded by adhesions, fixing it in the pouch of Douglas, and thus camouflaging it from view. In any of these instances, partial salpingolysis is possible, thus permitting more accurate assessment of the oviduct. If the terminal portion of the tube is free or is rendered accessible to inspection, then it is possible to establish whether the surgeon is confronted with an oviduct occluded by peritubal adhesions or with a true mural occlusion in the form of a hydrosalpinx. In the latter instance it is important to assess the following parameters which influence the prognosis subsequent to salpingostomy: distal ampullary diameter, thickness and rigidity of tubal wall.

This assessment is carried out concurrent with the transcervical injection of dilute methylene blue solution. The laparoscope is withdrawn to gain a panoramic view of the pelvis as a whole. The uterus is elevated into the anteverted position by pulling down on the uterine cannula so as to bring the Fallopian tubes into the visual field as much as possible. The chromopertubation solution is injected with a 20-ml syringe. Injection pressure is noted. Normally, the fluid enters the oviducts readily, distends them slightly, and then spills freely from the fimbriated ends into the cul-de-sac within seconds of injection. The passage of dye through each oviduct is studied in turn. If the utero-tubal junction is suspect, then it is essential to establish that optimal pressure has been reached. If the hysterosalpingography and, if performed, selective salpingography have

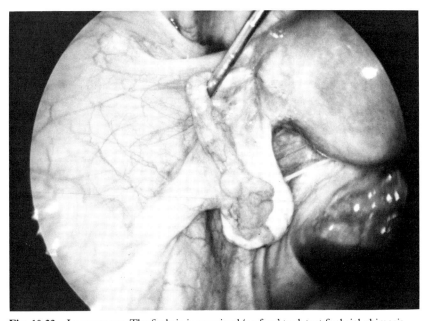

**Fig. 10.23** Laparoscopy. The fimbria is examined 'en face' to detect fimbrial phimosis or extraluminal and intraluminal adhesions (Gomel 1978).

depicted a tubal obstruction at the level of the cornua and there is lack of passage of dye into the oviduct despite high intrauterine pressures, then the diagnosis of proximal tubal obstruction is virtually certain. Injection of the dilute methylene blue solution may also lead to serosal staining — a finding consistent with salpingitis isthmica nodosa and lymphatic or vascular intravasation of dye in association with obstruction of the cornua. Throughout the midsection of the oviduct, healthy tubal tissues allow the dye solution to be seen in the ampulla. The ease with which the dye solution traverses the Fallopian tube and the ampulla may indicate the presence of midtubal pathology. With PID this takes the form of intraluminal adhesions, a feature that may have been demonstrated earlier at hysterosalpingography. The degree of patency of the fimbriated portion of the oviduct is demonstrated by the degree of distension of the ampulla in the prefimbrial region. Extreme distension associated with a slight trickle of methylene blue solution suggests a diagnosis of prefimbrial phimosis. Hydrosalpinx formation is associated with a total occlusion of the terminal portion of the Fallopian tube. When the distal wall is very thin, increased pressure within the oviduct may produce a crack in the wall through which the dye solution escapes.

In cases of reversal of sterilization, one cannot assume that the remaining portions of oviduct are healthy. The frequency of infertility of tubal origin in the community makes one realize that not all women requesting reversal of sterilization will have pristine tissues in the remaining sections of oviduct. Indeed, we have observed the presence of pathological features in the proximal tubal stumps in approximately 13% of our patients undergoing reversal (Gomel 1980a). For the proximal segment of tube the ease with which filling occurs, and thus turgidity is achieved, is noted. The lengths of proximal oviduct and distal oviduct (if present) are measured. In cases of tubal interruption, the ends (stumps) of the segment thus occluded are closely inspected to establish that they are free. Evidence of additional sutures, clips, fibrosis and other tissue distortions as well as the status of the fimbriated end (Fig. 10.24) are noted. If fimbriectomy has been performed, then

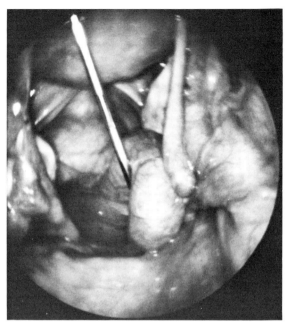

**Fig. 10.24**  Laparoscopy. Sterilization by surgical interruption of the proximal ampulla. Note that the distal segment of ampulla has become dilated (Gomel 1978).

the presence of a substantial portion of ampulla is sought.

If tuberculosis is suspected, then its presence may be judged likely from small calcified lesions on the peritoneal surfaces, severe fibrosis and distortion of the oviducts, by a tumor situated in the proximal ampulla, and by the presence of ascites that may later grow the bacillus.

Not all entities are as distinct as those of previous sterilization, presumptive PID, endometriosis, or tuberculosis. Nevertheless, at the end of the investigative phase of the laparoscopy the surgeon can correlate the laparoscopic findings with those of hysterosalpingography, and thus obtain a global picture of the evolution of the disease process.

## Operative laparoscopy

A diagnostic laparoscopy may be converted to an operative procedure, or, on the basis of the available investigations, an operative laparoscopy may be undertaken de novo to improve fertility or to treat a specific condition. Cases of periadnexal adhesions in the presence of tubal patency, fimbrial phimosis, hydrosalpinx, endometriosis and ovarian cysts may be dealt with laparoscopically under appropriate circumstances (Gomel 1975a, 1975b, 1977a,b, 1983a, 1983b, Semm & Mettler 1980, McComb & Paleologou 1991).

The prerequisites for operative laparoscopy include:

1. Adequate endotracheal anesthesia
2. Adequate pneumoperitoneum and Trendelenburg position
3. An empty bladder to permit access to the pelvis
4. Presence of a uterine cannula to allow uterine manipulation and intraoperative chromopertubation
5. Recognition of the structures
6. Functional operative instruments
7. Adequate surgical assistance
8. Appropriate training in operative laparoscopy

*Salpingo-ovariolysis*

Our primary approach to peritubal and periovarian adhesions has been via operative laparoscopy. Critics have stated that the accuracy of microsurgical lysis of adhesions cannot be achieved with the laparoscope, and this, from a purely technical viewpoint, is probably true. Nevertheless, laparoscopic surgery meets, and exceeds, the requirements of exquisite tissue care demanded by a microsurgical operation. Laparoscopic surgery deals with the pelvic organs in their own protected environment. Normal humidity, temperature, lack of contamination, and gentle handling of the tissues are all provided by laparoscopic surgery. It is also of interest that lysis of adhesions and other tissue incisions are attended by far less bleeding than at a formal laparotomy.

The key element to successful, and safe, laparoscopic salpingo-ovariolysis is the presence of space between adherent vital structures at the time of incision. The three-puncture technique allows a grasping forceps or suprapubic rod (or preferably alligator forceps) to steady the tissues and to introduce the laparoscopic scissors through a lower quadrant puncture. The adhesions are divided mechanically and electrocauterization

employed only for the larger vessels crossing the incision line; these are usually coagulated prior to division. The mechanical efficiency of the scissors should be excellent (Figs 10.25–10.27). Larger sheets of adhesions are excised and removed through the suprapubic trocar sleeve. Any fine bleeding points usually seal readily, but if any larger bleeding points persist then a low setting coagulation current through the bipolar electrode achieves effective hemostasis easily (Gomel 1983b). In practice, one finds that women who have patent Fallopian tubes with adhesion formation are most amenable to this surgery. However, the nature of the adhesions is critial to the outcome of laparoscopic division; for this to be undertaken, the adhesions should be relatively transparent or, if opaque, obviously fibrous and relatively avascular. When adhesions are dense and the pelvic organs are intimately adherent to one another, this form of surgery becomes hazardous, while the probability of adhesion reformation remains high. The experienced surgeon is well aware that dense adhesions are usually associated with other genital tract damage

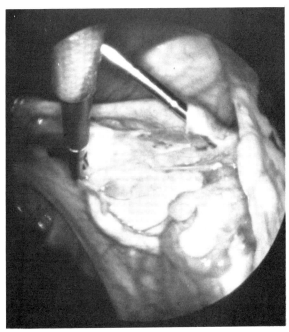

**Fig. 10.25** Laparoscopy. Lysis of periadnexal adhesions. Both the blunt probe and laparoscopic scissors are used to divide the adhesions at the level of the ovarian surface. Same patient as Fig 10.21 (Gomel 1978).

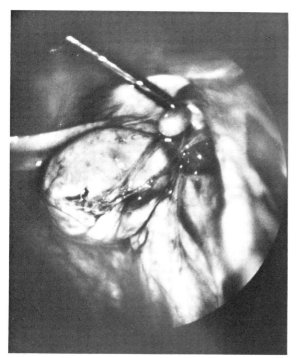

**Fig. 10.26**   Laparoscopy. Lysis of periadnexal adhesions. The adhesions are cut from the oviductal insertion (Gomel 1978).

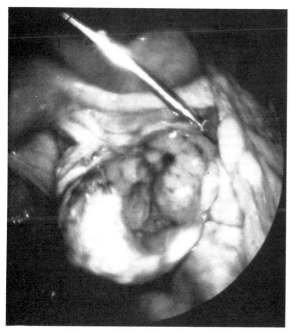

**Fig. 10.27**   Laparoscopy. Lysis of periadnexal adhesions. The pelvis is lavaged; hemostasis is excellent (Gomel 1978).

or hydrosalpinx formation that may require a formal laparotomy. If, indeed, a laparotomy is deemed necessary, it may be argued that the probability of pregnancy may be low enough to justify consideration of in vitro fertilization and embryo transfer as the primary therapy.

*Fimbrioplasty*

Fimbrioplasty can also be performed by laparoscopy. Terminal phimosis and even complete occlusion may be present due to the agglutination of the fimbriae. Otherwise the conglutination may be caused by a layer of adhesions covering and constricting the terminal end of the tube. If this is present, the serosal layer is incised with the laparoscopic scissors, and the fimbriae are thus freed. In cases of phimosis, the long-jawed 3-mm alligator forceps are inserted in the closed position past the phimosis and are then gently retracted with the jaws in the open position so as to stretch the phimotic ring. Alternatively, the ring can be released by judicious incision with fine laparoscopic scissors in avascular areas. These avascular areas are usually lines of scarification where the fimbriae have become agglutinated. Careful technique and gentleness are mandatory to avoid bleeding.

*Salpingostomy*

Operative laparoscopy has achieved sufficiently wide acceptance to permit salpingostomy to be performed at the initial laparoscopy in most cases of hydrosalpinx (and some would say all) that are considered operable. There is evidence to suggest that the major determinant in regards to subsequent pregnancy is the status of the oviduct. The surgeon no longer needs to predict (often fallibly) whether the repair of a hydrosalpinx will lead to fertility.

Salpingostomy by laparoscopy was first reported from our department (Gomel 1977b). The oviduct is immobilized by manipulating the uterus with the uterine cannula and with the use of a relatively atraumatic grasping forceps introduced through the second puncture. The terminal end of the oviduct is then distended with dilute methylene blue dye solution injected through the uterine cannula. The punctum of the hydros-alpinx is identified, and the laparoscopic scissors are used to cut along the lines of closure. The first incision is carried down towards the ovary to reconstruct the fimbriae ovaricae. Subsequent incisions, along the circumference of the stoma, are made viewing the tube from within. As a principle, many radial incisions of short length, made along the circumference of the tube avascular areas, will produce a better stoma than extending few incisions too far. Furthermore, with the former approach the amount of bleeding encountered is usually negligible. The fashioning of a neostomy can be effected mechanically using laparoscopic scissors, electrosurgically using a pointed electrode or with the use of laser energy.

A recent development led to a technique called 'intussusception salpingostomy' in which the ampullary mucosa is prolapsed through a small terminal ostium. Further, we have developed intracorporeal suture techniques that allow the use of 6–0 size suture (McComb & Paleologou 1991). The oviduct is immobilized. Usually only a single incision is made, and the antemesosalpingeal edge of the incision is then grasped with diamond-tipped forceps. Atraumatic grasping forceps hold the opposite edge of the incision and the opening is enlarged by gently pulling the two edges apart. Minor capillary bleeding usually ceases spontaneously. While the diamond-tipped forceps continue to hold the margin of the opening, the tip of the closed scissors pushes on the ampullary serosa in the direction of the opening to prolapse the ampullary mucosa out through the incision. This allows eversion of the distal ampullary mucosa to create a neo-ostium. The everted mucosa is usually held in place by the tension of the fibrous margin of the incision, but if the mucosa tends to invert again, it can be sutured in an everted position by placing one or two microsutures of absorbable material in the margins. Such laparoscopic techniques offer patency and pregnancy rates that approximate those obtained with microscopic techniques.

Rarely, one may encounter troublesome bleeding if the incision is carried too far towards the peripheral margin of the oviduct. Bleeding from the edge of the incision almost invariably stops spontaneously. Injection of a small amount of dilute solution of vasopressin (10 units in 100 ml) into the wall of the oviduct may be used as a hemostatic if this proves necessary. If compression, time and vasopressin prove unsuccessful one may resort to pinpoint electro-coagulation, preferably using a micro bipolar forceps.

### Laparoscopic management of endometriosis

In the past few years there has been a reappraisal of the significance of endometriosis in women presenting with infertility. While few authorities dispute the association of moderate and severe degrees of endometriosis with reduced fertility, the significance of mild and minimal stages remains controversial. This controversy notwith-standing, it remains our practice to attempt elimination of desposits of endometriosis, where possible, if these are found at laparoscopy in an infertile woman. Endometriosis in its mild forms is most amenable to laparoscopic excision or electrocoagulation (see also Chapter 20). In most instances a pointed electrode (Fig. 10.28) is used to fulgurate the endometriotic tissue located over safe areas. It is mandatory to bear in mind the proximity of the ureter and major pelvic vessels prior to electrocoagulation. As for all other forms

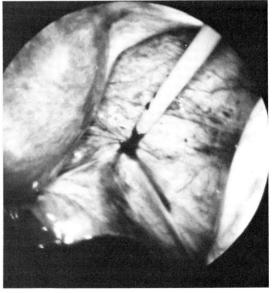

**Fig. 10.28** Laparoscopy. Electrocoagulation of endometriotic deposit in the cul-de-sac with a pointed electrode (Gomel 1979).

of laparoscopic coagulation, it is a wise maneuver to withdraw the laparoscope somewhat so as to achieve an overview of the coagulating instrument, to ensure that its insulated shaft is protruding adequately from the abdominal sheath, and that there is no other structure near to the shaft that would be endangered by the current. Adhesions associated with endometriosis can also be lysed. Laser photovaporization of deposits is a valid alternative, although it is recognized that laser therapy is less likely to be performed as an incidental procedure than is electrocoagulation. An alternative therapy is sharp excision of endometriotic deposits. When ablation (by electrosurgery or laser) is used primarily, biopsy specimens should also be obtained from the lesions, to confirm the diagnosis histologically.

In cases of suspected ovarian endometriosis, aspiration of the hemorrhagic content from an endometriotic cyst allows a diagnosis to be made, but only smaller endometriotic deposits can be dealt with definitively by ablation, either by laser vaporization or electrocoagulation. Laparoscopic excision of ovarian endometriomas has now become an acceptable form of management provided that the endometriotic cyst is of an acceptable size (usually 5 cm in diameter or less). For this procedure, the affected ovary should be mobile with a clearly defined endometrioma visible at the surface. Endometriosis affecting the ventral part of the ovary tends to extend to the ovarian fossa, and is more difficult to remove entirely. The ovary is stabilized by grasping and holding the ovarian ligament. The endometrioma is incised on its external surface, using either the scissors, needle-point electrocautery or laser. The contents of the cyst are drained—aided by irrigation with lactated Ringer's solution through a suction-irrigation cannula. When the cyst has been emptied and the cavity flushed, the margin of the cyst wall is identified in the incision and held with diamond-tipped grasping forceps. The cyst wall is teased away from the underlying ovarian stroma using the tips of the (closed) scissors; bands of fibrosis attached to the cyst wall can be divided. The cyst wall is removed intact, if possible. Bleeding points in the depths of the ovary can be injected with a dilute solution of vasopressin, or, if easily identifiable, can be

cauterized with needle-point cautery. The defect in the ovarian cortex left by removal of the endometrioma can either be left open (adhesions are rare subsequently if hemostasis is precise), or can be closed with one or two sutures of fine absorbable material, placed laparoscopically.

At the completion of the operative procedure, the scissors are replaced by a suction cannula through the third puncture site. Persistent bleeders, if any, are coagulated with the bipolar electrode that forms part of this suction cannula. Ringer's lactate solution is injected and then removed by suction. Finally, upon completion of lavage 150–200 ml of Ringer's lactate is left pooled in the pelvis.

*Authors' results of laparoscopic surgery*

**Salpingo-ovariolysis** Ninety-two infertility patients aged between 19 and 38 years who underwent laparoscopic salpingo-ovariolysis were followed up for at least 9 months. The duration of infertility was longer than 20 months for each couple. Most periovarian and/or peritubal adhesions were classified as severe, based on the international classification sanctioned by the International Federation of Fertility Societies (IFFS) (Gomel 1980b).

Of the 92 women, 54 (59%) ultimately achieved a term pregancy. In addition, there were two women who requested termination of pregnancy because of changes in their social circumstances. A further patient conceived an intrauterine pregnancy, which was aborted spontaneously. Four patients, although experiencing one spontaneous abortion, have achieved at least one term pregnancy. Five patients have had ectopic pregnancies; of these, two have later achieved a term delivery.

Of the 32 patients who have either failed to conceive or who have been lost to follow-up at the time of survey, two were using contraception and ten have undergone second-look laparoscopy. None have shown evidence of residual adhesions, whereas two have developed Stage I endometriosis (Gomel 1983b).

**Fimbrioplasty** Forty patients were followed up for at least 9 months after laparoscopic fimbrioplasty; 20 achieved (one or more) intrauterine pregnancies and 19 women live births (Gomel 1983a).

*Salpingostomy* Intrauterine pregnancy rates greater than 20% ensue after laparoscopic salpingostomy. This is notable because there may be less stringent selection of cases for laparoscopic procedures than for microsurgical laparotomy (McComb & Paleologou, 1991).

Laparoscopic surgery, then, is opportunistic in the sense that the surgeon cannot anticipate the exact circumstances within the pelvis. Often a diagnostic laparoscopy is transformed into an operative one to improve the potential of fertility of the women. It is necessary to be prepared for such surgery with proper investigation of the patient and with adequate equipment and adequate training.

The advantages of laparoscopic surgery are: therapy is provided at the time of diagnosis; it can be undertaken irrespective of the presence of other infertility factors; there is minimal discomfort; the hospital stay is brief; the cost is less than if laparotomy is undertaken; the results are satisfactory; and future laparotomy is not precluded if deemed necessary.

## CONTRAINDICATIONS TO RECONSTRUCTIVE SURGERY

The judicious use of hysterosalpingography and laparoscopy in a complementary manner, with ancillary investigations performed as indicated, allows a reasonable estimate to be made of the probability of pregnancy following surgical intervention. This figure must be discussed with the infertile couple, set in the context of the probability of pregnancy if no treatment is undertaken, and probability of pregnancy using assisted reproductive technology (usually IVF-ET). Thus, if surgery will not result in a significantly higher probability of intrauterine pregnancy than would be the case if no treatment were undertaken or if the couple underwent IVF-ET, it should not be undertaken. However, even if surgery is deemed to be the optimal management, there may be other reasons why it should not be undertaken; such reasons may be absolute or relative.

### Absolute contraindications

*Contraindications to pregnancy*

If maternal health would be jeopardized by pregnancy, then reconstructive surgery is contraindicated. Similarly, where there is a major risk of serious anomaly or disease in any offspring, the wisdom of undertaking surgery must be discussed with the couple and, if appropriate, with a geneticist.

*Pelvic tuberculosis*

Intrauterine pregnancy is a rarity with pelvic tuberculosis; it may occur occasionally if the disease process is diagnosed very early and treated medically (Palmer & Dalsace 1968, Boury-Heyler 1979, Gomel 1983a). Ectopic pregnancies have been reported after antituberculosis therapy and after reconstructive surgery for occlusions due to this condition. We therefore counsel patients who have evidence of previous or current tuberculosis not to undergo fertility surgery. Making a diagnosis of tuberculosis may be extraordinarily difficult. There may be no symptoms; conversely, metrorrhagia or pelvic pain have been described, as well as amenorrhea. A decreased menstrual flow or lack of uterine bleeding is secondary to endometrial destruction and/or synechiae formation. The most reliably consistent method of diagnosis is premenstrual curettage of the endometrial cavity, especially curettage of the cornual regions. A simple endometrial biopsy may miss the granulomatous lesions unless directed sampling of several areas is undertaken. The tissue should then be studied by direct smear and staining by the Ziehl-Nielsen method, prolonged culture and animal inoculation.

*Extensive pelvic adhesions—frozen pelvis*

Extremely dense adhesions may 'melt' the pelvic organs together. At laparoscopy, it may be difficult to discern where one portion of the reproductive tract begins and the other ends. Under such circumstances the denudation of the pelvic organs at the time of reconstructive surgery is so extreme that the adhesions inevitably return and fertility is rarely restored. In such circumstances, the use of IVF-ET has revolutionized management.

### Extensive intratubal adhesions

Occasionally at hysterosalpingography the intratubal lumen has loculations of the X-ray contrast, giving rise to a 'leopardskin' appearance. This reflects extensive adhesions of the endosalpingeal folds, one with the other. If it is confined to the distal ampulla, then resection of this portion of oviduct may be possible. Usually, however, most of the ampulla is involved and attempts at salpingoneostomy fail to reach any normal ampullary lumen. Attempted surgery therefore would result almost certainly in either failure or an unacceptable risk of tubal pregnancy.

### Absence of the fimbrial and ampullary segments

Attempts to perform an isthmic salpingostomy almost always meet with reocclusion of the Fallopian tube and infertility.

### Active pelvic infection

Surgical exploration in the presence of infection, even in a latent stage of the infection, will often cause an exacerbation and lead to failure. When a patient is encountered with a history of current active infection or infection in the recent past, then aggressive antibiotic therapy should be instigated and a full 6 months be allowed to elapse before undertaking reconstructive surgery.

### Unqualified surgeon

Reconstructive infertility surgery requires special training. Since the first attempt at this surgery represents the best chance for the women to conceive, it is essential that the operation be performed by a surgeon of special aptitude and training.

## Relative contraindications

### Bipolar tubal occlusion

Here the oviduct is blocked both at the cornual and the fimbrial extremities. Such a condition will require a more extensive surgical intervention involving both of these sites. Pregnancies have been reported following reconstructive surgery; therefore if the extent of disease is minor, there are no other identifiable abnormalities in the couple, and the option of IVF-ET has been discussed with the couple, then surgery may be considered. Otherwise, the standard approach is IVF (McComb et al 1991).

### Failed previous attempt

Prior surgical intervention that has failed is usually detrimental to the overall status of the pelvis and the function of the oviducts. If there is only a localized occlusion—for example, reocclusion of the terminal end of an oviduct that was found to be supple and not thickened or edematous at the initial surgery that was performed by conventional techniques; or the site of a failed attempt at reversal of sterilization—then this may be amenable to a further attempt. If, on the other hand, an extensive salpingo-ovariolysis and salpingostomy procedure undertaken with microsurgical techniques has met with failure, then the prognosis for a further procedure is extremely poor.

Therefore, the details of the previous surgery and a reappraisal of the pelvic anatomy and the couple's general fertility will determine whether a further attempt at surgery should be recommended.

### Tubal length

Pregnancy has ensued after reconstruction of Fallopian tubes measuring only 2.5 cm (measured from the cornu to the muco-serous junction at the fimbriae). Under such circumstances the fimbriae were intact, and the ampullary portion was at least 1.5 cm. The join was either at the level of the junction of the isthmus and interstitial oviduct or in the proximal isthmus. However, in cases of prior excision of the terminal oviduct it is necessary to have a much longer length of tube including the proximal half of the ampulla to

achieve a credible degree of success with reconstructive surgery.

## Age

Fertility potential declines significantly after 37 years of age. It may be reasonable, however, to perform a reversal of sterilization in a patient older than this, provided that the couple understands that there is an increased rate of obstetrical complications and fetal chromosomal anomalies. Pregnancy can be expected to occur relatively soon after reconstructive surgery for reversal of sterilization; however, the interval between surgery and pregnancy is likely to be significantly longer (up to several years) if the surgery performed was salpingostomy, and especially so if there was any degree of mucosal atrophy. In such a case, the age of the woman then becomes much more significant.

## Other absolute factors of infertility

In the event of an azoospermic or severely oligospermic partner, it is appropriate that therapeutic donor insemination (TDI) should be discussed and agreed upon before infertility surgery is undertaken. If there are other factors, such as anovulation resistant to therapy, then these too should be discussed and the various options for therapy presented to the patient.

## At the time of emergency laparotomy

Under the usual circumstances, emergency laparotomies for ectopic pregnancy, ruptured ovarian cyst or torsion of adnexal structures are usually performed outside the regular working hours. At this time the equipment, the surgical assistance available, and the disposition of the operating room staff is usually less than optimal for reconstructive infertility operations. For example, if a ruptured ectopic pregnancy is encountered in one oviduct and a hydrosalpinx is encountered in the other, then it is not appropriate to attempt a salpingostomy at this time. If, however, there are a few filmy adhesions encapsulating the contralateral adnexa then there is no contraindication to their excision.

## HYSTEROSCOPY

Hysteroscopy has been touted by some authors as a replacement for hysterosalpingography. However, it is quite clear that hysteroscopy can in no way evaluate the internal architecture of the oviduct except for the absolute junction of the oviduct with the endometrium of the uterus. Hysteroscopy's forte is the diagnosis of intrauterine adhesions, submucosal fibroids, abnormalities of the endometrium such as endometrial polyps, and occasional abnormalities of Müllerian duct development (Valle 1980). Where the indications exist, a hysteroscopy may be undertaken either as an office procedure or, if laparoscopy is necessary to complete the patient's investigation, hysteroscopy may be performed in combination with the laparoscopy (Cumming & Taylor 1980). Chromopertubation may be performed selectively using a catheter introduced through the operating hysteroscope into each oviduct, although this is now more likely to have been performed as an adjunct to hysterosalpingography.

Hysteroscopy has proven to be very useful in the division of uterine synechiae, under direct vision, with the use of hysteroscopic scissors introduced through the hysteroscopic sleeve. We have employed hysteroscopy when a diagnostic or therapeutic indication has been present, based on the patient's history (i.e. abnormal uterine bleeding) or hysterosalpingography findings (i.e. uterine anomalies, synechiae, filling defects).

## DEVELOPING TECHNIQUES IN EVALUATING TUBOPERITONEAL DISEASE

Evolving techniques in the evaluation of tuboperitoneal factors in infertility include both visualizing and imaging techniques. The majority of endoscopic procedures are now done with a camera attached to the eyepiece, allowing projection of the surgeon's endoscopic view on to a video screen. This facilitates both the surgeon's and assistants' functions, in that the surgery being performed is readily visible to all operating theatre personnel; the surgical assistant, in particular, benefits from seeing the surgeon's perspective.

In passing from endoscopic to microendoscopic procedures, the development of falloposcopy was probably predictable, yet the procedure remains largely experimental. Falloposcopy appears to be possible, using current techniques, in about 90% of appropriate cases (Kerin et al 1990). The procedure allows an assessment of the mucosal condition of the oviduct in women with suspected tubal factor infertility, although its therapeutic value is as yet untested.

The place of radionuclide hysterosalpingography (HSG) in the evaluation of tubal factor infertility also remains to be determined. In this procedure, albumin microspheres labelled with radioactive technetium-99 are introduced onto the cervix, and their subsequent passage into the upper genital tract and peritoneal cavity is monitored by a gamma camera. Discrepancies between the results of conventional HSG and radionuclide HSG suggest that fertility is a function more of oviductal mechanics (as yet, poorly defined) than of simple patency to the passage of dye (Brundin et al 1989).

Another imaging technique that is less invasive is color Doppler flow ultrasonography (Peters & Coulam 1991). This allows assessment of tubal patency although it cannot define intratubal architecture. It is useful for confirming tubal patency in such instances where tubal disease does not appear to be the cause of the infertility, as it is performed easily and without X-ray exposure. An example of such an instance would be an anovulatory woman requiring ovulation induction who has not had assessment of the Fallopian tubes.

Other imaging techniques, such as computerized tomography (CT), and magnetic resonance imaging (MRI), have found a very limited place in the evaluation of tuboperitoneal pathology. CT scanning has some use in evaluating adnexal masses, but it has less discriminatory value than ultrasonography in the pelvis. MRI has been shown to be of some value in distinguishing between adenomyosis and leiomyomas, but outside the uterus it has not, so far, proven useful in evaluating pelvic disease.

## SUMMARY

For women with tuboperitoneal disease, both hysterosalpingography and laparoscopy are needed to provide complementary information that will lead to a precise diagnosis of the site and severity of the tuboperitoneal disease. Hysteroscopy and selective tubal cannulation can provide useful supplementary information. Reconstructive tubal surgery can thereafter be performed appropriately, and is increasingly being performed laparoscopically. These investigations are also a necessary assessment before IVF procedures can be instigated.

It is hoped that in the near future the investigative armamentarium will include an assessment of the function of the oviduct afflicted by tuboperitoneal pathology. All of our contemporary investigations assess tubal morphology and patency, but not function; and prolonged infertility in the absence of tubal obstruction will usually be managed by performance of IVF-ET, thus bypassing tubal function. A valid assessment of Fallopian tube function would not only increase diagnostic acumen, but would also allow preoperative identification of those women likely to benefit from tubal surgery and those who would not. Making an accurate prediction of the outcome of management has become the goal for physicians managing infertility in the last decade of this century.

## REFERENCES

Boury-Heyler C 1979 La tuberculose tubaire, aspect actual en France. In: Oviduct et fertilite. Masson, Paris, p 219

Brundin A, Dahlborn M, Ahlberg-Ahre E, Lundberg H J 1989 Radionuclide hysterosalpingography for measurement of human oviductal function. Int J Gynecol Obstet 28: 53.

Cumming D C, Taylor P J 1980 Combined laparoscopy and hysteroscopy in the investigation of the ovulatory infertility female. Fertil Steril 33: 475

DeCherney A H, Kort H, Barney J B, De Vose G R 1980

Increased pregnancy with oil-soluble hysterosalpingography dye. Fertil Steril 33: 407

Gomel V 1975a Laparoscopic tubal surgery in infertility. Obstet Gynecol 46: 47

Gomel V 1975b Laparoscopic tubal surgery in infertility. Proceedings of the IVth European Sterility Congress in Reproduction, p 247

Gomel V 1977a Laparoscopy prior to reconstructive tubal surgery for infertility. J Reprod Med 18: 251

Gomel V 1977b Salpingostomy by laparoscopy. J Reprod Med 18: 265

Gomel V 1978 Recent advances in surgical correction of tubal disease producing infertility. Curr Prob Obstet Gynecol 1: 10

Gomel V 1980a Microsurgical reversal of female sterilization: a reappraisal. Fertil Steril 33: 587

Gomel V 1980b Classification of operations for tubal and peritoneal factors causing infertility. Clin Obstet Gynecol 28: 1259

Gomel V 1983a Microsurgery in female infertility. Little, Brown and Co., Boston

Gomel V 1983b Salpingo-ovariolysis by laparoscopy in infertility. Fertil Steril 40: 607

Gomel V, McComb P 1981 Unexpected pregnancies in women afflicted by occlusive tubal disease. Fertil Steril 36: 529

Gomel V, Taylor P J, Yuzpe A A, Rioux J E 1986 Laparoscopy and hysteroscopy in gynecologic practice. Year Book Medical, Chicago

Kerin J, Daykhovsky L, Segalowitz J, Surrey E et al 1990 Falloposcopy: a microendoscopic technique for visual exploration of the human fallopian tube from the uterotubal ostium to the fimbria using a transvaginal approach. Fertil Steril 54: 390

Lacey C G 1976 Laparoscopy: a clinical sign for intraperitoneal needle placement. Obstet Gynecol 47: 625

Leeton J, Salwood T 1978 The tortuous tube: pregnancy rate following laparoscopy and hydrotubation. Aust NZ J Obstet Gynaecol 18: 259

McComb P F, Paleologou A 1991 The intussusception technique for the therapy of distal oviductal occlusion at laparoscopy. Obstet Gynecol 78: 443

McComb P F, Rowe T C 1989 Salpingitis isthmica nodosa: evidence that it is a progressive disease. Fertil Steril 51: 542

McComb P F, Lee N H, Stephenson M D 1991 Reproductive outcome after microsurgery for proximal and distal occlusions in the same fallopian tube. Fertil Steril 56: 134

Mintz M, Cognat M 1973 Risques dela coelioscopie gynecologique. Acta Endoscopica Radiocinematograph 3: 62

Musset R 1979 An atlas of hysterosalpinography. Les Presses de 1'Universite Laval, Quebec

Novy M J, Thurmond A S, Patton P, Uchida B T, Rosch J 1988 Diagnosis of cornual obstruction by transcervical fallopian tube cannulation. Fertil Steril 50: 434

Palmer R, Dalsace J 1968 Le traitement chirurgical des sterilities tubaires. Bull Fed Soc Gynecol Obstet 20: 139

Peters A J, Coulam C B, 1991 Hysterosalpingography with color Doppler ultrasonography. Am J Obstet Gynecol 164: 1530–1534

Rowe T C, McComb P F 1987 Unknown intrauterine devices and infertility. Fertil Steril 47: 1038

Rozin S 1975 Genital tuberculosis. In: Behrman S J, Kistner R W (eds) Progress in infertility, 2nd edn. Little, Brown and Co., Boston

Semm K, Mettler L 1980 Technical progress in pelvic surgery via operative laparoscopy. Am J Obstet Gynecol 138: 121

Taylor P J 1977 Correlations in infertility; symptomatology, hysterosalpingography, laparoscopy and hysteroscopy J Reprod Med 18: 339

Valle R F 1980 Hysteroscopy in the evaluation of female infertility. Am J Obstet Gynecol 137: 425

Westrom L, Mardh P A 1982 Genital chlamydial infections In: Mardh P A, Holmes K K, Oriel J D (eds) Chlamydial infections. Elsevier Medical, New York, p 121

# Diagnosis of infertility (male)

# 11. Semen analysis

*Marek Glezerman   Benjamin Bartoov*

The most important single test in the evaluation of male infertility is the semen analysis. If performed skilfully and interpreted intelligently, it will provide a wide spectrum of information reflecting the spermatogenetic and steroidogenetic function of the testis and functional state of the secondary sex glands.

## COLLECTION OF THE EJACULATE

The only acceptable method for collection of the ejaculate is masturbation. Only this method permits complete collection of the specimen in a suitable container and best avoids contamination. The withdrawal technique is not very reliable, since some of the semen may be lost during withdrawal and vaginal secretions may contaminate the specimen.

Commercially available condoms should never be used for sperm collection since these are coated with spermicidal substances. If due to religious or psychological reasons masturbation is not acceptable, nonlubricated and nonmedicated condoms designed especially for this purpose may be used (Milex Limited). For some males, religious restrictions may prohibit ejaculation unless it is intravaginal. For these patients, even condom intercourse will present a form of unacceptable masturbation and a violation of the biblical injunction against 'spilling of the seed needlessly' (Genesis 38: 7–10). In these cases, a perforated 'Milex pouch' may be used. Since a very tiny hole will allow for a physical connection between penis and vagina but will virtually not affect the seminal volume, this simple technical procedure will relieve the conflict of conscience and is generally acceptable to both patient and religious authorities.

If a private area is available on the premises of the clinic or at the office, semen collection is best performed there since semen is then available for immediate evaluation. However, it may be less embarrassing for the patient to produce semen at his own home. This is acceptable if the semen can be delivered to the laboratory within less than 45 minutes (see below). If the patient's home is too far away and masturbation on the premises is not acceptable, we usually suggest renting a hotel room in the vicinity.

The specimen bottle, a wide-mouthed container, should be supplied by the laboratory. The jar must be completely dry before use since water will quickly kill sperm cells (Jequier 1986). It is advisable to use containers pretested by chemical and biological studies as to their effects on seminal parameters. Inchiosa (1965) demonstrated that toxic substances may leak through plastic and rubber material used in disposable syringes and Jaeger & Rubin (1970) showed that plastic bags used for blood storage may be similarly hazardous. Glass bottles are probably not necessarily better suited for collection of semen than tested plastic material. Calamera (1978) performed a study of spermatozoal motility and several plasma constituents in semen incubated in glass flasks and polyethylene plastic collectors at room temperature. No differences were observed.

In certain cases it might be necessary to obtain the ejaculate in fractions, so-called 'split-fractions' (see Chapter 25). Zaneveld & Polakoski (1977) have proposed a special tray consisting of three wide-mouthed plastic cups that are attached to each other and may be held by a 12-cm-long handle. A tray cover secures tight closing of the numbered specimen. Alternatively, the patient may be instructed to use two separate containers for the first and the following ejaculatory spurts respectively. The patient should receive written guidelines giving exact instructions concerning sexual abstinence, collection and transport of the sample.

## SEXUAL ABSTINENCE BEFORE COLLECTION OF THE EJACULATE

The period of continence preceding collection of the semen specimen has a remarkable influence on spermatozoal concentration and a lesser effect on motility (Freund 1962, 1963). Schirren (1972) has confirmed the correlation between sperm concentration and the number of days of abstinence (Table 11.1). For the sake of standardization, most laboratories specify a period of continence (usually 3–5 days).

Sperm output observed in longitudinal studies is far from uniform and may vary considerably even in fertile volunteers. Motility seems to be much less dependent on abstinence and remains relatively stable, at least within 5 days. Sauer et al (1988) used a method of automated videomicrography and measured five motility parameters in 10 fertile donors over a period of 120 h. Along this time period, no change in motility could be observed with change of ejaculatory frequency. However, prolonged abstinence will result in the output of ageing sperm cells from the epididimis

with resultant decreased motility (Mortimer et al 1982).

Paulsen (WHO 1987) has followed biweekly the sperm output in one individual for 2 years. This healthy donor had during that period no febrile illnesses nor did he receive any medication. Sperm concentrations fluctuated between 5 million sperm cells per ml and 170 million per ml. Thus, examination of a single semen specimen is of very limited usefulness for assessment of the quantitative gametogenic function of the tests. Since standardization is important in the evaluation of the infertile male, it is justified to perform at least two semen analyses prior to diagnosis and treatment. The semen samples are delivered at an interval of at least 2 weeks.

## EXAMINATION OF THE EJACULATE

Usually the color of the ejaculate is whitish-gray to yellowish and tends more to yellowish the longer the abstinence period is. Discoloration of the semen may point to genital tract infections if the specimen appears white or yellow (leukocytes) or to bleeding from some point along the tract if the semen is reddish (erythrocytes). Finally, certain drugs such as antibiotics may lead to discoloration.

The odor of semen has been compared to chestnut flowers and results probably from oxidation of spermine which originates from the prostatic gland. The odor of semen may remind obstetricians of amniotic fluid.

### Coagulation and liquefaction

Immediately after ejaculation, the liquid seminal fluid coagulates and subsequently liquefies within 5–40 min. The physiological function of this process remains unclear. The coagulation process differs basically from blood coagulation as far as coagulation factors are concerned. The coagulative enzyme in man originates in the seminal vesicle while the liquefying enzyme, seminine, is produced by the prostate gland.

The progress of coagulation or liquefaction may be disturbed. Azoospermia (i.e. complete absence of sperm cells in the semen sample) concomitant

**Table 11.1** Relationship between sexual abstinence and spermatozoal concentration. Note that there is no further increase of spermatozoal concentration after the 11th day of abstinence (Schirren 1972)

| Days of abstinence | Mean spermatozoal concentration ($\times 10^6$/ml) | Days of abstinence | Mean spermatozoal concentration ($\times 10^6$/ml) |
|---|---|---|---|
| 1 | 13 | 8 | 105 |
| 2 | 31 | 9 | 96 |
| 3 | 53 | 10 | 227 |
| 4 | 82 | 11 | 166 |
| 5 | 86 | 12 | 146 |
| 6 | 96 | 13 | 152 |
| 7 | 87 | 14 | 161 |

with complete lack of coagulation indicates agenesis of the seminal vesicle or occlusion of ejaculatory ducts. If the seminal coagulation fails to liquefy, probably due to poor prostate lytic activity, the persistent coagulum may trap spermatozoa and restrict motility. Thus, observation of coagulation and liquefaction is of considerable importance.

Following liquefaction, the seminal fluid achieves a viscous state. Hyperviscosity may also impair sperm transport. Usually, viscosity is estimated by observing the ability of the fluid to adapt to the form of the slowly rotated semen container (Zaneveld & Polakoski 1977) or by pouring it into another jar and observing its ability to fractionate (Amelar et al 1977). A more accurate method consists of measuring the time necessary for the seminal fluid to form a drop when released from a pipette (Eliasson 1973). A simple method involving centrifugation has been proposed by Boonsaeng (1981). Based on the observation that only liquefying semen produces supernatant during centrifugation and that the amount of produced supernatant is directly related to the volume of liquefying coagulum, this method permits quantitative assessment of the seminal liquefication.

## Volume and pH

Hypospermia and hyperspermia are terms describing semen samples with a volume of less than 1.5 ml and more than 5.5 ml respectively. A man is considered aspermic if sensation of orgasm is not accompanied by emission of semen. Seminal plasma serves as a vehicle and a dilutent for spermatozoa and as a buffering medium protecting sperm cells from the hostile vaginal environment; it contains sources of energy and serves to unlock energy-rich components of female genital secretions. These functions justify a deeper interest in seminal biochemistry.

Probably the only seminal parameter totally unrelated to other andrological parameters is the seminal volume (Dickerman et al 1988). Extremely low seminal volume may reduce the fertilizing capacity of a given semen sample by impairment of is vehicle function and biochemical interaction with sperm cells, and an extremely high volume may lead to dilution of sperm cells.

The normal volume of the seminal fluid averages 2–5 ml. Prolonged sexual abstinence or a high level of sexual arousal may result in a larger seminal volume. Furthermore, Duyck & Steeno (1990) have reported on a distinct entity of idiopathic high-volume semen. The prostatic and epididymal contributions to the seminal fluid usually do not exceed 1 ml. Thus, semen volume is mainly a function of the activity of the seminal vesicles. Inflammatory processes, mainly of this gland and to a lesser extent of the prostate, may lead to hyperspermia with resultant dilution of the cell content. Reduced seminal volume may result from androgen deficiency, may be the consequence of proximal occlusion of the ejaculatory ducts, or may simply reflect incomplete ejaculation or loss of parts of the specimen.

Determination of pH is easily performed using indicator paper. A pH exceeding 8.0 may suggest acute diseases of the seminal vesicles or may be due to delayed measurement. (Seminal plasma releases $CO_2$ continuously and consequently pH values increase). If the pH is below 7, it may be a sign of occlusion of the ejaculatory ducts or of contamination of the semen specimen by urine. Chronic inflammatory processes of the seminal vesicle may also be the reason for pH values of less than 7.2.

## Microscopic examination of the ejaculate

Before microscopic examination is performed, it is absolutely necessary to have a well-mixed specimen. The easiest and quickest way is to use a vortex mixer for about 10s at high speed. The sample should be checked microscopically after liquefication for debris, bacteria, and epithelial and blood cells. Indication for bacteriological studies should be decided upon at this stage. The presence of immature cells should be noted and special attention should be paid to any agglutination. Aggregation of sperm cells to cellular debris is not considered to be agglutination. If more than 10% of sperm cells show head–head, tail–tail or head–tail agglutination, infection or immunological problems may be suspected and specific tests should be performed.

*Sperm count*

A semen sample in which, after centrifugation, no sperm cells can be observed, is termed azoospermic. Aspermia describes a condition in which no seminal fluid is discharged during orgasm. Oligozoospermia, normozoospermia and polyzoospermia are terms which define semen samples containing less than normal, normal or higher than the normal concentrations of sperm cells respectively. There is no consensus, however, on where the limits should be set (Table 11.2). As mentioned earlier, biweekly sperm counts in a healthy subject have been shown to fluctuate between 5 million and 170 million sperm cells/ml, and variations in relation to abstinence have been observed by many investigators. Schwartz et al (1979) have found that each day of abstinence increases the sperm count in healthy donors by 13 million cells/ml. Polyzoospermia, too, is an ill-defined condition. Literature on polyzoospermia is scarce and the few studies dealing with this entity show a lack of standard criteria for diagnosis, different terms being used to describe semen samples with a sperm concentration considered to be higher than normal (Table 11.3). Patients with sperm concentrations above 250 million/ml seem to have impaired infertility. Glezerman et al (1982) studied 30 couples in whom the male partner presented with polysoozpermia. The spontaneous pregnancy rate was 38.7% and the spontaneous abortion rate was 25%. Sperm penetration tests revealed normal

**Table 11.3** Definitions of high density semen

| Authors | Term | Sperm density/ml ($\times 10^6$) |
|---|---|---|
| Joel 1969 | Hyperspermia | 120 |
| Singer et al 1979 | Polyspermia | 200 |
| Eliasson et al 1970 | Polyzoospermia | 250 |
| Glezerman et al 1982 | Polyzoospermia | 250 |
| Barnea et al 1980 | Polyspermia | 600($10^6$/total volume) |

mucus-penetrating ability in 29 out of 30 males studied. There is no convincing explanation for the obvious reduction in the reproductive performance of males with polyzoospermia.

Contemporary data reveal a peculiar downward shift in the average spermatozoal density in fertile men (Table 11.4). No study reported after 1974 showed an average sperm density above 100 million/ml in fertile men. James (1980) discussed probable reasons for this downward trend. He concluded that human error, counting techniques, psychological factors, social class and age of tested men, as well as sexual abstinence, probably played no significant role in this trend.

Leto & Frensilli (1981) also observed the changing parameters of donor semen and projected that, if the trend continues, no potential donor might meet in the future the current minimal standards (see Chapter 25). Looking at the range of sperm counts in fertile men, i.e. men whose wives were pregnant at the time of semen

**Table 11.2** Proposed normal values for sperm concentration

| Authors | Sperm cells/ml ($\times 10^6$) |
|---|---|
| Macomber & Sanders 1929 | 60 |
| MacLeod 1965 | 20 |
| Van Zyl 1972 | 10 |
| Schirren 1972 | 40 |
| Ludvik 1976 | 40 |
| Freund & Peterson 1976 | 40 |
| Eliasson 1977a | 20 |
| Amelar et al 1977 | 40 |
| Zaneveld & Polakoski 1977 | 50 |
| Zuckerman et al 1977 | 20 |
| Brotherton 1979 | 60 |
| Homonnai et al 1980 | 10 |
| Lunenfeld & Glezerman 1981 | 30 |
| Pryor 1981 | 40 |

**Table 11.4** Mean spermatozoal concentration in men of proved fertility

| Authors | Mean sperm count/ml ($\times 10^6$) | Men (no.) |
|---|---|---|
| Hotchkiss et al 1938 | 120 | 200 |
| Farris 1949 | 145 | 49 |
| Falk & Kaufman 1950 | 101 | 100 |
| MacLeod & Gold 1951 | 107 | 1000 |
| Nelson & Bunge 1974 | 48 | 390 |
| Rehan et al 1975 | 79 | 1300 |
| Sobrero & Rehan 1975 | 81 | 100 |
| Zuckerman et al 1977 | 63 | 4122 |
| Smith et al 1979 | 61 | 50 |
| David et al 1979a | 98 | 190 |
| Bahamondes et al 1979 | 68 | 186 |
| Hommonai et al 1980 | 84 | 627 |
| Abyholm 1981 | 89 | 51 |
| Jouannet et al 1981 | 95 | 324 |

analysis, men who have fathered at least two children and are applying for vasectomy, and fertile sperm donors, one finds sperm concentrations as low as 0.5 million/ml (Homonnai et al 1980). Bahamondes et al (1979) reported the lowest concentration to be 2 million/ml and Abyholm (1981) observed the same figure in his series. Nelson & Bunge (1974) studied semen samples in 390 men who applied for vasectomy and who had fathered at least two children. Four of these men were shown to be azoospermic. One should, of course, be realistic enough to accept the fact that some men who regard their children as proof of their fertility, are erroneous as far the cause–effect relationship is concerned. Yet, excluding azoospermia, there is probably no definite lower limit of sperm concentration below which all men are infertile. Glass & Ericsson (1979) reported on 16 couples who were thought to be infertile due to the male factor. Intrauterine insemination was performed in the female partners, but none conceived. Later, four couples reported pregnancies without treatment. They had been infertile for 2–6 years. Sperm counts in these males ranged from 0.3 million/ml to 30 million/ml. The normal variability of sperm concentration and exogenous factors which may temporarily reduce sperm counts should be taken into consideration when a statement about sperm count is made. Furthermore, any statement about semen analysis is true only for the time when the test has been made. Prognoses based on semen analysis certainly have much statistical value and are important to give probability values. They are, however, not a definite verdict.

The sperm concentration can be determined by using either a hemocytometer (Burker chamber, Neubauer chamber), by using the Makler chamber (Makler 1978a), or by electronic counting methods, such as Coulter counters (Brotherton 1979). Colorimetric and fluorometric methods for estimation of sperm concentration have also been proposed. In most centers the hemocytometric method is used. Prior to counting the sperm cells, the sample must be completely liquefied and thoroughly mixed. Sperm cells are diluted in a liquid in order to immobilize the cells. For this purpose one may use 5% triphenyltetrazoalium chloride in physio-logical saline, or 5 g Na $HCO_3$ + 1 g 35% formalin made up to 100 ml in distilled water, or simply distilled water, with subsequent placing of the test-tube in hot water for 5 min. The grade of dilution is chosen according to the estimated sperm count, e.g. 1:20 if high concentrations are anticipated, 1:10 for lower concentrations. For very low concentrations no dilution is made. Usually white blood cell pipettes are used for dilution. A drop of semen is added to both sides of the counting chamber (e.g. Neubauer) and the sperm cells are allowed to settle for some 20 min with the counting chamber placed in a moist environment. Sperm cells in the hemocytometer are then counted at a magnification of 100 × or 400 ×. Sperm concentration is expressed in number of sperm cells per millilitre. Total sperm count refers to the product of sperm concentration times total volume of the semen in millilitre. A hemocytometer possesses a grid containing five major squares, the central one being subdivided into 25 smaller squares. The major square is 5 mm long, 1 mm wide and 0.1 mm deep. The total number of sperm cells counted multiplied by the factor $10^4$ gives the actual sperm concentration per millilitre. If the sample has been diluted, say 1:20, then the formula for actual sperm concentration would be: number of sperm cells counted within the 25 small square × 10 000 × 20.

Makler (1978a) has designed a chamber which is only 0.01 mm deep and permits the observation of all sperm cells is one focal plane. Undiluted preheated semen can be counted easily in the grid, which measures exactly 0.033 $mm^2$. By multiplying the counted number of spermatozoa by the factor 3, the actual sperm concentration is obtained.

## Spermatozoal motility

Freshly ejaculated sperm cells move at a velocity of 75 $\mu$m/s while a high proportion of sperm cells from infertile men move at about 40 $\mu$m/s (Harvey 1960, Basco 1984).

For the critical process of fertilization, rather few sperm cells are required; however, they must be motile. Therefore, one of the most important parameters in semen analysis is spermatozoal motility.

Whatever method is used for motility determination, special care should be taken to evaluate motility under standardized temperature conditions, e.g. body temperature, 37°C. Janick & MacLeod (1970) have measured spermatozoal motility at different temperatures. There was a marked increase in the rate of forward progression in all 20 specimens examined when the temperature was raised from 23° to 37°C. Standardization at body temperature is therefore essential. The term 'room temperature', so often used, is not sufficiently defined and varies markedly between laboratories. Freund & Peterson (1976) reported data obtained from 35 different laboratories and found the room temperatures to range between 18° and 27°C. Furthermore, there were variations within each laboratory with season, geographical area and time of day. Temperature may also exert its influence on sperm motility in other aspects. Baker et al (1981) have observed a significant difference in sperm motility of asthenospermic, oligozoospermic and normospermic males when analysis was performed during winter or summer (low in winter, higher in summer). The magnitude of this difference was lower in semen donors who produced the specimen in the laboratory than in patients who usually collected the semen at home and transported it to the laboratory. The authors believe that exposure to different temperatures is the most likely explanation for this seasonal effect. The finding of higher motilities in semen samples collected later in the day is also consistent with this theory.

Traditionally, when evaluating motility, three parameters are assessed: the percentage of motile cells, the type of motility and longevity, i.e. the maintenance of spermatozoal motility as a function of time. A motility loss of 10–20% within 3 h is considered to be within the normal range. Table 11.5 gives the mean percentage of motile sperm cells in semen samples from men who had fathered a child, from men who had applied for vasectomy, having at least two children, and from fertile donors. The average percentage of motility in these studies ranged from 49% to 72%. Based on these data, a semen sample containing more than 50% progressively moving sperm cells is considered normal as far as motility is concerned. Asthenospermia is a

**Table 11.5** Mean percentage of motile sperm cells in semen samples of men with proved fertility

| Authors | Mean percentage of motile cells | Men (no.) |
|---|---|---|
| Falk & Kaufman 1950 | 61 | 100 |
| MacLeod & Gold 1951 | 58 | 1000 |
| Rehan et al 1975 | 65 | 1300 |
| Smith et al 1979 | 54 | 50 |
| Bahamondes et al 1979 | 66 | 185 |
| Homonnai et al 1980 | 49 | 627 |
| Abyholm 1981 | 53 | 51 |
| Jouannet et al 1981 | 72 | 324 |

term which describes semen samples in which the percentage of motile cells initially is below 50%. Motility is generally evaluated by direct microscopic observation of the semen. The simplest and most widely used technique for estimation of sperm motility is as follows: Immediately following liquefication, the semen sample is well mixed and a drop of undiluted semen is placed on a microscope slide and covered with a coverslip. Usually, bacteriological loops are used to produce standardized amounts of semen. The slide is examined immediately in order to avoid errors due to partial drying of the specimen. Quantitative motility is determined by counting 100 sperm cells (avoiding the edges of the coverslip). The percentage of motile cells is adjusted to the nearest 5% or 10%. When establishing the percentage of motile cells, progressively moving sperm cells are counted and the predominant type of movement is noted (e.g. poor, good, excellent). Abnormal patterns of motility (e.g. circular, shaking) are noted. After 3 h motility is again assessed for longevity. Although widely used and probably sufficient for routine purposes, this slide method has several drawbacks. The conventional method of evaluating spermatozoal motility is subjective and highly dependent on the skill and experience of the technician and no documentation can be kept. Furthermore, spermatozoal motility, assessed conventionally, is a composite term and includes proportion of motile cells and their estimated speed, described usually as 'fast', 'slow', 'poor', etc. Finally, quality control and quality assurance are very difficult if test results obtained by microscopic observation cannot be stored for re-evaluation. Much effort has therefore been invested in the development of computer-ized instrumentation in order to objectively assess seminal parameters, mainly motility.

*Automated semen analysis*

Janick & MacLeod (1970) measured the course of sperm cells per unit time on microfilm, Castenholz (1974) used the photokymographic approach, Jecht & Russo (1973) worked with a closed circuit method comprising video tape, digital data display, and a computer. Laser Doppler methods were used by Dubois et al (1974), turbidimetric methods by Sokoloski et al (1977) and Jouannet et al (1977) have proposed a method using light scattering determination of spermatozoal motility. Makler (1978b) has pointed out that in using the slide method the percentage motility is usually overestimated, since spermatozoa that move in and out of the micro-scopic field may be counted several times, while the number of nonmotile cells remains steady. Furthermore, the coverslip pressed on the drop without control does not become absolutely parallel with the lower slide. A relationship between thickness of the examined drop and sperm motility has been attributed to friction between sperm cells and surface of the slide. The

examination of different microscope fields may therefore give markedly varying results and lead to errors.

The Makler chamber provides standard condi-tions under which samples can be examined. Due to the special design of the chamber, vertical movement of cells and surface friction is elimi-nated while all cells are seen in one focal plane. Motility is measured by a multiple-exposure photographic technique (MEP) using a still camera and a stroboscope (Makler 1978c). Figure 11.1 demonstrates a typical semen specimen after six consecutive exposures during 1 s. Nonmotile sperm appear much brighter than motile sperm, which present as linked chains; the shape of the chain indicates direction. The distance travelled by each individual sperm and its progressive speed may be easily calculated from the direction, shape and length of the chains.

Makler et al (1980) have further improved their method by introducing a computer technique for semiautomatic tracing. The sperm track containing sheets are placed on a digitizer tablet and are followed with a sonic pen. The number of motile and immotile cells are counted and the percentage of abnormal cells is entered on the keyboard of a small computer which supplies results of sperm concentration, percentage of

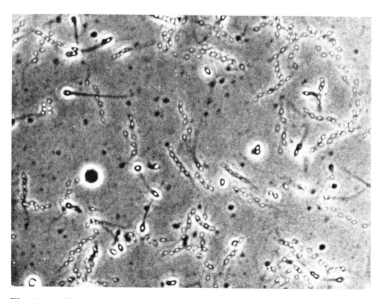

**Fig. 11.1**    Photomicrograph of sperm motility evaluation by the MEP method.

motile cells, mean velocity, and percentage of abnormal forms. Computerized semen analysers certainly offer a major advantage as far as characterization of motility is concerned. Sperm velocity (swimming speed) and linearity (ratio of curvilinear versus straight line velocity) may be important parameters and cannot be assessed by direct observation. The two most popular computerized semen analyzers are the CellSoft system (Cryo Resources Ltd) and the Hamilton Thorn system 2000 (Hamilton-Thorn Research).

The CellSoft system (CSS) recognizes sperm cells by relying on user-defined values for cell size and luminosity. A seminal constituent within the 'size gate' and moving within a range of preset speeds is defined by the computer as a sperm cell and is evaluated.

The Hamilton Thorn system (HTM) uses an infrared beam to identify sperm cells by motility assuming that any object which moves faster than $5\,\mu m/s$ is a sperm cell. The average size and luminosity is then calculated for all moving objects. These values are then used to determine if nonmoving objects are sperm cells. Size and luminosity are user definable.

Analyzed images provide data for concentration, motility, velocity and linearity. Furthermore, the systems evaluate lateral head displacement, circular motion and real-time images can be used for evaluation of morphology. Typically, slide methods for direct counts are used as standard against which computerized systems are evaluated. The Makler chamber (Sefi Medical Instruments) which provides a standardized depth of field is particularly suited for direct observation.

The image analysis technology used by CSS may have some sources of error which relate to the correct identification of sperm cells. Since the analysis is based on preset gates, clumped cells exceeding the preset parameters would be rejected from calculation. Sperm clumps consist typically of immotile cells and debris. Therefore concentration would be underestimated and motility overestimated. On the other hand, debris or other cells which fall in the range of preset gates would be identified as immotile sperm cells and included in the nonmotile cell count. The motile sperm fraction would also be increased by counting moving debris or immotile cells which flow after collison with sperm cells (Mortimer et al 1988). Knuth et al (1987) have assessed how parameter settings of the CSS affect the accuracy of results of automized semen analysis. Their results indicate that values obtained for concentration, percentage of motile sperm cells, velocity and linearity depend to varying degrees on the settings of the computer and may therefore not be comparable among different laboratories unless identical parameter settings are used.

Knuth & Nieschlag (1988) noted that the CSS system was unable to distinguish debris, leucocytes and other cellular matter from sperm cells when samples with less than $5 \times 10^6$ cells/ml were analyzed. The system overestimated sperm concentration in the lower range and underestimated concentration in the higher range. Others have also noted that the CSS is highly inaccurate when sperm concentration is in the lower range (Knuth & Nieschlag 1988, Mortimer et al 1988, Vantman et al 1988, Chan et all 1989).

The fertilizing capacity of a given semen sample is probably not affected by sperm concentration unless below $20 \times 10^6$/ml. The crucial limit seems to be in the range of $5 \times 10^6$/ml. It is therefore of concern that the evaluated system performed the poorest at precisely this range.

Gill et al 1988 compared sperm density using the CSS and the HTM against direct reading with the Makler chamber and a hemocytometer. The authors concluded that the HTM was superior to the CSS when sperm concentrations of less than $30 \times 10^6$/ml were evaluated, both systems default during analysis when counts exceed $200 \times 10^6$/ml and provide accurate and identical count when the average sperm concentration is $85 \times 10^6$/ml. Vantman et al (1988) reported a CV of 46% in samples with less than $10 \times 10^6$/ml when evaluated with the CSS.

A computerized semen analysis system offers a promising tool for standardization, quality control and assurance, and exciting research opportunities. At the time of writing, however, it seems too early to replace the traditional semen analysis as standardized by WHO (1987) by computerized systems. Only joint efforts by manufacturers and researchers which should be coordinated by panels of experts will optimize these systems, so that standardization of set-up parameters and correction of currently inherent methodological drawbacks will be achieved. Since the need is there, this will undoubtedly happen.

## Sperm viability

When evaluating sperm motility, the percentage of moving sperm cells is determined and the characteristics of motion described. Nonmoving sperm cells may be dead or just 'dormant'. This distinction is essential if one plans to use in vitro vitalizing methods for subsequent artificial insemination (see Chapter 25). Asssesment of sperm viability is based on supravital staining techniques. Several stains have been proposed, the most common of them being derivatives of fluorescein (eosin or erythrocin). Eosin in aqueous solution cannot penetrate living cells, and stained cells are therefore identified as dead. Background stains, such as nigrosin, are often used in addition to permit easier indentification of unstained (live) spermatozoa. Eliasson & Treichl (1971) have pointed out that the concentration of the background stain may influence the percentage of stained cells. They proposed the use of a 0.5% eosin Y solution in 0.15 M phosphate buffer at pH 7.4. Equal parts of the staining solution and semen (0.1 ml of each) are mixed thoroughly and after 1–2 min a drop of the mixture is transferred to a glass slide and allowed to air dry. Examination is performed by means of negative phase contrast microscope. Viable sperm cells are bluish and dead cells appear bright yellow. The eosin-negrosin method is performed as follows: semen and 0.5% bluish eosin (diluted in water) are mixed in equal parts. The mixture is added to an equal volume of 10% nigrosin (diluted in distilled water) and again thoroughly mixed. A drop of the mixture is transferred to a microscope slide, air dried and observed at a magnification of × 400. Viable sperm cells will remain unstained and appear against a red background, whereas dead cells will be stained red. The percentage of stained cells (i.e. dead cells) is expressed as the percentage of eosin-positive cells.

Supravital staining may also be useful to identify cellular elements in semen. Precursors of spermatozoa are often mistaken for pus cells by less experienced technicians. Unnecessary antibiotic therapy is often based on these erroneous tests. Phadke (1978) has reported a staining technique which permits easy identification of spermatocytes, spermiophages, leucocytes and trichomonas. The procedure is simple: one drop of 0.01% neutral-red (diluted in normal saline) is mixed with one drop of semen after liquefaction. One drop of the mixture is transferred to a microscope slide and covered with a coverslip. The edges are sealed with petroleum jelly. The slide remains at a temperature of 20–30°C for 1–2 h and examined at high magnification. Cellular elements can now be easily identified.

## Sperm morphology

The morphological phenotype of sperm cells present a historical picture of events occurring during germ cell production, epididymal sperm cell transport and storage. Evaluation of the sperm structure from the point of view of differentiation can help to diagnose a male factor of infertility with its possible etiology and to predict whether possible recovery to normal sperm cell production is likely. Because of the relationship between function and structure, the spermiogram may be also indicative for the future potential of the spermatozoa to undergo the different stages of the fertilization process.

Sperm morphology is considered a stable parameter as opposed to motility since it is less affected by the excretions of the accessory glands (Lindholmer 1974, Harrison et al 1978, Dott et al 1979). Furthermore, the sperm morphogram is independent of the number of spermatozoa, which is also a variable parameter. Information concerning the sperm morphogram was already available in the first quarter of this century when semen of selected bulls used for artificial insemination in cattle breeding was analysed (Blom 1950b, Blom & Birch-Andersen 1965). Major and minor sperm defects were defined in bull and boar spermatozoa and a clear correlation between sperm morphology and fertilization capacity was demonstrated (Blom 1968, 1972, Blom and Birch-Andersen 1975).

In man, assessment of sperm morphology is more complicated for two reasons: (a) the aniso-zoospermia phenomenon; and b) the difficulty of quantitatively assessing the fertility potential of a given semen sample.

Anisozoospermia is a term coined by Pollak (Blom 1950b) which expresses the morphological heterogeneity of the sperm population of fertile human semen which contrasts with the uniformity of form and structure of spermatozoa of any other species studied, including subhuman primates (Zamboni et al 1971). Human semen occasionally contains spermatozoa showing a single anomaly which, according to some investigators, will not affect fertility (Blom 1950b) and according to others is asssociated with infertility (Pedersen et al 1971, Schirren et al 1971, Ross et al 1973, Pedersen & Rebbe 1974). However, this uniformity is rare in humans. Usually human semen consists of sperm cells that include a combination of anomalies. This phenomenon made it difficult for morphologists to clearly define the limits of normality of human spermatozoa (Pedersen 1970, Koehler 1972, Flechion & Hafez 1976, Pedersen & Fawcett 1976) and, even more so, to establish a system of classification for the morphological anomalies in the spermatozoa of fertile and infertile men (Freund 1966, Smith et al 1979, David et al 1972, Hafez & Kanagawa 1973, Bartoov et al 1981). As many as 60 different morphological forms of human spermatozoa have been reported (Broecks & Keel 1979). In order to produce a workable morphogram, most laboratories dealing with routine semen analysis have adopted a simple classification system in which the sperm cell population is divided basically into normal and abnormal forms: the malformed spermatozoa are subdivided into about ten categories which can easily be defined with a certain degree of precision (duplicate head, tapering large and small head, multitail, etc.). Major sperm defects have been related to infertility in mammals (pear-shaped head, coiled tail defect and proximal cytoplasmic droplet). The remainder of the malformed cells are 'dumped' (classified) in the 'amorphous' category (David et al 1975, Zaneveld & Polakoski 1977, Van Zyl 1980, Eliasson 1981).

Thus, the frequency of normal spermatozoa (Fig. 11.2) and the malformed forms are the two

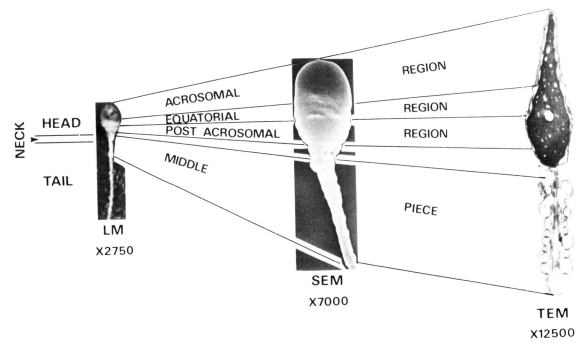

**Fig. 11.2**  Photomicrograph illustrating a normal sperm cell as observed by light microscopy (LM), scanning electron microscopy (SEM) and transmission electron microscopy (TEM).

principal categories obtained by the morphology of routine semen analysis using the light microscope. It has been demonstrated that semen of infertile patients contains a higher percentage of abnormal forms than semen of fertile men, and that morphological abnormalities may be due to infection, trauma, other testicular stress situations, certain drugs (e.g. nitrofurans), or hormonal imbalance (MacLeod 1970, David et al 1972). According to Zaneveld & Polakoski (1977), tapered sperm heads and immature sperm precursors are frequently associated with conditions such as varicocele, as well as with viral and bacterial infection. On the other hand, double-headed spermatozoa are more typical of varicocele than of infectious diseases. Allergic reaction causes a characteristic increase in amorphous and immature sperm cells and less in tapered forms. The presence of a large number of spermatozoa containing cytoplasmic droplets indicates that the sperm maturation process in the epididymis has been inadequate and thus points to epididymal pathology.

*Morphological evaluation*

As mentioned above, the percentage of normal forms were used for the assessment of the fertility capacity of the male. The normal percentage of normal spermatozoa was established by WHO (1987) to be 50%. However, in different laboratories normal values vary from 30% to 60%. This variance is probably due to the staining technique, the subjectivity of observation and the definitions of the malformations.

There are conflicting reports about the correlation between human sperm morphology and fertility. Zaini et al (1985) and Polansky & Lamb (1988) found no predictive value in sperm morphology, as well as other semen parameters, on the existence of male infertility factor even in computer-assisted measurements (Check et al 1990). On the other hand, higher proportions of sperm with normal morphology were found in fertile semen donors in AID programs (Edwinsson et al 1983, McGowan et al 1983). Francavilla et al (1990) have demonstrated that the percentage of normal forms is correlated with the pregnancy rate of couples with oligo-

zoospermic and asthenozoospermic semen and treated by intrauterine insemination.

Reduced fertility and a longer interval to first pregnancy was found to be associated with reduced percentage of normally configured sperm cells (Bartoov et al 1982, Bostole et al 1982). The contribution of sperm morphology to the asessment of the fertility capacity can be best demonstrated in a selected group of unexplained infertile couples in which sperm concentration and motility are within the normal range. Indeed, when this category of patients was examined by Aitken et al (1982) it appeared that semen of infertile men contained more abnormal forms than semen of fertile men. This finding established that isolated teratozoospermia is associated with male infertility. Although the correlation between the percentage of normal forms and the fertility status in the two groups was statistically significant ($r=0.31$), the predictive value of the sperm morphogram was poor. Recently we obtained similar results when we compared a group of 62 fertile males with 35 men with unexplained infertility with repeated unsuccessful IVF. The presence of an inherent seminal factor was assumed in the latter group when it was shown that ova obtained from their female partners underwent fertilization by donor semen. A significant positive correlation of 0.39 ($P<0.0001$) was obtained between the percentage of normal forms and fertility capacity. In order to improve the prognostic value of the prevalence of normal forms as a test for predicting fertility, it is necessary to define lower and upper limits within which fertility is more likely. The lower limit should be selected on the basis of maximum specificity i.e. correctly classsified infertile cases (true negative) with minimum fertile ones (false negative), and vice versa for the upper limits (sensitivity) i.e. corrcctly classified fertile cases (true positive) with minimum infertile ones (false positive). Figure 11.3 illustrates the relationship between the percentage of normal and abnormal forms in fertile and infertile cases in our study. Four per cent normal forms was found to be the lower limit, below which fertility was very unlikely (2% false negative). The upper limit of the 'gray zone' was chosen to be 45% normal forms (10% false positive). Within this

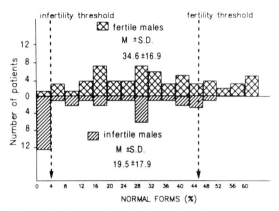

**Fig. 11.3** Distribution of fertile and infertile patients grouped according to the respective percentage of normally configurated sperm cells. Semen was obtained from 62 fertile men and 35 infertile men. The threshold values for normal sperm cells below which infertility was most common and above which fertility was most common are indicated by arrows.

zone, morphology was not a very good predictor of the fertility potential of a given semen sample and probably does affect fertility if more than 45% of sperm cells are normally configurated. Thus by assessing the percentage of normal forms as observed by light microscopy morphology it was possible to correctly predict fertility in 38% of the cases.

Similar results were reported when normal sperm morphology was correlated with the fertilization rate in vitro. Jeulin et al (1986) reported that the percentage of normal forms and abnormal acrosomes were related to IVF failure. Kruger et al (1986, 1988, Acosta et al 1988)

reported 14% of normal forms to be clear thresholds for high fertilization and pregnancy rate and 4% normal forms as the lower threshold for success in IVF. Therefore patients having less than 4% normal forms have a 'poor' fertility prognosis. Still, it seems that the prediction capability of the lower threshold is limited since fertilization and pregnancy rates per cycle of this category reported by Oehminger et al (1988) were 44.5% and 8.5% respectively.

The classical approach outlined above concentrates solely on the percentage of normal forms as a parameter for prediction of the fertility potential of a given semen sample. However, assessment of sperm morphology may provide additional information for prediction, namely the evaluation of specific malformations. Some malformations, such as slightly amorphous heads or elongated acrosomes, may be regarded as normal variations not impeding fertility and could be added to the percentage of normal forms. On the other hand, malformations such as tapered forms (Bartoov et al 1982; Table 11.6) may compete with normal sperm cells in ovum penetration. Since normal pronuclei formation might be unlikely in this situation, the presence of this type of abnormal forms impacts negatively on the fertility potential of a given semen sample. By the same token, one would expect a semen sample with a given percentage of abnormal forms to possses a higher fertility potential if the predominant malformation pattern relates to the sperm tail rather than to the sperm head. In the former

**Table 11.6** Unstandardized canonical discriminant weights of morphological discriminatory characteristics as observed by light microscopy (LM)

| Morphological characteristics (dimensions in μm) | Weight |
|---|---|
| Normal (head 6.0×3.0) (Fig. 11.2) | 0.053 |
| Long acrosomal region($\geq 4.0$) (Fig. 11.4a) | 0.323 |
| Short acrosomal region ($\leq 2.8$) (Fig. 11.4b) | −0.392 |
| Long postacrosomal region ($\geq 2.2$) (Fig. 11.4c) | −0.163 |
| Tapering (cigar) nuclear shape (>7.0 × <3.0) (Fig. 11.4d) | −0.069 |
| Neck disorder (Fig. 11.4e) | −0.257 |
| Constant | −1.851 |

$$\text{LM Morphology Score (LMS)} = \sum_{i=1}^{6} b_i \times \text{frequency} + \text{constant}.$$

The frequency of each one of the discriminatory characteristics, as was found in the patient, is multiplied by its weight. The score is calculated by summing up those multiplications, including the constant.

situation malformed sperm cells may be regarded as passive co-travellers, while in the latter situation they would actively compete with normal sperm cells for ovum penetration. Jeulin et al (1986) reported that the malformation criterion with the highest predictive value for fertilization in vitro relates to the acrosome. As far as morphology is concerned, we assess the fertility potential of a given semen sample by combining proportionally normal and abnormal sperm forms using an equation obtained by multifunctional statistical analysis. This equation yields a single score which is a weighed sum of the original malformation measurements and which is used to differentiate between a group of fertile men and suspected infertile one, and was computed using the statistical discriminate analysis method (Nie et al 1975). This makes irrelevant the questions pertinent to sperm morphology, such as: which malformations are compatible with male fertility; whether a specific malformation is an artifact of the preparation technique; and what percentage of defective spermatozoa results in infertility. Using this method, we were able to produce a light-microscope morphological score (LMS) which is based on the means, standard deviations and the correlations of the morphological discriminating characteristics obtained from 33 fertile men and 44 suspected infertile men (Table 11.6, Bartoov et al 1982).

The LMS enabled us to correctly predict 62% of the cases with an 'infertility' threshold of −1.0 and a 'fertility' threshold of +1.0. The remaining cases were in the 'unpredictable' zone. The morphometric approach might gain more attention in the near future when new image analysis technology improves and becomes easily available.

*Light microscopy (LM)*

A semen sample is prepared for LM observation by staining with the modified eosine-nigrosin method described by Blom (1950a). The examined semen is thoroughly mixed in a test-tube with a $180 \times$ shaker for a few minutes. A drop of the mixed semen is well mixed with one drop of filtered 1% (w/v) eosin B in saline solution, then mixed again with two drops of filtered 10% (w/v) nigrosin

solubilized in distilled water. The mixed specimen is prepared like a blood smear, air dried and observed under oil immersion at $\times$ 1000 magnification. If the concentration of spermatozoa is less than $20 \times 10^6$/ml, the sample is centrifuged at $1500 \times \mathbf{g}$ for 15 min and the smear is prepared from the precipitated spermatozoa. At least 100 spermatozoa are counted.

***Normal ultramorphology of sperm cells***
Mammalian spermatozoa consist of three regions, namely head, neck and tail. The sperm head is occupied mostly by the nucleus and acrosome but contains also cytoskeletal components and often very small amounts of cytoplasm (Fig. 11.2). The acrosome, which is a specialized lysosome, envelops the proximal part of the head and is located just beneath a plasma membrane. It covers about two-thirds of the nucleus in a cap-like fashion. The distal part of the nucleus is surrounded by cytoskeletal elements, situated between the nuclear envelope and the plasma membrane, the so-called postacrosomal lamina. The internal organelle of the head is the nucleus which contains highly condensed haploid chromatin.

The neck or connecting piece contains proximally the capitulum, which is a fibrous plate-like structure connected to the basal plate of the nuclear envelope by fine filaments. Distally the neck contains nine segmented columns which fuse into nine outer dense fibers and which extend throughout the flagellum.

The proximal portion of the sperm tail contains the mitochondrial sheet which is helically wrapped around the outer dense fibers of the middle piece. This concentration of mitochondria supplies the energy needed for sperm motility through an oxidative phospholinization process. The fibrous sheath which is most important for locomotion is a tapering cylinder and defines the extent of the principal piece of the flagellum. It contains two longitudinal columns attached to the outer dense fibers. The internal organnelle of the sperm tail is called axonema and consists of nine external and two central doublets.

Table 11.7 presents a LM morphogram containing normal form cells, and four regional malformed characteristics: head defect, middle piece defect, tail defect, cytoplasmic droplet.

**Table 11.7**   Means and standard deviation of the LM morphological characteristics in normal fertile male group ($n = 102$)

| Characteristics | Normal value (%) |
|---|---|
| Normal | $35 \pm 18$ |
| Head defects | $37 \pm 27$ |
| Middle piece defects | $4 \pm 1$ |
| Tail defects | $15 \pm 12$ |
| Cytoplasmic droplet | $1 \pm 1$ |

Results shown are mean ± SD.

Their average frequencies and standard deviation are derived from observations in 102 fertile males. For more objective morphogram analysis, a transparent grid divided into $2 \times 2$ μm should be applied in one of the oculars. This grid can be prepared easily by photographing a millimetric sheet reduced to one-half of the power of the ocular, and using the negative for preparing the grid. Using the eosin-nigrosin staining technique, normal sperm head length is between 5 and 6 μm and its width between 2 and 3 μm. The dimension of a small oval head is below $2.0 \times 5.0$ μm, and of a large one, above $3.0 \times 6.0$ μm. The length of the nuclear acrosomal region is $2.8-4.0$ μm. Therefore, a long acrosomal region, in order to be attributed a positive weight, should be equal to or above 4.0 μm (Fig. 11.4a); and a short acrosomal region, in order to be attributed a negative weight, should be below 2.8 μm (Fig. 11.4b).

The length of the post acrosomal head region is $1.7-2.1$ μm, therefore a 'long' postacrosomal region malformation is present if this part has a length equal or exceeding 2.2 μm (Fig. 11.4c). A 'tapering' head (Fig. 11.4d) is defined as 'agar shaped' if its length exceeds 7.0 μm in length and its width is less than 3.0 μm. Neck disorders are expressed as breakage of the axonema in the neck region or abaxial tail (Fig. 11.4e). From the fact that the 'long acrosomal region' parameter is assigned a positive weight and that the 'long postacrosomal' region parameter is assigned a negative weight, it can be concluded that the ratio of the acrosomal region to the postacrosomal region in the typical normal spermatozoa is above 1.5 which resembles that of ram and bull spermatozoa (Blom & Birch-Andersen, 1965). The extreme representatative malformation of this ratio could be the round headed spermatozoa which is believed to be a malformation associated with sterility (Pedersen & Rebbe 1974). The mean LMS of the fertile population was 1.17 with a standard deviation of 0.78. The resolution of the LMS to distinguish between the fertile and the suspected infertile men is above $+1.0$ and below $-1.0$, respectively. Between these two values there is an overlapping zone and the LMS is not discriminatory (Table 11.12).

An accurate assessment of normal spermatozoa can be routinely obtained by staining the seminal

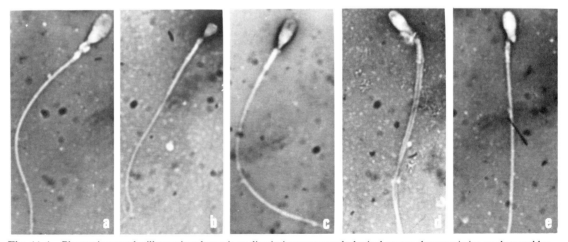

**Fig. 11.4**   Photomicrographs illustrating the various discriminatory morphological sperm characteristics as observed by light microscopy. **a** long acrosomal region; **b** short acrosomal region; **c** long postacrosomal region; **d** tapering cell; **e** neck disorder. ($\times 1500$)

fluid with fast staining techniques, such as eosin-nigrosin (Blom 1950a, Eliasson 1977), crystal violet (Broecks & Keel 1979) or commercially available prestained slides (Calamera & Vilar 1979). The Papanicolaou and Giemsa staining techniques for air-dried seminal fluid smear preparations are somewhat time consuming and can be better used (in case of observing too many round cells in the semen sample) for differentiating between immature sperm cells, white or red blood cells, bacteria, epithelial cells, etc. We prefer the nigrosin-eosin technique since it is uncomplicated, discriminates rather well between the different regions of the sperm cell without causing shrinkage of the sperm head, as often occurs when the Papanicolaou stain is used, and provides information on sperm viability.

The different categories of malformed sperm cells may be evaluated statistically by comparing the frequency and its standard deviation, as obtained from analysis of semen from a group of fertile men. Data should be obtained under the same conditions. The statistical comparison can be made only when each defect of a spermatozoon is recorded separately and expressed as a percentage. As a consequence, the percentage for 'normal' and the various 'abnormal' forms will be more than 100. Only when no malformation is detected in the entire cell is it defined as normal.

### Sperm ultramorphology

There is a variety of sperm defects and developmental abnormalities that may cause infertility and which cannot be identified by conventional methods of light microscopy. This is due to the fact that these methods are based on the classification and rating of morphological features relying exclusively on the overall appearance of head and tail of the sperm cell. The finer abnormalities, which exist in the organization of subcellular organelles, remain undetected. Therefore it is logical that the assessment of sperm morphology will be more accurate when ultrastructural methods of morphologic analysis are used (Zamboni 1987). Quantitative ultramorphological analysis (QUM) has been described by us previously (Bartoov et al 1982, 1990).

### Scanning electron microscopy (SEM)

The semen sample is prepared for SEM observation as described by Bartoov et al (1982). A SEM morphogram is obtained by examining randomly 50 cells at a magnification of about $\times$ 12 000. Table 11.8 presents a complete SEM morphogram containing 48 morphological characteristics, their average frequencies and standard deviations as they appeared in a group of 102 fertile men. The average percentage of normal spermatozoa as observed by high power magnification (Fig. 11.5) – was only 9.4%, which is one-third of that observed typically using LM. The preparation technique of semen samples for SEM causes a longitudinal shrinkage of the normal cell head to $3.40 \pm 0.40$ mm, while the sperm width remains $2.62 \pm 0.13$ mm. The length of the acrosomal region is $2.00 \pm 0.14$ μm. The equatorial region is $0.34 \pm 0.08$ μm and that of the short postacrosomal region is $1.06 \pm 0.17$ μm. Therefore, in SEM 'short' equatorial region is defined as measuring less than 0.2 μm and a 'short postacrosomal' region measures less than 0.7 μm. A sperm cell with a head length exceeding 4.2 μm is labelled 'tapering cigar shaped'.

### Transmission electron microscopy (TEM)

The semen sample is prepared for TEM observation as described by Bartoov et al (1982). Preparations sectioned along their longitudinal axis, revealing about 8 μm of the anterior part of the cell, including head, neck and middle

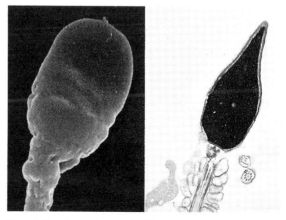

**Fig. 11.5** Photomicrographs illustrating normal sperm head and midpiece as observed by SEM (left) and TEM (right). (×6500)

**Table 11.8** Means and standard deviations of the SEM ultramorphological characteristics in normal fertile male group ($n = 102$)

| Characteristics | Normal (%) value* |
|---|---|
| Normal sperm cells | $94 \pm 7.4$ |
| Acrosome | |
|   Partial | $10.2 \pm 5.8$ |
|   Disorder | $8.3 \pm 5.8$ |
|   Lack | $1.4 \pm 1.4$ |
| Nucleus | |
|   Round | $0.1 \pm 0.5$ |
|   Large oval | $0.1 \pm 0.2$ |
|   Small oval | $5.3 \pm 5.2$ |
|   Pi | $4.0 \pm 4.4$ |
|   Amorphous | $6.0 \pm 4.9$ |
|   Tapering | $0.2 \pm 0.7$ |
|   Eggshape | $0.9 \pm 1.0$ |
|   Multinucleated | $0.2 \pm 0.5$ |
| Acrosomal region shape | |
|   Long | $2.7 \pm 2.8$ |
|   Short | $0.4 \pm 0.4$ |
|   Wide (pear form) | $1.4 \pm 1.2$ |
|   Narrow (arrowhead) | $0.3 \pm 0.8$ |
|   Disorder | $13.1 \pm 7.4$ |
| Equatorial region shape | |
|   Long | $0.1 \pm 0.2$ |
|   Short | $0.0 \pm 0.0$ |
|   Disorder | $1.3 \pm 1.8$ |
| Postacrosomal region shape | |
|   Long | $2.9 \pm 2.7$ |
|   Short | $1.5 \pm 1.9$ |
|   Wide (arrowhead) | $0.1 \pm 0.2$ |
|   Narrow (pear form) | $19.3 \pm 13.2$ |
|   Disorder | $0.5 \pm 1.0$ |
| Postacrosomal lamina | |
|   Partial | $1.5 \pm 1.7$ |

(*Continued*)

Table 11.8 (*contd*)

| Characteristics | Normal (%) value* |
|---|---|
|   Lack | $0.1 \pm 0.2$ |
| Posterior lamina | |
|   Partial | $2.7 \pm 2.8$ |
| Nuclear envelope | |
|   Postnuclear vesicles | $2.7 \pm 2.8$ |
| Neck | |
|   Disorder | $0.2 \pm 0.1$ |
|   Abaxial | $7.4 \pm 5.1$ |
| Mitochondrial sheath | |
|   Exposed | $0.2 \pm 0.1$ |
|   Agregation | $3.3 \pm 8.4$ |
|   Partial | $4.0 \pm 4.1$ |
|   Abscence | $0.4 \pm 0.9$ |
|   Narrow | $0.1 \pm 0.5$ |
|   Long | $0 \pm 0$ |
| Cytoplasm | |
| Droplet | $29.2 \pm 11.5$ |
| *Tail* | |
| Coiled towards head | $9.2 \pm 6.4$ |
| Coiled towards midpiece | $18.2 \pm 11.7$ |
| Coiled towards tail | $0.9 \pm 0.5$ |
| Breakage of axoneme | $2.7 \pm 3.0$ |
| Axoneme disorder | $0.5 \pm 1.1$ |
| Bending 90° | $0.7 \pm 1.4$ |
| Bending 180° | $0.1 \pm 0.4$ |
| Kinked | $0.3 \pm 0.7$ |
| Lack of tail | $0.3 \pm 1.4$ |
| Short tail | $0.7 \pm 1.4$ |
| Multitail | $1.0 \pm 0.7$ |
| Narrow tail | $0.1 \pm 0.2$ |
| Long tail | $0.2 \pm 0.2$ |

Results given mean one $\pm$ SD.

piece, are examined by TEM at a magnification of about $\times 15\,000$. The TEM morphogram is obtained by examining randomly 50 cells. Table 11.9 presents a complete TEM morphogram containing 25 morphological characteristics, their average frequencies and standard deviations as they appeared in a group of 102 fertile men. Examination of the fine internal structure of spermatozoa of fertile men further reduced the proportion of normal spermatozoa (Fig. 11.5) to an average of only 3.5%, which is a tenth of that observed using LM.

***Reliability and repeatability of QUM analysis*** To identify the within-sample reproducibility of malformed patterns, five different sperm samples were examined by the same technician. Each sample was observed five times blindly. A reliability test (R) performed after the examination had been completed, revealed a high correlation ($r > 0.5$) of 91% of morphological characteristics observed. The repeatability of detection of the malformed characteristics was examined by comparing two ultramorphograms of the same person made during a period of $3 – 9$ months, while no treatment was applied during this period. A correlation test made in ultramorphograms of 58 patients revealed that 84% of the morphological charactcristics had high correlation ($r > 0.5$) and the rest had lower reproducibility ($0.3 > r < 0.5$).

***Malformed patterns of the sperm cell organelles*** In order to assess the ultrastructural integrity of the different organelles of the sperm cell, namely, acrosome, postacrosomal lamina, nucleus, neck, mitochondrial sheath, fibrous sheath including outer dense fiber and the

**Table 11.9**　Means and standard deviations of TEM ultramorphological characteristics in normal fertile male group ($n = 102$)

| Characteristics | Normal (%) value* |
|---|---|
| Normal sperm cells | $3.5 \pm 4.0$ |
| Acrosome | |
| Irregular, vesiculated | $4.6 \pm 3.0$ |
| Partial | $0.6 \pm 1.2$ |
| Agenesis | $6.1 \pm 4.8$ |
| Lack | $11.1 \pm 8.4$ |
| Equatorial region disorder | $0.6 \pm 1.1$ |
| Nucleus regional disorder | |
| Acrosomal region disorder | $1.1 \pm 0.8$ |
| Equatorial region disorder | $1.4 \pm 0.6$ |
| Postacrosomal region disorder | $0.9 \pm 0.8$ |
| Caryoplasm | |
| Chromatin degradation | $2.9 \pm 2.5$ |
| Huge vacuoles | $5.2 \pm 4.6$ |
| Subcondensation | $9.0 \pm 6.7$ |
| Nuclear envelope | |
| Posterior nuclear vesicles | $1.4 \pm 2.2$ |
| Supernumerous membranes | $1.8 \pm 2.2$ |
| Postacrosomal lamina | |
| Lack | $3.9 \pm 3.9$ |
| Cytoplasm | |
| Droplet | $1.7 \pm 2.3$ |
| Around the head | $4.1 \pm 4.7$ |
| Subacrosomal space | $1.6 \pm 1.9$ |
| Axoneme | |
| $9+2$ disorder | $2.5 \pm 2.7$ |
| $9+0$ disorder | $0.7 \pm 0.3$ |
| Microtubules disorder | $0.0 \pm 0.0$ |
| ODF disorder | $0.7 \pm 1.3$ |
| Tail | |
| Kinked towards head | $2.5 \pm 2.9$ |
| Kinked towards midpiece | $2.0 \pm 2.5$ |

*Results given are mean $\pm$ SD. ODF, outer dense fibers.

axonema, one has to use the anatomical information obtained both externally by SEM and internally by TEM. These two sets of ultrastructural information complement each other and describe best the overall integrity of the organelles. Generally, the surface information is more accurate as far as the dimension of the organelle is concerned. On the other hand, the structural content of the organelle can be better described by the internal information. The different ultramorphological characteristics obtained can be condensed on an accumulative basis into four major malformation patterns: I, agenesis; II, incomplete genesis; III, damage; IV, degradation or loss. An illustration of these patterns in sperm acrosome and nucleus are depicted in Figures 11.6 and 11.7 respectively.

*Ultrastructural evaluation*

A detailed morphological analysis which includes the characteristics described above is important for identifying a specific anatomical malformation. However, from the aspect of sperm morphology, the male infertility factor is rarely expressed by a specific structural malformation but generally by a set of malformations. Thus, in order to evaluate the male factor of infertility, its possible etiology and prognosis, information has to be obtained on the level of the cell organelles. This 'organelle pattern' is an important body of information which permits two possible types of evaluation: etiological and prognostic.

The etiological evaluation is concerned mainly with the spermiogenesis process. Therefore agenesis of an organelle reflects a major failure of this process as compared with a damaged or a degraded organelle. From the prognostic point of view, agenesis or complete damage or loss of an organelle is of similar importance. Therefore, an ultrastructural malformational organellar index can be obtained for each of the sperm organelles, which is constructed from the frequencies of the morphological characteristics integrated into its malformed patterns multiplied by the evaluation factor.

An example of organelle and regional malformed indexes obtained from QUM analysis of 62 fertile males and 35 men with unexplained infertility based on prognostic evaluation is illustrated in Table 11.10 and Figure 11.7. Significant high negative correlations with fertility potential was obtained in five sperm organelle indexes — nucleus, acrosome, axonema, mitochondria and outer dense fibers (ODF) — as well as with head and tail regional malformations and with the total malformations of the sperm cell.

In order to optimize the organelle ultrastructural information as a prognostic tool of the fertility potential, a discriminate analysis was performed based on the above significantly correlated organelle indexes. A QUM score was obtained based on four organelles (Table 11.11). The specificity and sensitivity of the QUM fertility index (QFI) as predictor of fertility is illustrated in Figure 11.8. Using QFI <250 as a 'fertility' threshold, and >350 QFI as an

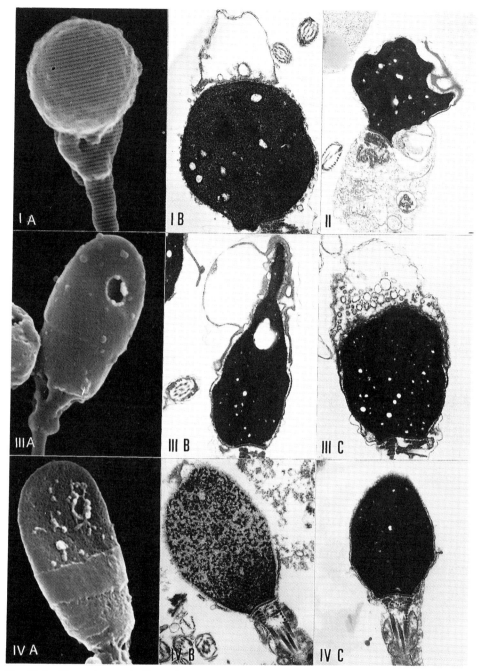

**Fig. 11.6** Photomicrographs illustrating malformed patterns of the acrosome. I, Agenesis (round form: A, SEM; B, TEM). II, Incomplete genesis (TEM). III, Damaged (partial: A, SEM; B, C, hyperplasia TEM). IV, Degradation or loss (A, SEM; B, C, TEM). (×8500)

'infertility' threshold it was possible to correctly classify 75% of the fertile male and 60% of the otherwise difficult to diagnose, unexplained infer-tile males with false-positives and negatives of 10% and 2% respectively, leaving only 26% of the cases in the unpredictable zone. Thus QUM

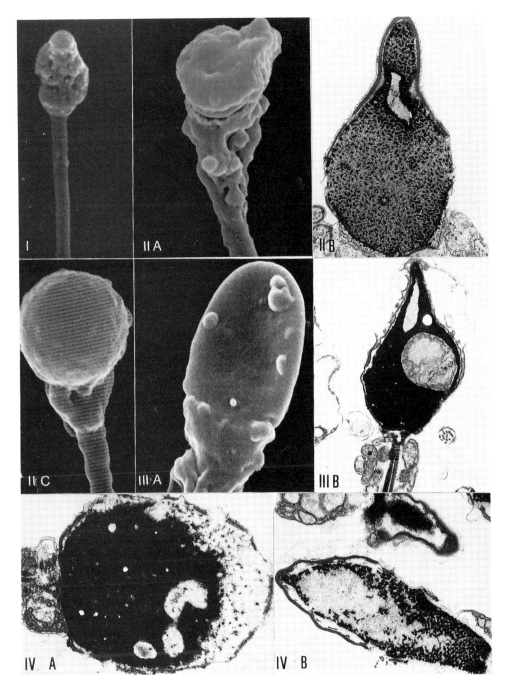

**Fig. 11.7**   Photomicrographs illustrating malformed patterns of the acrosome. (×8500)

analysis improves the predictive ability of sperm morphology as compared with the LM morphology based on percentage of normal forms (Table 11.12).

**Biochemical analysis**

Biochemical analysis of the secretory products of the accessory sex glands, a rationale which

**Table 11.10**   Statistical data of the organellar and regional malformational indexes in the fertile (FM) and infertile (IM) groups

| Organelle or region | FM (n=62) | | IM (n=35) | | r | P< |
|---|---|---|---|---|---|---|
| | Range (%) | Mean ± S.D (%) | Range (%) | Mean ± SD (%) | | |
| Nucleus | 47–239 | 125 ± 35 | 91–353 | 201 ± 51 | −0.67 | 0.001 |
| Acrosome | 12–128 | 65 ± 28 | 32–174 | 93 ± 35 | −0.47 | 0.001 |
| Postacrosomal lamina | 2–42 | 11 ± 8 | 2–36 | 15 ± 8 | −0.25 | 0.02 |
| Head | 182–928 | 515 ± 139 | 424–1434 | 804 ± 197 | −0.69 | 0.001 |
| Neck | 16–68 | 37 ± 12 | 8–64 | 33 ± 12 | 0.12 | NS |
| Axonema | 0–66 | 18 ± 13 | 9–115 | 41 ± 28 | −0.48 | 0.001 |
| Mitochondria | 0–66 | 13 ± 15 | 0–52 | 25 ± 15 | −0.37 | 0.001 |
| ODF | 2–70 | 22 ± 12 | 11–128 | 39 ± 20 | −0.46 | 0.001 |
| Tail | 22–275 | 112 ± 56 | 80–607 | 227 ± 110 | −0.57 | 0.001 |
| Cell | 386–2102 | 1143 ± 311 | 976–3220 | 1836 ± 450 | −0.67 | 0.001 |

r, correlation coefficient between the index and fertility.
NS, not significant.

**Table 11.11**   Standardized canonical discriminant weights of morphological discriminatory indexes observed by TEM and SEM

| Malformational indexes (%) | Weight |
|---|---|
| Nucleus | +0.78 |
| Fibrous sheath +ODF | +0.45 |
| Mitochondria sheath | +0.29 |

$$\text{Fertility score} = \sum_{i=1}^{3} (\text{weight} \times \text{frequency}).$$

The frequency of each one of the discriminatory indexes, as found in the patients, is multiplied by its weight. The score is calculated by summing up those multiplications.

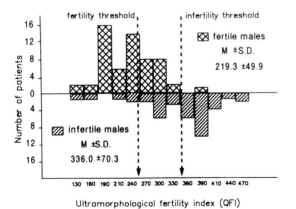

**Fig. 11.8**   Ultramorphological fertility index.

is undisputed in the study of thyroid, adrenal, pancreatic, placental, renal and hepatic functions, is still somehow neglected when it comes to epididymis, seminal vesicle and prostate gland (see also Chapter 7). Many sophicticated infertility clinics rely on rather narrow spectra of tests when it comes to semen analysis, and biochemistry of semen is not infrequently confined to fructose determination and measurement of pH. Although biochemistry of semen has been studied extensively, statements like 'The biochemical analysis … has little part to play in the routine investigation of an infertile man' (Pryor 1981) seem to relinquish a rather important tool for better understanding of semen analysis. The seminal plasma is a confluent of secretions from epididymes, seminal vesicles, ampoulles, the prostatic glands, and Cowper's and Littre's glands. A remarkable feature of the seminal plasma is the principal dependence of both its volume and chemical composition on the testicular hormone testosterone. In the rat other hormones, such as prolactin, may also exert some influence on the function of secondary sex glands (Dattatreymurty et al 1975). Body weight, fluid intake, etc., seem not to influence the functions of the secondary sex glands. On the other hand, testosterone secretion is partly controlled by supratentorial influences. Visual and olfactory stimuli and erotic fantasies have shown to increase testosterone production and consequently the activity of the secondary sex glands.

At the time of ejaculation specific interactions between the secretions of the various contributing glands ensue. For instance, the seminal vesicles

**Table 11.12**  Prognostic values of the different morphological indexes

| Index | Infertility threshold | Classification (%) | | Fertility threshold | Classification (%) | |
|---|---|---|---|---|---|---|
| | | Correct (IM) | False negative (FM) | | Correct (FM) | False positive (IM) |
| LM (% Normal) | < 4% | 37 | 2 | > 45% | 27 | 10 |
| LM (LMS)* | <−1.0 | 58 | 2 | >1.0 | 52 | 10 |
| EM (QFI)† | > 350 | 60 | 2 | < 250 | 75 | 10 |

LM, light microscope; EM, electron microscope
* Light microscope morphology score (Bartoov et al 1982).
† QUM fertility index.

secrete a coagulable protein and the prostate provides the necessary liquefying enzyme. The epididymis secretes glyceryl-phosphorylcholine and phosphorylcholine, and a prostatic phosphatase liberates free choline and inorganic phosphate. Spermine, derived from the prostate, forms crystals in a reaction with these phosphates.

One of the most notable peculiarities of the seminal plasma is the high concentration of some uncommon organic substances and enzymes, such as fructose, citric acid, inositol, glycerylphosphorylcholine, acid phosphatase, 5-nucleotidase and many others. It is beyond the scope of this presentation to discuss all the data that have accumulated concerning the composition of the seminal plasma. For an excellent and exhaustive review, see Mann & Lutvak-Mann (1981). The functions of some constituents of the seminal plasma are known; the role of most of them is still obscure. The origin of most substances have been defined, some of which may serve as important diagnostic tools for the evaluation of the functional state of the contributing glands. Yet, there are peculiar features of the seminal plasma for which we still do not have any explanation. In 1960 Rozin observed that seminal fluid from specimens containing highly motile sperm cells does stimulate poorly motile cells and that seminal plasma derived from specimens with decreased spermatozoal motility inhibits motility of sperm cells of other samples.

There is no doubt that the presence of seminal plasma is vital for spermatozoal motility. Lindholmer (1974) has demonstrated that epididymal sperm cells gain their motility only when immersed in seminal plasma (or albumin).

Basic biochemical analysis of seminal plasma should include the assessment of markers for the functional state of the secondary sex glands and examination of substances which might be directly related to the possible fertilizing ability of the spermatozoa.

We do not find it neccessary to perform seminal biochemistry at each follow-up semen analysis while managing an infertile couple. Seminal biochemistry provides, however, useful diagnostic information at the onset of an infertility evaluation and during specific treatment when information about seminal markers for the secondary sex glands is of value.

In this discussion we shall mention only a very selective and limited list of substances which should be assessed in a representative semen analysis. Specific tests, such as histochemical enzyme examination, tests for acrosin activity, trypsin inhibitors, immunological tests and others remain optional and may be used for special purposes.

*Epididymal semen*

Characteristic constituents of epididymal fluid are glycerylphosphorycholine (GPC) and carnitine. Free choline in seminal plasma is a product of the break down of phosphorylcholine derived mainly from the seminal vesicles. In man, GPC, the typical epididymal product, is not easily metabolized in semen after ejaculation and may therefore serve as a criterion for the assessment of epididymal function. Calamera & Lavieri (1974) compared GPC levels in semen obtained from 37 normal men and four patients in whom absence of vasa deferentia had been surgically confirmed. The concentration of GPC in the former group was 68.5 ± 3.3 mg% and 8.6 ± 0.7 mg% in the latter. In a similar study, Frenkel et al (1974) found 0.845 ± 0.1 µg/ml GPC in semen from 24 normal men as compared to 0.23 ± µg/ml in semen from seven vasectomized patients. Jeyendran et al (1989) have divided 52 men from an IVF program into one group of men whose sperm cells had fertilized ova and a second group where no fertilization had been observed. GPC concentrations were significantly higher in the first group than in the second, suggesting that GPC may influence the fertilizing ability of sperm cells.

Since, unlike those of most mammals, human seminal phosphatases are rather slow in metabolizing GPC, its physiological significance remains unclear. GPC can be measured by fluorimetric enzymatic analysis (Peterson & Freund 1971, Frenkel et al 1974), by paper chromatography and by measuring choline released by acid hydrolysis (Dawson et al 1957). The latter method is probably the easiest.

**Carnitine** L-Carnitine is a derivative of butyric acid and plays an important role in the transport of fatty acids through mitochondrial membranes (Fritz 1963) and in regulating sperm fructolysis. Cassilas (1973) has demonstrated that the carnitine content of bovine spermatozoa increases as they pass from the testis through the different parts of the epididymis. Carnitine may thus play a role in the maturation process of spermatozoa.

Frenkel et al (1974) measured free carnitine using a colorimetric method described by Marquis & Fritz (1966). They compared seminal levels from normal subjects and vasectomized men and noted no significant difference between epididymal and accessory gland concentrations. Lewin et al (1976), using a convenient rapid and inexpensive gas chromatographic method, found total carnitine levels to be extremely low (less than 100 µg/ml) only in patients in whom epididymis and seminal vesicles were defective. Intermediate concentrations (100–200 µg/ml) were found when one of these possibly contributing glands was defective, and levels above 250 µg/ml could be demonstrated when

both epididymis and seminal vesicles were in a normal functioning state. The authors concluded that carnitine is secreted by both glands and concomitant evaluation of other markers, such as fructose for the seminal vesicles, may be useful to detect functional disturbances in epididymis or seminal vesicles.

Wetterauer & Heite (1980) have reported their results obtained by an enzymatic-colorimetric method which specifically measures free carnitine. Contradicting both above-mentioned reports, the authors concluded that 94% of free carnitine originates in the epididymis.

In the light of these contradictions it seems that the role of carnitine as a specific epididymal marker is not sufficiently established and awaits further research. However, the suggested role of carnitine in the spermatozoal maturation process justifies its assessment in semen analysis.

*Inhibin*

The currently accepted view defines inhibin as a nonsteroid hormone which is produced by Sertoli cells under FSH control and in the presence of intact spermatogenesis. It regulates the synthesis and basal secretion of FSH and modulates the pituitary response to GnRH as far as FSH secretion is concerned (Steinberger & Steinberger, 1976, Bicsak et al 1987). A substance with inhibin-like activity has been isolated and characterized from pooled seminal fluid (Ramasharma et al 1984). Its complete amino sequence has been reported by Seidah et al (1984). A preparation believed to have a purity in the range of 10–30% has been described by Rivier et al (1986).

Inhibin is a heterodimer composed of an alpha and a beta subunit. The latter is actually formed by two subunits (A and B). Beta subunits may recombine as homodimers (A+A) or heterodimers (A+B). These substances are termed Activin A (homodimer) and Activin B (heterodimer). While inhibin inhibits the release of FSH secretion but not LH secretion, both activins are specific in exclusively stimulating the secretion of FSH. In human seminal plasma at least three molecular variants of inhibin have been described ranging from 1500 to 10 400 daltons (Arbatti & Sheth 1987).

Vaze et al (1980) have measured levels of inhibins in seminal plasma of oligospermic and normozoospermic semen and in normal human accessory reproductive organs. Seminal concentrations showed positive correlation with sperm concentration.

Interestingly to note, these authors were able to demonstrate notable amounts of inhibin in seminal vesicles and prostate glands. The significance of this finding is at this stage unclear.

In cases of azoospermia due to spermatogenetic failure inhibin is absent from the seminal plasma (Scott & Burger 1980). Assessment of inhibin may thus be a very valuable tool for prognosis of azoospermia: if, for instance, an azoospermic semen contains normal amounts of GPC but no inhibin, one may speculate that there is no obstruction but lack of spermatogenetic activity. The diagnosis of obstruction could be made if semen samples were found to be devoid of both GPC and inhibin. Normal gonadotropin levels, measured in blood plasma, could serve to confirm the diagnosis (see Chapter 12).

*Prostate gland fluid*

The fluid derived from the prostate gland is slightly acid (pH 6.5) and particularly rich in enzymes (acid phosphatase, β-glucoronidase, lysozyme, α-amylase, γ-glutamyl transferase, seminal proteinase-seminine, and others). Other typical substances derived from the prostatic fluid are citric acid, calcium, zinc, and spermine, the latter being responsible for the typical odor of spermatic fluid.

The ejaculatory process, initiated by contractions of the epididymis, is followed immediately by contractions of the prostate gland so that the first ejaculatory spurt, the so-called 'split', is composed of both epididymal and prostatic secretions.

**Zinc** Compared to other body fluids and tissues, the concentration of zinc in seminal fluid is very high (15–30 μg % as compared to 75–115 μg %). Marmar et al (1975) have measured zinc levels in fertile and infertile men and in patients with prostatitis. Patients with prostatitis had significantly lower zinc levels than healthy

controls and supplementary zinc caused a marked increase in the zinc concentration in their semen.

Seminal plasma contains several zinc binding ligands, and seems that some of them originate from the seminal vesicles (Arver 1980). It has been reported that zinc taken up by spermatozoa during contact of epididymal with prostatic secretions may be essential for an intrinsic sperm chromatin decondensation mechanism (Kvist 1980). Unsaturated zinc binding ligands from the seminal vesicle might decrease the bioavailability of zinc and thus decrease nuclear chromatin stability (Kvist & Eliasson 1980). High levels of zinc ligands from the seminal vesicles or low levels of available zinc may thus influence spermatozoal nuclear chromatin stability. Zinc may play an important role in the antibacterial activity of seminal plasma. However, various authors could not demonstrate statistically significant differences of zinc levels between fertile and infertile men (Umeyama et al 1986, Carrera & Mendoza 1990). While spermatozoal motility seems to require adequate concentrations of zinc in the semen, increased seminal zinc concentrations have been observed to correlate with reduced motility (Umeyama et al 1986, Carrera & Mendoza 1990). Zinc can be measured by atomic absorption spectroscopy. Since sperm cells are also rich in zinc, care should be taken that seminal plasma is devoid of sperm cells when tested for zinc.

**Citric acid** The physiological role of this substance, derived almost solely from the prostate, is still obscure. Mann (1964) has speculated that citric acid may be important in maintaining the osmotic equilibrium of the semen. The measurement of citric acid is usually colorimetric and based on the Furth–Hartmann reaction. Citric acid levels in seminal plasma reflect rather well the functional state of the prostate gland.

**Acid phosphatase (AP)** Several acid phosphatases can be distinguished in the human testis (Guha & Vanha-Perttula 1980). The major proportion of acid phosphatases, however, are secreted by the prostate gland and this substance is therefore a very reliable marker of prostatic function and has been used widely as a parameter for monitoring prostatic malignancies. One of the possible physiological functions of this enzyme is the breakdown of phosphorylcholine and the provision of free choline. No correlation between sperm count and motility, on the one hand, and AP, on the other hand, has been observed (Heite & Wetterauer 1979). Among numerous methods of analysis the method of choice is based on the enzymatic hydrolysis of the phosphate bond of *p*-nitrophenol (Polakoski & Zaneveld 1977).

## Seminal vesicles

Immediately following the ejaculation of the epididymal and prostatic spurt, the seminal vesicles contract rhythmically and provide the remaining ejaculatory spurts. Some 70% of the seminal fluid originates in the seminal vesicles. The fluid is alkaline. The two best-known specific products of the seminal vesicle are fructose and prostaglandins. Although the seminal plasma contains a variety of sugars such as glucose, ribose, fucose and others, fructose is the principal sugar providing a readily available exogenous energy source for sperm cells, and presents a very specific marker for the functional state of the seminal vesicles. Levels above 1200 ng/ml are considered normal. There does not seem to be a correlation between sperm count and motility and fructose levels (Videla et al 1981, Glezerman et al 1982). Among a variety of methods fructose can be measured by gas chromatography (Ludwig et al 1974), paper chromatography (Lewin & Beer 1975) and colorimetric methods based on the resorcinol reaction (Mann 1964). The latter method is probably the easiest and most widely in use.

## Prostaglandins

The techniques available for measurement of seminal prostaglandins are complicated and laborious. UV absorption, densitometry, enzymatic analysis, gas chromatography with spectrometry, and radioimmunoassay are examples of methods used. The determination of prostaglandins in seminal fluid is beyond the scope of the routine semen analysis. However, the importance of these substances justifies a short discussion. Prostaglandins have been demonstrated in the epididymis and testes but the principal source of these long-chain fatty acids is the seminal vesicles. The human seminal plasma possesses the highest concentration of prostaglandins of all body fluids. Some 17 prostaglandins (PG) have been identified in seminal plasma hitherto, the most important of them being $PGE_1$ and $PGE_2$ and their 19-OH derivatives. Normal values are 30–200 ng/ml ($PGE_1$ + $PGE_2$) and 90–260 ng/ml for the two derivatives (Cooper & Kelly 1975).

The physiological role of prostaglandins in human semen is poorly understood. PGE generally inhibits spontaneous contractions of the human uterus. Martin & Bydgeman (1975) stated that intrauterine instillation of $PGE_2$ increased uterine contractility during the proliferative and secretory phase but inhibited uterine contractions during menstruation. Pregnant uteri respond to PGE with contractions. The Fallopian tube is another target organ for prostaglandins. Sandberg et al (1964) have demonstrated that PGE contracts the quarter proximal to the uterus and relaxes the distal three-quarters. This action may influence spermatozoal and/or ovum transport.

PGE stimulate adenyl cyclase in most tissues. It is conceivable that seminal prostaglandins might raise the intraspermatozoal levels of cAMP, thus stimulating motility. Reduced prostaglandin levels in seminal fluid have repeatedly been associated with male infertility (Collier et al 1975).

## Cowper's and Littre's glands

The contribution of the secretions of these glands to the seminal volume is negligible. A physiological role beyond lubrication of the urethra is unknown for constituents of the secreted fluid and no specific marker has been defined.

## Prolactin

Sheth et al (1975) have demonstrated prolactin in the secretion of prostate and seminal vesicles. The levels of prolactin in seminal plasma is four- to seven-fold higher than in blood serum. The physiological significance of prolactin in seminal fluid is not clear. Prolactin may affect seminal sodium and potassium transport between spermatozoa and seminal plasma and thus influence sperm metabolism and motility. It has been stated that in rats, prolactin, in addition to testosterone, stimulates prostatic function (Dattatreymurty et al 1975). Analysis of prolactin is performed by radioimmunoassay and is usually not part of a standard semen analysis.

## IN VITRO MUCUS PENETRATION TEST AS A PARAMETER FOR SPERM ASSESSMENT

However sophisticated all methods for semen analysis may be, they describe and quantitate the behavior of sperm cells in their own medium, the seminal fluid. Marion Sims (1869) is credited for being the first to observe sperm cells in the cervical mucus after sexual intercourse. For almost 50 years this test was rarely utilized, being subject to moralistic attacks. Huehner, in 1913, again stressed its importance and the Sims–Huehner Test, or postcoital test, is now an integral part of every fertility survey. Yet, information gained from this test is limited. Its accuracy is influenced by environmental factors, such as pH of the vagina, composition of the cervical mucus, vaginal infections, coital technique, etc. Furthermore, only the interaction between husband's semen and wife's mucus can be evaluated and an abnormal test can be due to disturbances in the reproductive function of either partner (see also Chapter 13).

Consequently, Miller & Kurzrok (1932) proposed an in vitro method for evaluation of sperm–mucus interaction which permits cross-testing with donor sperm and donor mucus. A variety of in vitro sperm penetration tests have been developed since then. Diagnosis, classification and treatment of the cervical factor of infertility are discussed elsewhere in this volume (see Chapters 13 and 22). In the framework of this section on semen analysis we shall therefore focus on one question only: do the postcoital test (PCT) and the in vitro sperm penetration test provide additional information about the fertilizing potential of a given semen sample which cannot be obtained by routine semen analysis?

The PCT is based on the number of motile sperm cells per high-power microscopic field (HPF) in a mucus sample obtained some time after coitus or inseminating. In order for the test to be meaningful, cervical mucus has to possess the properties which are common at midcycle. This can be achieved by either performing the test during the preovulatory period or by administrating sufficient amounts of estrogen to the female partner. The physical properties of the cervical mucus are assessed using a scoring system (Insler et al 1972) and retrieved mucus is examined microscopically. Criteria for the assessment of the PCT have been defined in the WHO scientific group report (1976) (Table 11.13).

Giner et al (1974) found no correlation between quality of cervical mucus, number and degree of spermatozoal motility per HPF, the classification of the test, and occurrence of pregnancies. Harrison (1981) found no correlation between semen analysis and PCT in more than 20% of the cases. Since many different factors may influence the PCT, this test is certainly no substitute for semen analysis. However, the contact of seminal fluid and sperm cells with cervical mucus may permit the detection of immunological problems. Kremer & Jager (1976) performed PCTs in 19 couples in whom the male partners had circulating sperm agglutinins and normal semen analysis. They noted in 52 of 61 tests lack of progressive spermatozoal movement in the cervical mucus. The authors proposed a slide test which is aimed at differentiating between immunological and nonimmunological sperm agglutination. A positive sperm –

**Table 11.13** Grading system for postcoital test as proposed by WHO (1976)

| Definition | Observation (HPF) |
|---|---|
| Normal (A) | 7 sperm cells without agglutination Good progressive movement |
| Inconclusive (B) | 1–7 sperm cells without agglutination Good progressive movement |
| Suspected immunological factor (C) | Sperm agglutination regardless of total number of cells per HPF |
| Abnormal (D) | Nonmoving sperm cells only |
| Abnormal (E) | Absence of sperm cells |

cervical mucus-contact test (SCMC Test) is characterized by typical shaking movements of the sperm cells when they come in contact with cervical mucus in vitro. Persistent abnormal PCTs may, therefore, raise suspicion as to the existence of an immunological factor which would not have been suspected by semen analysis alone. Specific tests may then further clarify the situation.

The PCT is usually performed 12–16 h after coitus or insemination. If the test is inconclusive or abnormal, the examination is repeated several times while the coitus-sampling interval is gradually reduced.

Insler et al (1977) compared PCT and in vitro sperm penetration tests (SPT) in 166 infertile couples. Only in 95 of these cases (57%) was the PCT fully compatible with the penetration ability of husband's sperm in vitro. Thus, the SPT may provide additional information which is not obvious by PCT. In the same study, Insler et al (1977) reported on 56 men with an inherent defect indicated by reduced ability of sperm cells to penetrate both wife's and donor's cervical mucus. Ten of these men (18%) had normal sperm counts, sperm motility and morphology on routine semen analysis. In another study, Insler et al (1979) correlated seminal fluid analysis with mucus-penetrating ability of sperm cells in 100 infertile couples, 25 fertile donors, and 25 men with known sperm pathology. When semen analysis was abnormal, all SPTs showed abnormal results. In cases in which semen analysis was considered normal (semen donors), only two out of 25 semen samples showed poor results on in vitro penetration tests. In vitro penetration was influenced mostly by sperm motility and morphology and sperm count had a very limited influence. David et al (1979b) have come to the same conclusions.

Several techniques for in vitro SPTs have been proposed. Kremer (1965) has described a 'sperm penetration meter', a calibrated glass slide on which mucus-containing capillaries are glued. At one edge the slide has a small glass reservoir and the sperm penetration meter is incubated at 37°C for 30 min. After incubation, the sperm penetration meter is placed on the viewing table of a microscope for examination. The test permits evaluation of linear progression of sperm cells in cervical mucus and an estimate of their penetrating ability and longevity in a given mucus sample. Kremer & Kroeks (1975) have further improved their technique by replacing the round capillary with a flat one which permits easier observation through the microscope without the optical limitations posed by the circular shape. Mills & Katz (1978) have proposed a system containing flat capillaries, a loading manifold for drawing mucus or other highly viscous media into the tube, and a microscopic slide containing a sperm reservoir, similar to that proposed by Kremer. Reichman et al (1973) have used micro-hematocrit tubes filled with 3-cm-long columns of cervical mucus and placed vertically in semen samples. Following incubation for 90 min, sperm cells were counted in the upper 1 cm of the mucus. The test was classified as normal when at least five motile sperm cells were seen per HPF, inconclusive when the number was three to four, and poor when less than three sperm cells were observed.

The main problem of the in vitro SPTs is the availability of human cervical mucus. Therefore, surrogates for human cervical mucus have been proposed. Bisset (1980) used polyethlene glycol bisacrylate, which seems to possess rheological properties very similar to human midcycle mucus. The migration rate of sperm cells is similar in this artificial medium to that in human mucus. Gaddum-Rosse et al (1980) have used bovine

**Table 11.14**   Normal values of semen analysis

| | |
|---|---|
| Volume | 2–5ml |
| pH | 7.2–7.8 |
| Color | Gray-white-yellow |
| Liquefaction | Within 40 min |
| Fructose | >1200 µg/ml |
| Acid phosphatase | 100–300 µg/ml |
| Citric acid | >3 mg/ml |
| Inositol | >1mg/ml |
| Zinc | >75 µg/ml |
| Magnesium | >70 µg/ml |
| Prostaglandins ($PGE_1$ + $PGE_2$) | 30–200 µg/ml |
| Glycerylphosphorylcholine | >650 µg/ml |
| Carnitine | >250 µg/ml |
| Sperm count | 30–250 $10^6$/ml |
| Sperm motility | >50% after 1 h |
| | >40% after 3 h |
| Sperm morphology | >50% normal oval cells |
| Eosin-positive cells | 10% stained cells |

mucus and found it a suitable substitute for human cervical mucus. Lee et al (1981) have reported that bovine mucus may be stored for up to 4 weeks at 12°C without any change in its physical properties.

PCTs and particularly in vitro SPTs may be valuables additions to the routine semen analysis.

## NORMAL VALUES

Table 11.14 gives some guidance as to what should be considered normal in a given semen sample. It is important to stress that semen analyses should be performed under standardized conditions and normal values should be established for each laboratory.

## REFERENCES

Abyholm T 1981 An andrological study of 51 fertile men. Int J Androl 4: 646

Acosta A A, Kruger T F, Swanson R J et al 1988 The role of IVF in male infertility. In: Nogro-Vila A, Isidory A, Paulson J, Afdelmassih R, de Castro MPP, (eds) Andrology and human reproduction, Serono Symposia, vol 17. Raven, New York

Aitken R J, Best F S M, Richardson D W et al 1982 An analysis of sperm function in cases of unexplained infertility: conventional criteria, movement characteristics, and fertilizing capacity. Fertil Steril 30: 212

Amelar R D, Dubin L, Walsh PC 1977 Male infertility. Saunders, Philadelphia

Arbatti N J, Sheth A R 1987 Measurement of inhibin by immunoassay and receptor assay. In: Sheth A R (ed) Inhibins: isolation, estimation and physiology, vol I. CRC, Boca Raton, p 119

Arver S 1980 Zinc and zinc ligands in human seminal plasma. I. Methodological aspects and normal findings. Int J Androl 3: 629

Bahamondes L, Abdelmassih R, Dachs J N 1979 Survey of 185 sperm analyses of fertile men in an infertility service. Int J Androl 2: 526

Baker H W G, Burger H G, de Kretser M D, Lording D W, McGowan P, Rennie G C 1981 Factors affecting the variability of semen analysis results in infertile men. Int J Androl 4: 609

Barnea E R, Arronet G H, Weissenberg R, Lunenfeld B 1980 Studies on polyspermia. Int J Fertil 25: 303

Bartoov B, Fisher J, Eltes F, Langsam J, Lunenfeld B 1981 A comparative morphological analysis of abnormal human spermatozoa. In: Insler V, Bettendorf G (eds) Advances in diagnosis and treatment of infertility. Elsevier/North-Holland, Amsterdam, pp 355–373

Bartoov B, Eltes F, Langsam J, Snyder M, Fisher J 1982 Ultrastructural studies in morphological assessment of human spermatozoa. Int J Androl Suppl 5: 81

Bartoov B, Eltes F, Soffer Y et al 1990 Ultramorphologic characteristics of human sperm cells. In: Mashiah S, Ben Rafael Z, Laufer N, Schenker J G (eds) Advances in assisted reproductive technology. Plenum, New York

Basco L 1984 Clinical tests of sperm fertilizing capacity. Fertil Steril 41: 177

Bicsak T A, Vale W, Vaughan J, Tucker E M, Cappel S, Hsue A J W 1987 Hormonal regulation of inhibin production by Sertoli cells. Mol Cell Endocrinol 49: 211

Bisset D L 1980 Development of a model of human cervical mucus. Fertil Steril 33: 211

Blom E 1950a A one-minute live-dead sperm stain by means of eosin-nigrosin. Fertil Steril 1: 176

Blom E 1950b Interpretation of spermatic cytology in bulls. Fertil Steril 1: 223

Blom E 1968 A new sperm defect—'Pseudodroplets' in the middle piece of the bull sperm. Nord Vet Med 20: 279

Blom E 1972 The ultrastructure of some characteristic sperm defects and a proposal for a new classification of the bull spermiogram. VII. Symposio International di Zootechnia, Milona, pp 125 –139

Blom E, Birch-Anderson A 1965 The ultrastructure of the bull sperm. Nord Vet Med 17: 193

Blom E, Birch-Andersen A 1975 The ultrastructure of a characteristic spermhead defect in the boar. Andrologia 7: 199

Boonsaeng V 1981 A simple method to measure the liquefication rate of human semen. Andrologia 13: 342

Bostole E, Serup J, Raffe H 1982 Relation between morphologically abnormal spermatozoa and pregnancies obtained during a 20-year follow-up period. Int J Androl 5: 379

Broecks A, Keel B S 1979 The semen analysis: an important diagnostic evaluation. Lab Med 10: 686

Brotherton J 1979 Estimation of number, mean size and size contribution of human spermatozoa using a coulter counter. J Reprod Fert 5: 626

Calamera J C 1978 Spermatozoal motility and fructolysis—comparative study of samples obtained by masturbation and with plastic collectors. Andrologia 10: 169

Calamera J C, Lavieri J C 1974 Glycerylphosphorylcholine in human seminal plasma of normal subjects and sterile patients. Andrologia 6: 67

Calamera J C, Vilar O 1979 Comparative study of sperm morphology with three different staining procedures. Andrologia 11: 255

Carrera A, Mendoza C 1990 Zinc levels in seminal plasma of fertile and infertile men. Andrologia 22: 279

Casillas E R 1973 Accumulation of carnitine by bovine spermatozoa during maturation in the epididymus. J Biol Chem 248: 8227

Castenholz A 1974 Photokymographische Registriermethode zur Darstellung und Analyse der Spermatozoenbewegung. Andrologia 6: 155

Chan S Y W, Tsoi W L, Leung J, Ng V, Lo T, Wang C 1989 The accuracy of sperm concentration determination by the automated CellSoft semen analyzer before and after discontinuous Percoll gradient centrifugation. Anrologia 22: 55

Check J M, Shanis B, Bollendorf A 1990 Computer assisted analysis is not superior to routine analysis in distinguishing fertile from subfertile men. Arch Androl 13

Collier J G, Flower R J, Stanton S L 1975 Seminal prostaglandins in infertile men. Fertil Steril 26: 868

Cooper I, Kelly R W 1975 The measurement of E and 19-OH E prostaglandins in human seminal plasma. Prostaglandins 10: 507

Dattatreymurty B, Raghavan V P, Purandare T V, Sheth A R, Rao S S 1975 Synergistic action of prolactin with HCG on rat ventral prostate. J Reprod Fertil 44: 555

David G, Bisson J P, Jouannet P et al 1972 Les teratospermies. In: Thibault C (ed) La sterilite du male. Acquisitions recents. Paris, Masson et Cie, Paris

David G, Bisson J P, Cryglik F, Jaunet P, Genigon C 1975 Anomalies morphologiques du spermatozoide humain. 1. Proposition pour un systeme de classification. J Gynecol Obstet Biol Reprod 4 (suppl): 17

David G, Jouannet P, Martin-Boyce A, Spira A, Schwartz D 1979a Sperm counts in fertile and infertile men. Fertil Steril 31: 453

David M P, Amit A, Bergman A, Yedwab G, Paz G F, Homonnai Z T 1979b Sperm penetration in vivo: correlations between parameters of sperm quality and the penetration capacity. Fertil Steril 32: 676

Dawson R M C, Mann T, White I G, 1957 Glycerylphosphorylcholine and phosphorylcholine in semen and their relation to choline. Biochem J 65: 627

Dickerman Sagiv M, Segenreich E, Levinsky H, Singer R 1988 The evaluation of routine andrological parameters in human semen. Andrologia 20: 492

Dott H M, Harrison R A P, Foster G C A 1979 The maintenance of motility and the surface properties of epididymal spermatozoa from bull, rabbit and ram in homologous seminal and epididymal plasma. J Reprod Fertil 55: 113

Dubois M, Jouannet P, Berge P, David G 1974 Spermatozoa motility in human cervical mucus. Nature 252: 711

Duyck F, Steeno O 1990 High ejaculate volume: a distinct entity? Andrologia 22: 497

Edwinsson A, Bergman P, Steen Y, Nilsson S 1983 Characteristics of donor semen and cervical mucus at the time of conception. Fertil Steril 39: 327

Eliasson R 1973 Parameters of male fertility In: Hafez E S E, Evans T N (eds). Human reproduction. Conception and contraception. Harper & Row, New York, p 39

Eliasson R 1977 Supravital staining of human spermatozoa. Fertil Steril 28: 1257

Eliasson R 1981 Analysis of semen. In Burger H, de Kretser D (eds) The testis. Raven New York, pp 381–399

Eliasson R, Treichl L 1971 Supravital staining of human spermatozoa. Fertil Steril 22: 134

Eliasson R, Hellinga G, Luebcke F et al 1970 Empfehlungen zur Nomenklatur in der Andrologie. Andrologia 2: 186

Falk H C, Kaufman S A 1950 What constitutes a normal semen? Fertil Steril 1: 489

Farris E J 1949 The number of spermatozoa as an index of fertility in man. A study of 406 semen samples. J Urol 61: 1099

Flechion J E, Hafez E S E 1976 Scanning electron microscopy of human spermatozoa. In: Hafez E S E (ed). Human semen and fertility regulation in men. Mosby, St Louis, pp 76–82

Francavilla, Romano R, Santucci R, Poccia G 1990 Effects of sperm morphology and motile sperm count on outcome of intrauterine insemination in oligozoospermia and/or asthenozoospermia. Fertil Steril 53: 892

Frenkel G, Peterson R N, Davis J E, Freund M 1974 Glycerylphosphorylcholine and carnitine in normal human semen and in postvasectomy semen: differences in concentrations. Fertil Steril 25: 84

Freund M 1962 Interrelationships among the characteristics of human semen and factors affecting semen-specimen quality. J Reprod Fertil 4: 143

Freund M 1963 Effects of frequency of emission on semen output and an estimate of daily sperm production in man. J Reprod Fertil 6: 269

Freund M 1966 Standards for the rating of human sperm morphology. Int J Fertil 11: 97

Freund M, Peterson R N, 1976 Semen evaluation and fertility. In: Hafez E S E (eds). Human semen and fertility regulation in men. Mosby, St Louis, pp 344–354

Fritz I B 1963 Carnitine and its role in fatty acid metabolism. Adv Lipid Res 1: 285

Gaddum-Rosse P, Blaudau R J, Lee W I 1980 Sperm penetration into cervical mucus in vitro. I. Comparative studies. Fertil Steril 33: 636

Gill H S, Van Arsdalen K, Hypolite J, Levin R M, Ruzich J V 1988 Comparative study of two computerized semen motility analyzers. Andrologia 20: 433

Giner J, Merino G, Luna J, Aznar R 1974 Evaluation of the Sims–Huehner post-coital test in fertile couples. Fertil Steril 25: 145

Glass R H, Ericsson R J 1979 Spontaneous cure of male infertility. Fertil Steril 31: 305

Glezerman M, Berstein D, Zakut Ch, Misgav N, Insler V 1982 Polyzoospermia—a definite pathological entity. Fertil Steril 38: 605

Guha K, Vanha-Perttula T 1980 Acid phosphatases of the human testis. Int J Androl 3: 256

Hafez E S E, Kanagawa H 1973 Scanning electron microscopy and rabbit spermatozoa. Fertil Steril 24: 776

Harrison R A P, Dott H M, Foster G C 1978 Effect of ionic strength serum albumin and other macromolecules on the maintenance of motility and surface of mammalian spermatozoa in sample medium. J Reprod Fertil 52: 65

Harrison R F 1981 The diagnostic and therapeutic potential of the post-coital test. Fertil Steril 36: 71

Harvey C 1960 The speed of human spermatozoa and the effect on it of various dilutants with some preliminary observations of clinical material. J Reprod Fertil 1: 84

Heite H-J, Wetterauer W 1979 Zur Kenntnis der saueren Phosphatase im Seminal plasma—Bestimmungsmethode und diagnostische Bedeutung. Andrologia 11: 113

Homonnai Z T, Paz G, Weiss J N, David M P 1980 Quality of semen obtained from 627 fertile men. Int J Androl 3: 217

Hotchkiss R S, Brunner E K, Grenley P 1938 Semen analysis of two hundred fertile men. Am J Med Sci 196: 362

Huehner M 1913 Sterility in the male and female and its treatment. Pebman, New York

Inchiosa M A Jr 1965 Water-soluble extractives of disposable syringes. J Pharm Sci 54: 1379

Insler V, Melmed H, Eichenbrenner I, Serr D M, Lunenfeld B 1972 The cervical score—a simple semi-quantitative method for monitoring of the menstrual cycle. Int J Gynecol Obstet 10: 228

Insler V, Bernstein D, Glezerman M 1977 Diagnosis and classification of the cervical factor of infertility. In: Insler V, Bettendorf G (eds) The uterine cervix in reproduction. Thieme, Stuttgart, p 265

Insler V, Bernstein D, Glezerman M, Misgav N 1979 Correlation of seminal fluid analysis and mucus penetrating ability of spermatozoa. Fertil Steril 32: 316

Jaeger R J, Rubin R J 1970 Plasicizers from plastic devices: extraction, metabolism and accumulation by biological systems. Science 170: 460

Jamess W H 1980 Secular trend in reported sperm counts. Andrologia 12: 381

Janick J, MacLeod J 1970 The measurement of human spermatzoa motility. Fertil Steril 21: 140

Jecht E W, Russo J J 1973 A system for the quantitative analysis of human sperm motility. Andrologia 5: 215

Jequier A M 1986 Infertility in the male. Churchill Livingstone, Edinburgh

Jeulin C, Feruy D, Serres C et al 1986 Sperm factors related to failure of human in vitro fertilization. J Reprod Fertil 76: 735

Jeyendran R S, Van der Ven H H, Rosecrans R, Perez-Palaez M, AI-Hasani S, Zaneveld L J D 1989 Chemical constituents of human seminal plasma: relationship to fertility. Andrologia 21: 423

Joel C A 1969 Die Hyperzoospermie. Med Hyg 27: 1354

Jouannet P, Volochine B, Deguent P, Serres C, David G 1977 Light scattering determination of various characteristic parameters of spermatozoa motility in a series of human sperm. Andrologia 9: 36

Jouannet P, Czyglik F, David G, Mayaux M J, Moscato M L, Schwartz D 1981 Study of a group of 484 fertile men. I. Distribution of semen characteristics. Int J Androl 4: 440

Knuth U A, Nieschlag E 1988 Comparison of computerized semen analysis with the conventional procedure in 322 patients. Fertil Steril 49: 881

Knuth U A, Yeung C H, Nieschlag E 1987 Computerized semen analysis: objective measurement of semen characteristics is biased by subjective parameter setting. Fertil Steril 48: 118

Koehler J K 1972 Human sperm head ultrastructure. A freeze-etching study. J Ultrastruct Res 39: 520

Kremer J 1965 A simple sperm penetration test. Int J Fertil 10: 209

Kremer J, Jager S 1976 The sperm–cervical mucus contact test: a preliminary report. Fertil Steril 27: 335

Kremer J, Kroeks M V A M 1975 Modification of the in vitro spermatozoal penetration test by means of the sperm penetration meter. Acta Eur Fertil 6: 377

Kruger T F, Menkveld R, Stander F S H et al 1986 Sperm morphologic features as a prognostic factor in in vitro fertilization. Fertil Steril 44: 1118

Kruger T F, Acosta A A, Simmons K F, Swanson R J, Matla J F, Oehminger S 1988 Predictive value of abnormal sperm morphology in in vitro fertilization. Fertil Steril 49: 112

Kvist U, 1980 Importance of spermatozoal zinc as temporary inhibitor of sperm nuclear chromatin decondensation ability in man. Acta Physiol, Scand 109: 79

Kvist U, Eliasson R 1980 Influence of seminal plasma on the chromatin stability of ejaculated human spermatozoa. Int J Androl 3: 130

Lee W I, Gaddum-Rosse P, Slandau R J 1981 Sperm penetration into cervical mucus in vitro. III. Effects of freezing on estrous bovine cervical mucus. Fertil Steril 36: 209

Leto S, Frensilli F J 1981 Changing parameters of donor semen. Fertil Steril 36: 766

Lewin L M, Beer R, 1975 Semiquantitative paper chromatography assay for inositol and fructose: a method for evaluating prostatic and vesicular contributions to human seminal fluid. Isr J Med Sci 11: 523

Lewin L M, Beer R, Lunenfeld B 1976 Epididymis and seminal vesicle as sources of carnitine in human seminal fluid. the clinical significance of the carnitine concentration in human seminal fluid. Fertil Steril 27: 9

Lindholmer C H 1974 The importance of seminal plasma to human sperm motility. Biol Reprod 10: 533

Ludvik W 1976 Andrology. Thieme Verlag, Stuttgart

Ludwig G , Weigl H, Nuri M, Peters H J 1974 Vergleichende Bestimmung der Spermaplasma Fruktose nach der enzymatischen und der Duennschichtchromatograhischen Methode. Urologie 13: 177

Lunenfeld B, Glezerman M 1981 Diagnose und Therapie maennlicher Fertilitaetsstoerungen. Grosse, Berlin.

Mc Gowan M P, Baker M W G, Kosais G T, Rennie G 1983 Selection of high fertility donors for artificial insemination programmes. Clin Reprod Fertil 2: 269

MacLeod J 1965 The semen examination. Clin Obstet Gynceol 8: 115

MacLeod J 1970 The significance of deviation in human sperm morphology in the human testis. Adv Exp Med Biol 10: 481

MacLeod J, Gold R Z 1951 Semen quality in 1000 men of known fertility and 800 cases of infertile marriage. Fertil Steril 2: 115

Macomber D, Sanders M R 1929 The spermatozoa count. N Engl J Med 200: 981

Mahony M C, Alexanders N J, Swanson R J 1988 Evaluation of semen parameters by means by automated sperm motion analyzers. Fertil Steril 49: 876

Makler A 1978a A new chamber for rapid sperm count and motility estimation. Fertil Steril 30: 313

Makler A 1978b The thickness of microscopically examined seminal sample and its relationship to sperm motility examination. Int J Androl 1: 213

Makler A 1978c A new multiple exposure photography method for sperm motility determination. Fertil Steril 30: 192

Makler A, Tatcher M, Mohiliver J 1980 Sperm semi-autoanalyses by combination of the MEP and computer techniques. Int J Fertil 25: 62

Mann T 1964 The biochemistry of semen and of the male reproductive tract. Methuen, London

Mann T, Lutvak-Mann C 1981 Male reproductive function and semen. Springer, Berlin

Marmar N R, Katz S, Praisss D E, DeBeneticus T J 1975 Semen zinc levels in infertile and postvasectomy patients and patients with prostatitis. Fertil Steril 26: 1057

Marquis N R, Fritz I B 1966 Enzymological determination of free carnitine concentrations in rat tissues. J Lipid Res 5: 184

Martin J N, Bydgeman M 1975 The effect of locally administered PGE2 on on the contractility of the non-pregnant uterus in vivo. Prostaglandins 10: 253

Miller E G, Kurzrok R 1932 Biochemical studies of human semen: factors affecting migration of sperm through the cervix. Am J Obstet Gynecol 24: 19

Mills R N, Katz D F 1978 A flat capillary tube system for assessment of sperm movement in cervical mucus. Fertil Steril 29: 43

Mortimer D, Templeton A A, Lenton E A, Coleman R A 1982 Influence of abstinence and ejaculation-to-analysis delay on semen analysis: parameters of suspected infertile men. Arch Androl 8: 251

Mortimer D, Goel N, Shu M A 1988 Evaluation of the

Cellsoft automated semen analysis system in a routine laboratory setting. Fertil Steril 50: 960

Mueller B, Kirchner C 1978 Influence of seminal plasma proteins on motility of rabbit spermatozoa. J Reprod Fertil 45: 167

Nelson C M K, Bunge R G 1974 Semen analysis: evidence for changing parameters of male fertility potential. Fertil Steril 25: 503

Nie N H, Maldi Hull C, Jenkins J G, Steinberger K, Bent D H 1975 Statistical package for the social sciences. McGraw-Hill, New York, Ch 23

Oemhinger S, Acosta A A, Morshedi M et al 1988 Corrective measures and pregnancy outcome in in vitro fertilization in patients with severe sperm morphology abnormalities. Fertil Steril 50: 283

Pedersen H 1970 Ultrastructure of the ejaculated human sperm. In: Baccetti B (ed), Comparative spermatology. Academic, New York, pp 133–142

Pedersen H, Fawcett D W 1976 Functional anatomy of the human spermatozoa. In: Hafez E S F (ed) Human semen and fertility regulation in men. Mosby, St Louis, pp 65–75

Pedersen H, Rebbe H 1974 Fine structure of round-headed human spermatozoa. J Reprod Fertil 37: 51

Pedersen H, Rebbe H, Hamman R 1971 Human sperm fine structure in a case of severe asthenospermia-necrospermia. Fertil Steril 22: 156

Peterson R N, Freund M 1971 Glycolyis by human spermatozoa: levels of glycolytic intermediates. Biol Reprod 5: 221

Phadke A M 1978 Natural red supravital staining for cellular elements in the semen. Andrologia 10: 80

Polakoski K L, Zaneveld L J D 1977 Biochemical examination of the human ejaculate. In: Hafez E S E (ed) Techniques of human andrology. Elsevier/North Holland, Amsterdam, pp 265–286

Polansky F F, Lamb E J 1988 Do the results of semen analysis predict future fertility? A survival analysis study. Fertil Steril 49: 1059

Politoff L, Birkhauser M, Almendral A, Zorn A 1989 New data confirming a circannual rhythm in spermatogenesis. Fertil Steril 52: 486

Pryor J P 1981 Semen analysis. Clin Obstet Gynecol 8: 571

Ramasharma K, Sairam M R, Seidah N H et al 1984 Isolation, structure and synthesis of a human seminal plasma peptide with inhibin-like activity. Science 223: 1199

Rehan N E, Sobrero A J, Fertig J W 1975 The semen of fertile men: statistical analysis of 1300 men. Fertil Steril 26: 492

Reichman J, Insler V, Serr D M 1973 A modified in vitro spermatozoal penetration test. Int J Fertil 18: 232

Rivier J, McClintock R, Vaughan J et al 1986 Partial purification of Inhibin from ovine rete testis fluid. In: Zatuchni G J, Goldsmith A, Spieler J M, Sciarra J J (eds) Male contraception: advances and future aspects. Harper and Row, Philadelphia, p 401

Ross A, Christie S, Edmond P 1973 Ultrastructural tail defect in the spermatozoa from two men attending a subfertility clinic. J Reprod Fert 32: 243

Rozin S 1960 Studies on seminal plasma. I. The role of seminal plasma in motility of spermatozoa. Fertil Steril 11: 278

Sandberg F, Ingelman-Sundberg A, Ryden G 1964 The effect of prostaglandin E2 and E3 on the human uterus and the fallopian tubes in vitro. Acta Obstet Gynecol Scand 42: 269

Sauer M W, Zeffer K B, Buster J H, Sokol R Z 1988 Effect of abstinence on sperm motility in normal men. Am J Obstet Gynecol 158: 604

Schirren C G 1972 Praktische Andrologie. Hartmann, Berlin

Schirren C G, Holstein A F, Schirren C 1971 Ueber die Morphogenese rundkoepfiger Spermatozoen des Menschen. Andrologia 3: 117

Schwartz D, Laplanche A, Jouannet P, David G 1979 Within subject variability of human semen with regard to sperm count, volume, total number of spermatozoa and length of abstinence. J Reprod Fertil 57: 391

Scott R S, Burger H G 1980 Inhibin is absent from azoospermic semen of infertile men. Nature 285: 246

Seidah N G, Arbatti N J, Rochemont J, Sheth A R, Chretien M 1984 Complete amino acid equence of human seminal plasma-inhibin. FEBS 175: 349

Sheth A R, Mugtawala P P, Shah G V, Rao S S 1975 Occurrence of prolactin in human semen. Fertil Steril 26: 905

Sims M 1869 Sperm penetration test on the microscope as an aid in the diagnosis and treatment of sterility. NY Med J 8: 393

Singer S, Sagiv M, Barnet M et al 1979 High sperm densities and the quality of semen. Arch Androl 3: 197

Smith D, Dura C, Zamboni L 1970 Fertilizing ability of structurally abnormal spermatozoa. Nature 227: 79

Smith M L, Luqman W A, Rakoff J S 1979 Correlations between seminal radioimmunoreactive prolactin, sperm count and sperm motility in prevasectomy and infertility clinic patients. Fertil Steril 32: 312

Sobrero A J, Rehan N E, 1975 The semen of fertile men. II. Semen characteristics of 100 fertile men. Fertil Steril 26: 1048

Sokoloski J E, Blasco L, Storey B T, Wolf D P 1977 Turbidimetric analysis of human sperm motility. Fertil Steril 28: 1337

Steinberger A, Steinberger E, 1976 Secretion of an FSH inhibiting factor by cultured Sertoli cells. Endocrinology 99: 918

Umeyama T, Ishikawa H, Takeshima H, Hoshii S, Kioso K 1986 A comparative study of seminal trace elements in fertile and infertile men. Fertil Steril 46: 494

Van Zyl J A 1972 A review of the male factor in 231 infertile couples. S Afr J Obstet Gynecol 10: 17

Van Zyl J A 1980 The infertile couple. II. Examination and evaluation of semen. SA Med J: 485

Vantman D, Koukoulis G, Dennison L, Zinaman M, Sherins R J 1988 Computer assisted semen analysis: Evaluation of method and assessment of the influence of sperm concentration of progessively motile human spermatozoa. Gamete Res 30: 213

Vaze A Y, Thakur A N, Sheth A R 1980 Levels of inhibin in human semen and accessory reproductive organs. Andrologia 12: 66

Videla E, Blanco A M, Galli M E, Fernandez-Collazo E 1981 Human seminal biochemistry: fructose, ascorbic acid, citric acid phosphatase and their relationship with sperm count. Andrologia 13: 212

Wetterauer U, Heite H-J 1980 Carnitine in seminal plasma: its significance in diagnostic andrology. Arch Androl 4: 137

WHO Scientific Report Group 1976 Technical Report Series No. 514. WHO, Geneva

WHO 1987 WHO laboratory manual for the examination of

human semen and semen – cervical mucus interaction. Cambridge University Press, Cambridge

Zaini A, Jennings N G and Baker M W G 1985 Are conventional sperm morphology and motility assessments of predictive value in subfertile men? Int J Androl 8: 427

Zamboni L 1987 The ultrastructural pathology of the spermatozoan as a cause of infertility: the role of electron microscopy in the evaluation of semen quality. Fertil Steril 48: 711

Zamboni L, Zemjanis R, Stefanini M 1971 The fine structure of monkey and human spermatozoa. Analyl Rec 169: 129

Zaneveld L J D, Polakoski K L 1977 Collection and physical examination of the ejaculate. In: Hafez E S E (ed) Techniques of human andrology. Elsevier/North Holland, Amsterdam, pp 147–172

Zuckerman Z, Rodriguez-Rigau L J, Smith K D, Steinberger E 1977 Frequency distribution of sperm counts in fertile and infertile males. Fertil Steril 28: 1310

# 12. Diagnosis of male infertility

*Marek Glezerman    Bruno Lunenfeld*

## INTRODUCTION

Ideally the infertile couple should be diagnosed and treated as a unit. Evaluation should begin with a detailed marital, sexual and medical history. Throughout the course of evaluation and management the couple should be seen and counselled together periodically even if only one partner requires treatment. Treatment of infertility is based on a team approach involving reproductive endocrinologist, an andrologist and if necessary other professionals (e.g urologists). Specialized andrological clinics should ideally operate within the framework of an infertility unit with easy and informal access to other team members. Proper diagnosis and classification of patients is a sine qua non condition of effective and safe therapy. Moreover, comparison of the results obtained in various groups of patients at the same center or of patients treated at different centers is possible only if a well-defined and reproducible classification has been used. A classification is valuable as long as acceptable measurable and well-defined parameters are used and a reasonable compromise is achieved between the accuracy, the effort and cost required. For clinical purposes our group uses a simple classification based mainly on the medical history, physical examination, quantity and quality of sperm, biochemical characterization of the ejaculate and basic andrological tests.

Estimation of plasma follicle stimulating hormone (FSH) will help to differentiate between hypothalamic-pituitary and testicular failure in azoospermics or in patients with severe oligoasthenospermia. The estimation of leutenizing hormone (LH) and testosterone may help to identify and localize androgen deficiency. Prolactin estimation may become necessary if a space-occupying lesion in the hypothalamic-pituitary region is suspected or in the course of evaluation of impotence. The quantitative capability of the pituitary to secrete FSH in response to gonadotropin releasing hormone (GnRH) can be used as an indirect measure for inhibin, and thus as a semiquantitative parameter for the assessment of Sertoli cell function. An exaggerated excretion of FSH (more than 150% of base level) during the 90 min following injection of 100 µg of GnRH indicates inhibin deficiency and thus Sertoli cell insufficiency. Lack of sufficient response to GnRH indicates gonadotropic deficiency, either primary, due to pituitary, or secondary, due to hypothalamic insufficiency. This test has an important prognostic function in azoospermic patients scheduled for gonadotropic therapy (Lunenfeld et al 1981).

We feel that testicular biopsy may be useful only to confirm the diagnosis of obstruction of sperm-conveying structures in cases where seminal markers and/or hormone analysis are inconclusive. Otherwise this procedure is rarely indicated. Chromosonal analysis or search of cellular sex chromatin is indicated if aberrations are suspected.

On the basis of algorithmic schemes, infertile men can be classified into diagnostic groups, depending on the etiology and on localization of the disturbance. A number of surgical procedures and therapeutic agents and approaches, each acting through a different mechanism, are available today which, if used wisely and correctly, have a reasonable chance of enhancing fertility (see Chapters 4, 5 and 24) These algorithmic schemes enable choice of the appropriate management for each diagnostic group and the most suitable fertility-promoting method for those classified as amenable to treatment. The experience of the physician will allow for 'short cuts', for shifting centers of gravity and for addition of relevant extensions to the proposed scheme. Although it is essential that husband and wife should be assessed as a unit, for didactic clarity, evaluation of the male partner only will be described here.

Results of at least two spermiograms should be available at the first visit of the patient. This will permit a primary classification: aspermia, azoospermia, oligozoospermia, asthenospermia and teratospermia. The nature, volume, and biochemical characteristics of the semen permits assessment of the function of the accessory glands, and detection of signs of acute, chronic or postinflammatory processes (see Chapter 27).

## HISTORY AND PHYSICAL EXAMINATION

A general history of the couple provides information on age of both partners, duration of marriage, duration of unprotected coitus, previous use of contraceptive methods, adequate knowledge and use of the fertile period, past fertility of each of the partners during the present or previous unions, results of investigations already performed elsewhere, and previous or current treatment for infertility. Any diseases, treatments or surgery which might potentially influence fertility should be recorded. Surgical procedures which may seriously reduce fertility are listed in Table 12.1. For example, clamping or tearing of the vas

**Table 12.1**  Surgical operations in the male possibly associated with infertility

Urethral strictures or diverticulae
Hypospadias
Prostatectomy
Bladder neck operations
Vasectomy
Varicocele
Hydrocele
Inguinal hernia
Testicular torsion
Sympathectomy

deferens in very young patients undergoing repair of bilateral cryptorchidism or congenital hernia is a frequent traumatic cause of obstruction.

Since certain familiar diseases may affect fertility, it is essential that information concerning some typical diseases be recorded (diabetes mellitus, thyroid disorders, tuberculosis, hypertension, vascular diseases, dietrystilbestrol (DES) exposure).

The history of past illness should be as complete as possible and should include trivial longstanding infections and childhood illnesses. Alterations in spermatogenesis may be brought about by apparently harmless illnesses, such as measles and simple pneumonia, as well as by more serious infections such as typhoid fever. Infertility due to portal occlusion of sperm-conveying structures, or due to lesions within the epididymis may result in impaired final maturation of sperm cells. Lesions within the prostate or seminal vesicles may present as inadequate sperm coagulation, liquefaction or motility problems. All these may be related to sexually transmitted diseases. If there is a history of such, information must be collected regarding the number of episodes and months since the last episode. One should especially search for diseases such as syphilis, gonorrhea, mycoplasma and nonspecific urethritis, since these or their sequelae may be associated with impairment of semen. Any febrile disease or acute incident during the previous 6 months could result in a temporary decrease of quantity and quality of sperm. The age factor needs to be taken into consideration in the history. Prepubertal mumps orchitis is frequently benign and runs a reversible course. However, after puberty it may cause irreversible damage to the testes. Febrile or toxic damage to the spermatogenic system also seems to occur more frequently after puberty.

It should always be ascertained whether both testes have always been in the scrotum, and if not the type of treatment given to correct this condition should be noted. If there was a history of bilateral cryptorchidism in the past, fertility prognosis is extremely poor, independent of at what age surgery was performed. This must be differentiated from mobile testes, a condition where descent of testes was achieved by medical treatment alone. In this case prognosis is better. Corrected unilateral cryptorchidism does not usually affect fertility. Injury to the testes, epididymis-orchitis and urinary disease, may all be potential causes of infertility. Torsion of the testis, especially when diagnosis and detorsion were delayed, may lead to testicular atrophy and impaired fertility. However, patients who were operated within 8 h after the onset of symptoms have been found to have normally sized testes, and only slight changes in testicular morphology and sperm parameters. Thus, whenever testicular torsion has occurred in the past, the time element should be thoroughly investigated. Excessive consumption of alcohol (more than 60 g per day), tobacco, or narcotics, or regular use of hot baths or sauna may also lead to temporary infertility. Marshburn et al (1989) have noted that semen of infertile men is particularly sensitive to the toxic effects of smoking and coffee.

It has been reported that some types of respiratory diseases are associated with infertility. Patients with a history of fibrocystic disease of the pancreas may have congenital absence of the vas deferens, presumably resulting from a common genetic defect. Sometimes, a history of childhood bronchiectasis may be associated with azoospermia due to obstruction.

## Sexual history (Fig. 12.1)

Sexual history should cover at least frequency of intercourse, adequacy of penile penetration, information about ejaculatory function and orgasmic sensation.

Attention should also be given to the couple's knowledge of the fertile period.

## Urinary symptoms

The patient's history can make a significant contribution to the evaluation of impaired male fertility if it leads to detection of urinary symptoms of an inflammatory or obstructive nature. Patients with urethral stricture are more likely to notice their poor urinary stream than the retarded flux of their semen with its concomitant impaired disposition.

Equally, inflammatory symptoms of micturition

may be more rapidly, and more easily, registered as an unpleasant sensation by many patients, than occasionally slightly painful ejaculations, such as occurring in chronic recurrent vesiculoprostatitis. Further evaluation is then warranted.

Useful information may be gained by directed questioning. Often it is only after specific questioning that symptoms such as painful ejaculation, frank blood in the ejaculate or its brownish discoloration (hematospermia), or total absence of ejaculation are brought to light.

## History of drugs or exposure to exogenous chemicals

Attention has been drawn to the disturbance of spermatogenesis by various groups of pharmacological, physical and chemical agents. Little is known about how exogenous chemicals affect reproductive processes and alter their function. Leydig cell function appears to be much more resistant to the toxic effects of drugs than Sertoli cell function and spermatogenesis. A striking example of the effect of drugs on spermatogenesis is azoospermia provoked by cytostatic or antimitotic drugs used not only for their immunosuppressive properties but also for the treatment of a variety of noncancerous diseases (Table 12.2).

The intense mitotic activity of the postpubertal germinal epithelium of the testis is most highly

Table 12.2 Some diseases treated by antimitotic drugs

Connective tissue
  Rheumatoid arthritis
  Systemic lupus erythematosus
Neurological
  Multiple sclerosis
  Myasthenia gravis
Renal
  Nephrotic syndrome
  Glomerulonephritis
  Transplant rejection
Hematological
  Autoimmune hemolytic anemia
  Idiopathic thrombocytopenic purpura
  Circulating anticoagulants
Gastrointestinal
  Ulcerative colitis
  Chronic active hepatitis
Dermatological
  Psoriasis
  Pemphigus
  Pyoderma gangrenosum

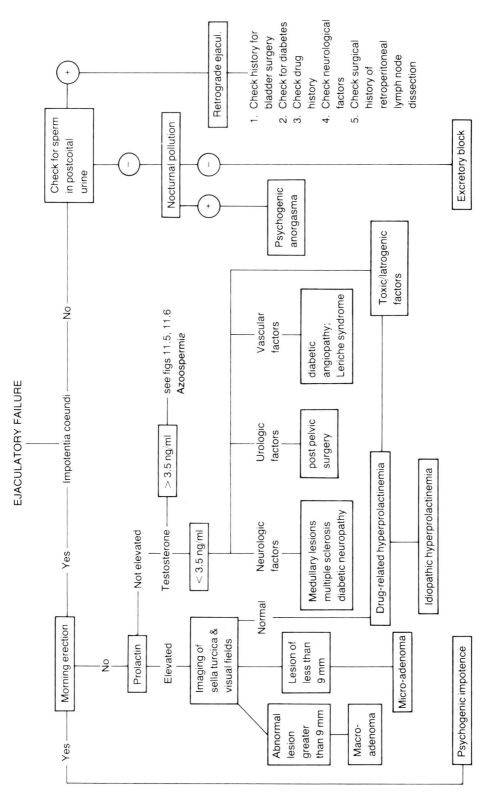

**Fig. 12.1**  Ejaculatory failure. In cases where erectory or ejaculatory insufficiency are accompanied by past or present signs of androgen deficiency, LH and testosterone determinations should be performed to assess the androgenic profile, and if androgen deficiency is confirmed, to localize its etiology. If LH is elevated in the presence of low or low-normal testosterone, primary Leydig cell insufficiency is most probably the cause. It should, however, be noted that elevated prolactin levels due to micro- or macro-adenoma may stimulate such a condition. If LH and testosterone are low, pituitary insufficiency, hypothalamic-pituitary dysfunction, or the rare fertile eunuch syndrome may be suspected.

prone to damage by these drugs, while Leydig cell function and testosterone secretion generally remain unimpaired.

Heindel & Treinen (1989) have estimated that over 100 chemicals have been delineated which have been shown to be toxic to the male reproductive system in rodents. Animal experiments have shed some light on chemicals which may affect the male reproductive system. Narcotics may affect the CNS and thus influence the brain-hypothalamus-pituitary-gonad axis (Smith & Gilbeau, 1985). Morris et al (1986) have shown that ethylene dimethane-sulfonate destroys Leydig cells in rat testes. Sprironolactone has also been shown to interface with Leydig cell function. Spironolactone used for the treatment of hypertension not only competes for the mineralocorticoid receptors, but also inhibits testosterone synthesis by reduction of testicular cytochrome P450 and 17α-hydroxylase activity. The main antiandrogenic action of spironolactone seems to be its capacity to inhibit the binding of dihydrotestosterone (DHT) to cytosol in nuclear receptors (Corval et al 1975, Rose et al 1977, Menard et al 1978). Acute and chronic alcohol consumption also appears to lower plasma testosterone synthesis. Van Thiel et al (1983) have demonstrated that ethanol acts as a Leydig cell toxin. Moreover, ethanol increases the metabolic clearance rate of testosterone concomitant with an increase in hepatic 5α-reductase activity and increased conversion of androgens into estrogens. Thus, testicular dysfunction may occur in patients prior to alcoholic liver cirrhosis (see also Chapter 29).

The insecticide DDT appears to have hormonal activity due to its contamination with *o*, *p*-dichlorodiphenyltrichlorethane (DDT = *p p* isomer). This substance competes for binding sites on the androgen receptor (Wakeling & Visek 1973) and may exert some estrogenic effects by binding to estrogen receptors (Bulger et al 1978). It also increases the catabolism of androgens. This may also be true for Dieldrin, herbicides such as the defoliant 2,4,5-trichlorophenoxyacetic acid and polychlorinated biphenyls used in plastics and lubricant industries, which may be easily absorbed through the skin. Sertoli cell function can be negatively affected by phtalate esters

(Creasy et al 1987) and dinitrobenzenes (Blackburn et al 1988). Two other insecticides, Kepone (decachlorooctahydro-1,3,4-2H-cyclobuta (cd) pentalen-2-one) and Mirex, which is converted up to 10% to Kepone, cause, in addition to neurological damage, testicular damage (Eroschenko 1978). These products are used against fire ants. The nematocide 1,2-dibromo-3-chloropropane has caused azoospermia and complaints of loss of libido in men working in a factory producing the product; however, testosterone and LH levels remained normal (Wharton et al 1979, Potashnik & Yanai-Inbar 1987). The closely related 2,3-dibromopropanol, a carcinogen which is detectable in urine of children who wear clothing impregnated with the Tris-BP flame retardant, causes testicular atrophy and sterility (Blum et al 1978). Benzene hexachloride, which is sometimes added to stored grain, has been reported to cause edema of testicular interstitial tissue.

Sperm cells may be selectively affected by various substances throughout the process of spermatogenesis and spermiogenesis. Busulphan has been known for 30 years to affect spermatogonia (Jackson et al 1962), glycol ethers are toxic for spermatocytes (Gray et al 1985) and spermatids are affected by ethane/methane compounds (Jackson et al 1961). Finally, sperm maturation in the epididymis is adversely affected by ornidazole (McLain & Downing 1988).

Thus, a careful and extensive history of habits, drugs and exposure to exogenous chemicals and/or irradiation is important in the evaluation of an infertile male.

**Physical examination**

Although often not feasible for technical reasons, ideally the patient should be naked, so that the physician can obtain a general impression of possible endocrine stigmata. The presence of Cushing's disease, hypogonadism or hypothyroidism may become obvious by observing the body habitus, the amount and distribution of body hair, the presence or absence of gynecomastia, and the pattern of fat distribution. Height, weight, blood pressure, any unusual length of extremities, and general nutritional status are noted. A test for anosmia is important in patients with hypogonadism in order to rule out Kallman's syndrome. If hyperprolactinemia is present a space-occupying lesion in the fossa turcica should be ruled out (visual fields, CT). In particular impotent patients should be checked neurologically. The thyroid gland is carefully palpated, and the breasts are carefully examined for gynecomastia. Abdominal palpation may reveal liver enlargement. Operative scars in the inguino–genital areas are noted (Table 12.1).

The examining room should be warm so that the scrotal dartos reflex will be relaxed, facilitating the examination of the genitalia. It is sometimes helpful to place a warm lamp near the scrotum during the examination. Urogenital examination includes inspection of the penis and the location of the urethral opening, and any abnormalities concerning the prepuce should be noted. Palpation of the scrotal content is performed in order to assess localization, consistency and possible tenderness of the testes. In order to measure the size of the testes, the scrotal skin is stretched over the testicle, and the contour of the testicle is defined by palpation and separated from the epididymal head. The size of the testicle is then compared to the corresponding ovoid on an orchidometer. Testicular size is an important clinical parameter for male infertility assessment. There is a good correlation between testicular volume and biological age. This is helpful to the pediatrician and endocrinologist in recognizing the onset of puberty, in differentiating between true and pseudosexual precocious puberty, and in evaluating whether a young man has delayed puberty or true hypogonadism. Men who have small and firm testes (volume less than 6 ml) may have Klinefelter's syndrome, a frequently overlooked chromosomal disorder. Testicular size of 15 ml or more is considered normal. Testicular size of less than 15 ml usually coincides with an abnormal spermiogram. The epididymis and vas deferens are carefully palpated when looking for cystic formations, tenderness or thickening which could confirm past, present or chronic inflammatory disease. The presence of scrotal swelling due to hernia, hydrocele or lymphocele is noted. With the patient standing upright, the presence of varicocele or of spermatic venous reflux during Valsalva maneuver is investigated. The formation of a varicocele results form pathological dilatation of the pampiniform plexus as a result of increased venous pressure when the patient is upright or his intraabdominal pressure is increased. This may be the consequence of absent or incompetent valves or of abnormal collateral communications of the internal spermatic veins. Another pathophysiological mechanism leading to the development of varicoceles has been suggested by Notkovitch (1955) and Sayfan et al (1984). Vascular anomalies of the superior mesenteric artery or the testicular artery may cause these vessels to impinge on the renal vein in the upright position. This, in turn may impede venous return through the renal vein and blood derived from kidney and adrenal glands may then flow back through the testicular vein and lead to its dilatation and the development of a varicocele. The term 'subclinical varicocele' is used when incompetent valves allow reflux of blood into the scrotum without clinically detectable venous dilatation.

The role of subclinical varicocele in infertility is not clear.

The clinical diagnosis of a varicocele is based on inspection and palpation. We have found the classification of Uehling (1968) rather useful:

Stage I: No varicocele on inspection and palpation, but palpable filling of the pampiniform plexus during a Valsalva maneuver.
Stage II: No varicocele on inspection but detectable varicocele by palpation.
Stage III: Varicocele clearly visible.

Other means for diagnosis of a varicocele are scrotal thermography, Doppler echography, venous scintigraphy and retrograde venography.

The groins are examined for lymphadenopathy, surgical or other scars. Finally, prostate and seminal vesicles are examined. The prostate gland is easily palpated by rectal digital examination unless the patient is markedly obese. The knee-chest position is helpful for examination of the obese patient. The prostate should be symmetrical, of firm consistency, normal in size, and not tender. Massage of the prostate is generally an uncomfortable procedure even to the normal male, and pain elicited by pressure to the prostate does not necessarily indicate that the gland is diseased. A prostate gland that is enlarged and boggy in consistency is often congested, infected, or both. Gentle massage of such a prostate may produce secretion which may reveal pus cells on microscopic examination.

The seminal vesicles are normally not palpated unless they are congested or diseased. The rust-colored semen occasionally noticed by patients is most often due to congestive seminal vesiculitis. Prostatic fluid and urine voided after prostatic massage should be examined microscopically.

## BLOOD ANALYSIS

Blood analysis should include screening for systemic diseases, such as anemia, signs of inflammation, liver and kidney disease. Measurement of prolactin is indicated in cases of sexual inadequacy. A striking correlation exists between elevated prolactin levels and impotency (Fronzo et al 1977). An elevated prolactin level may be a symptom of hypothalamic insufficiency to secrete the prolactin-inhibiting factor (PIF). On the other hand, various drugs increase plasma levels of prolactin (phenothiazine, reserpine, methyldopa, TSH), and elevated levels of this hormone may be an early sign of pituitary adenoma (see Chapter 17). Correlations between prolactin levels and sperm concentration are equivocal (Segal et al 1976, Fronzo et al 1977).

Testosterone should be determined in patients with a history or signs of deficient development of the secondary sex characteristics. Sometimes the only sign may be deficient sperm motility or abnormal sperm related to lack of epididymal sperm maturation. To determine the functional quality of the Leydig cells, the human chorionic gonadotrophin (hCG) stimulation test has been advised. The response to a single injection of 5000 IU is measured. Since in hypogonadal males a defined, however sometimes reduced, testosterone rise is observed within 48–96 h, (Smals et al 1979, Okuyama et al 1981, Forest & Roulier 1982), blood should be sampled at 72 h following a single hCG injection, with a repeated examination at 96 h to cover for individual variations. If an enzymatic defect in Leydig cell function is suspected, the simultaneous measurements of

androstendione and 17-hydroxyprogesterone levels will help to diagnose defects in 17 α-ketoreductase and 17–20 desmolase enzymes (Forest et al 1980).

Testosterone produced after hCG stimulation will affect seminal vesicles, epididymis and prostate, increasing their excretory products in seminal fluid. Increase of plasma testosterone and lack of any specific physiological markers in the ejaculate indicate a mechanical block at the respective level, or dysfunction or agenesis of the respective secondary sex gland.

Thus, the concomitant measurement of plasma testosterone and physiological markers in seminal fluid, following hCG stimulation (hCG seminal plasma test), may help to precisely localize the lesion and aid in the diagnosis.

FSH determination is necessary in patients with a sperm concentration of less than 5 million per ml. Elevated levels indicate germinal cell insufficiency and, in azoospermic men, primary germinal cell failure, Sertoli cell-only syndrome, or genetic conditions such as Klinefelter's syndrome. If the elevated levels are accompanied by elevated LH levels and subnormal testosterone, this indicates primary testicular failure, or 'andropause' (Lunenfeld et al 1982). Administration of GnRH may help to differentiate gonadotropic deficiency due to pituitary insufficiency or secondary to hypothalamic insufficiency. Since inhibin secreted by the Sertoli cells inhibits GnRH-stimulated pituitary secretion of FSH, exaggerated FSH titers after GnRH stimulation indicate lack of inhibin. This, in turn, reflects insufficiency of Sertoli cells and may also help to discover the patients with isolated primary germinal cell failure.

We administer 100 μg GnRH intramuscularly and measure FSH and LH levels twice prior to and at 15, 30, 90 and 120 min following injection.

Results of the GnRH test are classified as follows:

Type O: Neither FSH nor LH levels increase (pituitary failure).
Type I: FSH increases to less than twice the initial value and/or maximum FSH level does not exceed 3 mIU/ml (relative pituitary insufficiency).

Type II: FSH increases to less than three times the initial levels and maximum level does not exceed 9 mIU/ml. (This response is usually found in azoospermic patients with occlusion of sperm-conveying structures. Such a response justifies a testicular biopsy to verify the diagnosis).

Type III: FSH increases to more than three times basal levels and/or a maximum level > 9 mIU/ml.

This type of GnRH response is regarded as exaggerated and may be indicative of masked hypergonadotropic hypogonadism. It may also be a pattern indicating inadequate GnRH pulsatility by the hypothalamus.

It is obligatory for each laboratory to establish its own normal values in order to make this test a useful tool for diagnosis.

## SEMEN ANALYSIS (SEE CHAPTER 11)

The semen analysis is considered the most important single item in the evaluation of male infertility. Since some variations occur normally, at least two specimens should be examined before any judgment concerning semen analysis is made.

There is considerable controversy regarding what constitutes a 'normal' semen profile (see Chapter 11). With the exception of the absolutely azoospermic specimen, which may be classified as sterile, there is no sharp line of demarcation between fertility and infertility as far as the parameters of the semen quality are concerned. It may be best to group semen analysis results into potentially fertile and potentially subfertile. Statistical methods used in the analysis of data on 'fertile' or subfertile sperm have not kept pace with methodology used by demographers. Andrologists have based most of their recommendations on sperm data of fertile men (Table 12.3).

Data from 15 such publications (see Chapter 11), based on 8789 men with proven fertility, showed a mean value of sperm concentrations of 76.3 ± 18.6. If normality is defined as mean ± 2 SD, the often quoted figures of mean normal range 40–140 million/ml is confirmed. (For practical purposes, however, sperm concentra-

**Table 12.3**   Semen profile in fertile men (see Chapter 11)

| Property | Usual value* | $n$ |
|---|---|---|
| Sperm count ($\times 10^6$)/ml | 76.3 ± 18.6 | 8789 |
| Motility (%) | 60.5 ± 6.8 | 3637 |
| Normal forms (%) | | |
|    Bryan-Leisnman | 77.9 ± 9.7 | 602 |
|    Papanicolaou | 49.8 ± 18 | 76 |
|    Eosin-nigrosin | 58   ± 15 | |
|    SEM | 30   ± 21 | |
|    TEM | 14   ± 8 | |

* Results given are mean ± SD.

tions exceeding 20 million/ml are considered normal).

Counts below 10 million/ml are conventionally regarded as indicative of relative infertility (David et al 1979). The predictive value of this parameter has been called into question. However, when the fertility of the female partner is taken into account, about 50% of men with sperm counts below 10 million/ml can initiate a pregnancy (Smith et al 1977). Sperm concentration as an isolated parameter is probably not the most important parameter in a semen sample unless extremely low. Furthermore, there is a need for direct tests of the fertilizing capacity of an ejaculate in cases of oligozoospermia.

Data on morphology varies widely, probably due to methodology, classification and staining (Table 12.3). Motility is probably the single most important parameter of the semen analysis as far as fertility prediction is concerned (Dunphy et al 1989).

Even if rigid protocols are kept and sperm is examined as close as possible to the conception date of the female partner, this kind of analysis does not take into account the time factor or the number of trials. Furthermore, the multiple variables which may reduce the fertility capacity of the woman are not considered in this kind of analysis.

Statistical probability to predict the cumulative probability of conception over time is based on a certain monthly probability of fecundity. The life-table method is a statistical technique that corrects for varying lengths of follow-up and is used for assessment. We (Lunenfeld et al 1983) and other workers have used this method in assessing the success rate of fertility-promoting drugs in well-defined patient groups by comparing the 'normal cumulative pregnancy rate' to that of treated patients.

Using similar methodology we attempted to correlate some parameters of sperm analysis from sperm donors to cumulative conception rates of inseminated women in comparison to the cumulative conception rate in a normal population (Fig. 12.2). In this example, the cumulative conception rate of the inseminated women was higher than that of the normal population. The increased fecundity of this selected group may be due to the careful use of the fertile period, in fertile women. Thus, in order to better define

normal values for sperm parameters, a standard method of life-table analysis could be used. Such data may help to define the fecundability potential of defined groups of infertile couples. This permits assessment of results of therapy. However difficult this task may be, due to the multiple variables in both partners affecting fertility at present, it seems to be a worthwhile effort.

After a 3-day period of abstinence, the volume of seminal fluid averages between 2.0 and 4.0 ml. For practical purposes, 20 million sperm cells/ml are considered the lower limit of normality, provided that sperm motility and sperm morphology are normal. As the sperm count

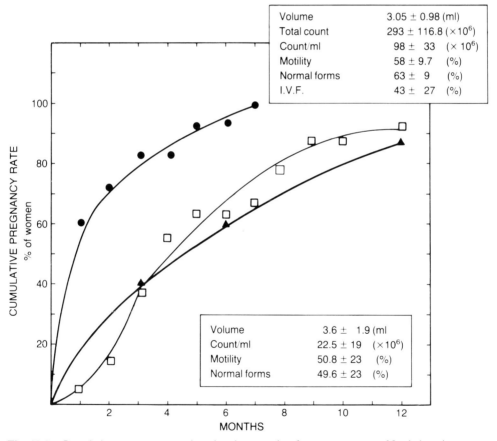

| | |
|---|---|
| Volume | $3.05 \pm 0.98$ (ml) |
| Total count | $293 \pm 116.8$ ($\times 10^6$) |
| Count/ml | $98 \pm 33$ ($\times 10^6$) |
| Motility | $58 \pm 9.7$ (%) |
| Normal forms | $63 \pm 9$ (%) |
| I.V.F. | $43 \pm 27$ (%) |

| | |
|---|---|
| Volume | $3.6 \pm 1.9$ (ml) |
| Count/ml | $22.5 \pm 19$ ($\times 10^6$) |
| Motility | $50.8 \pm 23$ (%) |
| Normal forms | $49.6 \pm 23$ (%) |

**Fig. 12.2** Cumulative pregnancy rate plotted against months of exposure. ▲——▲, North American women who had discontinued contraception (Tietze 1968). ●——● Israeli women exposed to donor insemination. (Means and standard deviation of some of the parameters of seminal analysis of the donors are given in the table A enclosed in the figure. The initial faster rate in this study is probably due to careful use of the fertile period.) □——□, Cumulative pregnancy rate of Israeli women whose hypogonadotropic azoospermic partners were treated with HMG/HCG, plotted against month of treatment. Means and standard deviation of some of the parameters of seminal analysis around time of fertilization are given in the table B enclosed in the figure. Note: start of semen analysis ~ 3 months after initiation of hMG/hCG treatment.

decreases, there is a corresponding decrease in the likelihood of conception, and when the sperm count is less than 5 million/ml, it is unlikely, but not impossible that pregnancy will occur. When observed within 1 h after ejaculation, at least 50% of the sperm cells should have vigorous motility with good forward progression and at least 50% of the sperm should be morphologically normal.

It is rare to see exceedingly low sperm counts accompanied by good sperm motility and morphology. However, such patients are often fertile, although time of exposure required is significantly longer. A typical example of such a situation is the hypogonadotropic-azoospermic patient treated with hMG/hCG (Lunenfeld et al 1983).

Occasionally, semen specimens of poor fertility potential are encountered in which count and motility are excellent and only the morphology is poor. A typical example for such a condition are sperm cells with lack of acrosome (round cells) or with lack or defects of acrosome, or sperm cells with defective DNA (Bartoov et al 1980, 1981).

It has been demonstrated by MacLeod (1965) and David et al (1972) that transient morphological abnormalities may be due to infection, trauma, varicocele and other testicular stress situations (Urry 1977), or hormonal imbalance. It has also been shown that semen of infertile patients contains a higher percentage of abnormal forms than semen of fertile men. This fact made morphology of sperm cells one of the major criteria for evaluating sperm quality in clinical investigations for fertility (see Chapter 11).

Human semen coagulates immediately following ejaculation, trapping and immobilizing spermatozoa in a tight fibrin matrix. Under normal circumstances, liquefaction occurs within several minutes and is usually complete after 5–40 min. Components of the coagulation system are added to the ejaculate as secretions from the seminal vesicles. The liquefaction factors, primarily plasminogen activators, originate from the secretions of the prostate glands. Modification of prostate gland fluids could eliminate or greatly reduce the rate of liquefaction of semen and thereby decrease fertility. This effect on the liquefaction rate has been observed in men with pathological conditions that result in delayed liquefaction of semen. A long-lasting coagulum could cause a significant reduction of fertility in the human, but whether increased coagulation time alone would result in consistent complete loss of fertility is doubtful. Spermatozoa normally bind several substances to their outer membrane; these substances, called sperm-coating antigens, are derived from the male genital tract fluid and are associated with sperm fertility inhibition usually by causing sperm agglutination. Examples of sperm-coating antigens are decapacitation factor and proteinase inhibitors. These binding substances normally block sperm fertility and are removed from the sperm head or are deactivated during the process of capacitation in the female genital tract. Antibodies against sperm-specific antigens, such as LDH, are known to inhibit fertility in females. Although the results are inconclusive, the agglutination of sperm by means of sperm-specific antibodies may be a possible cause of infertility (see Chapter 14).

Investigations into the biochemistry of fertilization have revealed some of the enzymes required for fertilization; of major importance are acrosin, hyaluronidase and corona–penetrating enzyme (CPE). In interpreting semen analysis data, it should be taken into account that the seminiferous epithelium is sensitive to various exogenous influences, e.g. heat, fever, allergic reactions, viral infection, and severe psychological stress. Infections or inflammations of the accessory genital glands can sometimes cause significant changes in the quality of semen. Since such infections may produce only minor symptoms, a careful clinical examination is necessary. A cytological examination of expressed prostatic fluid should be attempted if there is a suspicion of an infection or an inflammation in the accessory genital organs. When two or more of the following changes in semen analysis are present one should suspect an inflammation and/or infection in the accessory genital glands: (a) more than occasional leukocytes; (b) prolonged liquefaction time; (c) low sperm motility; (d) more than 25% coiled tails; (e) low concentrations of the organ-specific markers.

Comhaire et al (1989) have evaluated the accuracy of physical and seminal markers in semen to detect infections of the secondary sex glands. Men who had more than 10 000 aerobic pathogens in their semen also had significantly lower semen volume. The total output of citric acid was the most discriminating parameter between noninfected and infected males, followed by acid phosphatase.

Additional tests have been advocated to supplement the routine semen analysis. Common to these tests is the assumption that they measure a sperm function which cannot be detected by routine sperm analysis. In other words, apparently normal semen analysis may be associated with abnormal sperm performance in other tests.

## Sperm–mucus penetration test

Insler et al (1979) performed sperm–mucus penetration tests in 342 cases. An 'Inherent sperm defect', indicated by normal penetration of wife's mucus by donor sperm and reduced penetrating ability of husband's spermatozoa through both wife's and donor mucus, was found in 82 out of 342 examinations (24%). In 56 of these men, the seminal fluid analysis was performed within 60 days of the cervical factor evaluation. Judging by sperm count, motility and morphology, 50%, 77% and 71% of these males, respectively, would be considered to be fertile. However, only in 10 patients (18%) were all three seminal fluid parameters normal and in 48%, two or three parameters (count, motility or morphology) were definitely abnormal. In all these patients, sperm penetration through wife's and donor mucus was significantly reduced. This indicates an inherent biological deficiency of spermatozoa. Such a deficiency could not be detected by the routine seminal fluid analysis in 10 of the 56 males examined.

## Hypo-osmotic swelling test

The functional integrity of the sperm membrane cannot be measured by routine semen analysis. The hypo-osmotic swelling test has been designed by Jeyendran et al (1984) to address this question. Briefly, this test evaluates the percentage of sperm cells which demonstrate swelling when exposed by hypo-osmotic solutions. Check et al (1989) evaluated 135 infertile couples in whom no demonstrable cause of infertility was present in the female partner. Pregnancy rates were similar for women whose male partner's hypo-osmotic swelling tests showed 50% or more swelling regardless of results of semen analysis. In patients in whom this test produced abnormal results, no pregnancy was reported.

Coetzee et al (1989) reported only weak correlations of the hypo-osmotic swelling test and parameters of semen analysis, hamster penetration tests and human in vitro fertilization (IVF). The strongest correlation observed in this study was between percentage of swollen sperm cells and sperm viability.

## Hamster-penetration test

The hamster-penetration test has been introduced by Yanagimachi et al (1976) and has been used for many years to assess the in vitro fertilizing capacity of sperm cells into zone-free hamster ova. Margalioth et al (1989) followed prospectively 369 infertile couples for 2–5 years following infertility work-up. This included among others semen analysis and hamster-ova penetration tests (HOPT). There were no known causes for infertility in the female partners. After a median follow-up period of 44 months, 44% of couples reported pregnancies. There were significantly more pregnancies in couples whose male partners had normal semen analysis (39%) than in those with pathological semen analysis (21%). HOPT was significantly more specific to predict pregnancy than semen analysis. Using a cut-off point of 20% ova penetration, the authors reported that the positive and negative predictive power for the combined semen analysis and HOPT was 52% and 83% respectively.

The positive and negative predictive power for pregnancy using semen analysis alone was 37% and 79% respectively. Thus HOPT added to the predictive value of semen analysis.

## Tests for acrosome reaction

Calvo et al (1989) assessed the capability of sperm cells to undergo acrosome reaction when exposed to human follicular fluid. Sperm cells were obtained from men with proved fertility and those with unexplained infertility but normal semen analyses. Forty per cent of males with unexplained infertility produced sperm cells which were unable to undergo an acrosome reaction in the presence of follicular fluid. This lack of response could not be predicted from semen analysis. This test may therefore be useful as an adjunct to semen analysis since it also seems to measure sperm functions not measurable by routine semen analysis.

## Aspermia

After endocrine causes of aspermia have been excluded, i.e. eunuchoidism, the diagnostic pathway differs basically in cases in whom the ejaculatory deficiency occurs concomitantly with failure of erection, or in cases in whom erection is intact. In the latter case, one should primarily exclude retrograde ejaculation by examining postcoital urine samples (Glezerman & Lunenfeld 1976). If this syndrome has been excluded, the occurrence of nightly pollutions will point to psychogenic anorgasmia, while an excretory block at the prostate level may exist if nightly pollutions do not occur. Further endocrinological as well as urological evaluation, would then be necessary. Aspermia concomitant with erective failure may be due to psychogenic reasons, i.e. psychogenic impotence. In these cases, usually, no morning erections are reported. On the other hand, if erections do not occur under any circumstances and psychogenic impotence has been ruled out, then the reason for erective failure may be sought in neurological factors, e.g. multiple sclerosis, diabetic neuropathy, sequelae of pelvic surgery, and vascular factors such as diabetic angiopathy. Finally, iatrogenic and toxic influences, such as the use of certain antihypertensive drugs, should be considered.

## Azoospermia (see Fig. 12.3)

There are three distinct entities which are characterized by semen devoid of sperm cells: (a) spermatogenic failure; (b) obstruction at specific levels of the genital tract; (c) ejaculative failure leading to relative retrograde ejaculation. The easily performed postcoital urine examination will exclude the latter variety.

One may encounter normally developed males with azoospermia in whom no testes are palpable in the scrotum. After excluding iatrogenic androgenization in a castrate, the hCG test permits detection of ectopic testes. If no testosterone rise is observed in an eunuchoid patient following hCG injections, one may conclude that no testicular tissue is present. However, these patients will usually not be able to produce any ejaculate.

The presence of scrotal testes in azoospermic patients requires the differential diagnosis between obstruction and testicular failure. To a certain extent, one may rely on the presence of seminal markers for the sexual glands in order to exclude obstruction. Vasography may be indicated in some cases and others may require testicular biopsy in order to evaluate testicular spermatogenesis and, by inference, obstruction of sperm-conveying structures.

In most cases, determination of FSH levels will replace testicular biopsy. Elevated FSH levels indicate primary testicular failure, i.e. testicular atrophy, and chromosomal analysis may show a genetic syndrome, e.g. Klinefelter's syndrome. Negative genetic findings, concomitant with elevated FSH levels, will point to entities such as Sertoli-cell-only syndrome, germinal cell failure, focal tubular atrophy, or spermatogenic arrest. In these cases, no therapy being available, testicular biopsy would be of academic interest only. If FSH levels have been found to be normal or decreased, a GnRH test should be performed. Exaggerated response, in terms of FSH rise, is of the same diagnostic value as primary elevated FSH levels. If, on the other hand, FSH levels remain low or normal after GnRH administration, one may assume relative FSH deficiency which may be treated by exogenous gonadotropins. This diagnostic approach is basically identical in patients whose testes have been found to be altered in size or consistency, and who present with eunuchoid features. Low FSH levels in these patients point to secondary testicular insufficiency. One may differentiate between hypothalamic and pituitary failure using the GnRH test. If, following GnRH administration, no rise in FSH and LH levels occurs (type 0/I

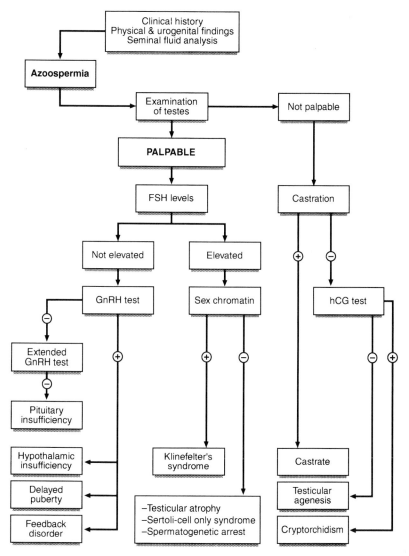

**Fig. 12.3**   Evaluation of the azoospermic male.

response) pituitary failure may be assumed. Adequate response to GnRH (type II) will point to hypothalamic failure. In both these conditions gonadotropic therapy gives excellent results (Lunenfeld & Berezin 1988).

## Abnormalities in sperm analysis

We have labelled a semen sample with a low concentration, poorly motile and morphologically abnormal sperm cells as oligo-terato-astheno-spermia syndrome (OTA syndrome). Although all three of the above pathologies of sperm usually occur concomitantly, the degree of severity of each can differ significantly in various patients.

### Oligozoospermia

For the purpose of this discussion, oligo-zoospermia is divided into mild oligozoospermia (10–20 million sperm cells/ml), moderate oligo-zoospermia, with a sperm count of 5–10 million sperm/ml or total sperm count of 15–30 million/ejaculate, and severe oligozoospermia, with sperm counts below 5 million/ml. Patients with moderate oligozoospermia demonstrated by repeated sperm analysis should be investigated for accessory gland infection, or immunological factors. In severe oligospermic patients FSH determinations should be performed. If elevated, then the diagnosis of partial chromosomal aberration or mixed forms of the Klinefelter type should be assessed by karyotyping. If the karyotype is normal, then a testicular biopsy will differentiate between partial obstruction and primary idiopathic testicular failure.

Severe oligozoospermia associated with elevated FSH levels and/or exaggerated response to GnRH is generally thought to reflect primary testicular failure. Patients in whom this pattern has been established are considered to suffer from hypergonadotropic hypogonadism ('overt' if base levels of FSH are elevated and 'masked' if FSH levels are normal, but GnRH elicits an exaggerated FSH response). Since it is believed that no effective treatment for restoration of spermatogenesis is available for this condition, patients are usually referred for artificial donor insemination. However, recent data indicate that this condition may also be caused by inadequate GnRH pulses and may be reversible. It has been shown in animal experiments that a disturbed pulse frequency of GnRH is followed by increased FSH levels. Furthermore, pilot studies have shown that pulsatile application of GnRH in oligozoospermic men who presented with elevated base levels of FSH was followed by normalization of FSH levels and increase of sperm count (Wagner et al 1985).

### Asthenospermia

In some patients, repeated seminal fluid analysis may show asthenospermia with a normal count and morphology (inherent motility deficiency). The lack of response to therapy in this category can be explained in some cases by sperm midpiece defects such as absence of mitochondria or by defective tail development (see Chapter 11). Lack of motility can also be seen in patients with Kartagener's syndrome. Furthermore, male accessory gland infection or immunological factors may also be responsible for low sperm motility. In vitro vitalization of spermatozoa by caffeine or kallikrein and subsequent insemination with the treated sperm has been attempted (Schill & Haberland 1979, Bedford & Elstein 1981). In some cases in which in vitro vitalization has failed, hCG or androgen therapy has been beneficial. In these patients, the diagnosis of relative androgen deficiency may be established post hoc. A positive eosin test, i.e. more than 20% eosin-stained cells, requires a re-evaluation of exogenous toxic influences. Accordingly, necrospermic patients can be classified in two groups, 'toxic' and 'idiopathic'. In 'dilution oligozoospermia' (semen volume 5 ml or more), split intercourse may enhance the chances of fertility. This is based on the observation that the first portion of the ejaculate derived from the epidydimis and prostate comprises about 75% of the total sperm cells to be ejaculated. Moreover, the first semen split usually contains spermatozoa endowed with the better motility. On the other hand, if the low concentration of sperm is similar in both portions of the ejaculate, hMG/hCG therapy may occasionally prove beneficial. Those who do not respond to hMG/hCG are classified as idiopathic oligo-asthenospermic.

### Teratospermia

An ejaculate which contains more than 70% abnormal sperm cells (severe teratospermia) may be due to chromosomal aberration. Meticulous evaluation of noxious environmental influences should nevertheless be carried out. However, in most instances, the medical history and physical examination do not reveal any abnormality. FSH, LH and testosterone levels are almost always in the normal range. The etiology of teratospermia can be found in the early and late stages of spermatogenesis (Bartoov et al 1980) or may be due to degenerative changes occurring during sperm maturation. Usually, human sperm consists of sperm cells that include a combination of anomalies. Since little is known about the mechanisms controlling the chromatin condensation system, acrosin formation, Golgi complex function, the mitochondrial organization process and the tail developing system, no specific therapy for teratospermia has been developed.

Occasionally, degenerative changes may occur in the epididymis due to phagocytosis by spermiophages (enhanced by infections or inflammation) or due to prolonged sojourn (neurological abnormalities or hormone imbalance). In this situation specific therapy may be attempted.

## REFERENCES

Bartoov B, Eltes F, Weissenberg R, Lunenfeld B 1980 Morphological characterization of abnormal human spermatozoa using transmission electron microscopy. Arch Androl 5: 305

Bartoov B, Fisher J, Eltes F, Langsam J, Lunenfeld B 1981 A comparative morphological analysis of normal human spermatozoa. In: Insler V, Bettendorf G (eds) Advances in diagnosis and treatment of infertility. Elsevier North Holland, Amsterdam, p 355

Bedford N A, Elstein M 1981 Effects of kallikrein on male subfertility, a double-blind cross-over study. In: Insler V, Bettendorf G (eds) Advances in diagnosis and treatment of infertility. Elsevier North Holland, Amsterdam, p 339

Blackburn D M, Gray A J, Lloyd S C, Sheard C M, Foster P M D 1988 A comparison of the effects of the three isomers of dinitrobenzene on the testis in the rat. Toxicol Appl Pharmacol 92: 54

Blum A, Gold M D, Ames B N et al 1978 Children absorb TRIS-BP flame retardant from sleepwear: urine containing the mutagenic metabolite 2, 3 dibromopropanol. Science 201: 1021

Bulger W H, Muccitelli R M, Kupfer D 1978 Interactions of chlorinated hydrocarbon pesticides with 8S estrogen binding protein in rate testes. Steroids 32: 165

Calvo L, Koukoulis G N, Vantman D et al 1989 Follicular fluid-induced acrosome reaction distinguishes a subgroup of men with unexplained infertility not identified by semen analysis. Fertil Steril 52: 1048

Check J H, Shanis B S, Epstein R, Wu Ch, Nowroozi K, Bollendorf A 1989 The hypoosmotic swelling test as a useful adjunct to the semen analysis to predict fertility potential Fertil Steril 52: 159

Coetzee K, Kruger T F, Menkveld R, Lombard C J, Swanson R J 1989 Hypoosmotic swelling test in the prediction of male fertility. Arch Androl 23: 131

Comhaire F H, Vermeulen L, Pieters O 1989 Study of the accuracy of physical and biochemical markers in semen to detect infectious dysfunction of the accessory sex glands. J Androl 10: 50

Corval P, Michaud A, Menard J, Freifeld M, Mahoudeau J 1975 Antiandrogenic effect of spirolactones: mechanism of action. Endocrinology 97: 52

Creasy D M, Beech L M, Gray T J B, Butler W H 1987 The ultrastructural effects of di-n-pentyl phtalate on the testis of the mature rat. Mol Cell Pathol 46: 357

David G, Bisson J P, Jouannet P et al 1972 Les teratospermies. In: Thibault C (ed) La Sterilite du Male. Acquisitions Recentes. Masson, Paris.

David G, Jovannek P, Martin-Boyce A, Spire A, Schwartz D 1979 Sperm counts in fertile and infertile men. Fertil Steril 31: 453

Dunphy B C, Neal L M, Cooke I D 1989 The clinical value of conventional semen analysis Fertil Steril 51: 324

Eroschenko V P 1978 Alterations in the testes of the Japanese quail during and after the ingestion of the insecticide Kepone. Toxicol Appl Pharmacol 43: 535

Forest M G, Roulier R 1982 Kinetics of steroidogenic responses to hCG in relation to age or previous gonadotrophin environment: induction of steroidogenic desensitization by pretreatment with hCG in hypogonadotropic hypogonadic (HH) adult men. Advance Miniposters of the Second European Workshop on the Testis, Rotterdam, The Netherlands, B9

Forest M G, Lecornu M, Peretti E 1980 Familial male pseudohermaphrodism due to 17–20 desmolase deficiency. In vivo endocrine studies. J Clin Endocrinol Metab 50: 826

Fronzo D, Sivieri R, Gallono G, Andriolo S, Angeli A, Ceresa F 1977 Effect of a prolactin inhibitor on libido, sexual potency and sex hormones in men with mild hyperproclactinemia, oligospermia and/or impotence. Acta Endocrinol (Copenh) 85 (Suppl 212): 142

Glezerman M, Lunenfeld B 1976 Zur Therapie der maennlichen Anorgasmie. Ein Fallbericht Akta Derm 2: 167

Gray T J B, Moss E J, Creasy D M, Gangolli S D 1985 Studies on the toxicity of some glycol ethers and alkoxyacetic acids in primary testicular cultures. Toxicol Appl Pharmacol 79: 490

Heindel J J, Treinen K A 1989 Physiology of the male reproductive system: endocrine, paracrine and autocrine regulation. Toxicol Pathol 17: 411

Insler V, Bernstein D, Glezerman M, Misgav N 1979 Correlation of seminal fluid analysis with mucus penetrating ability of spermatozoa. Fertil Steril 32: 316

Jackson H, Fox B W, Craig A W 1961 Antifertility substances and their assessment in the male rodent. J Reprod Fertil 2: 447

Jackson H, Parlington M, Fox B W 1962 Effects of busulphan (myleran) on the spermatogenic population of the rat testis. Nature (London, 194: 1184

Jeyendran R S, van der Ven H H, Perez Palacz M, Crabo B G, Zaneveld L J D 1984 Development of an assay to assess the functional integrity of the human sperm membrane and its relationship to other semen characteristics. J Reprod Fertil 70: 219

Lunenfeld B, Olchovsky D, Tadir Y, Glezerman M 1981 Therapie mit Gonadotropinen. Kriterien der Patientenauswahl. Muench Med Wschr

Lunenfeld B, Eshkol A, Glezerman M 1982 Male climacteric. In: Branhauer K, Frick J (eds) Handbook of urology, disturbances of male infertility, XVI edn. Springer Verlag, Berlin, p 421

Lunenfeld B, Berezin M, Sack J, Theodor R, Beer R, Weissenberg R 1983 Gonadotropic therapy in men with gonadotropic insufficiency. Results, tolerance and follow-up of children fathered by these patients. Excerpta Medica, Amsterdam International Congress Series 596: 13

Luinenfeld B, Berezin M 1988 Hypogonadotropic hypogonadism with gonadotropins. In: Garcia C,

Mastroianni L, Amelar R D, Dubin L (eds) Current therapy of infertility—3. Decker, Toronto, pp 187–193

MacLeod J 1965 Seminal cytology in the presence of varicocele. Fertil Steril 16: 735

Margalioth EJ, Mordel N, Feinmesser M, Bronson R A, Navot D 1989 The long term predictive value of the zona-free hamster ova sperm penetration assay. Fertil Steril 52: 490

Marshburn P B, Sloan C S, Hammond M G 1989 Semen quality and association with coffee drinking, cigarette smoking and ethanol consumption. Fertil Steril 52: 162

McLain R M, Downing J C 1988 The effect of ornidazole on fertility and epididymal sperm function in rats. Toxicol Appl Pharmacol 92: 488

Menard R H, Loriaux D L, Bartter F C, Gillette J R 1978 The effect of administration of spironolactone on the concentration of plasma testosterone, estradiol and cortisone in male dogs. Steroids 31: 771

Morris I D, Phillips D M, Bardin C W 1986 Ethylene dimethanesulfonate destroys Leydig cells in rat testes. Endocrinology 118: 709

Notkovitch H 1955 Testicular artery arching over renal vein. Br J Urol 27: 267

Okuyama A, Namiki M, Koide T et al 1981 A simple hCG stimulation test for normal and hypogonadal males. Arch Androl 6: 75

Potashnik G, Yanai-Inbar I 1987: Dibromochloropropane (DBCP): an eight year reevaluation of testicular function and reproductive performance. Fertil Steril 47: 317

Rose L I, Underwood R H, Newmark S R, Kirch E S, Williams G H 1977 Pathopysiology of spironolactone-induced gynecomastia. Ann Intern Med 87: 398

Sayfan J, Helvy A, Oland J, Nathan H 1984 Varicocele and left renal vein compression. Fertil Steril 41: 411

Schill W B, Haberland G L 1979 Kinin-enhancement of sperm motility. Hoppe Seylers Z Physiol Chem 355: 229

Segal S, Polishuk W Z, BenDavid M 1976 Hyperprolactinemic male infertility. Fertil Steril 27: 1425

Smals A G, Pieters G F F, Drayer J I M, Bernaad T J, Kloppenborg P W C 1979 Leydig cell responsiveness to single and repeated human chorionic gonadotropin administration. J Clin Endocrinol Metab 49: 12

Smith C G, Gilbeau P M 1985 Drug abuse effects on reproductive hormones. In: R L Dixon (ed) Endocrine toxicology. Raven, New York, pp 249–268

Smith K D, Rodriguez-Rigau L J, Steinberger E 1977 Relation between indices of semen analysis and pregnancy rate in infertile couples. Fertil Steril 28: 1314

Tietze Ch 1968 Fertility after discontinuation of intrauterine and oral contraception. Int J Fertil 13: 385

Uehling D T 1968 Fertility in men with varicocele. Int J Fertil 13: 58

Urry R L 1977 Stress and infertility. In: Cockett A K, Urry R L (eds) Male infertility. Grune and Stratton, New York p 145

Van Thiel D M, Gavaler J S, Cobb C F, Santucci L, Graham T O 1983 Ethanol, a Leydig cell toxin: evidence obtained in vivo and in vitro. Pharmacol Biochem Behav 18: 317

Wagner T O F, Brabant G, von zur Muehlen A 1985 Slow pulsing oligospermia. In: TOF Wagner (ed) Pulsatile LHRH therapy of the male. TM Verlag, Hameln, pp 111–117

Wakeling A E, Visek W J 1973 Insecticide inhibition of 5 dihydrotestosterone binding in the rat ventral prostate. Science 181: 659

Wharton D, Milby T H, Krauss R M, Stubbs H A 1979 Testicular function in DBCP exposed pesticide workers. J Occup Med 21: 161

Yanagimachi R, Yanagimashi H, Rogers B I 1976 The use of zona-free animal ova as a test system for the assessment of the fertilizing capacity of human spermatozoa. Biol Reprod 15: 471

# Diagnosis of infertility (male and female)

# 13. Diagnosis and classification of disturbed sperm–cervical mucus interaction

*Kamran S. Moghissi*

## INTRODUCTION

Evaluation of cervical factor and sperm–cervical mucus interaction are considered to be important steps in infertility investigation. Abnormalities of the cervix and its secretion are reported to be responsible for infertility in approximately 10–30% of women, but among carefully investigated couples and where the male factor has been adequately excluded, the true incidence is probably not greater than 5–10%.

During coitus 50–500 million spermatozoa are deposited in the cervix and posterior vaginal fornix. Human semen coagulates immediately after ejaculation and traps most sperm cells until seminal proteolytic enzymes bring about liquefaction. The first portion of the ejaculate, however, contains the highest concentration of spermatozoa (three-quarters in humans), which, under favourable conditions, promptly penetrate cervical mucus. The intermixing of the ejaculate and cervical mucus that is caused by penile movements and displacement of cervical mucus column may aid this process. Since sperm are rapidly destroyed by vaginal acidity, their entrapment in the coagulum until liquefaction takes place may be considered as a protective device to prevent their death.

In vitro studies have shown that nonliquefying semen samples are lysed when treated with an acid buffer. Thus, it is possible that vaginal acidity enhances liquefaction of the seminal coagulum. Indeed, complete liquefaction of the seminal clot in vivo appears to occur somewhat faster after ejaculation than in vitro.

Vaginal content is usually acid, with a pH of about 3–5. However, cervical secretion coats the upper part of the vagina and its fornices and considerably increases the alkalinity of the vaginal milieu, providing a favorable medium for spermatozoa, and apparently promoting their motility and longevity.

Seminal plasma, an alkaline fluid, also has a buffering effect upon the vaginal environment and alters the vaginal pH, thus smoothing the transition of sperm from the semen into the cervical mucus. Fox et al (1973) have measured vaginal pH during coitus continuously by telemetry and observed that 8 seconds after ejaculation the pH of the vagina rose from 4.3 to 7.2.

Sperm migration through the cervix involves three distinct but interrelated factors: (a) the ability of spermatozoa to penetrate the mucus by their intrinsic motility; (b) the fibrillar structure of cervical mucin enabling it to participate actively in the process of sperm transport; and (c) the morphological configuration of cervical crypts that contribute to the storage and preservation of spermatozoa in the cervical canal and their sustained and prolonged release to the upper tract.

Human sperm is endowed with intrinsic motility, a property essential for penetration of cervical mucus and subsequent fertilization. There is no convincing evidence that immotile or dead sperm can either pass through the human cervix or effect fertilization. Spermatozoa are highly active cells possessing metabolic, glycolytic and respiratory enzymes. They are capable of metabolizing a variety of exogenous and some endogenous substrates. Since spermatozoa possess a negligible reserve of endogenous glycogen, they must depend on extracellular carbohydrate for their energy requirements during their stay in or passage through the female reproductive tract. It is not known to what extent sperm survival and motility in cervical mucus are influenced by the amount of utilizable carbohydrates or other sperm nutrients present in cervical secretion. In vitro studies suggest that the viability of sperm is related to the glucose level of cervical mucus. Furthermore, a decrease in glucose concentration of cervical mucus has been found in many infertile patients (Kellerman & Weid 1970).

## CERVICAL SECRETION

Cervical mucus is a complex secretion produced constantly by the secretory cells of the endocervix. A small amount of endometrial, tubal and possibly follicular fluids may also contribute to the cervical mucus pool. In addition, cellular debris from uterine and cervical epithelia and leukocytes are present. Cervical mucus is a heterogeneous secretion that reveals a number of rheological properties such as viscosity, flow elasticity, spinnbarkeit, thixotropy, and tack or stickiness.

The most important constituent of cervical mucus is a hydrogel rich in carbohydrates and consisting of high molecular weight glycoproteins of the mucin type (Yurewicz & Moghissi 1981). Most of the physical properties of cervical mucus are due to these mucins. Several models have been proposed for the supramolecular organization of cervical mucin in the gel phase of cervical mucus. Earlier proposal of a relatively ordered micellar structure based on nuclear magnetic resonance studies (Odeblad & Rudolfsson 1973) has been challenged by an alternative model, based on laser light scattering data, suggesting a random network of entangled mucin molecules, a structure similar to that of raw rubber (Lee et al 1977).

Ovarian hormones regulate the secretion of cervical mucus; estrogen stimulates the production of copious amounts of watery mucus; and progesterone (or progestogens) inhibits the secretory activity of cervical epithelial cells. The physical properties and certain chemical constituents of cervical mucus show cyclic variations. Cyclic alterations in the constituents of cervical mucus may influence sperm penetrability,

nutrition and survival (Moghissi 1973a,b). Figure 13.1 shows serial determination of some important properties of human cervical mucus related to pituitary and ovarian hormones and sperm penetration in ten women during a normal menstrual cycle. These data clearly demonstrate that optimal changes of cervical mucus properties, such as greatest increase in quantity, spinnbarkeit, ferning, pH and decrease in viscosity and cell content occur immediately prior to ovulation and are reversed after ovulation. Preovulatory mucus is most receptive to sperm penetration (Moghissi et al 1964, 1972). It has been suggested that the proportion of saline in cervical secretion directly determines the consistency of the mucus and the rate of sperm penetration. Despite earlier reports to the contrary, recent studies have clearly demonstrated that the overall amino acid and carbohydrate composition of human cervical mucus remains unchanged during the menstrual cycle (Moghissi 1973b, Yurewicz & Moghissi 1981).

Sperm penetrability of human cervical mucus begins approximately on the ninth day of a normal cycle and increases gradually to a peak at ovulation. It is usually inhibited within 1–2 days after ovulation but may persist to a lesser degree for a longer period (Moghissi 1966). In some women sperm penetrability occurs only during a very limited period of the menstrual cycle. Individual variations are common (Moghissi 1966). Two phases of sperm migration through the cervix have been recognized: (a) a rapid phase during which the leading spermatozoa penetrate the central portion of cervical canal and advance in a line parallel to mucin fibrils originating in the vicinity of the internal os; and (b) a delayed phase. During the delayed phase sperm enter the cervical mucus around the periphery of the central core and are oriented by mucin fibrils originating from the crypts and colonize them. The latter process is responsible for the storage of sperm in the cervical crypts and their gradual release over an extended period into the uterus and oviducts.

The human uterine cervix is a thick-walled cylindrical structure that tapers off at its inferior extremity. The basic epithelial structure of the cervical mucosa is an intricate system of crypts that, grouped together, give an illusory impression

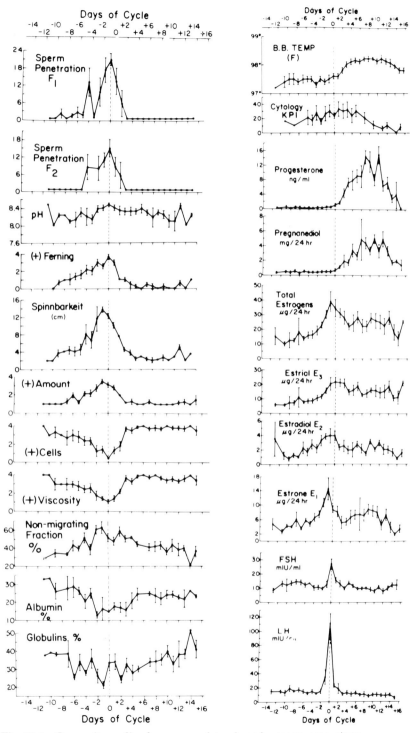

**Fig. 13.1**  Composite profile of serum gonadotropin and progesterone; urinary estrogens and pregnanediol; basal body temperature (BBT), karyopyknotic index (KPI) of vaginal cells; and cervical mucus properties throughout the menstrual cycle in ten normal women. Day 0, day of LH peak (dotted line). Vertical bars represent one standard error of the mean. $F_1$ and $F_2$ indicate the number of sperm in the first and second microscopic fields (200X) from interface, 15 min after the start of the in vitro sperm–cervical mucus penetration test (Moghissi et al 1972).

of glands (see Chapter 2). These crypts may run in an oblique, transverse or longitudinal direction but never cross one another, although they may bifurcate or extend downward (Fluhmann 1961). Cervical crypts are believed to act as a sperm reservoir (Jaszczak 1973, Tredway et al 1975, Insler et al 1981). Spermatozoa guided by the line of strain of cervical mucus are led to cervical crypts where they are stored and released to the upper tract for many hours following coitus (Moghissi 1979).

Insler et al (1981) showed that in estrogen-treated women the percentage of cervical crypts that were colonized with spermatozoa increased nine times compared with crypts in cervices of subjects treated with gestagens. Similarly, the sperm density in the crypts was also greater in estrogen-treated cervices.

Based on posthysterectomy histological cervical specimens of patients pretreated with estrogen

and inseminated with normal semen, Insler et al (1981) estimated the number of sperm stored in cervical crypts to be 150 000, 181 000 and 53 250 at 2, 24 and 48 h after insemination.

Spermatozoa reach the cervix within minutes after ejaculation (Sobrero & McLeod 1962). These sperm represent the most vigorous and morphologically normal ones within the ejaculate.

## INVESTIGATION OF CERVICAL FACTOR IN INFERTILITY

Spermatozoa are at all times suspended in a fluid medium. The interaction of sperm with female reproductive tract fluids is of critical importance for the survival and function of spermatozoa. Unfortunately there is no practical method for evaluation of human uterine and tubal fluids and the study of their effect on sperm. Cervical mucus, however, is readily available for sampling

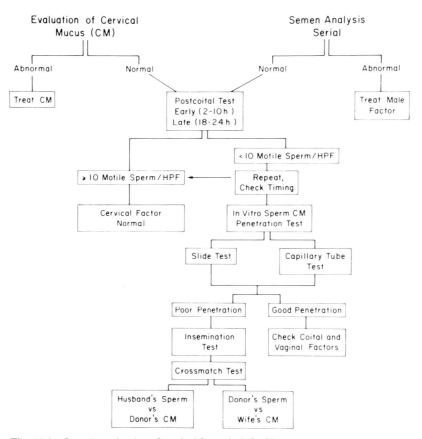

**Fig. 13.2**   Steps in evaluation of cervical factor in infertility.

and studies. Evaluation of sperm–cervical mucus interaction must therefore be included in infertility investigation. A stepwise plan for the evaluation of the cervical factor in infertility is shown in Figure 13.2. Semen analysis (see Chapter 11) and examination of cervical mucus should precede postcoital tests and more specific in vitro studies.

Many laboratories are unfamiliar with or ill prepared to analyse semen adequately. Information regarding semen volume and appearance, liquefaction time, sperm density, immediate and delayed motility, quality of motility, eosin stain, percentage of different morphological types (seminal cytology), and the presence of lenkocytes, agglutination, and other changes must appear on every report.

## EVALUATION OF CERVICAL MUCUS

The condition of cervical mucus greatly influences sperm receptivity; therefore it should be evaluated accurately before a postcoital test is performed. Preovulatory mucus receptive to sperm penetration is profuse, thin, clear, acellular and alkaline. It exhibits 4+ ferning (crystallization) and high spinnbarkeit. Figure 13.3 shows a scoring system that we have devised to evaluate the quality and adequacy of cervical mucus. This system takes into account five important properties of cervical mucus that are known to affect sperm cervical mucus penetration: amount, spinnbarkeit, ferning, viscosity and cellularity. Each item receives a score from 0 to 3. A score of 3 represents optimal changes. A maximum score of 15 indicates preovulatory cervical mucus that is receptive to sperm penetration. A score less than 10 is associated with relatively unfavourable cervical secretion, and a score less than 5 represents hostile cervical mucus usually impenetrable by the sperm (Moghissi 1977).

Several techniques for collection of cervical mucus have been described. Methods most

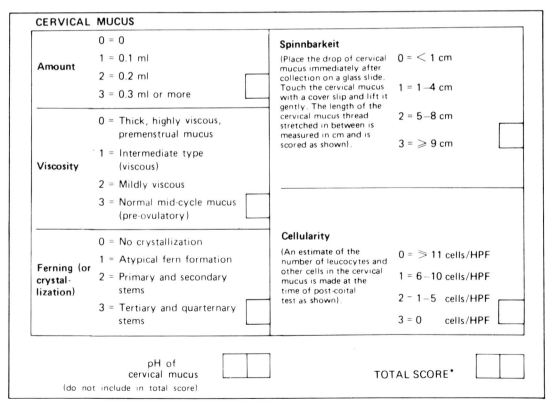

**Fig. 13.3** Cervical score. A composite of the amount, spinnbarkeit, ferning, viscosity and cellularity of cervical mucus. Maximum score is 15; scores less than 10 represent unfavorable mucus and less than five hostile cervical secretion.

commonly used consist of aspiration with a tuberculin syringe (without needle), pipette, polyethylene tube, or sampling with a mucus forceps. Cervical mucus should be collected and studied as close to the time of ovulation as possible. Clinical examination of cervical mucus includes determination of amount, viscosity, cellularity, pH, ferning, spinnbarkeit, and cultural studies if infection is suspected. Ferning (Figure 13.4) is performed by spreading cervical mucus on a glass slide and allowing it to dry. It is customarily graded from 0 to 4+, depending on the extent of crystal formation. Spinnbarkeit is measured by placing an adequate amount of cervical mucus on a microscope slide, covering it with a coverslip, and drawing the mucus between them. An estimate of spinnbarkeit (in centimeters) is made by measuring the length of the thread before it breaks. An alternative method is to pull a sample of cervical mucus from the cervix under direct observation, using a mucus forceps. The length of the mucus thread is estimated before it breaks (Insler et al 1972). This method is less accurate since it does not allow for the precise measurement of the mucus thread with a ruler. The pH of cervical mucus should be measured in situ or immediately following collection. Care should be taken to assay the pH of endocervical mucus correctly since the pH of the exocervical pool is always lower than that of the endocervical canal.

## POSTCOITAL TEST (SIMS–HUHNER TEST)

The postcoital test was described by Sims in 1866 who, recognizing the importance of sperm

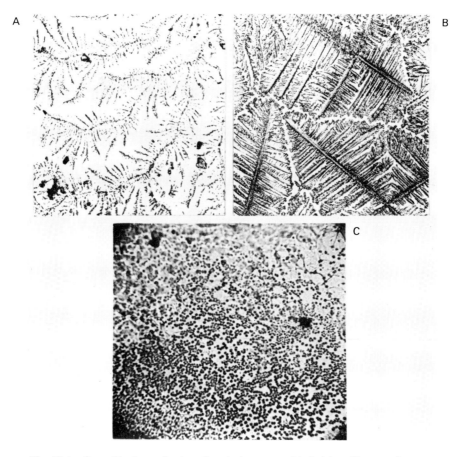

**Fig. 13.4**  Crystallization or ferning of cervical mucus. **a** 1+. **b** 4+. **c** Absence of ferning.

motility and timing of the test, performed immediate postcoital tests on many women, and found sperm in cervical mucus within a few minutes after coitus. He further observed the presence of live spermatozoa in the cervix from 36–48 h after intercourse. To Huhner, however, goes the credit for popularizing the test as an index of cervical mucus–sperm interaction. The Sims-Huhner test is now considered an integral part of infertility investigation, but despite its popularity there is a lack of standardization and disagreement remains on how to interpret the results.

## Timing

Postcoital tests should be performed as closely as possible to the time of ovulation, as determined by usual clinical means (basal body temperature (BBT), cervical mucus changes, vaginal cytology, Urinary LH and sonography). Each couple is instructed to abstain from sexual intercourse for 2 days prior to the test, which is performed approximately 6–10 h after intercourse (standard test). A satisfactory test may be followed by a 'delayed test' performed at a longer interval (18–24 h) when infertility persists. The presence in the endocervix of at least 10 motile spermatozoa per high power field ($\times$ 400) at this stage suggests favorable mucus and adequate survival of sperm in the cervix and would exclude cervical factor as a cause of infertility. When the initial standard test yields poor results, a second test is planned 1–3 h coitus (early test). A complete evaluation of cervical factor should be undertaken when both the standard and early tests are abnormal. It is also recommended that both cervical and male factors be reevaluated when the delayed PCT is abnormal or there is persistent unexplained infertility.

## Techniques of postcoital test

A nonlubricated speculum is inserted into the vagina, and a sample of the posterior vaginal fornix pool is aspirated with a tuberculin syringe (without needle), a mucus syringe, pipette or polyethylene tube. With a different syringe, samples of cervical mucus are obtained from the

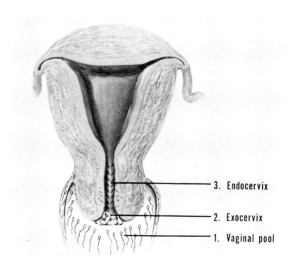

**Fig. 13.5**   For the postcoital test, using a tuberculin syringe (without needle), samples are obtained from: 1, the vaginal pool; 2, external cervical os and lower part of the endocervical canal; 3, endocervical canal.

3. Endocervix
2. Exocervix
1. Vaginal pool

exocervix and endocervical canal (Fig. 13.5). These are placed on a separate glass slide, covered with a coverslip, and examined under a microscope at $\times$ 200 and $\times$ 400. If exocervical mucus is covered with cells, debris and vaginal content, the area should be wiped dry with cotton prior to obtaining the endocervical specimen. Whenever possible, the quality of the mucus should be evaluated immediately upon collection.

## Interpretation

Interpreting the postcoital test requires an understanding of cervical mucus function and sperm transport. Cervical mucus protects sperm from the hostile environment of the vagina and from being phagocytosed. The mucus also may supplement the energy requirements of sperm, act as a filter to retain abnormal and sluggish sperm, and provide the proper milieu for sperm capacitation.

Within seconds ejaculated sperm enter midcycle cervical mucus. Subsequent migration through the cervical canal is accomplished principally by intrinsic motility. It may be influenced also by seminal plasma and sperm, phalanx formation, and orientation of strands of cervical mucin. The last phenomenon may be responsible for the storage of sperm in the cervical crypts and their gradual release over an extended period into the uterus and oviducts.

The function of the cervix as a sperm reservoir is of considerable importance in fertility. Only rarely does coitus occur at the time of ovulation. In most instances, union of gametes depends on a constant supply of sperm at the site of fertilization for some hours before and after ovulation. Following coitus a gradient is established within the cervix that is entirely time dependent. With increasing intervals between coitus and examination there is an orderly progression of sperm population from the lower to the upper part of the canal (Davajan & Kunitake 1969, K.S. Moghissi unpublished data).

On the basis of cervical mucus examination following artificial insemination, Tredway et al (1975) have suggested that the most appropriate time to perform a postcoital test is 2.5 h after intercourse, since they found the largest sperm population in the mucus at this time. The purpose of a postcoital test is not only determination of a sufficient number of active spermatozoa in cervical mucus but also evaluation of sperm survival and behavior many hours after coitus (reservoir role). Furthermore, there is a significant relationship between sperm survival for 48 h in cervical mucus and conception in donor artificial insemination cycles (Hanson et al 1982). Even after 48 h there is little change in motility of normal sperm in cervical mucus (Hanson & Overstreet 1981) or their penetration in the human zona pellucida or fusion with zona-free hamster oocytes (Gould et al 1984).

Therefore 6–10 h after coitus is a balanced time to determine both sperm density and longevity. Earlier timing may be reserved for those subjects who have negative or abnormal tests. With these facts in mind postcoital tests may be interpreted on a rational basis.

### Vaginal pool sample

Spermatozoa are usually destroyed in the vagina within 2–4 h and lose their fertilizing ability within a few hours (Frenkel 1961). The purpose of examining the vaginal pool sample therefore is to ensure that semen have actually been deposited in the vagina.

### Exocervical sample

The number of sperm in the lower part of the cervical canal varies with time elapsed after coitus. Within 2–3 h after intercourse there is a large accumulation of sperm in the lower part of the cervical canal (Davajan & Kunitake 1969, Moghissi 1973a, Tredway et al 1975). In a normal woman following coitus with a fertile man, more than 25 motile sperm (with 2–3+ motility) per high-power field (HPF) ($\times$ 400) are commonly observed in the exocervical specimen; 10 or more sperm per HPF with scores of 2–3+ motility are considered satisfactory. Less than 5 sperm/HPF, particularly when associated with sluggish or circular motion, is an indication of oligoasthenospermia or abnormality of cervical mucus (Elstein et al 1973).

Sperm motility in cervical mucus is graded from 0 to 3 as follows: 0 = immotile; 1 = in situ motility; 2 = sluggish motility; and 3 = vigorous forward motility.

Beginning 4 h after coitus the number of sperm in the exocervical pool gradually decreases. Thus, tests performed at intervals of 4 h or more following coitus may reveal fewer sperm in the mucus collected from the lower cervical canal.

### Endocervical sample

Sperm reach the level of the internal os rapidly after ejaculation. Their number, according to Tredway et al (1975), increases gradually and reaches a peak approximately 2–3 h later. Thereafter their number remains relatively constant for up to 24 h. Insler et al (1981) found that within 2 h after coitus the entire length of the cervix is colonized by sperm, but at 24 h the number of sperm, begin to decrease. At 6–10 h after intercourse, more than 10 sperm with adequate motility (score 3+) should normally be found per HPF. A similar number of sperm is usually detected in a delayed test (18–24 h after coitus).

## INTERPRETATION AND CAUSES OF NEGATIVE POSTCOITAL TEST

One negative postcoital test has little clinical

value and must be repeated. Controversy continues as to the signifinance of sperm found in cervical secretions several hours after coitus. Some investigators have suggested that they consist mainly of sperm populations of poor quality, which have failed their passage to the uterus. This conclusion is not supported by animal and human studies.

Grant compared the results of postcoital tests and endometrial aspirations in 920 women and found that motile sperm were present in the uteri of 10% although they could not be demonstrated in the cervical mucus (Grant 1958). An explanation of this finding may be that, in cases of oligospermia or when cervical mucus is relatively hostile, the more vigorous and healthier sperm penetrate the cervix and reach the uterine cavity shortly after coitus (rapid phase of transport). Other sperm, which are normally stored in cervical crypts and mucus, do not survive long enough to be detected (disturbed delayed phase of transport).

Most investigators believe that persistently negative postcoital tests indicate either an abnormality of the mucus or oligoasthenospermia. Recently the importance of the movement characteristics exhibited by the spermatozoa have been emphasized. It has been shown that the concentration of motile spermatozoa with a linear velocity and rolling mode of progression as determined by time exposure photomicrography or computer-assisted semen analysis (CASA) influence the number of spermatozoa penetrating the mucus (Aitkin et al 1986).

## Hostile cervical mucus

The most common cause of a negative or abnormal postcoital test is inappropriate timing (Table 13.1). Tests performed too early or too late in the cycle may be negative in an otherwise fertile woman. In some women the test may be positive for only 1 or 2 days in the entire menstrual cycle. When ovulation cannot be timed with a reasonable degree of accuracy, a luteinizing hormone (LH) home kit may be used to identify the LH surge. Alternatively, serial postcoital tests may be performed. In women with absent muccorhea or persistent hostile cervical mucus an

**Table 13.1** Etiological classification of abnormal sperm–cervical mucus interaction

_Female-related causes_
Inappropriate timing
Ovulatory disorders
  anovulation
  subtle anomalies of ovulatory process
Deposition problems
  dyspareunia
  prolapse
  congenital and anatomical anomalies
Anatomic and organic causes
  amputation or deep conization of the cervix
  deep cauterization or cryotherapy
  tumors: polyp, leiomyoma
  severe stenosis
  endocervicitis
Hostile cervical mucus
  increased viscosity
  increased cellularity (infection)
  acid mucus
  presence of sperm antibodies

_Male-related causes_
Deposition problems
  impotence
  retrograde ejaculation
  hypospadias
Semen abnormalities
  low concentration
  low motility
  high percentage of abnormal forms
  high volume (< 8 ml)
  low volume (< 1 ml)
  nonliquifying semen
Antisperm antibodies in semen and/or seminal plasma

artificial cycle might be induced by administration of ethinyl estradiol 50 μg daily beginning on day 5 of a normal menstrual cycle for a period of 3 weeks. The postcoital test may be performed 7–14 days after ingestion of ethinyl estradiol has begun. Postcoital tests are usually negative or abnormal in anovulatory cycles. Subtle anormalies of the ovulatory process, such as inadequate follicular maturation with low level preovulatory estrogen production, may also adversely affect cervical secretion and postcoital test results. Roumen et al (1982) found that repeated abnormal postcoital tests in a group of presumably ovulating infertile women were associated with lower preovulatory serum estradiol levels and higher serum FSH and prolactin levels. Similary, Sher & Katz (1976) evaluated a group of patients with idiopathic infertility and inadequate cervical mucus. Hormone investigation revealed that some of these women had low sex steroid profiles despite apparent ovulation. Treatment with ovulation-inducing agents was attempted to produce 'controlled' ovarian hyperstimulation and an improved cervical mucus and was followed by pregnancy in four of six patients. These data indicate that an optimal amount of circulating estrogen during a determined period of time prior to ovulation is required to stimulate the adequate quantity and quality of cervical secretion. Under normal circumstances the rise of preovulatory estradiol is sufficient to trigger the surge of LH and ovulation and to stimulate cervical mucus secretion. However, it is possible that in some instances the midcycle rise of estrogen would be sufficient to induce ovulation without causing concomitantly optimal cervical mucus secrection.

## Viscosity (consistancy) and cell content

The viscosity of cervical mucus is the greatest barrier to sperm penetration. There is no resistance to sperm migration in thin mucus, but viscous mucus, such as that observed in the luteal phase, pregnancy, and progestogen-treated women, forms an impenetrable barrier. Increased cervical mucus viscosity may also be induced occasionally as a result of treatment with clomiphene citrate. Viscous mucus diluted artificially with normal saline or 5% dextrose is more readily penetrated by sperm than undiluted mucus (Moghissi et al 1964).

Some relatively viscous samples of cervical mucus present a high degree of surface tension and thus appear to be initially impenetrable by sperm. When these samples are mixed with semen, sperm invasion may occur. This in vitro mixing test (M test) is a useful device to determine the ability of sperm to penetrate the mucus in vivo, particularly when it is realized that during coitus such mixing of cervical mucus and semen commonly takes place.

Cleanliness of cervical mucus appears to be a factor favoring sperm migration. Cellular debris and leukocytes impede the progress of sperm in mucus. Severe endocervicitis has been associated with reduced fertility. The precise relationship of mycoplasma infection to the postcoital test and to infertility remains to be determined.

## Effect of pH

Sperm are susceptible to changes in the pH of cervical mucus. Acid mucus immobilizes sperm, whereas alkaline mucus echances their motility. Excessive alkalinity of cervical mucus (over 8.5) may also adversely affect the viability of sperm. The optimal pH for sperm migration and survival in cervical mucus is between 7 and 8.5 (Moghissi et al 1964, Moghissi 1966). The pH ranges of normal midcycle cervical mucus have been reported to be between 6.3 and 8.5 (see also Chapter 22).

## Effect of immune antibodies

Human cervical mucus contains immunoglobulin A (IgA), secretory IgA, and occasionally traces of IgM. IgG is the most constant constituent and is found in almost all samples. The presence of IgG, IgA and IgM in the luminal contents of cervical crypts and basement membrane and in the interstitium has been demonstrated by immunological studies. Biosynthesis of IgG and IgA in the uterine, cervical and vaginal tissues of the rabbit and cervical tissues of women has been reported. Also agglutinating and immobilizing sperm antibodies are known to occur in cervical mucus (see Chapter 14). These antibodies may be found in the cervical mucus independent from those in the serum or may be associated with circulating antibodies. The postcoital test in majority of patients who have cervical mucus antibodies is either negative or grossly abnormal (Moghissi et al 1980). Kremer et al (1977) have also shown that when sperm antibodies are found in the cervical mucus or on the surface of sperm the ability of sperm to penetrate cervical mucus is impaired and sperm loose their progressive movements and show a local shaking motion. A sperm–cervical mucus contact test readily elicits this shaking phenomenon (See also Chapter 22).

The presence of antisperm antibodies on the sperm head may also prevent its penetration into otherwise normal appearing cervical mucus and be associated with a negative or poor postcoital test (Haas 1986). Interestingly, antibodies of similar isotype when directed against the sperm tail, may not impair mucus penetration (Wang et al 1985).

Circulating sperm antibodies, when not associated with cervical mucus antibodies, may also alter postcoital tests or in vitro sperm–cervical mucus penetration.

## Anatomical and organic causes

Amputation or deep conization of the cervix may result in total destruction of secretory epithelial cells lining the endocervix and cervical crypts and in an impairment of mucus production. The condition of 'dry cervix' is usually associated with considerable impairment of fertility since normal insemination and sperm migration cannot take place. Similar consequences may follow extensive cauterization, laser treatment or cryotherapy of the endocervix. The presence of a tumor, i.e cervical leiomyoma and polyp, may cause also a disturbance of mucus secretion. Cervical stenosis is usually secondary to previous operative procedures. When cervical stenosis is pronounced, no vaginal pool of mucus exists, and there is interference with the discharge of cervical secretion. This may have a deleterious effect on sperm survival in the vagina and sperm penetration in cervical mucus. Finally, in endocervicitis because of the presence of numerous leukocytes, exogenous proteins and bacterial toxins in cervical mucus, sperm migration in the mucus may be impeded.

## Miscellaneous causes

Poor coital techniques, vaginismus and dyspareunia may occasionally be associated with a negative postcoital test. A markedly anteflexed cervix may not come in contact with the semen pool (particularly when the volume of semen is scanty) and may be a cause of infertility. Vaginal infections and infestations are an uncommon cause of negative or abnormal postcoital tests.

## Male-related causes

A positive postcoital test results only when semen of good quality is deposited in the vagina. Conditions that prevent ejaculation, intromission or full penetration of the penis into the vagina are associated with a negative postcoital test. These include premature or retrograde ejaculation, operations on the prostate gland and bladder neck, hypospadias, and impotence. A common cause of a negative postcoital test is abnormal semen. Oligospermia, asthenospermia, a large number of morphologically abnormal spermatozoa, and delayed or abnormal liquefaction are known to be associated with absence or inadequate sperm penetration into cervical mucus.

The presence of sperm antibodies in the serum and/or semen also may be associated with an abnormal postcoital test. In these cases the sperm is coated with antibodies and may be unable to penetrate cervical mucus.

## THE SIGNIFICANCE OF THE POSTCOITAL TEST

Soon after ejaculation, spermatozoa are transferred from seminal plasma to female genital tract fluid in which they are suspended. The migration, survival and fertilizing potential of spermatozoa depend to a large extent on how they can adapt themselves to this new environment. The postcoital test provides valuable information on sperm–cervical mucus interaction.

A survey of published reports on postcoital tests indicates a great deal of controversy. Most investigators believe that postcoital tests correlate well with sperm concentration, morphology and motility in the semen as well as with in vitro studies (Davajan & Kunitake 1969). Substantial variance in all semen parameters over an extended period in humans has been observed. These changes affect the results of postcoital tests performed at different times (Poland et al 1985). Motile sperm have been observed in samples of cervical mucus obtained from the cervical os and canal 1.5–3 min following ejaculation and as long as 7 days after coitus (Sobrero & McLeod 1962). Under normal conditions, the percentage of motile and morphologically normal spermatozoa are usually higher in cervical mucus than in semen (Fredricsson & Bjork 1977, Hanson & Overstreet 1981). Attempts have been made to correlate the result of postcoital tests with the occurrence of pregnancy. Some studies show a positive relationship whereas others do not. Generally, in carefully performed studies that have excluded other causes of infertility, a positive postcoital test with a large number of sperm in cervical mucus ( > 10) is associated with a higher pregnancy rate (Hull et al 1982).

Serial postcoital tests have shown that the increased fluidity and spinnbarkeit of preovulatory cervical mucus coincides with a greater number of motile sperm being observed in mucus samples (Sujan et al 1963). After ovulation, the mucus becomes thick and few, if any, live sperm cells are found in it. Combined postcoital tests and endometrial aspirations have demonstrated that the greatest numbers of sperm in the endometrial cavity are found at or near the time of ovulation. Very few were found to be present in the uterus during the luteal or early follicular phases of the cycle (Frenkel 1961).

Studies performed by Ahlgren have shown that the number of sperm in cervical mucus and uterine cavity correlates well with that in the oviducts and pouch of Douglas (Ahlgren 1969). The greatest number of progressively motile sperm in these locations has been observed in the presence of a mature follicle in the ovaries. A significant decrease in the motile sperm population has been seen when ovaries contained corpora lutea. However, once the sperm reach the uterine cavity their further progression to the oviduct may not be influenced by the stage of ovarian cycle. The presence of sperm in the uterus correlates directly with high sperm density in the cervical mucus approximately 25–41 h after coitus.

The postcoital test has also been correlated with the occurrence of pregnancy. If the cervical mucus is good, and an adequate number of active motile sperm are found at the time of the postcoital test, the pregnancy rate is significantly greater than if poor sperm migration occurs with the finding of good cervical mucus (Buxton & Southam 1958). Jette & Glass (1972) found that the pregnancy rate in 555 infertile women was significantly higher in the presence of favorable cervical mucus and when there were more than 20 sperm/HPF in the mucus as demonstrated in postcoital tests. Giner et al (1974) were, however, unable to demonstrate such a relationship.

Moghissi (1977) performed a fractional postcoital test as a part of a complete infertility survey in 208 infertile women. The result of the best postcoital tests of 58 women who became pregnant was compared to that of 143 who did not. Excluded from the study were all women who had a definite impediment to fertility that could not be corrected and tests that were not timed to coincide with ovulation. Cervical scores were not significantly different in the two groups. As seen in Table 13.2, significantly larger numbers of sperm were found in postcoital tests of women who achieved pregnancy than in those who remained infertile. Since cervical scores in the two groups were comparable the data indicated that the greater number of sperm in cervical mucus was associated with a greater chance of pregnancy.

In another study, Hanson & Overstreet (1981) analysed the relationship of the number of motile sperm seen in cervical mucus 48 h after artificial insemination with donor sperm (AID) with subsequent fertility. They demonstrated a significant association between the occurrence of conception after AID and sperm survival for 48 h in the cervical mucus. Examination of their data suggested that when spermatozoa were consistently present in the mucus there was a significantly higher probability of conception in that insemination cycle.

The lack of correlation of postcoital test results with the occurrence of pregnancy has also been

**Table 13.2**  Results of best postcoital test in infertile women

| Group | No. | Cervical scores | Sperm/HPF exocervix | Sperm/HPF endocervix |
|---|---|---|---|---|
| I. Pregnant | 58 | $13.8 \pm 2.1$ | $12.8 \pm 10.8*$ | $16.8 \pm 11.7*$ |
| II. Persistent infertility | 143 | $14.05 \pm 1.56$ | $7.43 \pm 7.76$ | $7.1 \pm 8.28$ |

*Significant at $P < 0.001$ level compared to group II.

documented in some studies. For example, Harrison (1981) in a study of 423 couples found that the postcoital test was not a good indicator of fertility potential, since 24.5% of 98 women who had persistently negative postcoital tests achieved pregnancy.

To evaluate the validity of the postcoital test, Griffith & Grimes (1990) reviewed the English literature and found that the test suffers from a lack of standard methodology, lack of uniform definition of normal, and unknown reproducibility. Unfortunately, this effort was based on the premise that the postcoital test is of value only if it can predict pregnancy rather than assessing sperm transport. Also they compared studies using different methodology and criteria for normalcy rather than standards recommended by WHO (1987).

The findings of these studies could easily be explained and should not invalidate the usefulness of postcoital tests. It is now well recognized that sperm concentration, motility and morphology of most men are subject to considerable changes when serial semen analyses are performed (Poland et al 1985, WHO 1987). These alterations will be reflected in the results of postcoital or in vitro sperm–cervical mucus tests. Furthermore, timing of the tests, technical variation and other variables may alter the test results. Finally, it should be realized that pregnancy results only when various factors involved in the reproductive process, in addition to sperm–cervical mucus interaction, are in optimal functioning order.

## IN VITRO INVESTIGATIONS

Negative or abnormal postcoital tests are indications for in vitro cervical mucus–sperm penetration tests. Two different techniques have been used for in vitro investigation of sperm penetration of cervical mucus: the slide method and the capillary tube system. A good correlation has been found between the results obtained by these techniques (Kremer 1968). The results of in vitro sperm–cervical mucus penetration tests also compare fairly well with sperm concentration, motility and percentage of normal morphology in semen samples (Insler et al 1979, Keel & Webster

1988). Mortimer et al (1986) found that both the concentration of progressively motile spermatozoa and their movement characteristics are significant factors determining the outcome of homologous tests of human sperm–cervical mucus interaction. Finally, there is a significant correlation between the results of postcoital tests, in vitro tests, and semen analysis findings (Hayes et al 1984). The slide method as originally described by Miller & Kurzrok has been altered to provide quantitative results (Moghissi et al 1964) (Fig. 13.6).

In studies in vitro by the slide method a sharp boundary is observed separating human cervical mucus placed in juxtaposition to semen on a microscopic slide (Moghissi et al 1964) (Fig. 13.6). At the interface, finger–like projections or phalanges of seminal fluid develop within a few minutes and penetrate the mucus. Sperm usually fill these canals before entering the mucus. Most spermatozoa penetrate the apex of the phalangeal canal and enter the mucus. In most instances a single spermatozoon appears to lead a column of sperm into the mucus. After the initial resistance has been overcome by the leading sperm, others follow without difficulty. Once in the cervical mucus, sperm fan out and move at random. Some return to the seminal plasma layer, while most migrate deep into the cervical mucus until they

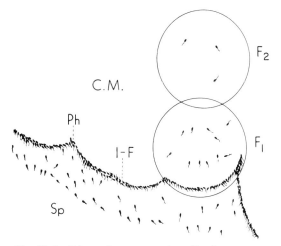

**Fig. 13.6** Schematic representation of in vitro sperm–cervical mucus penetration test by quantitative slide method. C.M., cervical mucus; Sp, sperm; I–F, interface; Ph, phalanges; $F_1$, first microscopic field; $F_2$, second field adjacent to $F_1$ (Moghissi 1966).

meet with resistance from cellular debris or leuko-cytes. They then either stop or change direction. Both phalanx and interface formation appear to be physical phenomena resulting from the contact of two biological fluids of differing viscosities and surface tensions.

To quantitate the test, the first microscopic field from the interface called $F_1$ is counted at various time intervals. The suggested times are 5 and 15 min after initiation of test. This is scored at $\times$ 200 and $\times$ 400 magnification. In order to study the depth of penetration, the second micro-scopic field adjacent to the first one, i.e. $F_2$, and the third ($F_3$) can also be evaluated and the number of spermatozoa in these fields can be counted and recorded (Fig. 13.6). In good tests at least 15 motile sperm/HPF in $F_1$ and at least 10 sperm/HPF in $F_2$ are recorded.

The capillary tube system measures the ability

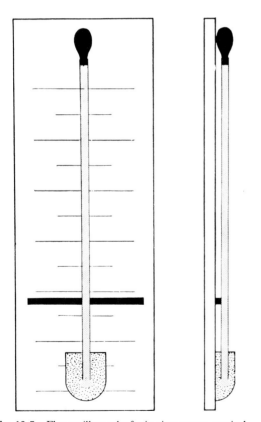

**Fig. 13.7**   Flat capillary tube for in vitro sperm–cervical mucus penetration test. The tube is filled with cervical mucus, sealed at the top and placed in a sperm reservoir (bottom). The entire system is mounted on a graduated slide (Kremer 1968).

of spermatozoa to penetrate a colum of cervical mucus in a flat capillary tube (Fig. 13.7). Sperm penetration in the capillary tube is assessed at 10 min, 30 min, 3 h or other intervals depending on the type of study. Both linear penetration and density of penetration should be recorded. A scoring system for the evaluation of sperm penetrability has been devised (Belsey et al 1980). The capillary tube system is particularly useful for evaluation of midcycle cervical mucus and to study depth of penetration (Kremer 1968). The slide method is applicable to a variety of cervical mucus samples, including those too viscous or too scanty to be studied by the tube technique. When both in vivo and in vitro tests are negative, normal donor sperm may be tested in vitro against the wife's cervical mucus, and preovulatory mucus obtained from a fertile donor should be tested with the husband's sperm (Fig. 13.2). This crossmatch test will determine whether the sperm or cervical mucus is respon-sible for abnormal results. With the introduction and popularity of modern techniques of intrauterine insemination (IUI), fewer in vitro tests are being performed by clinicians. These tests continue, however, to be an important research tool.

## THE USE OF BOVINE ESTRUS CERVICAL MUCUS FOR IN VITRO TESTS

Recently it has been shown that bovine estrus cervical mucus may be used as a substitute for human midcycle mucus (Moghissi et al 1982). Bovine estrus cervical mucus is biochemically and functionally similar to human mucus. The viscoelastic and rheological properties of the two secretions are also remarkably alike. Human spermatozoa can enter bovine cervical mucus (BCM) readily in vitro and maintain good motility and viability for several hours. Moghissi et al (1982) demonstrated that the pattern and depth of sperm penetration to human cervical mucus (HCM) and BCM were very similar. Human sperm appeared to migrate somewhat slower in BCM compared with HCM. Highly significant correlation was found between the depth of sperm penetration in HCM and BCM, particularly when both were of optimal quality. As expected, sperm count and motility showed significant correlation with the rate of sperm migration in both HCM and BCM. Greater sperm concentration and higher sperm motility were associated with greater depth of penetration in both HCM and BCM. However, BCM was more discriminating with regard to sperm form. Spermatozoa from ejaculates containing a higher percentage of abnormal cells did not migrate through the BCM as rapidly as they did in HCM.

In another study, Hayes et al (1984) compared the results of in vitro sperm penetration tests in HCM and BCM in 35 couples with the results of postcoital tests. Postcoital test results correlated significantly with in vitro sperm penetration. Furthermore, the concentration of morphologically normal motile sperm per ejaculate also correlated positively with the sperm penetration test and correlated more significantly with the postcoital test.

The results of these and several other studies indicate that BCM may indeed be used as a substitute for HCM to test in vitro sperm–cervical mucus interaction whenever difficulties are experienced to secure a sufficient amount of human material. Commercially prepared capillary tubes containing standardized samples of bovine mucus have now become available (Pentrak Kit, Serono, Bandolph, MA, USA). The use of bovine estrus mucus can considerably facilitate the testing of the ability of spermatozoa from a given man to penetrate normal cervical mucus and will provide a new dimension in evaluating the etiology of abnormal sperm–cervical mucus interaction.

## OTHER TESTS

When postcoital tests are consistently negative but in vitro tests show adequate sperm penetration in cervical mucus obtained from the female partner, the use of insemination test may be considered.

In this test the couple is instructed to abstain for a period of 2 days and report at the time of anticipated ovulation of the wife. The husband is required to provide a semen sample obtained by masturbation. The ejaculate is allowed to liquefy and the wife is artificially inseminated with this sample using intracervical technique of insemination. Approximately 1–2 h later, samples of mucus from the exocervix and endocervix are obtained and the concentration and quality of sperm are observed and recorded using the technique described for postcoital tests. In cases where large semen volume, oligospermia or liquefaction defects have been previously observed in the process of semen analysis, the first portion (or better portion ) of a split ejaculate may be used for this purpose.

The results of postinsemination tests are interpreted in a similar way to those of postcoital tests. If the postinsemination test shows at least 10 vigorously motile sperm/HPF, one should suspect the presence of factor(s) in the vagina, or alterations of buffering capacity of seminal plasma and/or cervical mucus contributing to early obstruction of sperm in the vagina. This situation may be encountered particularly when the volume of the ejaculate is small and cervical mucus is scanty.

The results of postinsemination tests may also be used as a guide for the management of the patient. If the result is favorable one may expect a good prognosis for attaining pregnancy with the use of homologous artificial insemination.

## CONCLUSIONS

The postcoital test determines the adequacy of sperm and receptivity of cervical mucus. It is the only test that evaluates the interaction between the sperm and the female genital tract fluids in vivo. The Sims–Huhner test should be an integral part of infertility investigation but must not be used as a substitute for semen analysis. Abnormal postcoital tests should be investigated with in vitro studies and insemination tests to determine whether anomalies of cervical mucus, sperm or both are responsible for the inability of sperm to penetrate the cervix. Since cervical mucus accurately reflects the ovarian cycle, the postcoital test is also a useful indicator of endocrine preparation of the female reproductive system.

REFERENCES

Ahlgren M 1969 Migration of spermatozoa to the fallopian tubes and the abdominal cavity in women, including some immunological aspects. Student literature, Lund, Sweden, p 11

Aitkin R J, Warner P E, Reid C 1986 Factor influencing the success of sperm–cervical mucus interaction in patients exhibiting unexplained infertility. J Androl 7: 3

Belsey M A, Eliassen R, Gallegos A J, Moghissi K S, Paulson C A, Prasad M R N 1980 Laboratory manual for examination of human serum and serum cervical mucus interaction. WHO , Geneva

Buxton C L, Southam A L 1958 Cervical physiology. In: Paul B (ed) Human infertility. Hoeber, New York

Davajan V, Kunitake G 1969 Fractional in vivo and in vitro examination of post–coital cervical mucus in the human. Fertil Steril 20: 197

Elstein M, Moghissi K S, Borth R 1973 Cervical mucus, present state of knowledge. In: Cervical mucus in human reproduction. WHO , Scriptor, Copenhagen, p 11

Fluhmann C F 1961 The cervix uteri and its disease, 3rd ed. Saunders, Philadelphia

Fox C A, Meldrum S J, Watson B W 1973 Continuous measurement by radiotelemetry of vaginal pH during human coitus. J Reprod Fertil 33: 69

Fredricsson B, Bjork G 1977 Morphology of postcoital spermatozoa in the cervical secretion and its clinical significance. Fertil Steril 28: 841

Frenkel D A 1961 Sperm migration and survival in the endometrial cavity. Int J Fertil 6: 285

Giner J, Meriono G, Luna J, Asnar R 1974 Evaluation of the Sims – Huhner postcoital test in infertile couples. Fertil Steril 24: 145

Gould J E, Overstreet J W, Hanson F W 1984 Assessment of human sperm function after recovery from the female reproductive tract. Biol Reprod 32: 888

Grant A 1958 Cervical hostility. Fertil Steril 9: 321

Griffith C S, Grimes D A 1990 The validity of the postcoital test. Am J Obstet Gynecol 162: 615

Haas G G 1986 The inhibitory effect of sperm–associated immunoglobulins on cervical mucus penetration. Fertil Steril 44: 334

Hanson F W, Overstreet J W 1981 The interaction of human spermatozoa with cervical mucus in vivo. Am J Obstet Gynecol 140: 173

Hanson F W, Overstreet J W, Katz D F 1982 A study of the relationship of motile sperm numbers in cervical mucus 48 hours after artificial insemination with subsequent fertility. Am J Obstet Gynecol 143: 85

Harrison R F 1981 The diagnostic and therapeutic potential of the postcoital test. Fertil Steril 36: 71

Hayes M F, Segal S, Moghissi K S, Magyar D, Agronow S 1984 Comparison of the in vitro sperm penetration test using human cervical mucus and bovine estrus cervical mucus with the postcoital test. Int J Fertil 29: 133

Hull M G, Savage P E, Bronham D R 1982 Prognostic value of the postcoital test. Prospective study based on time–specific conception rate. Br J Obstet Gynaecol 89: 299

Insler V, Melmed H, Eichenbrenner I, Serr D M, Lunenfeld B 1972 The cervical score. Int J Gynecol Obstet 10: 223

Insler V, Bernstein D, Glezerman M, Misgav N 1979 Correlation of seminal fluid analysis with mucus penetrating ability of spermatozoa. Fertil Steril 32: 316

Insler V, Glazerman M, Bernstein D, Zeidel L, Misgav N 1981 Cervical crypts and their role in storing spermatozoa In: Insler V, Bettendorf G (eds) Advances in diagnosis and treatment of infertility. Elsevier/North Holland, Amsterdam, p 195

Jaszczak S 1973 Migration of sperm in the cervix and uterus of non-human primates. In: Moghissi K S, Borth R (eds) Cervical mucus in human reproduction. Scriptor, Copenhagen p 33

Jette N T, Glass R H 1972 Prognostic value of the postcoital test. Fertil Steril 23: 29

Keel B A, Webster B W 1988 Correlation of human sperm motility characteristics with an in vitro cervical mucus penetration test. Fertil Steril 49: 138

Kellerman A S, Weid J C 1970 Sperm motility and survival in relation to glucose concentration: an in vitro study. Fertil Steril 21: 802

Kremer J 1968 The in vitro spermatozoal penetration test. In: Drukkerij Van Denderen N V (ed) Fertility investigation thesis. Groningen

Kremer J, Jager S, Kuiken J 1977 The meaning of cervical mucus in couples with antisperm antibodies. In: Insler V, Bettendorf G (eds) The uterine cervix in reproduction. George Thieme, Stuttgart

Lee W I, Verdugo P, Blandau R J, Gaddum–Rosse P 1977 Molecular arrangement of cervical mucus: a re-evaluation based on laser light-scattering spectrometry. Gynecol Invest 8: 254

Moghissi K S 1966 Cyclic changes of cervical mucus in normal and progestin treated women. Fertil Steril 17: 663

Moghissi K S 1973a Sperm migration through the human cervix. In: Elstein M, Moghissi K S, Borth R, (eds) Cervical mucus in human reproduction. Scriptor, Copenhagen p 128

Moghissi K S 1973b Composition and function of cervical secretion. In: Gripp R (ed) Handbook of physiology, endocrinology II, part 2, American Physiology Society, Washington DC Ch. 31 p. 25

Moghissi K S 1977 Significance and prognostic value of postcoital test. In: Insler V, Bettendorf G (eds) The uterine cervix in reproduction. Georg Thieme, Stuttgart p 146

Moghissi K S 1979 Sperm migration in the female genital tract. In: Zatucchini G I, Sobrero A J, Sspredel J J, Sciarra J J (eds) Vaginal contraception. Harper & Row, Maryland, USA, p 23

Moghissi K S, Dabich D, Levine J, Neuhaus O W 1964 Mechanism of sperm migration. Fertil Steril 15: 15

Moghissi K S, Syner F N, Evans T N 1972 A composit picture of the menstrual cycle. Am J Obstet Gynecol 114: 405

Moghissi K S, Sacco A G, Borin K S 1980 Immunologic infertility. I. Cervical mucus antibodies and postcoital test. Am J Obstet Gynecol 136: 941

Moghissi K S, Segal S, Meinhold D, Agronow S J 1982 In vitro sperm cervical mucus penetration: studies in human and bovine cervical mucus. Fertil Steril 37: 823

Mortimer D, Pandya J, Sawers R S 1986 Relationship between human sperm motility characteristics and sperm penetration to human cervical mucus in vitro. J Reprod Fertil 78: 93

Odeblad E, Rudolfsson C 1973 Types of cervical secretions: biophysical characteristics. In: Blandau R J, Moghissi K S (eds) The biology of the cervix. University of Chicago Press, Chicago p 267 Chicago

Poland M L, Moghissi K S, Giblin P T et al 1985 Variation of semen measures within normal men. Fertil Steril 94: 396

Roumen F J M E, Doesburg W H, Rolland R 1982 Hormonal patterns in infertile women with a deficient postcoital test. Fertil Steril 38: 42

Sher G, Katz M 1976 Inadequate cervical mucus —a cause of idiopathic infertility. Fertil Steril 27: 886

Sobrero A J, McLeod J 1962 The immediate post-coital test. Fertil Steril 13: 184

Sujan S, Danezis J, Sobrero A J 1963 Sperm migration and cervical mucus studies in individual cycles. J Reprod Fertil 6: 87

Tredway D R, Settlage D F, Nakamura R M, Motoshima M,

Umezaki C U, Mishell D R 1975 Significance of timing for postcoital evaluation of cervical mucus. Am J Obstet Gynecol 121: 387

Wang C, Baker H W G, Jennings M G, Burger H G, Lutjen P 1985 Interaction between human cervical mucus and sperm surface antibodies. Fertil Steril 44: 484

WHO 1987 Laboratory manual for examination of human semen and semen cervical mucus interaction. WHO, Geneva

Yurewicz E C, Moghissi K S 1981 Purification of human midcycle cervical mucin and characterization of its oligosaccharides with respect to size, composition and microheterogeneity. J Biol Chem 256: 11895

# 14. Immunological infertility and its diagnosis

*Norbert Gleicher*

## INTRODUCTION

As it is becoming increasingly apparent that endocrine and immune systems are closely inter-woven, it has also become increasingly more difficult to cover as broad a topic as suggested by this chapter title. This chapter will therefore *not* describe mutual influences of endocrine and immune systems on each other. For this purpose the reader is referred to an excellent recent review (Michael & Chapman 1990). *Nor* will this chapter address auto- and paracrine processes within the uterus and ovaries as they, regulated through the action of various cytokines, clearly can affect fertility. For that purpose the reader is referred to reviews by Toder & Shomer (1990) and Adashi (1990). Lastly, this chapter will *not* cover the so-called 'cervical factor' as it relates to immunolog-ical infertility since this topic is covered in the preceding chapter.

Rather, this chapter will concentrate on a number of *specific* immunological findings that have been directly associated with infertility in either female or male.

## ABNORMAL AUTOIMMUNE FUNCTION

Abnormal autoimmune function can affect fertility by preventing conception or, alternatively, by leading to pregnancy loss once a pregnancy has been established. It is actually quite surprising how long it has taken to recognize the effect of abnormal autoimmune function on reproductive processes. Table 14.1 summarizes a number of medical conditions which for decades have been known to be associated with excessive pregnancy loss. As we now know, all of these conditions have an autoimmune etiology. In fact, this author is

**Table 14.1** Medical conditions which historically have been associated with excessive pregnancy loss

Collagen vascular diseases
  Systemic lupus erythematosus
  Mixed connective tissue disease
  Systemic sclerosis
Dermatitis herpetiformis
Celiac disease
Herpes gestationis
Ulcerative colitis
Crohn's disease
Chronic active hepatitis
Thyroid disease
Diabetes mellitus
Endometriosis

Reproduced from Gleicher 1992 with permission

unaware of any medical condition historically linked with pregnancy loss which is not an autoimmune disease.

Considering this historical fact, one cannot be surprised by the initial observation of Lubbe's et al (1983) that associated the presence of lupus anticoagulant with the occurrence of pregnancy loss. Lupus anticoagulant is a still poorly defined apparent compendium of IgG, IgM and probably IgA phospholipid antibodies, which predispose affected patients to thromboembolic phenomena and pregnancy loss (Editorial 1984). It was this observation by Lubbe & associates which for the first time suggested that abnormal antibodies can affect reproductive processes. Lubbe's observa-tion was expanded by Gleicher & Friberg (1985), who demonstrated that aborting patients with lupus anticoagulant also demonstrated other immunoglobulin abnormalities, especially hyper-gammaglobulinemias. This again was an impor-tant observation because it suggested a broadly based *polyclonal* abnormality of B lymphocyte function in affected patients, later confirmed by many investigators. Moreover, this study suggested that total immunoglobulin levels could serve as a potential marker for abnormal B lymphocyte function in patients with reproductive failure. This has since been confirmed not only in patients with pregnancy loss (Gleicher et al 1989) but also in strictly infertile women with abnormal autoimmune function such as unexplained infertility (Gleicher et al 1989), endometriosis patients (Gleicher 1987), individuals with sperm antibodies (El-Roeiy et al 1988) and, most recently, in females with premature ovarian failure (Gleicher et al 1992a).

## Unexplained infertility

Unexplained infertility represents a paradoxical diagnosis because any relevant diagnostic finding actually disqualifies a patient from this diagnosis. If patients with so-called unexplained infertility are investigated for evidence of abnormal immunoglobulin production, a pattern is detected which proves to be typical for *all* patients with autoimmune associated reproductive failure. It consists of: (1) *total immunoglobulin abnormalities*, and (2) *autoantibody abnormalities* inclusive of phospholipid antibodies, though by no means exclusively of antiphospholipid specificity (Gleicher et al 1989). Table 14.2 summarizes findings in 26 patients with the diagnosis of unexplained infertility and, in comparison, in 24 patients with repeated pregnancy loss. As can be easily noted, the pattern of immunological abnormality is almost identical and can, as will be shown later, also be found in individuals with endometriosis, premature ovarian failure and sperm antibodies.

Similar results were also reported by Taylor et al (1989). In contrast to the preceding data, these authors also investigated tissue-specific autoantibodies. They reported significantly elevated autoantibody levels to smooth muscle, phospholipids as well as nuclear antigens.

**Table 14.2**   Immunological findings in 26 patients with unexplained infertility and 24 with repeated pregnancy loss

|  | Unexplained infertility | Repeated pregnancy loss | Control group |
| --- | --- | --- | --- |
| Total immunoglobulin (mg/dl) |  |  |  |
| IgG | 994 ± 380 | 1059 ± 300* | 708 ± 247 |
| IgM | 212 ± 75 † | 199 ± 66‡ | 130 ± 69 |
| IgA | 130 ± 56 | 189 ± 149 | 115 ± 66 |
| Autoantibodies (no. of positives)‖ |  |  |  |
| Phospholipids | 13 | 7 | — |
| Histones | 21 | 18 | — |
| Polynucleotides | 39 | 26 | — |
| Total | 73 | 28 | — |
| No. of abnormal autoantibodies per patient |  |  |  |
| 0 | 3 | 7 |  |
| 1 | 5 | 8 |  |
| 2 | 9 | 2 |  |
| 3 | 3 | 2 |  |
| 4 | 2 | 0 |  |
| 5 | 0 | 0 |  |
| 6 | 1 | 1 |  |
| 8 | 1 | 0 |  |
| 9 | 1 | 0 |  |
| 13 | 1 | 0 |  |
| 15 | 0 | 1 |  |

Modified from Gleicher et al 1989
\* Significantly different from control group (Student's t test).
† 10/26 patients demonstrated an IgM gammopathy (>210 mg/dl).
‡ 10/24 patients demonstrated an IgM gammopathy, two an IgA gammopathy (>182 mg/dl).
‖ Abnormalities were detected when patients were investigated for two phospholipid antibodies (cardiolipin, phosphatidyl-serine), total histone and four subfractions (H2A, H2B, H3, H4) and four polynucleotides (ssDNA, dsDNA, PolyI, Poly (dT).

## Endometriosis

In many ways endometriosis represents yet another form of unexplained infertility. While the disease is clearly associated with a decrease in fecundity and while with advanced stages of the condition, this infertility can be attributed to tubal factors, in mild stages of the disease the cause for the decrease in fertility is unknown. As in unexplained infertility, we have suggested that the impairment in fertility is due to autoantibody abnormalities (Gleicher 1987, El Roeiy et al 1988b).

Endometriosis patients exhibit the same immunological profile as previously described in women with unexplained infertility and repeated pregnancy loss. In fact, endometriosis is not only characterized by infertility but also by repeated and excessive pregnancy wastage. Its clinical presentation mimics that of an autoimmune disease, raising the question whether endometriosis is not, in fact, an autoimmune disease (Gleicher 1987).

Endometriosis demonstrates immunological abnormalities not only in respect to autoreactivity. Abnormalities in immune function have been widely reported in reference to almost any lymphocyte and macrophage function and, once again, the similarity to findings in patients with unexplained infertility is blatant (Hill & Anderson 1989). Abnormalities can be found in peripheral blood and especially prominently in peritoneal fluid (Halme et al 1984, Confino et al 1990).

Treatment of immunological abnormalities, and especially of autoantibody abnormalities, restores a level of fertility in endometriosis patients (El-Roeiy et al 1988b). Steinleitner et al (1991) also demonstrated in an animal model that non-specific immune modulation may improve fertility. Figure 14.1 graphically demonstrates our concept of the relationship between endometriosis, infertility and pregnancy loss, as they relate to autoantibody abnormalities.

## Pregnancy loss

As noted in the introduction to this chapter, the first observation between abnormal autoimmune function and reproductive failure was made in

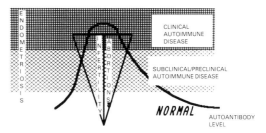

**Fig. 14.1** Graphic presentation of how endometriosis, infertility and pregnancy loss relate to autoantibody abnormalities. BAFS, reproductive autoimmune failure syndrome.

repeatedly aborting women (Lubbe et al 1983). Lubbe's observation led soon thereafter to the recognition that the immunological abnormalities in females afflicted by autoimmune problems were broadly based and exceeded the presence of lupus anticoagulant (Gleicher & Friberg 1985). In fact, as Table 14.2 demonstrates, autoantibody abnormalities in repeatedly aborting women are identical to those with unexplained infertility and endometriosis. This means that one can find a high incidence of gammopathies and autoantibody abnormalities not only among phospholipid antibodies but also among other autoantibody groupings such as antihistones and antipolynucleotides.

Unfortunately, this fact has *not* been recognized by many investigators in this field. Consequently, the literature is filled with reports which suggest that the investigation of lupus anticoagulant and/or of one or two phospholipid antibodies is adequate to diagnose affected patients. *This is incorrect!* Neither lupus anticoagulant or cardiolipin antibodies, nor antibodies to phosphatidylserine or phosphatidic acid, alone or in combination, represent adequate screening methods to detect affected patients. As Table 14.2 demonstrates quite well, only a broadly based screen of various autoantibody groupings will detect most (though never all) afflicted patients. In addition, we strongly recommend the investigation of total immunoglobulin levels, since at times only the presence of a gammopathy will be indicative of the diagnosis. Ten to fifteen per cent of affected females will demonstrate autoantibody abnormalities only when pregnant, while total immunoglobulin abnormalities are usually already detectable in the non-pregnant state. Table 14.3 demonstrates the autoantibody profile routinely evaluated at our Center. It is the summary of 45 separately evaluated and fully automated assays. Because of the automation, this autoantibody screen can be performed very economically at a cost almost equal to that of a single cardiolipin antibody determination.

Repeated pregnancy loss has also been associated with abnormal alloimmune function (Beer et al 1981). This has remained a highly controversial area, leading to a variety of immunization protocols which have utilized lymphocytes, trophoblast membranes, sperm, etc. Recently, the first properly controlled studies have been reported, leading increasingly to a consensus that immunizations probably do not increase pregnancy success (Hill 1990). Even though concern has been expressed, recent evidence actually does not suggest that lymphocyte immunizations may *increase* levels of abnormal autoantibodies (Kwak-Kim et al 1990).

## Premature ovarian failure

It has been convincingly demonstrated that premature ovarian failure in a high percentage of cases is due to an abnormal autoimmune response. Cohen & Speroff (1991) have reviewed these data and Coulam & Stern (1991) presented an overview of the proposed molecular mechanisms affecting folliculogenesis in the ovaries of affected patients.

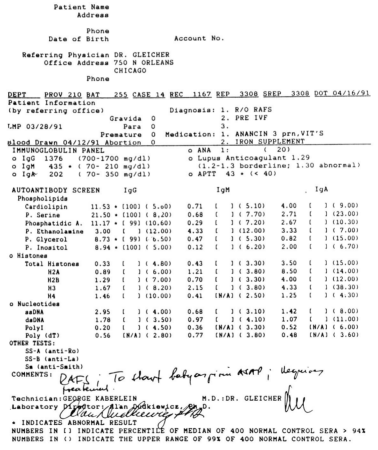

**Table 14.3** Autoantibody report. The Center for Human Reproduction investigates a broadly based autoantibody profile in affected patients rather than a single antibody such as cardiolipin.

It appears that a form of autoimmune oophoritis, not unlike the histological picture of autoimmune thyroiditis, precedes the occurrence of premature ovarian failure (Sedmark et al 1987, Biscotti et al 1989). Unfortunately, this phase of the disease occurs mostly insidiously. By the time patients are diagnosed, most will have reached an endstage of disease in which folliculogenesis has ceased and follicles within the ovaries are practically exhausted. At that point it is quite likely that the stimulating autoantigen(s) is (are) also exhausted. The immune response seen in patients with premature ovarian failure may therefore *not* be representative of the immune response during the active stage of the disease. This is supported by animal experience. For example, Miake et al (1988) demonstrated in a very elegant mouse model of premature ovarian failure an excellent correlation between levels of organ-specific anti-ovarian antibodies and ovarian histology, represented by autoimmune oophoritis and acute oocyte loss. Antibody levels decreased, however, as ovaries atrophied with increasing length of the autoimmune insult.

The diminution of the (auto)immune response over time may be the reason why the literature has remained somewhat contradictory in reference to autoantibody abnormalities in patients with premature ovarian failure (Coulam & Ryan 1985). More recently, it has been suggested that the autoimmune response is directed against the unoccupied luteinizing hormone/human chorionic gonadotropic receptor and hormone/receptor complex (Moncayo et al 1989). It thus appears that organ-specific and nonorgan-specific autoimmune responses occur in patients with premature ovarian failure (Mignot et al 1989), which is a quite characteristic finding in autoimmune diseases. In fact, premature ovarian failure behaves in many ways like any other classical autoimmune disease. As in other autoimmune conditions, premature ovarian failure is highly associated with other autoimmune diseases in the same individual. This applies especially to autoimmune thyroid disease, rheumatoid arthritis, Addison's disease and myasthenia gravis (Cohen & Speroff 1991), and in our experience also to endometriosis.

Premature ovarian failure, in fact, does demon-strate a very similar (though not identical) immunological profile as the three earlier discussed conditions unexplained infertility, endometriosis and repeated pregnancy loss. In a recent study (Gleicher et al 1992a), we were able to demonstrate that, as in those conditions, approximately three-quarters of patients demon-strated some organ-nonspecific autoantibody abnormalities. More remarkably, however, *all* patients demonstrated abnormalities in total immunoglobulin levels. It is therefore tempting to speculate that total immunoglobulin abnormali-ties may represent inexpensive and easy to obtain markers of an autoimmune attack on the ovary. In continuation with the previously discussed condi-tions, one consequently can conclude that the investigation of total immunoglobulin levels should probably represent an integral part of any infertility evaluation.

## Sperm antibodies

In the male the presence of sperm antibodies does represent 'auto'-immunity. Considerable evidence has accumulated which suggests that autoimmunity to sperm can reduce the fertility potential of males. The factors determining the appearance of sperm autoimmunity in appar-ently normal males have, however, remained unknown (Jones 1990). Investigation of this field has been further complicated by the utiliza-tion of a large variety of different sperm antibody assays which may often detect different antibody groupings with different clinical significance (Bronson 1990). As will be discussed in more detail in the following section on the impact of sperm antibodies on assisted reproductive technologies, a number of investigators have therefore suggested that more than one anti-sperm antibody test should be utilized when attempts are made to detect clinically relevant sperm antibodies.

The association of specific histocompatibility loci with sperm antibodies in males (Mathur et al 1983) and the finding of concomitantly elevated nonorgan-specific autoantibodies in those same males (El-Roeiy et al 1988a), suggest that autoim-munity to sperm does not differ from autoimmu-nity to other autoantigens.

Monoclonal antibodies to sperm have been demonstrated to interfere with sperm viability and its capability to penetrate and fertilize oocytes (Bronson 1990, Dor et al 1981). Similar to other autoantibodies, they often also have only limited specificity and may be highly cross-reactive with other autoantibodies (El-Roeiy et al 1988a).

Sperm antibodies in the male differ from those in the female. In general, antibody titers in the male are lower than in the female, and coexisting immunological parameters allow to a very high degree the correct prediction of the sex of the affected individual, thus suggesting that women and men respond differently to sperm antigens. The presence of a polyclonal B lymphocyte activation, as also seen in most other autoimmune conditions, is also documented by the by now well-recognized total immunoglobulin abnormalities in affected individuals, by the concomitant presence of a relatively high incidence of ANA-positivity and the presence of a multitude of autoantibodies (El-Roeiy et al 1988a).

Unfortunately, treatment options have remained limited and universally unsatisfactory. Recently, it has been suggested that inseminations with washed sperm will result in a relatively high fecundity rate (Confino et al 1986). Others have suggested other assisted reproductive technologies, though this approach has remained controversial, as will be discussed in more detail later.

## Autoimmunity to gonadal antigens

An abnormal autoimmune response against testicular and ovarian antigens can occur in otherwise apparently normal females and males. For example, antibodies to the zona pellucida have been noted in many females, inclusive of those with otherwise unexplained infertility, and have been utilized to produce contraceptive vaccines (Skinner et al 1990). At the same time, some authorities question the clinical significance of antibodies to the zona in females with otherwise unexplained infertility (Caudle et al 1987).

Experimental autoimmunity against ovarian and testicular antigens has been widely reported in the literature. The notion that a considerable portion of females with premature ovarian failure suffer from an autoimmune-induced process has

been earlier reviewed. It needs to be emphasized, however, that neither the existence of human autoimmune ovarian or testicular disease has been formally established.

## Autoimmunity to pituitary components

It has recently been suggested that autoimmune processes against tissue components of the anterior pituitary gland, its secretory products and receptors may cause infertility. Jones (1990) recently summarized a spectrum of antibody reactivity to various pituitary cell populations. It is likely that future investigations will, in analogy perhaps to thyroid autoimmune disease and myasthenia gravis, determine autoantibody reactivity against not only hormones but their receptor molecules. In fact, some authorities have suggested that autoimmune ovarian failure may represent such a receptor disease.

## Autoimmunity and assisted reproduction

The experience of patients with abnormal autoimmune function in assisted reproduction may shed additional light on the effect of abnormal autoimmunity on reproductive success. While reported data are limited, a few interesting observations have been made. First, it appears that patients in in vitro fertilization (IVF) programs demonstrate a highly increased incidence of autoantibody abnormalities (El-Roeiy et al 1987, Fisch et al 1991). Moreover, especially phospholipid antibodies appear to be concentrated within follicular fluid at excessive levels, even in correlation to excessive serum levels in affected patients. The latter observation thus strongly suggests that these phospholipid antibodies are produced locally within the ovary (El-Roeiy et al 1987). Lastly, preliminary evidence from the same study suggests that the presence of antiphospholipid antibodies in IVF patients adversely affects their pregnancy outlook.

## SPERM ANTIBODIES IN ASSISTED REPRODUCTION

We briefly reviewed sperm antibodies in males under the heading of abnormal autoimmune function. However, in the female, immunological reactivity to sperm does *not* represent autoimmunity. Sperm antibodies also deserve further discussion because this represents a continuously controversial area in diagnosis and management of infertility. Not only has the presence of antibodies to sperm been questioned but certainly their clinical significance.

The reasons for much of the confusion in this area are many. First and foremost, sperm antibody assays utilized in published studies often vary. Table 14.4 presents a selection of widely utilized sperm antibody assays. The specific correlation of sperm antibodies, detected with these greatly differing assays, to infertility not surprisingly varies greatly. Many experts in the field therefore suggest today that not only a single, but preferably two or three sperm antibody assays be utilized in parallel. At our Center we routinely utilize an isotype-specific immunobead assay in parallel to a standard agglutination test.

The field of assisted reproduction lends itself well to address a second difficulty in assessing the importance of immunity to sperm. Since patient populations vary greatly between reported studies and since infertility is frequently multifactorial, it has been difficult to establish the clinical significance of reactivity to sperm. In contrast, assisted reproduction provides a framework in which multifactorial causes of infertility can be controlled. Sperm antibody findings in couples undergoing assisted reproduction should therefore be generally applicable to an infertile population. The following is a summary of presently known facts about sperm antibodies in females

*and* males in reference to their impact on assisted reproduction.

## General aspects

Antibodies to sperm have been implicated as a causative factor of infertility as well as pregnancy wastage in animals and humans (Bell & McLaren 1979, Bronson et al 1984, Haas et al 1986). It is, however, still largely unknown how this infertility occurs. Various possibilities have been documented. They include interference with acrosome reaction and capacitation (Saling et al 1985), conversion of cervical mucus to an impermeable state (Wang et al 1985), interference of sperm–oocyte attachment (Bronson et al 1982) and oocyte penetration as well as oocyte fertilization (Kamada et al 1985).

The association between sperm antibodies and pregnancy wastage reported by Haas et al (1986) made us consider the possibility that individuals with sperm antibodies may also demonstrate other antibody abnormalities. After all, we never noted a *single* and *specific* antibody abnormality in any group of patients with reproductive failure, as has previously been noted. We therefore investigated a group of sperm antibody-positive females and males for the presence of other (and possibly related) immunological abnormalities (El-Roeiy et al 1988a). As Figure 14.2 demonstrates, in full concordance with other previously discussed conditions of reproductive failure, both

**Table 14.4** Selected sperm antibody assays in use

Immunobead assays
  Direct
  Indirect
Mixed agglutination reaction (MAR)
Radiolabelled antiglobulin assay
Immunofluorescense assays
Enzyme-linked immunoabsorbent assays (ELISA)
Sperm agglutination assays
  Microagglutination (Friberg test)
  Franklin–Dukes
  Kibrick
  Tray agglutination test (TAT)
  Tube-slide agglutination test (TSAT)
Complement dependent cytotoxicity assays

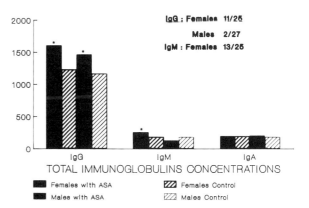

**Fig. 14.2** Immunoglobulin levels in sperm antibody-positive females and males. Asterisk (*) indicates statistically significant increase over controls. (Reproduced with permission from El-Roeiy et al 1988a).

sperm antibody-positive females as well as males demonstrated significantly elevated total immunoglobulin levels. Moreover, when sperm antibody-positive females and males were investigated for the presence of classical autoantibodies, such as phospholipid antibodies, antihistones and antipolynucleotides, a very significant range of positivity was noted in both sexes (Fig 14.3). Most of this reactivity was noted among antiphospholipid antibodies, though especially among IgM isotypes reactivity was also present among antipolynucleotides and antihistones.

These observations further convinced us that

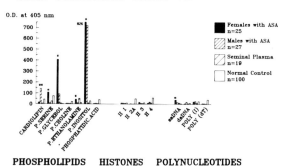

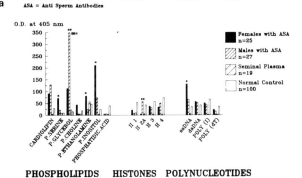

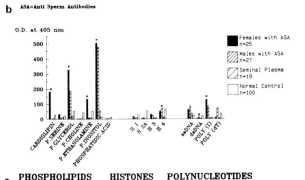

**Fig. 14.3** **a** IgG, **b** IgM, **c** IgA autoantibodies in sperm antibody positive females and males. (Reproduced with permission from El-Roeiy et al 1988a).

the immunological interruption of reproductive processes, while sometimes specific, universally is accompanied by a nonspecific polyclonal immune response. Since we are at present unable to confirm the presence of specific immune responses in affected individuals, it behoves us to search for the nonspecific immune response, characterized by abnormal total immunoglobulin levels and abnormal autoantibodies.

Further support for this concept in patients with sperm antibodies comes from the fact that sperm antibody activity can be absorbed with nonspecific autoantigens and that sperm antibody binding to nonspecific antigens can be inhibited with sperm (A. El-Roeiy & N. Gleicher unpublished data). To prove this point, we had the opportunity to work with a panel of human as well as mouse monoclonal sperm antibodies, kindly provided by P. Saling (Duke University, Durham, NC) and A. Menge (University of Michigan, Ann Arbor). Figure 14.4 demonstrates graphically that out of 30 monoclonal sperm antibodies, three were basically cross-reactive with nonorgan-specific autoantibodies. The figure also demonstrates that cross-reactivity was not only encountered with phospholipid antibodies but also with antibodies to polynucleotides. More interestingly, one of the cross-reactive monoclonal sperm antibodies (M37) has been previously shown by P. Saling to inhibit fertilization in the mouse model. This observation then strongly suggests that the cross-reactive nonorgan-specific autoantibody may have the same effect.

Figure 14.5a demonstrates how phospholipid micelles inhibit the binding of this M37 monoclonal mouse sperm antibody to mouse sperm. From a different vantage point, Figure 14.5b demonstrates how mouse sperm inhibits the binding of phospholipid antigens to M37 and, lastly, Figure 14.5c shows how this cross-reactivity between M37 and phospholipid antibodies can be tested through the inhibition of M37 binding with phospholipids by phospholipid micelles. The same cascade of experiments is demonstrated in Figure 14.6 though this time for a monoclonal sperm antibody called 20.D3, which demonstrated cross-reactivity to antipolynucleotides (all, A. El-Roeiy & N. Gleicher, unpublished data).

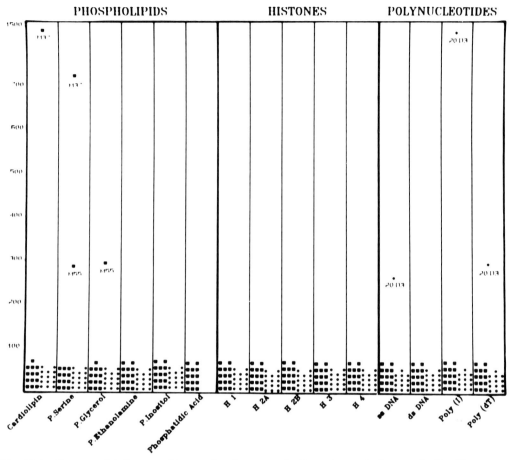

**Fig. 14.4** Cross-reactivity between 30 monoclonal sperm antibodies and a panel of autoantibodies. Two monoclonal sperm antibodies were reactive to phospholipids, cardiolipine, phosphatidylserine (X2) and phosphatidylglycerol, while one was reactive to polynucleotide ss DNA and Poly (dT).

These observations thus establish a link between the presence of sperm antibodies and the presence of other nonorgan-specific autoreactivities. This is further supported by the previously noted association of pregnancy loss with both nonorgan-specific autoantibodies and sperm antibodies. We believe that this association extends beyond the area of miscarriages into the area of infertility and therefore recommend the investigation of nonorgan-specific autoantibodies in sperm antibody-positive individuals and the investigation of sperm antibodies in autoantibody-positive patients.

### Sperm antibodies in the female

As noted earlier, assisted reproductive technolo-

gies (ART) lend themselves well to the investigation of the effect of sperm antibodies on fertility. Unfortunately, the investigation of sperm antibodies with ART presents some of the same problems outlined earlier. For example, Table 14.5 summarizes presently reported IVF experience in the presence of sperm antibodies in the female. From this table it will be quite clear that a large variety of sperm antibody tests have been utilized. If a trend can be detected, then one has to assume from these data that sperm antibodies in the female *possibly* adversely affect fertilization, embryo quality and pregnancy rates.

Vasquez-Levine et al (1991) reported recently what is so far the most comprehensive study on the topic. By investigating 33 females in 50 cycles who were sperm antibody positive

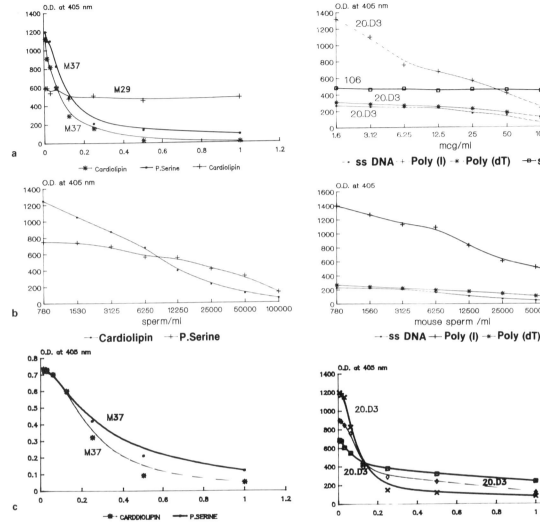

**Fig. 14.5** a–c demonstrate different binding experiments, all showing cross-reactivity between phospholipid antibodies and the monoclonal sperm antibody M37, previously demonstrated to inhibit fertilization in the mouse. For more detail see text.

**Fig. 14.6** a–c demonstrate similar binding experiments as shown in Figure 14.5 for the monoclonal sperm antibody 20.D3, which shows cross-reactivity with polynucleotide antibodies.

by immunobead assay, they noted a significant decrease in fertilization rate over 70 controls. Moreover, zygote cleavage rates were reduced, less advanced embryos developed and more unfavorable embryos were noted in sperm antibody-positive individuals. These observations strongly support an adverse effect of sperm antibodies in female IVF patients and thus provide further credence to the notion that sperm antibodies affect fertility adversely.

As most other studies on the subject, this one

too should be interpreted with caution. The authors were unable to demonstrate a correlation with a specific immunoglobulin class or with antibodies to a specific sperm region. Lastly, the authors reported many patients with IgM isotypes, in our experience a rather rare finding.

Clarke et al (1986) demonstrated that fertilization rates varied with the protein source utilized for media preparation: IgG and IgA sperm antibody-positive patient serum gave fertilization in 15%, while antibody-negative serum resulted in 69% fertilization. The same authors (Clarke et al

**Table 14.5**  Sperm antibodies in females

| Authors | Assay | Fertilization + | − | = | Embryo qual. + | − | = | Pregnancies + | − | = |
|---|---|---|---|---|---|---|---|---|---|---|
| Yovich et al 1984 | GAT, TSAT | | | X | | | X | | | X |
| Ackerman et al 1984 | AGGL, IMMOB | X | | | − | − | − | − | − | − |
| Clarke et al 1985 | ? | | | X | − | − | − | − | − | − |
| Pexieder et al 1985 | ELISA | X | | | | | X | | X | |
| Ausmanas et al 1986 | RAGT | | | X | | | X | | | X |
| Mandelbaum et al 1987 | IBA | X** | | | X** | | | ?X** | ?X** | |
| De Almeida et al 1987 | TSAT | | | X | | | X | | | X |

Assay: GAT, gelatin agglutination test; TSAT, tray slide agglutination test; RAGT, radiolabeled agglutination test; TBA, immunobead assay;
** Single case.
† For antibodies to spermhead *only*.

1988) reported in another publication that the random incubation of supernumerary oocytes from GIFT patients in sperm antibody-positive and -negative sera resulted in fertilization rates of 41% and 84%, respectively; a statistically significant difference. Serum that was most effective in preventing fertilization was the one with the highest IgG sperm antibody titers.

ART data on sperm antibodies in the female thus quite strongly suggest an adverse effect on fertility. Because of the previously noted cross-reactivity of some sperm antibodies with some nonorgan-specific autoantibodies, these data thus corroborate the earlier discussed potential effects of nonorgan-specific autoantibodies on fertility.

We therefore strongly support the investigation of sperm antibodies and of a panel of nonorgan-specific autoantibodies in all females with an infertility problem, and especially if they are to undergo an ART. In antibody-positive females undergoing ART, it appears beneficial to substitute their serum as a protein source. Whether further therapy is indicated has remained controversial. Some authors have suggested a clinical benefit from low dose corticosteroid therapy, though controlled trials are not available. We empirically treat antibody-positive females with low dose prednisone.

## Sperm antibodies in the male

The impact of sperm antibodies in the male has

been already alluded to in the section on abnormal autoimmune function. Table 14.6 summarizes the related ART experience. The reported experience allows only limited conclusions, probably even more so than in the female. Here, as well, it appears that sperm antibodies can affect fertility adversely. Van der Merwe et al (1990) have suggested that GIFT results in superior pregnancy rates in males with sperm antibodies. Why that should be is, at least on a theoretical basis, unclear.

Treatment of male infertility due to sperm antibodies has remained controversial. High dose corticosteroid levels for affected males appear of only limited or of no benefit. Since potential side-effects are abhorrent, this treatment approach has been largely abandoned. Danazol is now widely used in a variety of autoimmune diseases to reduce autoantibody levels, and we recently attempted to lower sperm antibodies in males through danazol therapy (Gleicher et al 1992b). In males with sperm antibodies it appeared ineffective.

One then is left with the mechanical approach of trying to 'wash off' sperm antibodies. Success of sperm washing will clearly depend on the affinity of a particular antibody to sperm. High-affinity antibodies can probably not be washed off. The validity of this approach is, however, suggested by quite satisfactory pregnancy rates in sperm antibody-positive males (and females) after intrauterine insemination with washed sperm (Confino et al 1986).

364 INFERTILITY: MALE AND FEMALE

**Table 14.6** Sperm antibodies in males

| Authors | Assay | Fertilization + | − | = | Embryo Quality + | − | = | Pregnancies + | − | = |
|---|---|---|---|---|---|---|---|---|---|---|
| Palermo et al 1989* | MAR | X | | | X | | | X | | |
| Junk et al 1986 | IBA | X[†] | | | − | − | − | − | − | − |
| Clarke et al 1985 | SIT | X[†] | | | X | | | X | | |
| Ausmanas et al 1986 | RAGT | | X | | X | | | X | | |
| van der Merwe et al 1990 | MAR | − | − | − | − | − | − | | | X[‡] |

Assay: MAR, mixed agglutination reaction (direct); IBA, immunobead assay; SIT, sperm immobilization test; RAGT, radiolabeled agglutination test.
\* Involved 25 couples treated with IVF, ZIFT, GIFT (32/313 cycles).
† Only if IgG and IgA antibodies present.
‡ GIFT cycles only.

## CONCLUSION

Immunological infertility is a relatively new concept, especially when one is willing to go beyond the concept of sperm antibodies. As the endocrine system and immune system appear increasingly interlinked, one can expect immunological concepts to assume increasing importance within the framework of normal as well as abnormal reproductive processes. It is hoped that this chapter provides an appropriate introduction.

## REFERENCES

Ackerman S B, Graff D, van Uem Jfhm, et al 1984 Immunologic infertility and in vitro fertilization. Fertil Steril 42: 474

Adashi E Y 1990 The potential relevance of cytokines to ovarian physiology: the emerging role of resident ovarian cells of the white blood cell series. Endocr Rev 11: 454

Ausmanas M, Tureck R W, Ben-Rafael Z et al 1986 Immunologic infertility and in vitro fertilization (IVF). Presented at the 42nd Meeting of the American Fertility Society and the 18th Meeting of the Canadian Fertility and Andrology Society, Toronto, Canada, 27 September – 2 October.

Beer A E, Quebbeman J F, Ayers J W T et al 1981 Major histocompatibility complex antigens, maternal and paternal immune responses and chronic habitual abortions in humans. Am J Obstet Gynecol 141: 987

Bell E B, McLaren R 1979 Reduction in fertility in female mice iso-immunized with a sub cellular sperm fraction. J Reprod Fertil 22: 345

Biscotti C V, Hart W R, Lucas J G 1989 Cystic ovarian enlargement resulting from autoimmune oophoritis. Obstet Gynecol 74: 492

Bronson R A 1990 Sperm antibodies. In: Gleicher N (ed) Reproductive immunology. Immunol Clin North Am 10: 165

Bronson R A, Cooper G W, Rosenfeld D L 1982 Sperm specific isoantibodies and autoantibodies inhibit the binding of human sperm to the human para pellucida. Fertil Steril 38: 724

Bronson R, Cooper G, Rosenfeld D 1984 Sperm antibodies: their role in infertility. Fertil Steril 42: 171

Caudle M R, Shivers C A, Wild R A 1987 Clinical significance of naturally occurring anti-zone pellucida antibodies in infertile women. Am J Reprod Immunol Microbiol 15: 119

Clarke G N, Lopata A, McBain J C, Baker H W G, Johnston W I H 1985 Effect of sperm antibodies in males on human in vitro fertilization (IVF). Am J Reprod Immunol 8: 62

Clarke G N, Lobata A, Johnson W I H 1986 Effect of sperm antibodies in females on human in vitro fertilization. Fertil Steril 46: 435

Clarke G N, Hyne R V, du Plessis Y, Johnston W I H 1988 Antibodies and human in vitro fertilization. Fertil Steril 49: 1018

Cohen I, Speroff L 1991 Premature ovarian failure: update. Obstet Gynecol Surv 46: 156

Confino E, Friberg J, Dudkiewicz A B, Gleicher N 1986 Intrauterine inseminations with washed spermatozoa. Fertil Steril 46: 55

Confino E, Harlow L, Gleicher N 1990 Peritoneal fluid and serum autoantibody levels in patients with endometriosis. Fertil Steril 53: 242

Coulam C B, Ryan R 1985 Prevalence of circulating antibodies directed toward ovaries among women with premature ovarian failure. Am J Reprod Immunol 9: 23

Coulam C B, Stern J J 1991 Immunology of ovarian failure. Am J Reprod Immunol 25: 169

De Almeida M, Herry M, Testart J et al 1987 In vitro fertilization results from thirteen women with anti-sperm antibodies. Hum Reprod 2: 599

Dor J, Rudak E, Aitken R J 1981 Antisperm antibodies: their effect on the process of fertilization studied in vitro. Fertil Steril 35: 535

Editorial 1984 Lupus anticoagulant. Lancet i: 1157

El-Roeiy A, Gleicher N, Friberg J, Confino E, Dudkiewicz A B 1987 Correlation between peripheral blood and follicular fluid autoantibodies and impact on in vitro fertilization. Obstet Gynecol 70: 163

El-Roeiy A, Valessini G, Friberg J et al 1988a Autoantibodies and common idiotypes in men and women with sperm antibodies. Am J Obstet Gynecol 158: 596

El-Roeiy A, Dmowski W P, Gleicher N, Radwanska E et al 1988b; Danazol but not gonadotropin-releasing hormone agonists suppresses autoantibodies in endometriosis. Fertil Steril 50: 864

Fisch B, Rikover Y, Shohat L et al 1991 The relationship between in vitro fertilization and naturally occurring antibodies: evidence for increased production of antiphospholipid autoantibodies. Fertil Steril 56: 718

Gleicher N 1987 Is endometriosis an autoimmune disease? Obstet Gynecol 70: 115

Gleicher N (ed) 1992 Autommunity. In:Principles and practice of medical therapy in pregnancy, 2nd edn. Appleton & Lange, New York, pp 413–421

Gleicher N, Friberg J 1985 IgM gammopathy and the lupus anticoagulant syndrome in habitual aborters. JAMA 253: 3278

Gleicher N El-Roeiy A, Confino E, Friberg J 1989 Reproductive failure because of autoantibodies: unexplained infertility and pregnancy wastage. Am J Obstet Gynecol 160: 1376

Gleicher N, Pratt D, Kaberlein G, Dudkiewicz A B 1992a Premature ovarian failure is characterized by gammopathies (submitted)

Gleicher N, Pratt D, Kaberlein G, Novotny M, Dudkiewicz A, 1992b Danazol does not suppress sperm antibodies in males. (submitted)

Haas G G, Kubota K, Queebman J F et al 1986 Circulating sperm antibodies in recurrently aborting women. Fertil Steril 45: 209

Halme J, Becker S, Wing R 1984 Accentuated cyclic activation of peritoneal macrophages in patients with endometriosis. Am J Obstet Gynecol 1487: 85

Hill J A 1990 Immunological mechanisms of pregnancy maintenance and failure: a critique of theories and therapy. Am J Reprod Immunol 22: 33

Hill J A, Anderson D J 1989 Lymphocyte activity in the presence of peritoneal fluid from fertile women and infertile women with and without endometriosis. Am J Obstet Gynecol 161: 861

Jones W R 1990 Infertility. In: Scott J S, Bird H A (eds) Pregnancy autoimmunity and connective tissue disorders. Oxford Medical Publications, Oxford, pp 279–300

Junk S M, Matson P L, Yovich J M, Bootsma B, Yovich J L 1986 The fertilization of human oocytes by spermatozoa from men with antispermatozoal antibodies in semen. J In Vitro Fert Embryo Transf 3: 350

Kamada M, Dactoh T, Hasebe H et al 1985 Blocking of human fertilization in vitro by serum with sperm immobilizing antibodies. Am J Obstet Gynecol 153: 328

Kwak-Kim J Y H, Bahar A M, Kim J H et al 1990 Antibodies to nuclear components and phospholipid epitopes are not induced or increased in women with recurrent spontaneous abortions (RSA) who are immunized with lymphocytes. Am J Reprod Immunol 22: 78 (abstr)

Lubbe W F, Butler W S, Palmer S J 1983 Fetal survival after prednisone suppression of maternal lupus anticoagulant. Lancet i: 1361

Mandelbaum S L, Diamond M P, DeCherney A 1987 Relationship of antisperm antibodies to oocyte fertilization in vitro fertilization—embryo transfer. Fertil Steril 47: 644

Mathur S, Genco P V, Williamson H O, Koopman Jr W R, Rust P F, Fudenberg H 1983 Association of human leucocyte antigens B7 and BW 35 with sperm antibodies. Fertil Steril 39: 343

Miake T, Taguchi O, Ikeda H et al 1988 Acute oocyte loss in experimental autoimmune oophoritis as possible model of premature ovarian failure. Am J Obstet Gynecol 158: 186

Michael S D, Chapman J C 1990 The influence of the endocrine system on the immune system. In: Gleicher N (ed) Reproductive immunology. Immunol Allergy Clin North Am 10: 215

Mignot M H, Shoemaker J, Kliengold M et al 1989 Premature ovarian failure. 1. The association with autoimmunity. Eur J Obstet Reprod Biol 30: 59

Moncayo H, Moncayo R, Bentz R et al 1989 Ovarian failure and autoimmunity: detection of autoantibodies against both the unoccupied luteinizing hormone/human chorionic gonadotropin receptor and the hormone – receptor complex of bovine corpus luteum. J Clin Invest 84: 1857

Palermo G, Devroey P, Camus M et al 1989 Assisted procreation in the presence of a positive direct mixed antiglobulin reaction test. Fertil Steril 52: 645

Pexieder T, Boillat E, Janecek P 1985 Antisperm antibodies and in vitro fertilization failure. J In Vitro Fert Embryo Transf 2: 229

Saling P M, Rons G, Waibel R 1985 Mouse sperm antigens that participate in fertilization. Inhibition of sperm fusion with the egg plasma membrane using monoclonal antibodies. Biol Reprod 33: 515

Sedmark D D, Hart W R, Tubbs R R 1987 Autoimmune oophoritis: A histopathologic study of involved ovaries with immunologic characterization of the mononuclear cell infiltrate. Int J Gynecol Pathol 6: 73

Skinner S M, Timmons T M, Schwoebel E D, Dunbar B S 1990 The role of zona pellucida antigens in fertility and infertility. In: Gleicher N (ed) Reproductive immunology. Immunol Allergy Clin North Am 10: 185

Steinleitner A, Lamberth H, Suarez M, Sedpa N et al 1991 Periovulatory calcium channel blockade enhances reproductive performance in an animal model for endometriosis-associated subfertility. Am J Obstet Gynecol 164: 949

Taylor P V, Campbell J M, Scott J S 1989 Presence of autoantibodies with unexplained infertility. Am J Obstet Gynecol 161: 377

Toder V, Shomer B 1990 The role of lymphocytes in pregnancy in reproductive immunology. Gleicher N (ed). Immunol Allergy Clin North Am 10: 65

van der Merwe J P, Kruger T F, Windt M L, Hulme V A, Menkveld R 1990 Treatment of male sperm autoimmunity by using the gamete intrafallopian transfer procedure with washed spermatozoa. Fertil Steril 53: 682

Vasquez-Levin M, Kaplan P, Guzman I, Grunfeld L, Garrisi G J, Navot D 1991 The effect of female antisperm antibodies on in vitro fertilization, early embryonic development, and pregnancy outcome. Fertil Steril 56: 84

Wang C, Baker H W G, Jennings M G et al 1985 Interaction between human cervical mucus and sperm surface antibodies. Fertil Steril 44: 484

Yovich J L, Kay D, Stanger J D, Boettcher B 1984 In-vitro fertilization of oocytes from women with serum antisperm antibodies. Lancet i: 369

# Treatment of infertility (female)

# 15. Gonadotropin releasing hormones

*Bruno Lunenfeld    Vaclav Insler*

## INTRODUCTION

Information arising in the central nervous system (CNS) or travelling through the bloodstream from other parts of the body culminates at the hypothalamus. The overall summation of these stimulatory and inhibiting signals results in the secretion of specific peptides from highly specialized hypothalamic neurons. These secretions, the releasing hormones, then stream along the neuron axon and are released at the nerve terminals located in the median eminence. There they are collected by the venous portal system and travel along the pituitary stalk to the anterior pituitary gland where they exert their action.

In 1971 the groups of Schally and of Guillemin isolated the luteinizing releasing factor (LHRF) and later described its amino acid content and sequence (Burgus et al 1971, Matsuo et al 1971, Schally et al 1971, Guillemin 1978).

It is still not clear whether the hypothalamus secretes only one peptide capable of inducing the release of both LH and FSH or there are two different releasing hormones, each for one gonadotropin. The belief in one releasing hormone is widely accepted since administration of the highly purified native hormone or its synthetic analogs causes the secretion of both luteinizing hormone (LH) and follicle-stimulating hormone (FSH) in vivo and in vitro (Schally et al 1971, Herbert 1976).

## CELLULAR MECHANISMS OF ACTION

The gonadotrophs comprise 10–15% of the total number of pituitary cells, and gonadotropin hormone releasing hormone (GnRH) binds selectively to these cells (Naor et al 1982).

The initial response of the gonadotroph to a GnRH stimulus is brisk and, as the signal fades, the cell stops releasing the hormone. This short stimulation is possible because of the rapid degradation of GnRH at the pituitary level.

The main stages of GnRH action upon the gonadotrophs are schematically presented in Figure 15.1. The decapeptide binds to specific receptors situated in the cell membrane. The hormone-receptor (H–R) complex is then internalized into the cell. It seems that a specific G-1 protein enchances this process by coupling with the H–R complex. G proteins probably play a role in signal transduction involving control of calcium and other second messengers. They also exert a function in regulation of cell growth and gating of ion channels.

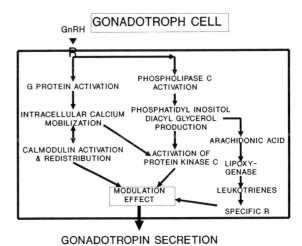

**Fig. 15.1** Schematic representation of molecular mechanism of GnRH action in the pituitary gonadotrope cell.

369

It seems that internalization of the H–R complex by itself does not mediate the biological response of the gonadotroph cell but rather serves as a means for ligand degradation and receptor recycling.

It has been postulated that several different substances such as calcium ions, inositol triphosphate (IP-3), arachidonic acid (AA) and diacylglycerol (DG) act as second messengers. This indicates that inside the gonadotroph cell GnRH activates simultaneously and/or sequentially a whole array of signals and functions which finally lead to gonadotropin synthesis and release.

One of the most important initial functions of GnRH is mobilization of intracellular calcium and opening of channels in the cell membrane enabling an influx of extracellular $Ca^{2+}$. This process is facilitated by activation and redistribution of calmodulin. It should be noted that an increase of intracellular calcium levels is capable of stimulating LH release even in the absence of GnRH receptor occupation. GnRH increases the rate of conversion of phosphatidic acid to phosphatidyl inositol (PI) and its further transformation into IP-3 and DG. This process is a result of activation of the phospholipase C system. Increased production of PIs in the gonadotroph cells does require the presence of GnRH bound to the receptor.

DG plays an important role in activation of protein kinase C (PKC). PKC is involved in LH-β mRNA production which indicates its role in stimulation of the LH β-subunit gene expression. There is, however, still no general agreement whether PKC is absolutely required for production and release of LH in all settings.

AA present in the gonadotroph cell may be metabolized by the lipoxygenases pathway into 5-hydroxyeicosatetraenoic acid (5-HETE) and a set of leukotrienes. These substances coupled to their specific receptors exert a modulating action on the effect of mobilization of calcium ions and phosphoinositide turnover, i.e. on the assembling and transfer of FSH- and LH-containing granules through the cell membrane and, consequently, secretion of these hormones into the blood-stream.

The mechanism of action of GnRH presented above has been intentionally simplified and compressed (for more extensive discussion see excellent reviews by Ben-Menahem et al 1990 and by Hawes & Conn 1990). It shows, however, that this simple decapeptide is capable of initiating multiple responses such as biosynthesis and release of FSH and LH, receptor regulation and cell responsiveness by simultaneous activation of a whole set of different but interdependent pathways.

GnRH has been shown not only to induce the secretion of gonadotropins but also to participate in their synthesis. Liu & Jackson (1978) showed in the rat that GnRH had an impact on the incorporation of carbohydrate residues (mainly sialic acid) into the molecule. They demonstrated that the carbohydrate content of LH released in response to GnRH stimulation differed from that released in the absence of exogenous GnRH and that there were two pools of secretable LH: stored and newly synthesized. The two could be differentiated by the carbohydrate content of their molecules. The newly synthesized releasable molecule contained more carbohydrate than the stored one and was biologically more active.

## PATTERN OF GnRH SECRETION

GnRH is secreted from the hypothalamus in a pulsatile fashion (i.e. short periods of abrupt secretion separated by longer periods of low or undetectable secretion). When the plasma levels of immunoreactive endogenous LHRH in women were measured by Elkind-Hirsch & colleagues (1982) they were found to be cyclic with a frequency approximating 1 pulse per hour.

The frequency and amplitude of the GnRH pulses are crucial for release of LH and FSH. Knobil's group (Pohl et al 1983) demonstrated that intermittent administration of exogenous GnRH to monkeys with arcuate nucleus lesions re-established the gonadotropin pulsatile secretion as indicated by peripheral plasma levels. In contrast, continuous administration of the releasing hormone at different infusion rates failed to restore gonadotropin secretion. Furthermore, in ovariectomized hypothalamic-lesioned monkeys, changing the GnRH pulse frequency itself or its amplitude had a direct influence on the secretion and relative amount of each of the gonadotropins. Thus, raising the frequency from the 'physiological' 1 pulse per hour rate to 3 or 5 pulses per hour reduced the secretion of both LH and FSH (Fig. 15.2). Lowering the frequency to 1 pulse every 3 h caused a variable decline in LH levels but not in FSH levels, which, in fact, rose (Fig. 15.3).

Lowering the exogenous GnRH pulse amplitude while keeping the pulse frequency at the 'physio-logical' rate resulted in a decline of both gonadotropins to undetectable levels. Raising the pulse amplitude under these conditions lowered the FSH levels but not the LH levels (Wildt et al

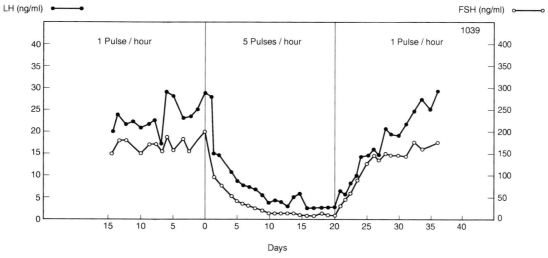

**Fig. 15.2** FSH and LH response to pulsatile GnRH administration. Suppression of gonadotropin secretion in a rhesus monkey bearing a hypothalamic lesion by increasing the frequency of GnRH infusion (1 mg min for 6 min) from 1 pulse/h to 5 pulse/h on day 0. Reinstitution of the standard frequency of 1 pulse/h 5 pulse/h on day 20 resulted in a graduate restoration in LH and FSH concentrations to control levels. (Reproduced with permission from Wildt et al 1981)

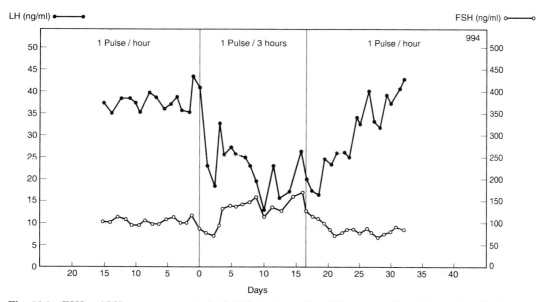

**Fig. 15.3** FSH and LH response to pulsatile GnRH administration. Effect on gonadotropin secretion of reducing the frequency of pulsatile GnRH administration in a rhesus monkey bearing a hypothalamic lesion from 1 pulse/h to 1 pulse/3 h on day 0. Note the dramatic fall of LH and the rise in FSH concentration during the experimental period. Reinstitution of the standard frequency of 1 pulse/h on day 16 resulted in a graduate restoration in LH and FSH concentrations to control levels. (Reproduced with permission from Wildt et al 1981)

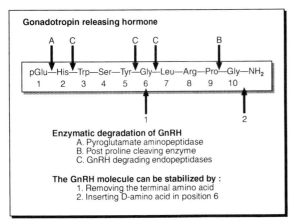

**Fig. 15.4**    Enzymatic degradation of GnRH.

1981). This experimental model indicates that the secretory reaction of the pituitary gland depends on the frequency and intensity of GnRH challenge.

## GnRH ANALOG: AGONISTS AND ANTAGONISTS

GnRH is a decapeptide. Its amino acids sequence is shown in Figure 15.4. The spatial structure of the molecule and its receptor binding characteristics are determined by the pyroglutamic acid in position 1 and by the amino acids in positions 4–10. The histidine and tryptophan acids in positions 2 and 3 are crucial in determining the molecular activity and substitution of these two amino acids, resulting in numerous analog that differ from the natural molecule by higher or lower activity.

A simple D-amino acid substitution in position

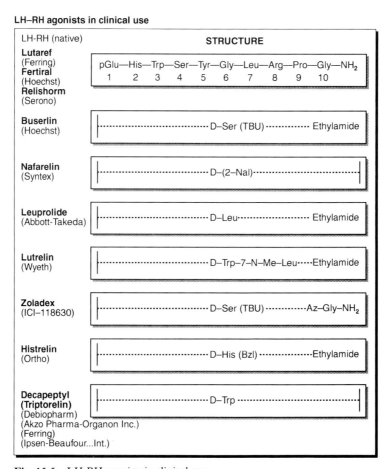

**Fig. 15.5**    LH-RH agonists in clinical use.

6 is common to most agonists. Many are nine amino acid peptides, the glycine in position 10 being replaced by an ethylamide group. These simple modifications impart an increase in binding affinity to pituitary GnRH receptors and/or an increased resistance to the proteolytic degradation that rapidly destroys native GnRH. Up until now more than 2000 GnRH analogs have been produced and more than a dozen are commercially available (Fig. 15.5). Modification in position 2 and substitution of several amino acids, or changing the GnRH by reducing the size of the amino acids chain, may produce materials with biological action opposite to that of the native hormone (GnRH antagonists). Further improvement in potency was then sought by modifications in various other positions. This led to potent GnRH antagonists which had about five of the original amino acids replaced by unnatural amino acid residues (Fig. 15.6).

The overall hydrophobicity and basicity of the original GnRH sequence are significantly increased in these antagonists. This combination of increased hydrophobicity and basicity has led to the problem of histamine release induced by most of the potent antagonists. This problem has previously been associated with a number of other peptides, e.g. substance P, which contain hydrophobic and basic residues (Dutta 1989). Recently analogs lacking in histamine-releasing activity have been synthesized and these can broadly be categorized into three types. The first approach involved switching the residues

between positions 5 and 6. The second and third approaches were based on reducing the overall hydrophobicity and shielding the side-chain basic groups. These were achieved by replacing the D-Trp$^3$ with D-Pal$^3$ and also by incorporating various substituents, e.g. isopropyl, nicotinyl or picolyl, on the side-chain amino groups in positions 5, 6 and 8 (Fig. 15.6).

GnRH is transported by the venous portal system to the pituitary where it exerts its action and is then degraded. Although the GnRH molecule appears to be designed for a rather long biological half-life because of the pyroglutamic residue blocking the amino end of the molecule to protect it from degradation by aminopeptidases and the amide function to protect the carboxyl end of the peptide from degradation by carboxypeptidases, native GnRH has a very short half-life. This is due to the fact that brain enzymes inactivate GnRH at the Gly$^6$ Leu$^7$ bond very rapidly (Hazum et al 1981, Goren et al 1990) (Fig. 15.5). GnRH is also metabolized in the kidney, as shown by in vivo studies with tritiated GnRH (Redding et al 1973) and the observation that the clearance rate of exogenous GnRH was calculated to be $1640 \pm 60$ ml per minute and the plasma half-life to be $5.5-8.0$ min in the normal subject (Pimstone et al 1977).

The portal vein concentration of GnRH was measured by Carmel & colleagues (1976) in the Rhesus monkey. During the early follicular phase they found basal levels of $66.0 \pm 6.6$ pg/ml interrupted by rapid rises in concentration (pulses) up to 200 pg/ml. In patients undergoing transsphenoidal surgery, they found levels ranging from undetectable to 1000 pg/ml.

## DIAGNOSTIC USE OF GnRH

GnRH acts directly on the pituitary and, when administered intravenously as a bolus, tests the size of the releasable pool of pituitary gonadotropin (Fig. 15.7). It is important to recognize that when the pituitary has not been previously primed by GnRH, this response to GnRH may not occur due to inadequate number or response capability of GnRH receptors. In such cases, continued stimulation with GnRH is called for prior to performing the standard GnRH test.

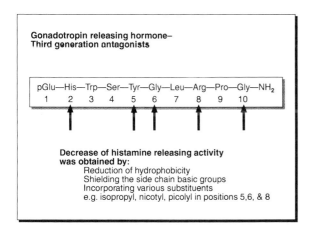

Fig. 15.6 GnRH third-generation antagonists

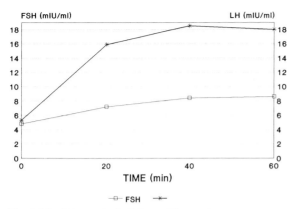

**Fig. 15.7**   Diagnostic GnRH test. The test is regarded as positive when intravenous or subcutaneous injection of a 100 µg bolus of GnRH results in a significant increase in FSH and LH within 20–40 min.

The standard test for adults is to administer 100 mg of GnRH intravenously in a bolus and then to obtain blood samples for gonadotropin assays every 15 min for 1 h. In adult females a variable response is observed depending on the phase of the menstrual cycle. In the early follicular phase, a three- to four-fold increase is observed in serum LH, while in the preovulatory period the increments can be much higher. Since LH release is modulated by estrogens, this difference in response is due to higher estrogen levels normally found in the latter part of the follicular phase. The test has some value in the localization of lesions in the hypothalamic-hypophyseal axis. However, it seems that the initial high hopes for the diagnostic value of GnRH in classifying amenorrheic patients into defined groups have not been fulfilled. Consensus has now been reached that amenorrheic women do not require a dynamic test with GnRH unless one is planning to induce ovulation by chronic intermittent infusion of this hormone. (The diagnostic use of GnRH in male infertility is discussed in Chapter 12.)

## THERAPEUTIC APPLICATIONS IN WOMEN

The use of GnRH can be considered for patients lacking endogenous gonadotropins who have a pituitary gland capable of responding to this medication. Thus, GnRH has a place in the treatment of hypothalamic amenorrhea.

In 1971 Kastin et al reported the use of GnRH to evoke sufficient LH secretion to induce ovulation in an amenorrheic patient after follicular growth and maturation was stimulated by human menopausal gonadotropin (hMG). The patient conceived and delivered a healthy baby. Since then a number of similarly induced ovulations and pregnancies have terminated in the births of healthy babies. It should be noted that all the women in this group exhibited endogenous estrogen activity before the commencement of the treatment. Administration of GnRH alone has been used for the treatment of infertility in hypothalamic amenorrhea and anorexia nervosa (Nillius & Wide 1979), however, its effectiveness has been limited.

Search of the early literature regarding the clinical use of nonpulsatile GnRH therapy revealed that in 218 trials only 67 ovulations and 14 conceptions occurred (Blankstein et al 1986).

Thus, the initial high hopes for GnRH therapy were not fulfilled, and the general interest in this treatment approach declined. Lack of the expected clinical responses to nonpulsatile administration of GnRH, even in high doses, is not surprising in view of the concept of down-regulation. Early experiments with GnRH agonist showed that initial stimulation of gonadotropin release was followed by return to baseline levels or below. Receptor binding studies showed that the latter effect was due to a decrease in the number of receptors on the cell and not to an alteration of the affinity of receptors for GnRH (Belchetz et al 1978). Following Knobil's (1980) demonstration that imitation of the physiological pulsatile pattern of GnRH could restore ovarian function in the hypothalamus-lesioned monkeys, interest in the therapeutic use of GnRH was again stimulated.

Leyendecker et al (1980) showed that it was possible to induce ovulation followed by pregnancy in an amenorrheic patient with hypothalamic failure by pulsatile intravenous administration of GnRH through a computerized infusion pump.

### Technique

GnRH is administered by a computerized

portable minipump attached to an indwelling intravenous or subcutaneous catheter. Frequent monitoring of the patient is necessary in order to detect whether there are any complications from the catheter (phlebitis, local inflammation, etc.) and to ensure that the pump functions well. The pulse frequency and dose are adjusted to the patient's response. Dosages and pulse frequencies used by various authors are shown in Table 15.1. Periodic measurement of serum FSH and LH can ascertain whether the pituitary responds normally and adequately to the pulsatile GnRH stimulation. The response to pulsatile administration of GnRH is reflected by the elevation of serum FSH and LH secretion and by an anatomical growth of follicles accompanied by biochemical changes mainly with respect to increased synthesis and secretion of steroid hormones. The follicular enlargement can be visualized by ultrasonographic measurements, and estrogen secretion can be measured directly by urine or blood assays, or indirectly by their effect on secondary targets such as the cervical mucus.

The patient is instructed to record basal body temperature (BBT) daily. This will permit detection of the day of presumed ovulation, allow an assessment of the length of the luteal phase, and help to determine the day when blood should be drawn for progesterone (day 5–8 post BBT nadir). It will also indicate whether a pregnancy can be suspected and when human charionic gonadotrophin (hCG) determination should be performed, as well as establish when treatment should be stopped. The cervical score (Insler et al 1972) should be estimated periodically from the fifth day on, in order to detect the initial estrogenic activity. This will assist in recognizing when the active phase of follicular growth started. When the cervical score is above 8 points, monitoring is continued by estrogen determination. When urinary estrogen levels reach about 80 µg/24 h, or serum estradiol is 250 pg/ml, ultrasonographic visualization of the ovaries should be undertaken. All these measurements enable assessment of the time of ovulation and a decision to be made on the optimal timing of coitus. At this point the patient is instructed to have sexual intercourse and to return to the clinic between 2 and 10 h thereafter. During this visit a cervical mucus sample is taken, the cervical score estimated, and a postcoital test performed. Treatment with GnRH may be interrupted whenever a satisfactory follicular diameter is reached and estrogen levels are in an acceptable range, at which time hCG is administered to induce ovulation. One or more additional hCG applications can be given in order to support the luteal function (Leyendecker et al 1980). Another possibility is to continue GnRH administration for both induction of ovulation and corpus luteum support (Martin et al 1990).

## Results

The results obtained by treatment with chronic

**Table 15.1**  Results obtained with intermittent GnRH at different doses and treatment schedules

| Author and year | Patients (no.) | Dose/pulse (µg) | Interval (min) | Route | Cycles (no.) | Ovulations | Pregnancies |
|---|---|---|---|---|---|---|---|
| Crowley & McArthur 1980 | 5 | 1.5–3.0 | 120 | SC | 3 | 3 | — |
| Leyendecker et al 1980 | 8 | 2.5 – 20 | 89 | IV | 26 | 26 | 6 |
| Nillius et al 1981 | 14 | 500 | 480 | SC | 14 | 11 | 2 |
| Schoemaker et al 1982 | 9 | 100 | 120 | IV | 8 | 5 | — |
| Schoemaker et al 1982 | 9 | 20 | 120 | IV | 20 | 17 | 5 |
| Schoemaker ct al 1982 | 9 | 20 | 96 | IV | 3 | 3 | 1 |
| Schoemaker et al 1982 | 9 | 10 | 90 | IV | 1 | 1 | — |
| Skarin et al 1982 | 6 | 20 | 90 | SC | 16 | 7 | 1 |
| Blankstein et al 1986 | 295 | 12.5–25 | 90 | IV | 516 | 405 | 135 |
| Berg et al 1983 | 27 | 20 | 90 | IV | 40 | 32 | 11 |
| Weber et al 1983 | 5 | 10–20 | 90 | IV | 5 | 4 | — |
| Coelingh-Bennink 1983 | 11 | 10– 40 | 90 | IV | 27 | 19 | 7 |
| Martin et al 1990 | 21 | 2.5–25 | 60–120 | IV | 76 | 73 | 19 |
| Hamburg et al 1989 | 118 | 15 | 90 | SC | 434 | 300 | 100 |

IV, intravenous; SC, subcutaneous.

intermittent (pulsatile) GnRH administration are summarized in Table 15.1. Schoemaker et al (1982) reported on different doses and different pulse intervals in 32 treatment cycles. By administering 100 μg of GnRH every 120 min, they achieved five ovulations in eight cycles, but no pregnancies. With this treatment regimen the authors found that the LH response showed a preovulatory dip and that both LH and FSH peaks were lower than those observed when 20 μg of GnRH were administered every 120 min. With the latter treatment regimen they achieved 17 ovulations in 20 cycles, and five pregnancies occurred. With 20 μg of GnRH every 96 min intravenously they achieved three ovulations in three cycles and one pregnancy. With 10 μg of GnRH each 20 min intravenously, one ovulation occurred, but no pregnancy resulted. From reviews of the available literature, it seems that doses between 3.4 and 20.0 μg, with pulse intervals between 62.5 and 120.0 min, are capable of eliciting pituitary response sufficient for follicular stimulation resulting in ovulation.

Martin et al (1990) summarized that the ovary is capable of tolerating a moderate range of GnRH-induced gonadotropin pulse frequencies for adequate follicular development and corpus luteum function. However, follicular phase frequencies slower than 90 min result in an abnormal midcycle LH surge and, consequently, in anovulation.

Reviewing 36 papers published between 1980 and 1984 (Blankstein et al 1986), 916 treatment cycles in 388 patients could be assessed. The conception rate was 56%, multiple gestation rate 7.3%, abortion rate 14.5% and hyperstimulation rate 1.1%. Homburg et al (1989) reported on 118 patients treated over 434 cycles resulting in 300 ovulations and 100 conceptions.

Martin et al (1990) reviewed the American experience with subcutaneous and intravenous pulsatile GnRH therapy for ovulation induction. In 300 cycles of subcutaneous pulsatile GnRH treatments, 75% resulted in ovulation and the conception rate was 30% per ovulatory cycle. Over 500 cycles of intravenous GnRH therapy resulted in an ovulation rate of 90%, the pregnancy rate, however, did not exceed 30% per ovulatory cycle.

## Side-effects

In principle all main complications of ovarian stimulation following clomiphene or gonadotropin therapy, such as multiple pregnancy, ovarian hyperstimulation and increased abortion rate, have also been observed after pulsatile GnRH application.

The multiple pregnancy rate after GnRH treatment is similar to that following clomiphene (5–8%) but significantly lower than that generated by gonadotropins (20–30%). Severe ovarian hyperstimulation is extremely rare and ovarian cysts (mild hyperstimulation) have been rather infrequent and resolved spontaneously after cessation of therapy (Schriock & Jaffe 1986). The abortion rate which is rather high with other types of ovulation-inducing therapy (15–25%) is very similar (29%) following GnRH treatment (Homburg et al 1989). One complication, i.e. the possibility of infection due to the indwelling intravenous catheter, is particular to the pulsatile application of GnRH. It seems, however, that this risk is not significant. Hopkins et al (1989) investigated 38 patients with 230 catheters in place for 4–52 days. The incidence of positive catheter tips cultures was 11%. Of 195 blood cultures obtained at the time of catheter removal, four were positive (2%). None of these four patients had any clinical signs of infection. Superficial phlebitis may occasionally be observed but disappears after withdrawal of the catheter. Although rather rare and without clinical consequences in healthy women, infection secondary to the indwelling intravenous catheter may present a tenable risk to women with mitral heart prolapse. Since many such women may be symptomless and not aware of the disease, it is advisable to perform a thorough cardiac examination in all candidates for pulsatile GnRH therapy. In patients suffering from mitral valve prolapse, the subcutaneous route of GnRH application or other ovulation-inducing therapy should be considered.

Failure due to mechanical defects was sometimes noted. Specifically, there were temporary interruptions of the pump function that resulted in periodic discontinuation of GnRH, causing luteal deficiencies expressed clinically by short luteal phases. Thus, in order to obtain optimal results with chronic intermittent administration of GnRH careful monitoring of pituitary and ovarian responses is necessary.

## GnRH ANALOG: AGONISTS AND ANTAGONISTS

Ever since the isolation, identification and synthesis of GnRH in 1971, the interest in the application of GnRH analogs has undergone an explosive growth rate. The potency of GnRH and its analogs as stimulators (when administered in a precise pulsatile fashion) or inhibitors of pituitary gonadotropin secretion (when administered chronically) permitted its exploration as a method of temporary gonadotropin-specific medical hypophysectomy. This ability permitted its exploitation as a method of reversible medical gonadectomy applied to treatment of diseases dependent on gonadal steroids. It served as a basis for developing four types of treatment modalities, based on different rationales (Lunenfeld & Insler 1991):

1. To suppress sex steroids in diseases in which development or progress is sex steroid dependent (metastatic prostatic cancer, hormone-dependent breast and endometrial cancer, uterine fibroids, and endometriosis).

2. To inhibit the precocious appearance of mature-type GnRH pulsatility (central precocious puberty) or to impede normal onset of pubertal GnRH pulsatility in order to postpone epididymal closure and thus permit growth to continue (slow-growing children).

3. To control the dynamics of gonadotropin secretion in induction of ovulation or superovulation (as adjunctive treatment of anovulation, polycystic ovary disease (PCOD) and assisted reproduction protocols.

4. To exploit possible local effects of GnRH agonists on tissues having GnRH receptors (some types of malignancies, uterine fibroids, etc.).

In the management of the infertile patient, where conventional treatment regimens had failed, GnRH agonists have been successfully utilized to suppress the pituitary ovarian axis, prior to stimulation of follicular growth and induction

of ovulation concomitantly with exogenous gonadotropins.

## GnRH agonists in the management of the infertile patient

In the management of the infertile patient, where conventional treatment regimens had failed, GnRH agonists have been successfully utilized to suppress the pituitary ovarian axis, prior to and concomitant with stimulation of follicular growth and induction of ovulation with exogenous gonadotropins.

It is well known that hypopituitary amenorrheic patients with low estrogens (Group I) respond better to gonadotropin therapy than normogonadotropic anovulatory, oligoovulatory women or patients with PCOD (Group II) (See Chapter 16). Some of these differences in response to stimulation seem to be inherent to the functional characteristics of the hypothalamic-pituitary-ovarian axis. Excessive LH during the follicular phase may interfere with normal follicular development, ovulation, fertilization or implantation. An untimely LH surge may cause luteinization of premature follicles or luteinization of an unruptured follicle (LUF syndrome) simulating the hormonal pattern of ovulation.

Laboratory synthesis of potent and/or long-acting analogs of GnRH makes it possible to efficiently reduce (down-regulate) the production and release of pituitary gonadotropins (Crowley et al 1981, Borgman et al 1982, Meldrum et al 1982, Yen 1983, Insler et al 1988a).

Treatment schemes combining pituitary suppression by GnRH analogs with ovarian stimulation by exogenous gonadotropins seemed therefore particularly attractive.

Bettendorf et al (1981) reported on preliminary results with this treatment module. They used the nasal spray of buserelin to suppress pituitary function and hMG/hCG to induce ovulation. However, in this trial the extent of pituitary down-regulation was ascertained by basal levels of FSH and LH only and not by dynamic tests. Moreover, in some cases, the GnRH analog was discontinued before the application of gonadotropins. Combined GnRH analog/gonadotropin therapy has been reinvestigated by several groups

(Bettendorf et al 1988, Fleming et al 1988, Hedon 1988). Our own experience with this type of treatment seems to be quite interesting (Insler et al 1988b, Lunenfeld 1988). Pretreatment with GnRH agonists reduces significantly the FSH levels within 14–21 days. The reduction of LH levels is also apparent but is significant only in cases in which the basic levels were relatively high. In the majority of cases treated with either daily or with monthly injections of decapeptyl or with nasal applications of buserelin, the levels of plasma estradiol and the pituitary response to estradiol benzoate stimulation was also significantly reduced. Ovarian stimulation by gonadotropins, when applied after down-regulation of the axis was achieved by GnRH agonist, required a higher hMG dose, a longer therapy and produced more follicles than the treatment by gonadotropins alone. However, these follicles

were probably smaller and less competent as indicated by the levels of estradiol, which were not significantly different in combined GnRH agonist/gonadotropin as compared to gonadotropin-alone therapy. Figure 15.8 shows a course of combined GnRH analog/gonadotropin therapy in a patient of Group II who was previously treated with repeated courses of clomiphene citrate and of hMG/hCG but failed to ovulate and/or conceive. The full potential of the combined pituitary suppression/ovarian stimulation therapy cannot yet be accurately assessed. To enable such an assessment, extensive and detailed information regarding the indications, the precise dosage and timing and the best monitoring parameters will have to be generated and critically analysed.

A relatively large subgroup of patients with hypothalamic pituitary dysfunction in whom the combined treatment with GnRH analogs and

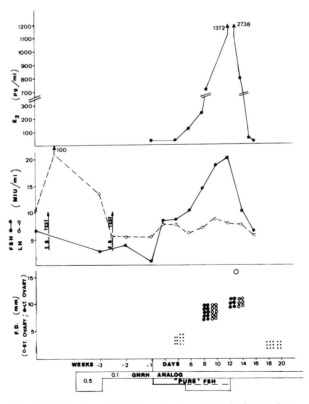

**Fig. 15.8** Combined GnRH analog/gonadotropin therapy in a patient belonging to WHO Group II. Note that in spite of an excessive amount of estradiol (over 2500 pg/ml), no LH surge was elicited.

FSH is of particular interest are those with PCOD. The term PCOD includes a state of ovarian abnormality and chronic hormonal imbalance which leads to multifactorial abnormalities in folliculogenesis and ovulation, rather than a single disease entity. Its characteristics are the marked variability in clinical, endocrine and morphological presentation and pathophysiology (see Chapter 26). Coutts et al in 1988 showed that in infertile PCOD patients the pregnancy rate achieved with this combined therapy was significantly higher (75%) than that obtained with hMG alone (38%). Preovulatory luteinization was totally eliminated by the combined therapy. Studies on PCOD patients treated with FSH showed that in those with relatively lower urinary LH output, the chances of obtaining high quality oocytes increased, giving rise to embryos which survived to implant. In women who conceived but had an early abortion, urinary LH output was significantly higher compared to those who continued their pregnancy. Further studies showed that women who had early miscarriage but later returned and successfully maintained the second pregnancy, had significantly lower LH output in the treatment leading to conception and normal outcome compared to the one leading to fetal loss. Trying to explain the high frequency of early abortions in hMG-treated women, Homburg et al (1988) proposed a further explanation suggesting that the presence of high tonic LH levels too soon in late follicular phase create early resumption of meiosis and consequently premature maturation of oocytes which may give rise to embryos which survive implantation but are lost in early pregnancy. All these facts seem to support the hypothesis that although GnRH agonists do not cure PCOD, prolonged administration may temporarily obscure the disease, and by improving the hormonal milieu may, in conjunction with FSH, allow follicular development to proceed normally. Following hCG administration ovulation will occur permitting fertilization of a mature egg with normal implantation.

## The use of GnRH agonists in IVF programs

The realization that FSH is capable of increasing the recruitment rate of new crops of small follicles, and is capable of stimulating multiple and normal follicular growth and development to the preovulatory stage with the yield of many fertilizable eggs, prompted the use of gonadotropins as the preferred treatment modality in most IVF programs. With the use of gonadotropins for induction of superovulation in normally ovulating women conceptual changes in our monitoring schemes had to be introduced. When attempting to induce ovulation, in anovulatory women the challenge was to imitate as much as possible the normal cycle and to aim at a single dominant follicle and prevent multiple follicular growth, multiple pregnancies and hyperstimulation. In IVF or GIFT programs in contrast the conceptual idea is to use a superphysiological dosage in order to obtain a large number of fertilizable eggs. For this purpose many different protocols have emerged each with its own merits and disadvantages and all using ultrasonographic procedures to estimate both the number and size of the growing follicles and estradiol assays to estimate their functional integrity (see Chapter 21). It is logical to assume that enlarging recruitment rate of follicles and deviating follicular developement from luteinization and atresia towards dominance will coincide with exaggerated estradiol levels. However, due to the asynchrony of follicular development, the increased production of estradiol will not always coincide with a similar production of 'inhibins' or other intraovarian regulators. Thus, in ovulatory women with a normal pituitary ovarian axis, the exaggerated estradiol levels provoke in about 15% of treatment cycles an untimely spontaneous LH surge leading to cancellation of ovum pick-up. The possibility of desensitizing the pituitary gland with superactive GnRH analogs and thus inhibiting its capability to respond to estradiol with an LH surge (Shadmi et al 1987), has prompted many investigators to use GnRH analogs prior to and in combination with hMG. This treatment regimen has already proven its merits in making logistics easier, significantly reducing cancellation rates and thus increasing the overall success rate in IVF programs. However, the temporary functional gonadotropic-specific hypophysectomy has introduced new challenges. It is possible to design stimulation protocols creating a predominantly FSH environment during the recruitment phase, eliminating an excessive endogenous LH environment which may interfere with normal follicular development. It should, however, be remembered that our knowledge regarding the optimal intra- and extrafollicular conditions required for full and synchronized maturation of follicle and ovum is still incomplete. For example, it is known that untimely repression of the meiosis-inhibiting factors provoke overaging of eggs with a significant reduction in their fertilization or implantation capacity. Treatment protocols available at present are, however, incompetent at exerting a fine-tuned control of ovum maturation.

Moreover, inhibition of endogenous gonadotropins following ovulation induction by hCG may, if not properly monitored, interfere with the luteal phase. The choice of the GnRH analog to be used depending on its delivery system, its mode of administration and its biological half-life will dictate the optimal gonadotropic treatment protocol considering follicular recruitment and development, ovulation induction and the corpus luteum function. The triphasic therapeutic regimen using GnRH agonists prior to and in combination with gonadotropins has been efficiently used for the stimulation of multiple follicular development in IVF programs. Its efficacy has been demonstrated already in 1986 from the data of the French IVF national register (FIVNAT, 1986, personal communication). At that time GnRH agonists in combination with hMG were used in 10.8% of the 5948 IVF cycles. The 21% pregnancy rate/cycle and 29.1% pregnancy rate/transfer was significantly higher than with clomiphene citrate (CC/hMG) (13% and 20.1% respectively) or with hMG (15.6% and 21.9%). The efficacy of GnRH agonist hMG combination therapy prompted its increased usage in France which reached 66% of all IVF cycles in 1988.

## ENDOMETRIOSIS

Endometriosis is a perplexing disease of unknown etiology and poorly understood histogenesis. It is characterized by ectopic, i.e. outside of the uterine cavity, growth of the endometrium. The growth and spread of endometriosis are controlled by the cyclic stimulation of ovarian hormones. After cessation of ovarian function, e.g. during the menopause, when ovarian estradiol and progesterone are no longer secreted, uterine as well as ectopic endometrium undergo atrophy and endometriosis resolves (see Chapter 20).

In view of the hormone dependency of endometriosis, the possibility of selectively suppressing the ovarian secretion of estrogens by repetitive GnRH administration is a new therapeutic approach to this disease. In the human, the main mechanism explaining the inhibitory effect of superactive GnRH agonist is a reversible down-regulation of gonadotropin secretion inducing a state of hypogonadotropic hypogonadism (pseudomenopause or medical castration).

An international multicentre trial (Kiesel et al 1989) was carried out using buserelin (900 µg/d, intranasally) for the treatment of endometriosis. Two hundred and seventy-five patients were included in the study and started treatment. The disorder was diagnosed by laparoscopy. Two hundred and thirty-nine women completed the treatment period of 6 months. After therapy, a second-look laparoscopy was performed in the majority of patients to determine the efficacy of this analog on endometriosis implants. In addition, endocrine parameters and changes of symptoms were monitored.

In 95% of all patients, serum estradiol levels were sufficiently suppressed during the 6-month treatment period. An improvement of implants according to American Fertility Society (AFS) classification occurred in 80%, and no change was observed in 69% of the patients. Of the 275 patients, 9% discontinued the treatment, but only 10 patients dropped out because of the side-effects experienced. The onset of ovulation was observed in 76% of the cases within 1 or 2 months after therapy. Of 90 infertile patients wanting children within a short term, 23% became pregnant in the first 6 months after treatment.

During therapy, dysmenorrhea, pelvic pain and dyspareunia improved considerably. Biochemical tests assessing electrolytes, liver function tests and hematology prior to initiation of therapy, at the end of therapy and at 6 months following termination of treatment revealed no significant differences.

This multicenter trial conducted in various countries provides important evidence of the efficacy or LHRH analogs in the treatment of endometriosis.

## UTERINE LEIOMYOMAS

Uterine leiomyomas or fibroids are neoplasms of smooth muscle found in approximately 20% of women older than 30 years. Fibroids are the most common tumors of the female genital organs and probably the most common tumor in women. Fibroids are commonly associated with infertility, menorrhagia and/or dysmenorrhea. Management of patients who have symptomatic uterine fibroids has traditionally been surgical: myomectomy for patients desirous of children or hysterectomy for women with very large or multiple fibroids or whose families are complete.

LHRH agonists by creating a hypoestrogenic environment provide for the first time a medical treatment for uterine fibroids. LHRH agonists significantly shrink these tumors in the majority of patients and cause them to clinically disappear in a minority of subjects. The potential impact of such treatment upon current gynecological care of patients with uterine fibroids may be significant. Such impact may be at various levels, especially with the pending availability of suitable implant systems of LHRH agonists for chronic gynecological disease such as fibroids or endometriosis. Preoperative use of LHRH agonists for uterine fibroids seems especially suited to women scheduled to undergo fibroid myomectomy. Patients less than 35 years old appear particularly suitable to preoperative LHRH-agonist treatment as shrinkage of fibroids is more consistent in this age group. Such patients are also more likely to complain of infertility and in these circumstances reduction of estrogen-dependent uterine blood flow, as well as the reduction in tumor size, are both important surgical advantages. GnRH analogs may also allow a less invasive surgical operation since 83% of uterine fibroids treated

with GnRH analogs will become smaller. GnRH agonists availability has also advanced understanding of the pathogenesis of the most common neoplasm in women. Chronic use of intranasal or subcutaneous LHRH agonists, or the pending widespread availability of biodegradable lactide-glycolide copolymers which can be injected as a single subcutaneous injection every 4 or 8 weeks provides a hypoestrogenic environment that distinguishes fibroids which are estrogen dependent for growth from those which are not. Furthermore, such medicines have been used in related tumors, such as benign metastasizing leiomyoma. Potential medical therapy not only for fibroids and other benign tumors, but also for leiomyosarcomas may now be possible, offering new options for gynecological tumors.

Wiznitzer et al (1988) showed that GnRH analogs can cause regression of uterine leiomyomas. This effect is thought to be mediated by the inhibition of gonadotropin release and steroid synthesis. They examined the possibility that these analogs may also act directly on uterine leiomyomas. Specific binding sites for GnRH are present in myoma membranes, as [125]I-labelled-buserelin binding was displaced with equal efficiency by the superagonists, buserelin and D-Trp[6]-GnRH, and by the antagonist Organon 30276, but not by unrelated peptides such as thyrotropin releasing hormone and oxytocin. A nonlinear Scatchard curve obtained for buserelin-specific binding suggests the presence of at least two binding sites, one of which exhibits a relatively high affinity for GnRH analogs (kDa of $10^{-8}$M). Western blotting with a specific GnRH receptor antibody revealed the presence of a 60-kDa protein in myoma membranes. This protein has a similar molecular weight to the purified pituitary GnRH receptor. These results indicate, for the first time, the presence of specific binding sites for GnRH in uterine leiomyomas, suggesting a direct effect of GnRH analogs on the tissue.

## POSSIBLE EFFECTS OF GnRH ANALOGS ON LIPID PROFILES AND BONE DENSITY

The possible adverse effects of repeated or long-term application of potent GnRH analogs to premenopausal women must be addressed. It has been established that hot flushes, vaginal dryness, excitability and lack of menstruation appear following approximately 6 weeks of therapy. All the above signs and symptoms vanish within 4–8 weeks after cessation of treatment.

It is well known that estrogens are involved in the control of lipid and bone metabolism. Temporary 'medical gonadectomy' caused by GnRH therapy obviously instigates a state of hypoestrogenism. It is clear that many clinicians have been anxious to obtain reliable data concerning the possible influence of this therapy on blood lipids and bone mineral content.

Dmowski et al (1989) found no change in total cholesterol during 6 months' treatment with buserelin. HDL cholesterol increased slightly from the baseline and LDL cholesterol did not change. Assessing the effect of GnRH analogs on bone turnover has proven to be difficult for several important reasons. Many of the currently available techniques of measuring bone have limitations which are well documented in the literature (Health and Public Policy Committee 1984, Davis 1987, Hall et al 1987, Ott et al 1987, Kelly et al 1988). These methods may encompass a broad range of normals and thus the detection of small changes in bone mass may be difficult (Ott et al 1987). Furthermore, a variety of techniques has been used in these studies including measurements of bone in the wrist and spine, as well as total body calcium (Cann et al 1986, Comite et al 1987, Barnes et al 1988, Johansen et al 1988). Unfortunately, these methods are not necessarily analogous, and the differences between measurements of the spine and wrist are an important consideration. The spine, unlike the wrist, is a weightbearing bone. Weightbearing bones can compensate for early bone loss by increasing the thickness of the primary (vertical) supporting trabeculae, to offset the loss of the secondary (horizontal) trabeculae (Singh et al 1970). This obscures the earlier loss of bone mass. Thus, this normal compensatory physiological response of the weightbearing bone in situations of altered bone turnover may partially explain reported differences in bone density between the spine, an axial bone, and nonweightbearing appendicular bones, like the wrist. This is, in fact, supported by the observa-

tion that Colles' fractures of the wrist, in contrast to hip and spine fractures which occur in late menopause, begin in the immediate postmenopausal period and the rate of fracturing increases quickly (Gallagher et al 1980). Thus, weightbearing bones may actually be less sensitive indicators of generalized changes in the skeleton in the premenopausal, perimenopausal and early postmenopausal years (Roberts et al 1982). For these reasons, it would be important to evaluate nonweightbearing sites such as the wrist, as well as the spine and hip, sites at which the longer term sequelae of a hypoestrogenic state may have a more pronounced deleterious impact but the outcome may not be evident until much later in life.

Several non-invasive methods are available for measuring bone mass. Single energy photon absorptiometry (SPA), dual energy photon absorptiometry (DPA), quantitative computed tomography (QCT) and neutron activation analysis (NA) have been extensively used (Laval-Jantet et al 1984, Jensen & Orphanoudakis 1985, Gotfredsen et al 1986, Davis 1987, Ott et al 1987), but their accuracy and correlation to the bone strength and ability to withstand fracture are still debated.

Although low bone mass is a significant risk factor for osteoporosis and potential fractures, other variables, such as protective muscle mass, the collagen matrix, ability to repair microfractures and biological variation, would ultimately be important to consider in evaluating the long-term risk of inducing alterations in bone turnover in the women exposed to GnRH analogs prior to menopause.

Bone changes during administration of GnRH agonist have been already fairly extensively studied. Some studies report no bone loss, while others found that some bone mass reduction appears, but the loss is reversible after discontinuation of GnRH therapy (Comite et al 1986, Kenigsberg et al 1987; Matta et al 1987 Comite & Jensen 1988, Tummon et al 1988). Some of the disagreement may be due to the variety of sites monitored as well as the differences in methods used. However, even with the same techniques findings were not necessarily comparable in different studies. While this may appear at first to be perplexing, this disagreement could be significant. First, there may be a decrease in bone mass but it may be small compared to the sensitivity of most of the techniques used. Nevertheless, small changes in bone turnover may be clinically significant.

The disparity in studies on the effect of GnRH analogs on bone could be important because it might imply that other factors could have been responsible for the outcome. A multitude of variables could differ in these studies. For example, the subjects could vary in response to GnRH analog treatment with regard to the degree and duration of hypoestrogenemia, caused by incomplete suppression. Alternatively, the occurrence of an intermittent 'agonist' or stimulatory effect with periodic release of estradiol might be responsible. This stimulatory or agonistic action might counteract the potential negative effect of an unrelenting hypoestrogenemia by periodic exposure to estrogen with its protective impact on bone turnover, effectively counter-balancing negative bone turnover. Individuals on GnRH analog might also have variable bone loss due to insufficient calcium intake. The occurrence of a relative hypoestrogenemia would result in decreased absorption of dietary calcium, together with the loss of the protective effect of estrogen upon parathyroid hormone (PTH). Suboptimal intake of calcium, coupled with increased mobilization of skeletal calcium and urinary excretion due to altered bone turnover might also lead to differences in the relative degree or absence of bone loss sustained on analog therapy. Furthermore, the underlying disorder for which the analog was given (i.e. endometriosis), as well as the age of the subject) (i.e. perimenopausal women) and the fact that individuals may lose or gain bone at different rates, may affect bone turnover. All the above factors may complicate the detection of any drug-induced impact. This is important if, as some of these studies have reported, this bone loss may be prevented (Comite et al 1987 Kenigsberg et al 1987; Matta et al 1987; Comite & Jensen 1988, Tummon et al 1988). Consequently, carefully designed prospective and longitudinal studies with controls for these variables to address these issues are essential.

## REFERENCES

Barnes R B, Mercer L J, Montner S 1988 Characterization of bone loss during treatment with a depot gonadotropin-releasing hormone agonist (GnRHa). The American Fertility Society, Atlanta, Georgia (abstr)

Belchetz P E, Plant T M, Nakai Y et al 1978 Hypophysial responses to continuous and intermittent delivery of hypothalamic gonadotropin-releasing hormone. Science 202

Ben-Menahem D, Dan-Cohen H, Naor Z 1990 Mechanism of action of gonadotropin releasing hormone: Interaction of $Ca^{2+}$ and protein kinase C. Isr J Obstet Gynecol 1: 49

Berg D, Mickan H, Michael S et al 1983 Ovulation and pregnancy after pulsatile administration of gonadotropin releasing hormone. Arch Gynecol 233: 205

Bettendorf G, Brendle W, Weise C, Poels W 1981 Effect of gonadotropin treatment during inhibited pituitary function In: Insler V, Bettendorf G (eds) Advances in diagnosis and treatment of infertility. Elsevier/North Holland, New York, p 43

Bettendorf G, Braendle W, Lichtenberg V, Lindner U K E 1988 Pharmacologic hypogonadotropism—an advantage for gonadotropin stimulation. Gynecol Endocrinol 2 (suppl 1): 66

Blankstein J, Mashiach S, Lunenfeld B 1986 Ovulation induction and in vitro fertilization. Year Book, Chicago

Borgman V, Hardt W, Schmidt-Gollwitzer M, Adenauer H, Nagel R 1982 Sustained suppression of testosterone production by the luteinizing hormone-releasing hormone agonist, Buserelin, in patients with advanced prostate carcinoma. Lancet i: 1097

Burgus R, Butcher M, Ling N et al 1971 Structure moleculaire du facteur hypothalamique (LRF) d'origine ovine controlant la secretion de l'hormone gonadotrope hypophysaire de luteinisation (LH). CR Acad Sci [D] (Paris) 273: 1611

Cann C E, Henzl M, Burry K, Andreko J, Hanson F, Adamson D, Trobough G 1986 Reversible bone loss is induced by GnRH Agonists. The Endocrine Society, Anaheim, California (abstr)

Carmel P W, Araki S, Ferin M 1976 Pituitary stalk portal blood collection in rhesus monkeys: evidence for pulsatile release of gonadotropin releasing hormone (GnRH). Endocrinology 99: 243

Coelingh-Bennink H J T 1983: Induction of ovulation by pulsatile intravenous administration of LHRH in polycystic ovarian disease. The 65th Annual Meeting of the Endocrine Society, San Antonio, Texas, 8–10 June

Comite F, Jensen P 1988 Bone density changes associated with GnRH analogs. International Symposium on GnRH Analogues in Cancer and Human Reproduction, Geneva, Switzerland

Comite F, Cassorla F, Barnes K M, Hench K D, Dwyer A, Skerda M C, Loriaux D L, Cutler G B, Pescovitz O H 1986 Luteinizing hormone releasing hormone analogue therapy for central precocious puberty: long term effect on somatic growth, bone maturation, and predicted height. JAMA, 255: 2613

Comite F, Jensen P, Lewis A, Hutchinson K, Polan M L,

DeCherney A H 1987 GnRH analog therapy in endometriosis: impact on bone mass. Society for Gynecologic Investigation, Atlanta, Georgia, (abstr)

Coutts J R T, Finnie S, Conaghan C, Black W P, Fleming R 1988 combined buserelin and exogenous gonadotrophin therapy for the treatment of infertility in women with polycystic ovarian disease. Gynecol Endocrinol 2 (suppl 1): 71

Crowley W F, McArthur J W 1980 Stimulation of the normal menstrual cycle in Kallman's syndrome by pulsatile administration of luteinizing hormone-releasing hormone. J Clin Endocrinol Metab 51: 173

Crowley W F, Comite F, Vale W, Rivier J, Loriaux D L, Cutler G B 1981 Therapeutic use of pituitary desensitization with a long-acting LH-RH agonist: a potential new treatment for idiopathic precocious puberty. J Clin Endocrinol Metab 52: 370

Davis M R 1987 Screening for postmenopausal osteoporosis. Am J Obstet Gynecol 156

Dmowski W P, Radvanska E, Binor Z, Tummon I, Pepping P 1989 GnRH agonists in the management of endometriosis: results of two randomized trials. In: Vickery B H, Lunenfeld B (eds) GnRH analogues in cancer and human reproduction, vol 2. Kluver Academic Publishers, Dordrecht, pp 7–15

Dmowski W P, Radwanska E, Binor Z, Tummon I, Pepping P 1990 GnRH agonists in the management of endometriosis: the results of two randomized trials. In: Vickery B H, Lunenfeld B (eds) GnRH analogues in reproduction and gynecology. Cluwer Academic, London, pp 7–15

Dutta A S 1989 Chemistry of GnRH analogues. In: Vickery B H, Lunenfeld B (eds) GnRH analogues in cancer and human reproduction, vol 1. Kluver Academic Publishers, Dordrecht, pp 33–43

Elkind-Hirsch K, Schiff I, Ravnikar V et al 1982 Determinations of endogenous immuno-reactive luteinizing hormone releasing hormone in human plasma. J Clin Endocrinol Metab 54: 602

Fleming R, Carter N, Jameson M E, Black W P, Coutts J T R 1988 Combined buserelin and exogenous gonadotropins (hMG/hCG) ovulation induction in infertile women with normal menstrual rhythm: results and implications. Gynecol Endocrinol 2(suppl 1): 69

Gallagher J C, Melton L J, Riggs B L, Bergstrath E 1980 Epidemiology of fractures of the proximal femur in Rochester, Minnesota. Clin Orthop, 150: 163

Goren A, Zohar Y, Fridkin M, Elhanati E, Koch Y 1990 Degradation of gonadotropin-releasing hormones in the gilthead seabream, *Sparus aurata*. I. Cleavage of native salmon GnRH and mammalian LHRH in the pituitary. Gen Comp Endocrinol 79: 291

Gotfredsen A, Nilas L, Riis B J, Thomsen K, Christiansen C 1986 Bone changes occurring spontaneously and caused by oestrogen in early postmenopausal women: a local or generalised phenomenon? Med J 292: 1098

Guillemin R 1978 Peptides in the brain: the new endocrinology of the neuron. Science 202: 390

Hall F M, Davis M A, Baran D T 1987 Bone mineral screening for osteoporosis. N Engl J Med 316: 212

Hawes B E, Conn P M 1990 GnRH mediated actions in the gonadotrope. In: Yen S C, Vale W W (eds) Neuroendocrine regulation of reproduction. Serono Symposia, Norwell, Mass, ch 21

Hazum E, Fridkin M, Baram T, Koch Y 1981 Degradation of gonadotropin releasing hormone by anterior pituitary enzymes. FEBS Lett 127: 273

Health and Public Policy Committee, American College of Physicians 1984 Radiologic methods to evaluate bone mineral content. Ann Intern Med, 100: 86

Hedon B 1988 Use of GnRH agonists for in vitro fertilization. Gynecol Endocrinol 2(suppl 1): 34

Herbert D C 1976 Immunocytochemical evidence that luteinizing hormones (FSH) are present in the same cell in the rhesus monkey pituitary gland. Endocrine 98: 1554

Homburg R, Armar N A, Eshel A, Adams J, Jacobs H S 1988 Influence of serum luteinising hormone concentration on ovulation, conception and early pregnancy loss in polycystic ovary syndrome. Br Med J 297: 1024

Homburg R, Eshel A, Armar N A et al 1989 One hundred pregnancies after treatment with pulsatile luteinising releasing hormone to induce ovulation. Br Med J 298: 809

Hopkins C C, Hall J E, Santoro N F, Martin K A, Filicori H, Crowley W F 1989 Closed intravenous administration of gonadotropin releasing hormone (GnRH): safety of extended peripheral intravenous catheterization. Obstet Gynecol 74: 267

Insler V, Melmed H, Eden E et al 1972 The cervical score: a simple semi-quantitative method for monitoring of the menstrual cycle. Int J Gynaecol Obstet 10: 223

Insler V, Lunenfeld E, Potashnik G, Levy J 1988a The effect of different LH-RH agonists on the level of immunoreactive gonadotropins. Gynecol Endocrinol 2: 305

Insler V, Potashnik G, Lunenfeld E, Meizner I, Levy J 1988b Ovulation induction with hMG following down regulation of the hypothalamic pituitary axis by LHRH analogs. Gynecol Endocrinol 2(suppl 1): 67

Jensen P S Orphanoudakis S C 1985 Clinical results from longitudinal determination of bone mass using quantitative computed tomography. J Comput Assist Tomogr 9: 627

Johansen J S, Riis B J, Hassager C, Moen M, Jacobson J, Christiansen C 1988 The effect of a gonadotropin-releasing hormone agonist analog (nafarelin) on bone metabolism. J Clin Endocrinol Metab 67: 701

Kastin A J, Zarate A, Midgley A R, Canales E, Schally A V 1971 Ovulation confirmed by pregnancy after infusion of porcine LHRH . J Clin Endocrinol Metab 33: 980

Kelly T L, Slovik D M, Schoenfeld D A, Neer R M 1988 Quantitative digital radiography versus dual photon absorptiometry of the lumbar spine. J Clin Endocrinol Metab 67: 839

Kenigsberg D, Hull M, Yasumura S, Cohn S, Ellis K 1987 Total body calcium (TBC) by neutron activation (NA) and osteocalcin (OC) in GnRH agonist (GnRHa) treated women with endometriosis. Society for Gynecologic Investigation, Atlanta Georgia (abstract)

Kiesel L, Thomas  K, Tempone A et al 1989 Efficacy and safety of buserelin in women with endometriosis—a multicenter open label study. Gynecol Endocrinol 3(suppl 2) : 5

Knobil E 1980 Neuroendocrine control of the menstrual cycle. Recent Prog Horm Res 36: 53

Laval-Jeantet M H, Roger B, Laval_Jeantet A M, Bergot C, Preteux F 1984 Anatomical basis of vertebral densitometry. In Fourth International Workshop on Bone and Soft Tissue

Leyendecker G, Struve T, Plotz E J 1980 Induction of ovulation with chronic intermittent (pulsatile) administration of LHRH in women with hypothalamic and hyperprolactinemic amenorrhea. Arch Gynecol 229: 177

Liu T C, Jackson G L 1978 Modification of luteinizing hormone biosyntehsis by gonadotropin releasing hormone, cycliheximide and actinomycin D. Endocrinology 103: 1253

Lunenfeld B 1988 Indication and management of GnRH analogues in ovulation induction protocols. Gynecol Endocrinol 2(suppl 1): 33

Lunenfeld B, Insler V 1991 The rationale and practice of GnRH therapy. In: Lunenfeld B  Insler V (eds). The curent status of GnRH analogues. Parthenon, Carnfarth, Lancashire UK, pp 13–17

Martin K, Santoro N, Hall J, Filicori M, Wierman M, Crowley W F 1990 Management of ovulatory disorders with pulsatile gonadotropin-releasing hormone. J. Clin Endocrinol Metab 71: 1081A

Matsuo H, Baba Y, Nair R M G, Arimura A, Schally A V 1971 Structure of the porcine LH and FSH releasing factor: I. The proposed amino acid sequence. Biochem Biophys Res Commun 43: 1334

Matta W H, Shaw R W, Hesp R, Katz D 1987 Hypogonadism induced by luteinizing hormone releasing hormone agonist analogues: effects on bone density in premenopausal women. Br Med J 294: 1523

Meldrum D R, Chang R J, Lu J, Vale W, Rivier J, Judd H L 1982 'Medical oophorectomy' using a long-acting GnRH agonist—a possible new approach to treatment of endometriosis. J Clin Endocrinol Metab 54: 1081

Naor Z, Childs G V, Leifer A M et al 1982 Gonadotropin releasing hormone binding and activation of enriched population of pituitary gonadotrophs. Mol Cell Endocrinol 25: 85

Nillius S J, Wide L 1979 Effects of prolonged luteinizing hormone-releasing hormone therapy on follicular maturation, ovulation and corpus luteum function in amenorrhoeic women with anorexia nervosa. Ups J Med Sci 84: 21

Nillius S J, Skarin G, Wide L 1981 Gonadotropin-releasing hormone and its agonists for induction of follicular maturation and ovulation. In: Insler V, Bettendorf G (eds) Advances in diagnosis and treatment of infertility. Elsevier North Holland, New York, p 5

Ott S M, Kilcoyne R F, Chestnut C H III 1987 Ability of four different techniques of measuring bone mass to diagnose vertebral fractures in postmenopausal women. J Bone Mineral Res 2: 201

Pimstone B, Epstein S, Hamilton S M et al 1977 Metabolic clearance and plasma half disappearance time of exogenous gonadotropin releasing hormone in normal subjects and in patients with liver disease and chronic renal failure. J Clin Endocrinol Metab 44: 356

Pohl C R, Richardson D W, Hutchinson J S et al 1983 Hypophysiotropic signal frequency and the functioning of the pituitary–ovarian system in the rhesus monkey. Endocrinology 112: 2076

Redding T W, Kastin A J, Gonzalez-Barcena D et al 1973 The half-life, metabolism and excretion of tritiated luteinizing hormone releasing hormone (LHRH) in man. J Clin Endocrinol Metab 37: 626

Roberts J G, DiTomasso E, Webber C E 1982 Photon scattering measurements of calcaneal bone density; results of in vivo cross-sectional studies. Invest Radiol 17: 20

Schally A V, Arimura A, Kastin A J et al 1971 Gonadotrophin releasing hormone: one polypeptide regulates secretion of luteinizing and follicle stimulating hormones. Science 173: 1036

Schoemaker J, Simons A H M, Burger C W 1982 Induction of ovulation with LH/FSH releasing hormone (LHRH). IVth Reinier de Graaf Symposium. Excerpta Medica, Amsterdam

Schriock E D, Jaffe R B 1986 Induction of ovulation with gonadotropin-releasing hormone. Obstet Gynecol Surv 41: 414

Shadmi A, Lunenfeld B, Bahari C, Kokia E, Pariente C, Blankstein J 1987 Abolishment of the positive feedback mechanism: a criterion for temporary medical hypophysectomy by LH- RH agonist. Gynecol Endocrinol 1: 1

Singh M, Nagrath A R, Maini P S 1970 Changes in the trabecular pattern of the upper end of the femur as an index of osteoporosis. J Bone Joint Surg 52A: 457

Skarin G, Nillius S J, Wide L 1982 Pulsatile luteinizing hormone-releasing hormone treatment for induction of follicular maturation and ovulation. IVth Reinier de Graaf Symposium. Excerpta Medica, Amsterdam

Tummon I A, Ali A, Pepping M A, Radwanska E, Binor Z, Dmowski W P 1988 Bone mineral density in women with endometriosis before and during ovarian suppression with gonadotropin-releasing hormone agonists or danazol. Fertil Steril 49: 5

Weber J M, Coelingh-Bennink H J T, Alsbach G P J, Thyssen J H H 1983 The effect of pulsatile intravenous administration of LHRH on gonadotropin secretion in polycystic ovarian disease. The 14th Acta Endocrinologia Congress, Stockholm, 23–30 June (abtr)

Wildt L, Haeusler A, Marshall G et al 1981 Frequency and amplitude of gonadotropin-releasing hormone stimulation and gonadotropin secretion in rhesus monkey. Endocrinology 109: 376

Wiznitzer A, Marbach M, Sharoni Y, Insler V, Levy, J, 1988 Gonadotropin-releasing hormone specific binding site in uterine leiomyoma. Gynecol Endocrinol 2: (suppl 1.): 184

Yen SSC 1983 Clinical applications of gonadotropin-releasing hormone and gonadotropin-releasing hormone analogs. Fertil Steril 39: 257

# 16. Human gonadotropins

*Vaclav Insler, Bruno Lunenfeld*

## HISTORICAL PERSPECTIVE

The path from the first recognition of the physiological role of gonadotropic hormones until development of preparations applicable for treatment of human infertility was long, difficult, and full of intellectual challenges and technical obstacles.

In the mid-twenties Zondek and Smith independently but almost simultaneously discovered that gonadal function was controlled by the pituitary gland. Zondek (1926) and Zondek & Ascheim (1927) demonstrated that implantation of anterior pituitary caused a rapid development of sexual organs in immature animals. At approximately the same time, Smith and his group showed that hypophysectomy resulted in a failure of sexual maturation in immature animals and in a rapid regression of sexual characteristics in adult animals (Smith 1926, Smith & Engle 1927).

During the 1930s and 1940s gonadotropin extracts from different animal materials were prepared and applied for stimulation of ovarian function in humans. It has been quickly realized, however, that these preparation were of very limited clinical value because nonprimate gonadotropins produced in the human a rapid immunological response neutralizing their therapeutic effect (Leethem & Rakoff 1948). This focused the scientific and technological efforts on extraction and purification of gonadotropins from human sources. Intensive research in this area was simultaneously carried out in Italy, England, Scotland, Switzerland and Sweden. In the late 1950s and early 1960s these efforts have been crowned by success.

Gemzell and his coworkers reported the first successful induction of ovulation using human pituitary gonadotropin in 1958 and the first pregnancy in 1960 (Gemzell et al 1958, 1960). At approximately the same time Bettendorf succeeded in extracting a potent gonadotropic agent from human pituitaries and reported on the first clinical experience with its use (Bettendorf et al 1961). Lunenfeld and his group, working with human menopausal gonadotropin, achieved ovulations and pregnancies in anovulatory women. Their results were reported at various scientific and medical meetings beginning in 1959 and later published in 1963 (Lunenfeld 1963).

Large-scale clinical studies were then undertaken in numerous centers throughout the world and their results reported in the literature. Of particular significance were the reports of Bettendorf (1963) and Gemzell (1964) who were able to induce ovulation and pregnancy in hypophysectomized women.

The introduction of rapid and reliable hormonal assays, and later the availability of ultrasound scanners enabling visualization and measurement of ovarian follicles, made monitoring of gonadotropin therapy accurate and objective and improved the results of treatment.

In the 1980s, the large scale in vitro fertilization (IVF) programs used the principles developed for and the experience gained from induction of ovulation in anovulatory women and added new important insights to the understanding of the mechanism of controlled ovarian hyperstimulation impelled by gonadotropins.

Table 16.1 describes shortly the most important milestones of a long and tedious way, which led from the discovery of the gonadotropic principle to IVF.

Induction of ovulation with human

**Table 16.1**   Milestones of developments leading to efficient treatment of female infertility

| | |
|---|---|
| 1926–27 | Discovery of the pituitary hormone controlling ovarian function |
| 1955 | Clinical use of urinary hormone assays (steroids and gonadotropins) |
| 1959 | Extraction and purification of gonadotropins from human pituitaries and menopausal urine |
| 1961 | Introduction of clomiphene citrate |
| 1965 | Widescale clinical use of gonadotropins and clomiphene |
| 1968 | Development of the first therapeutically oriented classification of anovulatory states |
| 1970 | Routine application of radioimmunoassays for estimation of hormone levels |
| 1971 | Isolation, determination of structure and laboratory synthesis of GnRH |
| 1972 | Introduction of prolactin assays |
| 1973–76 | Reports on pregnancies induced by GnRH therapy |
| 1974 | Development of prolactin-inhibiting drugs |
| 1978 | Discovery of pulsatile nature of GnRH secretion |
| 1979 | Ultrasound imaging of ovarian follicles |
| | Introduction of pulsatile GnRH therapy |
| | Delivery of the first test-tube baby |
| 1982 | Introduction of GnRH analogs for clinical use |
| | Introduction of purified FSH for ovulation-inducing therapy |
| 1984 | Routine clinical use of IVF-ET and GIFT programs |
| 1989 | New therapeutically oriented classification of anovulatory states. |
| 1990 | Induction of ovulation with combined growth hormone/gonadotropin therapy in poor responders. |
| 1991 | Introduction of recombinant gonadotropins |

gonadotropins has been an integral part of the routine work of many fertility clinics for more than 15 years. During that time numerous reports describing in great detail all aspects of gonadotropin therapy have been published (Thompson & Hansen 1970, Insler & Lunenfeld 1974, Lunenfeld & Insler 1978, Brown 1986). In the following chapter we will discuss the main principles of application and monitoring of gonadotropin treatment and summarize the results and complications of this therapy.

## CHEMISTRY PHARMACOKINETICS AND CLEARANCE

During the last 20 years, the major elements of the mechanism of action, control and regulation of secretion of gonadotropins have been elucidated, and more recently, their structure has been determined.

Gonadotropins are glycoproteins with molecular weights around 30,000 daltons and containing about 20% carbohydrates. The carbohydrate moieties in their molecules are fucose, mannose, galactose, acetylglucosamine and $N$-acetylneuraminic acid (Butt & Kennedy, 1971). The sialic acid content varies widely among the glycoprotein hormones, from 20 residues in human chorionic gonadotropin (hCG) and five in

follicle stimulating hormone (FSH) to only one or two in human luteinizing hormone (hLH). These differences are largely responsible for the variations in the isoelectric points of gonadotropins.

Different sialic acid content accounts for differences in molecular weight of the hormones isolated from various sources and in differences in biological activity determined in in vivo assays. The higher the sialic acid content, the longer the biological half-life. Thus, the increased amount of carbohydrate component in hCG is responsible for its significantly longer half-life than that of LH or FSH. Whereas the beta subunit of LH contains only one carbohydrate group, the beta subunit of hCG contains six. The function of the carbohydrates is not fully known, except for the fact that removal of the terminal neuraminic acid (sialic acid) residues drastically shortens the half-lives of the circulating hormones in blood. For this reason desialyated preparations of human luteinizing hormone (hLH), hCG and human follicle stimulating hormone (hFSH) show considerably reduced biological activity in vivo but retain activity in specific in vitro biological assays employing membrane receptors or isolated target cells. Attempting to measure these hormones by immunoassays or by in vitro bioassay procedures therefore do not express their actual bioactivity in vivo. Deglycosylated hormones can act in vitro as competitive antagonists of the actions of the intact hormone upon the cyclic AMP production and to a lesser extent on steroid hormone biosynthesis.

The gonadotropic hormones consist of two hydrophobic noncovalently associated alpha and beta subunits. The three-dimensional structure of each subunit is maintained by internally crosslinked disulfide bonds. Gonadotropic hormones can be dissociated into the individual subunits by denaturing agents (De la Llosa & Jutisz 1969). The subunits are practically without biological activity, but the hormonal activity is regenerated by recombination of the subunits. All the gonadotropins as well as thyroid-stimulating hormone (TSH) share a common alpha subunit of 92 amino acid residues in the same sequence with five disulfide bonds as well as two carbohydrate moieties. The beta subunits (of FSH, LH and hCG) are unique to each hormone and determine their biological specificity. They have amino acid chains of variable lengths (116–147 amino acid residues) and contain six disulfide bonds. There is only one known gene that codes for the beta chain of LH, while as many as six to eight genes or pseudogenes have been identified for the beta chain of chorionic gonadotropin (CG) (Talmadge et al 1983). It is not known how many of these CG genes are translated.

Methodologies which have allowed the analysis of the genes and gene products have shown that the two subunits of the gonadotropic hormones are translated from separate messenger RNAs (Fiddes & Goodman 1979) and both are synthesized as precursors. The nascent polypeptide alpha and beta subunits are then glycosylated in the Golgi apparatus by en bloc attachment of high mannose complex type oligosaccharide to two aspargine residues of each subunit (Fig. 16.1). Excess mannose and glucose residues are trimmed from the intermediates. Thereafter

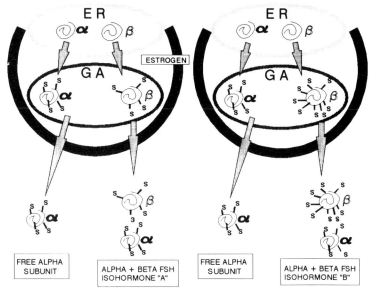

**Fig. 16.1** Simplified presentation of FSH synthesis in the pituitary cells. The alpha and beta subunits are translated from separate RNAs and synthesized as precursors in the endoplasmaic reticulum. The precursors are then glycosylated in the Golgi apparatus. The number and type of sugars attached depend on the intra- and intercellular environment in the pituitary gland resulting in production of several different FSH isohormones. In a high estrogenic environment the carbohydrate chains are shorter and, consequently, the clearance of the hormone is more rapid. In a low estrogenic environment the gonadotroph cells produce an FSH type with longer carbohydrate chains. This iso-hormone has a lower clearance rate and a longer half-life. ER, endoplasmic reticulum; GA, Golgi apparatus.

peripheral monosaccharides *N*-acetylglucosamine, galactose and *N*-acetylneuraminic acid are attached sequentially to complete the oligosacharide structures (Hussa 1980).

It has been shown that both pituitary FSH and LH exist in several different forms (iso-hormones) which exhibit charge heterogeneity and may thus be separated by isoelectric focusing. The various FSH and LH species differ from each other not only in their isoelectric point but also in their relative abundance, receptor binding activity, biological activity and plasma half-life (Ulloa-Aguirre et al 1988). Cook et al (1988) showed that human menopausal gonadotropin (hMG) also consists of up to five different FSH iso-hormones and up to nine LH species. These differences may cause differences in patients' response observed sometimes when using various lots of the same preparation.

The information regarding metabolism of gonadotropic hormones is scarce. It has been shown that purified preparations of hFSH, hLH and hCG injected intravenously into humans had serum half-lives (as determined by bioassays) of 180–240 min, 38–60 min and 6–8 h respectively.

The half-life of the alpha and beta subunit of LH was found to be only 16 min. The higher carbohydrate content of hCG (10%) is responsible for its significantly longer half-life, as compared to hFSH (5%) and hLH (2%).

Following intramuscular administration of Pergonal (containing FSH and LH derived from human menopausal urine) daily for 8 days, and testing blood levels twice a day, no increase in LH levels was observed. FSH which has an intermediate half-life longer than LH but shorter than hCG, even when given in low dose (150 IU), accumulated in the plasma and was still elevated above baseline level 3 days after the last injection (Diczfalusy & Harlin 1988). After intramuscular administration of hCG, peak serum levels were observed at 6–8 h. The level of the hormone was reduced to about 50% after 36 h and was still discernible after 6 days.

It is thus clear that hCG, when given as a substitution to LH, exerts a stronger and more prolonged biological effect due to its significantly longer half-life.

The mean metabolic clearance rate (MCR) of hFSH in women has been determined to be 14 ml/min and has not been determined in men. The MCR of hLH is 25–30 ml/min in women regardless of ovulatory state and is almost 50% higher in normal men. The disappearance curves for both hormones are multiexponential, indicating a distribution of these hormones in more than three mathematical compartments. In premenopausal women daily production rates of hLH are 500–1000 IU with a marked preovulatory rise, whereas production rates in postmenopausal women are 3000–4000 IU day. These values indicate that the pituitary content of hLH (and probably of hFSH) is turned over once or twice daily and that rapid biosynthesis of gonadotropins is necessary to maintain the normal levels of pituitary storage and secretion. Only 3–10% of the daily production of FSH and LH is excreted in the urine in a biologically active form, but nevertheless reflect the rate of gonadotropin secretion in physiological and pathological conditions. The recovery of exogenous gonadotropins in the urine of normal and infertile subjects is 10–20% of the administered hormone. Urinary excretion of gonadotropins accounts for only 5% of the MCR. The MCR of hMG in hypogonadotropic subjects is 0.4–1.7 ml/min.

The detailed information regarding the physiological processes involved in synthesis of gonadotropins by pituitary cells and development of recombinant DNA technology carries the possibility of producing pharmacologically active FSH preparations in huge quantities. Human pituitaries and postmenopausal urine have been until now the sole source for production of gonadotropin preparations (Lunenfeld at al 1981). These sources will obviously be insufficient to cover the steadily increasing demand in the near future. Thus, manufacturing of gonadotropin compounds using recombinant technology would cover an important need in the treatment of functional infertility.

The task of producing recombinant gonadotropin molecules has, however, proved to be extremely difficult. Whereas bacteria efficiently produce nonglycosylated peptides such as insulin, and yeast has been cloned for the production of certain vaccines, prokaryotic cells are incapable of correctly glycosylating the peptide subunits to produce biologically active gonadotropins. The glycosylation process is of primary importance in the synthesis of gonadotropins which are glycosylated heterodimeric peptides. The complex sugars are important for proper folding of the polypeptide backbone. The sites and extent of glycosylation determine tertiary structure, length of time of degradation, the regions of the molecule exposed to target cell receptors, and exposure of the molecule to mechanisms that regulate metabolism in vivo. Recombinant glycosylated peptides may be synthesized by certain mammalian cell lines. The Chinese hamster ovary cells are known to be suitable host cells for the production of glycosylated recombinant proteins; such cell lines were chosen for the expression of recombinant human FSH. To obtain this goal, cloned human FSH genes were inserted in an expression vector and transferred to the Chinese hamster ovary cell line. Specific cell clones have now been selected for large-scale production of recombinant FSH. The resultant preparations are very pure and have a high biological potency. It is hoped that in the near future recombinant FSH will substitute the gonadotropins obtained from human sources in therapies requiring gonadal stimulation in male or female patients.

## CLASSIFICATION OF PATIENTS

Gonadotropin treatment is primarily a substitution therapy and as such should be applied in patients lacking appropriate gonadotropin stimulation but having target organs (gonads) capable of normal response. In daily practice, however, gonadotropins are also used in other groups of patients.

In 1968 Insler et al proposed a simple treatment-oriented classification of patients selected for gonadotropin therapy. This classification has been modified and adopted by the WHO Scientific Group (WHO 1976) and is used in many centers. According to this classification gonadotropin treatment is applied in two main groups of women:

*Group I: hypothalamic-pituitary failure* Amenorrheic women with no evidence of endogenous estrogen production, nonelevated prolactin levels, normal or low FSH levels and no detectable space-occupying lesion in the hypothalamic-pituitary region.

*Group II: hypothalamic-pituitary dysfunction* Women with a variety of menstrual cycle disturbances including amenorrhea with evidence of endogenous estrogen production, and normal levels of prolactin and FSH. Patients with polycystic ovarian disease (PCOD) represent a distinctive variant of Group II, both because of the possible difference in the underlying pathophysiological mechanism(s) of the disease as well as due to some differences in response to ovarian stimulation.

In Group II gonadotropins are usually applied after other types of ovulation-inducing therapy have failed. It is theoretically plausible and clinically proven that the results of gonadotropin treatment are significantly better in Group I compared to Group II (Insler & Lunenfeld 1977). Amenorrheic women of Group I, however, represent only a small and ever-diminishing proportion of the infertility clinic population (Bettendorf et al 1981).

In recent years another group of patients, which is steadily growing in numbers, is being treated with human gonadotropins — women being subjected to in vitro fertilization (IVF) or to intrauterine insemination (IUI) combined with ovarian stimulation. Obviously, these patients differ from both Group I and Group II in having completely normal hormonal levels and competent hypothalamic-pituitary-ovarian feedback mechanisms.

The general principles of gonadotropin therapy applied to the above-mentioned three groups of patients are similar but the intensity of stimulation, course of treatment and hormonal patterns differ significantly. It may thus be summarized that, at present, four modes of gonadotropin treatment are used:

1. Substitution therapy—applied in patients of Group I
2. Stimulation therapy—given to patients of Group II
3. Regulation therapy—employed in women with PCOD
4. Hyperstimulation therapy—used in IVF,

gamete intrafallopian transfer (GIFT), tubal embyo transfer (TET) and IUI.

Each of the above therapeutic schemes may be used in conjunction with additional pharmaceutical agents enhancing the effect of gonadotropins or attenuating disturbing influences stemming from the ovary, the pituitary, the adrenal glands or other sources. The combined therapies will be discussed in another section of this chapter.

## THEORETICAL BASIS AND CLINICAL GOALS OF GONADOTROPIN THERAPY

The comprehensive basis of gonadotropin therapy is, of course, the knowledge of physiology of the reproductive ovulatory cycle (see Chapters 5 and 6). A detailed discussion of the principles of ovarian response to exogenous stimulation must, however, be focused on the events taking place in the ovary itself.

The experimental work of Hodgen and his group on primates (Goodman et al 1977, Hodgen 1983), the introduction of sonography for monitoring of follicular size and the IVF programs allowing for direct laparoscopic observation of the size and appearance of ovarian follicles concomitant with the appreciation of the maturity of ova, established a firm kernel of data concerning the sequence of ovarian changes leading to ovulation. According to Hodgen's work in primates, the sequence of events leading to ovulation is as follows:

***Recruitment of a follicular cohort*** is brought about by a slight but significant FSH rise observed during the preceding late luteal phase. This process is completed by the 3rd cycle day (Fig. 16.2a,b).

***Selection of the dominant follicle*** is a process by which one follicle of the cohort is endowed with the ability to mature earlier and/or quicker than all others (Fig. 16.2c). The exact mechanism of the selection process is not yet known. Baird (1987) stated that 'the follicle of the month' is selected by chance because it is at the right place at the right time. Our experimental work in the rat indicated that the 'assignment' of the follicle to be selected as the dominant one in

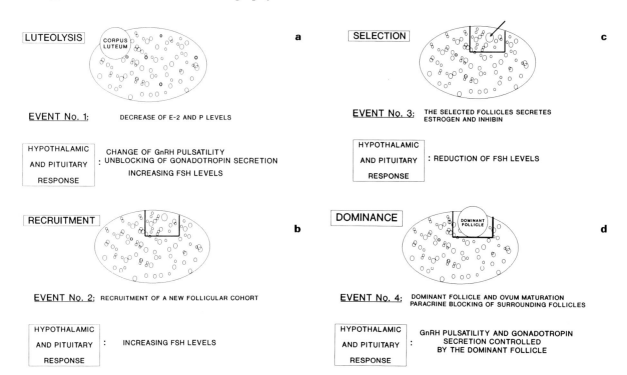

**Fig. 16.2    a–d** Schematic presentation of the sequence of events occurring in the ovary during a normal ovulatory cycle (for details see text).

the subsequent cycles is instigated by the rescuing action of the midcycle FSH peak in three consecutive previous cycles (Insler et al 1990). Gougeon (1986) determined that in the human, the progress from primordial to Graafian follicle takes at least 10 weeks. The process of selection of the dominant follicle is completed by the 7th cycle day.

**Dominance** is that part of the cycle when all the events such as the exponential rise of estrogen, negative feedback action upon the hypothalamus, modulation of pituitary secretion of gonadotropins, reduction of FSH secretion by inhibin and positive feedback evoking the midcycle LH surge are subordinated to the developmental rhythm of the dominant follicle. This controlling action of the dominant follicle lasts from the 8th cycle day until ovulation and persists also during the corpus luteum phase (Fig. 16.2d).

The basic principles of gonadotropin therapy were proposed by Insler & Lunenfeld (1974, 1977) following observation of the course of treatment in several hundreds of patients. Ovarian response can be elicited only when a certain dose of FSH-like material has been applied. This amount of gonadotropins is called *the effective daily dose*. Administration of gonadotropins at levels significantly below the effective daily dose does not evoke any measurable effect even when prolonged therapy is used.

Following the application of effective daily dose of gonadotropins a number of ovarian follicles is stimulated to begin growth and maturation. This period of gonadotropin therapy is called *the latent phase*. Since at this stage of follicular development appreciable amounts of estrogen are not yet secreted, the latent phase of therapy is clinically 'mute'. Recently, the introduction of high resolution vaginal sonography seems to enable detection of small antral follicles with a diameter of approximately 4–5 mm. This will probably permit identification of the beginning of ovarian response to stimulation. The latent phase begins with the application of the effective daily dose of gonadotropins and ends with the appearance of measurable ovarian response, i.e. rising estrogen levels and increasing follicular diameter. The second part of gonadotropin therapy, called *the*

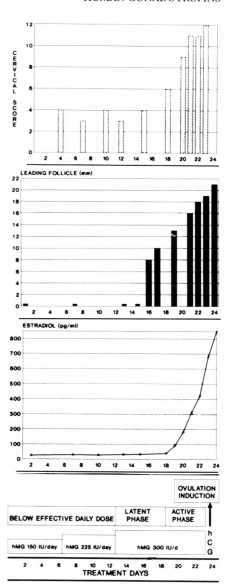

**Fig. 16.3** Ovarian stimulation by human gonadotropins— practical application of general principles. Administration of gonadotropins in insufficient quantities, i.e. below the effective daily dose (EDD), is not effective. In the case presented, the EDD was 300 IU of FSH and this dose was reached on day 13 of treatment. Follicular growth was observed on ultrasound 3 days later (day 16) but estrogens started to rise on day 18 of therapy, indicating the end of the latent phase. The active phase of therapy lasted 5 days (from day 18 until day 22). One day later the estrogen level was 690 pg/ml, the cervical score 12 points and the diameter of the leading follicle reached 21.5 mm. Ovulation was induced by 10 000 IU of hCG. The patient ovulated and conceived during this treatment cycle.

*active phase*, lasts from the initial estrogen rise until ovulation induction. It is characterized by an exponential rise of estrogen levels and steady growth of follicular diameter (Fig. 16.3).

The duration of the latent phase is 3–7 days and is significantly longer in patients of Group I than in women of Group II. The length of the active phase is 4–6 days and is similar in all patients.

The above principles, based on clinical observation and thorough analysis of patients' response, actually preceded by several years the theoretical considerations of the physiological events produced by experimental work (see above). The latent phase of gonadotropin therapy represents a 'telescoped-in' version of the recruitment and selection phases of the spontaneous cycle. The active phase of therapy corresponds to the period of dominance.

The question of differences of response observed in patients of Group I compared to those of Group II must now be briefly addressed. It is well known that in patients of Group II the effective daily dose is smaller, the latent phase is shorter and the response to treatment is less uniform (Insler & Lunenfeld 1977). It seems that

these differences in response to stimulation with exogenous gonadotropins may be explained by the state of the ovary at the beginning of treatment.

In women of Group I, at the initiation of each treatment course, the ovaries are at a quiescent state with almost all follicles at a low stage of development. The pharmacological dose of gonadotropins applied acts on a relatively uniform substrate (Fig. 16.4a – d). However this is not so in patients of Group II. In this group endogenous gonadotropins may cause a certain follicular development before or between treatments. Gonadotropin therapy is thus applied to an ovary containing already scores of follicles at various stages of development, provoking further growth of some of them, recruitment of additional ones and possibly preventing atresia of others. It is not surprising that the response to treatment is less uniform and more prone to hyperstimulation (Fig. 16.5a – d).

Gonadotropin therapy poses several interesting theoretical problems.

The exact size of the follicular cohort recruited

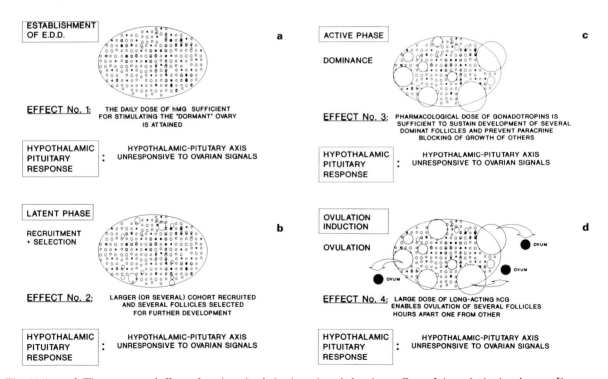

**Fig. 16.4  a–d** The sequence of effects of ovarian stimulation in patients belonging to Group I, i.e. substitution therapy. For details see text.

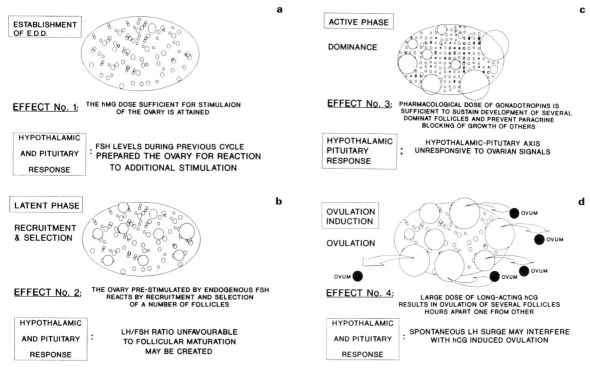

**Fig. 16.5  a – d** The sequence of effects of ovarian stimulation in patients belonging to Group II, i.e. stimulation or regulation therapy. For details see text.

in each cycle in the human is not known. It is thus impossible to know whether gonadotropin therapy, using unphysiological doses, provokes initial development of a larger cohort. Whatever the size of the initial cohort recruited, it seems that during the course of gonadotropin therapy additional follicles are stimulated and undergo partial or full maturation and others are rescued from atresia by the sustained high level of FSH. This process results in the development of several dominant follicles that reach full maturation hours or maybe even days apart one from the other (Figs 16.4d, 16.5d).

As indicated by the very low efficiency of single dose or 'trigger' schemes of therapy, to ensure follicular maturation during gonadotropin therapy relatively high FSH levels must be sustained throughout the treatment.

It is of interest to note that despite the rather high levels of estrogen occurring relatively early in the treatment, premature LH surges are rather rare (Garcia et al 1983). This is true in patients with hypothalamic-pituitary failure. In women

with hypothalamic-pituitary dysfunction, PCOD or in spontaneous ovulators undergoing super-ovulation therapy the premature luteinization episodes are, however, much more frequent (Flemming & Coutts 1990, see also Chapters 21 and 26).

When using human gonadotropins for induction of ovulation one has to accept the fact that some features of the spontaneous ovulatory cycle cannot be reproduced in the gonadotropin-induced cycles. These features are:

- Premenstrual recruitment and initial selection of follicles
- Feedback control of gonadotropin levels
- Balanced effect of intraovarian sex steroids
- Full maturation of one follicle only
- Exact synchronization of structural, functional and hormonal events throughout the entire genital system.

The ideal rationale of gonadotropin treatment is to provide gonadotropin levels of magnitude and timing similar to those observed in a normal ovulatory cycle and, consequently, to evoke recruitment of a follicular cohort, selection and full maturation of at least one dominant follicle, ovulation and sustained corpus luteum function.

Unfortunately, this goal has never been fully achieved. The FSH and LH levels and their ratios during gonadotropin-stimulated cycles are quite different from normal (Wu 1977, Healy & Burger 1983). Estrogen levels and their daily rate of ascent as well as progesterone values are not identical to those observed in spontaneous cycles (Insler & Potashnik 1983). The follicular fluid levels of estradiol and progesterone are lower and the level of inhibin is higher in preovulatory gonadotropin-stimulated cycles than in the dominant follicle of the natural cycle (Seegar-Jones et al 1985). Moreover, the pregnancy rate in gonadotropin-induced cycles with steroid profiles closely resembling those found in spontaneous ovulations is dismally low (Insler & Lunenfeld 1977). Thus, the theoretical rationale of gonadotropin therapy must be subordinated to its clinical aim which is: to obtain ovulation and pregnancy in all suitable cases while avoiding hyperstimulation.

Large-scale clinical experience indicates that this goal can be practically achieved. The unequivocal proof of the clinical efficiency of gonadotropin therapy are the thousands of babies born following gonadotropin-induced ovulations and conceptions.

## TREATMENT SCHEMES

A whole array of treatment schemes of gonadotropin therapy have been proposed and employed over the years. There are, however, only three essentially different types of therapy:

- Fixed dose regimens
- Individually adjusted schemes
- Combined therapy.

At the beginning of clinical trials two types of gonadotropin preparations were used: human pituitary gonadotropins (hPG) and human menopausal gonadotropins (hMG). Due to scarcity of human pituitaries, since the late seventies hMG preparations have been mainly employed. In the eighties a purified FSH prepara-

tion containing a negligible LH amount has been introduced. This preparation is at present used for the same indications as hMG and has also been proposed as the treatment of choice for patients with PCOD (see Chapter 26).

In the fixed dose regimens, a certain amount of hMG (or FSH) is administered on predetermined cycle days followed by hCG given one or more days after the last injection of hMG or pituitary gonadotropins (hPG). Although the dosages of gonadotropins and the days on which it was administered differed in various reports (Butler 1970, Crooke 1970, Marshall & Jacobson 1970), the general principle was identical. By using a fixed dose in each cycle, the patient's gonadotropin requirement (i.e. the effective daily dose) could be met only by successively increasing the dose in consecutive cycles. The individually adjusted treatment scheme (Rabau et al 1971) allows for successive increments of the gonadotropin dose according to the patient's response during the same cycle. It actually comprises the tests courses with the treatment course in one cycle, thus significantly increasing the efficiency of treatment (mean number of treatment courses per pregnancy). In some particularly sensitive cases, the individually adjusted treatment may avoid hyperstimulation which would have been brought about by using the fixed dose schedule.

The problem of the size of initial dose of hMG (or FSH) and of its increments as well as the ideal estrogen level to be arrived at before application of hCG is still a matter of discussion. We usually start with 2 ampules of hMG per day in patients of Group I and with 1 ampule in women belonging to Group II. The successive dose increments are usually by 1 ampule each and hCG is administered when urinary estrogen reaches a level of 75–300 μg/24 h or plasma estradiol attains a level of 300–1200 pg/ml and on ultrasound at least one follicle with a diameter exceeding 16 mm is observed (Figs. 16.6, 16.7).

It is interesting to note that with the advent of IVF programs, the whole circle of trial and error regarding the most efficient and safe treatment schemes of hMG was repeated. Different groups proposed fixed dose schedules not much different from those which were tried and discarded years

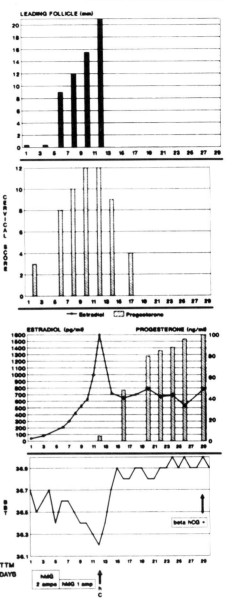

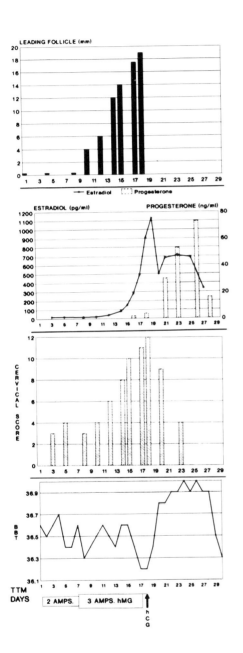

**Fig. 16.6** An example of gonadotropin substitution therapy. The EDD in this case was 3 amp/d, The duration of the latent phase was 5 days and of the active phase 6 days. On the day of hCG administration the estradiol level was 1120 pg/ml and the diameter of the leading follicle 19 mm. The patient ovulated as indicated by a sustained BBT high phase and progesterone peak levels of 75 ng/ml.

**Fig. 16.7** An example of gonadotropin stimulation therapy. The EDD was below 2 amp hMG/d, thus on the 5th treatment day the hMG dose was reduced to 1 amp/d. Under this stimulation an acceptable rate of follicular development as indicated by estradiol rise and follicular growth was achieved. Ovulation was induced by hCG on day 12, in the presence of estradiol levels of 1600 pg/ml and of a number of large follicles (leading one with a diameter of 21 mm). The patient conceived. Despite the very high progesterone levels during the luteal phase a singleton clinical pregnancy followed.

ago. Recently, however, more and more groups seem to adopt the individually adjusted treatment scheme, using some modifications suitable for the special purposes of an IVF program (Quigley 1985, Lopata et al 1986).

For the sake of completeness, one additional mode of ovulation induction using human gonadotropins should be mentioned here. In 1983 Kemmann et al described their initial experience with a portable infusion pump delivering subdermally a constant amount of hMG over a period on 18 h per day. The authors claimed that with this method of delivery a better response was obtained than with the standard intramuscular injection of hMG.

## COMBINED THERAPY

In the past most IVF programs used a combination of clomiphene citrate and hMG to stimulate a large enough crop of follicles ready for ovum pick-up. The claim was that this combination produced better, or at least more uniform, ovum maturation than hMG alone. In addition, clomiphene/gonadotropin combinations required smaller hMG doses, thus reducing the cost of treatment. This mode of treatment is being abandoned because of the long half-life of clomiphene citrate and the high incidence of untimely LH surges.

It is well known that patients of Group I respond better to gonadotropin therapy than women of Group II. The efficiency of treatment (mean number of treatment courses per pregnancy) and the pregnancy rate are significantly better in the former group compared to the latter (Lunenfeld & Insler 1978). Some of the reasons for this discrepancy are obvious. First, patients of Group II receive gonadotropin therapy only after they have failed to conceive when treated with other ovulation-inducing drugs. Secondly, the frequency of additional disturbances possibly affecting fertility such as endometriosis, tubal factors and polycystic ovaries are much more frequent in Group II.

There are, however, differences in response to stimulation between patients of Group I and Group II which seem to be inherent to the functional characteristics of the hypothalamic-pituitary-ovarian axis (see 'Theoretical basis and clinical goals of gonadotropin therapy' above). In other words, with regard to gonadotropin therapy

the presence of a functioning pituitary gland may be a disadvantage rather than an asset. Even with the best protocols for inducing ovulation in anovulatory patients and superovulation in in vitro procedures, a number of patients may not ovulate. Of those that do ovulate, some produce poorly fertilizable eggs and in others, poor implantation may be observed. It is conceivable that inappropriate endogenous LH secretion may be the dominant cause of failure in the majority of patients belonging to Group II. This disturbance may appear in two main forms: (a) elevated LH levels during the follicular phase, and (b) ill-timed LH surges.

### The effects of excessive LH in the follicular phase

It has been suggested that a high concentration of LH through the follicular phase causes early maturation of the developing oocyte producing at ovulation an egg that is physiologically aged (Homburg et al 1988a). These oocytes are unlikely to be fertilized or, if conception is achieved, may fail to implant or an early abortion may result. Several authors have reported that in IVF programs high concentration of LH in the few days before oocytes are collected were associated with reduced rates of fertilization and conception (Stanger & Yovitch 1985, Howles et al 1987, Punnonen et al 1988, McFaul et al 1989).

McFaul et al (1989) and Macnamee (1990) also demonstrated that if conception is achieved in a cycle in which the oocyte is prematurely exposed to elevated LH there is a significantly higher probability that an early abortion will result. This situation is particularly frequent in patients diagnosed as PCOD, where ovulation rates following ovulation induction are relatively high but pregnancy rate is low.

Johnson & Pearce (1990) support this concept and conclude that pituitary suppression by GnRH analog before induction of ovulation (by lowering LH levels) reduces the risk of spontaneous abortion in women with PCOD and in patients with primary recurrent spontaneous abortions following induction of ovulation.

The reports quoted above point to the conclusion that an excessive endogenous LH environment may interfere with normal follicular development and, might, by untimely inhibition of the meiosis-inhibiting factors, provoke overaging of eggs with a significant reduction in their fertilization or implantation potential. It has been shown (Macnamee 1990) that a definite correlation exists between mean LH levels in the follicular phase and the outcome of IVF.

## The effects of an untimely LH surge

Premature luteinization is a specific category of anovulation. This entity is frequently unrecognized, or misdiagnosed as unexplained infertility, or luteal phase defect.

This situation can occur if an untimely LH

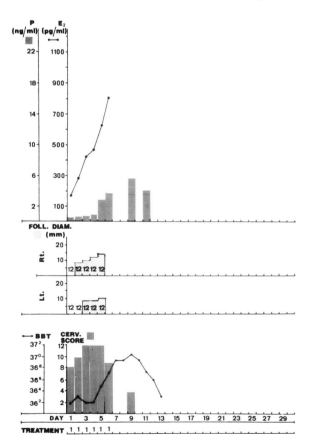

**Fig. 16.8** Gonadotropin treatment complicated by premature luteinization of follicles. Application of 1 amp/d of hMG over 6 days resulted in a steep peak. Although LH was not measured in this case, premature luteinization of follicles is evidenced by progesterone and BBT rise. Each ovary contained 12 follicles none of them reaching a diameter of 14 mm.

surge ensues in response to rising estrogen at a time when the follicle is still immature. It can be diagnosed if an LH peak is detected in the presence of relatively small (<14 mm) follicles demonstrated by ultrasonography (Fig. 16.8).

It is possible that the etiology of this entity is an exaggerated sensitivity of the pituitary to estrogen. Rising, but relatively low estradiol levels may trigger an LH surge. This assumption may explain the failure of clomiphene citrate or hMG to restore ovulation in such cases. Both agents cause multiple follicular development with an exaggerated estrogen rise, making the appearance of a premature LH peak even more likely.

A similar situation exists in ovulatory women with a normal pituitary-ovarian axis undergoing IVF, GIFT, zygote intrafallopian transfer (ZIFT), IUI or artificial insemination by donor (AID) procedures. They receive pharmacological doses of hMG (FSH) to induce superovulation. The exaggerated estradiol levels in response to this therapy provoke, in about 15% of treatment cycles, an untimely spontaneous LH surge leading to cancellation of ovum pickup or of the insemination procedure.

To overcome the possible interference of unbalanced and/or untimely endogenous gonadotropin secretion, combined therapy using agents suppressing hypothalamic-pituitary function together with hMG or a purified FSH preparation was recommended.

Ben-Nun et al (1984) generated pharmacological (drug-induced) hyperprolactinemia, causing a significant reduction of secretion and/or release of endogenous gonadotropins, and then stimulated the ovaries by exogenous hMG. They claimed that with this type of combined treatment ovulations and pregnancies could be obtained in several patients of Group II who previously failed to conceive when treated with hMG/hCG alone.

Laboratory synthesis of potent and/or long-acting analogues of gonadotropin-releasing hormone (GnRHa) makes it possible to efficiently reduce (down-regulate) the production and release of pituitary gonadotropins (Crawley et al 1982, Meldrum et al 1982, Yen 1983). Treatment schemes combining pituitary suppression by GnRH analogs with ovarian stimulation by exogenous gonadotropins seemed therefore particularly attractive (Fleming et al 1985, Shadmi et al 1987, Insler et al 1989, see also Chapter 15).

Several different protocols for the combined GnRHa and gonadotropins have been proposed. In the 'short' or 'ultrashort' protocols the GnRHa is administered either together with gonado-tropins or only a few days before the first gonadotropin dose and continued until indicated. This enables utilization of the initial flare-up effect of the analog, i.e. elevation of endogenous gonadotropin secretion. The treatment is shorter and the cost is lower, since less gonadotropins are required. On the other hand the initial relatively high LH levels (particularly in women with PCOD) may create a hormonal environment unfavorable to follicular development.

The long protocols are based on the concept that ovarian stimulation should begin only after the pituitary gland has been adequately suppressed by GnRH agonist. This effect can be achieved in the majority of cases within 14–21 days, depending on the type of GnRHa and patient's response.

Two main types of long protocols are used. According to one GnRH agonists are started in the midluteal phase and gonadotropins (hMG or FSH) are added after 10–14 days. It is claimed that this protocol is preferable, since in the hormonal environment of the luteal phase (relatively high estrogens and progesterone), the initial stimulatory effect of the agonist is attenu-ated and thus the LH levels and, consequently, androgen production are diminished (Fig. 16.9). The major problem with this protocol is the possi-bility of inadvertent application of GnRHa to patients with early pregnancy. There are no sufficient data to determine what, if at all, is the

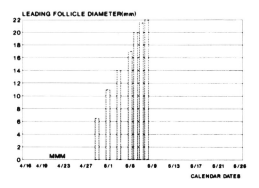

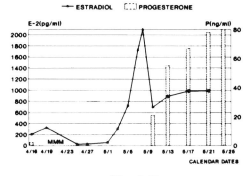

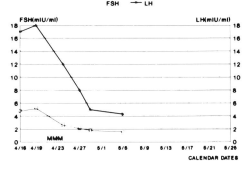

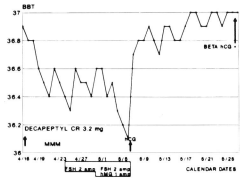

**Fig. 16.9** Combined GnRH/gonadotropin therapy in a woman with PCOD. The GnRH (3.2 mg of Decapeptyl CR (Ferring, Germany) was administered during the late luteal phase of the preceding cycle. The 'flare-up' effect was negligible. The endogenous LH and FSH were significantly suppressed 10 days following the GnRH injection and continued to decrease during the administration of exogenous gonadotropins ('pure' FSH Metrodin) and then FSH and hMG (Metrodin and Pergonal). The exponential rise of estrogens accompanied by steady growth of follicles indicated appropriate follicular growth and maturation. Following application of 10 000 IU of hCG she ovulated and conceived. M, menses.

effect of GnRH agonists upon pregnancy in the blastocyst or early nidation stage.

In the second version of long protocol the GnRHa is started on the first days of menstruation and gonadotropin stimulation is commenced when pituitary and ovarian function is suppressed as indicated by low FSH and LH levels and/or by estradiol values below 50 pg/ml and/or lack of presence of antral follicles (with diameter exceeding 4 mm) on sonographic ovarian scan. FSH/hMG administration in conjunction with the agonist is continued until at least one follicle reaches maturation, as judged by ultrasonography and estrogen levels. HCG is then administered to induce ovulation.

With either version of the long protocol of combined GnRHa/gonadotropin therapy protocol endogenous premature LH peaks are rare (less than in 1% of cycles). The gonadotropin dosage necessary for ovulation or superovulation induction and the duration of treatment are, however, significantly increased.

Both variants of the long protocol have already proven their merits. By making logistics easier and by significantly reducing cancellation rates in IVF programs, the overall success rate has been increased. The combined therapy allows design of stimulation protocols creating a predominantly FSH environment during the recruitment phase, and eliminating the interference of endogenous gonadotropins during the dominance and periovulatory phase. However, the temporary functional gonadotropin-specific hypophysectomy has introduced new challenges. Inhibition of endogenous gonadotropins following ovulation induced by hCG may, if not properly monitored, result in an inadequate luteal phase. This situation can be prevented by postovulatory periodic administration of hCG (Blumenfeld & Nahhas 1988).

The choice of the GnRH analog to be used should be based on a combination of factors including its delivery system, its mode of administration and its biological half-life. All the above criteria must be considered in designing the subsequent gonadotropin treatment protocol competent to stimulate follicular recruitment and development, timely ovulation induction and adequate corpus luteum function.

## Combined growth hormone/gonadotropin therapy

Even with the best protocols for inducing ovulation in anovulatory patients or superovulation for in vitro procedures, some patients need excessive amounts of gonadotropins and some remain 'poor' responders despite application of extremely high doses.

During the last few years the importance of intraovarian regulation via the potentiating effect of growth hormone-releasing hormone, growth hormone (GH) and growth factors and insulin on both the thecal cell response to LH and the granulosa cell response to FSH have been demonstrated (Adashi et al 1985a–c, 1990, Davoren & Hsueh 1986, Jia et al 1986, Ericson et al 1989). These findings may have a significant impact on the understanding of ovulatory disorders such as the polycystic ovarian syndrome, or on ovulation-inducing therapy and its main complication, the hyperstimulation syndrome.

Publications by Homburg et al (1988b) and Volpe et al (1989) claimed that GH added to hMG protocols significantly reduces the hMG dose necessary for follicular stimulation.

Ronnberg et al (1990), however, could not confirm these findings in a study of ovulatory patients undergoing a randomized stimulation protocol for IVF. Based on our past and present studies, we believe that we can reconcile the discrepancy between these publications. We have shown that some patients with decreased levels of GH (Blumenfeld & Lunenfeld 1989) or anovulatory, normoprolactinemic, nonPCOD patients who are 'bad responders' to gonadotropin stimulation and have a decreased level of GH reserve (Menashe et al 1990a,b) may benefit from the addition of GH to gonadotropin stimulation protocols. The results of a prospective study (Fig.16.10) demonstrated that patients who responded to clonidine or to arginine with elevation of GH, responded normally to hMG therapy with a mean effective dose of 1.5 amp/day (11.6 mean total dose) and patients who did not respond to clonidine with elevation of GH, either needed excessive amounts of gonadotropins (mean effective dose of 3 amp/day or a mean total dose of 36.5 amp) to obtain an acceptable

402

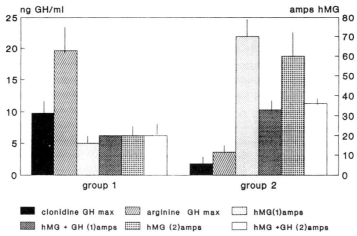

**Fig. 16.10** The gonadotropin dose requirement with and without addition of growth hormone in women responding (group 1) and not responding (group 2) to clonidine and arginine tests.

response, or, despite higher doses of hMG, responded inadequately as expressed by either low serum estradiol levels or lack of sufficient follicular development, or both. The combined administration of GH and hMG to clonidine-negative patients resulted in a good ovarian response despite a significantly lower dose of hMG. In clonidine-positive patients the addition of GH had no significant effect on response or hMG dosage.

This study also demonstrated that the clonidine test, might be a preliminary differentiating indicator of the relative sensitivity of patients to hMG. We think that it will help to select patients who might benefit from the concomitant GH-hMG therapy. One fact should, however, not be disregarded — the connection between patients' body weight and their response to clonidine. Lean women have normal GH pulsatility and GH rise following application of clonidine. Obese patients may show negligible GH pulses and lack of response to clonidine, probably due to excess of GH-binding protein. The usefulness of GH or growth hormone releasing factor (GRF) as adjunctive therapy with gonadotropins must not be overestimated, since insulin-like growth factor-I (IGF-I) is not mandatory for normal ovarian response. It has been shown (Laron et al 1968, Dor et al 1992) that a Laron-type dwarf (an autosomal recessive syndrome, characterized by elevated GH levels concomitant with negligible serum IGF-I levels), can spontaneously ovulate,

conceive and deliver. This same patient, due to secondary infertility, was recently superovulated with gonadotropins for IVF, which permitted us to investigate her ovarian response in detail (Dor et al 1992). Despite undetectable GH-binding protein, negligible IGF-I and elevated IGF-BP levels in her serum and follicular fluid, fertilizable eggs were obtained. This patient, who in effect provided an experiment of nature, together with IVF, permitted us to conclude that IGF-I is not obligatory for ovarian response, but seems to play a permissive modulating role in ovarian physiology. Whatever the exact role of growth hormone and different growth factors in the normal ovulation process, GH may serve as an important addition to the clinical armamentarium employed in the treatment of anovulation and infertility.

## MONITORING OF GONADOTROPIN THERAPY

Proper monitoring is crucial for the results of gonadotropin therapy, i.e. for achieving a high rate of conceptions while avoiding hyperstimulation and reducing the incidence of multiple pregnancy to an acceptable minimum.

Monitoring of the ovarian response to stimulation has four objectives:

1. To determine the size of the effective daily dose of gonadotropins (hMG or FSH)

2. To determine the length of gonadotropin application
3. To determine the size and timing of administration of the ovulatory dose of hCG
4. To determine the occurrence and time of ovulation and to evaluate the corpus luteum function.

Three different types of parameters are used in monitoring gonadotropin therapy:

- Clinical
- Ultrasonic.
- Hormonal

Clinical parameters include vaginal examination, basal body temperature (BBT) records and cervical mucus evaluation expressed as a semiquantitative cervical score (Insler et al 1972). Hormonal assays required for monitoring gonadotropin treatment consist of estrogen and progesterone estimations. The ultrasonic examinations are aimed at determining the number and size of ovarian follicles and, if possible, also at observing their postovulatory transformation into corpora lutea (Cabau & Bessis 1981, Hackeloer 1984, Ritchie 1985).

The latent phase of gonadotropin therapy is 'mute' to hormonal monitoring. At that time neither the clinical nor the hormonal parameters can give an objective measure of the ovarian response to stimulation. The role of monitoring at this stage is to establish the size of the effective daily dose of hMG. This is done empirically by successively increasing the daily dose of hMG (or FSH) by one ampule every 5–7 days until a distinct ovarian response begins as indicated by the initiation of steroidogenesis and by ultrasonically measurable follicular growth (Fig.16.6). The high resolution vaginal sonography permits detection of small antral follicles with a diameter not exceeding 3–4 mm. It can be speculated that in the near future it will be possible to recognize the initial recruitment of follicular cohorts(s) relatively early in the latent phase of therapy. This will permit a more accurate and earlier tailoring of the gonadotropin dose required in each individual treatment course and, consequently, improve the final results of therapy.

The main monitoring effort is centered at the active phase of treatment. The number of follicles developing and their growth rhythm must be established, and the time when at least one follicle is ready to receive the ovulatory LH stimulus must be determined as accurately as possible.

The lessons learned from IVF indicate that in order to carry out this complicated task it is best to use all three monitoring parameters (Fig.16.7): clinical, ultrasonic and hormonal. The number and diameter of follicles determined by ultrasound and the pattern of ascent of estrogen levels provide a good indication of the extant of follicular maturation. The clinical parameters (cervical score), in addition to being an indirect indicator of estrogen levels, reflect the functional state of the genital tract with regard to sperm transport.

It has been repeatedly shown that both plasma $17\beta$-estradiol as well as urinary total estrogen may be used for monitoring gonadotropin therapy with equal efficiency (Insler & Potashnik 1983, Brown 1986, Lequin et al 1986). A steady exponential rise of urinary or plasma estrogen is usually observed during the active phase of gonadotropin therapy. The ideal daily ascent rate is considered to be in the range of 40–100%. A slower ascent may reflect a suboptimal response and a steeper daily increase is a warning sign of an exaggerated response, possibly heralding hyperstimulation.

For many years, the dominant follicle was considered to be the main source of estrogen, the contribution of smaller follicles being regarded as marginal. IVF and ultrasound proved that this is true in monofollicular cycles only. In cycles with multifollicular development, peripheral estrogen levels reflect the sum total of steroidogenic activity of several leading follicles as well as of a number of 'runner up' follicles. Nitschke-Dabelstein et al (1981) showed that an excellent correlation between the $17\beta$-estradiol levels and the number and size of follicles observed on ultrasound could be found in monofollicular but not in multifollicular cycles. On the other hand, the follicular size as measured by ultrasound is inadequate as a sole parameter of follicular maturation, the functional integrity of the follicle being probably better expressed by its steroidogenic activity. This is the main reason for combining hormonal and sonographic parameters in monitoring gonadotropin therapy. A steady daily rise of estrogen levels concomitant with a constant growth of follicular diameter on ultrasound are the best indicators of successful ovarian stimulation as well as reasonably good predictors of hyperstimulation.

*Practical monitoring of gonadotropin treatment is carried out as follow:*

Patients are instructed to keep daily body temperature (BBT) records. Treatment is started between the 3rd and 5th day of spontaneous or induced bleeding. If combined GnRH analog/gonadotropins therapy is applied, the treatment is started when a complete pituitary-ovarian downregulation has been obtained (see under 'combined therapy' above). The initial hMG or FSH dose is usually 1 ampule per day in patients of Group II. In women of Group I and in patients receiving the combined therapy, treatment is usually started with 2 ampules per day. If the patient received gonadotropin therapy in the past, treatment is ordinarily commenced at the level of the effective daily dose (EDD) of the previous course. Prior to initiation of every course of treatment an ultrasonic scan of the pelvic region is performed in order to rule out the presence of abnormal follicular structures or cysts. Since such structures may interfere with ovarian response to stimulation, they should be punctured or the treatment should be delayed until their spontaneous disappearance.

Patients are examined every 1–3 days. This examination includes palpation of the ovaries, estimation of cervical score, postcoital tests when indicated, and a short interview with the patient regarding her general well-being. The dose of gonadotropins is adjusted according to the patient's response as indicated by estrogens, ultrasonography and clinical findings (Figs 16.6, 16.7). If estrogens are low and not rising, the initial dose of gonadotropins is continued for 5–7 days and then increased by 1 ampule. This procedure is repeated until the EDD, i.e the dose which causes a significant and steady estrogen rise, is achieved. In patients with low endogenous estrogens at initiation of therapy, cervical score estimations may replace estrogen assays for the estimation of EDD. From this day on the patient is examined daily or on alternate days. When estrogen levels reach or exceed 250 pg/ml, ultra-

sonography is performed. If estrogens increase too rapidly or the day-to-day difference exceeds the geometric rise, the dose is reduced by 1 ampule (75 IU FSH) and treatment is continued at this reduced dosage (Fig.16.7). If the estrogen rise is steady and not excessive, the same dose is continued until an estradiol level between 350 and 1200 pg/ml is reached. Since the duration of the active phase is 4–6 days, this level should be reached within this time limit. At this stage of therapy the third sonographic scan is performed. If, in both ovaries, the total number of measurable follicular structures does not exceed ten and between one and four follicles have a diameter exceeding 17mm, the ovulatory dose of hCG (10,000 IU) is administered. The patient is advised to have intercourse on three consecutive days starting on the day of hCG administration. After induction of ovulation the patient is examined 3–5 and 7–9 days following the hCG injection. Special care is taken not to overlook possible ovarian enlargement, abdominal pains, tenderness or distension, and weight gain exceeding 3kg. At least one blood sample is drawn and sent for progesterone assay. The patient is instructed to report back to the clinic if abdominal pains, nausea, vomiting or diarrhea appear. If a sustained high phase of BBT lasts for more than 14 days, an hCG and progesterone assay should be performed. Clinical research and experience showed that in gonadotropin therapy multifollicular and multiluteal cycles are a rule rather than an exception (Insler & Potashnik 1983). However, only a small proportion of the multiluteal cycles results also in multiple clinical pregnancies. Brown (1986) remarked that although multiple preovulatory follicles were seen by ultrasound in 50% of gonadotropin-induced cycles, the recorded multiple pregnancy rate was only 20%. O'Herlihy et al (1981) showed that multiple preovulatory follicles were found in 71% of clomiphene cycles, but the incidence of multiple pregnancy was only 14%. It is thus probable that in hMG-induced conception cycles a number of ova are usually released and possibly fertilized but only one or two of them are destined to produce a fetus.

The IVF programs introduced a very important contribution to the management of gonadotropin therapy, particularly when multiple follicles are stimulated. Some of the excessive follicles may be punctured under ultrasound control, thus reducing the estradiol levels, leaving a smaller number of follicles to be luteinized by the hCG administration and diminishing the chance of clinical hyperstimulation.

There is still no general agreement with regard to the integrity of corpus luteum function in stimulated cycles. Luteal insufficiency has been implied to be one of the major reasons for conception failure, nidation inadequacy or early clinical abortion. The problem is too complicated to be explained by analysis of steroid levels and their ratios or by examination of endometrial structure using light microscopy (and possibly also standard electron microscopy). In order to be able to determine whether the luteal function in stimulated cycles is normal we must compare it with a gold standard, i.e. the corpus luteum function in spontaneous ovulatory cycles. Unfortunately, this standard is not made of high purity gold. Landgren et al (1980) examined 68 meticulously selected spontaneously ovulating healthy women and found that the length of sustained high phase BBT was 13 days or less in 20% of cases. On day 8 after LH peak the difference between the lowest and highest levels of estradiol was fourfold and those of progesterone ninefold. Colston-Wentz (1980) examined 97 endometrial biopsies of presumably ovulating infertile women and reported that 33% of the samples showed an out of phase endometrium. Perez and his coworkers (1981) examined the corpus luteum and its function in 50 presumably ovulating infertile patients. They used four parameters: laparoscopy, progesterone values, endometrial biopsy and BBT. In 39 patients all four parameters were synchronized indicating adequate luteal function. However, in three cases, despite finding an apparently normal corpus luteum on laparoscopy, the other parameters were abnormal. In eight other women, laparoscopy did not reveal the presence of a recent corpus luteum, but three of them had a secretory endometrium. It thus seems that accurate evaluation of corpus luteum function in normal ovulatory cycles is difficult due to the following elements:

- Large variation of hormonal values between individuals

- High phase of BBT may be sustained by relatively low progesterone values
- Timing of endometrial biopsy may be false
- Standard histology of endometrium may not accurately represent its functional capacity.

Since most of the stimulated cycles are multifollicular and probably multiluteal, the problem is even more complicated. However, Laufer et al (1982) found that in stimulated, presumably ovulatory, cycles the estrogen and progesterone levels were significantly higher than in spontaneous ovulations, but in both groups steroid levels were similar in conceptional and nonconceptional cycles. Huang et al (1986) reported that in IVF cycles the individual variation of progesterone levels during the luteal phase was large, but cycles with pregnancy did not significantly differ from those without pregnancy. Nylund et al (1990) studied 57 IVF cycles from which 15 resulted in clinical pregnancy and 42 in unsuccessful implantation. The values of estradiol, progesterone, testosterone and sex hormone binding globulin (SHBG) were not different in the two groups. The reports on endometrial structure in stimulated (or IVF) cycles are controversial. Search of the scientific literature of the last decade showed that some authors found frequent endometrial abnormalities (Garcia et al 1981, Cohen et al 1984, Sterzik et al 1988, Paulson et al 1990), while others reported that in stimulated and hyperstimulated cycles the endometrium was fully in phase, despite the high levels and/or abnormal ratios of sex steroids (Frydman et al 1982, Dehou et al 1987, Barash et al 1992).

Considering the methodological and objective difficulties in assessment of the corpus luteum function in stimulated cycles which are usually multifollicular, it is obvious that no consensus has been reached with regard to exogenous hormonal support of the corpus luteum function following induction of ovulation. Some authors advise to support the corpus luteum by administering intramuscular injections or vaginal suppositories of progesterone (Leeton et al 1985, Yovich et al 1985). Others suggest 2 or 3 booster injections of 2500–5000 IU of hCG on days 5 and 7 after ovulation induction (Buvat et al 1990, Hutchinson-Williams et al 1990, Yovich et al 1991). The final conclusion as to the frequency and extent of corpus luteum insufficiency in stimulated cycles and the impact of this condition on the results of therapy cannot be established at this time. Consequently, the luteal phase support is not considered an integral part of ovulation (or superovulation) inducing therapy.

## RESULTS OF GONADOTROPIN THERAPY

Conception rates following gonadotropin therapy are dependent on the following factors (in order of importance):

- Selection of patients
- Type of monitoring
- Treatment scheme.

In women with hypothalamic-pituitary failure (Group I), substitution therapy with gonadotropins is very efficient in inducing ovulation and pregnancy. Gonadotropin treatment applied as stimulation or regulation therapy in patients having some, albeit deranged, hypothalamic-pituitary-gonadal function (Group II), is by far more complicated and less efficient see also 'Treatment schemes' above).

While in patients of Group I pregnancy rates of up to 82% were achieved, in Group II conception rates varied between 20% and 35% (Lunenfeld & Insler 1978, Lunenfeld et al 1985, Australian Department of Health 1981, Bettendorf et al 1981). The same discrepancy was also seen when cumulative pregnancy rates were calculated using

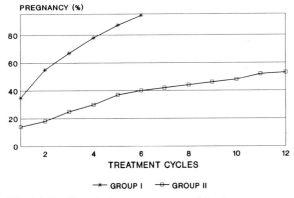

**Fig. 16.11** Cumulative pregnancy rates following gonadotropin therapy (without IVF, GIFT or TET procedures) in patients of Group I and Group II, Women of Group II received gonadotropin treatment after failure of other treatment modalities. In order to reduce the possible bias, women over 35 years old were excluded.

the life table analysis method. In Group I, after six cycles of therapy, the cumulative pregnancy rate exceeded 90%. In contrast, patients of Group II required 12 cycles of therapy in order to reach a cumulative conception rate of less than 60% (Fig. 16.11).

Age of the patients also influences the outcome of treatment markedly. Women over 35 years of age had a significantly reduced conception rate regardless of the type of diagnosis and treatment (Insler et al 1981). The duration of amenorrhea, on the other hand, had no bearing on the results of gonadotropin therapy. The treatment was as efficient in women being amenorrheic for 1 year only as in those who suffered from amenorrhea for 10 years or more.

Table 16.2 shows the results of gonadotropin therapy as reported by 18 different groups working independently on four continents. This list does not purport to include all data on gonadotropin therapy published so far. It shows, nevertheless, the overall dimension of this therapy and its importance in the therapeutic armamentarium of fertility clinics throughout the world. The list includes over 23 000 treatment courses given to 8399 women and 2933 conceptions. Since the majority of entries deals with rather large groups of patients, this summary represents the results of gonadotropin treatment in unselected material typical to busy fertility clinics.

The pregnancy rates (per patient) varied between 23.1% and 82.5%, with an average of 34.2%. Pregnancy rates per cycle ranged from 7.1% to 21.8%. The intensity of treatment (the mean number of treatment courses per patient) fluctuated from 2.0 to 4.2. By knowing the pregnancy rate per cycle specific to each clinic, one can easily calculate the overall prognosis and cost of this treatment.

During the last few years hMG stimulation has been used in spontaneously ovulating women with unexplained infertility or subfertility of the male partner. In this group the ovarian stimulation (or controlled hyperstimulation) is usually combined with IUI. The aim of these experiments has been to determine whether in this category of patients gonadotropin therapy combined with IUI is equally efficient as IVF-ET, GIFT or TET procedures. The results presented in Table 16.2

**Table 16.2** Conception rates following gonadotropin therapy

| Author | Patients | Cycles | Pregnancies | | |
|---|---|---|---|---|---|
| | | | No. | % Cycles | % Patients |
| Australian Department of Health 1981 | 1056 | 4008 | 552 | 13.8 | 52.3 |
| Bettendorf et al 1981 | 756 | 1585 | 224 | 14.1 | 29.6 |
| Butler 1970 | 134 | 438 | 31 | 7.1 | 23.1 |
| Caspi et al 1974 | 101 | 343 | 62 | 18.1 | 61.4 |
| Ellis & Williamson 1975 | 77 | 332 | 43 | 13.3 | 55.8 |
| Gemzell 1970 | 228 | 463 | 101 | 21.8 | 44.3 |
| Goldfarb et al 1982 | 442 | 1098 | 118 | 10.7 | 26.7 |
| Healy et al 1980 | 40 | 159 | 33 | 20.7 | 82.5 |
| Kurachi 1983 | 2166 | 6096 | 523 | 8.6 | 24.2 |
| Lunenfeld et al 1985 | 1107 | 3646 | 424 | 11.6 | 38.3 |
| Potashnik et al 1986 * | 262 | 580 | 85 | 14.6 | 32.4 |
| Spadoni et al 1974 | 62 | 225 | 26 | 11.5 | 41.9 |
| Thompson & Hansen 1970 | 1190 | 2798 | 334 | 11.9 | 28.1 |
| Tsapoulis et al 1974 | 320 | ? | 163 | | 50.9 |
| CUMULATIVE (subtotal) | 7941 | | 2719 | | 34.2 |
| Serhal et al 1988 | 48 | 77 | 5 | 6.5 | 15.6 |
| Welner et al 1988 | 97 | 388 | 12 | 3.1 | 12.4 |
| Martinez et al 1991 | 48 | 77 | 5 | 6.5 | 15.6 |
| Chaffkin et al 1991 | 266 | 695 | 85 | 12.2 | 31.9 |
| CUMULATIVE (subtotal) | 458 | 1243 | 114 | 9.2 | 24.9 |
| CUMULATIVE (total) | 8399 | | 2933 | | 34.9 |

*Potashnik G, Glassner M, Holzberg G, Insler V unpublished data. Ovulatory women treated for unexplained or male infertility. hMG stimulation combined with timed intercourse or IUI.

seem to be promising. With a relatively low mean number of courses per patient (2.7), 24.9% of women achieved conception.

## Outcome of pregnancies

The course of gestation following induction of ovulation with hMG appeared to be normal. Analysis of the mode of delivery showed a high incidence of interventions, breech extraction, vacuum extraction, forceps delivery, and cesarean sections. The high incidence of obstetrical intervention may be explained by elevated multiple pregnancy rate, primiparity ratios, relatively high maternal age and by psychological factors involved in delivering a 'premium child' in patients of long-standing infertility.

Our study (Ben-Rafael et al 1986) showed that the sex ratio (M/F) of the single births was 1.06 (54% boys) and of the twins 0.72 (42% boys). The numbers of triplets were too small to analyse. In 1976 Caspi reported 32 males and 50 females in the single births (39%), with a twin M/F ratio of 0.78 (Caspi et al 1976a,b). In the series

reported by Bettendorf et al (1981) the incidence of male children in single pregnancies was 51.8%. However, in the above author's series the incidence of male children in twins and triplets was 53.8% and 66.7% respectively. The normal secondary sex ratio at 28 weeks is considered to be 106 boys to 100 girls (Tricomi et al 1960, Serr & Ismajovich 1963).

The sex ratio (M/F) for twins was found by Nichols (1952) to be 1.043, for triplets 1.007 and for quadruplets 0.940. The high incidence of girls in our twin series and the high incidence of male children in twins and triplets in the series of Bettendorf et al (1981) are probably due to the rather small numbers involved. By combining all the three series, one approaches the expected sex ratios indicating clearly the importance of sufficiently large number in order to estimate similarities or divergence in sex ratio.

## Congenital malformations

Table 16.3 shows the rate of congenital malformations found in a combined series of 941 babies

**Table 16.3**  Congenital malformations after ovulation induction with human gonadotropins

| Author | No. | Major | Minor |
|---|---|---|---|
| Kurachi et al 1985 | 509 | 9 | 1 |
| Hack & Lunenfeld 1978 | 209 | 4 | 4 |
| Caspi et al 1976b | 157 | 4 | 11 |
| Harlap 1976 | 66 | 1 | 5 |
| Total | 941 | 18 (1.91%) | 21 (2.23%) |
| Normal population | | (1.27%) (0.31–2.25) | (7.24%) |

born after induction of ovulation with hMG/hCG. The incidence was 22.3/1000 and 19.1/1000 of minor and major malformations respectively. The incidence of congenital malformations in normal populations has been reported to be 12.7/1000 after 28 weeks' gestation, with a range of 3.1–22.5 (McKeown 1960, Stevenson et al 1966). There is a further rise to 23.1/1000 by the age of 5 years. Hendricks (1966) reported a rate of 3% in the neonatal period, with twice as many malformations in twin births, mostly monozygotic twins. Shoham et al (1991a,b) reviewed a large number of reports dealing with congenital malformations in children born after induction of ovulation and concluded that clomiphene citrate, hMG/hCG or the association of these drugs with IVF-ET and GIFT procedures do not carry an increased risk for congenital malformations as a whole, nor is there any specific malformation that has an increased incidence that is related in any way with the use of those drugs. It can thus be summarized that, at present, the clinical evidence does not indicate that babies born after hMG/hCG ovulation induction are at any greater risk of malformation than the general population.

## COMPLICATIONS OF GONADOTROPIN THERAPY

All complications of gonadotropin treatment are essentially due to ovarian stimulation, follicular development and luteinization or ovulation. To the best of our knowledge direct side-effects to the drug itself have not been reported.

The main complications of gonadotropin treatment are:

1. Ovarian hyperstimulation syndrome
2. High incidence of multiple pregnancy
3. Abortion rate higher than in spontaneous conceptions

## Ovarian hyperstimulation

### Incidence of hyperstimulation

Analysis of several large series encompassing 10 929 treatment cycles showed that the incidence of moderate and severe hyperstimulation was 3.4% and 0.84% respectively (Table 16.4) It should be noted that all the above reports included cases treated without sonographic monitoring. The possible influence of patients' selection, treatment schedules and monitoring methods on the relative risks of hyperstimulation have been discussed in previous sections of this chapter. It is true that only some of the patients who received hCG, despite inappropriate rise or excessive levels of estrogen, develop ovarian hyperstimulation. It is certain, however, that all women who did develop the syndrome had abnormally high preovulatory estrogen levels. Only future statistical analysis will demonstrate if the additional use of sonography will enable a further reduction in the rate of hyperstimulation or multiple births.

### Classification

Ovarian hyperstimulation is the most serious

**Table 16.4**  Incidence of hyperstimulation following ovulation induction with human gonadotropins

| Author | Treatment cycles (no.) | Mild hyper stimulation (%) | Severe hyper stimulation (%) |
|---|---|---|---|
| Australian Department of Health 1981 | 4008 | 3.7 | 0.9 |
| Caspi et al 1976a | 343 | 6.0 | 1.2 |
| Ellis & Williamson 1975 | 322 | 5.0 | 0.6 |
| Spadoni et al 1974 | 225 | 4.4 | 1.8 |
| Thompson & Hansen 1970 | 2798 | ? | 1.3 |
| Lunenfeld et al 1985 | 3232 | 3.1 | 0.25 |
| Total | 10929 | 3.4 | 0.84 |

complication of ovulation induction therapy. The syndrome (OHSS) occurs when ovulation-inducing treatment results in the growth of multiple large follicles followed by the development of follicular and luteal cysts. A comprehensive classification of hyperstimulation into six grades was originally proposed by Rabau et al (1967) and was later modified into three grades (WHO 1976).

Grade I (mild hyperstimulation) is characterized by variable ovarian enlargement with cysts measuring up to 5 cm in diameter. Laboratory findings include urinary estrogen over 150 μg/24 h and pregnanediol excretion exceeding 10 mg/24 h. With measurements of steroids in blood this would correspond to estradiol values greater than 1500 pg/ml and progesterone levels over 30 ng/ml in the early luteal phase.

Grade II (moderate hyperstimulation) is characterized by ovarian cysts accompanied by additional symptoms such as abdominal distension, nausea, vomiting and diarrhea. A sudden weight increase exceeding 3000 g may be an early sign of moderate hyperstimulation.

Grade III (severe hyperstimulation) is defined by the presence of large ovarian cysts, ascites and sometimes hydrothorax. Severe hemoconcentration is usually also observed and may, in extreme cases, result in blood hypercoagulation. Tulandi et al (1984) found the pregnancy rate in hyperstimulated cycles to be three times greater than in nonhyperstimulated cycles. It is generally agreed that mild hyperstimulation (multifollicular development) is associated with an increased pregnancy rate. However, we have shown that in severe hyperstimulation, the abortion rate is significantly higher.

*Pathogenesis*

Ovarian hyperstimulation is the result of massive follicular luteinization. It therefore occurs only following hCG administration or following an endogenous LH peak induced by the elevated estrogen production of multifollicular growth. In the former case, clinical symptoms usually appear 5–10 days following the first dose of hCG. In the latter case, hyperstimulation is extremely rare because the intraovarian regulatory mechanisms

and endogenous negative feedback are usually able to prevent an endogenous LH surge of sufficient height and duration to cause massive luteinization. Ovarian enlargement (with or without cyst formation) and ovulation may occur. Thus, preventing ovulation by withholding hCG is an effective method of avoiding hyperstimulation in overstimulated ovaries.

Hyperstimulation appears when a large number of follicles is recruited and sustained by the pharmacological dose of gonadotropins. According to our observations (unpublished data), it seems that multiple relatively small follicles are more prone to generate hyperstimulation than the fully matured ones. The mean number of follicles was significantly greater in hyperstimulated than in nonhyperstimulated cycles (Fig.16.12). However, the mean follicular diameter was larger in nonhyperstimulated cycles (Fig.16.13), indicating that in treatment courses which eventually could develop hyperstimulation,

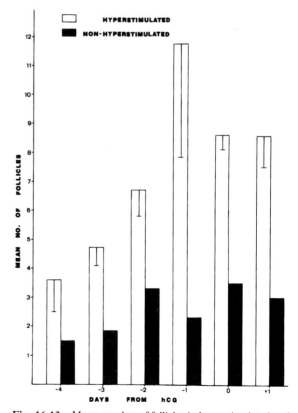

**Fig. 16.12** Mean number of follicles in hyperstimulated and nonhyperstimulated gonadotropin treatments.

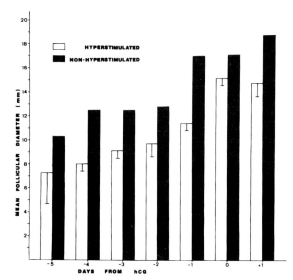

**Fig. 16.13**   Mean follicular diameter in hyperstimulated and nonhyperstimulated gonadotropin treatments.

the majority of follicles did not reach full maturity.

The fact that ovulation (luteinization) is a precondition necessary for hyperstimulation to occur suggested the involvement of ovarian (luteal) secretions in the pathogenesis of this syndrome. Polishuk & Schenker (1969) found that high-dose hMG treatment caused no complications in male rabbits while all hyperstimulated female rabbits, including a group with extraperitonealized ovaries, displayed ovarian enlargement and ascites. They concluded that ovarian secretion is responsible for increased capillary permeability causing an extraperitoneal fluid shift. In fact, high levels of hormones have been detected in severe cases of clinical hyperstimulation, including estradiol, estriol, progesterone, 17-OH-progesterone, pregnanediol, pregnanetriol, testosterone, 17-hydrocorticosteroids, 17-ketosteroids and aldosterone (Engel et al 1972, Schenker & Weinstein 1977).

The exact factors responsible for enhanced capillary permeability are the subject of debate. Prostaglandins, histamine and estrogens have been mentioned (Davis 1960, Engel et al 1972, Schenker & Polishuk 1976). More recent studies (Navot et al 1987) seem to indicate that some compounds belonging to the angiotensin system may damage the integrity of capillaries. Tollan &

her coworkers (1990) studied transcapillary fluid dynamics in 10 women during ovarian stimulation using the 'wick' method for measuring the interstitial colloid osmotic pressure and the 'wick in needle' approach for estimating the interstitial hydrostatic pressure. Plasma colloid osmotic pressure decreased and interstitial colloid osmotic pressure increased during the course of stimulation, with a corresponding rise of plasma estrogen levels. These findings imply a reduced transcapillary colloid osmotic gradient, probably due to increased capillary permeability to plasma proteins. This report adds to our understanding of the mechanism of abnormal fluid compartmentalization during ovarian hyperstimulation. It does not, however, identify the factor which unsettles the functional integrity of the capillary walls. Koos (1991) reported that a paracrine angiogenic factor, called the vascular endothelial growth factor (VEGF), and its specific mRNA were found in granulosa cells. He also observed that following ovulation the vascular growth rate as expressed by the ovarian endothelial cells proliferation is higher than that in rapidly growing malignant tumors.

Vascular neogenesis is a condition sine qua non of the normal follicular growth. In ovarian hyperstimulation syndrome this process is both enhanced and disturbed, resulting in incompetent capillary function, which leads to recompartmentalization of body fluids and consequently to reduction of intravascular volume and formation of ascites and/or hydrothorax and general edema. Figure 16.14 illustrates schematically the sequence of events leading to the ovarian hyperstimulation syndrome.

Regardless of its exact etiology, the increased capillary permeability results in massive ascites and hypovolemia which Engel et al (1972) term the 'cardinal events' in the pathogenesis of the OHSS. Hypovolemia is associated with hemoconcentration, decreased central venous pressure, low blood pressure, and tachycardia. Severe hypovolemia also causes decreased renal perfusion leading to increased reabsorption of sodium and water in the proximal tubule (Polishuk & Schenker 1969) causing oliguria and low urinary sodium. Exchange of hydrogen and potassium for sodium in the distal tubule is reduced resulting in

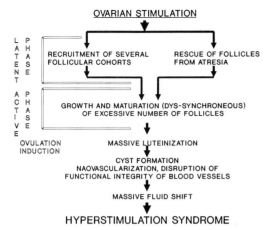

OVARIAN STIMULATION

LATENT PHASE

RECRUITMENT OF SEVERAL FOLLICULAR COHORTS

RESCUE OF FOLLICLES FROM ATRESIA

ACTIVE PHASE

GROWTH AND MATURATION (DYS-SYNCHRONEOUS) OF EXCESSIVE NUMBER OF FOLLICLES

OVULATION INDUCTION

MASSIVE LUTEINIZATION

CYST FORMATION

NAOVASCULARIZATION, DISRUPTION OF FUNCTIONAL INTEGRITY OF BLOOD VESSELS

MASSIVE FLUID SHIFT

HYPERSTIMULATION SYNDROME

**Fig. 16.14** Schematic presentation of the pathogenesis of ovarian hyperstimulation syndrome (OHSS). The process essentially begins during the latent phase of therapy by recruitment of an excessive number of follicles. Continuation of pharmacological dosage of gonadotropins during the active phase enables the support of growth and maturation of a large number of follicles. Induction of ovulation by hCG results in massive luteinization of both mature and immature follicles. The luteinized follicles trigger a neovascularization process of immense proportion, accompanied by disruption of functional integrity of blood vessels. This results in recompartmentalization of fluids followed by other clinical symptoms of OHSS.

an accumulation of $H^+$ and $K^+$ causing hyperkalemia and a tendency to acidosis (Engel et al 1972). The extensiveness of ascites is reflected in the patients' weight gain. Patients with severe OHSS can gain as much as 15–20 kg.

A quite dangerous although extremely rare side-effect of OHSS is the occurrence of thromboembolic phenomena. The connection between hMG treatment and clotting abnormalities was first reported by Mozes et al (1985). While the cause of thromboembolic phenomena is still not fully established, it is probably related to hemoconcentration (and to elevated estrogen levels). Phillips et al (1975) reported high levels of factor V, platelets, fibrinogen, profibrinolysin, fibrinolytic inhibitors and increased thromboplastin generation in patients with OHSS.

## Treatment

As hyperstimulation is a self-limiting disease, its treatment should be symptomatic and conservative even though the severity of its symptoms would seem to demand radical, surgical care. Treatment is generally medical, with laparotomy

reserved for cases of an abdominal catastrophe (i.e. ovarian torsion or rupture and internal hemorrhage). The ovarian cysts are so large and brittle that surgical attempts at a palliative procedure usually result in oophorectomy.

Medical treatment of severe hyperstimulation is aimed at: (1) maintaining blood volume while correcting the disturbed fluid and electrolyte balance, (2) preventing thromboembolic phenomena, and (3) relieving secondary complications of ascites and hydrothorax. The patient should be monitored by fluid intake/output records, weight, and frequent measurements of the degree of hemoconcentration as indicated by hemoglobin and hematocrit estimation. In very severe cases, constant measurement of central venous pressure may be indicated. Plasma expanders such as dextran and plasma supplemented with appropriate electrolytes should be administered early. Diuretic agents are contraindicated since fluid in the third space is unavailable for diuresis and most diuretics influence the distal tubule with minimal effect on the proximal tubule (Engel et al 1972). Thus, the artificially induced diuresis may further diminish the intravascular volume but be unable to cause reduction of the ascites or hydrothorax.

Anticoagulant therapy is usually unnecessary if the aforementioned steps are employed promptly. However, because of the danger of disseminated intravascular clotting, blood coagulation should be monitored and if severe hypercoagulability is present, heparin treatment may be considered. Since in such cases miniheparinization is not effective, full heparinization (according to patient's response) should be applied. It should, however, be remembered that in early pregnancy heparin may cause retrotrophoblastic bleeding and lead to abortion.

The third goal of treatment is relieving pulmonary and/or abdominal symptoms. Pleural effusions should be drained, and Rabau et al (1967) proposed paracentesis for alleviating breathing difficulty. Schenker & Weinstein (1977) argue against paracentesis because of the danger of puncturing cysts and causing intraperitoneal hemorrhage. In our hands, paracentesis did not cause intraperitoneal hemorrhage. Needless to say, puncture of the abdominal cavity and/or of ovarian cysts should be performed under sonographic control.

## Abortions

The abortion rate in conceptions following gonadotropin therapy is around 21%. Brown (1986) compiled and reviewed a series of 1712 pregnancies and found that the combined abortion and perinatal deaths rates fluctuated from 10% to 28% in different reports.

There was no significant difference in the abortion rate in relation to diagnostic groups. The rate was 26% in patients of Group I and 32.6% in women of Group II respectively (Blankstein et al 1986). However, the abortion rate in the first conception cycle (28.8%) was significantly higher then in the second or third gestation (12.8%). The main reasons for increased abortion rates in conceptions resulting from induction of ovulation have been presumed to be: (a) structural and functional inadequacy of the endometrium to ensure proper and timely nidation of the embryo; (b) functional incompetence of the corpus luteum preventing it from a proper reaction to the pregnancy signal, i.e. the initial increase of hCG produced by the trophoblast; (c) multiple pregnancy, and (d) emotional factors. An in-depth analysis of the literature seems, however, to indicate that the dominant cause for early pregnancy wastage in conceptions resulting from ovarian stimulation is the quality of ova, which, in turn, depends on the nature of follicular environment during follicular maturation. This conclusion is also strongly supported by analysis of the fate of spontaneous pregnancies. According to Chard (1991) only 30% of natural conceptions produce a term pregnancy.

## Multiple pregnancy

Multiple pregnancy is rather frequent following gonadotropin therapy. Brown (1986) reviewed 1712 pregnancies resulting from ovulation induction by human pituitary or menopausal gonadotropins and found that the average multiple pregnancy rate was 24.4%, fluctuating between 21% and 33%. As expected, small series showed a lower incidence of multiple gestations than large series. The causes of multiple conceptions following induced cycles are very similar to those causing ovarian hyperstimulation, i.e. the pharmacological stimulation of multifollicular development. Thus, the risk factors and the possibilities to avoid (or at least reduce the incidence of) both complications are similar (see 'Ovarian hyperstimulation' above). Insler & Potashnik (1983) reported that in 26% of gonadotropin-induced cycles three or more functional corpora lutea were produced and that mean plateau progesterone levels were higher in the conceptional than in the nonconceptional cycles. Further analysis of the above data indicated that in hMG treatment cycles conception occurs in most cases in the presence of more than one corpus luteum, and in one-quarter of cases in the presence of three or more functioning corpora lutea. Since only around 25% of gonadotropin-induced pregnancies result in twins and only 5% produce three or more fetuses, and since the mean plateau progesterone levels are similar in single and multiple hMG-induced pregnancies, it could be speculated that in the majority of hMG conceptions a number of ova are released and fertilized but only one of them is destined to produce a living fetus. The others perish before reaching the uterine cavity or are absorbed or extruded prior to implantation.

If, however, a quadruplet, quintuplet, etc., pregnancy reaches the gestational age of 7–8 weeks, its further development may represent a severe danger to the fetuses because of a very high probability of extreme prematurity, a considerable medical complication to the mother, and a pronounced psychological, social and financial burden to the family. The technique of fetal reduction under sonographic control has been developed. Breckwoldt et al (1988) reported a case of gonadotropin-induced pregnancy with nine gestational sacks present in the uterus. Six of the fetuses were eliminated under sonographic guidance. This technique, although medically simple and logical, is still controversial for ethical, legal and religious reasons.

## CONCLUDING REMARKS

During the last two decades human

gonadotropins have become an integral part of therapy of functional infertility. Introduced as a substitution therapy for hypogonadotropic hypogonadism, the indications for this modality have been gradually amplified to the treatment of other types of fertility disturbances such as anovulation, oligoovulation, PCOD, etc. Finally, the concept of achieving superovulation by controlled ovarian hyperstimulation (COH) in spontaneous ovulators has been instigated. This, in combination with IVF, GIFT, IUI and other assisted reproduction techniques, demanded the use of gonadotropins in the treatment of mechanical, male and unexplained infertility. The number of patients treated grew over the years to such proportions that supply shortages of the drug have become imminent. Production of human FSH and LH by genetic engineering techniques seems to be within reach and will probably cover the growing demand in the near future.

## REFERENCES

Adashi E Y, Carol H, Resnick A, D'Ecole J, Svoboda E M, Van Wyk J J 1985a Insulin-like growth factors as intraovarian regulators of granulosa cell growth and function. Endocrinol Rev 6: 400

Adashi E Y, Resnick A, Svoboda E M, Van Wyk J J 1985b Somatomedin C synergizes with FSH in the acquisition of projection biosynthetic capacity by cultured rat granulosa cells. Endocrinology 116: 2135

Adashi E Y, Resnick A, Svoboda E M, Van Wyk J J 1985c Somatomedin C enhances induction of LH receptors by FSH in cultured rat granulosa cells. Endocrinology 116: 2369

Adashi E Y, Resnick C E, Hernandez E R et al 1990 The ovarian IGF-1 system as a paradigm for putative intra-ovarian regulators. In: Yen S S C, Vale W W (eds) Neuroendocrine regulation of reproduction, Serono Symposia. Norwell, MA, pp 185–194

Australian Department of Health 1981 Results of hMG therapy. Australian Department of Health, Canberra

Baird D T 1987 A model for follicular selection and ovulation: lessons from superovulation. J Steroid Biochem 27: 15

Barash A, Czernobilsky B, Insler V, Borenstein R, Rosenberg M, Fink A 1992 Endometrial morphology and hormonal profiles in in vitro fertilization patients. Eur J Obstet Gynecol 44: 117–121

Ben-Nun I, Lunenfeld B, Ben-Aderet N 1984 Prevention de la lutcinisation prematuc du follicule par hyperprolactinemie iatrogene volontaire au cours des traitements par HMG Hormons. Reprod Med 5: 54–57

Ben-Rafael Z, Matalon A, Blankstein J, Serr D M, Lunenfeld B, Mashiach S 1986 Male to female ratio after gonadotropin-induced ovulation. Fertil Steril 45: 36

Bettendorf G 1963 Human hypophyseal gonadotropin in hypophysectomized women. Int J Fertil 8: 799

Bettendorf G, Apostolakis M, Voigt K D 1961 Darstellung hochaktiver Gonadotropin Fraktionen aus menschlichen Hypophysen und deren Anwendung beim Menschen. Procs Int Fed Gynecol Obstet 1: 76 (abstr)

Bettendorf G, Braendle W, Sprotte C H, Weise C H, Zimmerman R 1981 Overall results of gonadotropin therapy. In: Insler V, Bettendorf G (eds) Advances in diagnosis and treatment of infertility. Elsevier/North Holland, New York, pp 21–26

Blankstein J, Mashiah S Lunenfeld E 1986 Ovulation induction and in vitro fertilization. Year Book, Chicago

Blumenfeld Z, Lunenfeld B 1989 The potential effect of growth hormone on follicle stimulation with human menopausal gonadotropin in a panhypopituitary patient. Fertil Steril 52: 328

Blumenfeld Z, Nahhas F 1988 Luteal dysfuction in induction of ovulation: the role of repetitive human chorionic gonadotropin supplementation during luteal phase. Fertil Steril 50: 403

Breckwoldt M, Neulen J, Wieacker P, Schillinger H 1988 Induction of ovulation by combined GnRH -A/hMG/hCG treatment. In: Lunenfeld B (ed) Symposium on GnRH analogues in cancer and human reproduction. Parthenon, Casterton Hall, pp 58–58

Brown J B 1986 Gonadotropins. In: Insler V, Lunenfeld B (eds) Infertility: male and female. Churchill Livingstone, Edinburgh pp 359–396

Butler J K 1970 Oestrone response patterns and clinical results following various Pergonal dosage schedules. In: Butler J K (ed) Developments in the pharmacology and clinical uses of human gonadotrophins. G.D.Searle, High Wycombe, UK, pp 42–46

Butt W R, Kennedy J F 1971 Structure–activity relationships of protein and polypeptide hormones. In: Margoulis M, Greenwood P C (eds) Protein and polypeptide hormones. Excerpta Medica, Amsterdam, p 115

Buvat J, Marcolin G, Guittard C, Herbaut J C, Louvet A L, Dehaene J L 1990 Luteal support after luteinizing hormone-releasing hormone agonist for in vitro fertilization: superiority of human chorionic gonadotropin over oral progesterone. Fertil Steril 53: 490

Cabau A, Bessis R 1981 Monitoring of ovulation induction with human menopausal gonadotropin and human chorionic gonadotropin by ultrasound. Fertil Steril 36: 178

Caspi E, Levin S, Bukovsky J, Weintraub Z 1974 Induction of pregnancy with human gonadotropins after clomiphene failure in menstruating ovulatory infertility patients. Isr J Med Sci 10: 249

Caspi E, Ronen J, Schreyer P et al 1976a Pregnancy and infant outcome after gonadotropin therapy. Br J Obstet Gynaecol 83: 967

Caspi E, Ronen J, Schreyer P, Goldberg M D 1976b The outcome of pregnancy after gonadotrophin therapy. Br J Obstet Gynaecol 83: 967

Chaffkin L M, Nulsen J C, Luciano A A, Metzger D A 1991 A comparative analysis of the cycle fecundity rates associated with combined human menopausal gonadotropin (hMG) and intrauterine insemination (IUI) versus either hMG or IUI alone. Fertil Steril 55: 252

Chard T 1991 Frequency of implantation and early pregnancy loss in natural cycles. Baillieres Clin Obstet Gynaecol 5: 179

Cohen J J, Debache C, Pigeau F, Mandelbaum J, Plachot M, de-Brux J 1984 Sequential use of clomiphene citrate, human menopausal gonadotropin, and human chorionic gonadotropin in human in vitro fertilization. II. Study of luteal phase adequacy following aspiration of the preovulatory follicles. Fertil Steril 42: 360

Colston-Wentz A 1980 Endometrial biopsy in the evaluation of infertility. Fertil Steril 33: 121

Cook A S, Webster B W, Terranova P F, Keel B A 1988 Variation in the biologic and biochemical characteristics of human menopausal gonadotropin. Fertil Steril 49: 704

Crawley W F, Comite F, Vale W, Rivier J, Loriaux D L, Cutler G B 1982 Inhibition of serum androgen levels by chronic intranasal and subcutaneous administration of a potent luteinizing hormone-releasing hormone (LH-RH) agonist in adult men. Fertil Steril 27: 1240

Crooke A C 1970 Comparison of the effects of pergonal and pituitary follicle stimulating hormone. In: Butler J K (ed) Developments in the pharmacology and clinical uses of human gonadotrophins. G.D. Searle, High Wycombe, UK, pp 36–41

Davis J S 1960 Hormonal control of plasma and erythrocyte volume of rat uterus. Am J Physiol 199: 841

Davoren J B, Hsueh A J W 1986 Growth hormone increased ovarian levels of immunoreactive somatomedin C/insulin-like growth factor I in vivo. Endocrinology 118: 888

De La Llosa P, Jutisz M 1969 Protein and polypeptide hormones. In: Margoulis M (ed) Protein and polypeptide hormones. Exerpta Medica, Amsterdam, pp 229–234

Dehou M F, Lejeune B, Arijs C, Leroy F 1987 Endometrial morphology in stimulated in vitro fertilization cycles and after steroid replacement therapy in cases of primary ovarian failure. Fertil Steril 48: 995

Diczfalusy E, Harlin J 1988 Clinical-pharmacological studies on human menopausal gonadotrophin. Hum Reprod 3: 21

Dor J, Ben-Shlomo I, Lunenfeld B et al 1992 Insulin like Growth Factor-I (IGF-I) may not be essential for ovarian follicular development: evidence from IGF-I deficiency. J Clin Endocrinol Metab 74: 539–542

Ellis J D, Williamson J G 1975 Factors influencing the pregnancy and complication rates with human menopausal gonadotropin therapy. Br J Obstet Gynaecol 82: 52

Engel T, Jewelewicz R, Dyrenfurth I 1972 Ovarian hyperstimulation syndrome. Am J Obstet Gynecol 112: 1052

Ericson G F, Garzo V G, Magoffin D A 1989 Insulin-like growth factor-I regulates aromatase activity in human granulosa and granulosa luteal cells. J Clin Endocrinol Metab 69: 716

Fiddes J C, Goodman H M 1979 Isolation, cloning and sequence analysis of the cDNA for the alpha-subunit of human chorionic gonadotropin. Nature 281: 351

Fleming R, Coutts J R T 1990 The use of exogenous gonadotrophins and GnRH-analogues for ovulation induction in PCO syndrome. Res Clin Forums 11: 77

Fleming R, Haxton M J, Hamilton R 1985 Successful treatment of infertile women with oligomenorrhoea using a combination of an LHRH agonist and exogenous gonadotropins. Br J Obstet Gynaecol 92: 369

Frydman R, Testart J, Giacomini P, Imbert M C, Martin E,

Nahoul K 1982 Hormonal and histological study of the luteal phase in women following aspiration of the preovulatory follicle. Fertil Steril 38: 312

Garcia J, Jones G S, Acosta A A, Wright G L 1981 Corpus luteum function after follicle aspiration for oocyte retrieval. Fertil Steril 36: 565

Garcia J E, Jones G S, Acosta A A, Wright G 1983 Human menopausal gonadotropin/human chorionic gonadotropin in follicular maturation for oocyte aspiration. Phase I. Fertil Steril 39: 167

Gemzell C A 1964 Treatment of infertility after partial hypophysectomy with human pituitary gonadotropins. Lancet i: 644

Gemzell C A 1970 Recent results of human gonadotropin therapy. In: Bettendorf G, Insler V (eds) Clinical application of human gonadotropins. G. Thieme Verlag, Stuttgart, pp 6–20

Gemzell C A, Diczfalusy E, Tillinger G 1958 Clinical effect of human pituitary follicle stimulating hormone. J Clin Endocrinol Metab 18: 138

Gemzell C A, Diczfalusy E, Tillinger G 1960 Human pituitary follicle stimulating hormone. 1. Clinical effect of a partly purified preparation. Ciba Found Coll Endocrinol 13: 191

Goldfarb A F, Schlaff S, Mansi M L 1982 A life-table analysis of pregnancy yield in fixed low-dose menotropin therapy for patients in whom clomiphene citrate failed to induce ovulation. Fertil Steril 37: 629

Goodman A L, Nixon W E, Johnson D L, Hodgen G D 1977 Regulation of folliculogenesis in the rhesus monkey: selection of the dominant follicle. Endocrinology 100: 155

Gougeon A 1986 Dynamics of follicular growth in the human: a model from preliminary results. Hum Reprod 1: 81

Hack M, Lunenfeld B 1978 The influence of hormone induction of ovulation on the fetus and newborn. Pediatr Adoles Endocrinol 5: 191

Hackeloer B J 1984 The role of ultrasound in female infertility management. Ultrasound Med Biol 10: 35

Harlap S 1976 Ovulation induction and congenital malformations [letter]. Lancet ii: 961

Healy D L, Burger H G 1983 Serum FSH, LH and PRL during the induction of ovulation with exogenous gonadotropins. J Clin Endocrinol Metab 56: 474

Healy D L, Kovacs G T, Pepperell R J, Burger H G 1980 A normal cumulative conception rate after human pituitary gonadotropin. Fertil Steril 34: 341

Hendricks C H 1966 Twinning in relation to birth weight mortality and congenital malformations. Obstet Gynecol 27: 47

Hodgen G 1983 The dominant follicle. Fertil Steril 38: 281

Homburg R, Armar N A, Eshel A, Adams J, Jacobs H S 1988a Influence of serum luteinising hormone concentration on ovulation, conception and early pregnancy loss in polycystic ovary syndrome. Br Med J 297: 1024

Homburg R, Eshel A, Abdallah H I, Jacobs H S 1988b Growth hormone facilitates ovulation induction by gonadotropins. Clin Endocrinol 29: 113

Howles C M, Macnamee M C, Edwards R G, Goswamy R, Steptoe P C 1987 Effect of high tonic levels of luteinising hormone on outcome of in vitro fertilisation. Endocrinol Rev 1: 268

Huang K E, Muechler E K, Schwarz K R, Goggin M, Graham M C 1986 Serum progesterone levels in women treated with human menopausal gonadotropin and human chorionic gonadotropin for in vitro fertilization. Fertil Steril 46: 903

Hussa R O 1980 Biosynthesis of human chorionic gonadotrophin. Endocr Rev 1: 268

Hutchinson-Williams K A, DeCherney A H, Lavy G, Diamond M P, Naftolin F, Lunenfeld B 1990 Luteal rescue in in vitro fertilization-embryo transfer. Fertil Steril 53: 495

Insler V, Lunenfeld B 1974 Application of human gonadotropins for induction of ovulation. In: Campos da Paz A, Hasegave T, Notake Y, Hayashi M (eds) Human reproduction. Igaku Shoin, Tokyo, pp 25–38

Insler V, Lunenfeld B 1977 Human gonadotropins. In: Philip E, Barnes J, Newton M (eds) Scientific foundations of obstetrics and gynaecology. Heineman, London, pp 629–649

Insler V, Potashnik G 1983 Monitoring of follicular development in gonadotropin stimulated cycles. In: Beier H M, Lindner H M (eds) Fertilization of the human egg in vitro. Springer Verlag, Berlin, pp 111–122

Insler V, Melmed H, Mashiah S, Monselise M, Lunenfeld B, Rabau E 1968 Functional classification of patients selected for gonadotropin therapy. Obstet Gynecol 32: 620

Insler V, Melmed H, Eichenbrenner I, Serr D M, Lunenfeld B 1972 The cervical score—a simple semiquantitative method for monitoring the menstrual cycle. Int J Obstet Gynecol 10: 223

Insler V, Potashnik G, Glassner M 1981 Some epidemiological aspects of fertility evaluation. In: Insler V, Bettendorf G, Geissler K H (eds) Advances in diagnosis and treatment of infertility. Elsevier/North Holland, New York, pp 165–178

Insler V, Potashnik G, Lunenfeld E, Meizner I, Levy J 1989 The combined suppression/stimulation therapy in IVF-ET programmes: expectations and facts. Gynecol Endocrinol 4 (suppl): 47

Insler V, Kleinman D, Sod-Moriah U 1990 Role of midcycle FSH surge in follicular development. Gynecol Obstet Invest 30: 228

Jia XC, Kalmijin J, Hsueh A J W 1986 Growth hormone enhances FSH induced differentiation of cultured rat granulosa cells. Endocrinology 118: 1401

Johnson P, Pearce J M 1990 Recurrent spontaneous abortion and polycycstic ovarian disease: comparison of two regimens to induce ovulation. Br Med J 300: 154

Kemmann E, Brandeis V T, Shelden R M, Nosher J L 1983 The initial experience with the use of a portable infusion pump in the delivery of human menopausal gonadotropins. Fertil Steril 40: 448

Koos R D 1991 Angiogenesis in the ovary. Abstracts of the Eric Fernstrom Symposium on Local Regulation of Ovarian Function, June 1991, Luund, Sweden, p 31

Kurachi K 1983 Problems concerning ovulation induction. Nippon Sanka Fujinka Gakkai Zashi 35: 1127

Kurachi K, Aono T, Suzuki M, Hirano M, Kobayashi T, Kaibara M 1985 Results of HMG (Humegon)-HCG therapy in 6096 treatment cycles of 2166 Japanese women with anoculatory infertility. Eur J Obstet Gynecol Reprod Biol 19: 43–51

Landgren B M, Unden A L, Diczfalusy E 1980 Hormonal profile of the cycle in 68 normally menstruating women. Acta Endocinologica 94: 89

Laron Z, Pertzelan A, Karp M 1968 Pituitary dwarfism with high serum levels of growth hormone. Isr J Med Sci 4: 883

Laufer N, Navot D, Schenker J G 1982 The pattern of luteal phase plasma progesterone and estradiol in fertile cycles. Am J Obstet Gynecol 143: 808

Leethem J H, Rakoff A E 1948 Studies on antihormone specificity with particular reference to gonadotropic therapy in the female. J Clin Endocrinol Metab 8: 262

Leeton J, Trounson A, Jessup D 1985 Support of the luteal phase in in vitro fertilization programs: results of a controlled trial with intramuscular Proluton. J In Vitro Fert Embryo Trans 2: 166

Lequin L, Mendels E, Trimbos-Kemper G et al 1986 Oestrogens in urine or plasma to monitor ovarian response to exogenous gonadotropins. Serono Symposium on the Control of Follicular Development, Ovarian and Luteal Function: Lessons From in Vitro Fertilization (abstr)

Lopata A, Gronow M J, Johnston W I H, McBain J C, Speirs A L, Leung P S 1986 In vitro fertilization and embryo implantation. In: Insler V, Lunenfeld B (eds) Infertility: male and female, Churchill Livingstone, Edinburgh, p 496

Lunenfeld B 1963 Treatment of anovulation by human gonadotropins. Int J Obstet Gynecol 1: 153

Lunenfeld B 1990 Past present and future of gonadotropins. In: Mashiah S, Ben-Rafael Z, Laufer N, Schenker J G (eds) Advances in assisted reproductive technologies. Plenum, New York, pp 39–44

Lunenfeld B, Insler V 1978 Diagnosis and treatment of functional infertility. Grosse Verlag, Berlin

Lunenfeld B, Serr D M, Mashiah S et al 1981 Therapy with gonadotropins: where are we today. In: Insler V, Bettendorf G, Geissler K H (eds) Advances in diagnosis and treatment of infertility. Elsevier/North Holland, New York, pp 27–31

Lunenfeld B, Mashiah S, Blankstein J 1985 Induction of ovulation with human gonadotropins. In: Shearman R (ed) Clinical reproductive endocrinology. Churchill Livingstone, Edinburgh pp 523

Macnamee M C 1990 The role of in vitro fertilization in polycystic ovarian disease. Res Clin Forums 11:89

Marshall J R, Jacobson A 1970 A technique of dose selection in ovulation induction with HMG. In: Butler J K (ed) Development in the pharmacology and clinical uses of human gonadotrophins. GD Searle, High Wycombe, UK, pp 141–150

Martinez A R, Bernardus R E, Voorhorst F J, Vermeiden J P W, Schoemaker J 1991 Pregnancy rates after timed intercourse or intrauterine insemination after human menopausal gonadotropin stimulation of normal ovulatory cycles: a controlled study. Fertil Steril 55: 258

McFaul P B, Traub A I, Thompson W 1989 Premature luteinization and ovulation induction using human menopausal gonadotropins or pure follicle stimulating hormone in patients with polycystic ovary syndrome. Acta Eur Fertil 20: 157

McKcown J 1960 Malformations in a population observed for five years. In: Ciba Foundation Colloqia on Congenital Malformations. J&A Churchill, London, p2

Meldrum D R, Chang R J, Lu J, Vale W, Rivier J, Judd H L 1982 Medical oophorectomy using a long-acting GnRH agonist—a possible new approach to treatment of endometriosis. J Clin Endocrinol Metab 54: 1081

Menashe Y, Lunenfeld B, Pariente C, Frenkel Y, Mashiach M 1990a Can growth hormone increase, following clonidine administration, predict the dose of human menopausal hormone needed for induction of ovulation? Fertil Steril 53: 432

Menashe Y, Lunenfeld B, Pariente C, Mashiach M 1990b

Effect of growth hormone on ovarian responsiveness. Gynecol Endocrinol 4: 6

Mozes M, Bogokovsky H, Anteby E et al 1965 Thromboembolic phenomena after ovarian stimulation with human gonadotrophins. Lancet ii: 1213

Navot D, Margalioth E J, Laufer N et al 1987 Direct correlation between plasma renin activity and severity of the ovarian hyperstimulation syndrome. Fertil Steril 48: 57

Nichols J B 1952 Statistics of births in the USA, 1915–1948. Am J Obstet Gynecol 64: 376

Nitschke-Dabelstein S, Sturm G, Prinz H, Buchholz R 1981 Plasma 17 beta-estradiol and plasma progesterone as indicators of cyclic changes in the follicle-bearing ovary. In: Insler V, Bettendorf G (eds) Advances in diagnosis and treatment of infertility. Elsevier/ North Holland, New York, pp 57–64.

Nylund L, Beskow C, Carstrom K et al 1990 The luteal phase in successful and unsuccessful implantation after IVF-ET. Hum Reprod 5: 40

O'Herlihy C, Pepperell R J, Brown J B, Smith M A, Sandri L, McBain J C 1981 Incremental clomiphene therapy: a new method for treating persistent anovulation. Obstet Gynecol 58: 535

Paulson R J, Sauer M V, Lobo R A 1990 Embryo implantation after human in vitro fertilization: importance of endometrial receptivity. Fertil Steril 53: 870

Perez R J, Plurad A V, Palladino V S 1981 The relationship of the corpus luteum and the endometrium in infertile patients. Fertil Steril 35: 423

Phillips L L, Gladstone W, Vande-Wiele R 1975 Studies of the coagulation and fibrinolytic systems in hyperstimulation syndrome after administration of human gonadotropins. J Reprod Med 14: 138

Polishuk W Z, Schenker J G 1969 Ovarian hyperstimulation syndrome. Fertil Steril 20: 443

Punnonen R, Ashorn R, Vilja P, Heinonen P K, Kunjansuu E, Tuohimaa P 1988 Spontaneous luteinizing hormone surge and cleavage of in viro fertillized embryos. Fertil Steril 49: 479

Quigley M M 1985 Selection of agents for enhanced follicular recruitment in an in vitro fertilization and embryo replacement treatment program. Ann N Y Acad Sci 442: 96

Rabau E, Serr D M, Mashiach S et al 1967 Current concepts in the treatment of anovulation. Br Med J Clin Res 4: 446

Rabau E, Lunenfeld B, Insler V 1971 The treatment of fertility disturbances with special reference to the use of human gonadotropins. In: Joel C H (ed) Fertility disturbances in men and women. Karger, Basel, pp 508–540

Ritchie W G M 1985 Ultrasound in the evaluation of normal and induced ovulation. Fertil Steril 43: 167

Ronnberg L, Martikainen H, Tapanainen J 1990 Is there any benefit to use growth hormone in ovarian hyperstimulation? Gynecol Endocrinol 4: 27

Schenken R S, Hodgen G D 1983 Follicle-stimulating hormone induced ovarian hyperstimulation in monkeys: blockade of the luteinizing hormone surge. Gynecol Endocrinol 57: 50

Schenker J G, Polishuk W Z 1976 The role of prostaglandins in ovarian hyperstimulation syndrome. Eur J Obstet Gynecol Reprod Biol 6: 47

Schenker J G, Weinstein D 1977 Ovarian hyperstimulation syndrome: current survey. Fertil Steril 30: 255

Seegar-Jones GEA-A, Garcia J E, Rosenwaks Z 1985 Specific effects of FSH and LH on follicular development and oocyte retrieved as determined by a program for in vitro fertilization. Ann N Y Acad Sci 442: 119

Serhal P F, Katz M, Little V, Woronowski H 1988 Unexplained infertility—the value of Pergonal superovulation combined with intrauterine insemination. Fertil Steril 49: 602

Serr D M, Ismajovich B 1963 Determination of the primary sex ratio for human abortions. Am J Obstet Gynecol 87: 63

Shadmi A L, Lunenfeld B, Bahari C, Kokia E, Pariente C, Blanstein J 1987 Abolishment of the positive feedback mechanism: a criterion for temporary medical hypophysectomy by LHRH agonist. Gynecol Endocrinol 1: 1

Shoham Z, Patel A, Jacobs H S 1991a Polycystic ovarian syndrome: safety and effectiveness of stepwise and low-dose administration of purified follicle-stimulating hormone. Fertil Steril 55: 1051

Shoham Z, Zosmer A, Insler V 1991b Early miscarriage and fetal malformations after induction of ovulation by Clomiphen citrate and or human menopausal gonadotropins in in vitro fertilization, and gamete interfallopian transfer. Fertil Steril 55: 1

Smith P E 1926 Hastening of development of female genital system by daily hemoplastic pituitary transplants. Proc Soc Exp Biol Med 24: 131

Smith P E, Engle E T 1927 Experimental evidence of the role of anterior pituitary in development and regulation of gonads. Am J Anat 40: 159

Spadoni L R, Cox D W, Smith D C 1974 Use of human menopausal gonadotropin for the induction of ovulation. Am J Obstet Gynecol 120: 988

Stanger J D, Yovitch J L 1985 Reduced in vitro fertilization of human oocytes from patients with raised basal luteinizing hormone levels during the follicular phase. Br J Obstet Gynaecol 92: 385

Sterzik K, Dallenbach Ch, Schneider V, Sasse V, Dallenbach-Hellweg G 1988 In vitro fertilization: the degree of endometrial insufficiency varies with the type of stimulation. Fertil Steril 50: 457

Stevenson A C, Johnson H A, Stewart P M I 1966 Congenital malformations: a report of a study of a series of consecutive births in two centers. Bull WHO 34: 9

Talmadge K, Boorstein W R, Fiddes J C 1983 The human genome contains seven genes for the beta sub-unit of chorionic gonadotropin but only one gene for the beta sub-unit of luteinizing hormone. DNA 2: 279

Thompson L R, Hansen L M 1970 Pergonal (menotropin): a summary of clinical experience in the induction of ovulation and pregnancy. Fertil Steril 21: 844

Tollan A, Holst N, Forsdahl F, Fadnes H O, Maltau J M 1990 Transcapillary fluid dynamics during ovarian stimulation for in vitro fertilization. Am J Obstet Gynecol 162: 554

Tricomi V, Serr D M, Solish G 1960 The ratio of male and female embryo as determined by sex chromatin. Am J Obstet Gynecol 75: 504

Tsapoulis A D, Zourlaz P A, Comninos A C 1974 Observations on 320 infertile patients treated with human gonadotropins (human menopausal gonadotropin/human chorionic gonadotropin). Fertil Steril 29: 492

Tulandi T, McInnes R A, Arronet G H 1984 Ovarian hyperstimulation following ovulation induction with human menopausal gonadotropin. Int J Fertil 29: 113

Ulloa-Aguirre A, Espinoza R, Damian-Matsumura P, Chappel S C 1988 Immunological and biological potencies of the different molecular species of gonadotrophins. Hum Reprod 3: 491

Volpe A, Coukos G, Barreca A et al 1989 Ovarian response to combined growth hormone gonadotropin treatment in patients resistant to induction of superovulation. Gynecol Endocrinol 3: 125

Welner S, DeCherney A H, Polan M L 1988 Human menopausal gonadotropins: a justifiable therapy in ovulatory women with long-standing idiopathic infertility. Fertil Steril 158: 111

WHO 1976 WHO Technical Report Series, no, 514. Geneva, WHO

Wu C 1977 Plasma hormones in human gonadotropin induced ovulation. Obstet Gynecol 49: 308

Yen S S C 1983 Clinical applications of gonadotropin-releasing hormone and gonadotropin-releasing hormone analogs. Fertil Steril 39: 257

Yovich J L, McColm S C, Yovich J M, Tuvik S 1985 Early luteal serum progesterone concentrations are higher in conception cycles. Fertil Steril 44: 185

Yovich J L, Edirisinghe E R, Cummins J M 1991 Evaluation of luteal support therapy in a randomized controlled study within a gamete intrafallopian transfer program. Fertil Steril 55: 131

Zondek B 1926 Ueber die Funktion des Ovariums. Zeitschrift Geburtshilfe Gynaekologie 90: 327

Zondek B, Ascheim S 1927 Das Hormon des Hypophysenvorderlappens; Testobject zum Nachweis des Hormons. Klin Wochenschr 6: 248

# 17. Ergot derivatives in the management of infertility

*E. del Pozo*

## PATHOPHYSIOLOGY OF HYPERPROLACTINEMIA

### Mechanism of cyclic disturbances induced by hyperprolactinemia

In women, galactorrhea may be found in the presence of ovulatory cycles and normoprolactinemia, but increasing plasma concentrations of prolactin are accompanied by cyclic disturbances ranging from irregular menstrual bleeding or inappropriate luteal function to anovulatory periods and cessation of menses. The mechanisms by which hyperprolactinemia exerts its anovulatory effect are complex. In some instances a variety of menstrual disturbances such as anovulatory periods, oligomenorrhea and menometrorrhagia can be found in the presence of moderate hyperprolactinemia indicating that a certain periodic activity can subsist in hyperprolactinemic states. In the author's experience, values above 70 ng/ml are usually associated with amenorrhea. Thus, initial interference with ovarian function followed by a suppressive effect at the level of the cycling center seems a likely mechanism for subfertility in hyperprolactinemia.

The output of the prolactin-regulating system is considered to consist of two hypothalamo-hypophyseotropic messengers, a prolactin secretion-releasing factor (PRF) and an inhibiting factor (PIF). In mammals regulation of prolactin secretion is predominantly inhibitory. Thus it has long been known that section of the pituitary stalk increases prolactin secretion in experimental animals, and this mechanism has also been confirmed in humans. This would suggest the presence of a PIF at suprasellar level. There is also experimental evidence for the existence of a PRF

(Hyde & Ben-Jonathan 1989). More insight into the mechanism governing the secretion of PIF by the hypothalamus was obtained after characterization of the tuberoinfundibular system (Hökfelt & Fuxe, 1972), and its identification as a part of complex mechanisms regulating the secretion of prolactin by the anterior pituitary. This system presumably acts at the level of the median eminence to release PIF, utilizing dopamine (DA) as the neurotransmitter. Any stimulation of the synthesis of dopamine, e.g. the administration of L-dopa which is endogenously transformed into dopamine, would in turn increase PIF and subsequently reduce prolactin secretion from the pituitary galactotropes. Mechanisms leading to the opposite effect, namely, a block of dopamine (DA) effect at the level of the lactotrope cell will elevate serum prolactin. Since it is known that in pathological hyperprolactinemia the response to dopaminergic blockade and to thyroid-releasing hormone (TRH) stimulation are blunted or absent (del Pozo et al 1974, Malarkey 1975, Archer & Josimovich 1976, Healy et al 1977), a deficiency in hypothalamic dopamine or a disturbance in the mechanisms governing its synthesis or release can be assumed.

### Blood sampling for prolactin determinations

Circulating prolactin is subjected to circadian oscillations that may influence clinical interpretation of basal values recorded in the morning hours. In the author's experience, specimens collected at 9 a.m. are reliable enough and no cannulation is required, since it was shown that the prolactin concentration of samples collected via an in situ needle at 30-min intervals was on

419

average reduced by only 18%, which is within clinical tolerance. The prolactin-stimulating effect of protein intake (Carlson 1989) can be considered to be negligible for clinical purposes. Substances known to elevate basal circulating prolactin are listed in Table 17.3 in the section corresponding to the hyperprolactinemia syndrome. Also the molecular heterogeneity of prolactin, e.g. the presence of the glycosylated form in variable amounts (Hashim et al 1990, Haro et al 1990), may not be relevant for the interpretation of results of plasma prolactin measurements in regard to diagnosis and therapy. However, it should be pointed out that maintained fertility with elevated circulating prolactin may be due to the presence of biologically inactive fractions of high molecular weight, so called big-big prolactin (Whittaker et al 1981).

## Effect of hyperprolactinemia on gonadotropin release

Excessive prolactin secretion is frequently associated with amenorrhea, and delayed puberty or primary amenorrhea may result when hyperprolactinemia has been present before menarche (Kleinberg et al 1977). That this effect of prolactin is exerted at suprasellar level is demonstrated by the normal to exaggerated LH response found after GnRH administration in such patients (Zarate et al 1973, del Pozo et al 1974).

Bohnet et al (1974) were the first to show that hyperprolactinemia induced with TRH would disturb LH pulsatility in normal women, since a fluctuating gonadotropin pattern is essential for ovulation to occur. Indeed, idiopathic hyperprolactinemia is characterized by impaired rhythmicity in the secretion of LH (Bohnet et al 1976, Moult et al 1982), probably due to intermittent reduction in endogenous GnRH bursts. Indeed, Sauder et al (1984) found no changes in mean circulating LH and a reduction in pulse amplitude following treatment with bromocriptine in four of five hyperprolactinemic patients who resumed menses, whereas LH pulse frequency was significantly increased.

Hyperprolactinemia is characterized by a reduced sensitivity of central mechanisms to estrogen or estrogen receptor blockade. Several investigators (Glass et al 1975, Aono et al 1976) have reported a lack of LH response to an estrogen challenge in these patients in comparison with normally cycling women. Prolactin normalization with bromocriptine restores positive estrogen feedback in hyperprolactinemic patients (Aono et al 1979). Insensitivity of estrogen receptors is further documented by the failure to elicit an LH surge after clomiphene stimulation in many hyperprolactinemic women (Thorner et al 1974, Healy et al 1977, Zarate et al 1978, Glass et al 1979). Indeed, clomiphene resistance was recorded in 64 (87%) of 74 cases reviewed by the author. However, it should be mentioned that March et al (1979) have reported a high rate of ovulation in hyperprolactinemic women in the higher plasma estrogen range. The defective episodic hypothalamic activity and the resistance to an estrogen challenge can be brought to a common denominator in the light of experimental work provided by Knobil's group (Knobil et al 1980, Wildt et al 1981). These authors clearly demonstrated that the positive feedback action of estradiol on gonadotropin secretion was exerted at the level of the pituitary gland under the permissive effect of pulsatile discharges of GnRH. Lacking or reduced episodic hypothalamic stimulation would therefore disturb the stimulatory effect of estrogen on pituitary gonadotropes. In hyperprolactinemia, it could be assumed that pulsatile hypothalamic activity is obstructed by exposure of central structures to elevated circulating prolactin. This interference would prevent the pituitary response to an estrogen challenge and can be tentatively assumed responsible for the resistance to clomiphene characteristic of hyperprolactinemia. Indeed, the induction of pulsatile GnRH waves by intermittent exogenous administration of this peptide can normalize ovarian function in women with hyperprolactinemia (Leyendecker et al 1980). Also, treatment with bromocriptine has re-established pituitary response to estrogen and rendered central mechanisms sensitive to clomiphene (Aono et al 1979). Certainly this would imply that a disturbed hypothalamic function is a general characteristic of the disease. It would, however, differ from classic estrogen-sensitive hypothalamic amenorrhea, probably owing to distinct central inhibitory properties of prolactin, or to more extensive estrogen receptor blockade by the latter.

## Effect of hyperprolactinemia on the ovary

There is experimental and clinical evidence for an action of prolactin on the corpus luteum. This lactogenic hormone has been found to be necessary for the maintenance of luteal function in experimental animals (Döhler & Wuttke 1974). Studies by McNatty et al (1974) have helped in understanding the regulatory role of prolactin on progesterone synthesis by the corpus luteum. In vitro work by these authors has shown that synthesis of progesterone by human granulosa cells is dependent on the prolactin concentration in the culture medium. The inhibitory effect of this lactogen on human luteal function has been documented by Delvoye et al (1974) and L'Hermite et al (1979) in experiments conducted in normally menstruating women. Elevation of plasma prolactin concentrations induced with neuroleptic drugs caused a shortening of the hyperthermic phase and a reduction in progesterone synthesis by the corpus luteum. In agreement with these findings del Pozo et al (1976, 1979) reported that short luteal phase and low progesterone secretion may be associated with elevated plasma prolactin concentrations in some infertile women.

The relationship between prolactin and ovarian estrogen synthesis in the galactorrhea syndromes is not completely understood. As judged by the near normal plasma estrogen levels exhibited by some of these patients, a certain degree of follicular maturation can be assumed. There is, however, a negative correlation between prolactin and estrogen production (Kandeel et al 1979). Data by McNatty et al 1979 collected from human antral follicles indicate that exposure to increasing prolactin concentrations in the medium does not modify estrogen synthesis by the cultured cells, whereas progesterone production is impaired. Indeed, ovarian response to exogenous gonadotropin stimulation is maintained in hyperprolactinemic amenorrhea (del Pozo et al 1975b, Archer & Josimovich 1976). More recently, Caro & Woolf (1980) were able to show that the estradiol elevation that follows the gonadotropin surge induced by exogenous GnRH was not different in normal and hyperprolactinemic women. Finally, it should be mentioned that low circulating prolactin may decrease ovarian progesterone synthesis through 'oversuppression' of PRL secretion with bromocriptine (Schulz et al 1978).

## Psychogenic factors in hyperprolactinemia

Despite the advent of sensitive laboratory techniques to measure human plasma prolactin and with the confirmation of the causative role of this lactogen in the galactorrhea-amenorrhea syndromes, little attention has been paid to the possible etiological implication of psychogenic factors. A correlation between dopaminergic pathways, prolactin and mental illness has been well established. This is, however, a negative one since neuroleptic drugs enhance prolactin secretion via dopamine receptor blockade and at the same time improve the mental condition of schizophrenic subjects. On the other hand, hyperprolactinemia has been connected with psychogenic overlay (Zacur et al 1976), and bromocriptine, a potent dopamine agonist, has been found to possess antidepressive properties (Theohar et al 1981). Furthermore, it was recently demonstrated that normalization of prolactin secretion with bromocriptine administered concomitantly with neuroleptic drugs did not interfere with the antipsychotic effect of the latter (del Pozo 1982). There are also clinical observations indicating that plasma prolactin concentrations are not directly connected with the underlying physiopathology of mental disease. For example, the elevation of circulating prolactin that follow dopaminergic blockade does not modify the therapeutic effect of neuroleptic drugs, whereas psychotic changes associated with idiopathic hyperprolactincmia will regress after normalization of plasma prolactin via dopamine receptor stimulation (Zacur et al 1979).

## Effect of hyperprolactinemia in male subjects

Although prolactin circulates in male blood in appreciable concentrations, its physiological role has not been clarified. Certainly the chronic ingestion of dopamine antagonists or estrogens may lead to sustained hyperprolactinemia; the same effect can be expected in male subjects on chronic estrogen therapy for prostatic cancer or transsexualism (Frantz 1973, del Pozo 1982). Indeed, male-to-female transexuals have been found not only to exhibit elevated circulating prolactin but to have enlarged pituitaries as a consequence of long-term stimulation by exogenous estrogens (Gooren et al 1985). A possible relationship between prolactin and pubertal gynecomastia seems questionable. Normal plasma prolactin has been reported in this situation (Turkington 1972) and the self-limiting character of the condition in adolescent subjects makes the study of a causal relationship difficult.

Testicular androgen synthesis is usually reduced in hyperprolactinemic males. The central inhibitory effect of prolactin can be localized at suprasellar level, since a positive LH response to exogenous GnRH has been recorded in idiopathic (Franks et al 1978, Carter et al 1978) or provoked hyperprolactinemia (Falaschi et al 1978). The degree of response, however, can be reduced in the presence of prolactinomas (Nagulesparen et al 1978). A disturbance of endogenous control of GnRH can be assumed on the basis of experimental animal data but the primary central mechanism causing gonadal insufficiency remains uncertain. Most male patients with hyperprolactinemia show normal basal plasma LH (Thorner et al 1974), although altered LH pulsatility has also been reported (Winters & Troen 1984), nor have its secretory rhythms been studied. Similar to that of hyperprolactinemic women, the male prolactin responses to a TRH challenge and to dopamine blockade are blunted, probably due to a primary hypothalamic dopamine disturbance or to prolactin itself via a short-loop mechanism (del Pozo 1982). It is interesting to note that Thorner & Besser (1977) found no changes in the plasma gonadotropin hourly profiles in hyperprolactinemic males after normalization of prolactin secretion following bromocriptine therapy, compared with untreated profiles. Despite experimental evidence of a direct action of prolactin at the level of the gonad, this effect has not been clearly demonstrated in men. Hypoandrogenic males with elevated plasma prolactin usually exhibit adequate sex steroid responses to exogenous chorionic gonadotropin (Friesen et al 1973, Carter et al 1978, Franks et al 1978). Diminished response rates can be expected in subjects with low basal plasma testosterone levels and reduced functional capacity of the Leydig cells. Therefore, absolute androgen increases after stimulation with chorionic gonadotropin in hyperprolactinemia should be considered cautiously when compared with levels in normal subjects, since these exhibit higher basal androgen production and accordingly higher reserve capacity. A direct effect of prolactin on spermatogenesis seems unlikely, and limited experience by the author in male hyperprolactinemia indicates probable androgen dependency in defective sperm maturation (del Pozo 1982). There is no clear evidence that prolactin plays a role in oligospermia accompanied by

**Table 17.1** Effect of inappropriately increased prolactin secretion

| *Females* | |
|---|---|
| Clinical | Failure to enter menarche |
| | Galactorrhea with ovulatory cycles |
| | Short luteal phase |
| | Menometrorrhagia |
| | Anovulatory cycles |
| | Amenorrhea* |
| | Hirsutism |
| Biochemical | Elevated plasma prolactin concentrations |
| | Lack of sleep-related prolactin elevations |
| | Altered LH pulsatility |
| | Lack of positive estrogen feedback on LH |
| | Low basal estrogens† |
| | Elevated androgenic adrenal steroids† |
| | Positive pituitary and ovarian response to exogenous stimulation |
| | Clomiphene resistance |
| *Males* | |
| Clinical | Failure to enter puberty |
| | Galactorrhea+ |
| | Oligoaspermia, subfertility |
| | Signs of androgen failure, decreased potency |
| Biochemical | Elevated plasma prolactin concentrations |
| | Lack of prolactin elevation during sleep |
| | Low androgen production |
| | Defective LH pulsatility |
| | Positive pituitary and testicular response to exogenous stimulation |

\* Not necessarily associated with galactorrhea.
† Subjected to variance.
+ Less frequent in males probably due to reduced mammary tissue mass.

**Table 17.2**  Pathology associated with hyperprolactinemia

| Condition | Mechanism |
|---|---|
| Chiari–Frommel syndrome | Postpartum failure of hypothalamus to return to nonpregnant cyclic activity |
| Argonz–Ahumada–del Castillo syndrome | Idiopathic hypothalamic dysfunction |
| Forbes–Albright syndrome | Pituitary tumor (prolactinoma): <br> a. autonomous prolactin secretion? <br> b. secondary to hypothalamic dysfunction? |
| Drug-induced: antidepressants, neuroleptics, estrogenic contraceptives, etc. | Provoked through alteration of hypothalamic regulatory control (dopamine blockade or direct stimulation of pituitary lactotrophs) |
| Hyperprolactinemia after thoracic injury or thoracic herpes | Mechanism unknown: neural stimulation? |
| Hyperprolactinemia associated with irregular menses or shortened luteal phase | Probably direct interference with ovarian progesterone synthesis |
| Hyperprolactinemia after pituitary surgery for treatment of metastasizing diseases or diabetic retinopathy | Severance of hypothalamo-pituitary connections |
| Hyperprolactinemia associated with other endocrinopathies: hypothyroidism, hyperthyroidism, acromegaly, Cushing's syndrome or Nelson's syndrome | Mechanism unknown: secondary to hypothalamic dysfunction or disruption of pituitary connections? Disturbed pituitary adrenal feedback? |
| Hyperprolactinemia secondary to infectious disease | Functional pituitary disconnection in herpes zoster, encephalitis, meningitis, sarcoidosis, etc.? |
| Ectopic prolactin secretion | Hypernephroma, lung cancer? |
| Hyperprolactinemia in the polycystic ovary syndrome | Caused by elevated circulating estrogens probably favored by enhanced synthesis of androgen precursors |
| Hyperprolactinemia with secondary hypogonadism without galactorrhea | Cause of refractoriness of mammary tissue to prolactin unknown: downregulation of mammary receptors possible |
| Hyperprolactinemia of advanced renal disease | Mechanism unknown but likely to be a factor present in renal tissue |
| Hyperprolactinemia of advanced liver disease | Mediated by elevated estrogen production? |

normal testosterone and lactogen levels. This is supported by the poor response following prolactin inhibition.

## Biological effect of hyperprolactinemia

The clinical and biological effects of hyperprolactinemia are summarized in Table 17.1. Female hyperprolactinemia can present with a number of intermediate clinical pictures ranging from the occurrence of regular cycles with inability to conceive, short luteal phases, oligomenorrhea and metrorrhagia, to the complete cessation of cyclical activity and amenorrhea. The existence of hyperprolactinemia before puberty produces in both sexes pubertal retardation. As a consequence of the central disturbance, hypoestrogenism and hypoandrogenism develop. The circadian secretory rhythm of prolactin is abolished and the sleep-related plasma elevation is missing.

## Inappropriate prolactin secretion: a syndrome

The clinical picture of the galactorrhea-amenorrhea syndromes had been known for more than a century before their endocrine background was elucidated. In 1855 Chiari et al described a syndrome of persistent postpartum lactation and amenorrhea accompanied by uterine involution. The clinical symptoms and signs of this syndrome were clarified further by Frommel in 1882. Argonz & del Castillo (1953) reported on a similar condition unrelated to pregnancy, and Forbes et al (1954) described a syndrome of galactorrhea and amenorrhea with pituitary tumors. Thus, the presence of a radiologically normal sella and the absence of neurological lesions are generally thought to favor the diagnosis of hypothalamic dysfunction rather than of pituitary tumors. However, the reliability of these criteria is doubtful, since lesions which appear clinically hypothalamic may evolve to frank pituitary adenomas (see also Chapter 9). Conditions characterized by excessive prolactin secretion and the underlying mechanisms are presented in Table 17.2. In general, four mechanisms can be viewed responsible for hyperprolactinemia: increased autonomous secretion, estrogen effect, disturbances of dopaminergic control and exacerbation of neural reflexes. A deficiency in dopamine would in theory correspond to a 'physiological' separation of lactotrope cells from their hypothalamic control corresponding to anatomical severance of the pituitary stalk. Substances in clinical use known to interfere with dopamine, directly or via catecholamine metabolism, are listed in Table 17.3. For a more detailed description the reader is referred to Flückiger et al 1982.

**Table 17.3** Substances in clinical use inducing hyperprolactinemia

Neuroleptics
  Phenothiazines
  Butyrophenones
  Diphenyl-butylpiperidine
  Sulpiride
Antidepressant drugs
  Dibenzazepine derivatives*
Antihypertensives
  alpha-Methyldopa
  Reserpine
Hormones
  TRH
  Estrogens
Opiates
  Morphine
  Metenkephalin
Other
  Domperidon
  Metoclopramide†
  Histamine blocking agents+

*Weak prolactin stimulator.
†Structurally related to the neuroleptic sulpiride.
+Hyperprolactinemic effect not confirmed on chronic administration.

## USE OF ERGOT DERIVATIVES IN THE MANAGEMENT OF INFERTILITY

### Structural characteristics

Numerous ergot compounds alter anterior pituitary function via dopaminergic stimulation, but most information available on their effect on prolactin secretion is restricted. With very few exceptions, which are not of importance in this

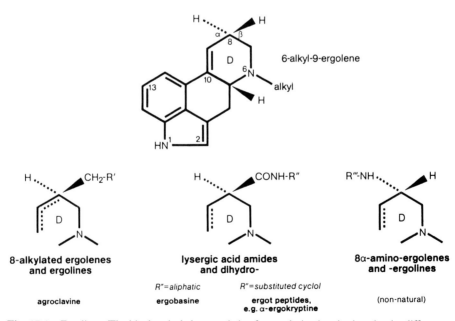

**Fig. 17.1** Ergolines. The biochemical characteristic of ergot derivatives is given by the different side-chains to the 8 position to form three groups: clavines, lysergic acid amides and 8 α-aminoergolines.

context, these compounds belong to one of three ergot families indicated in Figure 17.1. Ergot compounds are made up of either a 6-alkyl-9-ergolene or a 6-alkyl-ergolene with different side-chains to position 8 of the tetracyclic moiety. The various compounds may have further substituents, which can be important for the pharmacological profile of a particular drug. Of the three families, the 8α-amino-ergolines do not have natural representatives (alkaloids). In 1972 it was shown that bromocriptine, a potent dopamine agonist, would reduce plasma prolactin in normal subjects (del Pozo et al 1972) and that its administration to hyperprolactinemic women would restore ovulatory cycles (Besser et al 1972, del Pozo et al 1972) and suppress postpartum lactation (Brun del Re et al 1973). Later on, other ergot derivatives were reported to exhibit prolactin-inhibiting properties and have been successful in the management of galactorrhea-amenorrhea. In the following section the clinical profile of ergot derivatives possessing these properties will be outlined.

## Bromocriptine

A considerable therapeutic advance was obtained with the introduction of bromocriptine, a lysergic acid derivative, in the management of galactor-rhea-amenorrhea. Its chemical structure is presented in Figure 17.2. The compound is usually administered orally in doses of 1.25–2.5 mg two or three times daily. In rare instances a dosage increase to 10–15 mg or more daily is required in order to reestablish normal ovulatory mechanisms. The potent dopaminergic

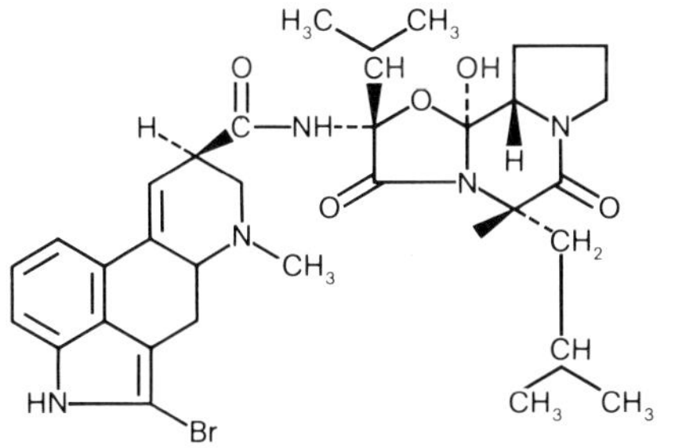

**Fig. 17.2** Chemical structure of bromocriptine (Parlodel). The compound belongs to the ergopeptine subgroup of the lysergic acid amides.

agonistic effect of the drug may induce hypotension, nausea and occasionally vomiting in sensitive subjects. This can be prevented by increasing the dosage gradually after initiating therapy with 1.25 mg or less, the drug being taken after meals. In many instances intolerance symptoms will subside spontaneously after medication has been continued for several days. It is noteworthy that Polatti et al (1978) restricted the administration of the drug to the period prior to and around the presumed ovulation time and obtained results equivalent to those of continuous treatment. Bernal & Villamizar (1982) reduced therapy to 1.25 or 2.5 mg administered as a single daily dose in the evening. With this regimen ovulations were recorded in 16 out of 18 cases. More recently, a retarded injectable form of bromocriptine has been developed. Pharmacokinetics of this new galenic formulation have shown that a single intramuscular injection of 50 mg of a microcapsulated form (polylactic-acid) would provide adequate prolactin suppression for more than 30 days in normal volunteers (del Pozo et al 1986). In the following sections the clinical effect of the drug will be illustrated in a series of case reports.

The effectiveness of bromocriptine in hyperprolactinemic anovulation in galactorrhea-amenorrhea has been amply demonstrated (del Pozo et al 1974, Rolland et al 1974, Thorner et al 1974, 1975, Bohnet et al 1976, Canales et al 1976, Fossati et al 1976, Jacobs et al 1976, Rjosk et al 1976, Badano et al 1977, Gomez et al 1977, Kleinberg et al 1977), also for the long-acting injectable form (Ciccarelli et al 1989, Schettini et al 1990). Overall response rates for oral administration in a collective of 187 cases are presented in Table 17.4.

The sequence of clinical and biological findings following bromocriptine treatment in this conditions is illustrated in Figure 17.3. A 26-year-old nulliparous woman reported amenorrhea of 12 months' duration after discontinuation of an oral contraceptive. Plasma prolactin was slightly elevated and urinary estrogens were low. Onset of treatment with bromocriptine, 2.5 mg twice daily, was followed by rapid restoration of menstrual cycles and normal ovulatory mechanisms as demonstrated through the biphasic pattern of basal body temperature, plasma progesterone

**Table 17.4**   Overall results of bromocriptine treatment in infertility due to hyperprolactinemia in a collection of 187 cases

|  | n | Ovulation | Desired pregnancy | Obtained pregnancy |
|---|---|---|---|---|
| Amenorrhea without radiological evidence of tumor | 167 | 158 | 116 | 89 |
| Amenorrhea in the presence of a prolactinoma | 8 | 4* | 5 | 3 |
| Inadequate luteal function | 12 | 10 | 6 | |

\* In two of eight cases persistence of anovulation thought due to postsurgical condition.

elevations in the middle of the hyperthermic phase, and an endometrial biopsy showing a secretory phase at the onset of vaginal bleeding. Urinary excretion of estrogen increased to within the normal range. It is interesting to note that ovulation took place shortly after initiation of therapy, an effect observed by other investigators (Bernal & Villamizar 1982), suggesting that some follicles had already reached a certain stage of maturation and that development to the preovulatory stage can occur with a relative short period. Strauch et al (1977) and Pepperell et al (1977) have followed the hormonal kinetics in the early stages of treatment and found that ovulation is frequent in the first cycle of bromocriptine therapy. In some cases, anovulation persisted due to incomplete prolactin suppression but follicle rupture occurred after dosage increase. LH pulsatility is restored by this treatment (Bohnet et al 1976).

Thorner et al (1974) and Darragh et al (1976) recorded clinical and hormonal changes compatible with premature menopause in some hyperprolactinemic women. Treatment with bromocriptine led to restoration of ovulatory

cycles. Thus, the possibility of a prolactin-mediated effect should be considered before the diagnosis of early menopause can be established with certainty in a woman with amenorrhea-galactorrhea, low estrogens and elevated plasma FSH. Moderately elevated PRL levels may be associated with luteal inadequacy (Seppälä 1976a, del Pozo et al 1976, Fredricsson et al 1977) and treatment with bromocriptine can restore fertility (del Pozo et al 1979). A typical response pattern is presented in Figure 17.4. The role of PRL in the etiology of normoprolactinemic luteal inadequacy remains controversial. Whereas Diedrich et al (1978) and Mühlenstedt et al (1979) reported a favorable effect following the use of bromocriptine, Saunders et al (1979) found no action, in agreement with a recent report showing no correlation between the circadian PRL secretory

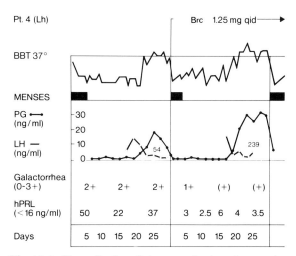

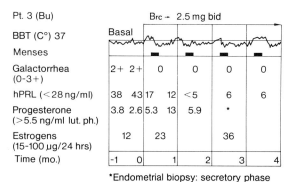

**Fig. 17.3**   Response to bromocriptine in a case of hyperprolactinemic amenorrhea (explanation in text). Brc, bromocriptine.

**Fig. 17.4**   Normalization of plasma prolactin and restored luteal function in an infertile woman with a hyperthermic phase of the cycle of 7.5 days on the average. The luteal index (integral of progesterone profile) increased from 54 (normal >107) to 239. The patient conceived in the second cycle of treatment. Brc, bromocriptine.

pattern and luteal inadequacy in normopro-lactinemic infertility (Soules et al 1991).

The absence of milk secretion in hyperpro-lactinemic amenorrhea is not uncommon. The following case report will remind the clinician that the absence of galactorrhea does not exclude hyperprolactinemia as the cause of amenorrhea (Fig. 17.5). A 25-year-old woman was first seen because of a history of oligomenorrhea and cessa-tion of menses 2 years prior to the consultation. The physical examination was unremarkable and no milk could be obtained from her breasts by manual expression. The biochemical data showed moderate hyperprolactinemia and low estrogen. Treatment with bromocriptine, 5 mg daily in divided doses, promptly normalized the hormonal picture and reestablished ovulation. A careful analysis of the discordant patterns of hyperpro-lactinemia and galactorrhea in secondary amenor-rhea has been published by Seppälä et al (1977). More difficult to explain is the association of galactorrhea and metrorrhagia. A rapid response to bromocriptine has been reported in this condi-tion (del Pozo et al 1974, Jaszmann & Sternthal 1974). Here a possible mode of action can be postulated by the blocking effect of elevated prolactin concentrations on vascular reactivity as proposed by Horrobin et al (1976).

Concerning lactation after delivery in the presence of pathological hyperprolactinemia, liberal guidelines have now replaced more conser-vative behavior of earlier times. It was feared that the suckling stimulus would augment prolactin secretion and possibly contribute to the growth of an existing tumor. Data collected in the postpartum period (del Pozo, unpublished) have shown that breast feeding does not substantially modify prolactin secretion and that the elevated basal plasma lactogen levels are able to maintain adequate milk secretion. Thus, postpartum hyperprolactinemic women are encouraged to breast feed if they wish to do so.

*Miscellaneous effects of bromocriptine on reproduction and other systems*

The effect of bromocriptine on normopro-lactinemic anovulation has also been tested. A positive effect has been reported in some instances but controlled studies in larger series of euprolactinemic patients have failed to show clear differences between placebo and drug treatment. Nevertheless, Seppälä et al (1976a) found a number of bromocriptine responders with normo-prolactinemic anovulation. Van der Steeg & Coelingh Bennink (1977) reported ovulations after treatment with bromocriptine in 74% of women with postpill anovulation. The authors attributed the favorable effect to the dopaminergic action of the drug facilitating the release of GnRH from the hypothalamus. This mechanism would be independent of the prolactin-lowering effect and also would explain the positive results reported by other authors (Hirvonen et al 1976, Wolf & del Pozo 1979, Moggi et al 1979, Coelingh Bennink 1979, Koike et al 1981) in 'converting' euprolactinemic antiestrogen-resis-tant patients to sensitivity. Thus, the concomitant treatment with bromocriptine and antiestrogens led to ovulatory cycles in women previously resis-tant to the latter agents alone, as shown by Suginami et al (1986) in normoprolactinemic women with excessive nocturnal prolactin surges and hyperresponse to dopamine blockade. Although the basic mechanism of this effect remains uncertain, the bromocriptine-induced elevation of plasma estrogen reported by Seppälä et al. (1976b) in normoprolactinemic amenorrhea may have sensitized the hypothalamus to the action of the antiestrogen. Also the stimulation of testosterone aromatization into estradiol may have played a role in the induction of this phenomenon (Martikainen et al 1989). Lenton et

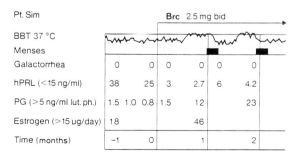

**Fig. 17.5**  Hyperprolactinemic amenorrhea in the absence of galactorrhea (explanation in text). Brc, bromocriptine.

al (1977) recorded a 63.4% pregnancy rate in apparently ovulating women unable to conceive after treatment with clomiphene or a progestogenic agent. The authors speculated that the favorable effect of bromocriptine might be mediated by mechanisms other than suppression of prolactin secretion alone. Indeed, Kort et al (1980) demonstrated by ultrasound scanning that bromocriptine treatment would induce follicular enlargement paralleling plasma estradiol increases in normoprolactinemic anovulatory patients. The opposite effect has also been described, i.e. ovulatory response to simultaneous administration of clomiphene and bromocriptine in hyperprolactinemic women failing to ovulate on bromocriptine alone (Turksoy et al 1982).

Sexual function is often impaired in patients on maintenance hemodialysis. This disturbance can undoubtedly have many causes involving both psychological and hormonal factors. Basal plasma prolactin has been found to be higher than normal in this condition which is also associated with reduced libido and sexual activity (Flückiger et al 1982). In a controlled trial conducted by Bommer et al (1979), the effect of bromocriptine on sexual activity was studied in male hemodialysis patients. Plasma prolactin concentrations were consistently reduced while sexual function, assessed by appropriate questionnaires, was markedly improved. Treatment with bromocriptine has been found to relieve mastodynia accompanying fibrocystic disease of the breast (Zippel et al 1977, Mansel et al 1978). Martin-Comin et al (1976) were also able to substantiate a positive effect on such breast lesions by radiological examinations. In other studies, Schulz et al (1975) and Palmer & Monteiro (1977) demonstrated a reduction in premenstrual breast engorgement and mastalgia in normally ovulating women. These favorable results have recently been confirmed and extended in a multicenter study (Mansel & Dogliotti 1990). The mechanism of pain relief is not clear. Histochemical and morphological studies in breast-tissue biopsies have failed to show significant changes after prolonged treatment with bromocriptine (Zippel et al 1977). It can be speculated that the fall in circulating prolactin led to a reduction in ductal pressure and subsequently to an improvement in mastodynia.

***Effect of bromocriptine on LH: its usefulness in the management of infertility.*** Dopaminergic stimulation with bromocriptine has been found to lower plasma LH after single administration (Lachelin et al 1977). Although this effect may not be relevant in the presence of normal steroid feedback conditions to the hypothalamic-pituitary system (del Pozo et al 1975a, Schulz et al 1978), it could become important in situations of estrogen dominance such as in the syndrome of polycystic ovaries (PCO). Quigley et al (1981) were able to show increased LH sensitivity to dopamine in this condition. Indeed, Rocco et al (1979) reported restoration of cyclicity in some PCO patients treated with bromocriptine and, more recently, Falaschi & del Pozo (1982) could explain this effect by recording a significant reduction in LH fluctuations and in the response to GnRH in PCO patients treated with this compound. The presence of normal dopaminergic mechanisms in the control of prolactin in this syndrome would rule out a mechanism involving inhibition of prolactin secretion (Falaschi et al 1980). The same authors could demonstrate that the damping of LH secretion by bromocriptine in PCO was independent of the existence or nonexistence of hyperprolactinemia (Falaschi & del Pozo 1982) but a positive effect was only observed in cases previously selected by a fall in circulating androgens on bromocriptine therapy (Falaschi et al 1986).

***Treatment of male hyperprolactinemia with bromocriptine.*** Carter et al (1978), treating 11 out of 22 hyperprolactinemic male patients with bromocriptine, observed a major decline in plasma prolactin and an improvement in potency. Plasma testosterone increased from a mean of 135 ng% to 396 ng%. It is interesting to note that in two subjects who had remained impotent after testosterone replacement therapy potency returned when hyperprolactinemia was reduced with bromocriptine. In another series of 29 patients, Franks et al (1978) also noted a return of potency in subjects treated with bromocriptine, and similar results have been reported by Fossati et al (1976) and Spark et al (1980). These findings have been amply confirmed (Spark et al 1982, Buvat et al 1985, Hulting et al 1985). It is striking that, in symptomatic males, pituitary lesions seem to be far more advanced and mean plasma prolactin levels substantially higher than in hyperprolactinemic women (del Pozo et al 1983). This is probably due to the absence in men of the alarm signal of cessation of cyclic activity which makes lesions clinically apparent in women at an earlier stage of development. More difficult to assess is the relationship between oligospermia and prolactin in normoprolactinemic individuals without other signs of endocrine abnormality. In a study of 18 oligospermic patients screened by the author all had normal plasma prolactin concentrations. A careful survey of the literature (del Pozo 1982) has failed to show a clear relationship between low sperm productions and plasma prolactin levels. The same can be stated for changes in potency, despite isolated communications showing favorable results following bromocriptine therapy.

*Impact of bromocriptine treatment on pregnancy and fetal development.* So far, information has been collected from 1410 patients conceiving during therapy with bromocriptine (Turkalj et al 1982). The mean daily drug intake was 5 mg (range 1–40 mg), and the duration of treatment was between 1 and more then 8 weeks. In 157 women (11.1%) spontaneous abortion occurred, and pregnancy was interrupted in 28 women for different reasons. The incidence of spontaneous termination is within the range recorded in the nontreated population (Turkalj et al 1982). There was a great variability in the time interval between discontinuation of bromocriptine intake and the occurrence of spontaneous abortion, suggesting a lack of dependency between treatment and course of gestation. In addition, treatment with daily doses between 5 and 32 mg throughout pregnancy in eight cases failed to modify its course and produced no alterations in fetal development.

The multiple pregnancy rate in the collective of 1236 live births studied was 2.5%. Major and minor malformations occurred in the bromocriptine series in 3.5% of cases. Smithells (1976) cites a frequency of 2.7% spontaneous malformations for a collective of over 600 000 control mothers. A higher incidence of fetal malformation in newborn infants (major malformations 4.1% and minor malformations 6.5%) was reported by Drew et al

(1977) after reviewing the world literature covering 20 million births. In the USA the Collaborative Perinatal Project studied 50 282 pregnancies and recorded 6.5% malformations (Heinonen et al 1977). It can be concluded that the incidence of congenital malformations in bromocriptine-treated pregnancies lies within normal limits.

### Lisuride

Zikan & Semonsky reported in 1960 on the synthesis of an 8α-amino ergoline derivative stereochemically related to D-isolysergic acid (Fig. 17.6). This compound is presently marketed under the name Lisuride as the hydrogen maleate. It was first characterized as a serotonin antagonist (Votava & Lamplova 1961), but Horowski & Wachtel (1976) found that is possessed dopaminergic properties in experimental animals. This was confirmed in humans after the drug was shown to reduce plasma prolactin under basal conditions and in stimulatory tests (Horowski et al 1978, Delitala et al 1979). Clinically Lisuride is usually administered twice daily in doses ranging from 50 to 200 µg. At the higher dosage strength, signs of dopaminergic overstimulation such as drowsiness and nausea have been recorded (Delitala et al 1979).

The efficacy of Lisuride in hyperprolactinemic anovulation and in luteal insufficiency was tested by De Cecco et al (1978) and Bohnet et al (1979). Lengthening of the hyperthermic phase of the cycle was observed in women with a previous diagnosis of luteal insufficiency, and prolonged treatment lowered plasma prolactin in nine out of 11 cases exhibiting elevated plasma prolactin. Ovulatory cycles could be restored in eight. These

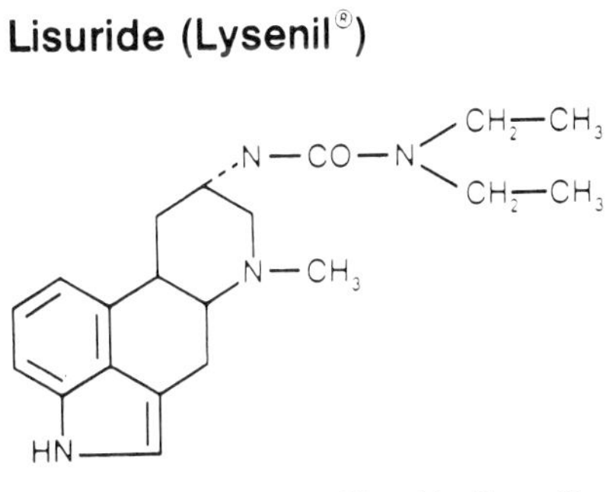

### Lisuride (Lysenil®)

**Fig. 17.6** Chemical structure of lisuride (Lysenil).

favorable results were confirmed and extended later by De Cecco et al (1983) and by Dallabonzana et al (1985, 1986).

## Cabergoline

A new ergot derivative, cabergoline (1-[(6-allylerg-olin-8β-yl) carbonyl] 1-[3-(dimethylamino) propyl] 3-ethylurea) (Fig. 17.7), has been recently developed on the basis of its prolonged action following single oral administration (Ferrari et al 1986, Pontiroli et al 1987). A dose-related prolactin inhibitory effect has been observed in normally cycling women, in puerperae and in hyperprolactinemic patients (Mattei et al 1988). Thus, single weekly oral doses of 0.3–1.2 mg were able to restore normal prolactin plasma levels and to reestablish cyclic activity in a large number of patients. Investigators have claimed for this compound a low incidence of side-effects and a lack of action on circulating GH, TSH, LH and cortisol following acute administration (Pontiroli et al 1987).

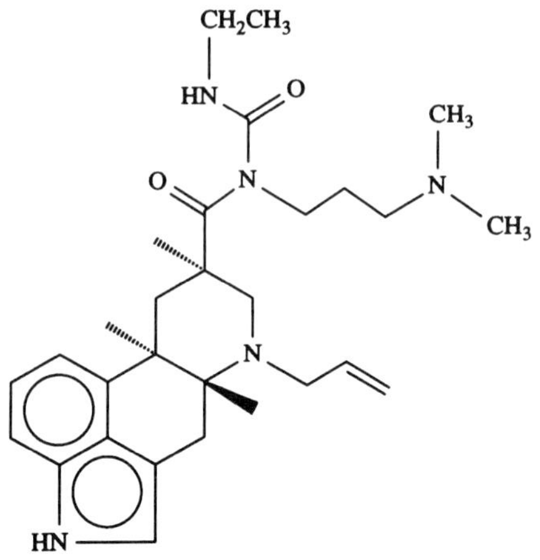

## Hydergine

Prolactin inhibition is inherent to the molecular structure of ergolines. Previous exhaustive studies have shown an action gradient involving high and low molecular weight derivatives (Flückiger & del Pozo 1980). Thus, ergonovine, a compound known to stimulate uterine contractions, has a weak and short-lasting prolactin-suppressing effect, whereas methysergide, a substance characterized as a serotonin antagonist, exerts a somewhat more marked prolactin inhibition.

**Fig. 17.7**   Chemical structure of cabergoline.

Hydergine, a combination of four alkaloids, also reduces circulating prolactin at higher doses than classic prolactin-inhibitors. Recently, Tamura et al (1989) reported a favorable effect of hydergine on hyperprolactinemic anovulation when basal plasma prolactin values were below 100 ng/ml. Daily doses of 6 mg failed to restore ovulatory cycles in women with circulating prolactin above this limit, indicating that this compound is also a weak dopamine-blocking agent.

### Non-ergot prolactin inhibitors

The search for prolactin inhibitors unrelated to the ergot molecule have led to the synthesis of compound CV 205–502 (Nordmann & Petcher 1985), an octahydrobenzo-[g]-quinoline, with structural similarities to apomorphine (Fig. 17.8). This substance has been characterized as a potent

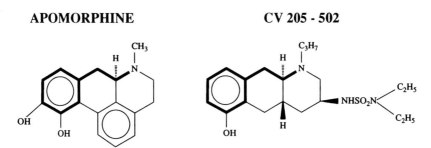

**Fig. 17.8**   Chemical structure of compound CV 205–502 (Norprolac) in comparison with apomorphine.

$D_2$ agonist (Closse et al 1988) and studies conducted in normal volunteers have shown that single oral doses of 0.06 mg effectively suppressed prolactin secretion for 36 h (Gaillard & Brownell 1988). First clinical trials have demonstrated its effectiveness and good tolerance in the management of hyperprolactinemic syndromes in daily doses between 0.150 and 0.450 mg (Rasmussen et al 1987, Vance et al 1990, van der Lely et al 1991). In addition, the transient and mild side-effects recorded in a minority of patients render CV 205–502 a worthy alternative for patients showing intolerance to bromocriptine therapy (van der Lely et al 1991).

## REFERENCES

Aono T, Miyake A, Shioji T, Kinugasa T, Onishi T, Kurachi K 1976 Impaired LH release following exogenous estrogen administration in patients with amenorrhea-galactorrhea syndrome. Clin Endocrinol (Oxf) 42: 696

Aono T, Miyake A, Shioji T, Yasuda M, Koike K, Kurachi K 1979 Restoration of oestrogen positive feedback effect on LH release by bromocriptine in hyperprolactinemic patients with galactorrhea-amenorrhea. Acta Endocrinol Copenh 91: 591

Archer D F, Josimovich J B 1976 Ovarian response to exogenous gonadotropins in women with elevated serum prolactin. Obstet Ginecol Latinoam 48: 155

Argonz J, del Castillo E B 1953 Syndrome characterized by estrogenic insufficiency, galactorrhea and decreased urinary gonadotropin. J Clin Endocrinol Metab 13: 79

Badano A R, Arcangeli O A, Mirhn A et al 1977 La bromocriptina en el tratamiento del sindrome de amenorrea e hiperprolactinemia. Obstet Ginecol Latinoam 35: 325

Bernal M, Villamizar M 1982 Restoration of ovarian function by low nocturnal single daily doses of bromocriptine in patients with the galactorrhea-amenorrhea syndrome. Fertil Steril 37: 392

Besser G M, Parke L, Edwards C R W, Forsyth I A, McNeilly A S 1972 Galactorrhea: successful treatment with reduction of plasma prolactin levels by brom-ergocryptine. Br Med J 3: 669

Bohnet H G, Dahlen H G, Schneider H P G 1974 Hyperprolactinemia and pulsatile LH fluctuation. Acta Endocrinol Copenh 184: 109

Bohnet H G, Dahlen H G, Wuttke W, Schneider H P G 1976 Hyperprolactinemic anovulatory syndrome. J Clin Endocrinol Metab 42: 132

Bohnet H G, Hanker J P, Horowski R, Wickings E J Schneider H P G 1979 Suppression of prolactin secretion by lisuride throughout the menstrual cycle and in hyperprolactinemic menstrual disorders. Acta Endocrinol Copenh 92: 8

Bommer J, Riu E, del Pozo E, Bommer G 1979 Improved sexual function in male haemodialysis patients. Lancet ii: 496

Brun del Re R, del Pozo E, de Grandi P, Friesen H, Hinselman M, Wyss H 1973 Prolactin inhibition and suppression of puerperal lactation by a Br-ergocryptine (CB 154). Obstet Gynecol 41: 884

Buvat J, Lemaire A, Buvat-Herbaut M, Fourlinnie J C, Racadot A, Fossati P 1985 Hyperprolactinemia and sexual function in men. Horm Res 22: 196

Canales E S, Forsbach G, Soria J, Zarata A 1976 Infertility due to hyperprolactinemia and its treatment with ergocryptine. Fertil Steril 27: 1335

Carlson H E 1989 Prolactin stimulation by proteins is mediated by amino acids in humans. J Clin Endocrinol Metab 69: 7

Caro J F, Woolf P D 1980 Pituitary-ovarian axis responsivity to prolonged gonadotropin-releasing hormone infusion in normal and hyperprolactinemic women. J Clin Endocrinol Metab 50: 999

Carter J N, Tyson J E, Tolis G, Van-Vliet S, Faiman C, Fiessen H G 1978 Prolactin-secreting tumors and hypogonadism in 22 men. N Engl J Med 299: 847

Chiari J, Braun K, Späth J 1855 Klinik der Geburtshilfe und Gynäkologie, Erlangen

Ciccarelli E, Miola C, Avataneo T, Camanni F, Besser G M, Grossman A 1989 Long-term treatment with a new repeatable injectable form of bromocriptine, Parlodel LAR, in patients with tumorous hyperprolactinemia. Fertil Steril 52: 930

Closse A, Camps M, Wanner A, Palacios J M 1988 In vivo labeling of brain dopamine D2 receptors using the high-affinity specific D2 agonist [³H]CV 205–502. Brain Res 440: 123

Coelingh Bennink H J T 1979 Intermittent bromocriptine treatment for the induction of ovulation in hyperprolactinemic patients. Fertil Steril 31: 267

Dallabonzana D, Liuzzi A, Oppizi G et al 1985 Effect of the new ergot derivative terguride on plasma PRL and GH levels in patients with pathological hyperprolactinemia and acromegaly. J Endocrinol Invest 8: 147

Dallabonzana D, Liuzzi A, Opizzi G et al 1986 Chronic treatment of pathological hyperprolactinemia and acromegaly with the new ergot-derivative terguride. J Clin Endocrinol Metab 63: 1002

Darragh A, O'Kelly D A, Browne A D H, del Pozo E 1976 Restoration of fertility in prolactin-induced premature menopause. Irish J Med Sci 145: 231

De Cecco L, Foglia G, Ragni N, Rossato P, Venturini P L 1978 The effect of lisuride hydrogen maleate in the hyperprolactinemia-amenorrhoea syndrome: clinical and hormonal responses. Clin Endocrinol (Oxf) 9: 491

De Cecco L, Venturini P L, Ragni N, Valenzano M, Constantini S, Horowsh R 1983 Dopaminergic ergots in lactation and cycle disturbances. In: Calne D B, Horowski R, McDonald R J, Wuttke W (eds) Lisuride and other dopamine agonists. Raven, New York, p 291

Delitala G, Wass I A H, Stubbs W A, Jones A, Williams S, Besser G M 1979 The effect of lisuride hydrogen maleate, an ergot derivative, on anterior pituitary hormone secretion in man. Clin Endocrinol (Oxf) 11: 1

del Pozo E 1982 Hyperprolactinemia in male infertility. In: Bain J, Schill W-B, Schwarestein L (eds) Treatment of male infertility. Springer Verlag, Berlin

del Pozo E, Brun del Re R, Varga L, Friesen H 1972 The

inhibition of prolactin secretion in man by CB 154 (2-Br-ergocryptine). J Clin Endocrinol Metab 35: 768

del Pozo E, Varga L, Wyss H et al 1974 Clinical and hormonal response to bromocriptine (CB 154) in the galactorrhea syndromes. J Clin Endocrinol Metab 39: 18

del Pozo E, Goldstein M, Friesen H, Brun del Re R, Eppenberger U 1975a Lack of action of prolactin suppression on the regulation of the human menstrual cycle. Am J Obstet Gynecol 123: 719

del Pozo E, Varga L, Schulz K D et al 1975b Pituitary and ovarian response patterns to stimulation in the postpartum and in galactorrhea-amenorrhea. Obstet Gynecol 46: 539

del Pozo E, Wyss H, Lancranjan I, Obolensky W, Varga L 1976 Prolactin-induced luteal insufficiency and its treatment with bromocriptine: preliminary results. In: Crosignani P G (ed) Proceedings on 'ovulation in the human', Freiburg. Academic, London, p 297

del Pozo E, Wyss H, Tolis G, Alcaniz J, Campana A, Naftolin F 1979 Prolactin and deficient luteal function. Obstet Gynecol 53: 282

del Pozo E, Gerber L, Hunziker S 1983 Response to bromocriptine therapy in 115 prolactinoma cases. In: Tolis G, Stefanis C, Mountokalakis T, Labrie F (eds) Prolactin and prolactinomas. Raven, New York

del Pozo E, Schlüter K, Nüesch E, Rosenthaler J, Kerp L 1986 Pharmacokinetics of a long-acting bromocriptine preparation (Parlodel LA) and its effect on release of prolactin and growth hormone. J Clin Pharmacol 29: 615

Delvoye P, Taubert H-D, Jürgensen O, L'Hermite M, Delogne J, Robyn C 1974 Serial measurements of gonadotrophins and progesterone in the luteal phase of the menstrual cycle during hyperprolactinaemia induced by sulpiride. C R Acad Sci Paris 279: 1463

Diedrich K, Leindenberger F, Lehman F, Bettendorf G 1978 Klinisch experimentelle Studie zur Therapie ovarieller Funktionsstörungen mit 2-Br-α -Ergocryptin. Geburtshilfe Frauenheilk 38: 716

Döhler K D, Wuttke W 1974 Total blockage of phasic pituitary prolactin release in rats: effect of serum LH and progesterone during the estrous cycle and pregnancy. Endocrinology 94: 1595

Drew J, Parkinson P, Walstab J E, Beischer N A 1977 Incidences and types of malformations in newborn infants. Med J Aust 2: 945

Falaschi P, del Pozo E 1992 Effect of bromocriptine on LH secretion in the polycystic ovary syndrome: role of prolactin. In: Calne D B, Horowski R, McDonald R, Wuttke W (eds) Lisuride and other dopamine agonists: basic mechanisms and endocrine and neurological effects. Raven, New York, p 325

Falaschi P, Frajese G, Sciarra F, Rocco A, Conti C 1978 Influence of hyperprolactinaemia due to metoclopramide on gonadal function in men. Clin Endocrinol (Oxf) 8: 427

Falaschi P, del Pozo E, Rocco et al 1980 Prolactin release in polycystic ovary. Obstet Gynecol 55: 579

Falaschi P, Rocco A, del Pozo E 1986 Inhibitory effect of bromicriptine treatment on LH secretion in polycystic ovary syndrome. J Clin Endocrinol Metab 62: 348

Ferrari C, Barbieri C, Caldara R et al 1986 Long-lasting prolactin-lowering effect of cabergoline, a new dopamine agonist, in hyperprolactinemic patients. J Clin Endocrinol Metab 63: 941

Flückiger E, del Pozo E 1980 Ergot derivatives and pituitary hormones. In: Müller E E (ed) Neuroactive drugs in endocrinology. Elsevier, Amsterdam, p 169

Flückiger E, del Pozo E, von Werder K 1982 In: Labhart A (ed) Prolactin—physiology, pharmacology and clinical findings. Springer-Verlag, Berlin

Forbes A P, Hennemann P H, Griswold G C, Albright F 1954 Syndrome characterized by galactorrhea, amenorrhea and low urinary FSH. J Clin Endocrinol 14: 265

Fossati P, Strauch G, Tourniaire J 1976 Etude de l'activite de la bromocriptine dans les etats d'hyperprolactinemie. Resultats d'un essai cooperatif chez 135 patients. Nouv Press Med 5: 1687

Franks S, Jacobs H S, Martin N, Nabarro J D N 1978 Hyperprolactinemia and impotence. Clin Endocrinol (Oxf) 8: 277

Frantz A G 1973 The regulation of prolactin secretion in humans. In: Ganong W F, Martini L (eds). Frontiers in neuroendocrinology. Oxford University Press, New York, p 337

Fredricsson B, Bjork G, Carlstrom K 1977 Short luteal phase and prolactin. Lancet i: 1210

Friesen H G, Tolis G, Shiu R, Hwang P 1973 Studies on human prolactin: chemistry, radioreceptor assay and clinical significance. In: Pasteels J L, Robyn C (eds) Human prolactin. Excerta Medica, Amsterdam, p 11

Frommel R 1882 Ueber puerperale Atrophie des Uterus. Z Geburtshilfe Gynaekol 7: 305

Gaillard R C, Brownell J 1988 Hormonal effects of CV205–502 a novel octahydrobenzo[g] quinoline with potent dopamine agonist properties. Life Sci 43: 1355

Glass M R, Shau R W, Butt W R, Logan Edwards R, London D R 1975 An abnormality of oestrogen feedback in amenorrhea-galactorrhea. Br Med J 3: 274

Glass M R, Shaw R W, Butt W R, Logan Edwards R, London D R 1979 Oestrogen-gonadotropin feedback abnormalities in hyperprolactinaemic amenorrhoea demonstrated by the response to clomiphene administration. Br J Obstet Gynaecol 86: 64

Gomez F, Reyes F I, Faiman C 1977 Nonpuerperal galactorrhea and hyperprolactinemia. Clinical findings endocrine features and therapeutic responses in 56 cases. Am J Med 62: 648

Gooren L, Van der Veen E A, van Kessel H 1985 Follow-up PRL levels in long-term oestrogen-treated male-to-female transsexuals with regard to prolactinoma induction. Clin Endocrinol 22: 201

Haro L S, Lee D W, Singh R N P, Bee G, Markoff E, Lewis U J 1990 Glycosylated human prolactin: alterations in glycosylation pattern modify affinity for lactogen receptor and values in prolactin radioimmunoassay. J Clin Endocrinol Metab 71: 379

Hashim I A, Aston R, Butler J, McGregor A M, Smith C R, Norman M 1990 The proportion of glycosylated prolactin in serum is decreased in hyperprolactinemic states. J Clin Endocrinol Metab 71: 111

Healy D L, Peppperell R J, Stockdale J, Bremner W J, Burger H G 1977 Pituitary autonomy in hyperprolactinemic secondary amenorrhea: results of hypothalamic-pituitary testing. J Clin Endocrinol Metab 44: 809

Heinonen O P, Slone D, Shapiro S 1977 Birth defects and drugs in pregnancy. Publishing Sciences Group, Littleton

Hirvonen E, Ranta T, Seppälä M 1976 Prolactin suppression stimulates clomiphene responsiveness. Int J Fertil 21: 255

Hökfelt T, Fuxe K 1972 Effects of prolactin and ergot alkaloids on the tuberoinfundibular dopamine (DA) neurons. Neuroendocrinology 98: 100

Horowsh R, Wachtel H 1976 Direct dopaminergic action of

lisuride hydrogen maleate, and ergot derivative, in mice. Eur J Pharmacol 36: 373

Horowski R, Wendt H, Gräf K H 1978 Prolactin-lowering effect of low doses of lisuride in man. Acta Endocrinol Copenhagen 87: 234

Horrobin D F, Mtabaji J P, Manku M S 1976 Physiological cortisol levels block the inhibition of vascular reactivity produced by prolactin. Endocrinology 99: 406

Hulting A L, Muhr C, Lundberg P O, Werner S 1985 Prolactinomas in men: clinical characteristics and the effect of bromocriptine treatment. Acta Med Scand 217: 101

Hyde J E, Ben-Jonathan N 1989 The posterior pituitary contains a potent prolactin-releasing factor: in vivo studies. Endocrinology 125: 736

Jacobs L S, Franks S, Murray M A F, Hull M G R, Steele S J, Nabarro J D N 1976 Clinical and endocrine features of hyperprolactinaemic amenorhea. Clin Endocrinol (Oxf) 5: 439

Jaszmann L, Sternthal V 1974 Advances in the treatment of the galactorrhea-amenorrhea syndrome: induction of ovulation and inhibition of lactation with 2-Br-alpha-ergocryptine. Geburtshilfe Frauenheilk 34: 59

Kandeel F R, Butt W R, Rudd B T, Lynch S S, London D R, Logan Edwards R 1979 Oestrogen modulation of gonadotrophin and prolactin release in women with anovulation and their responses to clomiphene. Clin Endocrinol (Oxf) 10: 619

Kleinberg D L, Noel G D, Frantz A G 1977 Galactorrhea: a study of 235 cases, including 48 with pituitary tumors. N Engl J Med 196: 589

Knobil E, Plant T M, Wildt L, Belchetz P E, Marshall G 1980 Control of the rhesus monkey menstrual cycle permissive role of hypothalamic gonadotropin-releasing hormone. Science 207: 1371

Koike K, Aono T, Miyake A, Tsutsumi H, Matsumoto K, Kurachi K 1981 Induction of ovulation in patients with normoprolactinemic amenorrhea by combined therapy with bromocriptine and clomiphene. Fertil Steril 35: 138

Kort H I, Obbins J C, Decherney B V 1980 Ovarian function and morphology following treatment with bromoergocryptine. Fertil Steril 33: 236

Lachelin G C L, Leblanc H, Yen S S C 1977 The inhibitory effect of dopamine agonists on LH release in women. J Clin Endocrinol Metab 44: 728

Lenton E A, Sobowale O S, Cooke I D 1977 Prolactin concentrations in ovulatory but infertile women: treatment with bromocriptine. Br Med J 2: 1179

L'Hermite M, Michaux-Duchene A, Robyn C 1979 Tiapride-induced chronic hyperprolactinaemia: interference with the human menstrual cycle. Acta Endocrinol Copenh 92: 214

Leyendecker G, Struve T, Plotz E J 1980 Induction of ovulation with chronic intermittent (pulsatile) administration of LHRH in women with hypothalamic and hyperprolactinemic amenorrhea. Arch Gynäkol 229: 177

Malarkey W B 1975 Nonpuerperal lactation and normal prolactin regulation. J Clin Endocrinol Metab 40: 198

Mansel R E, Dogliotti L 1990 European multicenter trial of bromocriptine in cyclical mastalgia. Lancet 335: 190

Mansel R E, Preece P E, Hughes L E 1978 A doubleblind trial of the prolactin inhibitor bromocriptine in painful benign breast disease. Br J Surg 65: 724

March C M, Dvajan V, Mishell D R 1979 Ovulation induction in amenorrheic women. Obstet Gynecol 53: 8

Martikainen H, Rönneberg L, Puistola U, Tapanainen J, Orava M, Kauppila A 1989 Prolactin suppression by bromocriptine stimulates aromatization of testosterone to estradiol in women. Fertil Steril 52: 51

Martin-Comin J, Pujol-Amat P, Cararach V, Davi E, Robyn C 1976 Treatment of fibrocystic disease of the breast with a prolactin inhibitor: 2-Br-alpha-ergocryptine (CB 154). Obstet Gynecol 48: 703

Mattei A M, Ferrari C, Baroldi P et al 1988 Prolactin-lowering effect of acute and once weekly repetitive oral administration of cabergoline at two dose levels in hyperprolactinemic patients. J Clin Endocrinol Metab 66: 193

McNatty K P 1979 Follicular determinants of corpus luteum function in the human ovary. Adv Exp Med Biol 112: 465

McNatty K P, Sawers R S, McNeilly A S 1974 A possible role for prolactin in the control of steroid secretion by the human Graafian follicle. Nature 250: 654

Moggi G, Giampietro O, Chisci R, Brunori I, Simonini N 1979 Pregnancy induction after bromocriptine-cyclofenil treatment in some normoprolactinemic anovulatory women. Fertil Steril 32: 289

Moult P J A, Rees L H, Besser G M 1982 Pulsatile gonadotrophin secretion in hyperprolactinaemic amenorrhoea and the response to bromocriptine therapy. Clin Endocrinol (Oxf) 16: 153

Mühlenstedt D, Meissner M, Shneider H P G 1979 Prolaktin und Lutealphasendefekt. Geburtshilfe Frauenheilk 39: 580

Nagulesparen M, Ang V, Jenkins J S 1978 Bromocriptine treatment of males with pituitary tumours, hyperprolactinaemia, and hypogonadism. Clin Endocrinol (Oxf) 9: 73

Nordmann R, Petcher T J 1985 Octahydrobenzo-[g]quinolines: potent dopamine agonists which show the relationship between ergolines and apomorphine. J Med Chem 28: 367

Palmer B V, Monteiro J C M P 1977 Bromocriptine for severe mastalgia. Br Med J 1: 1083

Pepperell R J, Evans J H, Brown J B et al 1977 A study of the effects of bromocriptine on serum prolactin, follicle stimulating hormone and luteinizing hormone and on ovarian responsiveness to exogenous gonadotropins in anovulatory women. Br J Obstet Gynaecol 84: 456

Polatti F, Bolis P F, Ravagni-Probizer M F, Baruffini A, Cafalleri A 1978 Treatment of hyperprolactinemic amenorrhea by intermittent administration of bromocriptine (CB 154). Am J Obstet Gynecol 131: 792

Pontiroli A E, Viberti G C, Mangili R, Cammelli L, Dubini A 1987 Selective and extremely long inhibition of prolactin release in man by 1-ethyl-3-(3'-dimethylamino-propyl)-3-(6'-allylergoline-8'-β-carbonyl)-urea-diphosphate (FGCE 21336). Br J Clin Pharmacol 23: 433

Quigley M E, Rakoff J S, Yen S S C 1981 Increased luteinizing hormone sensitivity to dopamine inhibition in polycystic ovary syndrome. J Clin Endocrinol Metab 52: 231

Rasmussen C, Bergh T, Wide L, Brownell J 1987 CV 205–502: a new long-acting drug for inhibition of prolactin hypersecretion. Clin Endocrinol (Oxf) 26: 321

Rjosk H K, von Werder K, Fahlbusch R 1976 Hyperprolaktinämische Amenorrhoe. Geburtshilfe Frauenheilkd 36: 575

Rocco A, Falaschi P, Pompei P, del Pozo E, Franjese G 1979 Chronic anovulation in polycystic ovary syndrome: role of hyperprolactinemia and its suppression with bromocriptine. In: Zichella L, Pancheri P (eds) Psychoneuroendocrinology in reproduction. Elsevier North Holland, Amsterdam, p 387

Rolland R, Schellekens L A, Lequin R M 1974 Successful treatment of galactorrhea and amenorrhea and subsequent restoration of ovarian function by a new ergot alkaloid 2-brom-alpha-ergo-cryptine. Clin Endocrinol (Oxf) 3: 155

Sauder S E, Frager M, Case G D, Kelch R P, Marshall J C 1984 Abnormal patterns of pulsatile luteinizing hormone secretion in women with hyperprolactinemia and amenorrhea: response to bromocriptine. J Clin Endocrinol Metab 59: 941

Saunders D M, Hunter J C, Haase H R, Wilson G R 1979 Treatment of luteal phase inadequacy with bromocriptine. Obstet Gynecol 53: 287

Schettini G, Lombardi G, Merola B et al 1990 Rapid and long-lasting suppression of prolactin secretion and shrinkage of prolactinomas after injection of long-acting repeatable form of bromocriptine (Parlodel LAR). Clin Endocrinol 33: 161

Schulz K-D, Del Pozo E, Lose K H, Künzig H J, Geiger W 1975 Successful treatment of mastodynia with the prolactin inhibitor bromocriptine (CB 154). Arch Gynäkol München 220: 83

Schulz K-D, Geiger W, del Pozo E, Kunzig H J 1978 Pattern of sexual steroids, prolactin, and gonadotropic hormones during prolactin inhibition in normally cycling women. Am J Obstet Gynecol 132: 561

Seppälä M, Hirvonen E, Ranta T 1976a Bromocriptine and luteal insufficiency. Lancet i: 229

Seppälä M, Hirvonen E, Ranta T 1976b Bromocriptine treatment of secondary amenorrhea. Lancet i: 1154

Seppälä M, Lehtovirta P, Ranta T 1977 Discordant patterns of hyperprolactinemia and galactorrhoea in secondary amenorrhoea. Acta Endocrinol Copenh 86: 457

Smithells R W 1976 Environmental teratogens of man. Br Med Bull 32: 27

Soules M R, Bremmer W J, Steiner R A, Clifton D K 1991 Prolactin secretion and corpus luteum function in women with luteal phase deficiency. J Clin Endocrinol Metab 72: 986

Spark R F, White R A, Connolly P B 1980 Impotence is not always psychogenic. Newer insights into hypothalamic-pituitary-gonadal dysfunction. JAMA 243: 750

Spark R F, Wills C A, Oreilly G, Ransil B J, Bergland R 1982 Hyperprolactinaemia in males with and without pituitary macroadenomas. Lancet ii: 129

Strauch G, Balcke J C, Mahoudeau J A, Bricaire H 1977 Hormonal changes induced by bromocriptine (CB 154) at the early stage of treatment. J Clin Endocrinol Metab 44: 588

Suginami H, Hamada K, Yano K, Kuroda G, Matsuura S 1986 Ovulation induction with bromocriptine in normoprolactinemic anovulatory women. J Clin Endocrinol Metab 62: 899

Tamura T, Satoh T, Minakami W, Tamada T 1989 Effect of hydergine in hyperprolactinemia. J Clin Endocrinol Metab 69: 470

Theohar C, Fischer-Cornelssen K, Akesson H O et al 1981 Bromocriptine as anti-depressant: double-blind comparative study with imipramine in psychogenic and endogenous depression. Curr Ther Res 30: 830

Thorner M O, Besser G M 1977 Hyperprolactinaemia and gonadal function: results of bromocriptine treatment. In Crosignani P G, Robyn C (eds) Prolactin and human reproduction. Academic, London, p 285

Thorner M O, McNeilly A S, Hagan C, Besser G M 1974 Long-term treatment of galactorrhea and hypogonadism with bromocriptine. Br Med J 2: 419

Thorner M O, Besser G M, Jones A, Dacie J, Jones A E 1975 Bromocriptine treatment in female infertility: report of 13 pregnancies. Br Med J 4: 694

Turkalj I, Braun P, Krupp P 1982 Surveillance of bromocriptine in pregnancy. JAMA 247: 1589

Turkington R W 1972 Serum prolactin levels in patients with gynectomasia. J Clin Endocrinol Metab 34: 62

Turksoy R N, Biller B J, Farber M, Cetrulo C, Mitchell G W 1982 Ovulatory response to clomiphene citrate during bromocriptine-failed ovulation in amenorrhea galactorrhea and hyperprolactinemia. Fertil Steril 37: 411

Vance M L, Lipper M, Klibanski A, Biller B M K, Samean N A, Molitch M E 1990 Treatment of prolactin-secreting pituitary macroadenomas with the long-acting non-ergot dopamine agonist CV 205–502. Ann Intern Med 112: 668

Van der Lely A J, Brownell J, Lamberts S W 1991 The efficacy and tolerability of CV205–502 (a non-ergot dopaminergic drug) in macroprolactinoma patients and in prolactinoma patients intolerant to bromocriptine. J Clin Endocrinol Metab 72: 1136

Van der Steeg H J, Coelingh Bennink H J T 1977 Bromocriptine for induction of ovulation in normoprolactinemic post-pill anovulation. Lancet i: 502

Votava Z, Lamplova 1 1961 Antiserotonin activity of some ergolenyn and isoergolenyl derivatives in comparison with LSD and the influence of monoamine inhibition on this antiserotonin effect. In: Rothlin E (ed) Neuropsychopharmacology, vol 2. Elsevier, Amsterdam, p 68

Whittaker P G, Wilcox T, Lind T 1981 Maintained fertility in a patient with hyperprolactinemia due to big-big prolactin. J Clin Endocrinol Metab 53: 863

Wildt L, Hausler A, Hutchinson J S, Marshall G, Knobil E 1981 Estradiol as a gonadotropin releasing hormone in the rhesus monkey. Endocrinology 198: 2011

Winters S J, Troen P 1984 Altered pulsatile secretion of luteinizing hormone in hypogonadal men with hyperprolactinaemia. Clin Endocr 21: 257

Wolf A S, del Pozo E 1979 Conversion of clomiphene response by bromocriptine therapy in normoprolactinemic amenorrhea. Acta Endocrinol Copenh 25: 186

Zacur H A, Chapanis N P, Lake C R, Ziegler M, Tyson J E 1976 Galactorrhea-amenorrhea: psychological interaction with neuroendocrine function. Am J Obstet Gynecol 125: 859

Zarate A, Jacobs H S, Canales E S et al 1973 Functional evaluation of pituitary reserve in patients with the amenorrheagalactorrhea syndrome utilizing luteinizing hormone releasing hormone (LH-RH), L-Dopa and chlorpromazine. J Clin Endocrinol Metab 37: 855

Zarate A, Canales E S, Forsbach G, Fernandez-Lazala R 1978 Bromocriptine. Clinical expenience in the induction of pregnancy in galactorrhea-amenorrhea. Obstet Gynecol 52: 442

Zikan V, Semonsky M 1960 Mutterkornalkaloid XVI. Einige n-lD-6-methyl-isoergolenyl-8/-N/D-6-methyl-ergonyl-8/'und ND-6-methyl-erogolin-v-y'-8/NI-substitineste Harnstoffe. Colln Czech Chem Commun 25: 1922

Zippel H H, Schulz K-D, del Pozo E 1977 Morphological studies in human proliferating mammary tissues under treatment with the prolactin inhibitor bromocriptine (CB 154). Acta Endocrinol Copenh 84: 42

# 18. Steroids and steroid-like compounds

*H.-D. Taubert    H. Kuhl*

## INTRODUCTION

Sex steroids, in particular estradiol–17β and progesterone, are intricately involved in the regulation of follicular maturation, ovulation, gonadotropin release, ripening of the oocyte, tubal transport of the zygote, implantation, maintenance of pregnancy, and many other features of the reproductive process. As many of these facets seem to present themselves as possible targets for the treatment of functional causes of infertility, considerable efforts have been made in the past five decades to use natural sex steroids, their synthetic derivatives, and non-steroidal analogs therapeutically (Tables 18.1, 18.2).

The reports of a few cases published in 1932 by the late Carl Kaufmann and his coworker Bickel of the Charité in Berlin have to be considered as being the starting point of therapy with sex steroids in gynecology (Kaufmann, 1932, Kaufmann & Bickel 1932). Kaufmann was the

**Table 18.1** Steroids and steroid-like substances used in the therapy of female functional infertility

| Type | Generic name | Mode of application | Therapeutic indication |
|------|--------------|---------------------|------------------------|
| Estrogens | Ethinylestradiol | Oral | Cervical dysmucorrhea |
| | Estradiol valerate | Oral/parenteral | Combination with ovulation inducers |
| | Estradiol benzoate | Parenteral | |
| | Estriol | Oral | |
| | Epimestrol | Oral | Anovulation, luteal phase defect |
| Progestogens | Nortestosterone derivatives: | | |
| | Allylestrenol | Oral | |
| | Ethynodiol di-acetate | Oral | |
| | Norethynodrel | Oral | |
| | Norethisterone acetate | Oral | Withdrawal bleeding |
| | Lynestrenol | Oral | Endometriosis |
| | 17α-Hydroxyprogesterone derivatives | | |
| | Chlormadinone acetate | Oral | |
| | Medroxyprogesterone acetate | Oral | |
| | Medrogestone | Oral | |
| | 17α-Hydroxyprogesterone caproate | Parenteral | |
| | Retroprogesterone: | | |
| | Dydrogesterone | Oral | Luteal phase defect |
| | Progesterone | Parenteral/vaginal | Threatened or habitual abortion |
| Stilbenes | Clomiphene citrate | Oral | Anovulation |
| | Cyclofenil | Oral | Luteal phase defect |
| | Tamoxifen | Oral | Luteinized, unruptured follicle |
| Corticosteroids | Dexamethasone | Oral | Anovulation with hyperandrogenemia |
| Antiandrogens | Spironolactone | Oral | Anovulation with hyperandrogenemia |
| Androgens | Danazol | Oral | Endometriosis |

435

**Table 18.2**   Chronology of the development of endocrine therapy in gynecology

| | |
|---|---|
| 1929/30 | Isolation and synthesis of estrone and estriol |
| 1930 | First therapeutic application of PMS (pregnant mare's serum) |
| 1932 | Kaufmann scheme: first sequential therapy with an estrogen and a progesterone preparation |
| 1934 | Structure and synthesis of progesterone |
| 1936 | Structure and synthesis of estradiol |
| 1938 | First orally effective sex steroids: ethinyl estradiol and ethisterone |
| 1938 | Estrogenic effect of DES (diethylstilbestrol) |
| 1958 | hPG (human pituitary gonadotropin) |
| 1960 | hMG (human menopausal gonadotropin) |
| 1961 | Ovulation-inducing effect of clomiphene citrate |
| 1965 | Cyclofenil |
| 1968 | Epimestrol |
| 1969 | Cyproterone acetate |
| 1971 | Structure and synthesis of LH-RH |
| 1972 | Prolactin-suppressing effect of bromocriptine |
| 1974 | LH-RH analogs |
| 1974 | Tamoxifen |
| 1977 | Danazol |
| 1979 | Pulsatile therapy with LH-RH |

first to succeed in inducing proliferation of an atrophic endometrium followed by full secretory transformation and menstrual bleeding in a woman devoid of ovarian function.

The complete substitution of ovarian function was achieved by a sequential regimen employing first an estrogen (Progynon benzoate), and thereafter a progesterone preparation.

The second and equally important milestone was the synthesis of the first orally effective estrogen, ethinylestradiol, and the first oral progestogen, ethisteron, in 1938 by Inhoffen & Hohlweg. In the same year, Dodds et al recognized the estrogenic potential of diethylstilbestrol, a stilbene derivative without direct structural relationship to steroids.

When compared to the treatment of amenorrhea and of menstrual irregularities, the impact of oral and injectable estrogens and progestogens on the management of functional infertility was not very great. Even though it had been recognized as early as 1932 (Hohlweg & Junkmann 1932) that the ovary partakes in the regulation of ovulation by triggering the preovulatory LH surge through a positive feedback effect of estrogen upon the anterior pituitary, most attempts to induce ovulation by the injection of estrogens were doomed to failure. As a consequence, the use of estrogens and progestogens in the treatment of female infertility remained more or less limited to:

• Substitutional therapy with progesterone and progestogens in luteal phase defect, and for the prevention of threatened and habitual abortion
• Stimulation of the cervical mucus in cases of cervical sterility due to dysmucorrhea
• Suppression of the proliferative action of estrogens in endometriosis.

A real therapeutic breakthrough occurred in 1961 when Greenblatt et al made the epochal discovery that a nonsteroidal analog of estradiol, clomiphene citrate (Fig. 18.1), exerts a stimulatory effect on ovarian function in many women with anovulatory infertility.

Even though several other ovulation-inducing agents (Table 18.2) were subsequently introduced into clinical practice, it may safely be stated that treatment with clomiphene has probably helped more infertile women to conceive than any other infertility therapy.

Before clomiphene became generally available, a fair success rate had been achieved by some investigators (Jones et al 1953, Perloff et al 1965, Toaff et al 1978) by treating anovulatory women with corticosteroids. As some women with anovulation undoubtedly produce more androgens than normally seen—and these may be produced in part by the adrenals—there is still a certain place for the use of corticosteroids in the treatment of

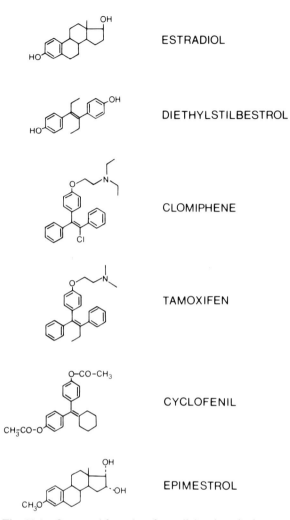

ESTRADIOL

DIETHYLSTILBESTROL

CLOMIPHENE

TAMOXIFEN

CYCLOFENIL

EPIMESTROL

**Fig. 18.1** Structural formulas of estradiol and synthetic estrogen analogs.

anovulation. Later reports indicated that even spironolactone, an aldosterone antagonist with marked antiandrogenic properties, appears to be of promise in some of these cases.

## The clinical spectrum of ovarian dysfunction

Functional infertility is often due to faulty function of the ovary which, again, can be caused by a disturbance of the hypothalamus, the pituitary, the ovary, or the adrenals. Ovarian dysfunction is a cause of infertility in women, as they either fail to ovulate, or fail to develop an adequately functioning corpus luteum subsequent to ovulation. Luteal dysfunction is believed to

jeopardize the process of implantation and early embryonal development, resulting eventually in abortion.

## Ovulation-inducing agents

The close temporal relationship between the estrogen surge in the late follicular phase of the cycle and the preovulatory LH peak suggests a functional role for estradiol in triggering ovulation via the release of LH. There is ample evidence from animal experiments to support this assumption. Figure 18.2 shows that the administration of 200 µg ethinylestradiol to women brings about a temporary decrease in serum LH followed by a rise to a level in excess of the initial values. This 'positive feedback' effect was used by Kupperman (1963), almost 30 years ago, to induce ovulation by injecting anovulatory women approximately 2 weeks after a progesterone-induced withdrawal bleeding with 20 mg equine estrogens (Premarin). In 44% of the certainly well-selected cases, ovulation occurred and most of the ovulating patients actually conceived. Even though a favorable response may occasionally be achieved, a placebo-like effect is difficult to exclude, and the problem of choosing the right moment for the injection appears formidable. Even if a follicle would develop, it is usually not possible to influence with estrogens the more or less disturbed or arrested follicular development which is present in a large proportion of anovulatory women with oligomenorrhea and amenorrhea. Consequently, ovulation induction with estrogens was superseded by the use of a new and more effective class of agents which have become known as ovulation inducers.

Subsequent to the recognition of the estrogenic potential of diethylstilbestrol (DES) by Dodds et al (1938), a large number of structurally related compounds was synthetized, which were either estrogenic such as chlorotrianisene (TACE), hormonally inactive like triparanol, or active antiestrogens like clomiphene. The latter compound and two similar subtances, tamoxifen and cyclofenil, were found to be singularly suitable for the treatment of anovulation in women with normoestrogenic, dysgonadotropic oligomenorrhea and amenorrhea. This group of nonsteroidal ovulation inducers was comple-

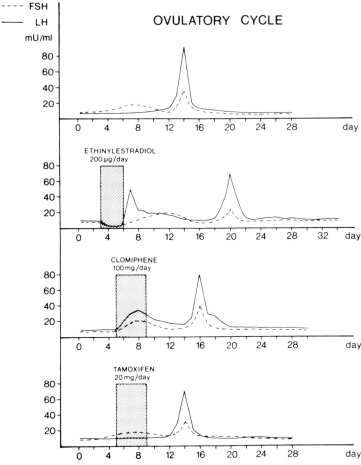

**Fig. 18.2** Differing effects of ethinyl estradiol, clomiphene, and tamoxifen upon serum FSH and LH in women with normal ovulatory cycle. (Adapted from Tsai & Yen 1971, Vandenberg & Yen 1973, Groom & Griffiths 1976).

mented by epimestrol which is a derivative of the natural estrogen estriol.

## ANTIESTROGENS

### CLOMIPHENE-CITRATE

**Pharmacology and biological activity**

Clomiphene, cyclofenil and tamoxifen are nonsteroidal agents bearing a certain structural relationship to the potent estrogen DES (Fig. 18.1). Although these compounds are not steroids but triphenylethylenes, their steric configuration shows a remarkable structural similarity to estradiol, and consequently allows the binding to estrogen receptors.

Epimestrol differs from the other ovulation inducing agents in that it is actually a steroid, 3-methoxy-epiestriol (Fig. 18.2). The common denominator of these compounds is their 'janus face-like' ability to elicit estrogenic or antiestrogenic effects in animals or in man depending on tissue, species, duration of treatment, and the estrogenic milieu (Katzenellenbogen et al 1979). Even though it is mainly an antiestrogen, clomiphene can exert a weak estrogenic effect in animals with estrogen deficiency. Clomiphene stimulates the growth of the uterus of oophorectomized rats, and increases water and glycogen content. On the other hand, it interferes with the growth-promoting effects of estradiol when administered concomitantly to oophorectomized rats. This may reflect some differences in the interaction of ovulation-inducing agents with the estrogen receptor at the cytoplasmic and nuclear level.

Another important property with respect to their mode of action in the human is the relative long-acting effect of estrogen antagonists. Orally ingested, clomiphene is readily resorbed and undergoes enterohepatic circulation, and only one-half of the dose is excreted within 5 days. Early reports indicated that even after 6 weeks clomiphene or its metabolites are demonstrable in the faeces (Swyer 1965); this has, however, been refuted by more recent evidence (Geier et al 1987). Although the binding affinity of clomiphene to the cytoplasmic estrogen receptor is weaker compared to that of estradiol, the prolonged circulation in the organism and the protracted retention in the nucleus of target cells provide for the pronounced estrogen-antagonistic effectiveness of this compound.

*Pharmacology*

Clomiphene citrate is available as a racemic mixture of Zu- (*cis-*) and En-(*trans-*) clomiphene citrate. The former is biologically much more active than the latter. Each of the two isomers has its own pharmacological and pharmacokinetic profile. The En to Zu ratio was found to be 1:1 two hours after the ingestion of a single dose of the racemic mixture, but 1:6 after 24 h. After intake of 50 mg of a mixture of En-clomiphene (62%) and Zu-clomiphene (38%), a peak level of Zu-clomiphene of 7.5 ng/ml is reached after 7 h, and of En-clomiphene of 4.2 ng/ml on average after 4 h (Mikkelson et al 1986). As Zu-clomiphene is the more estrogenic of the two isomers, the response of the target tissue should vary according to the relative affinities and concentrations of the isomers at the relevant estrogen receptor. These time-dependent changes in the ratio of the two isomers might have a significant impact both on the pulsatile pattern of gonadotropin release and on the quality of the cervical mucus. It is remarkable that there is a subject-to-subject difference in the blood level of the En-isomer and its metabolites (Mikkelson et al 1986).

The blood level of estrogen-receptor binding material has been studied in women devoid of functioning ovaries after ingestion of clomiphene citrate. A 4-hydroxy metabolite of clomiphene citrate present in the serum bound competetively and with higher affinity to the rat uterine receptor than the parent substance. The maximum was reached after 4–5 h. The half-life time varied between 4.5 and 10 h. In patients receiving clomiphene citrate from days 5 to 9 of the cycle, ligands were demonstrable between days 14 and 22, but none at day 60 (Geier et al 1987). This indicates that there is no accumulation when the accepted criteria for the use of clomiphene are being observed, as formerly believed.

In consideration of the pharmacological disparities between the two isomers and possible differences in the galenic preparation of different brands of clomiphene, a comparison appeared legitimate. Diamond et al (1986) could actually show that serum estradiol levels were greater in Clomid-treated women compared to those using Serophene. Otherwise there was no difference of clinical significance.

*Mode of action*

The principal mechanism of action of clomiphene is an increase in the release of GnRH from the hypothalamus into the hypothalamic-pituitary portal circulation with a resultant increase in pituitary luteinizing hormone secretion resulting in the release of more LH per pulse (Archer et al 1989).

The earliest event in the response of a target cell to estradiol is the binding of the steroid to the receptor in the nucleus. The formation of the complex involves an allosteric change of the receptor configuration which interacts preferentially with a small number of specific binding sites on the genome. Beyond this, there are also nonspecific interactions of the receptor protein with DNA (Yamamoto & Alberts 1974). The result of these processes is a series of metabolic activities, i.e. increase of RNA, enzyme induction, and protein synthesis which reflect the hormonal effect.

The linear relationship between binding of the steroid and the reaction suggests that the only limiting factor in the response is the amount of receptor available (Katzenellenbogen et al 1979). The slower an estrogen dissociates from the receptor complex, the longer is the duration of nuclear retention, and the greater the biological effect (Weichmann & Notides 1980).

The full sequence of estrogen response of a target cell requires that a minimal number of estrogen–receptor complexes are retained in the nucleus for several hours.

The differences in the action of the various estrogens seem to be correlated with differential stimulation of nuclear binding sites with high affinity and low capacity, and those with low affinity and high capacity (Markaverich et al 1981). The varying distribution of both types of nuclear binding sites is responsible for the differing response of several target organs to the administration of estradiol, estriol or the anti-estrogens.

In contrast to estradiol, an estrogen antagonist, although complexed with estrogen receptor in the nucleus, seems to be incapable of inducing the adequate allosteric configuration of the complex. As a consequence, its nuclear interaction is different from that of estrogens, and it initiates only some of the known estrogenic responses. In certain tissues, it does not appear to evoke any estrogen-like response at all (Sutherland 1981).

The most important aspect of the action of antiestrogens is that they do not seem to be capable of inducing the synthesis of estrogen receptors. Moreover, their dissociation from chromatin is impaired, and they remain in the nucleus for a longer period of time blocking the interaction of receptors with estrogens (Katzenellenbogen et al 1979). Therefore, clomiphene and the other ovulation inducers are estrogen antagonists because they cause, to a certain extent, a state of estrogen insensitivity of the target cell.

### Endocrine effects

It appears to be very likely that a reduction in the negative feedback of endogenous estrogens is a key event in ovulation induction by antiestrogens. Antiestrogens have been demonstrated to inhibit the uptake of tritiated estriol into the hypothal-amus and the pituitary (Kato et al 1968, Schulz-Amling et al 1973) and to cause a prolonged depletion of hypothalamic and pituitary estrogen receptors (Kahwanago et al 1970, Etgen 1979). Consequently, the reduction of the negative feedback effect of estrogens results in an increase of GnRH release and an elevation of gonadotropin secretion (Igarashi et al 1967, Baier & Taubert, 1969a, Vaitukaitis et al 1971, Kuhl et al 1977, Miyake et al 1980). This rise in LH and FSH levels which is initiated during treatment is followed by an enhancement of follicular activity (Kjeld et al 1975, Swyer et al 1975, Wu 1977).

When clomiphene is applied during the early follicular phase to ovulating women, an increase of LH and—to a much lesser degree—of FSH can be observed (Fig. 18.2) (Vandenberg & Yen 1973). This suggests a decrease in the feedback inhibition of the hypothalamic-pituitary axis by estradiol. This positive effect on LH release by clomiphene is enhanced by administration during the late follicular phase. Contrary to that, clomiphene has no effect on gonadotropin secre-tion during the luteal phase (Vandenberg & Yen 1973). After treatment of cyclic women with clomiphene citrate, the LH pulse frequency was accelerated, and mean LH, FSH and estradiol were increased, while the response of the pituitary to gonadotropin releasing hormone (GnRH) remained unchanged. Naloxone did not have an effect on LH pulsatility or pituitary response to GnRH (Judd et al 1987). This was interpreted to mean that at least in the early follicular phase clomiphene exerts its action at the hypothalamic GnRH pulse generators and does not depend on the activity of opioid neurons.

During the application of clomiphene, a rapid stimulation of estradiol biosynthesis takes place which continues to increase markedly after cessa-tion of clomiphene ingestion until a maximum is reached the day before the preovulatory LH surge (Vandenberg & Yen 1973). This continuous enhancement of follicular estradiol synthesis is, however, independent of serum gonadotropin level suggesting a direct effect of the antiestrogen upon the ovary (Fig.18.3).

It has also been demonstrated that the synthesis of estradiol by human ovaries is enhanced by a factor of three even in the absence of

EARLY FOLLICULAR PHASE    LATE FOLLICULAR PHASE    LUTEAL PHASE

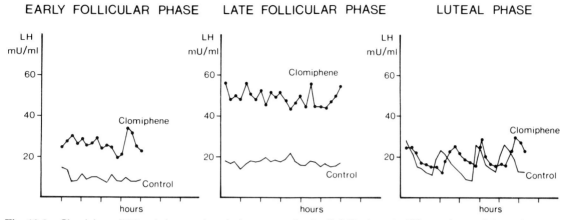

**Fig. 18.3**    Clomiphene (100 mg) does not impair the pattern of pulsatile LH release in different phases of the ovulatory cycle but increases the amplitude. (Adapted from Vandenberg & Yen 1973).

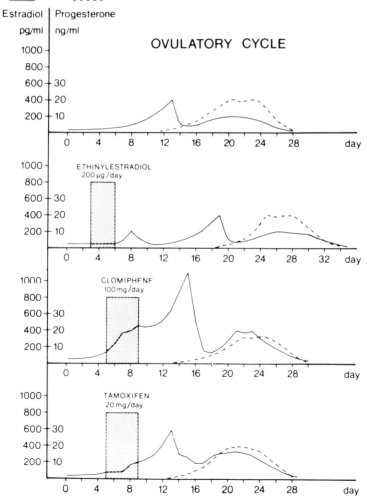

**Fig. 18.4**    Differing effects of ethinyl estradiol, clomiphene and tamoxifen on serum estradiol and progesterone in women with normal ovulatory cycle. (Adapted from Tsai & Yen 1971, Vandenberg & Yen 1973, Groom & Griffiths 1976).

gonadotropins when a perfusion is carried out with androstendione and clomiphene (Stähler et al 1975). The relative independency of follicular maturation from LH release is corroborated by the enhancement of estradiol production during the follicular and luteal phase when tamoxifen is applied from day 5 to 9 of a normal ovulatory cycle, although gonadotropin levels seem to be unaltered (Figs. 18.2, 18.4) (Groom & Griffiths 1976).

A marked increase in serum LH over that of FSH can be shown to occur when ethinyl estradiol and clomiphene are administered during the early follicular phase to ovulatory women. This is not demonstrable when taxomifen is given (Fig.18.2). This temporary change in the ratio of LH to FSH seems to bring about some impairment of follicular maturation, resulting in delayed ovulation when the former compounds are being used.

It is obvious that the induction of ovulation by antiestrogens cannot only be explained by a withdrawal of the inhibitory effect of endogenous estrogens on gonadotropin release. Although the development of tertiary follicles is dependent on LH and FSH, the individual differences in the internal hormonal environment indicate a certain intrafollicular regulation of hormone levels in the antral fluid and of steroid synthesis (McNatty & Baird 1978). The alterations of LH, FSH, estradiol and androgen concentration in the follicular fluid during the process of maturation do not only control steroid production but also oocyte development. Just before ovulation, the concentration of estradiol in the follicular fluid may reach a level about 3000-fold higher than that in serum. Estradiol is capable of increasing FSH and LH receptors, and thus of stimulating follicular maturation (Goldenberg et al 1972, Richards et al 1976). Besides the long-loop feedback regulation of the hypothalamic-pituitary-ovarian axis, an internal short-loop feedback control within the follicles appears to be responsible for the individual hormonal 'microclimate' of the follicular fluid. This was recently corroborated by the finding of Zhuang et al (1982) that estradiol as well as clomiphene augments the gonadotropin-stimulated estrogen production in cultured granulosa cells from immature rat follicles. The direct

positive feedback effect of clomiphene could be responsible for the in vitro stimulation of estradiol synthesis in perfused ovaries (Stähler et al 1975), and for the fourfold estrogen concentration in follicular fluid during clomiphene treatment as compared to normal ovulatory cycles (Smith & Kistner 1963), and for the gonadotropin-independent enhancement of serum estradiol in women under clomiphene treatment (Vandenberg & Yen 1973). The marked rise in the intrafollicular estradiol level leads to a relative autonomy from gonadotropins of the maturing follicle until ovulation.

Such a process of accelerated estradiol accumulation and autonomy of the follicle with respect to the control by gonadotropins could account for clomiphene-induced overstimulation of the ovary, and for the failure of high doses of ethinyl estradiol to interfere with clomiphene-induced ovulation (Taubert & Dericks-Tan 1976a,b). On the other hand, the direct action of clomiphene on the ovary can only take place when follicular development has reached a certain stage of maturation. This is confirmed by the clinical observation that ovulation can only be induced by clomiphene in women having endogenous estrogens.

The complex nature of action of clomiphene depends to a large degree on the functional stage of the follicles, as it counteracts the estrogen effect in more mature follicles in vitro (Laufer et al 1982), while it stimulates aromatase activity in immature follicles (Zhuang et al 1982). En- and Zu-clomiphene were found to inhibit dose-dependently the LH-stimulated synthesis of estradiol in cultured human granulosa cells obtained from women stimulated with clomiphene/human menopausal gonadotropin (hMG) and human chorionic gonadotropin (hCG). As the inhibition was reversible, a toxic effect of clomiphene could be excluded, even though a concentration 10–100 times higher than normally found in tissue or blood after administration in vivo was used (Olson & Granberg 1990). Similar findings were obtained in the monkey: clomiphene use brought about a rise in gonadotropins and a fall in estradiol indicating a direct effect of clomiphene upon the ovary (Marut & Hodgen 1982).

The treatment with clomiphene of anovulatory

or oligoovulatory women who show a certain degree of follicular activity and a functionally responsive hypothalamic-pituitary-ovarian axis, results in a significant rise in LH and, to a lesser extent, in FSH (Jacobson et al 1968a,b, Yen et al 1970). After termination of clomiphene administration, the LH levels generally increase for 1 or 2 more days. Thereafter, LH decreases gradually until the time of the preovulatory LH surge which occurs in most cases between days 13 and 20 after the beginning of clomiphene therapy. There is a concomitant rise in serum estradiol (Kjeld et al 1975, Taubert & Dericks-Tan 1976a,b, Wu 1977), which continues into the preovulatory surge of a higher level than normally seen.

A comparison of estradiol and progesterone levels between clomiphene and hMG-stimulated cycles revealed significant differences (Dlugi et al 1985). Stimulation with clomiphene resulted in a lower estradiol level in the early and mid luteal phase as compared to hMG, and serum progesterone was lower after treatment with hMG. This seems to be caused either by differences in the follicular maturation process under the influence of both compounds, or it is the expression of a direct inhibitory effect of clomiphene on follicular steroidogenesis.

It is often overlooked that the success of clomiphene therapy does not only depend on a sufficient stage of follicular maturation but also on body weight which should not be less than 81% of the ideal weight (Marshall & Fraser 1971), as patients with anorexia nervosa fail to respond.

### Antifecundity effects of clomiphene citrate

It had already been noticed in the first clinical trials of clomiphene citrate that there was a marked discrepancy between the ovulation rate and the percentage of women who actually conceived, the former exceeding the latter by a factor of 2. The tenet has widely been accepted that this is due to the antiestrogenic effect of clomiphene citrate which may interfere at least to some degree with conception by:

- Impeding the ascent of the spermatozoa through the cervical mucus by altering its quality in an unfavorable fashion

- Inhibiting the nidation of the blastocyst by interfering with the proper development of the endometrium
- Disturbing implantation by a direct action on the fertilized ovum.

There are conflicting data on the antifecundity effect of clomiphene citrate in women and in experimental animals. When intrafollicular oocytes were exposed to clomiphene citrate which had been added to an ovarian perfusate, there was a significant reduction in the pregnancy rate after the transfer of ova ovulated and fertilized in vitro in the rabbit (Yoshimura et al 1988). The same group of investigators had already reported in 1986 that 65% of inseminated ova from clomiphene citrate-treated ovaries showed signs of degeneration as compared to 37% in the controls. The percentage of fertilized ova which reached the morula stage was 15% in the clomiphene citrate-treated group as compared to 49% in the control group (Yoshimura et al 1986). It was concluded that this loss in developmental capacity may explain at least in part the discrepancy observed between the rate of ovulation and conception in anovulatory women.

While clomiphene citrate has been used effectively in the treatment of histologically proven luteal phase insufficiency (Murray et al 1989, Guzick & Zeleznik 1990), adverse effects have also been found in the endometrium of anovulatory women after ovulation induction with clomiphene citrate. Deficient luteal phases have been observed after induction of ovulation by clomiphene (Cook et al 1984), which may be caused by inadequate stimulation of the ovary during the follicular phase (Garcia et al 1977), but may also be due to a direct negative effect upon the ovary (Adashi 1984). A premature epithelial secretory pattern has been observed in the follicular phase following clomiphene citrate. This may reflect a functional desynchronization which could possibly have an impact on the preimplantation period (Birkenfeld et al 1986). Similarly, clomiphene citrate appeared to impair endometrial receptivity for mouse blastocysts, possibly by a direct effect, since there were practically no pregnancies in animals which had received such treatment (Nelson et al 1990).

Even though clomiphene citrate has, at least in vitro, an estrogenic effect on the human endometrium (Markiewicz et al 1988), it seems to have a dual capacity to express both estrogenic and antiestrogenic effects. This should be considered since it may alter the proper estrogen/progesterone ratio necessary for successful implantation. The serum estradiol level is higher during the 5 days preceding ovulation than in spontaneous cycles when clomiphene citrate is used. The normal increase in uterine volume and in endometrial thickness as shown by ultrasound is conspicuously absent in clomiphene-induced cycles. This indicates that the antiestrogenic effect of clomiphene citrate inhibits the preovulatory growth of the uterus. It is not yet known whether this effect contributes to the discrepancy between ovulation and conception rate in clomiphene-treated women (Eden et al 1989). There is, however, some evidence that the 'endometrial factor' may not be as important with respect to the discrepancy between ovulation and pregnancy rate as it has previously been presumed.

The difference between the number of women ovulating in response to treatment with clomiphene citrate and those actually conceiving becomes much less substantial when analysed according to the lifetable method. In addition, the diagnosis of luteal phase insufficiency — be it spontaneous or induced — is difficult, and the condition is probably overdiagnosed in clinical practice (Hecht et al 1989a).

## Indications

If an ovulation-inducing agent such as clomiphene is expected to be clinically effective, the following preconditions need to be fulfilled:

1. The patient should produce a sufficient amount of estradiol to allow withdrawal bleeding to occur in response to treatment with an oral progestogen.
2. The hypothalamo-pituitary-ovarian axis should be potentially intact, particularly with respect to the positive feedback effect of estradiol.

As a consequence, clomiphene is indicated for the treatment of infertile women with anovulation who either bleed spontaneously at regular or irregular intervals, or upon the administration of a progestogen (WHO Group II), and who are normoprolactinemic. Contrary to that, patients who do not react to a challenge with a progestogen with bleeding (WHO Group I, VI) are poor candidates for therapy with clomiphene, and respond much better to hMG and bromocriptine, respectively (see Chapters 9, 16 and 17).

## The use of clomiphene versus other ovulation inducers

Even though there are few valid comparisons between the therapeutic efficacy of clomiphene, cyclofenil, tamoxifen and epimestrol, it may safely be stated that clomiphene is more effective than the other compounds, tamoxifen being a possible exception. A just appraisal of the therapeutic value of epimestrol is difficult to make, as there are quite variable results which have been reported by different investigators. On the other hand, there seem to be few if any objectionable side-effects, like those which have been reported for clomiphene. Epimestrol may even offer some advantage if a close follow-up of treatment is difficult or not possible at all, and when the anti-estrogenic effect of clomiphene upon the cervical mucus should be avoided.

## Treatment of anovulation

Although a great and at times confusing variety of treatment schemes has been proposed, there is no final proof that the eventual success rate depends on a particular dose of clomiphene or a certain duration of therapy. Nevertheless, it is generally agreed upon to begin clomiphene therapy with relatively low doses.

Treatment is usually begun by advising the patient to take 50 mg of clomiphene per day for 5 days beginning 5 days after the onset of spontaneous or progesterone-induced bleeding.

When clomiphene citrate therapy was started on day 2, 3, 4 or 5, the outcome in terms of ovulation rate, luteal phase defects or pregnancies was comparable (Wu & Winkel 1989). Day 5 seems to be optimal for inducing superstimulation. Consequently, it seems to be the ideal day for initiating clomiphene therapy in in vitro fertilization (IVF) programs, but not for anovulatory patients wishing a singleton pregnancy (Marss et al 1984). The patient is then advised to have intercourse approximately every other day beginning at day 9 or 10 after the first day of bleeding until a rise in the basal body temperature (BBT) demonstrates that ovulation has occurred.

The further mode of application of clomiphene depends on whether the patient ovulates or fails to do so.

*Ovulatory response* When a patient responds to treatment with 50 mg of clomiphene per day with ovulation, the therapy is usually continued at this dose until pregnancy ensues or a different course has to be taken, e.g. in a case where the postcoital test reveals hostility of the cervical mucus to spermatozoa, or the luteal phase subsequent to induction of ovulation proves to be inadequate.

*Persistent anovulation* Should ovulation fail to be induced as indicated by a monophasic BBT, a persistently positive ferning pattern of the cervical mucus, and the absence of a luteal phase progesterone value, the dose of clomiphene is raised in the following cycle to 100 mg/day given again from day 5 through 9. If there is no bleeding within 5 weeks, a progestogen is prescribed for 5–10 days to induce withdrawal bleeding, in order to avoid an unnecessary delay in the continuation of treatment.

In order to predict the time of ovulation the timing of the LH surge in spontaneous cycles is useful. When LH rose in control cycles on day 16 or earlier, clomiphene citrate delayed it; if the normal LH surge occurred on day 18 or later, clomiphene advanced it (Hecht et al 1989b). A substantial number of anovulatory women who do not respond to the standard regimen of clomiphene therapy can be made to ovulate when its dose is raised, the period of treatment extended beyond the customary 5 days, and other hormonal agents are used to provide an additional stimulus. This will be described in the section on 'Extended and combined therapy' below.

## Monitoring of clomiphene therapy

Ovulation is presumed to have occurred when the

BBT has risen by 0.3° to 0.5°C, and remains elevated at this level for 12 days or more. When there is any doubt whether or not ovulation really took place, a blood specimen for the measurement of progesterone is obtained approximately 2 weeks after the last tablet of clomiphene has been taken. A value of 3–10 ng/ml progesterone is generally accepted as evidence of ovulation having occurred (Israel et al 1972, Landgren et al 1980). It has to be emphasized that the BBT will not show the usual hyperthermic shift in some women even though a corpus luteum secreting progesterone is present (Johansson et al 1972, Moghissi 1976). Moreover, a single postovulatory value of progesterone does definitely not preclude the existence of an inadequate luteal phase subsequent to induced ovulation.

At the time the blood sample is obtained for the assay of progesterone (or 1 week later), a pelvic examination is performed to assess ovarian size in order to rule out overstimulation of the ovary. This is supplemented by a sonographic examination whenever indicated, particularly in the presence of adnexal pain or tenderness to palpation and a cystic enlargement of one or both ovaries. Whenever ovarian overstimulation is noted, further treatment with clomiphene should be withheld until the cysts have completely disappeared. (Refer to 'Adverse reactions' below).

The patient should be instructed prior to the initiation of therapy to observe and report any side-effects (blurring of vision, hot flushes, nausea, etc.), and signs of overstimulation of the ovaries such as abdominal pain.

The application of clomiphene or any of the other ovulation inducers should not be repeated unless it is absolutely certain that the patient has not already conceived in the preceding treatment cycle, as there have been anecdotal reports on the occurrence of malformations (Biale et al 1978) when clomiphene was taken inadvertently during the earliest stages of pregnancy. The patient should therefore be instructed to abide by the following rules:

Clomiphene should only be taken again when—
• the BBT has returned to the usual level of the follicular phase

- the intensity and duration of the last menstrual period was normal
- there were no signs and symptoms of ovarian enlargement.

Should there be any doubt, treatment should be postponed until a pregnancy has been ruled out by a sensitive hCG assay in urine (Brandau 1978) or serum (Younger et al 1978, Dericks-Tan & Taubert 1979). Whenever the BBT remains at or above a level of 37°C for 12 days or more, conception is likely to have taken place. The diagnosis of pregnancy should be attempted at the earliest possible date, as a rise in serum hCG (doubling time in serum 2.5 days) can be used to demonstrate the vitality of the conceptus at a very early stage.

Treatment with clomiphene may fail for several reasons. Even when the accepted criteria for its use are fulfilled, approximately one out of five women with anovulatory infertility will not ovulate upon being treated with clomiphene. Moreover, only one-half of those who do so will eventually succeed in conceiving. Ultimately, only four out of five pregnancies will result in the birth of a healthy child, as the abortion rate in this group of women is higher than in a fertile population.

A practical method for the assessment of a clomiphene cycle with respect to further treatment was described by Shoham et al (1989). FSH and LH were determined on days 5 and 9, estradiol on day 14, and progesterone on day 23 after 100mg of clomiphene had been given daily from days 5 to 9. Spontaneously ovulatory women served as controls. In addition, ultrasound measurements were done daily from day 9 until ovulation; the cervical score (Insler et al 1972) was recorded on day 14. Clomiphene brought about an elevation of FSH, LH on day 9, and of estradiol on day 14. There were more follicles in this group, but the cervical score was lower than in the control group. In 3/15 patients there was a discrepancy between the cervical score and the serum level of estradiol. The authors suggest that by these means patients can be identified who require different modes of stimulation such as hMG/hCG or pulsatile GnRH rather than clomiphene.

## Extended and combined therapy

Ovulation has been successfully induced in infertile women who were resistant to the standard therapy with clomiphene when the treatment scheme was altered by raising the dose, extending the time of application, or adding other hormonal agents.

### Extended dosage schemes

Though it is not recommended by the manufacturer to administer clomiphene in doses exceeding 100 mg per day and for longer periods of time than 5 days, there is now sufficient evidence that larger doses than usually used are needed to induce ovulation in otherwise refractory patients (Adams et al 1972, Rust et al 1974, Drake et al 1978), particularly those being overweight (Shepard et al 1979). When Shepard et al (1979) treated their patients by the dosage scheme of Rust et al (1974), they achieved an ovulation rate of 80.6%, and of those nearly all conceived.

The effect of obesity on the response to clomiphene does not seem to be related to tissue uptake and storage of the drug. Obese, anovulatory women have been shown to have an elevated level of circulating estrone (but not of estradiol!) that can be compared to the midfollicular phase of normal-weight eumenorrheic women (Shepard et al 1979), and a lower than normal concentration of sex hormone binding globulin (SHBG) (Plymate et al 1981, Lobo et al 1982b). It is therefore conceivable that clomiphene has to be increased in order to compete with estrogens for hypothalamic receptors, and the low level of SHBG may increase free testosterone, and thus bring about an impediment of follicular maturation (see Chapters 4 and 5). Dehydroepiandrosterone sulfate (DHEA-S) is often elevated in anovulatory women. Clomiphene citrate was generally shown to be effective in women with high androgen levels. When the serum level of DHEA-S exceeds 5000 ng/ml, the response may, however, be decreased unless a corticosteroid is used as well (Hoffman & Lobo 1985).

The use of large doses of clomiphene for the induction of ovulation gained considerable interest when O'Herlihy et al (1981) reported that the otherwise unavoidable switch to hMG/hCG could largely be avoided in a case of apparent failure of clomiphene, when high doses are used in an incremental manner, and the success of therapy is monitored by daily measurements of estrogens and of follicular size by ultrasound.

Thirty patients who had remained anovulatory when subjected to the standard therapy, and had not shown a follicular reaction, were treated with clomiphene continuously with rising doses until a response was obtained. Treatment was started with a daily dose of 50 mg. Thereafter, the dose was increased by 50 mg approximately every 5 days unless the total urinary estrogens increased by more than 20 µg per 24 h. The maximal daily dose was 250 mg. The duration of treatment was arbitrarily limited to 25 days. When the largest follicle has reached a diameter of 18–19 mm, hCG was injected as an adjunct.

The authors repeated this treatment in up to three cycles. Twenty-one out of 30 patients ovulated, and nine of these became pregnant. It is remarkable that there were only a few side-effects. Hyperstimulation of the ovaries was observed only once. As all ovulating patients had done so by day 21 of treatment, a period of more than 3 weeks therapy does not seem to improve upon the results.

Similarly, Lobo et al (1982a) were successful in inducing ovulation in eight out of 13 women with 250 mg clomiphene per day given for 8 days, and an injection of 10 000 IU hCG on day 14. None of these women had previously ovulated when 250 mg clomiphene had been administered for 5 days.

As the peremptory use of clomiphene in doses exceeding 100 mg per day (Weise et al 1982b) does not seem to improve the overall results in a very impressive manner as compared to the combination with hCG and the treatment schemes of O'Herlihy et al (1981) and Lobo et al (1982a), the latter should be employed in cases of apparent clomiphene failure.

The problem of choosing the right dosage scheme for a particular patient was emphasized by the observation of Jones & de Moraes-Ruehsen (1967) that smaller than the usually used doses can be of therapeutic value, and may be associated with fewer adverse reactions. This observation was confirmed by Barrett & Hakim (1974) who achieved a good pregnancy rate in a group of 60 apparently well-selected patients by starting treatment with unusually low doses of clomiphene. At first, each patient was given a single dose of 100 mg clomiphene on day 5 after the onset of bleeding. When there was no ovulatory response to this, the dose was raised to 100 mg to be taken on days 5 and 7. When this also failed, 50 mg was given daily from days 5 to 9, and this was eventually followed by 100 mg on days 5, 7 and 9. In a few patients, this had to be increased to 100 mg daily from days 5 to 9. It is quite noteworthy that all of these 60 patients conceived. None the less, it remains to be proven whether or not such a spectacular result can only be attributed to the careful use of dose increments. Careful selection of the patients, exclusion of other infertility factors or their appropriate treatment, and the close follow-up required for the conduct of such a study provide favorable conditions, the impact of which upon the end-result should not be understimated.

As it may be assumed that the tissue-specific antiestrogenic effect of clomiphene is to a certain degree dose-dependent, the problem of poor penetration of the cervical mucus by spermatozoa after application of clomiphene should be lessened when ovulation can be induced by the use of a minimal dose.

It is strongly suggested to carry out an endometrial biopsy in the late luteal phase when treating patients with clomiphene citrate for ovulation induction, as an out-of-phase endometrium has been observed in approximately one out of four cases. Once the diagnosis of induced luteal phase insufficiency has been made, the dose of clomiphene citrate is raised, hCG injections are added, or a switch is made to vaginal progesterone suppositories (Keenan et al 1989).

*Clomiphene and hCG*

It had already been pointed out by Kistner (1966) that some patients who do not ovulate when being treated with clomiphene will do so when an injection of hCG is given 5–7 days after cessation of clomiphene therapy. Nearly 80% of anovulatory patients respond to clomiphene citrate with folliculogenesis, an endogenous LH peak and ovulation. A subgroup of women which fails to ovulate can easily be identified by demonstrating the persisting follicle by means of ultrasound. Hormonal evaluations are not helpful in distinguishing between responders and nonresponders in such a situation, but ultrasound will be of help to find the patients who fail to ovulate on clomiphene citrate but will do so ultimately within 36 h after an injection of 10 000 IU hCG (Prough et al 1990).

When a daily dose of 100 mg clomiphene alone is not sufficient to induce ovulation, it has been widely practised to inject 5000 IU to 10 000 IU hCG intramuscularly approximately 1 week after the last dose of clomiphene has been taken. This is often followed by another injection of 5000 IU hCG 5 days later, or 3 doses of 2500 IU each, given every 3 days, to stimulate the function of the corpus luteum as a means to avoid luteal phase defect after induced ovulation.

Other investigators, such as Gysler et al (1982), withhold the addition of hCG to the therapeutic regimen until the daily dose of clomiphene has been increased to 250 mg.

The pregnancy rate obtained by such a combination of clomiphene and hCG has, however, been at times disappointing (Swyer et al 1975). Sutaria et al (1980) did not see any increase in the ovulation rate when 5000 IU hCG was given either after treatment with 50 or 150 mg clomiphene. The relatively low pregnancy rate of 31.4% was possibly in part due to the problem of timing the injection of hCG. Although hCG induces ovulation within 34–40 h when administered in the presence of a mature follicle (O'Herlihy et al 1981), it may favor atresia and thus inhibit ovulation when not given at the peak of follicular activity (Williams & Hodgen 1980). It was shown by O'Herlihy et al (1982) by real-time ultrasound that follicular growth occurs in induced cycles at a faster rate than in spontaneous ones, but the diameter of the follicle at the time of ovulation was similar to that observed on normal ovulatory cycles. When this information was used to time the administration of hCG after clomiphene, 14 out of 21 patients, who had previously failed to ovulate upon treatment with

clomiphene, conceived. This result becomes even more impressive when the fact is considered that five out of the seven patients, who did not become pregnant, were found to have endometriosis at laparoscopy. Similarly, Bryce et al (1982) found that a follicular diameter of 20 mm was a good predictor of ovulation.

As O'Herlihy et al (1981) achieved ovulation in all patients with the dose of 5000 IU, and larger doses are known to entail the risk of hyperstimulation of the ovaries, and of multiple gestation, the use of 10 000 IU hCG or more, as suggested by Kistner (1975), cannot be recommended any longer.

*Clomiphene and hMG*

Although many patients who fail to respond to clomiphene will ovulate when treated with hMG/hCG, the use of gonadotropins is fraught with certain risks such as ovarian enlargement, multiple pregnancy and the hyperstimulation syndrome, and is quite costly and time consuming (Chapter 16). As clomiphene seems to augment the reactivity of the ovary to hMG, possibly by a direct effect, repeated attempts have been made to reduce the dose of hMG and the duration of its application by administering clomiphene and hMG in a sequential fashion. The feasibility of such an approach had been advocated by Crooke et al (1969) who demonstrated that clomiphene augmented the activity of pituitary FSH preparation by a factor of 1.73. The clinical effectiveness of such a combination can be deduced from data provided by March et al (1976b). The dose of hMG could be reduced by about 50% in normogonadotropic and normoestrogenic women. This type of treatment has been used with particular success for superstimulation of the ovary and timing of ovulation in preparation for in vitro fertilization and embryo transfer (IVF-ET).

Clomiphene has been given as a pretreatment in different doses: 50 mg/day for 5 days (Robertson et al 1977), 100 mg/day for 7 days (Kistner 1976), and 200 mg/day for 5 days (March et al 1976b). This was followed in each case by the injection of hMG (usually starting with 2 ampoules daily), the dose of which was raised in certain intervals in accord with the reaction of the individual patient, i.e. the rise in urinary or serum estrogens, an increase in the cervical score (Insler et al 1972), and ovarian enlargement.

There are somewhat contradictory data as to the therapeutic effectiveness of this combined regimen. Taymor et al (1973) failed to observe any pregnancies even though all patients appeared to have ovulated. Kistner (1976) reported that 23 out of 80 patients became pregnant. An even higher pregnancy rate of 49% was achieved by Robertson et al (1977). In this group, however, 11 multiple births, including two triplets and three quadruplets occurred. Contrary to that, there were only two sets of twins amongst the 23 successfully treated patients of Kistner (1976). Recently, a multiple pregnancy rate of 7.7% has been reported when clomiphene was given in combination with hMG, which is in the range known for clomiphene alone (Ron-El et al 1989).

In summary: the combined use of clomiphene and hMG may be considered as an alternative to a classical regimen of hMG/hCG, provided the course of treatment is carefully monitored to avoid overstimulation and multiple pregnancies. Should a patient fail to ovulate upon treatment with either one of the methods described above, the use of hMG/hCG (Chapter 16) should be considered.

*Clomiphene and LH-RH (GnRH)*

Even though a large number of studies have been carried out on the induction of ovulation by LH-RH in anovulatory women (Chapter 15), relatively few reports have yet appeared on the combined use of LH-RH and clomiphene. Ovulation has been induced in previously unresponsive women by the infusion of 50 μg LH-RH, and the application of large doses of LH-RH by the nasal route after priming with clomiphene (Keller 1972, Taubert & Dericks-Tan 1976a). This showed that LH-RH can be used in the place of hCG to provide an additional ovulatory stimulus. Similarly, Bohnet et al (1976) succeeded in bringing about ovulation in clomiphene-resistant patients by applying large doses (100 μg subcutaneaously, three times a day) for 10–20 days prior to treatment with

clomiphene. More recently, Phansey et al (1980) reported that five out of eight previously non-responsive women ovulated after receiving 100 mg clomiphene from days 5 to 9, and 0.6–1.2 mg LH-RH three times a day as nasal drops from days 11 to 14. Moreover, three of these five women conceived, and there were no side-effects such as hyperstimulation of the ovaries. Similar results have recently been reported by Ulrich et al (1990): clomiphene citrate-resistant women were treated 3 times daily with 25 μg LH-RH from days 5 to 7 followed by 100 mg of clomiphene citrate per day from days 10 to 14. Thirteen out of 20 patients ovulated, and six of these conceived. This outcome was comparable to that of Kotsuji et al (1988), who injected previously clomiphene-resistant hypogonadotropic women three times per week with 100 μg of GnRH for 4 weeks. As this type of treatment does not seem to require any intensive monitoring by ultrasound or the measurement of estradiol, and is completely self-administered, it could possibly be developed into an effective alternative to the combination of clomiphene and hCG. Ovulation has also been induced by pulsatile administration of LH-RH in anovulatory women unresponsive to clomiphene citrate. Sixteen out of 19 patients ovulated in 16/73 cycles, and there were three pregnancies (Molloy et al 1985).

Similarly, anovulatory women with clomiphene-resistant polycystic ovarian disease ultimately responded to a pure FSH preparation after the GnRH agonist buserelin had been injected (0.5 mg subcutaneously twice a day) for 4 weeks, and five out of nine patients conceived (Remordiga et al 1989).

*Clomiphene and bromocriptine*

The use of bromocriptine for ovulation induction in normoprolactinemic women is controversial, but Koike et al (1981) reported on combined therapy in a small group of anovulatory women who had previously not responded to treatment with 150 mg clomiphene per day for 3 days. Combined therapy with clomiphene (50 mg three times a day) and bromocriptine (2.5 mg/daily) for 10 days evoked an ovulatory response in 61% of these patients. The pregnancy rate was, however, disappointingly low (13.3%). The suppression of prolactin seems to enhance the responsiveness of the hypothalamic-pituitary-ovarian axis towards clomiphene (Hirvonen et al 1976). It remains to be shown whether this is due to a direct effect of bromocriptine on the ovary, or an enhancement of the secretion of LH-RH and gonadotropins, possibly by suppression of prolactin. As prolactin is involved in the regulation of progesterone production by human granulosa cells (at least in vitro), the suppression by bromocriptine should not be too extensive (McNatty 1977).

When women with normoprolactinemic amenorrhea, who had been unresponsive to clomiphene citrate, were treated with bromocriptine, nearly 30% ovulated. When bromocriptine was combined with clomiphene citrate, however, the ovulation rate rose to 50% (Porcile et al 1990). It was, therefore suggested to treat patients unresponsive to clomiphene citrate with this combination before resorting to hMG/hCG; it is less complex and costly, and there is no risk of ovarian hyperstimulation and multiple birth.

It should be mentioned parenthetically that clomiphene (and clomiphene combined with hCG) has been found to be effective in the treatment of some patients with hyperprolactinemic anovulation (Radwanska et al 1979, Turksoy et al 1982).

### Clomiphene and estrogens

Estrogens have been used in combination with clomiphene in various ways to improve the quality of the cervical mucus and to induce an LH surge. It was shown by Canales et al (1978) that an LH surge will occur within 72 h after the injection of 1 mg of estradiol benzoate intramuscularly 7 days after the last dose of a 5-day course of 100 mg of clomiphene per day had been taken. Thirteen out of 22 anovulatory women, who had failed to respond to treatment with clomiphene alone, ovulated after the addition of the estrogen to the therapeutic regimen, and 10 out of these 13 conceived. An enhancement in serum prolactin was elicited by the estrogen but appeared to be of little consequence. None of the patients had galactorrhea, hirsutism, or ovarian enlargement.

A similar beneficial effect of estrogens had also been observed when a sequential preparation (2 mg estradiol valerate, 11 days; 2 mg estradiol valerate, and 50 µg levonorgestrel, 10 days) was administered for 3 months to clomiphene-resistant women. When clomiphene was given again, 11 out of 19 women ovulated and conceived (Gitsch et al 1977).

The same type of favorable response was observed when clomiphene was given in conjunction with a sequential preparation (clomiphene citrate, 100 mg days 5–9; sequential preparation, days 5–25).

Huber & Schneider (1984) achieved pregnancies in women who had responded to clomiphene citrate but did not conceive within 6 months, when 0.02–0.04 mg of ethinyl estradiol were given for 5 days after the last tablet of clomiphene citrate. Patients with a low serum estradiol level and a cervical score of 7 or less were found to respond to exogenous estrogen in a more favorable manner than those with high serum levels of estradiol and a low cervical score (Insler et al 1972, Kokia et al 1990).

The effectiveness of exogenous estrogen therapy for treatment of clomiphene citrate-induced cervical mucus abnormalities was, however, questioned by Bateman et al (1990). Oral micronized estradiol (2 mg), conjugated estrogens (5 mg) or a placebo was administered from days 9 to 14 subsequent to a 5-day course of 50–150 mg clomiphene citrate. The cervical score was examined within 48 h of ovulation; it was found that treatment with the estrogen preparations did not improve the quality of the cervical mucus.

It should be noted in this context that symptoms of ovarian overstimulation of considerable severity were observed in some women who were treated by a sequential scheme of clomiphene (days 5–9) and estrogen (days 8–12) (Taubert & Dericks-Tan 1976b).

### Clomiphene and corticoids

Hyperandrogenism of either ovarian, adrenal or mixed ovarian/adrenal origin can be an important cause of anovulatory infertility, since androgens interfere by means of their antiestrogenic effect with the regulation of ovulation (see Chapters 5 and 6).

In the presence of clinical signs of hyperandrogenism such as hirsutism, acne, clitoral enlargement and polycystic ovarian disease, a thorough appraisal of the androgen status of the patient should, therefore, be obtained before clomiphene is administered. In addition, repeated determinations of serum testosterone should be performed between the time of clomiphene administration and ovulation even in patients who have previously not shown any clinical signs of hyperandrogenemia, as serum testosterone may rise considerably in response to stimulation of ovarian steroidogenesis by clomiphene. It is of utmost importance to recognize this transient type of hyperandrogenism as well as the chronic one, since both groups of patients have a fairly good chance of responding with ovulation when clomiphene is given in combination with a glucocorticoid. Lisse (1980) succeeded in inducing ovulation in eight out of 13 clomiphene-resistant patients when clomiphene (200 mg/day from days 5 to 9) was combined with dexamethasone (2 mg/day from days 5 to 14); and all ovulating patients conceived.

Similarly, Fayez (1976) reported that particularly women with androgen excess of adrenal or mixed ovarian/adrenal origin responded better to a combination of clomiphene and dexamethasone than to the former alone, while patients thought to have ovarian androgen excess reacted very well to clomiphene alone (pregnancy rate 61%).

The interval type of dexamethasone therapy as described by Lisse (1980) appears preferable to a continuous one, as the number and severity of side-effects are reduced when compared to a continuous application of a glucocorticoid. If the combination of clomiphene and dexamethasone fails to bring about the desired result, the use of antiandrogens, gonadotropins or wedge resection of the ovaries should be considered. (see Chapter 26).

### Failure to conceive

When a patient with functional infertility appears to respond well to treatment with clomiphene but fails to conceive, the following additional causes of infertility have to be taken into consideration.

At first, the postcoital test should be repeated after treatment to evaluate a possible deleterious effect of clomiphene upon the cervical mucus. Should serial determinations of the cervical score (Insler et al 1972), and well-timed postcoital test reveal persistently poor cervical mucus, and mainly immotile spermatozoa, the use of estrogens has to be considered.

The diagnosis of dysmucorrhea (see Chapter 13), either spontaneous or clomiphene induced, should, however, not be made unless the quality of the cervical mucus has been checked up to the time of presumed ovulation. Serum progesterone has been found to be elevated in clomiphene-stimulated cycles during the 3 days preceding ovulation. It has been postulated that this may be one of the causes of a low cervical score seen in some cases following clomiphene (Fidele et al 1989c).

The use of estrogens in combination with clomiphene as a means of improving the quality of the cervical mucus remains a controversial issue. Although an improvement can be brought about by estrogens, this effect is not demonstrable in all cases, and it is unproven whether a genuine improvement in the total pregnancy rate can really be achieved (Wentz et al 1976).

The following treatment schemes have been used:

1. Estriol, 1–2 mg/day, taken from days 5 to 14. This regimen is widely used, as estriol does not interfere with the ovulation-inducing action of clomiphene, but the effect on mucus production by the endocervical glandular tissue is, in our experience, not very impressive.
2. More effective seems to be treatment with ethinyl estradiol (60 μg/day or more), estradiol valerate (1–2 mg/day), and conjugated estrogens (7.5 mg/day) from days 8 to 15 (Taubert & Dericks-Tan 1976b).

Even though estrogens do not seem to interfere with ovulation and conception, delayed ovulation has been observed by us.

If the penetration of the cervical mucus by spermatozoa does not improve after treatment with estrogens in combination with clomiphene, artificial insemination with husband's sperm may be attempted (Chapters 22 and 25).

The chances for conception appear to be quite low when at laparoscopy no spermatozoa can be recovered from the peritoneal fluid subsequent to insemination (Templeton & Mortimer 1980, Möslein-Rossmeissel et al 1989).

Although progesterone is often higher in induced ovulatory cycles than in spontaneous ones, the luteal phase following ovulation induction with clomiphene is often short and functionally deficient (Van Hall & Mastboom 1969). This could possibly be explained by an antiestrogenic effect of clomiphene upon the endometrium. In the absence of other causes of infertility (particularly the tubal and male factor), this should be investigated by an endometrial biopsy. The endometrial specimen is obtained approximately 10 days after the presumed date of ovulation after a pregnancy has been excluded. In a case of inadequate or delayed secretory transformation of the endometrium (especially if progesterone is also lower than expected) (Kjeld et al 1975), hCG should be given in the manner described above. Otherwise, the administration of hMG has to be resorted to. It has not been uncommon to prescribe a progestogen to be taken during the luteal phase subsequent to clomiphene to prevent luteal phase defect. The efficacy of this practice has, to our knowledge, not been proven.

In some cases, the ovum may become trapped in a follicle which became luteinized in response to clomiphene but did not rupture. It has recently been questioned, however, whether laparoscopic demonstration of the stigma as a sign of ovum release is really a reliable diagnostic parameter (Vanrell et al 1982).

The possible role of IVF in the treatment of this group of patients is discussed in Chapter 21.

Many authors suggest hMG/hCG therapy should be applied in all women in whom anovulation is the main cause of infertility and who were extensively and appropriately treated with clomiphene but failed to conceive (see Chapters 16 and 23).

## Results of treatment

When clomiphene is given at a standard dose of 50–100 mg per day for 5 days during each treatment cycle, approximately 70% of properly selected patients (WHO Group II) can be expected to ovulate (WHO 1973). The majority will respond to either dose, although some will require more clomiphene or a combination of clomiphene with hCG, bromocriptine, corticosteroids, estrogens or hMG. The relationship between the necessary dose of clomiphene and the percentage of responding patients is shown in Figure 18.5. About one-half of those women who eventually ovulate will do so in response to 50 mg, and again half of the nonresponders will eventually respond to the dose of 100 mg. Only a few will require treatment by doses in excess of 100 –150 mg per day. Patients with anovulatory cycles or oligomenorrhea seem to ovulate and conceive more readily than those with amenorrhea (93% vs 59%: Gysler et al 1982).

The overall pregnancy rate varies from 25% to 35% when the standard regimen is employed, and does not differ much between patients with primary and secondary infertility (WHO 1973, Weise et al 1982b). Some investigators report much lower, and others considerably higher pregnancy rates, the estimates ranging between 11% and 50% (Whitelaw et al 1970). Schmidt-Elmendorff & Kaemmerling (1977) found clomiphene not to be more effective than other ovulation inducers, as the pregnancy rate (20%) did not exceed that obtained by administration of epimestrol or cyclofenil. The other extreme

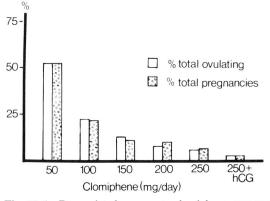

**Fig. 18.5** Dose-related response to clomiphene: percentage of women ovulating in response to various doses of clomiphene (white bars), and of women conceiving (shaded bars). (Adapted from data of Gysler et al 1982.)

is represented by Barrett & Hakim (1974) who reported a 100% success rate employing a mode of treatment with incremental doses. Since the selection of patients, the diagnostic and therapeutic approach, the intensity and monitoring of treatment and, last but not least, the extent of psychological guidance accompanying treatment differ widely, the number of variables affecting the ultimate rate of success is too large to allow a meaningful appraisal of these differences.

Most patients conceive during the first three ovulatory cycles (Fig. 18.6), albeit a small but none the less important group will finally become pregnant when treatment is continued for longer periods of time, even for 29 cycles as reported by March et al (1976a).

It was recently emphasized by Weise et al (1982b) that the conception rate decreases considerably when patients receiving treatment with clomiphene are older than 30 years of age. Even though the age-dependent decrease in fertility should not be lightly dismissed as being a

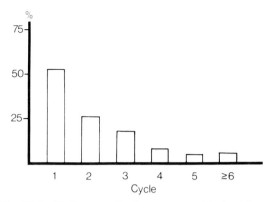

**Fig. 18.6** Ovulatory cycle after treatment with clomiphene in which pregnancy occurred. (Adapted from data of Gysler et al 1982.)

factor to be reckoned with, therapeutic nihilism does not seem to be justified in patients under the age of 40 years. It is shown in Figure 18.7 that the percentage of patients with functional infertility who conceived after treatment with clomiphene or other hormonal agents did not

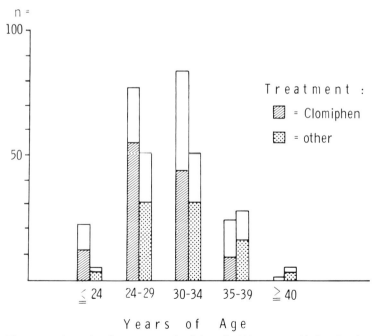

**Fig. 18.7** Age-related response to clomiphene in 208 women with functional infertility. The percentage of women per age group who conceived after having been treated with clomiphene or other hormonal agents (hMG, hCG, progestogens, etc.) is shown.

differ greatly between age groups, and 10 out of 24 women aged 35–39 years conceived after having been treated with clomiphene.

## Outcome of pregnancy

All patients undergoing treatment with clomiphene should be informed that there is clearly an increased risk for abortion to occur after induced ovulation and conception.

A comparison of the excretion of hCG and pregnandiol-3α-glucuronide in pregnant women, who had either ovulated spontaneously or in response to clomiphene citrate, during the first trimester failed to show any difference, but the latter excreted more estrone-3-glucuronide (Strigini et al 1986). This could possibly mean that estrogen synthesis is set at a higher level than usually seen in early pregnancy when treatment with clomiphene citrate has been carried out for ovulation induction.

Even though abortion rates of less than 10% have been reported (Gorlitzky et al 1978), there is consensus that a fetal wastage of 20–25% has to be expected (Hammond & Talbert 1982, Jewelewicz 1975, Garcia et al 1977, Weise et al 1982b). In addition, the further course of pregnancy may be complicated by intrauterine fetal death, premature delivery, isthmo-cervical insufficiency, and a higher than normal rate of cesarean section. These complications of the second and third trimester of pregnancy are certainly not specific for clomiphene-treated patients but are common to the infertile population as a whole. Patients with anovulation and luteal phase inadequacy constitute often an inordinately high proportion of all infertile women seeking medical help (Wernicke et al 1975).

As a consequence, all pregnancies occurring after treatment with clomiphene should be considered as being exposed to a special risk, and, therefore, subjected to particularly intensive prenatal care. Even though it has been claimed that more boys than girls are born to the wives of male patients who had been treated for infertility with clomiphene citrate, the significance of such findings has been dismissed (Rönnberg & Passoja 1986).

## Treatment of luteal phase insufficiency

It is widely accepted that luteal phase insufficiency can be caused by a deficiency of FSH secretion in the particular phase resulting in inadequate proliferation of the granulosa cells and ultimately in the formation of a corpus luteum with a reduced mass of luteal tissue and inadequate capacity for the production and secretion of progesterone (for review see Rothchild 1983). As a consequence ovulation-inducing drugs such as menotropins and clomiphene citrate have been used as a therapeutic alternative to hCG and progesterone (Insler et al 1983). The dosage schemes and the monitoring of therapy do not differ from the principle described in the chapter on ovulation induction. The midluteal concentration of progesterone rises by a factor of 3 when clomiphene citrate is used in the treatment of luteal phase insufficiency. The drug seems to be most effective in severe cases (Guoth 1987).

A comparison of the capacity of clomiphene citrate and vaginal progesterone suppositories to normalize an out-of-phase endometrium in women with luteal phase insufficiency proved both modalities to be equal when calculated according to the lifetable method (Murray et al 1989).

The efficacy of treatment seems to depend to a large degree on the number of preovulatory follicles induced by clomiphene citrate. Guzick & Zeleznik (1990) reported that 10/18 patients with histologically proven luteal phase insufficiency had subsequently to therapy more than one follicle of 15 mm diameter, while the remaining eight had just one. The endometrial deficiency was corrected in eight of ten women of the former group, but only in two of eight women with a single preovulatory follicle. This seems to indicate that endometrial deficiency benefits from the development of more than one follicle.

Clomiphene citrate given from days 5 to 9 of the cycle to normally cycling women increases the number of corpora lutea and their weight, the concentration of LH/hCG receptors, and the total tissue content of progesterone and 17α-hydroxyprogesterone. These effects may be the basis for efficacy of clomiphene citrate in increasing midluteal phase progesterone levels, of responsiveness to hCG stimulation, and in correcting luteal phase insufficiency (Yeko et al 1990).

## Ectopic pregnancy

A twofold risk of ectopic pregnancy had been observed by Korow & Payne as early as 1968 in women who had become pregnant following clomiphene citrate. More recently, Marchbanks et al (1985) calculated a relative risk of 10.0 for ectopic pregnancy in patients who had used clomiphene citrate. Four out of five patients had been given clomiphene citrate for luteal phase insufficiency, only one for anovulation. It is imaginable that this is a risk factor independent of clomiphene citrate. Contrary to that, Corson & Batzer (1986) reported five ectopics in 274 clomiphene-induced gestations. This does not seem to be very different from what would have been expected in the general population.

There seem to be two possible risk factors: polyovulation and the excessively high estrogen level following clomiphene citrate. If there is more than one ovum, one may become lodged in the tube and implant. It has been shown in animal experiments that high estrogen levels can cause tubal dysfunction resulting in isolation of the ovum in a segment of the tube. Similarly, post-coital interception with high doses of estrogen, when not efficient in preventing nidation, has been shown to result in approximately 10% of the cases in an ectopic pregnancy (Morris & van Wagenem 1973).

## Clomiphene citrate treatment of ovulating women

During the last decade clomiphene citrate has been used more and more in the treatment of infertile women whose ovarian function has to be considered as normal, as they ovulate and have a normal luteal phase. There is certainly a rationale for such an approach in women undergoing courses of IVF, GIFT and IUI in order to program ovulation as nearly as possible. Ovarian stimulation is usually initiated by clomiphene citrate, and this is followed by injections of hMG

or FSH until the follicle can be brought to rupture by a single injection of hCG. There was no difference in follicular response, cycle day for hCG, the number of oocytes recovered, and the number of dropped cycles when pure FSH rather than hMG was used. Moreover, the former is much more costly than hMG (Quigley et al 1988).

Intentional superstimulation of the ovaries has been recommended as a treatment of peritubal and periovarian adhesions in women having at least one patent tube before microsurgery is carried out. The ovarian enlargement caused by superstimulation with clomiphene citrate and hMG seems to change the spatial arrangement between the ovaries and the Fallopian tubes in a beneficial manner. Aboughar et al (1989) succeeded in inducing superstimulation in 82.5% of their patients, and 28/42 conceived (including four extrauterine pregnancies).

Even though the conception rate in couples with male or idiopathic factors was significantly increased by IUI carried out in spontaneous cycles, treatment with clomiphene citrate did not improve the results in the experience of Martinez et al (1990) . Contrary to that, couples with either unexplained infertility or surgically corrected endometriosis were treated with clomiphene citrate and IUI or were just observed. There were 14 pregnancies in 148 treatment cycles (fecundity = 0.095), and five pregnancies in 150 untreated cycles (fecundity = 0.033) (Deaton et al 1990). This seems to indicate that clomiphene citrate in combination with IUI improve fecundity in couples with unexplained infertility or surgically corrected endometriosis.

When women with unexplained infertility were given clomiphene citrate, there was a 66% rise in mean midluteal progesterone level. The fertility increased within 3 months of treatment by 54% as compared to the use of a placebo (Glazener et al 1990). The rise in progesterone does not necessarily explain the enhanced fertility, as even large follicles may be impaired after treatment with clomiphene citrate. Testart et al (1990) reported that treatment with clomiphene citrate increased the cumulative pregnancy within 3 months from 14.6 to 22.3%. Nothing seems to be gained by intermittent therapy, as there does not seem to be a carryover effect. Women with more than 3 years of unexplained infertility derived the greatest benefit from therapy with clomiphene citrate, as the conception rate rose from 2.9% when a placebo was used for 3 months to 14.4% after treatment with clomiphene. This leads to the conclusion that clomiphene citrate should be offered to all women with unexplained infertility of more than 3 years' duration. Those with a shorter duration of infertility do not seem to gain anything from this type of therapy.

## Adverse reactions

Hyperstimulation of the ovaries with cystic and at times painful enlargement does occasionally occur after the administration of clomiphene, but the incidence is rather low. Gysler et al (1982) observed palpable ovarian enlargement in only 5.1% of their patients. Most were unilateral and none exceeded the diameter of 10 cm. When abdominal discomfort and pain, or a palpable enlargement of one or both ovaries make it likely that hyperstimulation has occurred, the extent of cyst formation should be established by ultrasound and the determination of serum estradiol. Most of these cysts will regress without therapy other than bedrest. In an exceptional case (Taubert & Jürgensen 1972), acute abdominal symptoms may require laparotomy. It is important to realize that the cystic ovary may actually increase in size when it becomes exposed to hCG secreted from the trophoblast of an early pregnancy. As a consequence, hCG should only be given as an additional ovulatory stimulus after it has been determined that there is no ovarian enlargement and tenderness. Cyclic administration of clomiphene should not be resumed before the symptoms have completely disappeared and the ovaries have returned to their normal size. There is no evidence that future chances for fertility are jeopardized by an episode of hyperstimulation (Kincses & Sas 1975).

The sensitivity of the ovaries may vary from cycle to cycle to a considerable degree, even though the same dose of clomiphene is given. A single incidence of hyperstimulation does not necessarily mean that the ovary will overreact again in subsequent treatment cycles (Bailer et al 1980).

Other adverse reactions are not common. Approximately one out of ten patients will complain about hot flushes of varying intensity and dizziness. Occasionally, visual disturbances such as blurred vision or decreased acuity, due to the mydriatic action of the drug, will appear. These will clear as soon as the medication is discontinued.

## Multiple pregnancies

The frequency of multiple gestation can approach 6–7% (WHO 1973), although other investigators report clearly smaller numbers (Ruiz Velasco et al 1979, Gorlitzky et al 1978) and, occasionally, a higher incidence (Hull et al 1979: 17.8%). In a report by Merrell National Laboratories (1972), the majority were twins, although the incidence of triplets (0.5%), quadruplets (0.3%) and of quintuplets (0.13%) was considerably higher than in spontaneous conceptions. High conception rates are usually associated with an increased number of multiple births (Schenker et al 1981). It has been suggested that clomiphene brings about multiple ovulation by repeated suboptimal stimulation of the ovaries resulting in several follicles reaching a critical stage (Healy & Burger 1978). A subsequent greater ovulatory stimulus then causes multiple ovulation.

When clomiphene is used in combination with hCG, the number of multiple gestations appears to be higher than that subsequent to clomiphene with or without the addition of other drugs, but less than with hMG and hCG (Schenker et al 1981). Robertson et al (1977) reported a reduction of the rate of multiple births from 34% to 8% when clomiphene was given prior to hMG.

There is no evidence that the number of multiple births is raised when clomiphene is used in combination with bromocriptine (Schenker et al 1981).

## Teratogenic effects

Although there are casuistic reports on the association of clomiphene with hydatidiform mole and anencephaly (Biale et al 1978), there is no evidence that congenital anomalies occur at a greater rate than seen in a normal population

(3%, Hendricks 1966). Another stilbene derivative, diethylstilbestrol (DES), has been linked to the development of adenocarcinoma of the vagina in the female and of genital malformations in the male offspring of women treated with high doses of this synthetic estrogen for prolonged periods of time during pregnancy (Gunning 1976). Recently, a case of superfetation secondary to ovulation induction with clomiphene citrate has been reported (Beat & Sehoud 1987). This emphasizes the tenet that particular care should be taken to instruct the patient on the proper use of clomiphene, in order to avoid the intake of the drug within the first weeks of an unrecognized pregnancy, even though there is no basis to assume that clomiphene might have a tumorogenic or teratogenic effect.

**Psychic alterations**

There have been only scattered reports on psychopathological events during treatment with clomiphene citrate. They are exemplified by a recent report on an acute bout of the illness in a 25-year-old manic depressive woman during treatment with clomiphene citrate (Kapfhammer et al 1990). The rapid changes in serum estradiol seen during therapy with clomiphene citrate were presumed to be an eliciting factor for such a psychopathological reaction which appears to be similar to episodes occuring in women during the postnatal period, during premenstrual recurrences of puerperal psychotic attacks, and while taking estrogens for postmenopausal substitution.

**Comment**

It has frequently been stated that there is a disturbing discrepancy between the ovulation rate in clomiphene-treated, anovulatory women, and the number of those who finally become pregnant and are eventually delivered of a healthy child.

In recent years, a number of clinical studies have been reported which permit us to question the validity of that dogma, and to take a less fatalistic view. Satisfying pregnancy rates have been obtained by using clomiphene according to novel dosage schemes or in combination with other hormones. In addition, at least one of the other ovulation-inducing agents, tamoxifen, has been shown to be possibly a true alternative to clomiphene. Moreover, it has been pointed out by Gorlitzky et al (1978) that approximately 50% of the patients who ovulate on clomiphene become pregnant within 3 months. This compares well with the fertile population, as Guttmacher (1956) showed that 57% of pregnant women had conceived after 3 months of exposure. This leads to the conclusion that a 50% conception rate with clomiphene does not present a discrepancy between ovulation rate and the number of pregnancies, as it mirrors the results obtained in the general population (Gorlitzky et al 1978). As it actually should be expected, the success rate with clomiphene becomes, however, quite low (6–12%) when a pelvic or cervical infertility factor coexists with anovulation, or the husband is subfertile (Gysler et al 1982).

Even though various treatment schemes have been shown to be clinically effective, the problem of definition of the diagnostic criteria for the use of unorthodox modes of treatment with clomiphene has not yet been solved. An outstanding example for this is the work of O'Herlihy et al (1982) which provides a sound basis for a rational and effective use of hCG by means of ultrasound indicating the best time of injection. Similarly, the combined use of clomiphene and dexamethasone appears justified in hyperandrogenic women not responding well to clomiphene alone, or those showing a rise in serum androgens as a sequel to clomiphene treatment.

Although clomiphene has been widely used for 30 years, and an enormous amount of basic research and clinical data has been accumulated, no large-scale study has yet been carried out comparing different modes of treatment. As a consequence, it is impossible to incorporate all the modifications which have been successfully employed into a grand design which could serve as a generally applicable blueprint for therapy. Moreover, any endocrine therapy of functional infertility has to be carried out in cognizance of the fact that ovarian dysfunction is often causally linked to psychological conflicts and to psychopathology, which will hardly become evident during a cursory interview. In view of this it does not come as a surprise that the rate of spontaneous remission is high in patients with anovulatory infertility. This is exemplified by the results of a study by Evans & Townsend (1976) who treated 352 patients with anovulatory infertility of differing etiology with a carefully designed plan, which began with the administration of a placebo, continued with the administration of sex steroids, and finally clomiphene or gonadotropins. Each of these steps was separated from the other by a therapy-free interval of 3 months. It is remarkable that 40% of the patients ovulated, and 20% conceived after the use of a placebo. On the other hand, the wish to beget a child may serve as a powerful alibi to compensate unresolved conflicts and problems concerned with sexuality and an ambiguous attitude towards motherhood and pregnancy (Anthony & Benedek 1970). It is mandatory to recognize this type of situation before a clomiphene-induced pregnancy brings about a profound change in the life of the patient or a prolonged and unsuccessful course of therapy aggravates the conflicts.

There is no reliable standard for length and intensity of treatment. In each individual case the attending physician has to carefully weigh whether to encourage the infertile couple to continue treatment, or to advise temporary or final termination of therapy.

## CYCLOFENIL

Even though the number of experimental and clinical studies on the mode of action and therapeutic efficacy of cyclofenil is much smaller than those concerned with that of clomiphene citrate, there are some reports indicating that this agent has a certain place in the treatment of functional infertility.

### Chemistry and mode of action

Cyclofenil (bis(acetoxyphenyl)-cyclohexylidenemethane) is chemically related to clomiphene citrate (Fig. 18.1) in that it is not a steroid but a triphenyl ethylene derivative. It is a weak estrogen, its potency being only 1/1000 that of DES in the vaginal cornification and uterine weight test in the rat. It is similar to clomiphene citrate in its biological activity. When given to spayed mice, it will interfere with the growth-inducing effect of estradiol on the uterus. In the estrogen-progesterone blocked, oophorectomized rat, cyclofenil brings about a release of gonadotropins which is mediated by the hypothalamus (Baier & Taubert 1969). Similarly, a rise in serum LH is induced in humans (for review see Matsumoto 1973). The mode of action of cyclofenil involves in all probability both an effect upon the hypothalamic-pituitary axis and the ovary. In the organism, it is quickly converted into the corresponding diphenol and circulates as such (Person 1965), the half-life of a single dose of 200 mg being between 18 and 29 h (Borgström 1981). It is metabolized via hydrolysis of the acetic ester, undergoes some enterohepatic circulation, and is eliminated as a glucuronide.

### Indications

Cyclofenil may be prescribed for the same indications as clomiphene citrate, i.e. the treatment of anovulation in normoestrogenic and normoprolactinemic women (WHO Group II), and in cases of luteal phase defect, provided that the limited therapeutic efficacy of this compound when compared to that of clomiphene is taken into consideration.

A special indication for its use is that cyclofenil does not appear to have a deleterious effect upon the quality of the cervical mucus, as is seen occasionally with clomiphene.

### Treatment

Cyclofenil is usually given in a dose of 200 mg three times a day between days 3 and 7 or 5 and 9 of spontaneous or progesterone-induced bleeding. The administeration of this regimen may be repeated several times when ovulation seems to have occurred, as far as this can be deduced from a biphasic BBT and the well-timed measurement of progesterone in serum. The overall situation of the patient will have to be taken into consideration to decide whether cyclofenil therapy should be continued or replaced by that with another ovulation inducer.

When cyclofenil fails to induce ovulation, the switch to a more effective method of treatment should not be delayed.

The use of a combined therapeutic regimen of cyclofenil followed by an injection of hCG, or a combination with hMG (75 IU hMG days 1–7; cyclofenil 800 mg per days 3–7) has been tried with apparent success. An ovulation rate of 70% and a pregnancy rate of 50% has been reported in infertile women formerly not responding to cyclofenil alone, when the latter was combined with hMG (Soutone & Jalatte 1972).

An interesting observation has been contributed by Moggi et al (1979). They treated 13 normoprolactinemic infertile patients, who had not reacted to any type of treatment with ovulation-inducing agents before, with a combination of 2.5 mg bromocriptine (days 5–26) and 600 mg cyclofenil (days 5–12). It is quite remarkable that 10 out of these 13 women conceived within two treatment cycles. Although it remains to be clarified how these two compounds interact, it has been proposed that the beneficial effect is due to an enhancement of serum estradiol by bromocriptine to nearly normal levels, making the gonadostat more receptive to the action of cyclofenil.

## Monitoring of therapy

Patients who are being treated with cyclofenil should be subjected to the same type of supervision as those receiving clomiphene citrate, even though only few side-effects have been reported so far. The patients should be thoroughly instructed as to how to avoid taking the compound inadvertently during the earliest week of an unrecognized pregnancy.

## Side-effects

Treatment with cyclofenil seems to be remarkably free from undesirable side-effects. Some minor disturbances such as blurring of vision do occur, but the incidence is low (about 3%). Moreover, hyperstimulation of the ovaries is quite uncommon, and there is no increase in the number of twin gestations (Matsumoto 1973).

## Results

The presently available body of evidence shows clearly that cyclofenil is not as effective an ovulation inducer as clomiphene, particularly when the pregnancy rate rather than the percentage of ovulating patients or ovulatory cycles are taken as a point of reference. Neale et al (1970) reported having been able to induce ovulation in one-third of a group of 90 anovulatory patients, four of whom eventually conceived. A low pregnancy rate as compared to a rather impressive ovulation rate has also been reported in a large, cooperative study involving several institutions (Matsumoto 1973). A total of 1195 patients were treated with cyclofenil in 2413 cycles, and 52.6% of these women ovulated. The pregnancy rate was, however, disappointingly low (17.9%). This is in close agreement to the experience Schmidt-Elmendorff & Kaemmerling (1977) gained in a comparative study on the effectiveness of epimestrol, cyclofenil and clomiphene citrate. The conception rate after treatment with cyclofenil was 20.4% and with epimestrol 18.3% It should be noted that in this series an unusually low pregnancy rate was also obtained with clomiphene citrate (18.9% only).

The rate of abortions is within the range observed in pregnant women after ovulation induction with clomiphene.

## Comment

The overall efficacy of any drug used in the treatment of infertility does not only reflect its pharmacological qualities and the absence of objectionable side-effects, but to a certain degree, the confidence of the prescribing physician that this type of treatment will work in a particular patient. The use of cyclofenil has been burdened by a reputation of being a second or even third choice after clomiphene. This is certainly not going to encourage many physicians to emphasize its use as much as that of a more proven method of treatment, and will eventually lead to a negative selection of patients. It is very regrettable that there are as yet only a very few studies comparing the effectiveness of cyclofenil, epimestrol, tamoxifen and clomiphene. Such a study should include an evaluation of the cervical factor. Until this has been achieved, cyclofenil should be reserved for those cases where valid reasons for not employing clomiphene as a first mode of treatment are present.

## TAMOXIFEN

A promising addition to the gamut of fertility-promoting agents seems to have been made by the discovery of tamoxifen, an inducer of ovulation, with effectiveness comparable to that of clomiphene.

### Chemistry and mode of action

Tamoxifen, $p$-($\beta$-dimethylaminoethoxyphenyl)-1, 2-diphenyl-but-1-ene, is structurally related to clomiphene citrate and seems to act in a similar manner (Fig. 18.1). Like clomiphene, there are two geometric isomers of tamoxifen. While trans-(Z)-tamoxifen is a potent antagonist of estrogens, cis-(E)-tamoxifen is an estrogen agonist. After intake, both isomers are transformed to the 4-hydroxy metabolites which have a much higher affinity for the estrogen receptor than the parent compounds. As compared to estradiol (100%), the affinity of trans-(Z)-tamoxifen is 2%, of trans-(Z)-4-hydroxy-tamoxifen 285%, of cis-(E)-tamoxifen 0.2%, and of cis-(E)-4-hydroxy-tamoxifen 5% (Robertson et al 1982). In all probability, the trans-(Z)-4-hydroxy-tamoxifen which is accumulated in the nucleus, is responsible for the antagonistic action of tamoxifen. The cis-(E) isomer of 4-hydroxy-tamoxifen was demonstrated to be partly converted to the potent antiestrogen trans-(Z)-4-hydroxytamoxifen (Jordan et al 1988).

Tamoxifen has been widely used in the therapy of metastasizing and inoperable mammary cancer, as it inhibits the binding of estradiol to the receptor in mammary and uterine tissue (McGuire & dela Garza 1973). In the rat, tamoxifen interferes with the estrogen-induced increase in uterine weight, delays ovulation, and inhibits implantation. As has been pointed out with reference to clomiphene citrate, its fertility-promoting effect involves in all probability more than one target organ. Although Groom & Griffiths (1976) found no increase in serum gonadotropins after treatment of normal, premenopausal women with tamoxifen, a direct effect on the pituitary gonadotropins is likely. In addition, a direct effect upon the ovarian follicle may contribute to the marked increase in serum estradiol at the time of the preovulatory rise, and of estradiol and progesterone during the luteal phase observed in infertile women after tamoxifen treatment (Senior et al 1978). The enhanced secretion of progesterone reflects probably an increase in the size and secretory activity of the preovulatory follicle, which leads to larger luteal mass as compared to control cycles.

### Indications

The presently available evidence suggests that tamoxifen is a genuine alternative to clomiphene in the treatment of women with functional infertility.

Although it has been postulated that tamoxifen might be more effective in oligomenorrheic women (Gerhard & Runnebaum 1979), and certainly has worked in some women unresponsive to clomiphene citrate (Klopper & Hall 1971), no definite suggestion can be made as yet as to when tamoxifen should be used in the place of clomiphene. Most of the clinical publications report on the treatment of anovulatory women only.

Fukushima et al (1982) demonstrated the usefulness of tamoxifen in the treatment of luteal phase deficiency. Therapy with tamoxifen increased the previously lower than normal progesterone concentration. Moreover, the midcycle estradiol peak was about twice that observed in the cycle preceding treatment, and the glycogen content of endometrial tissue at the midluteal phase was significantly enhanced. The improvement of endometrial function is attested to by the fact that six out of 17 patients treated for a total of 40 cycles became pregnant.

### Pretreatment work-up

The diagnostic work-up of infertile women scheduled to undergo treatment with tamoxifen is identical to that described for clomiphene citrate therapy.

## Treatment

Tamoxifen is administered in a dose of 20 mg per day beginning on day 3 after a spontaneous or progestogen-induced vaginal bleeding. There are as yet no reports on experiences with varied dosage schemes or a combination with other fertility-promoting agents such as hCG, hMG or bromocriptine. Since tamoxifen has been given in cases of metastasizing mammary cancers for prolonged periods of time, and the number and severity of side-effects was low, there is no obvious reason why the compound should not be given for 6 or more cycles, as is customarily done with clomiphene citrate, provided that there are no other possible causes of infertility.

## Monitoring of therapy

Hyperstimulation has so far not been of major concern in most reports, but in one series of 30 patients, ovarian enlargement of mild to moderate degree was noted in 20% of cases (Gerhard & Runnebaum 1979). Consequently, the same criteria with respect to follow-up of the patients should be applied as in therapy with clomiphene citrate.

## Side-effects

There are considerable differences in the reports on frequency and severity of side-effects. Some investigators reported on an absence of any significant side-effects, while Gerhard & Runnebaum (1979) stated that 16 out of 30 women treated with tamoxifen complained about one or more of the following symptoms: hypermenorrhea, acne, weight gain, dizziness, flushes and headaches.

In women with estrogen deficiency, tamoxifen acts as a weak estrogen. Treatment with 30 or 40 mg daily increased the serum levels of SHBG and other hepatic proteins, and decreased those of FSH and prolactin to a similar extent as 2 mg estradiol (Fex et al 1981, Helgason et al 1982).

## Results

When assessing the therapeutic efficacy of tamoxifen one has to keep in mind that the number of clinical studies reported as yet is rather small when compared to clomiphene citrate. It may, however, be safely stated that approximately 60–80% of the patients will ovulate in response to a 5-day course of treatment (Klopper & Hall 1971, Williamson & Ellis 1973, Gerhard & Runnebaum 1979). There is less certainty with respect to the pregnancy rates, as considerable differences have been reported, i.e. 10% by Gerhard & Runnebaum (1979) and 56% by Williamson & Ellis (1973). Multiple gestations have not been reported yet. The rate of abortion appears to be in the usual range.

## ESTROGENS

### Ovulation induction

Estradiol exerts a positive feedback effect upon gonadotropin release when its serum level exceeds a critical threshold for a limited period of time (Karsch et al 1973). This results in an enhanced LH release. Estradiol thus provides a decisive stimulus for the steep rise of serum LH in midcycle, which in turn induces follicular rupture (see Chapters 5 and 6). Considerable effort has been directed towards therapeutic utilization of this physiological finding.

The daily application of 200 µg of ethinyl estradiol orally during the early follicular phase of the cycle leads within 8–16 h to a suppression of LH and, much more pronounced, of FSH (Tsai & Yen 1971) (Fig.18.2). About 36 h after the cessation of estrogen treatment, a rebound-type increase of LH (but not FSH) above pretreatment levels can be observed. This suggests that the acute drop in serum estrogen may act as a triggering event. In contrast, FSH recovers slowly and does not exceed the pretreatment level (Tsai & Yen 1971). This dichotomy in the effect of exogenous estrogen upon LH and FSH release reflects the as yet unsolved problem of using estrogens therapeutically in functional infertility. Ethinyl estradiol in a dose of 200 µg/day obviously causes a transitory disturbance in the normal sequence of follicular maturation, and the follicular phase is clearly prolonged. A period of 13–15 days has been observed to elapse between the termination of estrogen treatment and the delayed occurrence of the LH peak in women with normal ovulatory cycles (Tsai & Yen 1971, Yen & Tsai 1972). Considering this, it does not come as a surprise that ovulation induction with intravenous injections of conjugated estrogens proved to be rather disappointing.

An intriguing approach to the solution of this question was described in 1976 by Evans et al. Amenorrheic and oligomenorrheic women who had been observed without treatment for at least 4 months, were treated with ethinyl estradiol and ethynodiol diacetate, in a cyclic manner, and with doses adjusted in a stepwise fashion in order to imitate as nearly as possible the physiological fluctuations occurring during the cycle. It is quite remarkable that 25 out of 50 patients treated ovulated after having been exposed to this regimen twice, and nine became pregnant. The authors conceded that a placebo effect might have played a role, even though these patients had preciously not responded to a placebo.

Although the unorthodox approach of Evans et al (1976) probably deserves some re-evaluation, the use of estrogens in ovulation induction is at present more or less limited to that of an adjunct to clomiphene when there is spontaneous or induced dysmucorrhea.

## EPIMESTROL

Although it is debatable whether epimestrol (3-methoxy-epi-estriol; Fig. 18.1) acts in the organism as an estrogen or antiestrogen, it differs from the synthetic antiestrogens such as clomiphene structurally and in its pharmacological effects to such a degree that it appears justifiable to include it in the section dealing with the fertility-promoting effects of estrogens.

As a derivative of the natural estrogen estriol, epimestrol is the only ovulation inducer (apart from hMG/hCG) which is not a stilbene but a steroid. Its estrogenic effect is only 1/100 to 1/200 that of ethinyl estradiol. It is eliminated from the organism as a glucuronide. As it has been noted to improve—unlike clomiphene—the quality of the cervical mucus and thus favor its penetration by

spermatozoa, it is assumed to act as a weak estrogen rather than an antiestrogen. Epimestrol differs from the stilbene-type ovulation inducers and DES in that it fails to induce any change in plasma FSH and pituitary gonadotropin content when injected intravenously into oophorectomized, estrogen-progesterone-blocked rats (Baier & Taubert 1969b). Contrary to that, epimestrol was, however, found to induce a significant rise in serum LH and prolactin in anovulatory women within 24 h when 5 mg were given orally every 6 h. The rise in serum FSH occurred in a more protracted manner, and did not become significant before the fourth day of treatment. The elevated hormone levels returned to pretreatment value within 24 h after discontinuation of treatment but the pituitary response to LHRH remained enhanced for at least 36 h after the last tablet had been taken (Genazzani et al 1978). Although its exact mode of action needs to be elucidated, these results were interpreted to mean that with respect to the release of LH and prolactin epimestrol acts upon the hypothalamic-pituitary axis like a weak estrogen.

## Indications

Treatment with epimestrol should be limited to women with anovulatory infertility who respond to a challenge with a progestogen by vaginal bleeding (WHO Group II). Moreover, its use appears to be of some promise for the treatment of luteal phase defect, as Bohnet et al (1980a,b) had reported that a defective luteal phase could be normalized by treatment with epimestrol in ten out of 17 cases.

Epimestrol is not quite as effective in inducing ovulation as clomiphene. On the other hand, its use is not encumbered by the serious side-effects reported for the latter. It is, therefore, quite difficult to establish guidelines which would help to decide in the individual case whether it would be preferrable to use a more potent compound. Its lack of undesirable side-effects, and the beneficial effect upon the quality of the cervical mucus could be an advantage in patients who had previously experienced ovarian hyperstimulation, or were found to have dysmucorrhea, particularly after having been treated with clomiphene.

Whenever it is preferred over the latter, the patient should be informed why the use of clomiphene is going to be postponed in favor of a therapeutic trial with epimestrol. As all of the patients treated by Villalobos et al (1975) with epimestrol showed an increase in the spinnbarkeit and the volume of the cervical mucus, the question arises whether or not this compound might be suitable for the treatment of dysmucorrhea.

### Pretreatment work-up

Before epimestrol is administered, at least for a longer period of time, tubal patency should be tested by an appropriate method. A spermiocytogram of the husband's semen is obtained, and a postcoital test is carried out.

### Treatment

Epimestrol is usually given at a dose of 5 mg per day between days 3 and 12 or days 5 and 14 following the onset of spontaneous or progestogen-induced bleeding. The treatment may be continued for approximately six cycles (Erb 1975). If the patient ovulated but has not become pregnant by then, a thorough reevaluation of the situation should be carried out (including laparoscopy) before a change to another ovulation inducer is contemplated. When ovulation fails to be induced by epimestrol in two or three cycles, its use should be discontinued in favor of clomiphene. The combination of epimestrol with clomiphene ( 50 mg per day for the first 5 days of epimestrol therapy) did not improve upon the results obtained with either agent alone (Villalobos et al 1975).

### Results

There are very conflicting reports on the therapeutic efficacy of epimestrol, with the ovulation rate ranging from 12.5% (Sharf et al 1971) to 86% (Köhler 1980), whilst the number of pregnancies varies between 18% (Schmidt-Elmendorff & Kaemmerling 1977) and 61% (Köhler 1980). Obviously, the lower figure is more representative than the higher. Generally speaking, the number of pregnancies is about one-half of that achieved by treatment with clomiphene.

The incidence of abortions does not seem to exceed that seen after administration of other ovulation inducers (13–33%; Sas & Resch 1973, Erb 1975, Villalobos et al 1975, Meckies et al 1976, Schmidt-Elmendorff & Kaemmerling 1977). Sas & Resch (1973), in a small group of 23 pregnant women, noted signs and symptoms of threatened abortion in ten cases.

### Side-effects

Overstimulation of the ovaries seems to be rather uncommon (Sas & Resch 1973). Accordingly, there are no reports of a higher incidence of multiple gestations (Sas & Resch, 1973, Benz & Litschgi 1975, Schmidt-Elmendorff & Kaemmerling 1977). Side-effects of moderate to mild degree such as hot flushes, hypermenorrhea, nausea and headaches are rarely seen, and do not affect more than about 3% of the patients (Sas & Resch 1973, Schmidt-Elmendorff & Kaemmerling 1977).

### Comment

The therapeutic use of epimestrol is beset by the same problem as that of cyclofenil. There is a marked discrepancy between the apparent effectiveness with respect to alterations of gonadotropin release on the one hand, and the disappointingly low conception rate on the other. When compared to the huge amount of scientific data which has been amassed on the modus operandi and efficacy of clomiphene, the information on epimestrol and its mode of action is minuscule. Until this deficit has been corrected by studies delineating the mode of action of this estrogen derivative and the reason for its less than satisfying clinical performance, its use should be recommended with some reservation.

## PROGESTOGENS

The progestogens used in the treatment of female infertility are structurally a rather heterogeneous group of compounds (Table 18.1), which include:

- Natural progesterone
- Stereoisomers of progesterone (retroprogesterones)
- Derivatives of $17\alpha$-hydroxyprogesterone
- Derivatives of nortestosterone.

Although widely divergent with respect to side-effects, all progestogens have in common the capacity: (1) to bind to the progesterone receptor in the endometrium and myometrium, and (2) to induce secretory transformation of a proliferative endometrium. The binding affinity to the progesterone receptor does not always correlate well with the clinical effectiveness of a progestogen, and some widely used preparations such as lynestrenol, norethynodrel and ethynodiol diacetate neither bind nor exert any effect before being transformed metabolically into norethisterone. As estrogens induce the production of the progesterone receptor in the endometrium, progestogens cannot act upon the uterus or other target organs unless they have been primed by endogenous or exogenous estrogen. As a consequence, withdrawal bleeding can be brought about by a progestogen only in those amenorrheic women who are producing some estrogen. Depending on their molecular structure, progestogens are capable of eliciting various side-effects, some of which are of clinical concern, e.g. high-dose preparations with inherent androgenic properties (e.g. norgestrel).

All progestogens with the exception of the retroprogesterones have a hyperthermic effect, i.e. they elevate the BBT by a direct effect upon the temperature centre. This pharmacological effect should be taken into consideration when a substitutional therapy is carried out in a case of luteal phase defect in a spontaneous or clomiphene-induced ovulatory cycle.

## Therapeutic indications

The use of a progestogen may be considered for the following indications:

- Induction of withdrawal bleeding in oligo/amenorrhea
- Correction of a progesterone deficit in luteal phase defect
- Prevention of threatened or recurrent abortion
- Suppression of endometriosis (See Chapter 20).

## Withdrawal bleeding

When a progestogen is given to an oligomenorrheic or amenorrheic women for 10 days, the endometrium will undergo full secretory transformation comparable to that seen in a normal, ovulatory cycle, provided that the endometrium had been previously exposed to an adequate stimulus of endogenous or exogenous estrogen inducing proliferation. After the last tablet has been taken, the endometrium undergoes changes similar to those occurring physiologically during the days of waning function of the corpus luteum. Menstruation-like bleeding begins as a rule 2–4 days after the last tablet has been taken, i.e. the progestogen has been withdrawn. When an injectable preparation has been used, the onset of bleeding is less predictable.

Withdrawal bleeding can also be induced by a shorter course of treatment, e.g. of 5 days' duration, or by daily injections of 10 mg of progesterone in oil for 5 days (Riley 1960). Under these circumstances, bleeding will occur from an endometrium which had not undergone full secretory transformation. Occasionally, withdrawal bleeding may be delayed by as much as 8–10 days when ovulation occurred during the application of the progestogen. In a case like that, the progesterone secreted by the corpus luteum maintains the endometrium up to the end of the luteal phase, even though the application of the progestogen has already been discontinued for some time. There is a certain basis for the assumption that ovulation is induced in some anovulatory women when they are treated with a synthetic progestogen. Such an effect could possibly be due to the antiestrogenic properties of progesterone which, to a certain extent, are comparable to that of clomiphene in that it interferes with the replenishment of the cytoplasmic estrogen receptor (Koligian & Stormshak 1977). This leads to a decrease in the number of hypothalamic and pituitary binding sites, e.g. for the negative feedback effect of endogenous estradiol. It appears, therefore, conceivable that in some cases a rebound-like phenomenon can be brought about by the cyclic administration of a progestin resulting in ovulation, provided there is a ripe follicle. As such an effect is certainly neither common nor predictable, and difficult to distinguish from spontaneously occurring ovulation, and does not offer any basis for rational use in the treatment of anovulatory infertility. In accord with this, the use of retroprogesterones, particularly of trengestone (Taubert & Jürgensen 1969, Dapunt & Windbichler 1970), as ovulation-inducing agents has more or less been abandoned, as the original expectations raised by reports on ovulation rates approximating 45% failed to be fulfilled.

### Luteal phase defect

Luteal phase defect (syn. corpus luteum insufficiency, luteal phase insufficiency) is a relatively rare cause of infertility which affects approximately 3–10% of infertile women (for review see Taubert 1978, Wentz et al 1990). It is particularly prevalent in women suffering repeated abortions (Grant et al 1959, McDonough et al 1978), in patients with intermittent or moderate hyperprolactinemia (Seppälä et al 1976, Coelingh-Bennink 1979), in perimenopausal, still ovulating patients (Sherman & Korenman 1975), and subsequent to ovulation induction with clomiphene (Van Hall & Mastboom 1969, Garcia et al 1977). It should, however, be kept in mind that atypical hyperthermic shifts suggestive of luteal phase defect have been observed in 18% of cycles in women with proven fertility.

Being a disorder of the ovulatory cycle, luteal phase defect is characterized by incomplete or delayed secretory transformation of the endometrium rendering a poor substrate for the implantation of the blastocyst.

The faulty secretory transformation of the endometrium is caused either by insufficient stimulation by progesterone secondary to a malfunction of the corpus luteum, or by an inherent defect of the endometrium (Keller et al 1979). There are various causes for subnormal secretion of progesterone: delayed onset of luteinization (Koninckx et al 1978), inadequate stimulation by LH (Dreykluft et al 1971, van der Kerckhove & Dhont 1972, Jürgensen et al 1973, Lepoutre et al 1973), interference with its action by prolactin (Mühlenstedt et al 1978, Del Pozo et al 1979, Mühlenstedt et al 1979, Saunders et al 1979), or—probably in the majority of cases—improper follicular maturation subsequent to a relative FSH deficit in the early follicular phase (DiZerega & Hodgen 1981a,b, Strott et al 1970, Koninckx et al 1978).

### Choice of therapy

As a result of the heterogeneous nature of luteal phase inadequacy quite differing forms of therapy have been used with success. When hyperprolactinemia and hyperandrogenemia can be excluded as etiological factors (Seppälä et al 1976, Soules et al 1977, Coelingh-Bennink 1979, Rodriquez-Rigau et al 1979b), a decision has to be made whether to improve luteal function by:

- Stimulation of follicular development with oral ovulation inducers or with hMG/hCG
- Stimulation of corpus luteum function by injection of hCG (5000–10 000 IU intramuscularly after ovulation, followed by 5000 IU 5 days later; or every 2–3 days 2500 IU intramuscularly for the duration of the hyperthermic phase)
- Substitution of a progesterone deficit by application of progesterone or of a progesterone ester.

Ovulation inducers are the treatment of choice when an unruptured, luteinized follicle is suspected, when substitutional therapy with progestogens or stimulation of the corpus luteum by hCG have failed, and when low FSH values in the early follicular phase associated with low estradiol values indicate inadequate follicular development.

The treatment of luteal phase inadequacy due to hyperprolactinemia with bromocriptine is described in Chapter 17, and that due to hyperandrogenism with glucocorticoids in a later section of this chapter.

## Treatment of luteal phase defect

### Progesterone

A deficiency in progesterone production by the corpus luteum can be corrected by the injection of 12.5–25 mg progesterone in oil every 24 h (Jones 1973). As daily injections are impractical and would be declined by most patients, the use of vaginal suppositories containing 25 mg of progesterone may be preferable. Table 18.3 supplies the composition of such suppositories if they have to be prepared by a pharmacist. Progesterone is readily absorbed through the vaginal mucosa (Jones 1973, 1976). Either way of administration may result in normalization of the progesterone values in serum (Nillius & Johansson 1971), the dose should, however, not be exceeded (Wentz 1980), as progesterone exerts a negative feedback upon its own receptor (Haukkamaa & Lukkainen 1974, Bayard et al 1978), and exogenously administered progestogens have been shown to produce luteal phase deficiencies in women (Aksel & Jones 1974).

Treatment is begun 3 days after ovulation is judged to have occurred on the basis of a typical rise of the BBT, or a rise in urinary or serum LH measured by a rapid assay (Brandau 1978, Younger et al 1978). The dose is: 1 suppository containing 25 mg of progesterone every 12 h for at least 10 days, or until bleeding ensues, or a positive pregnancy test has been obtained. This can be achieved by measuring hCG in serum or urine before the menstrual period is being missed (Dericks-Tan & Taubert 1979).

Although it appears to be reasonable to continue the application of progesterone beyond the point at which the diagnosis of pregnancy has been made, treatment is often limited to a substitution for the duration of the luteal phase. This

approach is supported by the findings of Soules et al (1981), that 17α-hydroxyprogesterone and hCG were normal after treatment of luteal phase defect with progesterone, even though luteal function was enhanced to a considerable degree when clomiphene has been used instead.

It was, however, pointed out by Soules et al (1977) that a continuation of progesterone treatment into the early weeks of pregnancy was probably preferable. This issue has not yet been finally resolved.

When progesterone is given beyond the date of the next menstrual period, a state of pseudopregnancy is induced, and the onset of bleeding is delayed. As the patient is likely to interpret this as a sign of pregnancy, disillusionment will be hard to avoid.

Once the decision has been made to substitute progesterone in the early weeks of pregnancy, an injection of 250 mg of 17α-hydroxyprogesterone caproate is given once a week until the 16th week of pregnancy (Wentz 1980). This type of treatment is carried on well into the third trimester when there is a history of premature deliveries, repeated miscarriages, or the hCG assay and other diagnostic means indicate the presence of a twin gestation. The rationale of using progestogens as a means for prevention of repeated abortions (see below) is still a controversial issue.

### Synthetic progestogens

The use of certain synthetic progestogens for the treatment of luteal insufficiency (Fig. 18.8) has resulted in pregnancy rates which are comparable to those achieved with other modes of treatment (for review see Taubert 1978). It is debatable, however, whether they offer any advantage over progesterone suppositories or treatment with gonadotropins and ovulation inducers, except for the fact that progesterone suppositories are somewhat inconvenient to use and are not commercially available in many countries.

It is noteworthy in this context that progesterone and its derivatives induce some typical ultrastructural alterations in the endometrial cell, the most conspicuous of which are the formation of a nucleolar channel system, of giant mitochondria, and an accumulation of glycogen (Kohorn et

**Table 18.3** Prescription for 25 prosterone vaginal suppositories (each containing 25 mg of progesterone)

| | |
|---|---|
| Progesterone | 0.63g |
| Polyethyleneglycol 400 | 29.8g |
| Polyethyleneglycol 6000 | 19.8g |

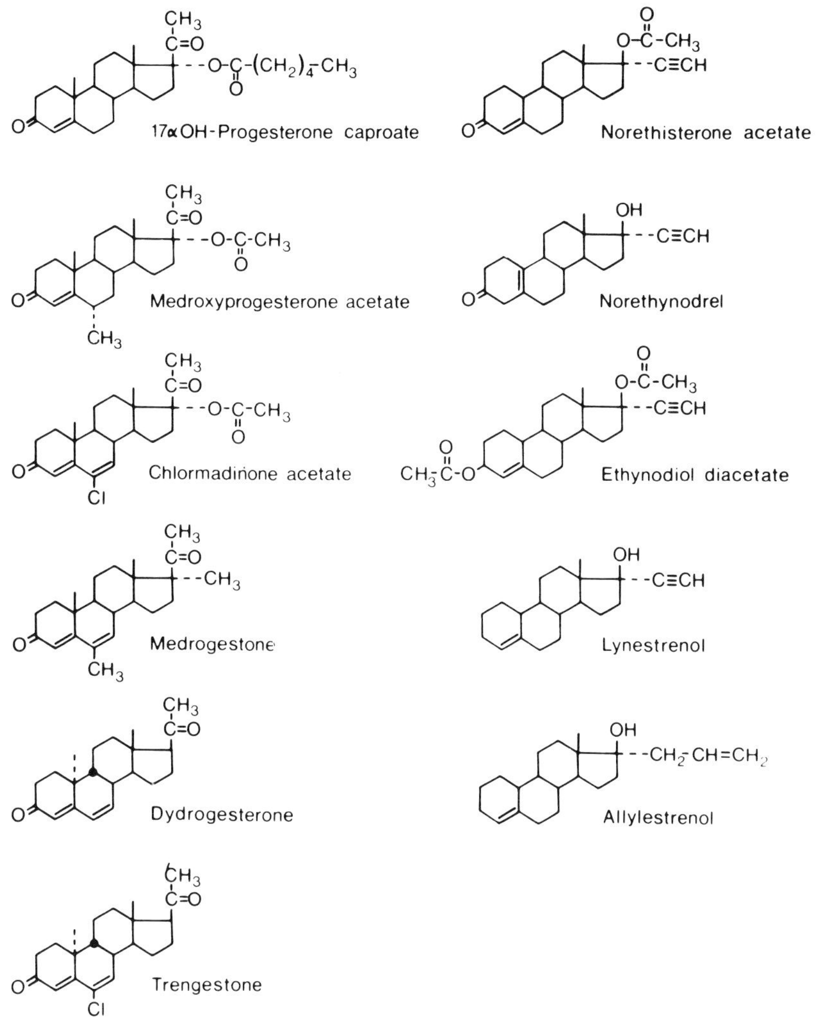

**Fig. 18.8**  Structural formulas of progesterone and synthetic progestogens.

al 1972). Moreover, these compounds are capable of maintaining pregnancy in oophorectomized rodents, and are devoid of any androgenic side-effect. The latter features are lacking in the nortestosterone derivatives such as lynestrenol, norethisterone, norgestrel and ethynodiol diacetate, and they do not induce the nucleolar channel system. Moreover, the use of nortestosterone derivatives has been tainted by the stigma of having caused masculinization of female embryos when used in high dosages and for prolonged periods in early pregnancy (Heinonen et al 1977). In order to avoid possible teratogenic effects, the use of synthetic progestogens is not

recommended any more during early pregnancy, and this should include the conception cycle.

Contrary to that, a retroprogesterone, i.e. a stereoisomer of natural progesterone (Fig. 18.8), dydrogesterone, has been, and still is widely used in the treatment of luteal phase insufficiency. It does not cause an elevation of the BBT, does not suppress the production of progesterone by the corpus luteum as do other progestogens (Johansson 1971, Bishop et al 1962, Saure et al 1975), but may cause considerable alterations in the normal cyclic pattern of hormones (Jaffe et al 1969). It was recently shown by Balasch et al (1982) that treatment of luteal phase defects with dydrogesterone resulted in a success rate of 68%, i.e. similar to that of therapy with vaginal suppositories of progesterone.

Treatment is initiated 3 days after presumed ovulation and is carried out for 10–12 days as it has been described for progesterone suppositories. A serum sample for the assay of hCG may be obtained when the BBT maintains a level of 37°C or higher on the last day of therapy. When a hCG level indicating early pregnancy has been obtained, a decision has to be made whether to continue therapy with dydrogesterone or an injectable depot preparation (Table 18.1).

Rather than administering dydrogesterone orally once or twice a day, a depot preparation may be given between days 17 and 18 of the cycle (250 mg 17α-hydroxyprogesterone caproate possibly in combination with 5 mg estradiol valerate). This type of treatment releases the patient from the responsibility of administering the progestogen orally or vaginally in a regular manner, but has a certain disadvantage because it does not assure a steady blood level of the drug. The possibility of menstrual irregularity (delayed menses) due to the depot-type preparation must also be considered.

As the final pregnancy rate depends to a great extent on the selection of patients for substitutional therapy with progestorone and progestogens, and on the presence or absence of other infertility factors; there is a considerable divergency between the results reported by different investigators. A pregnancy rate of 59% has been reported (Soules et al 1977) and Rosenberg et al (1980) demonstrated that nine out of 13 women suffering from luteal phase defect not complicated by other abnormalities conceived when treated with vaginal suppositories for 6 months, and seven of these carried the pregnancy to term. When dydrogesterone was given at a dose of 10 mg/day from day 17 through 26 of the cycle, 15 out of 48 women with luteal phase defect became pregnant (Taubert et al 1969), and the abortion rate did not exceed that commonly seen.

A similar rate of success was recorded by Weise et al (1982a) who injected on day 20 of the cycle 40 mg of progesterone and 4 mg estradiol benzoate in oil intramuscularly and obtained a pregnancy rate of 31%.

## Threatened and repeated abortion

Even though progesterone depresses myometrial activity in the pregnant uterus, there is no good evidence for the assumption that the use of oral progestogens (dydrogesterone), or of injectable preparations (17α-hydroxyprogesterone caproate) substantially reduces the incidence of first-trimester abortions. It has clearly been shown in double-blind studies that the protective effect does not exceed that of a placebo (Goldzieher 1964, Alling-Moller & Fuchs 1965, Govaerts-Videtzky et al 1965, Klopper & Mac Naughton 1965, Berle & Behnke 1977). This has to be expected in a condition which is caused in up to 59% of the cases by a genetic disturbance (for review see Nocke 1979). Some evidence has, however, been presented indicating that injections of 17αOH-progesterone caproate started in the 16th week of pregnancy may be effective in reducing the incidence of premature labor (Johnson et al 1975).

In view of the fact that the efficacy of progestogen therapy in the prevention of threatened and repeated abortions has never been proven, and since these compounds have been suspected of having been responsible for the occurrence of birth defects in the offspring of mothers treated in the early weeks of pregnancy, the indication for such supportive therapy should at least be demonstrated by showing a progesterone deficit in the luteal phase of a preconceptional cycle.

The ineffectiveness of progestogens in preventing embryonal demise does not preclude that the onset of bleeding may be delayed for a considerable period of time. The vitality of the conceptus should, therefore, be closely monitored by repeated measurements of hCG in serum, and —beginning in the 7th to 8th week of pregnancy —by sonography. Whenever the serum level of hCG is found to be too low for the chronological age of the pregnancy, and if it fails to rise normally (doubling time 2.5 days), irreversible damage of the conceptus has occurred with certainty.

## Teratogenic effects

The ripe Graafian follicle and the tubal fluid

contain a very high concentration of progesterone. As a consequence, the oocyte is physiologically exposed to a level of progesterone exceeding that in serum by a factor of 1000 (Ross 1976). It may be deduced from this that a defective output of progesterone by the preovulatory follicle and/or by the corpus luteum creates an unfavorable environment for oocyte maturation, fertilization, and implantation. This implies that the absence rather than the presence of progesterone is harmful for embryonal development. In rodents, progesterone has even been shown to offer a certain protective effect against some teratogens such as ergocornine and actinomycine (Carpent & Desclin 1969).

Synthetic progestogens, however, have been implicated as being the cause of congenital malformations in children born to women who were exposed to progestogen therapy in the first 4 months of pregnancy (Chez 1978). Similar claims have been raised with respect to estrogens, anti-estrogens, and combined preparations. However, the presently available evidence for a teratogenic effect of synthetic progestogens or of progesterone is at best contradictory. Nevertheless, some authorities, e.g. the FDA, have issued repeated warnings against the use of synthetic progestogens in early pregnancy.

## Comment

Luteal phase insufficiency is by definition a disorder of the ovulatory cycle which can be caused by a whole set of different endocrine disturbances. The common denominator is the inadequate secretory transformation of the glandular and stromal compartments of the endometrium as a consequence of faulty functioning of the corpus luteum. This fault does not seem to be a very constant phenomenon as cycles with what appears to be a deficient luteal phase have been shown to alternate in an unpredictable fashion with apparently ovulatory or anovulatory cycles.

Luteal phase inadequacy has not only been observed in women with short and atypical hyperthermic phase of the BBT, but also amongst those having a perfectly normal follicular phase followed by normal periovulatory events (Grunfeld et al 1989). Moreover, luteal phase inadequacy does not necessarily persist in the same individuum.

In clinical practice, the diagnosis of luteal phase insufficiency is usually made by measuring progesterone in serum or the histological evaluation of an endometrial biopsy taken during the late luteal phase. It is widely accepted that the latter is a better indicator of luteal function than serial determinations of progesterone in serum obtained in the midluteal phase (Balasch et al 1986), or, as suggested by Daya (1989), on day 25 or 26 of the cycle.

Consequently, the endometrial biopsy was reemphasized as a means for a structured approach to the diagnosis and treatment of luteal phase insufficiency by Witten & Martin in 1985. Infertile women with glandular/stromal asynchrony of the endometrial compartments shown by endometrial biopsy were treated either with clomiphene citrate or progesterone vaginal suppositories. In cases of asynchrony, clomiphene citrate brought about a cumulative pregnancy rate of 60% compared to 40% when progesterone was used; vice versa progesterone was more effective (cumulative pregnancy rate 66%) than clomiphene when the development of the glandular and stromal compartments was synchronous. In addition, there was no association between serum progesterone levels and the discrepancies shown by biopsy.

Even though these criteria seem to provide a basis for a rational approach to the treatment of luteal phase insufficiency, it is quite difficult to establish a cause-and-effect relationship between a certain method of treatment and the eventual outcome. Wentz et al (1990) summarized years of experience in diagnosing and treating luteal phase insufficiency by stating two salient factors. No woman was diagnosed as having luteal phase inadequacy as the single fertility factor. In addition, the incidence of this disorder in the infertile population is probably as low as 5%, and there are no differences in the fecundity of patients diagnosed to have luteal phase inadequacy or not. Indeed, luteal phase inadequacy still remains a diagnostic and therapeutic enigma.

## CORTICOSTEROIDS

Hyperandrogenism may result in infertility by causing anovulation or luteal phase defect (Steinberger et al 1979, Diamant & Evron 1981). The serum androgens testosterone, androstendione and DHEA are not exclusively of adrenal origin, but are also secreted by the ovary. Similarly, ACTH does not only stimulate the production of androgens by the adrenal cortex, but also, to a lesser degree, that of ovarian androgens (Schwartz et al 1981). Conversely, the secretion of ovarian androgens is decreased to a certain extent by dexamethasone (Abraham 1974): The administration of 0.5 mg dexamethasone four times a day throughout the cycle was shown to result in a reduction of serum testosterone by 50%, dihydrotestosterone (DHT) by 50%, androstendione by 30–50%, DHEA by 80% and DHEA-S (the latter being almost exclusively of adrenal origin) by more than 90%. Moreover, it could clearly be shown that the production of androgens could be stimulated by hCG not only in the ovary, but also in the adrenals (Schwartz et al 1981). Glucocorticoids seem to affect the release of gonadotropins by a direct action upon the pituitary, as dexamethasone was found to lower serum LH and FSH, and to blunt the response of the pituitary gonadotropins to exogenous LHRH in normally cyclic women (Sowers et al 1979).

The fertility-inhibiting effect of hyperandrogenemia is probably mediated by several mechanisms. A local inhibition of aromatization and of peripheral conversion of ovarian and adrenal androgens to estrone (Louvet et al 1975) may result in elevated intraovarian androgen levels, leading to an arrest of follicular maturation, increased atresia (Louvet et al 1975) or a deficiency of corpus luteum function (Rodriquez-Rigau et al 1979b). Moreover, the enhancement of androgen secretion by ovulation induction with clomiphene or gonadotropins is probably an important cause of the relatively low pregnancy rate and increased number of abortions (Dupon et al 1973, Schumert et al 1975).

As a consequence, the suppression of elevated androgen levels by means of glucocorticoids (Fig. 18.2) should be considered when hyperan-drogenemic women with anovulatory infertility or luteal phase defect do not respond to therapy with clomiphene or other inducers of ovulation.

### Diagnostic considerations

When hyperandrogenism is suspected as being one of the possible causes of infertility, a measurement of the serum androgens should be carried out, particularly in the presence of physical signs of hyperandrogenemia such as hirsutism, seborrhea, temporal alopecia and polycystic enlargement of the ovaries (see Chapter 26). As the serum level of the androgens may fluctuate during the day to a considerable extent, the diagnosis of hyperandrogenemia should be based on at least three separate measurements of testosterone, DHEA-S (and possibly DHT, and free testosterone) obtained during the morning hours on three separate occasions or at intervals of 20–30 min. When there are elevated values, an overnight suppression test and an ACTH stimulation test should be carried out to rule out Cushing's syndrome and adrenal hyperplasia. Testosterone values in excess of 2 ng/ml and a DHEA-S level of more than 7000 ng/ml are strongly suggestive of the presence of an androgen-producing tumor in the ovary or adrenal gland, and an appropriate search should be initiated before any treatment with ovulation-inducing agents is contemplated.

When treatment with clomiphene does not result in ovulation, or there is a failure to conceive even though ovulation appears to have been induced, interference by androgens should be ruled out by measuring testosterone and DHEA-S repeatedly between the application of the compound and the time ovulation is expected to occur. When there is a marked rise in serum androgens in cases of clomiphene-resistant anovulation, the addition of dexamethasone or of an equivalent dose of another glucocorticoid to the therapeutic regimen is justified.

### Treatment

The efficacy of cortisone in the treatment of follicular phase defect was first described by Jones et al in 1953. Although this therapeutic approach to the treatment of functional infertility was largely superseded by ovulation inducers in the past two decades, the value of androgen suppression by glucocorticoids (Fig. 18.9), e.g. dexamethasone in a dose of 0.5 mg/day, has been confirmed by others (Perloff et al 1965, Toaff et al 1978).

This is exemplified by a report of Rodriquez-Rigau et al (1979a) who treated 106 women with clinical and laboratory evidence of hyperandrogenism with a daily dose of 7.5–10 mg prednisone. Thirty-six per cent of the amenorrheic women and 91% of the anovulatory women resumed ovulation. In all of the remaining 81 women, prednisone therapy resulted in a shortening of the follicular and a lengthening of the luteal phase, even though the duration of the intermenstrual span was not changed.

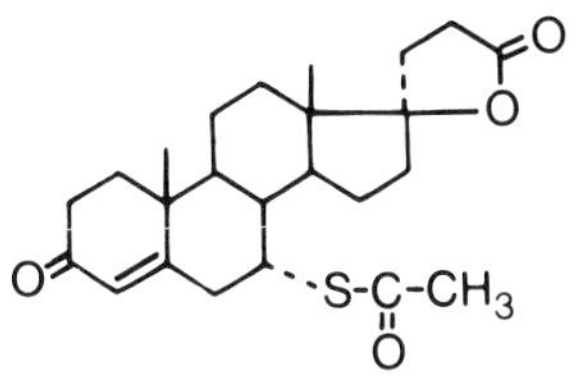

**Fig. 18.9** Structural formulas of glucocorticoids and danazol.

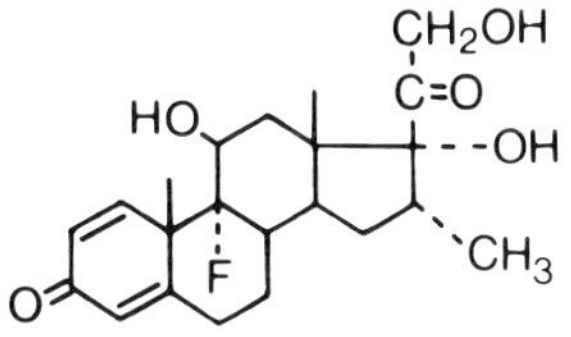

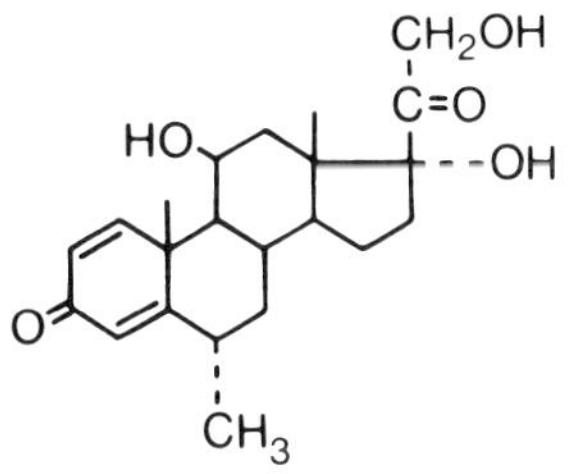

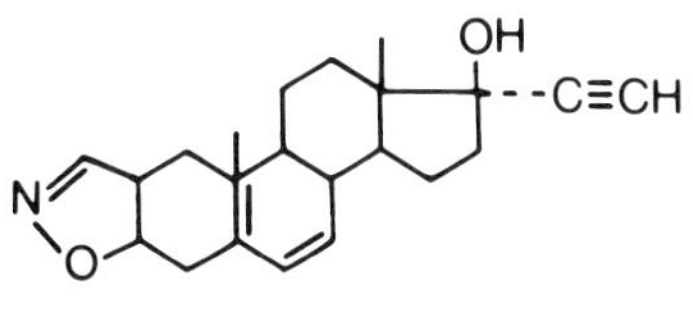

The combined use of clomiphene and a glucocorticoid in well-chosen cases appeared particularly promising, when either compound alone did not succeed in inducing ovulation (Diamant & Evron 1981). Undesirable side-effects of glucocorticoid therapy can be reduced when the administration of dexamethasone or prednisone is limited to 10 days per cycle, the treatment scheme being as follows: clomiphene, 100–200 mg/day from day 5 through 9 after the onset of bleeding, 2 mg dexamethasone from day 5 to 14. Nine out of 13 anovulatory women not responding to clomiphene in doses up to 200 mg per day became pregnant after having been treated with such a combination of clomiphene and dexamethasone (Lisse 1980).

In some cases of hyperandrogenism, treatment with spironolactone has been reported as being successful (see below).

## ANTIANDROGENS

As hyperandrogenism plays an important etiological role in many cases of functional infertility, particularly in patients responding poorly to ovulation inducers (Dupon et al 1973, Schumert et al 1975), the use of antiandrogens has lately been suggested as a possible, novel therapeutic approach (Evron et al 1982).

The aldosterone antagonist spironolactone (aldactone; Fig. 18.9) which is widely used as an antihypertensive agent, especially in cases of primary hyperaldosteronism, has been shown to be a potent antiandrogen. In contrast to another potent antiandrogen, cyproterone acetate, it is devoid of any progestational effect and could be applied during the follicular phase.

The antiandrogenic effect of spironolactone is apparently conveyed by several pathways: testosterone biosynthesis is suppressed at the step of $17\beta$-hydroxylation (Schumert et al 1975), the conversion of androgens in the periphery is enhanced (Rose et al 1977), and the compound inhibits the binding of DHT to the receptors (Rifka et al 1978). In vitro studies using human fetal liver cells did not show any effect of spironolactone in therapeutic concentrations on aromatase activity (Carr 1986). The effect seems rather to be mediated by decreasing

$17\alpha$-hydroxylase- and 20,21-desmolase activity. Shapiro & Evron (1980) were the first to show that hirsutism of hyperandrogenic women could be decreased by treatment with spironolactone. This favorable response encouraged the application of this new therapeutic principle to the treatment of hyperandrogenic women with anovulatory dysfunction. Spironolactone was administered in a dose of 100–150 mg/day from day 1 through day 21 of the cycle. This regimen resulted in a decrease of previously elevated LH level via a suppression of testosterone, and in a depression of previously normal prolactin. As evidenced by the measurement of progesterone in serum, 85% of the patients ovulated and had normal, regular cycles.

No serious side-effects, except of mild forms of polyuria and polydipsia, were observed, probably as a result of the intermittent application of spironolactone.

Even though ovulation induction with spironolactone is still in the experimental stage, the results of Evron et al (1982) justify further clinical studies, provided a teratogenic effect can be safely excluded. Reference should, however, be made to isolated reports of mammary cancer being observed in a few women who had been treated continuously for a prolonged period of time with spironolactone. A causal relationship cannot be ruled out with certainty, particularly as mastodynia is a frequent side-effect during therapy with spironolactone (Hammerstein 1977).

## DANAZOL (see also Chapter 20)

### Chemistry and mode of action

Danazol is a weakly androgenic derivative of $17\alpha$-ethinyltestosterone which interferes with gonadal function in a complex manner ultimately causing atrophy of estrogen-dependent tissues. It is bound by the androgen, estradiol and progesterone receptor (Barbieri et al 1979). No estrogenic or progestational effects could, however, be demonstrated, and the function of the adrenals is not influenced.

Danazol inhibits slightly FSH but not LH, even though it prevents the preovulatory LH surge and thus ovulation. The serum estradiol and progesterone remain at the early follicular phase levels. The reduced estrogen level causes atrophy of the endometrium (Davison et al 1976).

In addition to its effect upon the pituitary, danazol may exert a direct inhibitory action on target tissues, reducing the sensitivity to steroid hormones by competing for the binding with steroid receptors, but without exerting any estrogenic or progestational effect. Danazol is also capable of inhibiting a number of enzymes involved in ovarian and adrenal steroid biosynthesis (Jenkin 1980).

After ingestion of 400 mg of danazol, maximal serum levels of 80–100 ng/ml were found within 1–2 h, the half-life being 4.5 h. There is no evidence that accumulation occurs to a significant extent.

### Therapy

When danazol, which actually defies classification into any of the known categories of steroids, is taken in a dose of 200 mg three times a day, menstrual function becomes completely suppressed. This effect is utilized in the treatment of endometriosis and of fibrocystic disease of the breast.

There is no indication for the use of danazol in the treatment of functional causes of infertility.

As danazol has considerable androgenic and anabolic side-effects (i.e. weight gain), GnRH agonists such as buserelin (Dmowski et al 1989) and nafarelin (Burry et al 1989), and progestogens such as gestrinone (Rose et al 1988, Fedele et al 1989b), and the combination of cyproterone acetate and ethinyl estradiol (Fedele et al 1989a) have been used as alternatives. These drugs have been shown to be equally effective in providing women suffering from endometriosis with symptomatic relief and at least partial resolution of endometrioid lesions. Moreover, there is no difference in the rate of recurrence of symptoms after the treatment has been discontinued. The pregnancy rates after discontinuation of treatment are roughly comparable, too. It has recently been claimed (Telimaa 1988) that postoperative treatment of endometriosis with danazol (and with medroxyprogesterone acetate) does not lead to an improvement of the results if infertility is the main complaint. The rate of fecundation appeared actually delayed when these drugs were used.

## Side-effects

Danazol decreases the concentration of high-density liprotein (mainly $HDL_2$), increases low density cholesterol, and causes slight, transient and reversible liver damage (Heikkinen et al 1988), whereas the GnRH agonists do not (Burry et al 1989, Dmowski et al 1989). On the other hand, the hypoestrogenic state induced by GnRH agonists can be associated with a measurable amount of bone loss such as seen in postmenopausal women (see also Chapter 15). On the contrary, danazol but not GnRH treatment is effective in lowering the level of autoimmune antibodies (against phospholipids, histones and polynucleotides) which are found in about 50% of women suffering from endometriosis and seem to be associated with infertility and pregnancy wastage (El-Roeiy et al 1988).

## REFERENCES

Aboughar M A, Mansour R T, Serour G I, 1989 Ovarian superstimulation in the treatment of infertility due to peritubal and periovarian adhesions. Fertil Steril 51: 834

Abraham G E 1974 Ovarian and adrenal contribution to peripheral androgen during the menstrual cycle. J Clin Endocrinol Metab 39: 340

Adams R, Mishell D R, Israel R 1972 Treatment of refractory anovulation and corpus luteum function using measurements of plasma progesterone. Obstet Gynecol 39: 562

Adashi E Y 1984 Clomiphene citrate mechanism(s) and site(s) of action—a hypothesis revisited. Fertil Steril 42: 331

Aksel S, Jones G 1974 Effects of progesterone and 17-hydroxyprogesterone caproate on hormonal corpus luteum function. Am J Obstet Gynecol 118: 466

Alling-Møller K J, Fuchs F 1965 Double-blind control trial of 6-methyl-17-acetoxyprogesterone in threatened abortion. J Obstet Gynaecol Br Commwlth 72: 1042

Anthony E J, Benodek T (eds) 1970 Parenthood: its psychology and psychopathology. Little Brown, Boston

Archer D F, Hofmann G, Brzyski R et al 1989 Effects of clomiphene citrate on episodic luteinizing hormone secretion throughout the menstrual cycle. Am J Obstet Gynecol 161: 581

Baier H, Taubert H D 1969a The effect of clomiphene upon plasma FSH-activity and hypothalamic FSH-RF content in ovariectomized, estrogen-progesterone blocked rats. Endocrinology 84: 946

Baier H, Taubert H D 1969b Investigations on the effects of epimestrol and stilbestrol upon release of FSH and LH. Horm Metab Res 1: 309

Bailer P, Gips H, Rauskolb R, Korte K, 1980 Serumkonzentrationsverhalten von Östradiol-17β und Progesteron bei durch Clomiphene überstimulierte Ovarien. Geburtshilfe Frauenheilkd 40: 72

Barbiere R L, Lee H, Ryan K J 1979 Danazol binding to rat androgen, glucocorticoid, progesterone, and estrogen receptors: correlation with biologic activity. Fertil Steril 31: 182

Balasch J, Vanrell J A, Marquez M, Burzaco I, Gonzales-Merlo J 1982 Dydrogesterone versus vaginal progesterone in the treatment of the endometrial luteal phase deficiency. Fertil Steril 37: 751

Balasch J, Creus M, Vanrell J A, 1990 Luteal function after delayed ovulation. Fertil Steril 45: 342

Barrett C A, Hakim C A 1974 Low-dosage clomiphene therapy in the treatment of infertility due to defective ovulation. Afr Med J 48: 1456

Bateman B G, Nunley W C, Kolp L A 1990 Exogenous estrogen therapy for treatment of clomiphene citrate induced cervical mucus abnormalities: is it effective? Fertil Steril 54: 577

Bayard F, Damilano S, Robel P, Baulieu E E 1978 Cytoplasmic and nuclear estradiol and progesterone receptors in human endometrium. J Clin Endocrinol Metab 46: 635

Beat F A, Sehoud M A-F 1987 Superfetation secondary to ovulation induction with clomiphene citrate: a case report. Fertil Steril 47: 515

Benz J J, Litschgi M 1975 Epimestrol: Eine ovulationsauslösende Substanz. Geburtshilfe Frauenheilkd 35: 194

Berle B, Behnke K 1977 Über Behandlungserfolge der drohenden Fehlgeburt. Geburtshilfe Frauenheilkd 37: 139

Biale Y, Leventhal H, Altaras M, Ben-Aderet N 1978 Anencephaly and clomiphene-induced pregnancy. Acta Obstet Gynecol Scand 57: 483

Birkenfeld A, Navot D, Leivj I S et al 1986 Advanced secretory changes in the proliferative human endometrial epithelium following clomiphene citrate treatment. Fertil Steril 45: 462

Bishop P M F, Borell U, Diczfalusy E, Tillinger K G 1962 Effect of dydrogesterone on human endometrium and ovarian function. Acta Endocrinol 40: 203

Bohnet H G, Dahlén H G, Keller E et al 1976 Human pituitary gonadotropin index II. LH-RH test and clomiphene response before and after LH-RH stimulation. Clin Endocrinol 5: 25

Bohnet H G, Hilland U, Hanker J P, Schneider H P G 1980a Epimestrol in der Behandlung der normoprolaktin-ämischen Corpus-luteum-Insuffizienz. Geburtshilfe Frauenheilkd 40: 926

Bohnet H G, Hanker J P, Hilland U, Schneider H P G 1980b Epimestrol treatment of inadequate luteal progesterone secretion. Fertil Steril 34: 346

Borgström L 1981 Plasma levels and pharmacokinetics of cyclofenil after oral administration to man. Eur J Clin Pharmacol 19: 213

Brandau H 1978 Measurement of LH in urine by HI-Gonavis test for the predetermination of ovulation. Geburtshilfe Frauenheilkd 38: 1047

Bryce R L, Shuter B, Sinosich M J, Stiel J N, Picker R H, Saunders D M 1982 The value of ultrasound, gonadotropin, and estradiol measurements for precise ovulation detection. Fertil Steril 37: 42

Burry K A, Patton P E, Illingworth D R 1989 Metabolic changes during medical treatment of endometriosis: nafarelin acetate versus danazol. Am J Obstet Gynecol 160: 1454

Canales E S, Cabezas A, Vazquez-Matute L, Zarate A 1978 Induction of ovulation with clomiphene and estradiol benzoate in anovulatory women refractory to clomiphene alone. Fertil Steril 29: 496

Carpent G, Desclin L 1969 Effects of ergocornine on the mechanism of gestation and on fetal morphology in the rat. Endocrinology 84: 315

Carr B R 1986 The effect of spironolactone on aromatase activity. Fertil Steril 45: 655

Chez R A 1978 Proceedings of the Symposium 'Progesterone, progestins, and fetal development'. Fertil Steril 30: 16

Coelingh-Bennink H J T 1979 Intermittent bromocriptine treatment for the induction of ovulation in hyperprolactinemic patients. Fertil Steril 31: 267

Cook J L, Schroeder J A, Yussman M A, Sanfilippo J S 1984 Induction of luteal phase defect with clomiphene citrate. Am J Obstet Gynecol 149: 613

Corson S L, Batzer F R 1986 Letter to the editor. Fertil Steril 45: 307

Crooke A C, Hansotia M D, Bertrand P V 1969 Joint action of clomiphene citrate and human pituitary gonadotropins. Lancet i: 587

Dapunt O, Windbichler H 1970 Behandlungsergebnisse mit dem Retrosteroid 'Ro 48347' bei endokriner Sterilität. Wien Med Wochenschr 82: 58

Davison C, Banks W, Fritz A 1976 The absorption, distribution and metabolic fate of Danazol in rats, monkeys, and human volunteers. Arch Int Pharmacodyn Ther 221: 294

Daya S 1989 Optimal time in the menstrual cycle for serum progesterone measurement to diagnose luteal phase defects. Am J Obstet Gynecol 161: 1009

Deaton J L, Gibson M, Blackmer K M, Nakajima S T, Badger G J, Brumsted J R 1990 A randomized, controlled trial of clomiphene citrate and intrauterine insemination in couples with unexplained infertility or surgically corrected endometriosis. Fertil Steril 54: 1083

Del Pozo E, Wyss H, Alcaniz J, Camapana A, Naftolin F 1979 Prolactin and deficient luteal function. Obstet Gynecol 53: 282

Dericks-Tan J S E, Taubert H D 1979 Radioimmunologischer Schnelltest für HCG bei normaler und gestörter Frühschwangerschaft. Dtsch Med Wochenschr 104: 1179

Dericks-Tan J S E, Taubert H D 1988 Die laboranalytische Früherkennung von Störungen der ersten Schwangerschaftshälfte. Festschrift Prof Dr Otto Käser: Ausgewählte kapitel aus der Geburtshilfe und Gynäkologie, Herausg D. Da Rugna Schwabe Verlag, Basel, pp 203–216

Diamant Y Z, Evron S 1981 Induction of ovulation with combined clomiphene citrate and dexamethasone treatment in clomiphene citrate non-responders. Eur J Obstet Gynecol Reprod Biol 11: 335

Diamond M P, Herbert C M, Maxson W S, Wentz A C 1986 Comparison of two brands of clomiphene citrate for stimulation of follicular development in a program for in vitro fertilization. Fertil Steril 45: 522

DiZerega G S, Hodgen G 1981a Follicular phase treatment of luteal phase dysfunction. Fertil Steril 35: 428

DiZerega G S, Hodgen G D 1981b Luteal phase dysfunction: a sequel to aberrant folliculogenesis. Fertil Steril 35: 489

Dlugi A M, Laufer N, Botero-Ruiz W et al 1985 Altered follicular development in clomiphene citrate versus human menopausal gonadotropin stimulated cycles for in vitro fertilization. Fertil Steril 43: 40

Dmowski W P, Radwanska E, Bino Z, Tummon I, Pepping P 1989 Ovarian suppression induced with buserelin or danazol in the management of endometriosis: a randomized comparative study. Fertil Steril 51: 395

Dodds E C, Golberg L, Lawson W, Robinson R 1938 Estrogenic activity of alkylated diethylstilbestrol. Nature 142: 34.

Drake T S, Treadway D R, Buchanan G C, 1978 Continued clinical experience with an increasing dosage regimen of clomiphene citrate administration. Fertil Steril 30: 274

Dreykluft R, Magnus U, Zielske F, Hommerstein J 1971 Normal and disturbed function of the corpus luteum as reflected by hormonal analysis in blood. Acta Endocrinol Suppl 152: 69

Dupon C, Rosenfield R L, Cleary R F 1973 Sequential changes in total and free testosterone and androstenedione in plasma during spontaneous and clomid induced ovulatory cycles. Am J Obstet Gynecol 115: 478

Eden J, Place J, Carter G D, Jones J, Alaghband-Zadeh J, Pawson M 1989 The effect of clomiphene citrate on follicular phase increase in endometrial thickness and uterine volume. Obstet Gynecol 73: 187

E1-Roeiy A, Dmowski W P, Gleicher N et al 1988 Danazol but not gonadotropin-releasing hormone agonists suppress autoantibodies in endometriosis. Fertil Steril 50: 864

Erb H, 1975 Zur Ovulationsauslösung mit Epimestrol. Gynäkol Rundsch 15: 171

Etgen A M 1979 Antiestrogens: effects of tamoxifen, nafoxidine, and CI-628 on sexual behaviour, cytoplasmic receptors, and nuclear binding of estrogen. Horm Behav 13: 97

Evans J, Townsend L 1976 The induction of ovulation. Am J Obstet Gynecol 125: 321

Evans J H, Taft H P, Brown J B, Adey F D, Johnstone J W 1976 Induction of ovulation by cyclical hormone therapy. J Obstet Gynec Br Cmmwth 74: 367

Evron S, Shapiro G, Diamant Y Z 1982 Induction of ovulation with spironolactone (aldactone) in anovulatory oligomenorrhoeic and hyperandrogenic women. Fertil Steril 36: 468

Fayez J A 1976 Selection of patients for clomiphene citrate therapy. Obstet Gynecol 47: 671

Fedele L, Arcani L, Bianchi S, Baglioni A, Vercellini P 1989a Comparison of cyproterone acetate and danazol in the treatment of pelvic pain associated with endometriosis. Obstet Gynecol 73: 1000

Fedele L, Bianchi S, Viezzoli T, Arcaini L, Canadiani G B 1989b Gestrinone versus danazol in the treatment of endometriosis. Fertil Steril 51: 781

Fedele L, Brioschi D, Marchini M, Dorta M, Parracini F, 1989c Enhanced preovulatory progesterone levels in clomiphene-induced cycles. J Clin Endocrinol Metab 69: 683

Fex G, Adielsson G, Mattson W 1981 Oestrogen-like effects of tamoxifen on the concentrations of proteins in plasma. Acta Endocrinol 97: 109

Fukushima T, Tajima C, Fukuma K, Maeyama M 1982

Tamoxifen in the treatment of infertility associated with luteal phase deficiency. Fertil Steril 37: 755

Garcia J, Jones G S, Wentz A C 1977 The use of clomiphene citrate. Fertil Steril 28: 707

Geier A, Lunenfeld B, Pariente C et al 1987 Estrogen receptor binding material in blood of patients after clomiphene citrate administration by a radioreceptor assay. Fertil Steril 47: 778

Genazzani A R, Fachinetti F F, DeLeo V et al 1978 Effect of epimestrol on gonadotropin and prolactin plasma levels and response to luteinizing-hormone releasing hormone/thyrotropin-releasing hormone in secondary amenorrhea and oligomenorrhea. Fertil Steril 30: 654

Gerhard I, Runnebaum B 1979 Comparison between tamoxifen and clomiphene therapy in women with anovulation. Arch Gynecol 227: 279

Gitsch E, Schneider W H F, Spona J 1977 Optimisation of clomiphene effect by oestrogen-progestogen pre-treatment. 9th World Congress on Fertilily Steril Miami.

Glazener C M A, Coulson C, Lambert P A et al 1990 Clomiphene treatment for women with unexplained infertility: placebo-controlled study of hormonal responses and conception rate. Gynecol Endocrinol 4: 75

Goldenberg R L, Vaitukaitis J L, Ross G T 1972 Estrogen and follicle hormone interactions on follicle growth in rats. Endocrinology 90: 1492

Goldzieher J W 1964 Double-blind trial of a progestin in habitual abortion. JAMA 188: 651

Gorlitzky G A, Kase N G, Speroff L 1978 Ovulation and pregnancy rates with clomiphene citrate. Obstet Gynecol 51: 265

Govaerts-Videtzky M, Martin L, Hubinont P O 1965 A double-blind study of progestogen treatment in spontaneous abortion. J Obstet Gynaecol Br Cwth 73: 1034

Grant A, McBride W G, Noyes J M 1959 Luteal phase defects in abortion. Int J Fertil 4: 323

Greenblantt R B, Barfield W E, Jungck E C, Ray A W 1961 Induction of ovulation with MRL/41. JAMA 178: 101

Groom G V, Griffiths K 1976 Effect of the antiestrogen tamoxifen on plasma levels of luteinizing hormone, follicle-stimulating hormone, prolactin, estradiol, and progesterone in normal premenopausal women J Endocrinol 70: 421

Grunfeld L, Sandler B, Fox J, Boyd C, Kaplan P, Navot D 1989 Luteal phase deficiency after completely normal follicular and periovulatory phases. Fertil Steril 52: 919

Gunning J E 1976 The DES story. Obstet Gynecol Surv 31: 827

Guoth J 1987 Clomiphene citrate response is predictable in corpus luteum deficiency. Eur J Obstet Gynecol Reprod Biol 24: 563

Guttmacher A F 1956 Factors affecting normal expectancy at conception. JAMA 161: 655

Guzick D S, Zeleznik A 1990 Efficacy of clomiphene citrate in the treatment of luteal phase deficiency: quantity versus quality of preovulatory follicles. Fertil Steril 54: 206

Gysler M, March C M, Mishell D R, Bailey E J 1982 A decade's experience with an individualized clomiphene treatment regimen including its effect on the postcoital test. Fertil Steril 37: 161

Hammerstein J 1977 Spironolactoner-Therapie. Mitteilung der Kommission Steroid-Toxikologie der Deutschen Gesellschaft für Endokrinologie. Endokrinologie-Information 1: 162

Hammond M G, Talbert L M 1982 Clomiphene citrate

therapy in infertile women with low luteal phase progesterone. Obstet Gynecol 59: 275

Haskins A L 1966 In: Greenblatt R B (ed) Ovulation: stimulation, suppression, detection. Lippincott, Philadelphia, p 158

Haukkamaa M, Lukkainen T 1974 The cytoplasmic progesterone receptor of human endometrium during the menstrual cycle. J Steroid Biochem 5: 477

Healy D L, Burger H G 1978 A hypothesis of high multiple pregnancies after clomiphene. Aust NZ J Obstet Gynecol 18: 242

Hecht B R, Khan-Dawood F S, Dawood M Y 1989a The luteinizing hormone surge: timing and characteristics in the plasma and urine after clomiphene citrate treatment. Fertil Steril 52: 402

Hecht B R, Khan-Dawood F S, Dawood M Y 1989b Peri-implantation phase endometrial estrogen and progesterone receptors: effect of ovulation induction with clomiphene citrate. Am J Obstet Gynecol 161: 1688

Heikkinen J, Rönnberg L, Kirkinen P, Sotaniemi A 1988 Serum bile acid concentration as an indicator of liver dysfunction induced during danazol therapy. Fertil Steril 50: 761

Heinonen O P, Slone D M, Monson R R, Hook E B, Shapiro S 1977 Cardiovascular birth defects and antenatal exposure to female sex hormones. N Engl J Med 296: 67

Helgason S, Wilking N, Carlström K, Damber M-G, von Schoultz B 1982 A comparative study of the estrogenic effects of tamoxifen and 17 β-estradiol in postmenopausal women. J Clin Endocrinol Metab 54: 404

Hendricks C H 1966 Twinning in relation to birth weight and congenital malformation. Obstet Gynecol 27: 47

Hirvonen E, Ranta T, Seppälä M 1976 Prolactin suppression stimulates clomiphene responsiveness. Int J Fertil 21: 255

Hoffman D, Lobo R A 1985 Serum dehydroepiandrosterone sulfate and the use of clomiphene citrate in anovulatory women. Fertil Steril 45: 196

Hohlweg W, Junkmann K 1932 Die hormonal-nervöse Regulierung der Funktion des Hypophysenvorderlappens und der Keimdrüsen. Klin Wochenschr 11: 321

Huber H, Schneider W H F 1984 Additive Therapie bei Ovulationsindikation mit clomiphene. Geburtshilfe Frauenheilkd 44: 233

Hull M G R, Savage P E, Jacobs H S 1979 Investigation and treatment of amenorrhea resulting in normal fertility. Br Med J 1: 1257

Igarashi M, Ibuki Y, Kubo H et al 1967 Mode and site of action of clomiphene. Am J Obstet Gynecol 97: 120

Inhoffen H H, Hohlweg W 1938 Neue per os wirksame weibliche Keimdrüsen-hormon-Derivate: 17-Äthinylöstradiol und Pregnenin-on-3-ol-17. Naturwissenschaften 26: 96

Insler V, Melmed H, Eichenbrenner J, Serr D M, Lunenfeld B 1972 The cervical score—a single semiquantitative method for monitoring the menstrual cycle. J Gynecol Obstet 10: 223

Insler V, Holcsberg G, Goldstein D, Levy J, Potashnik G 1983 Treatment of luteal insufficiency by induction of ovulation. In: H-D Taubert & Kuhl (eds) The inadequate luteal phase. MTP, Lancaster, pp 175–182

Israel R, Mishell D R, Stone S C, Thorneycroft I H, Moyer D L 1972 Single phase luteal progesterone assay as an indication of ovulation. Am J Obstet Gynecol 112: 1043

Jacobson A, Marshall J R, Ross G T 1968a Plasma luteinizing hormone during clomiphene-induced ovulatory cycles. Am J Obstet Gynecol 101: 1025

Jacobson A, Marshall J R, Ross G T 1968b Plasma gonadotropins during clomiphene-induced ovulatory cycles. Am J Obstet Gynecol 102: 284

Jaffe R B, Midgley A R, Goebelsmann U 1969 Regulation of human gonadotropins: V. Effect of dydrogesterone on serum levels of FSH and LH in women. Am J Obstet Gynecol 104: 1031

Jenkin G 1980 Review: the mechanism of action of danazol, a novel steroid derivative. Aust NZ J Obnecol Gynecol 20: 113

Jewelewicz R 1975 Management of infertility resulting from anovulation. Am J Obstet Gynecol 122: 909

Johansson E D B 1971 Depression of progesterone levels in women treated with synthetic gestagen after ovulation. Acta Endocrinol 68: 779

Johansson E D B, Larsson-Cohn U, Gemzell C 1972 Monophasic basal body temperature in ovulatory menstrual cycles. Am J Obstet Gynecol 113: 933

Johnson W C, Austin K L, Jones G S, Davis G H, King T M 1975 Efficacy of 17 α-hydroxyprogesterone caproate in the prevention of premature labor. N Engl J Med 293: 675

Jones G S 1973 Luteal phase insufficiency. Clin Obstet Gynecol 16: 255

Jones G S 1976 The luteal phase defect. Fertil Steril 25: 351

Jones G S, deMoraes-Ruehsen M, 1967 Clomiphene citrate for improvement of ovarian function. Am J Obstet Gynecol 99: 814

Jones G S, Howard J E, Langford H 1953 The use of cortisone in follicular phase disturbances. Fertil Steril: 49–62.

Jordan V C, Koch R, Langan S, McCague R 1988 Ligand interaction at the estrogen receptor to program antiestrogen action: a study with nonsteroidal compounds in vitro. Endocrinology 122: 1449

Judd S C, Alderman J, Bowden J, Michailow L 1987 Evidence against the involvement of opioid neurons in mediating the effect of clomiphene citrate on gonadotropin-releasing hormone neurons. Fertil Steril 47: 574

Jürgensen O, Hildebrandt H, Fritz I, Kronauer J, Taubert H-D 1973 Plasma LH und Progesteron in normalen und gestörten Zyklen. Arch Gynäkol 214: 418

Kahwanago I, Heinrichs W L, Herrmann W L 1979 Estradiol 'receptors' in hypothalamus and anterior pituitary gland: inhibition of estradiol binding by SH-group blocking agents and clomiphene citrate. Endocrinology 86: 1319

Kapfhammer H F, Messer T, Hoff P 1990 Psychotische Erkrankung während einer Behandlung mit Clomifen. Deutsch Med Wschr 115: 936

Karow W G, Payne S A 1968 Pregnancy after clomiphene citrate treatment. Fertil Steril 19: 351

Karsch F J, Weick R F, Butler W R et al 1973 Induced LH surges in the rhesus monkey: strength-duration characteristics of the estrogen stimulus. Endocrinology 92: 1740

Kato J, Kobayashi T, Villee C A 1968 Effect of clomiphene upon the uptake of estradiol by the anterior hypothalamus and hypophysis. Endocrinology 82: 1049

Katzenellenbogen B S, Bhakoo H S, Ferguson E R et al 1979 Estrogen and antiestrogen action in reproductive tissues and tumors. Recent Progr Horm Res 35: 259

Kaufmann C 1932 Umwandlung der Uterusschleimhaut einer kastrierten Frau aus dem atrophischen Stadium in das der sekretorischen Funktion durch Ovarialhormone Zentralbe Gynäkol 56: 2059

Kaufmann C, Bickel L 1932 Über die Behandlung genitaler Blutungen mit Corpus-luteum-Hormon. Zentralbe Gynäkol 56: 1329

Keenan J A, Herbert C M, Bush R J, Wentz A C 1989 Diagnosis and management of out-of-phase endometrial biopsies among patients receiving clomiphene citrate for ovulation induction. Fertil Steril 51: 964

Keller D W, Wiest W C, Askin F B, Johnson L W, Strickler R C 1979 Pseudocorpus luteum insufficiency. J Clin Endocrinol Metab 48: 127

Keller P D 1972 Induction of ovulation by synthethic luteinizing-hormone releasing-factor in infertile women. Lancet ii: 570

Kinces L, Sas M 1975 Fertilität nach vorangegangener Ovarium-Überstimulierung. Fort schr Med 93: 323

Kistner R W 1966 Use of clomiphene citrate, human chorionic gonadotropin, and human menopausal gonadotropin for induction of ovulation in the human female. Fertil Steril 17: 569

Kistner R W 1975 Induction of ovulation with clomiphene citrate. In: Behrman S J, Kistner R W (eds) Progress in infertility. Little Brown, Boston pp 509–536

Kistner R W 1976 Sequential use of clomiphene citrate and human menopausal gonadotropin in ovulation induction. Fertil Steril 27: 72

Kjeld J M, Harsoulis P, Nader S, Kuku S F, Fraser T R 1975 Hormonal responses to a first course of clomiphene citrate in women with amenorrhea. Br J Obstet Gynecol 82: 397

Klopper A, Hall M 1971 New synthetic agent for the induction of ovulation: preliminary trial in women. Br Med J 1: 152

Klopper A, MacNaughton M 1965 Hormones in recurrent abortion. J Obstet Gynecol Br Cwlth 72: 1022

Köhler R F 1980 Epimestrol bei kinderloser Ehe Dtsch. Med Wschr 105: 1250

Kohorn E I, Rice S I, Hemperly S, Gordon M 1972 The relation of the structure of progestional steroids to nucleolar differentiation in human endometrium. J Clin Endocrinol Metab 34: 257

Koike K, Aono T, Miyake A, Tsutsumi H, Matsumoto K, Kurachi K 1981 Induction of ovulation in patients with normoprolactinemic amenorrhea by combined treatment with bromocriptine and clomiphene. Fertil Steril 35: 138

Kokia E, Bider D, Lunenfeld B, Blankstein J, Mashiach S, Ben-Rafael Z 1990 Addition of exogenous estrogens to improve cervical mucus following clomiphene citrate medication. Acta Obstet Gynecol Scand 69: 139

Koligian K B, Stormshak F, 1977 Nuclear and cytoplasmic estrogen receptors in ovine endometrium during the estrous cycle. Endocrinology 101: 524

Koninckx P R, Heyns W J, Corvelyn P, Brosens I A 1978 Delayed onset of luteinization as a cause of infertility. Fertil Steril 29: 266

Kotsuji F, Saoo T, Kamitani N, Tominaga T, Kitaguchi M, Okamura Y 1988 The efficacy of every-other-day administration of gonadotropin-releasing hormone in women with hypothalamic amenorrhea: gonadotropin releasing hormone treatment can induce clomiphene responsiveness. Obstet Gynecol 17: 615

Kuhl H, Hock H, Taubert H-D 1977 Acute effects of low doses of clomiphene upon LH release in ovariectomized, estrogen-progesterone treated rats. Endocrinol Exp 11: 49–55.

Kupperman H S 1963 Human Endocrinology. Davis Philadelphia, pp 344–345

Landgren B M, Unden A L, Diczfalusy E, 1980 Hormonal profile of the cycle in 68 normally menstruating women. Acta Endocrinol 94: 89

Lappöhn R E, Bogelchelman D H 1989 The relation of fertility and ovarian histology after bilateral wedge-resection. Fertil Steril 52: 221

Laufer N, Reich R, Braw R, Shenker J G, Tsafiri A 1982 Effect of clomiphene citrate on preovulatory rat follicles in culture. Biol Reprod 27: 463

Lepoutre L, Dhont M, van der Kerckhove D 1973 LH and progesterone in the menstrual cycle. Further observations on the relationship with the length of the luteal phase. Ann Endocrinol 34: 327

Lisse K 1980 Kombinierte Clomiphen-Dexamethason-Therapie bei Clomiphen-Resistenz. Zentralbl Gynäkol 102: 645

Lobo R A, Granger L R, Davajan V, Mishell D R 1982a An extended regimen of clomiphene citrate in women unresponsive to standard therapy. Fertil Steril 37: 762

Lobo R A, Gysler M, March C M, Goebelsmann U, Mishell D R 1982b Clinical and laboratory predictors of clomiphene response. Fertil Steril 37: 168

Louvet J P, Harman S M, Schreiber J R, Ross G T 1975 Evidence of a role of androgen in follicular maturation. Endocrinology 97: 366

March C M, Israel R, Mishell D R 1976a Pregnancy following 29 cycles of clomiphene citrate therapy: a case report. Am J Obstet Gynecol 124: 209

March C M, Tredway D R, Mishell D R, 1976b Effect of clomiphene citrate upon amount and duration of human menopausal gonadotropin therapy. Am J Obstet Gynecol 125: 699

Marchbanks P A, Coulam C B, Annegers J F 1985 An association between clomiphene citrate and ectopic pregnancy: a preliminary report. Fertil Steril 44: 268

Markaverich B M, Williams M, Upchurch S, Clark J H 1981 Heterogeneity of nuclear estrogen-binding sites in the rat uterus: a simple method for the quantitation of Type I and Type II sites by ($^3$H) estradiol exchange. Endocrinology 109: 62

Markiewicz L, Laufer N, Gurpide E 1988 In vitro effects of clomiphene citrate on human endometrium. Fertil Steril 50: 772

Marshall J C, Fraser T R 1971 Amenorrhoea in anorexia nervosa: assessment and treatment with clomiphene citrate Br Med J 1: 590

Marss R P, Vargyas J M, Shangold G M, Ylee B 1984 The effect of time of initiation of clomiphene citrate on multiple follicle development for human in vitro fertilization and embryo replacement procedures. Fertil Steril 41: 682

Martinez A R, Bernardus R E, Voorhorst F J 1990 Intrauterine insemination does and clomiphene citrate does not improve fecundity in couples with infertility due to male or idiopathic factors: a prospective, randomized, controlled study. Fertil Steril 53: 847

Marut E L, Hodgen G D 1982 Antiestrogenic action of high-dose of clomiphene in primates: pituitary augmentation but ovarian attenuation. Fertil Steril 38: 100

Matsumoto S 1973 Use of cyclofenil (sexovid) to induce ovulation. Int J Fertil 18: 209

McDonough P G, Tho P T, Byrd J R 1978 Evaluation of reproductive failure in 101 couples. 30 Fertil Steril 30 (suppl): 720 (abstr)

McGuire W L, de la Garza M, 1973 Similarity of the oestrogen receptor in human and rat mammary carcinoma. J Clin Endocrinol Metab 36: 548

McNatty K P 1977 Prolactin and ovarian steroidogenesis. Acta Endocrinol Suppl 212: S21

McNatty K P, Baird D T 1978 Relationship between follicle-stimulating hormone, androstendione and oestradiol in human follicular fluid. J Endocrinol 76: 527

Meckies J, Leo-Rossberg I, Felhart R, Moltz L, Hammerstein J 1976 Behandlung steriler Frauen mit Epimestrol: Erfahrungsbericht über 143 Patientinnen mit 30 Graviditäten. Dtsch Med Wochenschr 47: 1711

Merell 1972 Merell National Laboratories Product Information Bulletin.

Mikkelson T J, Kroboth P D, Cameron W J, Dittert L W, Chungi W, Manberg P J 1986 Single-dose pharmacokinetics of clomiphene citrate in normal volunteers. Fertil Steril 4: 392

Miyake A, Aono T, Minnagawa J, Kawamura Y, Kurachi K 1980 Changes in plasma LH-RH during clomiphene-induced ovulatory cycles. Fertil Steril 34: 172

Möslein-Rossmeissl S, Baumann R, Rücker K, Taubert H-D 1989 Nachweis von Spermatozoen in der Peritonealflüssingkeit nach intrauteriner Insemination. Fertil Steril 5: 68

Moggi G, Giampietro O, Chisci R, Brunori I, Simonini N 1979 Pregnancy induction after bromocriptine-cyclofenil treatment in some normoprolactinemic anovulatory women. Fertil Steril 32: 289

Moghissi K S 1976 Accuracy of basal body temperature for ovulation detection. Fertil Steril 27: 1415

Molloy B G, Hancock K W, Glass M R, 1985 Ovulation reduction in clomiphene nonresponsive patients: the place of pulsatile gonadotropin-releasing-hormone in clinical practice. Fertil Steril 43: 26

Morris J M, van Wagenem G, 1973 Interception: The use of postovulatory estrogens to prevent implantation. Am J Obstet Gynecol 115: 101

Mühlenstedt D, Bohnet H G, Hanker J P, Schneider H P G 1978 Short luteal phase and prolactin. Int J Fertil 23: 213

Mühlenstedt D, Meissner M, Schneider H P G 1979 Prolactin and luteal phase defect. Geburtshilfe Frauenheilkd 39: 580

Murray D L, Reich L, Adashi E Y 1989 Oral clomiphene citrate and vaginal progesterone suppositories in the treatment of luteal phase dysfunction: a comparative study. Fertil Steril 51: 35

Neale C, Bettendorf G, Treu F 1970 Clinical studies of bis-(p-acetoxyphenyl)-cyclohexylidenemethane (Sexovid) and on 6-chloro-9β, 10α–pregna-1,4,6-triene-3,20-dione (Ro 48347). Bull Schweiz Akad Med Wiss 25: 545

Nelson L M, Hershlag A, Kurl R S, Hall J L, Stillman R J 1990 Clomiphene citrate directly impairs endometrial receptivity in the mouse. Fertil Steril 53: 727

Nillius S J, Johansson E D B 1971 Plasma level of progesterone after vaginal, rectal or intramuscular administration of progesterone. Am J Obstet Gynecol 110: 470

Nocke W 1979 Verursacht die Gabe von Östrogenen und/oder Gestagenen in der Frühschwangerschaft congenitale Mißbildungen? Endokrinol Information 1: 11

O'Herlihy C, Pepperell R J, Brown J B, Smith M A, Sandri L, McBain J C 1981 Incremental clomiphene therapy: A new method for treating persistent anovulation. Obstet Gynecol 58: 535

O'Herlihy C, Pepperell F J, Robinson M 1982 Ultrasound timing of HCG administration in clomiphene-stimulated cycles. Obstet Gynecol 59: 40

Olsson J-H, Granberg S, 1990 Effect of clomiphene isomers on oestradiol synthesis in cultured human granulosa cells. Hum Reprod 5: 928

Perloff W H, Smith K D, Steinberger E 1965 Effect of prednisone on female infertility. Int J Fertil 10: 31

Persson B H 1965 Clinical effect of bis-(acetoxyphenyl)-cyclohexlidene-methane (Compound F 6066) on menstrual disorders. Acta Soc Med Ups 70: 71

Phansey S A, Barnes M A, Williamson H O, Segel J, Nair R M G 1980 Combined use of clomiphene and intranasal luteinizing-hormone releasing-hormone for induction of ovulation in chronically anovulatory women. Fertil Steril 34: 448

Plymate S R, Farriss B L, Bassett M L 1981 Obesity and its role in polycystic ovary syndrome. J Clin Endcrinol Metab 52: 1246

Porcile A, Gallardo E, Venegas E 1990 Normoprolactinemic anovulation nonresponsive to clomiphene citrate: ovulation induction with bromocriptine. Fertil Steril 53: 50

Prough S G, Aksel S, Yeoman R 1990 Luteinizing hormone bioactivity and variable responses to clomiphene citrate in chronic anovulation. Fertil Steril 54: 799

Quigley M M, Collins R L, Blankstein J 1988 Pure follicle stimulating hormone does not enhance follicular recruitment in clomiphene citrate/gonadotropin combinations. Fertil Steril 50: 562

Radwanska E, McGarrigle H H, Little V, Lawrence D, Sarris S, Swyer G I M 1979 Induction of ovulation in women with hyperprolactinemic amenorrhea using clomiphene and hCG or bromocriptine. Fertil Steril 32: 187

Remordiga V, Venturini P L, Anserini P, Lanera P, De Cecco L 1989 Administration of pure follicle-stimulating hormone during gonadotropin-releasing hormone agonist therapy in patients with clomiphene-resistant polycystic ovarian disease: hormonal evaluation and clinical perspectives. Am J Obstet Gynecol 160: 108

Richards J S, Ireland J J, Rao M C, Bernath G A, Midgley A R, Reichert L E 1976 Ovarian follicular development in the rat: hormone receptor regulation by estradiol, follicle stimulating hormone and luteinizing hormone. Endocrinology 99: 1562

Rifka S M, Pita J C, Vigersky R A, Wilson Y A, Loriaux D L 1978 Interaction of digitalis and spironolactone with human steroid receptors. J Clin Endocrinol Metab 46: 338

Riley G M 1960 Gynecologic endocrinology. P B Hoeber, New York, p 117

Robertson S, Birrell W, Grant A 1977 Fewer multiple pregnancies using clomiphene/human gonadotropin sequence. Fertil Steril 28: 294 (abstr)

Robertson D W, Katzenellenbogen J A, Long D J, Rorke E A, Katzenellenbogen B S 1982 Tamoxifen antiestrogens. A comparison of the activity, pharmacokinetics, and metabolic activation of the cis and trans isomers of tamoxifen. J Steroid Biochem 16: 1

Rodriguez-Rigau L J, Smith K D, Tcholakian R K, Steinberger E 1979a Effect of prednisone on plasma testosterone levels and on duration of phases of the menstrual cycle in hyperandrogenic women. Fertil Steril 32: 408

Rodriguez-Rigau L J, Steinberger E, Atkins B J, Lucci J A 1979b Effect of testosterone on human corpus luteum steroidogenesis in vitro. Fertil Steril 31: 448

Rönnberg L, Passoja A 1986 Sex ratio and male clomiphene treatment (Letter to the Editor). Fertil Steril 46: 1171

Ron-El R, Soffer Y, Langer R, Herman A, Weintraub Z, Caspi E 1989 Low multiple pregnancy rate in combined clomiphene citrate human menopausal gonadotropin treatment for ovulation induction or enhancement. Hum Reprod 4: 495

Rose L I, Underwood R T, Newmark S R, Risch E S, Williams G H 1977 Pathophysiology of spironolactone-induced gynecomastia. Ann Intern Med 87: 398

Rose G L, Dowsett M, Mudge J E, White J O, Jeffcoate S L 1988 The inhibitory effects of danazol, danazol metabolites, gestrinone, and testosterone on the growth of human endometrial cells in vivo. Fertil Steril 49: 224

Rosenberg S M, Luciano A A, Riddick D H 1980 The luteal phase defect: the relative frequency of, and encouraging response to, treatment with vaginal progesterone. Fertil Steril 34: 17

Ross G T 1976 On intraovarian control of oogenesis in the human. In: Crosignani P G, Mishell D R, (eds) Ovulation in the human. Academic, London, pp 127–140

Rothchild I, 1983 Pathophysiology of the inadequate corpus luteum. In: H-D Taubert H-D, Kuhl H (eds) The inadequate luteal phase. MTP, Lancaster, pp 21–31

Ruiz-Velasco V, Rosas-Arceo J, Matute M M 1979 Chemical inducers of ovulation: comparative results. Int J Fertil 24: 61

Rust L A, Israel R, Mishell D R 1974 An individualized graduated therapeutic regimen for clomiphene citrate. Am J Obstet Gynecol 120: 785

Sas M, Resch B 1973 Der Schwangerschaftsverlauf nach Epimestrol-induzierten Ovulationen. Geburtshilfe Frauenheilkd 33: 506

Saunders D M, Hunter J C, Haase H R, Wilson G R 1979 Treatment of luteal phase inadequacy with bromocriptine, Obstet Gynecol 53: 287

Saure A, Karjalainen O, Tervävainen T, 1975 Effect of synthetic gestagen on progesterone formation in the human corpus luteum in early pregnancy. Acta Endocrinol Suppl 199: 161

Schenker J G, Yarkoni S, Granat M 1981 Multiple pregnancies following induction of ovulation. Fertil Steril 35: 105

Schmidt-Elmendorff H, Kämmerling R 1977 Vergleichende klinische Untersuchungen von Clomiphen, Cyclofenil und Epimestrol. Geburtshilfe Frauenheilkd 37: 531

Schulz-Amling W, Abraham R, Taubert H-D 1973 Untersuchungen über den Wirkungsmechanismus von Clomifen: Hemmung der Östradiolaufnahme in Hypothalamus und Hypophyse, Arch Gynäkol 214: 125

Schumert Z, Spitz E, Diamant Y Z, Polyshuk W Z, Rabinowith D 1975 Elevation of serum testosterone in ovarian hyperstimulation. J Clin Endocrinol Metab 40: 889

Schwartz U, Sörensen R, Moltz L 1981 Long term effects of oral contraceptive and glucocorticoid suppression of ovarian and adrenal vein steroids in normal women. Acta Endocrinol Suppl 243: 264

Senior B E, Cawood L M, Oakley R E, Mc Kiddie J M, Siddle D R 1978 A comparison of the effects of clomiphene and tamoxifen treatment on the concentrations of oestradiol and progesterone in the peripheral plasma of infertile women. Clin Endocrinol 8: 381

Seppälä M, Hirvonen E, Ranta R 1976 Hyperprolactinemia and luteal insufficiency. Lancet i: 229

Shapiro G, Evron S 1980 A novel use of spironolactone: treatment of hirsutism. J Clin Endocrinol Metab 51: 429

Sharf M, Graff G, Kuzminsky T 1971 Combined therapy
  with quinestrol and clomiphene in functional sterility.
  Obstet Gynecol 37: 260
Shepard M K, Balmceda J P, Leija C G 1979 Relationship of
  weight to successful induction of ovulation with clomiphene
  citrate. Fertil Steril 32: 641
Sherman B M, Korenman S G 1975 Hormonal characteristics
  of the human menstrual cycle throughout reproductive life.
  J Clin Invest 55: 699
Shoham Z, Lidor A, Lunenfeld B 1989 The assessment of a
  cycle with clomiphene as an indicator for further treatment.
  J Endocrinol Invest 12: 9
Smith G V, Kistner R W 1963 Action of MER-25 and of
  clomiphene on the human ovary. JAMA 184: 878
Soules M R, Wiebe R H, Aksel S, Hammond C B 1977 The
  diagnosis and therapy of luteal phase deficiency. Fertil
  Steril 28: 1033
Soules M, Hughes C L jr, Aksel S, Tyrey L, Hammond C B
  1981 The function of the corpus luteum of pregnancy in
  ovulatory dysfunction and luteal phase deficiency. Fertil
  Steril 36: 31
Soutone J H, Jallatte S-S, 1972 Le cyclofenil en pratique
  gynécologique. Rev Fr Gynecol 67: 343
Sowers J R, Rice B F, Blanchard S 1979 Effect of
  dexamethasone on LH and FSH response to LH-RH and
  to clomiphene in the follicular phase of women with normal
  menstrual cycles. Horm Metab Res 11: 478
Stähler E, Sturm G, Daume E, 1975 Einwirkung von
  Clomiphen auf das Ovar, untersucht am in vitro
  perfundierten menschlichen Ovar. Arch Gynäkol 219: 585
Steinberger E, Smith K D, Tcholakian R K, Rodriguez-Rigau
  L J 1979 Testosterone levels in female partners of infertile
  couples. Am J Obstet Gynecol 133: 133
Strigini F, Collins W P, Whitehead W I, Melis G B, Fioretti
  P, Campbell S 1986 Hormone excretion during early
  pregnancy following spontaneous and clomiphene citrate-
  induced ovulation. Fertil Steril 46: 209
Strott C A, Cargille C M, Ross G T, Lippsett M B 1970 The
  short luteal phase. J Clin Endocrinol Metab 30: 246
Sutaria U T, Crooke A C, Bertrand P V, Hodgson C 1980
  Clomiphene and human chorionic gonadotropin in the
  treatment of anovulatory infertility. Int J Gynaecol Obstet
  18: 435
Sutherland R L 1981 Estrogen antagonists in chick oviduct:
  antagonist activity of eight synthetic triphenylethylene
  derivatives and their interaction with cytoplasms and
  nuclear estrogen receptor. Endocrinology 109: 2061
Swyer G I M 1965 Clomiphene. In: Austin C R, Perry J A
  (eds) Biology Council Symposium on aspects affecting
  fertility, 1965. Churchill, London, pp 180–190.
Swyer G I M, Radwanska E, McGarrigle H H G 1975 Plasma
  oestradiol and progesterone estimation for the monitoring
  of induction of ovulation with clomiphene and chorionic
  gonadotrophin. Br J Obstet Gynaecol 82: 794
Taubert H D 1978 Luteal phase insufficiency. In: Keller P J
  (ed) Contributions to gynecology & obstetrics, vol IV.
  Karger, Basel, p 108
Taubert H D, Dericks-Tan J S E 1976a Induction of
  ovulation by clomiphene citrate in combination with high
  doses of estrogens or nasal application of LH-RH. In:
  Crosigniani P G, Mishell D R Jr (eds) Ovulation in the
  human. Academic, London, pp 265–273
Taubert H D, Dericks-Tan J S E, 1976b High doses of
  estrogens do not interfere with the ovulation-inducing effect
  of clomiphene citrate. Fertil Steril 27: 375

Taubert H D, Jürgensen O 1969 The treatment of
  monophasic cycles with the retroprogesterone RO 4 8347.
  Bull Schweiz Akad Med Wiss 25: 503
Taubert H D, Jürgensen O 1972 Behandlung der
  anovulatorischen Sterilität mit Clomiphen. Zentralbl
  Gynäkol 94: 1043
Taubert H D, Jürgensen O, Becker H 1969 Clinical
  observations on luteal phase insufficiency. Bull Schweiz
  Akad Med Wiss 25: 586
Taymor M L, Berger M J, Nudemberg F 1973 The combined
  use of clomiphene citrate and human menopausal
  gonadotropin in ovulation induction. In: Haregana T,
  Hayashi M, Ebling F J G, Henderson I W (eds) Fertility
  and sterility, Proceedings of the VIIth World Congress,
  Tokyo Kyoto. Excerpta Medica, Amsterdam, Int Congr
  Series 278, p 658.
Telimaa S 1988 Danazol and medroxyprogesterone acetate
  inefficacious in the treatment of infertility in endometriosis.
  Fertil Steril 50: 872
Templeton A A, Mortimer D 1980 Laparoscopic sperm
  recovery in infertile women. Br J Obstet Gynaecol 87: 1128
Testart J, Castanier M, Feinstein M C, Frydman R, 1990
  Pituitary and steroid hormones in the preovulatory follicle
  during spontaneous or stimulated cycles. In: Rolland R, van
  Hall E V, Hillier S G et al (eds) Follicular maturation and
  ovulation. Excerpta Medica, Amsterdam, pp 193–201
Toaff T, Toaff M F, Gould S, Chayen R 1978 Role of
  androgenic hyperactivity in anovulation. Fertil Steril
  29: 407
Tsai C C, Yen S S C 1971 The effect of ethynyl estradiol
  administration during early follicular phase of the cycle on
  the gonadotropin level and ovarian function. J Clin
  Endocrinol Metab 33: 917
Turksoy R N, Biller B J, Farber M, Cetrulo C, Mitchell G W
  1982 Ovulatory response to clomiphene citrate during
  bromocriptine-failed ovulation in amenorrhea-galactorrhea
  and hyperprolactinemia. Fertil Steril 37: 441
Ulrich U, Nehmzow M, Krause B, Göretzlehner G 1990
  Ovulation induktion durch Clomifenkonversion. Zentralbl
  Gynäkol 112: 501
Vaitukaitis J L, Bermudez J A, Cargille C M, Lippsett M B,
  Ross G T 1971 New evidence for an anti-estrogenic action
  of clomiphene citrate in women. J Clin Endocrinol Metab
  32: 503
Vandenberg G, Yen S S C 1973 Effect of anti-estrogenic
  action of clomiphene during the menstrual cycle: evidence
  for a change in the feedback sensitivity. J Clin Endocrinol
  Metab 37: 356
van der Kerckhove D, Dhont M 1972 The relationship
  between plasma LH levels, as determined by RIA, and the
  life-span of the corpus luteum. Ann Endocrinol 33: 205
van Hall E V, Mastboom J L 1969 Luteal phase insufficiency
  in patients treated with clomiphene. Am J Obstet Gynecol
  103: 165
Vanrell J A, Balasch J, Fuster J S, Fuster R 1982 Ovulation
  stigma in fertile women. Fertil Steril 37: 712
Vargyas J M, Marrs R P O, Kletzky O A, Mishell D R 1982
  Correlation of ultrasonic measurement of ovarian follicle
  size and serum estradiol levels in ovulatory patients
  following clomiphene citrate for in vitro fertilization. Am J
  Obstet Gynecol 144: 569
Villalobos H, Canales E S, Velazquez N, Zarate A, Soria J
  1975 Assessment of the therapeutic effect of epimestrol
  associated with clomiphene in female sterility. Int J Fertil
  20: 41

Weichman B M, Notides A C 1980 Estrogen receptor activation and the dissociation kinetics of estradiol, estriol and estrone. Endocrinology 106: 434

Weise W, Shönijahn A, Prügel P 1982a Behandlungsergebnisse bei funktioneller weiblicher Sterilität. I. Mitteilung: Kombinierte Östrogen-Gestagen Therapie. Zentralbl Gynäkol 104: 2

Weise W, Honza A, Prügel P 1982b Behandlungsergebnisse bei funktioneller weiblicher Sterilität. II. Mitteilung: Clomiphentherapie. Zentralbl Gynäkol 104: 9

Wentz A C 1980 Progesterone therapy of the inadequate luteal phase. In: Givens J R (ed) Clinical use of sex steroids. Year Book Medical Publisher, Chicago pp 189–210

Wentz A C, Garcia S C, Kingensmith G J, Migeon C, Jones G S 1976 Gonadotropin output and response to LH-RH administration in congenital adrenal hyperplasia. J Clin Endocrinol Metab 42: 239

Wentz A C, Kossoy L R, Parker R A 1990 The impact on luteal phase inadequacy in an infertile population. Am J Obstet Gynecol 162: 937

Wernicke K, Jürgensen O, Maischein M, Halberstadt E, Taubert H D, 1975 Schwangerschafts- und Geburtsverlauf bei erfolgreich behandelten Sterilitätspatientinnen. Arch Gynäkol 219: 295

Whitelaw M J, Kalman C F, Grams L R 1970 The significance of the high ovulation rate versus the low pregnancy rate with clomid. Am J Obstet Gynecol 107: 865

WHO 1973 Agents stimulating gonadal function in the human. Technical report no 154. WHO, Geneva, pp 15–19

Williams R F, Hodgen G D 1980 Disparate effects of human chorionic gonadotropins during the late follicular phase in monkeys: normal ovulation, follicular atresia, ovarian acyclicity and hypersecretion of follicle-stimulating hormone. Fertil Steril 33: 64

Williamson J G, Ellis J D 1973 The induction of ovulation by tamoxifen. J Obstet Gynaecol Br Cwlth 80: 844

Witten B I, Martin S A 1985 The endometrial biopsy as a guide to the management of luteal phase defect. Fertil Steril 44: 460

Wu C 1977 Plasma hormones in clomiphene citrate therapy. Obstet Gynecol 49: 443

Wu C, Winkel C A 1989 The effect of therapy initiation day on clomiphene citrate therapy. Fertil Steril 52: 564

Yamamoto K R, Alberts B 1974 On the specificity of the binding of the estradiol receptor protein to deoxyribonucleic acid. J Biol Chem 249: 7076

Yeko T R, Khan-Dawood F S, Dawood M Y 1990 Luteinizing hormone and human chorionic gonadotropin receptors in human corpora lutea from clomiphene citrate-induced cycles. Fertil Steril 54: 601

Yen S S C, Tsai C C 1972 Acute gonadotropin release induced by exogenous estradiol during the mid-follicular phase of menstrual cycle. J Clin Endocrinol Metab 34: 298

Yen S S C, Vela P, Ryan K J 1970 Effect of clomiphene citrate in polycystic ovary syndrome: relationship between serum gonadotropin and corpus luteum function. J Clin Endocrinol Metab 31: 7

Yoshimura Y, Hosoi Y, Atlas S J, Wallach E D 1986 Effect of clomiphene citrate on in vitro ovulated ova. Fertil Steril 45: 800

Yoshimura Y, Hosoi Y, Atlas S J, Dharmajaran A M, Adashi T, Wallach E D 1988 Effect of the exposure of intrafollicular oocytes to clomiphene citrate on pregnancy outcome in the rabbit. Fertil Steril 50: 153

Younger J B, Boots L R, Coleman C 1978 The use of a one-day luteinizing hormone assay for timing of artificial insemination in infertility patients. Fertil Steril 30: 648

Zhuang L Z, Adashi E Y, Hsueh J W 1982 Direct enhancement of gonadotropin-stimulated ovarian estrogen biosynthesis by estrogen and clomiphene citrate. Endocrinology 110: 2219

# 19. Reconstructive tubal surgery in the female

*Victor Gomel    Patrick Taylor*

## INTRODUCTION

For the successful establishment of human pregnancy in vivo the gametes must meet within the ampulla of the fallopian tube. Peritubal or periovarian adhesive disease may inhibit oocyte pick up and tubal occlusion, due to either pathological processes or surgical interruption following sterilization, will effectively preclude the fusion of the sperm and oocyte. Until the advent of in vitro fertilization (IVF) and embryo transfer in the human (Steptoe & Edwards 1978), surgical repair of the damaged oviducts offered the only realistic hope of pregnancy in women suffering from tubal and/or peritoneal lesions. The use of traditional reconstructive techniques yielded disappointingly low success rates (Gomel 1980a).

Swolin (1975) used magnification and a technique designed to minimize surgical trauma in the peritoneal cavity, in the correction of distal tubal occlusion. Despite reduction of postoperative adhesions and the improved tubal patency rates yielded by the application of microsurgical principles, the rate of viable pregnancy was not significantly better than that obtained by conventional methods. Microsurgery has found its optimal application in tubal anastomosis where magnification enables proper alignment of the tubal segments and precise apposition of the tissue planes with fine inert suture material. Magnification also permits the observation of subtle morphological details enhancing the recognition of tubal abnormalities even in the presence of patency. Microsurgery allowed the introduction of tubo-cornual anastomosis for the treatment of proximal tubal occlusion (Gomel 1974, 1977a).

Tubal reconstructive microsurgery became an integral part of infertility practice. The assimilation of microsurgical principles into gynecology made gynecologists much more conscious of the effects of peritoneal trauma and postoperative adhesions. It fostered a conservative approach to interventions for benign pelvic disease in women wishing to preserve fertility (Gomel 1980a, 1983a).

It is the purpose of this chapter to discuss basic microsurgical principles, the instruments used, and the application of magnification. While the general investigation of the infertile couple, which is no less relevant in cases of tubal infertility, will not be described in detail, those investigations pertaining to the tubes and pelvic peritoneum will receive due attention. Since the early days of microsurgery a broader spectrum of therapeutic options has become available. These options and their selection will be discussed. As this chapter specifically addresses the subject of microsurgery, the procedures that should be performed using these techniques will be described in detail. The place of adjuvant therapy, and the postoperative management of these patients will be considered.

## BASIC PRINCIPLES OF TUBAL MICROSURGERY

There is nothing mystical about the use of an operating microscope. It will not miraculously transform the clumsy surgeon into a virtuoso. Microsurgery, as in any other discipline, requires training and the application of certain fundamental principles, which can be mastered by most competent gynecologists. Furthermore, these principles designed to reduce tissue trauma can be used in routine gynecological surgery.

The term 'pelvic courtesy' encompasses all that the microsurgeon should strive to achieve. This courtesy is displayed by showing a profound respect for the tissues, by reducing trauma to a minimum, obtaining meticulous pinpoint hemostasis, and using delicate instruments and fine inert sutures.

The microscope: (1) permits identification of abnormal morphological changes, and thus enables, when necessary, complete excision of the affected tissues; (2) facilitates fine tissue dissection using microscissors or electrosurgery with a microelectrode that also enables precise hemostasis to be achieved; (3) enables precise approximation of tissue planes with the accurate placement of the fine microsutures (Gomel 1978a). The microscope is not used, as some less respectful junior staff have suggested, simply so that the senior surgeon with failing eyesight can find the operative field.

The pelvic peritoneum is exquisitely susceptible to the effects of trauma, responding with an intense inflammatory reaction, the end result of which will be adhesion formation. Trauma can be caused by any insult, be it chemical, thermal, abrasive or bacterial. The surgeon must avoid introducing any foreign material into the peritoneal cavity. Gloves must be washed free of any powder prior to making the incision. Abdominal packs should be of a nonabrasive material and soaked in Ringer's lactate (Ringer's irrigation USP) or heparinized Ringer's lactate solution before they are used. Tissue handling should be gentle and performed with wet gloved fingers or Teflon-coated rods. Where the use of forceps is unavoidable they should be of a special design. Because swabbing causes tissue abrasion it is replaced by irrigation. Hemostasis is obtained electrosurgically using a 100 μ insulated electrode with a pointed tip. Bleeding points are exposed under a jet of irrigation and precisely electrocoagulated, avoiding significant damage to adjacent areas (Gomel 1977b).

Fibrinogen is contained in inflammatory exudate, and in the serum. Once converted into fibrin it adheres to traumatized surfaces forming a matrix upon which fibroblast proliferation can occur. This is the basis of adhesion formation. Peritoneal surfaces may be damaged due to the desiccation caused by exposure to the operating room atmosphere and surgical lights. This can largely be prevented if the tissues are kept moistened by constant irrigation with Ringer's lactate solution. Addition of 5000 units of heparin to each litre of the Ringer's lactate (irrigation solution) will also reduce clot formation and facilitate the removal of clots and fibrin from the peritoneal cavity at the end of the procedure (Gomel 1978a).

In summary, reducing trauma to a minimum, irrigation, meticulous hemostasis, accurate tissue approximation with fine inert sutures and the use of delicate instruments are the basic principles of microsurgical technique. Magnification, best obtained with an operating microscope that also provides coaxial lighting, facilitates the application of these principles.

## The instruments

A very large selection of instruments is available to the microsurgeon. Few are required for successful performance of most procedures. Indeed the less cluttered the instrument tray, the more smoothly will the surgery proceed. The following will provide a short description of those instruments that we have found to be most valuable.

Teflon-coated rods of two lengths and configuration, one of which has a cylindrical and the other a conical tip, are invaluable for retraction and elevation of adhesions. They can be used as protective backstops over which adhesions can be divided by electrosurgery and while performing a fimbrioplasty or salpingostomy. It should be added that although some surgeons favor the laser, there is no evidence to date that its use facilitates the procedure or yields any better results than electrosurgery. Also, the equipment for performing electrosurgery is much cheaper and more readily available.

The Valley Lab (Force II) electrosurgical generator (Valley Lab, Boulder, CO, USA), which is standard equipment in most operating rooms, is suitable for all microsurgical work. It delivers pure cutting, pure coagulating, or blended currents at steady low levels. We usually employ blended current for transection and pure coagulating current to achieve hemostasis. Although our preference is to carry out the whole procedure using an insulated microelectrode, referred to earlier, microbipolar jewellers forceps are available to coagulate larger individual vessels. The microelectrode is mounted in an insulated, hand-held pencil grip. A rocker switch mounted on this handle allows delivery of current in either a cutting or coagulating mode. When the Valley Lab unit is set to the 'blend' mode, it will deliver blended current when 'cut' is depressed, and pure coagulating current when 'coag' is activated.

Microscissors, both toothed and plain platform microforceps, and a microneedle holder will be required (Fig. 19.1). In addition, straight scissors of a similar configuration to the iris scissors used in ophthalmology are necessary. They are used primarily for transecting the tube. The forceps should possess rounded tips. The shafts should be designed so that they, like the scissors and needle holder, can be comfortably grasped like a pen between the dominant thumb and two forefingers. The toothed forceps should be used only to steady tissue which will be excised, or occasionally the muscular layer of the tube. The nontoothed are used to grasp gently or retract the serosa or tissue which will remain after the operation has been concluded. Strong toothed forceps, such as the St Martin-Gomel* forceps, permit grasping of larger or firmer tissue that requires excision, as is the case with the excison of a tubal segment in either tubo-tubal or tubo-cornual anastomosis.

The needle holder also has a blunt tip. Sharp points can inadvertently tear tissue. We prefer a configuration where the inside surface of one jaw is concave while the other is convex. This provides a more secure grasp and facilitates positioning the needle in the holder.

Irrigation can be provided using an intravenous catheter connected to a standard intravenous line. A fingertip-controlled device (Gomel irrigator) inserted between the catheter and the line is commercially available and provides more accurate irrigation. A stainless steel collar at the distal end can be slid up or down over the barrel, thus stopping or starting the flow of fluid.

Finally attention should be paid to the microsutures and the needles upon which they are swaged. Unless there are specific reasons to use nonabsorbable sutures, synthetic absorbable ones are to be preferred. To keep needle trauma to a minimum the needles should be of a fine tapercut pattern. Although fine sutures will give the best results, there is no need to use ones smaller than 8-0 calibre mounted on a 130-$\mu$m 4-mm or 5-mm tapercut needle (available from Ethicon Inc., Somerville, NJ, USA). This is the optimal suture for most gynecological microsurgical procedures.

## Magnification

Magnification can be provided by the use of loupes or from an operating microscope. Loupes, which can be mounted on spectacle frames or on a head band, will provide focal distances ranging from 20-40 cm (8-16 in). Magnifications vary from 2× to 8×. It is difficult to work with loupes that provide greater magnification than 4×. While loupes are certainly cheaper than a microscope, they are only suitable for use in short simple procedures and for dividing adhesions which are deep within the pelvis. Maintaining one's head at a fixed distance from the operative field can be tiring in the extreme.

The operating microscopes are versatile, and provide excellent magnification and coaxial illumination. Magnifications range from 2× to 40× and fields of view from 5 mm to 100 mm. An objective lens with a focal length of 275 mm is available which is ideal for use during operative gynecological procedures. Microscopes may be floor, wall or ceiling mounted. Focusing and zoom capabilities may be manual or motorized and controlled with foot pedals. Many are equipped with beam splitters which permit the fitting of two pairs of binocular eyepieces so that the surgeon and the assistant can simultaneously observe the procedure. A miniature television camera may also be fitted to a beam splitter enabling the operating room personnel to follow the surgery, and video recordings of the procedure to be made.

This section has discussed the technical

---

* All of the microsurgical instruments described here are available from Martin, Tuttlingen, Germany.

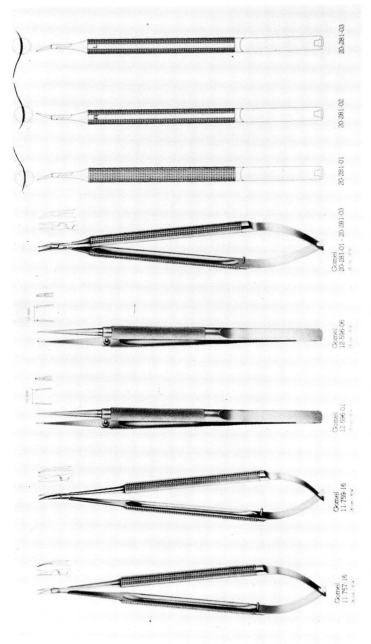

**Fig. 19.1**   Basic microsurgical instruments: Scissors, plain and toothed forceps, needle holder.

principles of gynecological microsurgery. The mark of a good surgeon is not knowing how to operate, but when to operate, and it is to the latter issue that attention will now be directed.

## INVESTIGATION AND SELECTION OF THE APPROPRIATE THERAPEUTIC OPTION

In all branches of medicine it is a mistake to divorce the purely technical considerations from the needs of the patients. This is particularly true when the desired outcome, the birth of a healthy child, cannot be assured, as in the case of an infertile couple or a woman requesting reversal of a previously performed tubal sterilization. It is incumbent upon the physician who is caring for such patients to establish a plan of investigation and management where the probable outcomes and options are accurately described so that patients can become actively involved in the decision-making process. If, despite all reasonable efforts, the couple remain childless, they are much more likely to achieve some degree of resolution of this conflict if they are satisfied that they have been able to exert a great degree of control over the events leading to this unfortunate conclusion.

For the couple in whom infertility is due to tuboperitoneal causes, or to a previously performed sterilization, there are only two realistic options by which pregnancy may be achieved: tubal reconstruction or IVF. To complicate issues further, microsurgery is no longer the only method by which tubal reconstruction can be effected. Laparoscopically directed tubal reparative surgery, or tubal cannulation, may offer alternative avenues of approach. Neither surgical attempts to effect tubal repair nor IVF should be regarded as competitors, but rather as complementary options towards achieving the desired goal. It is the purpose of this section to suggest how both nontechnical and purely technical considerations will influence the choice of treatment.

### Non-technical considerations

Irrespective of the nature of the tubal damage,

three other factors must be taken into consideration:

- Cost
- The age of the woman
- The wishes of the couple.

The influence of cost should not be underestimated, and will depend largely upon whether or not a given service is insured in the country in which the couple live. In Canada, for example, the health care service in most provinces will pay for any tubal reparative procedure if the lesion is 'natural', but will not subsidize reversal of a previous sterilization, or IVF. The impact of these sorts of financial constraints upon decision making can be very important.

The age of the woman is critical. Multivariate analysis (Collins & Rowe 1989) has identified this single factor as one of the most important determinants of outcome in all cases of infertility. In simple terms, the older the woman, once she has passed her thirtieth birthday, the poorer the results. This effect becomes most noticeable once she enters her fifth decade. A 'take home baby rate' of 45% has been reported in women of 40 years of age or more following reversal of sterilization (Trimbos-Kemper 1990). This is considerably less than that noted in women who are younger.

When the results of IVF are examined, the impact is even more noticeable. Between ages 40 and 41 a take home baby rate of 8.3% per oocyte recovery is reported. This falls to 2.4% thereafter (FIVNAT 1990). At first sight it might seem reasonable to perform tubal repair (unless contraindicated) as the initial treatment, reserving IVF as the court of last appeal for those in whom the repair has not resulted in a pregnancy. This is usually the case in younger women. After age 38, given the rapid rate of decay in the success rate per single cycle of IVF, an argument can be sustained for considering IVF first. Those who do not conceive may still wish to consider tubal surgery given the fact that this approach should offer multiple cycles during which conception may occur.

It is now becoming clear that opportunities to conceive can be improved in the older woman if donor oocytes taken from a younger woman are used (Abdalla et al 1990). This subject is beyond the scope of this chapter.

In every instance the wishes of the individual couple must be paramount. The final decision will rest with them, and will be influenced by their perception of the facts and their own internal value system. This does not mean that the physician's own value system is not worthy of respect. The responsible doctor will not accede to requests to perform treatment with essentially no likelihood of success.

If the couple's decision is to be influenced by their perception of the facts, it is incumbent upon the physician to provide them with information which is as accurate as humanly possible. This should be based on a clear understanding of the technical considerations which allow rational choices to be made between treatment options (Gomel & Taylor 1992). A discussion of these technical considerations follows.

**Technical considerations**

There are circumstances where any form of tubal repair is contraindicated and IVF represents the only therapeutic option. Absent tubes, prior tuberculous salpingitis, tubal damage of such severity as to render surgery impossible, and tubal disease coincident with another important infertility factor (Gomel 1978a, 1983b) are obvious examples. In other situations tubal reconstruction will offer the best chance of success. For these patients a logical sequence of treatment might be tubal repair followed by IVF if the former proves to be unsuccessful.

Deciding upon the proper course of action involves a critical appraisal of both IVF and tubal reparative procedures within the context of the situation of each couple. This information can only be provided after a thorough investigation (Gomel & James 1990).

Outcomes following IVF can be discussed. The most important figures are the take home baby rate after one cycle of IVF and the cumulative rates after repeated cycles. As the optimum number of IVF cycles is unknown, it would seem reasonable to discuss the cumulative pregnancy rate after four cycles, a number of attempts which

will usually strain the financial resources of all but the most affluent. The effect of frozen embryo replacement upon the cumulative pregnancy rates must be taken into account. The potential complications of the procedure and the multiple pregnancy, abortion and ectopic pregnancy rates must also be considered. This is the information which will help the couple to make logical choices when similar information with respect to tubal reparative procedures, in their particular case, is presented. Such figures with respect to both IVF and tubal repair should reflect the local experience, which may be better or worse than that reported by other centres. For the sake of this discussion, internationally reported data will be used, although in a somewhat modified form.

Most registries report all relevant rates based upon those cycles in which oocytes were recovered. While this is an excellent form of scientific communication, it does not provide an individual couple with the answer to their question 'What are our chances of taking a baby home if we decide to undergo one or more cycles of IVF?' The material that follows reflects rates calculated upon cycles initiated and includes those that did not go to oocyte recovery.

Medical Research International (1991) has reported the collected USA results for 1989. The delivery rate per oocyte pickup cycle (OPU) was 14%, but 15.5% of cycles were cancelled prior to OPU. Thus the delivery rate per cycle initiated was 11.8%. The pregnancy rate remains fairly constant in successive cycles (Cohen 1991). This suggests that if the American figures are used a cumulative delivery rate of 40% might be expected after four cycles. A small further increase in the success rate can be achieved if excess embryos are cryopreserved. The net effect is small. Not all cycles yield sufficient embryos nor do all embryos survive the freezing and thawing process. Those that do survive and are replaced yield a clinical pregnancy rate of 11% and a delivery rate of 8% (Medical Research International 1991).

IVF, particularly in stimulated cycles, is not without risk. Ovarian hyperstimulation syndrome, infection and bleeding can occur. Triplets or higher order multiple pregnancies account for 4%

of deliveries. The twin pregnancy rate is approximately 20%. Premature delivery and delivery of babies of low birth weight are natural consequences of these multiple gestations. Perinatal mortality is just less than 10%. The abortion rate of IVF pregnancies lies between 20% and 25%, and 6% of clinical pregnancies will be ectopic. Regrettably in the very patients, those with tubal disease, who must choose between tubal surgery and IVF, ectopic pregnancy can occur in as many as 12% of conceptions which follow IVF (Zouves et al 1991). When choosing, the couple can use this information to compare with the potential risks and benefits of tubal repair.

The overall risks of tubal reparative procedures, be they carried out by laparotomy, laparoscopy or tubal cannulation techniques, are small and include the recognized complications common to any surgical or anesthetic intervention. Furthermore, procedures via laparoscopy are carried out on a day-care basis and those via laparotomy are admitted to hospital for 1 day (they are discharged on the first postoperative day). If anatomically successful, such approaches offer multiple cycles during which conception can occur, and the opportunity to have more than one pregnancy. The abortion and multiple pregnancy rates in those patients who conceive do not differ from those of the normal population. The live birth and ectopic pregnancy rates are dependent upon the specific nature of the tubal disease and the extent of tubal damage. Both of these factors can only be evaluated after the completion of suitable investigations.

## Investigation

Whether the couple is complaining of infertility, or requesting reversal of a previously performed tubal sterilization, attention should be paid to all other factors which might prejudice the outcome. The investigation of fertility potential and of tuboperitoneal factors are dealt with elsewhere in this book and will not be described in detail here. Suffice to say that the findings may have an important impact upon the selection of treatment. Evidence of severe seminal abnormalities or defects of ovulation would tilt the scales in favour of IVF, even though in the case of seminal

defects the results of IVF will be less satisfactory.

Hysterosalpingography and laparoscopy are complementary methods in the investigation of tubal and peritoneal factors. Hysterosalpingography should be the initial investigation, by this method any uterine abnormalities can be identified, although their exact nature may need to be clarified by hysteroscopy and/or laparoscopy. Cornual occlusion and nonocclusive proximal tubal lesions can be detected. The presence of distal tubal occlusion and the condition of the tubal endothelium can be evaluated (Gomel 1978a, 1983c). The information yielded by hysterosalpingography is important during the subsequent laparoscopy if reparative procedures are undertaken. It also assists the surgeon in booking an appropriate length of operating-room time for the laparoscopy.

In cases of reversal of sterilization, attention to the history and examination of the previous operative report and, where available, the pathology report should provide information regarding the status of the tubes at the time of the procedure, and the reversal potential. Hysterosalpingography will provide information about the uterine cavity and the proximal tubal segments. Those women who were sterilized with clips or rings and whose tubes were normal at the time of the procedure will be excellent candidates for repair and would require only hysterosalpingography as further investigation. If it is unclear how the previous procedure was performed, and, particularly in women sterilized by electrosurgical means, evaluation of the tubes should include both hysterosalpingography and laparoscopy (Gomel 1983c). Thirty per cent of such patients for whom the previous operative report suggested a good prognosis were found to have irreparable tubes (Taylor & Leader 1982).

Corrective surgery can be performed laparoscopically in many instances (see Ch. 10). Prior knowledge that tubal disease exists will allow the surgeon to book an adequate amount of time to carry out such procedures. In addition, secure in the knowledge that the uterine cavity, cornua and intratubal architecture are normal, the surgeon who discovers unsuspected periadnexal disease and/or tubal phimosis at the time of laparoscopy can proceed with laparoscopic salpingo-ovariolysis and tuboplasty with confidence (Gomel & Taylor 1986). Before leaving the subject of the hysterosalpingography, it is worth repeating that while a properly performed tubal X-ray can be invaluable, one that has been poorly carried out is of little use to either the physician or the patient.

Hysterosalpingography has its limitations. It is not a very sensitive tool in the diagnosis of periadnexal adhesive disease. While it will identify the proximal segments of previously interrupted tubes, it gives no information about the all-important distal segment. Finally, the false-positive rate of diagnosis of proximal occlusion is high.

The final evaluation of the tubes must always be carried out laparoscopically with the exception of those previously sterilized patients described earlier in this section. Details of the performance of the laparoscopic survey have been discussed in Chapter 10.

## Selection

Once the nature of the tubal disease and degree of tubal damage have been identified, the most appropriate approach must be selected. The outcome of tubal reconstruction will in part depend on attributes over which the surgeon can exert some degree of control, and in part on the inherent properties of the cases which were operated upon.

The skill of the surgeon is of major importance. The first procedure performed is the one most likely to be successful. Selection of cases will greatly influence cumulative pregnancy rates. If difficult cases have not been attempted, apparently excellent results will accrue. Classification of the cases also rests with the reporting surgeon. They must be classified on the basis of the adnexa with least damage. Finally, cases lost to follow-up must be reported as 'not pregnant', otherwise the results will have an erroneously favorable skew.

Inherent to the individual cases are: (1) the nature and extent of the pelvic adhesions, (2) the severity and extent of the disease process affecting the tube, (3) the extent of tubal damage, (4) the final length of the reconstructed oviduct, (5) the presence or absence of additional pelvic disease,

and (6) the concurrent presence of other factors which might prejudice fertility (Gomel 1980b,c, Gomel & Swolin 1980). These caveats must be borne in mind when reviewing any published series. This section will discuss the outcome of surgical treatment of specific tubal lesions.

### Periadnexal adhesive disease and fimbrial phimosis

Periadnexal adhesive disease may exist alone or in conjunction with tubal occlusion. If it is the sole lesion laparoscopic salpingoovariolysis should be performed at the time of the diagnostic laparoscopy. In these circumstances the live birth rate will be approximately 50-60% within 24 months. Five per cent of these patients will experience an ectopic pregnancy.

On occasion, although complete distal occlusion does not exist, the fimbria are agglutinated or prefimbrial fimosis will be noted. Laparoscopically performed fimbrioplasty should give a live birth rate of 40-48% with no change in the rate of ectopic pregnancy (Gomel 1975, 1983e,f, Bruhat et al 1983, Fayez 1983, Dubuisson et al 1990).

### Distal tubal occlusion

Distal tubal occlusion almost always is accompanied by periadnexal adhesive disease. It can be treated laparoscopically or by formal microsurgical means. Live birth rates following microsurgical salpingostomy range from 19%-35% (Table 19.1), and ectopic pregnancy rates from 5% to 18% (Swolin 1975, Gomel 1978b, 1980b, 1983g, Gomel & Swolin 1980, Larsson 1982, Verhoeven et al 1983, Tulandi & Vilos 1985, Boer-Meisel et al 1986, Donnez & Casanas-Roux 1986a, Kosasa & Hale 1988). Satisfactory results can be achieved laparoscopically (Gomel 1977c, Daniell & Herbert 1984, Dubuisson et al 1990, Canis et al 1991, McComb & Paleoulogou 1991). The factors which will affect the outcome of salpingostomy include: the distal tubal diameter, large hydrosalpinges being associated with a worse prognosis; the nature of the tubal endothelium at the neostomy site; the extent of periadnexal adhesions; and the type of the adhesions. A

**Table 19.1**  Results of microsurgical salpingostomy

| Reference | Patients | Intrauterine pregnancy | Viable births | | Ectopic pregnancy |
|---|---|---|---|---|---|
| | (no.) | (no.) | No | % | (no.) |
| Swolin 1975* | 33 | 9 | 8 | 24 | 6 |
| Gomel 1978b† | 41 | 12 | 11 | 26.8 | 5 |
| Gomel 1980b† | 72 | 22 | 21 | 29.2 | 7 |
| Larsson 1982‡ | 54 | 21 | 17 | 31.5 | 0 |
| Verhoeven et al 1983 | 143§ | 34 | 28 | 19.6 | 3 |
| Tulandi & Vilos 1985 | 67‖ | 15 | NS | | 3 |
| Boer-Meisel et al 1986 | 108 | 31 | 24 | 22.2 | 19 |
| Donnez & Casanas-Roux 1986a | 83 | 26 | NS | | 6 |
| Kosasa & Hale 1988 | 93 | 37 | 34 | 36.6 | 13 |

NS = not stated.
* Long term follow-up.
† Follow-up period more than 1 year.
‡ Follow-up period more than 4 years.
§ Twenty-three of these were iterative procedures, among which only three (13%) had live births.
‖ Thirty-seven of these procedures were performed using $CO_2$ laser.

scoring system has been developed which permits the surgeon to predict the probable outcome with reasonable accuracy (Gomel 1988).

Patients whose adnexa produce a poor score should be discouraged from undergoing surgery and encouraged to consider IVF. In those deemed to have a favorable outlook, salpingostomy can be carried out at the time of the diagnostic laparoscopy. Only in a few cases today will laparotomy and microsurgical repair be indicated.

*Proximal occlusion*

The diagnosis of proximal occlusion is fraught with pitfalls. Patent tubes may be present despite positive findings at the time of both hysterosalpingography and laparoscopy. Selective salpingography and fallopian tube cannulation can be carried under hysteroscopic or ultrasonographic guidance (Jansen & Anderson 1987) and may serve to clarify the situation. Reports are now appearing describing treatment of proximal tubal obstruction using transcervically introduced catheters (Platia & Krudy 1985, Confino et al 1986, Daniell & Miller 1987). Simpson (1991) has reviewed this subject in detail. Postprocedure patency rates of 70-90% have been reported, and among those in whom at least one tube remains open, pregnancy rates of 30-50% can occur.

Since obstruction of the proximal tubal segment with viscous, jelly-like material has been reported (Gomel 1983h), it is likely that tubal cannulation may be dislodging such mucus plugs or breaking down cornual synechiae (Kerin et al 1991). Both selective salpingography and tubal cannulation can clarify the false-positive results observed at hysterosalpingography, usually poorly performed. In our center where hysterosalpingography is performed using a meticulous technique, selective salpingography and tubal cannulation have not yielded the success rates that have been reported in the literature. This is confirmed in a recent report by Letterie & Sakas (1991). Selective salpingography and tubal cannulation may overcome spasm or inspissated mucus which might have resolved spontaneously. Unfortunately no randomized studies have appeared comparing this approach with simple expectancy. Until such research is completed it is reasonable to attempt tubal cannulation in cornual occlusion as an initial therapeutic measure. Almost invariably when true pathological occlusion exists at the cornua, as in extensive postinflammatory fibrosis, salpingitis isthmica nodosa and endometriosis of the tube, and tubal cannulation fails, IVF or microsurgery are the only remaining options.

Microsurgical correction of these true causes of proximal occlusion can yield live birth rates of between 37% and 58% and ectopic pregnancy rates of between 5% and 7% (Gomel 1977a, 1980b, 1983i, McComb & Gomel 1980, Donnez & Casanas-Roux 1986b, McComb 1986). It would seem that microsurgery would offer a better chance of success than IVF.

### Previous sterilization

Laparoscopic techniques by which to repair previously interrupted tubes are under development. Presently microsurgical repair still offers the best chance of success. Live birth rates of 60-80% can be achieved provided that the reconstructed tube is longer than 4 cm, of which the distal ampulla must be more than 1 cm (Gomel 1977a, 1978a, 1980b, 1980c, 1983j, Winston 1980, DeCherney et al 1983, Silber & Cohen 1984, Paterson 1985, Boeckx et al 1986, Spivak et al 1986, Rock et al 1987, Pei Xue and Yuen-Yu 1989, Putman et al 1990). Tubal pregnancy rates are usually low (Table 19.2). Clearly, in most cases of prior sterilization, microsurgical repair would be the primary approach as it offers an excellent chance of success (Gomel & James 1990).

If a fimbriectomy has been performed, live birth rates of approximately 30% can be achieved

provided that at least 50% of the ampulla has been preserved (Gomel 1983k).

### Unusual circumstances

There is no place, now that IVF is readily available, for repeated attempts to repair pathologically damaged tubes. If the first salpingostomy has been unsuccessful it is highly improbable that a second attempt will succeed. If there is obstruction at both the proximal and distal ends of the tube the results of combined salpingostomy and cornual anastomosis are sufficiently disappointing to suggest that IVF should be the treatment of choice.

If a reversal of sterilization has failed because of demonstrable reocclusion, then if sufficient healthy tube remains and the patient is willing to undergo a second anastomosis the outcome in these cases should be gratifying.

While the number of choices facing the couple with tubal infertility or requesting reversal of a previous tubal sterilization appear to be confusing, attention to both the nontechnical factors and those technical factors described in this section should permit most couples to make informed choices. In this way their best chances of a successful outcome can be assured, and for

**Table 19.2**   Results of microsurgical tubo-tubal anastomosis for reversal of sterilization

| Reference | Patients (no.) | Intrauterine pregnancy (no.) | Viable births | | Ectopic pregnancy (no.) |
|---|---|---|---|---|---|
| | | | no. | % | |
| Gomel 1974 | 11 | | 8 | 73 | 1 |
| Gomel 1980c | 118 | | 76 | 64 | 1 |
| Winston 1980 | 105 | 63 | NS | | 3 |
| Gomel* 1983j | 118 | | 93 | 79 | 2 |
| DeCherney et al †1983 | 124 | | 72 | 58 | 8 |
| Silber & Cohen ‡ 1984 | 48 | | 31 | 66 | 2 |
| Henderson 1984 | 95 | | 51 | 54 | 5 |
| Paterson 1985 | 147 | | 87 | 59 | 5 |
| Spivak et al § 1986 | 68 | | 34 | 51 | 6 |
| Boeckx et al 1986 | 63 | 44 | NS | | 3 |
| Rock et al 1987 | 80 | | 49 | 61 | 10 |
| Pei Xue & Yuen-Yu ‖ 1989 | 117 | | 95 | 81 | 2 |
| Putman et al 1990 | 86 | 64 | 55 | 64 | |

NS = not stated.
*   Resurvey of 1980 series; follow-up period more than 18 months.
†  Follow-up period more than 18 months.
‡  Follow-up period more than 4 years.
§  Follow-up period more than 1 year.
‖  Follow-up period more than 3.5 years.

those who do not conceive their active involvement in the decision-making process may help to ease their inevitable disappointment.

It is clear that in correctly selected cases microsurgery still has an important role to play. The next section will describe specific microsurgical procedures in detail.

## IMMEDIATE PREOPERATIVE PREPARATION AND ABDOMINAL INCISION

Although the operating room staff are highly trained professionals, it is to the surgeon's advantage to ensure that all is in readiness prior to the arrival of the patient in the operating room. The microsurgical instrument set should be reviewed with the scrub nurse to ensure that all the necessary pieces of equipment are present and that those with moving parts are functioning properly. The availability of other auxilliary surgical equipment including the proper electrosurgical unit should be noted. The microscope should be examined to confirm that all the moving parts do so, that the illumination system is working, and that any video equipment is set up and functioning smoothly.

Once the patient is brought into the operating room, placed on the operating table and anaesthetized, a Foley catheter is inserted into the bladder and a paediatric Foley catheter introduced into the uterus through which intraoperative chromopertubation is performed. So that this can be achieved smoothly the patient is placed in the frog-leg position. The usual aseptic precautions are observed. The cervix is exposed with a speculum and grasped with a tenaculum. A number 8 or 10 Foley catheter is passed into the uterine cavity with the aid of uterine packing forceps, and the balloon is inflated. A sterile extension tube is connected to the catheter and to a 20-ml syringe containing a dilute methylene blue solution. The patient's legs are extended.

The abdomen is washed and draped and the syringe placed on top of the drapes so as to be easily accessible to the surgeon or assistant. Prior to commencing the procedure the scrubbed operating room personnel must wash their gloves free of powder and wipe them. The abdominal incision is made, a wound protector introduced, and a self-retaining retractor (Dennis-Brown) applied. The bowel is packed off with nonabrasive swabs which have been soaked in the irrigation solution. The patient is placed in 10 degrees of Trendelenburg position. When necessary, the table may be tilted 10–15 degrees towards the surgeon. While the microscope may be draped, we have not found this to be necessary, particularly if it is remote controlled. The microscope is swung into position and focused. Finally the surgeon, assistant and scrub nurse ensure that they are comfortably seated.

### Abdominal incision

We have been performing tubal reconstructive procedures via laparotomy using a small (minilaparotomy) incision. The length of the incision is determined on the basis of the prior findings. The subcutaneous fascia is infiltrated with 0.25% bupivacaine (Marcaine) solution and the incision is made. Prior to incising the fascia, the rectus muscles are also infiltrated with the same solution. This procedure is repeated prior to abdominal closure. A transverse suprapubic skin incision is made; the subcutaneous fat is dissected upwards and downwards over the fascia which is incised vertically in the midline. The recti are separated in the midline and the peritoneum is also incised vertically. The small incision and infiltration with local anesthetic reduces postoperative discomfort and analgesic requirements; it permits prompt mobilization and discharge from hospital on the first postoperative day. This approach also markedly reduces the postoperative recovery period.

## SURGICAL TECHNIQUE

The following procedures may be performed microsurgically:

- Tubo-tubal anastomosis for reversal of sterilization
- Tubo-cornual anastomosis to repair proximal tubal disease

- Tubo-tubal anastomosis to repair mid-tubal disease
- Repair of distal tubal occlusion or phimosis
- Salpingo-ovariolysis
- Unusual procedures.

A detailed description of each follows.

## Tubo-tubal anastomosis to repair a previous sterilization

Simply stated, repair of a previous sterilization is achieved by excising the occluded portions of both the distal and proximal tubal remnants until healthy tissue is identified (Fig. 19.2). Once hemostasis has been secured, anastomosis is performed in a way to achieve proper alignment of the tubal segments and precise apposition of the lumina.

The tube is not of uniform diameter (especially with regard to luminal calibre) and so the details of technique will vary somewhat depending upon the prior sterilization procedure which determines the type of anastomosis. Tubo-tubal anastomosis may be:

- Intramural–isthmic
- Intramural–ampullary
- Isthmic–isthmic
- Isthmic ampullary
- Ampullary–ampullary
- Ampullary–infundibular

Many of the steps of the procedure are the same. This section will address the steps which are shared, and will consider the variations necessary to deal with specific types of anastomosis.

An earlier section described opening the abdomen and placing the retractor. Once the pelvic organs have been exposed they are inspected. Any periadnexal adhesions are divided (as will be discussed when salpingo-ovariolysis is described). The uterus and adnexa are elevated by placing them on sponges previously soaked in the irrigation solution. Small sponges are placed to stabilize the tube to be repaired. The other adnex is covered with a wet sponge to prevent desiccation. The microscope head is swung into position.

The proximal tubal stump is distended by transcervical chromopertubation. The occluded distal end of the proximal tubal segment is grasped with a strong toothed forceps (St Martin-Gomel) and traction exerted. Using fine straight scissors the tube is transected from the antimesosalpingeal border, the incision being halted at the mesosalpinx thus avoiding the subtubal vascular arcade. Fluid will be seen to spurt from the lumen. The microelectrode is used to excise the occluded distal portion from the mesosalpinx. The transection line must remain close to the tube to avoid section of the vessels cited earlier. The tubal mucosa is examined to ensure that it is healthy. This examination is carried out at a magnification of 20× to 25×.

The tube is held gently between the thumb and forefinger, bleeders are exposed under a jet of irrigation fluid and hemostasis secured with the microelectrode. These tiny vessels are located between the serosa and the muscularis, and precise pinpoint hemostasis will not damage the tube. More significant vessels such as those that may be (inadvertently or by necessity) divided in the mesosalpinx may be electrocoagulated by the use of the bipolar jewellers forceps. Bleeding from the mucosa will stop spontaneously and should not be electrocoagulated for fear of adversely affecting future tubal function. Assuming no great disparity in diameter, the distal tubal segment is prepared in a similar fashion. Patency of this segment is confirmed by retrograde injection of irrigation solution.

The first approximating 8–0 suture is placed at 6 o'clock. Accurate placement of this suture in the muscularis is essential for proper alignment of the two segments of tube. The suture is inserted in such a way as to ensure that the knot is exterior. While in principle we have avoided inclusion of the mucosa, there are data to suggest that this is not essential (Pei Xue & Yuen-Yu, 1989). Depending on the tubal calibre at the site of anastomosis, three or more additional sutures are next placed to complete the first layer of the anastomosis. While three additional sutures placed at cardinal points are usually sufficient for an isthmic–isthmic anastomosis, more are needed in an ampullary–ampullary anastomosis. The additional sutures are placed three or four at a time as a continuous series of loops, including the muscularis and submucosa (or mucosa) of the

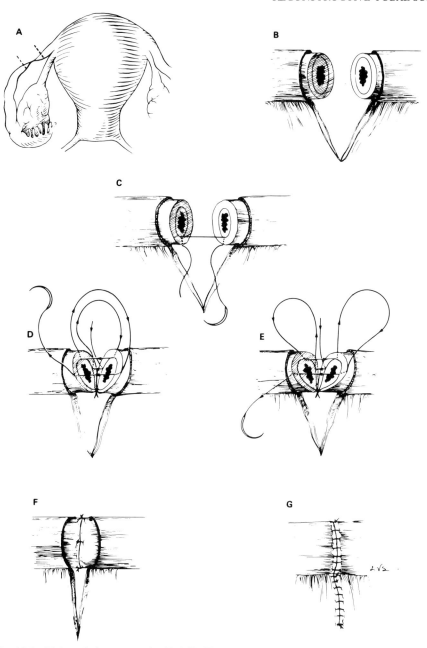

**Fig. 19.2** Tubo-tubal anastomosis: (**A & B**) The occluded ends of both proximal and distal segments of tube are excised; (**C**) The first suture (approximating muscularis and mucosa) is placed at 6 o'clock position; (**D & E**) Subsequent sutures are placed using a single strand of suture. Each suture is tied individually after division of the loop between successive sutures; (**F**) The muscularis and mucosa already approximated; (**G**) Approximation of the serosa and mesosalpinx complete the anastomosis. (From Gomel V, Rowe T C. Microsurgery in gynecology 1987. In: Current obstetrics and gynecologic diagnosis and treatment. Pernoll M L, Benson R C (Eds) Appleton & Lange, Norwalk Conn. With permission.)

two segments. This step is repeated ensuring appropriate distance between adjacent sutures.

The sutures are tied one at a time after the loop between two successive sutures has been divided.

Splinting of the lumen is not necessary and may cause endothelial damage. In our view splinting hinders rather than facilitates placement of sutures. The novice may stain the serosa with methylene blue or indigo carmine solution to accent visibility.

The serosa is joined with two continuous sutures, each beginning at the antimesosalpingeal border (12 o'clock position) of the tube. One of these sutures is run anteriorly and the other posteriorly. Finally the defect in the mesosalpinx is repaired with interrupted or continuous sutures. Chromopertubation should demonstrate tubal patency and a watertight anastomotic site.

These fundamentals will need to be varied depending upon the type of anastomosis.

*Intramural–isthmic anastomosis*

Even in the apparent absence of a proximal tubal segment, either a tiny portion of isthmus or at least the intramural portion will be available. The presence of short isthmic stumps may not be evident when they adhere to the uterus, as is frequently the case after electrocoagulation of the tubes. This is the result of desiccation and retraction of the adjacent mesosalpinx. Transcervical chromopertubation will erect the proximal tubal segments, the presence of which should be suspected from the prior hysterosalpingography, or, by distending the uterus, indicate the site where the intramural segment should be sought. Isthmic stumps adherent to the uterus can be freed by careful dissection that avoids transection of any significant vessels. In the absence of an isthmic stump, it is necessary to establish the precise site of the intramural segment. The sites of insertion into the uterus of the round and ovarian ligaments provide useful referral points which together with the distension of the uterus by transcervical chromopertubation point to the appropriate area of the cornual region which is dissected to identify the intramural segment. The muscularis of the intramural segment is dissected from the surrounding uterine muscularis for a millimeter or so and the tube transected, at which point the dilute dye solution should exit from the lumen. As the cornual area is very vascular, injection with a 30-gauge needle of 1.5–2 ml of dilute

vasopressin solution (10 units diluted in 60–100 ml of normal saline) may facilitate the procedure by significantly decreasing the oozing. The vasopressin solution is injected in a circular manner, 1 cm medial to the site of dissection, and under the serosa of the uterus. Once the tubal lumen has been identified it must be examined at high magnification to ensure that the tissues are healthy. The distal isthmic segment is prepared as previously described.

To reduce tension while performing the anastomosis, a stay suture of 7–0 or 8–0 Vicryl may be placed immediately below the tube approximating the mesosalpinx to the cornual region. The anastomosis is then performed as previously described. After the approximation of the inner layer (muscularis and mucosa), the serosa of the tube is approximated to the serosa and superficial muscle of the uterus. The defect in the mesosalpinx is repaired by joining the mesosalpinx to the serosa of the lateral edge of the uterus. Splinting of the lumen, which can cause endothelial damage, is not necessary, and in our view hinders rather than facilitates the placement of sutures.

*Intramural–ampullary anastomosis*

The intramural segment is prepared as described above. The proximal stump of the ampullary segment is exposed by a blunt probe which is gently introduced through the infundibular end of the tube, or simply by distending it with either irrigation fluid or dilute methylene blue solution introduced through the fimbriated end. The serosa over the tip of the stump is incised in a circular fashion and dissected free from the underlying muscularis using microscissors. A small incision is made over the tip of the ampullary stump to enter the lumen, and enlarged in such a fashion as to create an opening which will correspond in size to the lumen of the intramural portion. A two-layer anastornosis is then performed.

*Isthmic-isthmic anastomosis*

The technique for performing this type of repair, where the lumina are of comparable diameter, is that which was described as basic technique in the introductory paragraphs.

*Isthmic-ampullary anastomosis*

The isthmic stump is prepared as previously described. Inevitably there will be considerable disparity between the isthmic and ampullary lumina. Under most circumstances the proximal part of the ampullary stump will be occluded, but amenable to opening in the manner described above under intramural-ampullary anastomosis. If such is the case it will be possible to create a lumen which approximates that of the isthmic portion. While the muscularis of the ampulla is considerably thinner than that of the isthmus, this usually poses no problem in approximating the submucosa or mucosa and muscularis of the two segments. The serosa and mesosalpinx are then joined in the fashion which has been described.

The ampullary stump may be occluded by a suture or clip, the removal of which may lead to the creation of an opening into the ampullary lumen which is much larger than the isthmus and through which lush folds of mucosa will prolapse. The disparity can be partly overcome by enlarging the isthmic lumen. A 2-3 mm slit is made with scissors at its antimesosalpingeal border. The corners so created are partially excised. An ovoid opening will have been created. To approximate the first layer the 6 o'clock suture is inserted first and tied. Usually five additional sutures are required, and these are placed as described earlier. The 12 o'clock stitch incorporates the muscularis and submucosa of the ampulla to identical tissues of the isthmus at the apex of the slit. The procedure is completed by approximation of the serosa and mesosalpinx.

*Ampullary–ampullary anastomosis*

In this type of anastomosis the major difficulty to be overcome is the propensity of the ampullary mucosa to prolapse. While some authors advocate excision of these fronds (Winston 1980), we recommend against such an approach for fear of subsequent intratubal adhesion formation at this site. The folds can be replaced with pressure from the irrigating solution or with the tip of the nontoothed microforceps while tying the successive sutures of the first layer. The entire thickness of the muscularis, together with the mucosal edge (and not the mucosal fronds), is included in the primary layer of sutures. Because of the greater diameter of the ampulla, approximation of this layer will require many more interrupted sutures than in an isthmic-isthmic anastomosis.

## Tubo-cornual anastomosis to repair proximal disease

True cornual or proximal tubal occlusion may result from a number of pathological processes. Madlenat et al (1977) performed a histological evaluation on tissues excised from 131 cases. The following lesions were identified; salpingitis isthmica nodosa 45 (34%), endometriosis 25 (19%), inflammatory sclerosis 25 (19%), scarring sclerosis 17 (12.9%), ectopic gestation 6 (4.5%), tuberculosis 5 (3.5%), and in 8 (6.1%) no lesions were noted.

In cases of pathological occlusion, some healthy intramural tube is usually spared thus permitting the conservation, rarely of all and frequently of part, of the intramural segment. In a small percentage of cases the whole of the intramural segment is involved in the disease process. Fortunately in such cases microsurgery permits an anastomosis to be performed between the healthy portion of distal tube and the uterine tubal ostium (Fig. 19.3). The key to achieving a successful outcome is the excision of the affected portion of tube until healthy tissues are identified. To do so requires examination of the cut surface of the tube under magnifications of 20× to 25×.

Dilute pitressin solution is injected into the cornual region. This is done as previously described in a circular manner, 1 cm medial to the uterotubal junction, along the circumference of the cornua. The serosa and the muscularis of the uterus are incised at the level of the utero-tubal junction. Examination under high magnification permits evaluation of the status of the cut surface while concurrent transcervical chromopertubation permits assessment of tubal patency. If the intramural tube is found to be abnormal or occluded at this site the tubal muscularis is dissected from the surrounding uterine muscle for

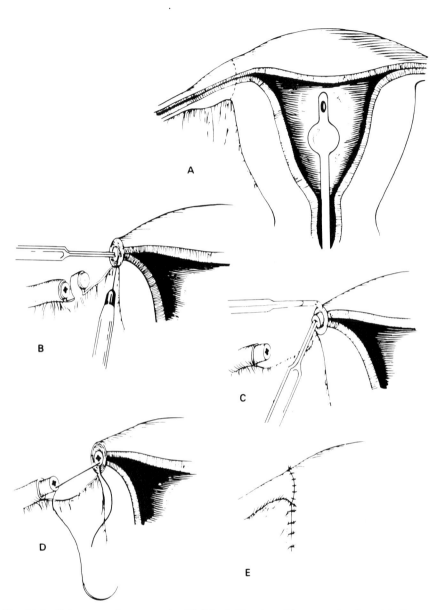

**Fig. 19.3**   Tubo-cornual anastomosis: (**A**) After infiltration of the cornual region with dilute vasopressin solution the tube is transected at the uterotubal junction; (**B**) The isthmus is serially transected until normal and patent tube is reached. The occluded portion of intramural tube is dissected from the surrounding uterine musculature and; (**C**) excised using a curved blade. The abnormal isthmic segment is excised; (**D**) The muscularis and mucosa of the two segments of tube are approximated with interrupted sutures the first of which is placed at 6 o'clock position; (**E**) The sero-muscularis of the cornu is approximated to the serosa of the isthmus, and the mesosalpinx is joined to the uterus. (From Gomel V, Rowe T C 1987 Microsurgery in Gynecology. In: Current obstetric and gynecologic diagnosis and treatment. Pernoll M L, Benson R C (Eds). Appleton & Lange, Norwalk Conn. With permission.)

a few millimetres (depending on the findings of the prior hysterosalpingography) towards the uterine cavity. The tube is then transected. If the tube is still occluded or appears abnormal, the intramural segment is dissected further, 1 mm at a time, and transected until patent and normal tube is reached. The dye solution will spurt from the open lumen. However, it is essential to scrutinize the cut surface at high magnification in order to detect any abnormalities.

The distal oviduct is prepared by making serial cuts over the isthmus starting at the utero-tubal junction until normal and patent tube is reached. This is accomplished with the iris-type scissors, stopping the incision each time just before the mesosalpinx. The abnormal tubal segments are excised from the mesosalpinx electrosurgically, avoiding the vessels that form the arcade beneath the tube.

The initial suture is placed at the 6 o'clock position and approximates the mucosa and muscularis of the two segments. The suture is held. Because of the cornual crater that results from the excision of a portion of intramural tube, tying the first suture would make the placement of the subsequent sutures difficult if not impossible. The subsequent sutures are placed using a continuous strand of suture as described before. The 6 o'clock suture is tied first. If there is tension, it is necessary to hold the distal tubal segment near the intramural segment while tying this suture. Alternatively a 7-0 Vicryl suture is placed just below the tube through the mesosalpinx and the lateral border of the uterus near the cornual crater. This suture is tied in order to reduce tension while tying the anastomotic sutures. After the approximation of the muscularis of the tube, the seromuscularis of the uterus is approximated to the serosa of the tube.

### Tubotubal anastomosis to repair mid tubal disease

Midtubal occlusion as a result of pathological reasons is rare. Such lesions include endometriosis, carneous moles (the end-result of some undiagnosed or expectantly treated tubal pregnancy) or congenital absence of a tubal segment. Another cause is tuberculosis which is not amenable to surgical repair (Gomel & Filmar 1987, Urman et al 1992). A tubal pregnancy treated by linear salpingotomy or with methotrexate may result in a tubal occlusion in the gestational implantation site and surgical treatment by segmental excision will leave the tube in two segments. In the case of the latter,

reconstruction is carried out in a manner similar to that used in reversal of sterilization (Gomel 1983l). Occlusions can be treated by excision of the diseased mid-portion of the tube, taking care to ensure that all the unhealthy tissue has been removed. Patency of the proximal and distal segments is confirmed as described before. Microsurgical anastomosis is then performed as described under reversal of sterilization for the specific type of anastomosis.

### Reconstructive surgery for distal tubal occlusion

Distal tubal occlusion is usually caused by pelvic inflammatory disease. Salpingitis may result in either partial (tubal phimosis) or complete (hydrosalpinx) distal tubal occlusion. Both conditions may be associated with varying degrees of periadnexal adhesive disease. In other instances the ovary, the tube (especially the fimbriated end) although patent, or both may be encapsulated by broad adhesions that obviate oocyte capture by the tube. Periadnexal disease in the presence of radiologically patent, relatively normal appearing tubes usually results from periadnexal infections. It may be reasonable to argue that if any of these conditions is not amenable to laparoscopic correction the patient should be advised to consider IVF seriously. While our primary approach to periadnexal disease and/or tubal phimosis has been laparoscopic salpingo-ovariolysis and fimbrioplasty, there may still be a place for microsurgical salpingostomy in selected cases.

Treatment of distal tubal occlusion (salpingo-ovariolysis, fimbrioplasty and salpingostomy) may be carried out laparoscopically. When performing such procedures it is imperative to observe the proven microsurgical tenets (Fig. 19.4). Operative laparoscopy for such conditions offers several advantages: corrective treatment may be carried out during the initial diagnostic laparoscopy without significantly increasing the morbidity of the procedure and irrespective of the presence of other infertility factors; when compared to laparotomy there is significantly reduced postoperative discomfort, hospital stay and recovery period. In addition, the reported results appear comparable and there may be savings in health-care costs.

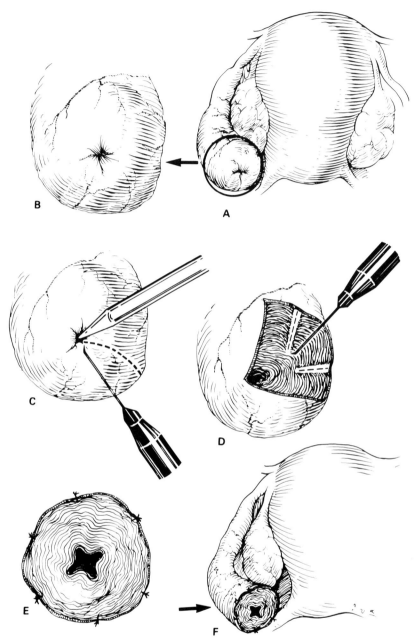

**Fig. 19.4**  Salpingostomy: (**A**) Salpingo-ovariolysis is completed first;
(**B**) Under magnification the distal end of the hydrosalpinx exhibits a series of
pale avascular lines that radiate from a central dimple; (**C**) The central point is
entered and the incision extended toward the ovary over an avascular line; (**D**)
Viewing the tube from within additional incisions are placed along the circumference
of the tube over avascular areas, between mucosal folds; (**E**) Once a satisfactory stoma
has been fashioned, the flaps are tacked back and secured to the ampullary sero-
musculosis; (**F**) The completed salpingostomy. (From Gomel V, Rowe T C 1987
Microsurgery in gynecology. In: Current obstetric and gynecologic diagnosis and
treatment. Pernoll M L, Benson R C (Eds). Appleton & Lange, Norwalk Conn. With
permission.)

The technique of laparoscopic salpingo-ovari-olysis, fimbrioplasty and salpingostomy and associated results have been discussed in Chapter 10 and will not be repeated here.

*Salpingo-ovariolysis*

Salpingo-ovariolysis is often an integral part of other microsurgical procedures. There are usually three steps in salpingo-ovariolysis: liberation of the adnexa, excision of the adhesions, and, occasionally, reperitonealization.

The adhesions must first be freed from their distal attachments to enable mobilization and elevation of the adnexa to permit accurate lysis at the level of the tube and ovary. Omentum and/or loops of bowel that are adherent to the pelvic organs are freed using sharp dissection. Bowel and omentum are displaced into the upper abdominal cavity and kept in place with abdominal pads soaked in the irrigation solution.

Loupes with a long focal length frequently offer greater flexibility than the microscope in permitting visualization of the distal insertion of adhesions deep within the pelvis. Adhesions are lysed at the level of their distal attachments. A long Teflon rod is placed behind the adhesion along the division line and elevated. Division is effected electrosurgically using a microelectrode on an elongating adaptor, or mechanically with fine long scissors. Any large vessels along the line of transection are electrocoagulated. It is very important that care is taken to avoid traumatizing or denuding the healthy parietal peritoneum. Once the adhesions are totally divided at their distal margin the adnexa becomes liberated from its attachments and may be elevated along with the uterus on packs soaked in the irrigation solution. Elevation of the adnexa permits the surgeon to carry out the remainder of the procedure more comfortably.

The microscope is now brought into place over the operative field and both the surgeon and assistant sit down for the remainder of the surgical procedure. Adhesions are now excised from their attachments to the adnexa. They are exposed, one layer at a time. Each is grasped with toothed forceps and put on the stretch to expose the demarcation line between adhesions and serosa or ovary. A fine Teflon rod placed under the incision line facilitates exposure. The area is irrigated and division effected with the microelectrode. Shallow adhesions between the tube and ovary or uterus are exposed and simply divided. Damage to the tubal serosa or ovarian surface may be avoided by keeping the transection line 1 mm away from these surfaces.

If defects have been made in the healthy serosa these denuded areas may be reperitonealized provided peritoneal edges can be brought together without tension. Depending on the size and the site of the defect, 6-0 to 8-0 gauge synthetic absorbable sutures are used. Although use of peritoneal grafts to cover large raw areas has been proposed, it is probable that such grafts tend to be avascular and may themselves predispose to further adhesion formation.

*Fimbrioplasty*

Partial distal occlusion may be due to agglutination of the fimbriae. In addition, the fimbriated end of the tube may be covered by fibrous tissue which requires incision or excision to allow access to the tubal tissues. In occasional circumstances the stenosis is at the level of the abdominal tubal ostium located at the apex of the infundibulum (prefimbrial phimosis). In the event of fimbrial agglutination reconstruction may be effected simply by introducing a closed mosquito forceps through the fimbriated end, opening the jaws within the tubal lumen, and gently withdrawing the instrument. This movement is repeated a few times varying the direction in which the jaws of the forceps are opened. Bleeding is usually negligible. If this simple procedure is ineffective it may be necessary to separate the fimbria mechanically or electrosurgically using a Teflon rod in the lumen as a backstop. One or two 8-0 sutures may need to be placed to maintain patency.

With prefimbrial phimosis the fimbria may appear normal; however, during chromopertubation, the ampullary portion of the tube will distend prior to any exit of dye solution. Our approach is to introduce a thin Teflon probe into the tube and place an incision at the antimesosalpingeal edge of the tube from the infundibulum, past the stenotic portion, to the distal ampulla. The edges of the two flaps thus created are folded back and secured to the adjacent ampullary serosa with absorbable 7-0 or 8-0 sutures. With all of these variations there may also be a significant degree of peritoneal adhesive disease which must be removed first.

*Salpingostomy*

Once salpingo-ovariolysis is complete the tubes are distended with dye by transcervical chromopertubation. When examined at magnification the distal end of the hydrosalpinx will be seen to demonstrate a series of pale avascular lines which radiate centrifugally from a central dimple. The microelectrode is used to make the first incision through this dimple. Dye will escape. An incision is made from the dimple along one of the avascular lines toward the ovary to fashion a fimbria ovarica. Once the tube has been opened in this fashion it is possible to view the tube from within and place further incisions in the avascular lines between large mucosal folds. These incisions made along the circumference of the tube lead to the creation of small flaps which are tacked back to the tubal serosa with a few interrupted 8-0 Vicryl sutures.

We have described earlier the prognostic factors in salpingostomy: tubal diameter, tubal wall thickness, percentage of the well-preserved mucosal folds and nature of adhesions (Gomel 1988). Once the distal tube has been opened, it is obviously possible to assess the status of the tubal endothelium at this site. It is also possible to assess the epithelium of the ampulla by performing tuboscopy. We have for several years routinely inspected the ampulla by using a hysteroscope during salpingostomy procedures. Once the initial opening into the tube is made, the hysteroscope is introduced with its sheath. The ampulla is examined while the tube is simultaneously distended with the irrigation solution.

*Salpingostomy for reversal of fimbriectomy*

A 'fimbriectomy' sterilization results in the removal of varying portions of distal Fallopian tube. A medioampullary salpingostomy may be recommended for restoration of fertility if at least one-half of the ampullary segment is present. This can be determined by hysterosalpingography. The procedure is similar to terminal salpingostomy. The tube is distended and entered at the occluded end. We usually employ electrosurgery using a microelectrode to perform the procedure. The initial incision is extended towards the ovary. Further incisions are made along the circumference of the tube between the folds while viewing the tube from within. The resulting flaps are tacked back with a few interrupted 7−0 or 8−0 sutures.

## Some unusual procedures

Rare sets of circumstances may be encountered which are amenable to microsurgical correction. A patient has on one side a healthy proximal segment of tube which is devoid of an ampullary-infundibular portion, whereas on the other side the opposite pertains. The problem is to construct one healthy tube from the remnants which are present on opposite sides of the pelvis. A single healthy tube may exist on the opposite side of the pelvis to the patient's only ovary. A healthy tube and ovary may be present on the contralateral side of a unicornuate uterus devoid of ipsilateral tube and ovary.

Plastic reconstruction of one functional tube from two contralateral remnants can be achieved by anastomosis of the two segments behind the uterus, maintaining the physiological relationship between infundibulum and ovary. In the presence of both ovaries, the utero-ovarian ligaments are first approximated with interrupted nonabsorbable 4-0 or 5-0 sutures. This brings the ovaries together and helps reduce tension with the subsequent tubal anastomosis. Shapiro & Haning (1979) have reported successful delivery following such a procedure.

When a single ovary exists on the opposite side from the patient's only tube, simple approximation of the fimbriated extremity of the tube to the ovary may be possible. The ovary is mobilized and the meso-ovarium is fixed to the posterior surface of the uterus with nonabsorbable sutures. The oviduct is mobilized and the mesosalpinx sutured to the posterior aspect of the uterus. The nonabsorbable sutures are placed on the mesosalpinx about 1 cm from the tube. This will effectively place the infundibulum in close proximity with the ovary. Alternatively the ovary may be transposed to the contralateral side with its vascular pedicle kept intact (Gomel 1983m).

In the face of a unicornuate uterus without an ipsilateral tube and ovary and a contralateral adnexa, the tube and ovary may be transposed preserving their vascular pedicle. An anastomosis can then be performed between the tube and intramural segment in the unicornuate uterus. We have reported such a case (Gomel & McComb 1985). The woman subsequently delivered three healthy children. There have been occasional reports of tubo-ovarian transposition since then, the most recent from Pabuccu et al (1991).

## CONCLUSIONS

The evolution of the management of tuboperitoneal causes of infertility has moved very rapidly in the past 20 years. A wide range of options is available, including tubal microsurgery, laparoscopic surgery and IVF. The decisions about which option to select as the primary approach must be based on an accurate evaluation of the fertility potential of the individual couple and the Fallopian tubes, ovaries and pelvic peritoneum.

Nontechnical considerations which include the cost, age of the woman, and above all the wishes of the couple must be factored into the decision-making process. The technical aspects of the risks, and pregnancy rates, including ectopic pregnancy rates, must be fully understood by both the surgeon and patients and should be based on local experience.

This chapter has discussed the basic principles of tubal microsurgery. The investigation and methods whereby therapeutic options may be chosen have been explored. The steps of each microsurgical procedure have been described in detail. Examination of the outcomes of tubal microsurgery leads to the conclusion that it still remains an integral part of the treatment of tubal infertility.

## REFERENCES

Abdalla H I, Barber R, Kirkland A et al 1990 A report on 100 cycles of oocyte donation; Factors affecting outcome. Hum Reprod 5: 352

Boeckx W, Gordts S, Buysse K, Brosens I 1986 Reversibility after female sterilization. Br J Obstet Gynecol 93: 839

Boer-Meisel M E, teVelda E R, Habbema J D F, Kardaum J W P F 1986 Predicting the pregnancy outcome in patients treated for hydrosalpinx: a prospective study. Fertil Steril 45: 23

Bruhat M A, Maage G, Manhes H, Soualhat et al 1983 Laparoscopy procedures to promote fertility ovariolysis and salpingolysis results to 93 selected cases. Acta Eur Fertil 14: 476

Canis M, Mage G, Pouly J L, Manhas H et al 1991. Laparoscopic distal tuboplasty: report of 87 cases and a 4 year experience. Fertil Steril 56: 616

Cohen J 1991 The efficiency and efficacy of IVF and GIFT. Hum Reprod 6: 613

Collins J A, Rowe T C 1989 Age of the female partner is a prognostic factor in unexplained infertility: a multicentre study. Fertil Steril 52: 15

Confino E, Friberg J, Gleicher N 1986 Transcervical balloon tuboplasty. Fertil Steril 46: 963

Daniell J, Herbert C M 1984 Laparoscopic salpingostomy utilizing the $CO_2$ laser. Fertil Steril 41: 558

Daniell J M F, Miller W 1987 Hysteroscopic correction of cornual occlusion with resultant term pregnancy. Fertil Steril 48: 490

DeCherney A H, Mezer H C, Naftolin F 1983 Analysis of failure of microsurgical anastomosis after midsegment, non-coagulation tubal ligation. Fertil Steril 39: 618

Donnez J, Casanas-Roux F 1986a Prognostic factors of fimbrial microsurgery. Fertil Steril 46: 200

Donnez J, Casanas-Roux F 1986b Prognostic factors influencing the pregnancy rate after microsurgical cornual anastomosis. Fertil Steril 46: 1089

Dubuisson J B, Borquet de Jolinere Aubriot F X et al 1990 Terminal tuboplasties by laparoscopy: 65 consecutive cases. Fertil Steril 54: 401

Fayez J A 1983 An assessment of the role of operative laparoscopy in tuboplasty. Fertil Steril 39: 476–479

FIVNAT 1990 et bilan general 1986–1989 Contr Fertil Sexual 18: 588

Gomel V 1974 Tubal reconstruction by microsurgery. Presented at the Eighth World Congress on Fertility and Sterility, November 3 to 9, 1974, Buenos Aires, Abstract 39

Gomel V 1975 Laparoscopic surgery in tubal infertility. Obstet Gynecol 46: 47

Gomel V 1977a Tubal reanastomosis by microsurgery. Fertil Steril 28: 59

Gomel V 1977b Reconstructive surgery of the oviduct. J Reprod Med 18: 181

Gomel V 1977c Salpingostomy by laparoscopy. J Reprod Med 18: 265

Gomel V 1978a Recent advances in surgical correction of tubal disease producing infertility. Curr Probl Obstet Gynecol 1: (10) 3–60

Gomel V 1978b Salpingostomy by microsurgery. Fertil Steril 29: 389

Gomel V 1980a The impact of microsurgery in gynecology. Clin Obstet Gynecol 23: 1301

Gomel V 1980b Clinical results of microsurgery in female infertility. In: Crosignani P G, Rubin B L (eds) Microsurgery. Academic, London pp 77–93

Gomel V 1980c Microsurgical reversal of sterilization: a reappraisal. Fertil Steril 33: 587

Gomel V 1983a An odyssey through the oviduct. Fertil Steril 39: 144

Gomel V 1983b Microsurgery in female infertility. Little, Brown & Co, Boston, pp 129–134

Gomel V 1983c Microsurgery in female infertility. Little, Brown & Co, Boston, pp 111–124

Gomel V 1983d Microsurgery in female infertility. Little, Brown & Co, Boston, pp 225–229

Gomel V 1983e Salpingo-ovariolysis by laparoscopy in infertility. Fertil Steril 34: 607

Gomel V 1983f Microsurgery in female infertility. Little, Brown & Co, Boston, pp 143–144

Gomel V 1983g Microsurgery in female infertility. Little, Brown & Co, Boston, pp 230–233

Gomel V 1983h Microsurgery in female infertility. Little, Brown & Co, Boston, pp 171–172

Gomel V 1983i Microsurgery in female infertility. Little, Brown & Co, Boston, pp 235–237

Gomel V 1983j Microsurgery in female infertility. Little, Brown & Co, Boston, pp 237–242

Gomel V 1983k Microsurgery in female infertility. Little, Brown & Co, Boston, p 233

Gomel V 1983l Microsurgery in female infertility. Little, Brown & Co, Boston, p 199

Gomel V 1983m Microsurgery in female infertility. Little, Brown & Co, Boston, p 214

Gomel V 1988 Distal tubal occlusion. Fertil Steril 49: 946

Gomel V, Filmar S 1987 Arrested tubal pregnancy. Fertil Steril 48: 1043

Gomel V, James C 1990 Restauration de la fertilite apres sterilisation tubaire anastomose tubo-tubaire contre fertilisation in vitro. Contracep Fertil Sexual 18: 439

Gomel V, McComb P 1985 Microsurgical transposition of the human fallopian tube and ovary with subsequent intrauterine pregnancy. Fertil Steril 43: 804

Gomel V, Swolin K 1980 Salpingostomy: microsurgical techniques and results. Clin Obstet Gynecol 23: 1243

Gomel V, Taylor P 1986 Endoscopy in the infertile patient. In: laparoscopy and hysteroscopy in gynaecological practice. Chicago, Year Book Medical, pp 75–94

Gomel V, Taylor P J 1992 Reconstructive microsurgery versus in vitro fertilization/JARGE, in press

Henderson S R 1984 The reversibility of female sterilization with the use of microsurgery: a report on 102 patients with more than one year of follow-up. Am J Obstet Gynecol 149: 57

Jansen R P S, Anderson J C 1987 Catheterization of the fallopian tubes from the vagina. Lancet ii: 309

Kerin J F, Surrey E S, Williams D B, Daykhovsky L, Grundfest W S 1991 Falloscopic observations of endotubal isthmic plugs as a cause of reversible obstruction and their histologic characterization. J Laparoendoscop Surg 1: 103

Kosasa T S, Hale R W 1988 Treatment of hydrosalpinx using a single incision eversion procedure. Int J Fertil 33: 319

Larsson B 1982 Late results of salpingostomy combined with salpingolysis and ovariolysis by electromicrosurgery in 54 women. Fertil Steril 37: 156

Letterie G S, Sakas E L 1991 Histology of proximal tubal obstruction in cases of unsuccessful tubal canalization. Fertil Steril 56: 831

McComb P 1986 Microsurgical tubocornual anastomosis for occlusive cornual disease: Reproductive results without the need for tubouterine implantation. Fertil Steril 46: 571

McComb P, Gomel V 1980 Cornual occlusion and its microsurgical reconstruction. Clin Obstet Gynecol 23: 1229

McComb P, Paleoulogou A 1991 The intussusception salpingostomy technique for the therapy of distal oviductal occlusion at laparoscopy. Obstet Gynecol 78: 443

Madlenat P, DeBrux J, Palmer R 1977 L'etologie des obstructions tubaires proximales et son role dans le pronostic des implantations. Gynecologie 28: 47

Medical Research International, Society for Assisted Reproductive Technology, The American Fertility Society 1991 In vitro fertilization-embryo transfer (IVF-ET) in the United States: 1989 results from the IVF-ET registry. Fertil Steril 55: 14

Pabaccu R, Ulgenalp I, Baser I, Orhon E, Dilek S 1991 Microsurgical transposition of the human fallopian tube. Gynecol Obstet Invest 31: 51

Paterson P J 1985 Factors influencing the success of microsurgical tuboplasty for sterilization. Clin Reprod Fertil 3: 57

Pei Xue, Yuen-Yu Fa 1989 Microsurgical reversal of female sterilization: long term follow-up of 117 cases. J Reprod Med 34: 451

Pernoll M L, Benson R C (eds) 1987 Microsurgery in gynecology. In: Current obstetric and gynecologic diagnosis and treatment, 6th edn. Appleton and Lange, Norwalk, CT, Ch 57

Platia M, Krudy A G 1985 Transvaginal fluoroscopic recanalization of a proximally occluded oviduct. Fertil Steril 44: 704

Putman J M, Holden A E C, Olive D L 1990 Pregnancy rates following tubal anastomosis: Pomeroy partial salpingectomy versus electrocautery. J Gynecol Surg 6: 173

Rock J A, Guznick D S, Katz E, Zacur H A, King T M 1987 Tubal anastomosis: pregnancy success following reversal of Falope ring or monopolar cautery sterilization. Fertil Steril 48: 13

Shapiro S S, Haning R V 1979 Tubal anastomosis of a fimbrial segment pedicle graft. Fertil Steril 32: 478

Silber S J, Cohen R 1984 Microsurgical reversal of tubal sterilization: factors affecting pregnancy rate, with long term follow-up. Obstet Gynecol 64: 679

Simpson C W 1991 Transcervical fallopian tube catheterization. J SOGC 13: 37

Spivak M M, Librach C L, Rosenthal D M 1986 Microsurgical reversal of sterilization: a six-year study. Am J Obstet Gynecol 154: 355

Steptoe P C Edwards R G 1978 Birth after reimplantation of a human embryo. Lancet ii: 366

Swolin K 1975 Electromicrosurgery and salpingostomy: long term results. Am J Obstet Gynecol 121: 418

Taylor P J, Leader A 1982 Reversal of female sterilization. How reliable is the operative report? J Reprod Med 27: 246

Trimbos-Kemper T C M 1990 Reversal of sterilization of

women over 40 years of age: a multicenter survey in the Netherlands. Fertil Steril 53: 575

Tulandi T, Vilos G A 1985 A comparison between laser surgery and electrosurgery for bilateral hydrosalpinx: a two year follow-up. Fertil Steril 44: 846

Urman B, Gomel V, McComb P, Lee N 1992 Midtubal occlusion: etiology management, and outcome. Fertil Steril 57: 747

Verhoeven H C, Berry H, Frantzen C, Schlosser H W 1983 Surgical treatment for distal tubal occlusion: a review of 167 cases. J Reprod Med 28: 293

Winston R M L 1980 Reversal of sterilization. Clin Obstet Gynecol 23: 126

Zouves C, Erenus M, Gomel V 1991 Tubal ectopic pregnancy after in vitro fertilization and embryo transfer: a role for proximal occlusion or salpingectomy after failed distal tubal surgery. Fertil Steril 56: 691

# 20. Treatment of endometriosis

*Melvin R. Cohen    Frank D. DeLeon*

Endometriosis, first reported in the 19th century by von Rokitansky (1860), has become an enigmatic disease of the 20th century. Why this frustrating disease—the growth and proliferation of misplaced endometrial glands and stroma—has become almost epidemic in the USA is unknown.

## INCIDENCE OF ENDOMETRIOSIS

Endometriosis has been reported as occurring in approximately 20–50% of laparotomies and in 30% of diagnostic laparoscopies for infertility. Bayly & Gossack (1956) found the rate of endometriosis to be 22.4% in 1177 laparotomies. Kistner (1962) recorded an incidence of 18%. In a report from the Mayo Clinic, William & Pratt (1977) reported a prospective study of the incidence of endometriosis in 1000 consecutive laparotomies: 50% of patients had endometriosis. Semm (1979) stated that 51% of infertile patients in whom diagnostic or operative pelviscopy (laparoscopy) was performed had endometriosis. He reported genital endometriosis in 26% of 6232 pelviscopies (laparoscopies) performed for different indications (Semm 1981).

At the Fertility Institute from 1975 through 1980, 2012 laparoscopies were performed for unexplained infertility; in this series there were 291 patients with mild, moderate or severe endometriosis, an incidence of 14.5%.

Greenblatt et al (1971) stated that endometriosis is the most frequent cause of tubal infertility. This has not been our experience.

## THE IMPACT OF LAPAROSCOPY

Prior to the reintroduction of gynecological laparoscopy in the USA (Cohen 1967), asymptomatic endometriosis was diagnosed infrequently. Currently the simplicity of laparoscopy with visualization of the internal genitalia plus biopsy when feasible, has enabled the gynecologist to make a definitive diagnosis of endometriosis early in the progress of this disease.

Diagnostic laparoscopy enables the gynocologist to discover minute foci of the disease process. When the laparoscope is inserted close to suspected lesions there is magnification for better identification of foci of endometriosis. Further, all gynecologists are urged to obtain photographs at the time of laparoscopy. In many cases when these photographs are carefully examined, small foci of endometriosis are discovered which had been apparently missed at the time of laparoscopy.

## PATHOGENESIS

There are four principle theories concerning the pathogenesis of endometriosis:

### Theory of implantation

Sampson (1925) attributed the histogenesis of endometriosis to retrograde menstruation wherein fragments of viable endometrium are refluxed through the oviducts and implanted on the pelvic viscera. In support of this theory is the following:

1. At laparoscopy and at laparotomy, performed during menstruation, blood can be seen escaping from the fimbria into the cul-de-sac. Such cul-de-sac blood contains endometrial

cells and microscopic examination of these cells suggests that they are viable.

2. Patent Fallopian tubes are usually present in mild or moderate endometriosis. When obstructed tubes are found to coexist with endometriosis, it is usually a late phenomenon associated with severe endometriosis.

3. Experimental production of endometriosis was achieved by Jacobsen (1922), who transplanted bits of uterine mucosa in the rabbit peritoneal cavity and reproduced lesions resembling endometriosis. TeLinde & Scott (1950) showed that pelvic endometriosis could be induced in the Rhesus monkey by surgically inverting the uterus so that intra-abdominal menstruation occurred. Endometriosis occurred in six of the ten animals so treated, though it took a long period of time to effect these changes. Ridley & Edwards (1958) demonstrated that, in the human, endometrium shed during menstruation could be implanted into the skin prior to laparotomy with the production of endometriosis.

Further, there have been reports of congenital atresia of the uterine cervix, a rare Müllerian anomaly frequently associated with pelvic endometriosis (Nunly & Kitchin 1980).

## Theory of metaplasia

Iwanoff (1898) and Meyer (1903) suggested that the peritoneal mesothelium could be stimulated to produce functioning endometrium by metaplasia. This stimulation could come from reflux of menstrual detritus plus inflammation. In other words, according to Iwanoff and Meyer, viable endometrium need not be present to induce endometriosis.

## Theory of precursor cells

Fetal rests could possibly be reactivated to undergo abnormal proliferation in response to cyclical ovarian hormone production.

## Metastatic theory

This theory is necessary to explain endometriosis occurring in distant organs such as the lungs, pleura, extremities and pelvic lymph nodes. Halban (1924) even suggested that all ectopic areas of endometriosis, wherever found, could be explained by metastatic growths originating in the endometrium and reaching their destination via lymphatics. Metastases could occur should such tissues reach the lumen of a lymph channel or vein. In this way, bits of tissue could be set free to be carried by the bloodstream to distant sites.

## THE IMPACT OF ENDOMETRIOSIS ON INFERTILITY

### Mechanical factors

In moderate to severe endometriosis there are sufficient mechanical factors (e.g. adhesions to adnexa with interference in ovum pickup) which could account for the deleterious effects of endometriosis on fertility. However, frequently even in moderate to severe endometriosis, there is patency of the Fallopian tubes and although the ovary may be adherent to the posterior leaf of the broad ligament, for example, there is still sufficient ovarian surface to enable a follicle to develop with expulsion of an egg, and fertility. Indeed, we do see patients with moderately severe endometriosis who conceive.

### Ovulatory dysfunction

In early endometriosis, when the disease is typically evidenced by superficial lesions of the pelvic peritoneum or wherein there would be a few spots of superficial ovarian endometriosis, one wonders whether the endometriosis is merely coincidental or whether there is indeed an effect upon ovulatory dysfunction. Ovulatory dysfunction, for example luteal phase insufficiency, has been well documented as a factor in infertility and usually these reports have not implicated the presence or absence of endometriosis. Dmowski et al (1980) could not substantiate the hypothesis postulated by some investigators that the luteinized unruptured follicle (LUF) syndrome could be the cause of infertility in women with endometriosis. In this laparoscopic study of 199 women, all had evidence of ovulation as judged by dated endometrial biopsies and/or elevated levels of plasma progesterone or urinary pregnanediol.

Schenken & Asch (1980), in an animal study in the rabbit, surgically implanted endometrium from one uterine horn into the peritoneum. Adipose tissue implanted in another group of animals served as a control. They found that the induction of endometriosis significantly impaired fertility rates. Further, they found that the decrease in fertility was independent of adhesions formation and primarily due to a defect in ovulation.

## Patterns of pregnanediol and LH excretion in endometriosis

In a preliminary study Cheesman et al (1982) investigated the urinary secretion patterns of LH and pregnanediol in patients with endometriosis, both untreated and danazol treated. The presence or absence of endometriosis was confirmed by laparoscopy; endometrial biopsies, plasma progesterone, and daily urinary LH and pregnanediol were obtained for each patient. Infertile patients without endometriosis served as controls. In these patients all endometrial biopsies were in phase and plasma progesterones were normal. Control patients ($n=10$) had a single midcycle urinary LH peak followed by a rapid rise in pregnanediol. Patients with untreated endometriosis ($n=14$) had a double peak of urinary LH; the first (midcycle) peak was normal in height, but was followed by a smaller peak either 2 or 3 days later. Urinary pregnanediol concentrations did not begin to rise in these patients until the time of the second LH surge, rather than rising immediately after the first surge. Peak concentrations of pregnanediol were lower and the duration of elevation was shorter than in controls. In four patients who were treated with danazol, three had only a single LH peak and a rise in pregnanediol that was not significantly delayed from that of the control group. It appears from this preliminary data that RIA of morning

| Classification | Characteristics |
|---|---|
| Mild | 1) Scattered, fresh lesions (i.e., implants not associated with scarring or retraction of the peritoneum) in the anterior or posterior cul-de-sac or pelvic peritoneum<br>2) Rare surface implant on ovary, with no endometrioma, without surface scarring and retraction and without periovarian adhesions<br>3) No peritubular adhesions |
| Moderate | 1) Endometriosis involving one or both ovaries, with several surface lesions, with scarring and retraction, or small endometriomata<br>2) Minimal periovarian adhesions associated with ovarian lesions described<br>3) Minimal peritubular adhesions associated with ovarian lesions described<br>4) Superficial implants in the anterior and/or posterior cul-de-sac with scarring and retraction, some adhesions, but not sigmoid invasion |
| Severe | 1) Endometriosis involving one or both ovaries with endometrioma > 2×2 cm (usually both)<br>2) One or both ovaries bound down by adhesions associated with endometriosis, with or without tubal adhesions to ovaries<br>3) One or both tubes bound down or obstructed by endometriosis, associated adhesions or lesions<br>4) Obliteration of the cul-de-sac from adhesions or lesions associated with endometriosis<br>5) Thickening of the uterosacral ligaments and cul-de-sac lesions from invasive endometriosis with obliteration of the cul-de-sac<br>6) Significant bowel or urinary tract involvement. |

**Fig. 20.1** A proposed classification of pelvic endometriosis (Acosta et al 1973).

urine for LH and for pregnanediol may be diagnostically useful in explaining the mechanism of ovulatory dysfunction in endometriosis.

## Prostaglandin synthesis in endometriosis

A great deal of attention has been paid to the formation of prostaglandins (PGs) and related compounds by endometriotic tissue. Drake & associates (1981) have shown that metabolites of thromboxane $A_2$ ($TXA_2$) and prostacyclin ($PGI_2$) are present in elevated concentrations in peritoneal fluid. The fluid volume is also increased, making the total production of these products even greater in patients with endometriosis. How these compounds effect reproductive function is not known, but the role of related prostaglandins in ovulation has been studied. Using the platelet cell as a model, it may be hypothesized that $TXA_2$ and $PGI_2$ interact at receptors for $PGF_{2\alpha}$ and $PGE_2$ respectively (Moncada & Vane 1979). In support of this relationship, $PGI_2$ and $PGE_2$ are both found to cause relaxation of Fallopian tubes and $PGF_{2\alpha}$ stimulates their contraction (Goldberg & Ramwell 1975, Drake et al 1981). When ovulation is inhibited by perfusion of indomethacin in animal previously given hCG, subsequent addition of $PGF_{2\alpha}$ to the perfusion medium will promote ovulation in the rabbit (Hamada et al 1979) or monkey (Wallach et al 1975). $PGF_{2\alpha}$ had little effect in promoting ovulation of follicles in animals not given gonadotropin and indomethacin, but $PGE_2$ was strongly inhibitory (Hamada et al 1977). The greater formation of $PGI_2$ in peritoneal fluid of patients with endometriosis (Drake et al 1981) would, in the balance, exert a net inhibitory effect on ovulation.

| | |
|---|---|
| Stage I | Areas of endometriosis are present on the posterior pelvic peritoneum (cul-de-sac, uterosacral ligaments) or on the surface of the broad ligaments but do not exceed 5 mm in diameter. Avascular adhesions may involve the tubes, but the fimbriae are free. The ovaries may show a few avascular adhesions, but there is no ovarian fixation. The surfaces of the bowel and the appendix are normal. |
| Stage IIa | Areas of endometriosis are present on the posterior pelvic peritoneum (cul-de-sac, uterosacral ligaments) and the broad ligaments but do not exceed 5 mm in diameter. Avascular adhesions may involve the tubes, but the fimbriae are free. Ovarian involvement by endometriosis has been subclassified as follows: <br> IIa1: Endometrial cyst or surface area 5 cm or less <br> IIa2: Endometrial cyst or surface area over 5 cm <br> IIa3: Ruptured endometrioma <br> The bowel and the appendix are normal |
| Stage IIb | The posterior leaf of the board ligament is covered by adherent ovarian tissue. The tubes present adhesions not removable by endoscopic procedures. The fimbriae are free. The ovaries are fixed to the broad ligament and show areas of endometriosis over 5 mm in diameter. The cul-de-sac presents multiple implants but there is no adherent bowel nor is the uterus in fixed position. The bowel and the appendix are normal. |
| Stage III | The posterior leaf of the broad ligament may be covered by adherent tube or ovary. The tubal fimbriae are covered by adhesions. The ovaries are adherent to the broad ligament and the tube and may or may not show surface endometriosis or endometriomas. The cul-de-sac shows multiple areas of endometriosis, but there is no evidence of adherent tubes or uterine fixation. The bowel and the appendix are normal. |
| Stage IV | Endometriosis involves the bladder serosa, and the uterus is in fixed, third-degree retroversion. The cul-de-sac is covered by adherent bowel or is obliterated by the fixed uterus. The bowel is adherent to the cul-de-sac, uterosacral ligaments, or uterine corpus. The appendix may be involved by the endometriotic process. |

**Fig. 20.2**  Suggested classification of endometriosis (Kistner et al 1977).

The source of peritoneal fluid prostaglandins includes direct secretion by endometriotic implants, as well as possible secretion by macrophages and peritoneal surface. Recent work has revealed that implants can produce significantly higher levels of $PGF_{2\alpha}$ and $PGE_{2\alpha}$ than normal adjacent peritoneum (DeLeon et al 1988). There is also evidence that 'fresh, petechial' lesions make significantly greater amounts of prostaglandins than 'burned out' implants (Vernon et al 1986). Certainly the beneficial effect of antiprostaglandins in the treatment of dysmenorrhea associated with endometriosis is very suggestive that prostaglandins do play a role in the patient with endometriosis.

## Autoimmune response in infertility associated with endometriosis

In a review article, Weed & Arquembourg (1980) postulated that there could be autoimmune mechanisms present in the Müllerian system to combat antigens foreign to the host. These would involve IgA, IgG and IgM. Perhaps endometriosis creates an antigen from the host's own endometrial proteins which is recognized by the host as foreign. This immune response may cause the host to become infertile by causing the rejection of early embryo implantation or by interfering with sperm transport.

## SIGN AND SYMPTOMS

Early endometriosis is usually asymptomatic except for the presence of infertility. Signs and symptoms of endometriosis vary from patient to patient. There may be but one presenting symptom or a combination of several. Acquired dysmenorrhea, dyspareunia and pelvic pain would suggest moderate to severe endometriosis. More severe endometriosis may be associated with metrorrhagia, rectal bleeding and hematuria. It is our opinion that whenever there is unexplained infertility, endometriosis should be suspected.

## CLASSIFICATION OF ENDOMETRIOSIS

Initially, for the purpose of our clinical studies, we

utilized the classification of Acosta et al (1973) (Fig. 20.1). Later Kistner et al (1977) (Fig 20.2) presented a rather complicated classification useful in evaluating patients requiring laparotomy. We have now adopted the classification of the American Fertility Society (Fig. 20.3).

## DIAGNOSIS OF ENDOMETRIOSIS

Endometriosis may be suspected by a history of acquired dysmenorrhea, pelvic pain (typically premenstrual), dyspareunia (chiefly at times of deep penetration), as well as bleeding irregularities plus pelvic findings of cul-de-sac nodularity, a fixed retroversion, and possible adnexal masses. However, though a diagnosis of endometriosis may be suspected by a history and pelvic examination, laparoscopy or laparotomy is necessary to prove the existence of this disease (Figs. 20.4–20.6).

## DIAGNOSTIC LAPAROSCOPY

When laparoscopy is performed, the use of a second puncture suprapubically with the introduction of a probe is essential to manipulate the adnexa and uterus so that all surfaces of all pelvic organs may be carefully examined. Gross examination of the organs usually suffices to determine whether endometriosis exists, although confirmatory biopsy, when feasible, is indicated. Ectopic endometriosis implants appear as brown, purplish or black hemorrhagic areas. Even if implants are not immediately visible, endometriosis should be suspected whenever pelvic adhesions involve the ovaries but not the tubes.

## Atypical endometriosis

Classical endometriosis has been described as having a typical bluish-black appearance with 'powder burns' often associated. It is now clear that endometriosis can present with a variety of unusual lesions. Jansen & Russel (1986) described in great detail atypical presentation of 'nonpigmented' peritoneal endometriosis. Lesions included white opacified lesions, red flame-like lesions, glandular lesions, yellow-

## AMERICAN FERTILITY SOCIETY CLASSIFICATION OF ENDOMETRIOSIS

Patient's name _____

| | |
|---|---|
| Stage I | (Mild) | 1–5 |
| Stage II | (Moderate) | 6–15 |
| Stage III | (Severe) | 16–30 |
| Stage IV | (Extensive) | 31–54 |

Total _____

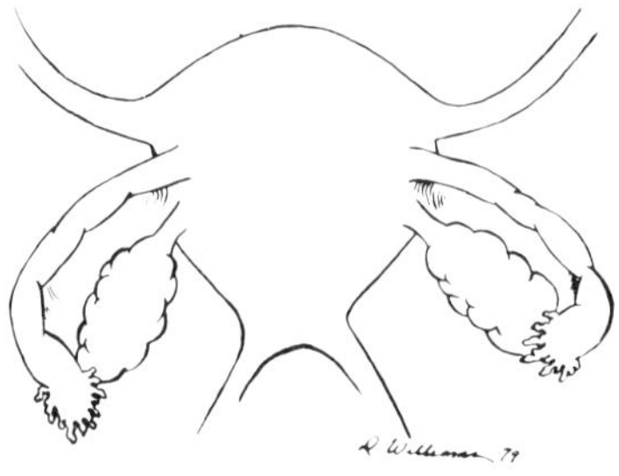

| | | | <1 cm | 1–3 cm | >3 cm |
|---|---|---|---|---|---|
| PERITONEUM | ENDOMETRIOSIS | | <1 cm | 1–3 cm | >3 cm |
| | | | 1 | 2 | 3 |
| | ADHESIONS | | filmy | dense w/ partial cul-de-sac obliteration | dense w/ complete cul-de-sac obliteration |
| | | | 1 | 2 | 3 |
| OVARY | ENDOMETRIOSIS | | <1 cm | 1–3 cm | >3 cm or ruptured endometrioma |
| | | R | 2 | 4 | 6 |
| | | L | 2 | 4 | 6 |
| | ADHESIONS | | filmy | dense w/ partial ovarian enclosure | dense w/ complete ovarian enclosure |
| | | R | 2 | 4 | 6 |
| | | L | 2 | 4 | 6 |
| TUBE | ENDOMETRIOSIS | | <1 cm | >1 cm | tubal occlusion |
| | | R | 2 | 4 | 6 |
| | | L | 2 | 4 | 6 |
| | ADHESIONS | | filmy | dense w/ tubal distortion | dense w/ tubal enclosure |
| | | R | 2 | 4 | 6 |
| | | L | 2 | 4 | 6 |

Associated Pathology:

**Fig. 20.3**   Classification of endometriosis (American Fertility Society).

brown patches, circular defects and peritoneal defects. After reviewing over 120 biopsies the frequency of microscopically proven endometriosis ranged between 45% and 82%, depending on the specific lesion described. It is likely that if we only recognize and treat classical appearing endometriosis, we may in fact be missing the diagnosis in some patients. Patients with atypical endometriosis may be erroneously labelled as having unexplained infertility. Furthermore, without properly treating atypical endometriosis, it is possible that persistence of symptoms and worsening of disease is likely. In Jansen's study of atypical endometriosis, he opted to follow six patients with observation but no medical or surgical treatment. All of the lesions initially described as atypical progressed to the typical pigmented endometriosis lesions within 6–24 months, confirming the existence of a biological continuum between nonpigmented and pigmented endometriosis lesions.

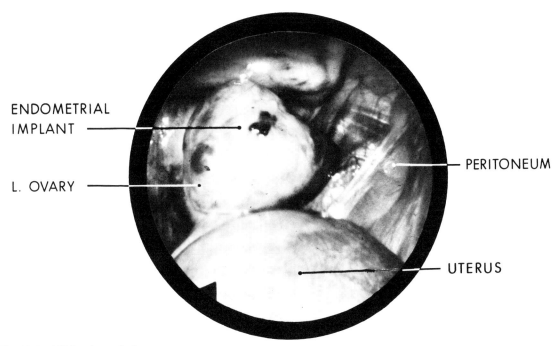

**Fig. 20.4** Mild endometriosis.

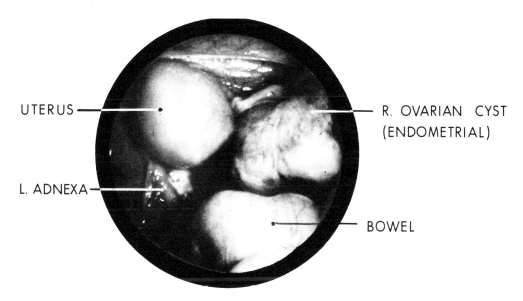

**Fig. 20.5** Moderate endometriosis.

## Microscopic endometriosis

Besides atypical or nonpigmented endometriosis lesions, it is extremely likely that normal appearing peritoneum in patients presenting with clinical symptoms of the disease may be harboring microscopic lesions. To answer this question Murphy et al (1986) evaluated grossly normal peritoneum and endometriotic implants by scanning electron microscopy in patients being

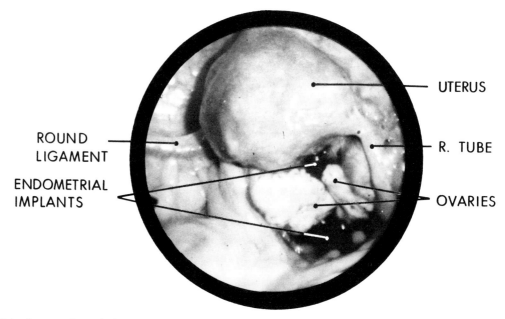

ROUND LIGAMENT

ENDOMETRIAL IMPLANTS

UTERUS

R. TUBE

OVARIES

**Fig. 20.6**   Severe endometriosis.

treated by conservative surgery. Evaluation of biopsies revealed 26% of 'normal peritoneum' harbored endometriosis whereas 80% of the grossly evident implants were noted to be positive for the disease.

Although in this study scanning electron microscopy of peritoneum was performed only in patients who had grossly evident disease, it is possible that microscopic disease may also be present in many patients who are symptomatic but have not yet developed grossly evident disease. Thus, the true incidence of endometriosis is probably underestimated. This study suggests, furthermore, that surgical treatment of endometriosis is primarily cytoreductive and in most instances recurrence of disease after surgical treatment may be due to persistence of disease which becomes grossly evident with time.

## DIFFERENTIAL DIAGNOSIS

Endometriosis must be differentiated from the following conditions:

1. All causes of acquired dysmenorrhea, pelvic pain and dyspareunia. This would include pelvic inflammatory disease — acute, subacute and chronic. Chronic inflammatory disease with bilateral pelvic masses is rarely confused with endometriosis. Such patients will give an adequate history of a preceding episode following the use of an intrauterine device or possibly an induced or spontaneous abortion with a febrile course. A hysterosalpingogram, utilizing aqueous contrast media, would be contraindicated in the presence of an acute or subacute salpingitis, but may be judiciously used in the presence of chronic pelvic inflammatory disease. The presence of a bilateral hydrosalpinx, for example, usually excludes the presence of endometriosis.

2. All causes of pelvic masses in addition to pelvic inflammatory disease. This would include adnexal tumors and cysts.

3. All causes of a fixed retroversion. If this retroversion is unassociated with cul-de-sac nodularity or tenderness, there would be the possibility of simple pelvic adhesions not associated with pelvic endometriosis.

4. All causes of an acute surgical abdomen. An acute pelvic episode may occur should an ovarian endometrial cyst rupture. This must be differentiated from an acute appendicitis, an ectopic pregnancy, twisted ovarian cyst or a ruptured Graafian follicle with intraperitoneal blood.

5. Bowel pathology, such as tumors or diverticulitis, may be a differential problem, and appropriate methods of diagnosis, such as barium studies, proctoscopy and /or sigmoidoscopy might be necessary.

6. Urinary tract problems such as hematuria, dysuria or pelvic pain due to ureteral involvement must be investigated.

## RATIONALES FOR MEDICAL THERAPY: PSEUDOPREGNANCY AND PSEUDOMENOPAUSE

Following the observation that endometriosis regresses during pregnancy, Kistner (1959) described estrogen-progestogen 'pseudopregnancy' therapy in the treatment of endometriosis.

A high dosage level of a predominantly progesterone-loaded oral contraceptive can be administered continuously for a number of months. Such tablets contain norethynodrel, norethindrone, norethindrone acetate, norgestrel or ethynodiol diacetate plus mestranol or ethinyl estradiol, and are prescribed in doses two to four times the amount needed for contraception. This will produce a negative feedback effect on the pituitary directly blocking FSH and LH production. Full estrogen production and ovulation are prevented and without the corpus luteum, no progesterone is produced. Without hormonal cyclicity, anovulation occurs and endometrial tissue is not stimulated by periodic hormonal surges. Amenorrhea occurs and implants regress and atrophy. Necrotic tissue is absorbed by the body as part of the normal healing process. Upon completion of therapy, there is generally a return of ovulation and cyclic menstrual bleeding. This type of therapy is called pseudopregnancy.

Pseudopregnancy treatment initially causes endometrial hypertrophy and decidual changes before atrophy occurs, hence symptoms commonly worsen before there is a response to treatment. Additional untoward effects — thromboembolism, hypertension, nausea, depression, etc.—may be seen with this type of therapy.

Menopause, whether spontaneous or surgically induced, also improves or cures endometriosis. However, waiting for the onset of menopause can be of value only to the older patient who is willing for this to happen. Radical surgery to induce a menopausal state is unfortunately sometimes necessary in the patient with extensive disease both within and outside the pelvis.

Medical therapy to produce a temporary menopausal state with prompt return to normal menses and ovulation would be an acceptable mode of treatment of endometriosis, provided that side reactions to such therapy were minimal. It is hoped that danazol (Danocrine), introduced by Greenblatt et al (1971), will prove to be a drug specifically tailored for treatment of endometriosis.

## WHAT IS DANAZOL?

Danazol (see also Chapter 18) was synthesized at the Sterling-Winthrop Research Institute by Manson et al (1963) by the addition of the isoxazole moiety to the A ring of the steroid ethisterone (Fig. 20.7). It is an orally active pituitary gonadotropin inhibitory agent devoid of estrogenic and progestational activity, with weak, impeded androgenic activity (Dmowski et al 1971). Separate studies have established that danazol is antiprogestational and antiestrogenic. It is unique in exhibiting a pituitary gonadotropin inhibitory activity completely separate from overt sex hormone activity. In addition to suppressing gonadotropins, it is anabolic, and extensive toxicological studies have established its safety in the laboratory animal.

Endocrine changes induced by danazol (800 mg daily) in normally cycling women result in amenorrhea within 8 weeks. There is inhibition of ovulation, inhibition of ovarian steroidogenesis, hypoestrogenic changes in the vaginal cytology, and atrophic changes in the endometrium. At

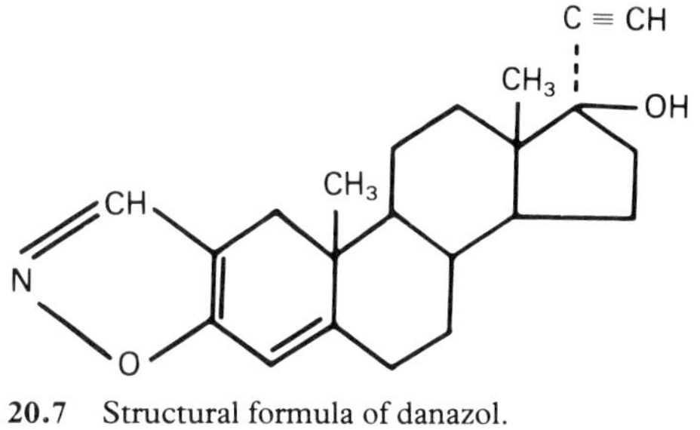

**Fig. 20.7**   Structural formula of danazol.

times, hot flushes, sweats and other symptoms suggesting menopause (pesudomenopause) occur. Side-effects are due to the anabolic and mild androgenic properties of this steroid.

Danazol acts on endometriosis primarily by suppressing the rise of serum FSH and the surge and midcycle rise of LH with resulting suppression of ovarian function.

Recent experiments in monkeys show that danazol induces short luteal phases and decreased progesterone production due to a direct effect at the gonadal level. Other data in mice demonstrate that it directly inhibits gonadal steroidogenesis. Danazol suppresses all endogenous stimuli to the endometrium, allows spontaneous healing and atrophy of the disease, and by itself exerts no stimulatory effects on the endometrium, as is the case with the newer progestins.

## Results of treatment with danazol

In a previous study, danazol was administered to 39 patients with endometriosis that had been diagnosed at laparoscopy and confirmed by laparoscopic biopsy (Dmowski & Cohen 1975). None of the patients had undergone surgical resection of the lesions prior to this treatment. While they were receiving the drug, all patients developed evidence of ovarian suppression. The results were evaluated by repeat laparoscopy, biopsy, and laparoscopic photography before and after treatment. Each patient was treated with 800 mg danazol daily for an average of 6 months. There was marked decrease in the extent of endometriosis after treatment; 59% of the patients having no evidence of the disease, 26% having peritoneal adhesions and hemosiderin deposits but no active endometriosis, and 15% exhibiting residual endometriosis. Histological studies in the last group revealed atrophic changes in the uterine ectopic endometrium and evidence of a healing process.

In an exhibit on danazol presented at the American Medical Association, Dmowski & Cohen (1978) reported on an augmented series of 103 patients with proven endometriosis who had received a full course of danazol (800 mg daily). They were able to evaluate 99 (96%) of these patients. The duration of tretment varied between 3 and 18 months, with a mean of 6 months. These patients were re-evaluated at the end of treatment and again about 37 months later (range 27–52 months). Ninety patients were infertile prior to treatment, and the pregnancy rate after treatment was 46.4%. When patients with absolute sterility due to tubal factors or male factors were deleted, there was a corrected pregnancy rate of 72.2%. The results of treatment according to extent of disease are shown in Figure 20.8. Although one thinks of suppression of endometriosis as effective

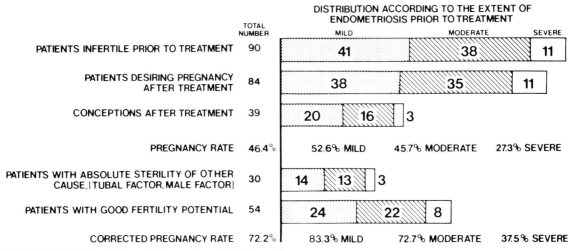

**Fig. 20.8**   Infertility before and after treatment with danazol.

only in mild disease, conceptions did occur following treatment of moderate and severe disease. The majority of conceptions occurred within 6 months after termination of treatment. There was a recurrence rate of 39% within 37 months following therapy. Side-effects included acne in 34% of the patients, sweats and hot flushes in 17%, voice changes in 2%, and hirsutism. Hirsutism is a very serious side-effect unless reversible. In this series, it was reported by only one patient and there was marked improvement after discontinuation of therapy.

Dmowski & Cohen concluded that the results of treatment with pseudomenopause have been very encouraging. Relief of symptoms during treatment was reported by all patients, and in 86% pelvic examination provided clinical evidence of improvement.

## Low-dosage danazol therapy

In a publication from Sterling-Winthrop Research Institute (1981) a double-blind study as a single multicenter investigation has been reported. The study consisted of 11 separate trials with an identical protocol. Of 136 patients, 106 qualified for symptom analysis. All patients had a pretrial laparoscopy which served to establish the baseline extent of their endometriosis. A second laparoscopy, carried out upon completion of 6 months of therapy, served to provide a visual measure of change in extent of the disease. The dosage regimes followed were 100, 200, 400 and 600 mg danazol daily, administered in two divided doses. Endometriosis was graded as severe, moderate, minimal or none. They concluded that regardless of dosage schedule, treatment was effective with successes being scored for 69–76% of patients. No differences were seen amongst the four daily dosages of 100, 200, 400 or 600 mg. This study showed that there was a dose-related suppression of menstrual function. For example, after 6 months of treatment with 600 mg daily, 88% of patients were amenorrheic. On the 100-mg regimen, 21% were amenorrheic and 42% continued to have menses on a monthly basis. Significantly, there were adverse reactions at all dose levels, though the side reactions were neither grave nor life-threatening. They concluded that danazol administered in a daily dosage of 100–600 mg for a period of 6 months is a safe and effective treatment for endometriosis. Because of this data, the Federal Drug Administration (FDA) has permitted a dose change. In the past the FDA would only permit a dose regimen of 800 mg daily for 3–9 months as therapy for endometriosis. As part of this study group, Biberoglue & Behrman (1981) reported their double-blind study on 32 patients. They found that the pregnancy rate was 45% and concluded that lower than maximum doses of danazol produced similar beneficial effects in the treatment. With low doses, however, they did not achieve freedom from side-effects. The average symptomatic recurrence rate was 36% with a mean duration of 19 months of follow-up and was apparently dose dependent.

Moore et al (1981) reported their double-blind study in 38 women. They found an overall pregnancy rate of 28%; 51% of the women had recurrence of symptoms within 1 year of discontinuation of danazol. Dmowski et al (1982) also reported on the effects of low-dose danazol. Clinical improvement was variable from just over 50% on 100-mg dose to 83% on 600-mg dose. Laparoscopic improvement in the extent of endometriosis was noted in all patients, but residual disease was common. After the completion of treatment, seven patients required operations for residual endometriosis or for its early recurrence. Six of 15 infertile patients conceived spontaneously within 6 months after treatment. They concluded that danazol was less effective in doses lower than the standard 800 mg daily. However, individual downward adjustment of the dose may be attempted based on the development of amenorrhea and clinical improvement.

It is our opinion that a dose sufficient to create amenorrhea is essential in the management of endometriosis. Two variations in treatment schedules could be suggested: (a) begin with a very small dose, such as 100 mg daily, and should menses occur, double the dose until amenorrhea is achieved; or (b) reverse the procedure starting with 800 mg daily and after amenorrhea is achieved, gradually reduce the dose to 600, 400,

200 and even 100 mg daily provided that break-through bleeding or menses do not occur.

## GONADOTROPIN-RELEASING HORMONE (GnRH) AGONIST THERAPY FOR ENDOMETRIOSIS

The most recent medical treatment for endometriosis involves the use of GnRH agonists. These agonist analogs are synthesized by chemically altering one or more of the ten amino acids of the natural GnRH structure. Initially believed to enhance fertility because of their prolonged half-lives and biological potency, they were named agonists. It is clear now that the initial stimulation of gonadotropins and estradiol is followed by a continuous suppression of ovarian steroids similar to that seen in oophorectomized women. This is due to the loss of available pituitary gland receptors as well as refractoriness of available receptors (desensitization) to further stimulation. This paradoxical effect of GnRH agonists resulting in castrate levels of estradiol has been referred to as 'medical oophorectomy' by Meldrum et al (1982).

In a recent large, randomized, double-blind study Henzl et al (1988) compared the efficacy of GnRH agonist to danazol for treatment of endometriosis. In this study 213 patients with documented endometriosis were randomly assigned to receive nafarelin acetate nasal spray (400 or 800 μg per day) or 800 mg per day of danazol. After 6 months of treatment a second-look laparoscopy was performed to document the extent of endometriosis. All three groups were found to have significantly less disease after medical treatment. When the three groups were compared to each other, however, there was no statistical difference among them, meaning that all three groups were equally successful. Similar benefits among the three groups were observed for pain relief during therapy. Pregnancy outcome after therapy consisted of 52% for the 800-μg group, 30% for the 400-μg group, and 36% for those treated with danazol. The main differences among the GnRH and danazol groups involved side-effects. The GnRH group complained of more hot flashes, 90% versus 68% among the danazol group, as well as decreased libido, and vaginal dryness. All of these side-effects are most likely due to hypoestrogenism. The danazol group reported more complaints of weight gain, edema, and myalgia than the GnRH group.

This excellent study clearly demonstrates similar efficacy of GnRH analogs and danazol for treatment of endometriosis. Its value when compared to other medical therapies available seems to be in its acceptability by the patient due to lessened side-effects. More studies are needed to evaluate the effect of GnRH on bone loss (see also Chapter 15). At this time there are three main routes of administration of GnRH analogs: intranasal, subcutaneous and intramuscular.

## SURGICAL LAPAROSCOPY

Surgical laparoscopy, or minisurgery by electrocautery, is a very rewarding procedure. In our opinion, the release of adhesions and the release of an endometrioma between an ovary and the posterior leaf of the broad ligament, enables a patient with moderate endometriosis, theoretically amenable only to conservative surgery, to respond to medical management. Furthermore, minisurgery is very effective for lysing adhesions in patients with severe endometriosis who have been pretreated successfully with danazol or GnRH analogs.

## LASER OPERATIVE LAPAROSCOPY

The laparoscope, initially used only as a diagnostic tool, has allowed us a port of entry for sophisticated surgical instruments, unipolar, bipolar cautery and most recently a variety of surgical lasers. Conservative surgery for endometriosis formerly performed by laparotomy can now be performed via small laparoscopic incisions by experienced laparoscopic surgeons. The goals of operative laparoscopy are similar to those performed by laparotomy, mainly to restore normal anatomy and eliminate pelvic pain. The advantage of laser operative laparoscopy is that patients can be treated at the same time that the diagnosis is made. The extent of surgery that can be performed in this manner is proportional to the experience of the laparoscopist.

Several laser systems are available for laparoscopic surgery and treatment of endometriosis. The most common include the $CO_2$, argon, and neodymium:yttrium aluminium garnet (Nd:YAG). Each laser has its unique advantages and disadvantages.

## $CO_2$ laser

Of the various lasers available, the $CO_2$ laser is the most versatile, and is extremely safe due to its limited depth of penetration (2–4 mm) and lateral thermal damage (0.5 mm). This allows use of the $CO_2$ laser in delicate areas where bipolar cautery would be unsafe such as the bladder, lateral side wall near the ureter, and bowel serosa. Besides vaporization, the $CO_2$ laser can also be used for excision or incision by increasing the power density.

The pregnancy rate in patients with endometriosis treated by $CO_2$ laser laparoscopy is comparable to results previously reported with conservative laparotomy (Table 20.1).

Disadvantages of the $CO_2$ laser include focusing of the He-Ne beam, as well as production of smoke 'plume' which needs frequent evacuation to allow adequate visualization of the target area.

## KTP – argon lasers

The KTP and argon lasers have similar wavelengths, 532 mm and 514 mm respectively, and are delivered via a fiberoptic fiber. They produce an intense green-blue light and can be transmitted through different diameter fibers (400 and 600 µm), thus changing the spot size. The advantages of these lasers over the $CO_2$ include: (1) a selective absorption by hemoglobin, (2) less plume production, and (3) an easy delivery system which uses lower power settings in the range of 5–10 watts. The main disadvantage is the need to wear special glasses which distort the view of the pelvis and make it difficult to visualize small implants of endometriosis. Keye et al (1987) have reported pregnancy rates following argon laser treatment of mild, moderate and severe endometriosis to be 38%, 30% and 20%, respectively.

## Nd:YAG laser

Although the Nd:YAG laser has been used primarily for intrauterine surgery, its use with sapphire tips for treatment of endometriosis has been reported. (Corson et al 1989).

Its main drawback is that without the sapphire tips there is very deep tissue penetration (2–6 mm). With the use of sapphire, the depth of penetration is limited and a pregnancy rate of 47% has been reported by Corson et al. Unfortunately, there is a need to continuously cool the sapphire tips during surgery. Several deaths have been reported when using air or $CO_2$ as the cooling medium for intrauterine surgery (Baggish & Daniell 1989). Because of this, this laser system has not been as popular as the $CO_2$ or KTP–Argon systems for treatment of endometriosis.

Table 20.1   Pregnancies by stage of endometriosis as an isolated factor

| Author | All stages(no.) total Pregnant* | | Mild(no.) total Pregnant* | | Moderate(no.) total Pregnant* | | Severe/extensive(no.) total Pregnant* | |
|---|---|---|---|---|---|---|---|---|
| Feste 1985 | 60 | 42(70) | 44 | 31(70) | 14 | 10(71) | 2 | 1(50) |
| Adamson 1986 | 34 | 21(62) | 27 | 17(64) | 6 | 4(70) | 1 | 0(0) |
| Martin1986 | 34 | 23(67) | 13 | 9(69) | 11 | 6(55) | 10 † | 8(80) |
| Nezhat 1986 | 102 | 65(64) | 24 | 18(75) | 51 | 32(63) | 27 ‡ | 15(56) |
| Paulsen 1986 | 144 | 107(74) | 91 | 70(76) | 53 | 37(70) | 0 | 0 |
| Total | 374 | 258(69) | 199 | 145(73) | 135 | 109(66) | 40 | 24(60) |

* Figures in parentheses are percentages.
† Suppression with 800 mg/day Danacrine.
‡ No suppressive therapy.
Reproduced from Martin 1986.

## Technique

The use of the laser allows several procedures to be performed. Lysis of adhesions can be accomplished safer than with electrocautery. Several punctures may be needed, since operative forceps and a suction-irrigator are a must to clearly visualize the pelvic field. When the pelvis is clear of adhesions, the peritoneal and ovarian endometriosis are treated by either excision or ablation depending on the effect desired. Excision of tissue requires higher power density. Small bleeders (<0.2mm) can be coagulated by defocusing the beam and decreasing the power density. More profuse bleeding may require bipolar coagulation.

Endometriomas can be treated by drainage, or preferably by drainage and coagulation of the remaining cyst wall. At this time we prefer the complete removal of the cyst wall to avoid possible recurrence. This procedure, in our hands, is 50–60% effective, thus requiring coagulation of the base at least half of the time. Patients with ovarian endometriomas are treated postoperatively with chemical suppression for 6 months' duration.

Another advantage of the $CO_2$ laser over cautery is its relative safety in using it over peritoneum covering the ureter, bladder and in some cases superficial bowel serosa. By defocusing the beam and lowering the power density the penetration can be limited, preventing injury.

Nezhat et al (1989) reported the results of 243 patients with infertility associated with endometriosis ranging from mild to extensive treated with the $CO_2$ laser laparoscopically. One hundred and sixty-eight (69.1%) achieved pregnancy. These included 71.8% in 39 patients with stage I disease, 69.8% in 86 patients with stage II disease, 67.2% of 67 patients with stage III disease, and 68.6% in 51 patients with stage IV disease. They conclude that videolaseroscopic treatment of endometriosis with infertility, in experienced hands, is at least as efficacious as other forms of therapy for mild and moderate disease, but appears to be more successful than laparotomy for more severe and extensive stages of endometriosis.

Patients with severe dysmenorrhea and endometriosis may be candidates for laparoscopic uterine nerve ablation. Several investigators have used either bipolar current (Lichten & Bombard 1987) or laser (Feste 1985) to transect the uterosacral nerves at the time of laparoscopy with 60–80% of the patients reporting improvement of menstrual pain when followed up for 1 year. Although this procedure is relatively easy to perform there are potential complications including ureteral injury, uterine artery bleeding and uterine prolapse.

## CONSERVATIVE LAPAROTOMY FOR ENDOMETRIOSIS

An adequate surgical exposure, with careful hemostasis, is necessary. Our preference is the Maylard transverse incision with incision of the recti muscles. To insure good hemostasis, we employ the Shaw hot knife. If a laser is available, the abdominal incision may be performed by laser surgery. A wound protector, a circular plastic device which prevents seepage from the abdominal incision, is very advantageous inasmuch as the field must be carefully kept bloodless and irrigated with lactated Ringer's solution.

Presacral neurectomy is never done as a primary procedure for dysmenorrhea, but it is certainly very valuable as an adjuvant when conservative surgery for endometriosis is employed.

Careful lysis of adhesions should involve the use of a micro needle. The unipolar technique is employed; however, at laparotomy it is possible to mobilize the bowel and protect it with moist sponges.

Excision or cautery of all endometriotic foci must be done. Ovarian resection should be performed to remove endometriomas. Unilateral oophorectomy may be necessary for a large endometrioma, provided the other ovary can be salvaged.

Careful peritonization with, for example, 6–0 Dexon suture, is necessary. Peritoneal patches are very important should there be any raw surface on the uterus or posterior cul-de-sac that cannot be peritonized.

Uterosacral plication should be done, with

nonabsorbable suture such as # 3 silk. Plication of the round ligaments may be advantageous as a temporary procedure, for example to suspend the adnexa out of the pelvis.

Postoperatively, the peritoneum should be irrigated with copious amounts of lactated Ringer's.

Instillation of 50–200 ml of 35% Dextran 70 is apparently valuable in the prevention of adhesions.

Postoperative care with prophylactic antibiotics plus dexamethasone, according to the Horne technique (Horne et al 1973), will ensure a smooth postoperative recovery, though there is no proof that this therapy improves the prognosis in the surgical treatment of severe endometriosis.

## SEMM (1981): THREE-STEP THERAPY OF GENITAL ENDOMETRIOSIS

This innovative though radical approach to the management of endometriosis involves the following three steps.

### First therapeutic step: surgical

Pelviscopy (laparoscopy) permits both reliable diagnosis and surgical therapy in one procedure (Semm 1976).

Semm uses a method of tissue coagulation at 100°C, which enables effective destruction of the ectopic endometrium sites as well as elimination of endometriotic foci on the bladder dome. He prefers this therapeutic modality rather than monopolar or bipolar high frequency coagulation. Further, if a chocolate cyst is found, it may be punctured and enucleated by endoscopic techniques. He also advocates the use of a loop ligator. He claims that following surgical laparoscopy plus a few months of hormonal treatments, near normal ovaries with fine brain-like convolutions are usually found. He advocates the use of a hook-shaped scissors or, if possible, a point coagulator only for endometrial implants in uterosacral ligaments. He further completes 'adhesio-, salpingo- and ovario-lysis'. He does not, however, perform fimbriolysis or salpingostomy at the first step.

### Second therapeutic step: hormonal

Semm states that initial laparoscopy may leave small implants undetected or insufficiently coagulated. To eliminate these small lesions hormonal therapy with antigonadotropins (danazol) or gestagens is administered over a period of 4–8 months. He claims that in his patients hormonal treatment after surgical therapeutic laparoscopy has resulted in a 95% healing rate of endometriosis.

### Third therapeutic step: surgical

Pelviscopy is used for final repair of the Fallopian tubes. Tubal surgery must not be performed during the first step pelviscopy. On initial endoscopy, coagulation of implants and periadnexal adhesions prepare for the third step which is directed towards surgical repair of distal tubal pathology, by fimbriolysis or salpingostomy.

Using his three-step approach, he reported a pregnancy rate of 41% in a group of 246 patients with tubal damage caused by endometriosis.

## ROLE OF DRUGS STIMULATING OVULATION

Because endometriosis will recur unless the patient becomes pregnant or menopausal, anything that can be done to promote pregnancy will, in effect, prevent recurrence of endometriosis. It is the impression of many that there is some ovulatory dysfunction in the patient with even mild to minimal endometriosis. Attempts are made at laparoscopy to document anovulation or ovulatory dysfunction by observing the presence or absence of a corpus leteum and noting whether a stigma is present. In addition, endometrial biopsy studies and plasma progesterone may disclose poor luteal function.

We have found that clomiphene citrate (Clomid, Serophene) either alone or in association with human chorionic gonadotrophin (hCG) has been very rewarding in the promotion of conception. Inasmuch as clomiphene frequeently induces ovulation but creates hostile cervical secretions, we frequently perform AIH utilizing

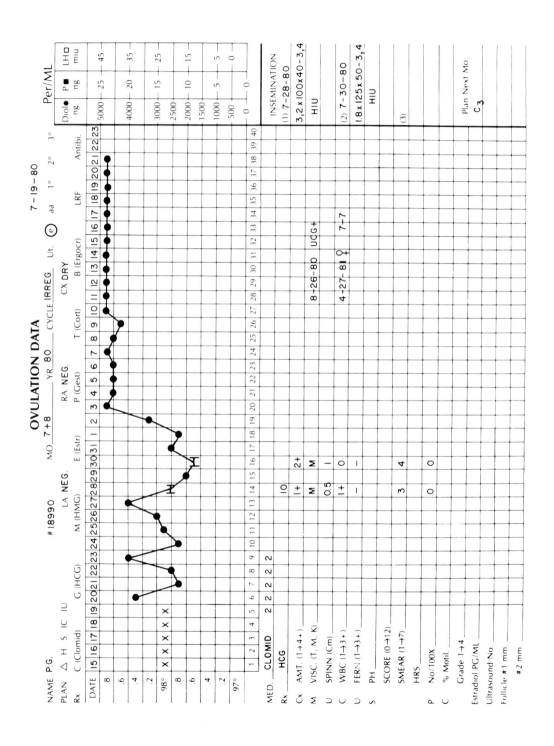

**Fig. 20.9**  Ovulation data sheet—patient P.G. with arrested endometriosis and anovulation successfully treated with clomiphene citrate plus human chorionic gonadotropin (hCG) and husband insemination (AIH)

Cycle represents the average menstrual cycle.

The date and pelvic examination as indicated:

  e, erect uterus; aa, acutely anteflexed uterus; 1° 2° 3°, degrees of retroversion; L A, left adnexa; R A, right adnexa; CX, cervix

Rx, treatment as indicated:

  C, clomid; G, human chorionic gonadotropin; M, human menopausal gonadotropin, E, estrogen; P, gestogen; T, corticoids; B, ergocryptine; LRF, releasing factor; Antibi., antibiotics

Per ML, Urinary pregnanediol

  P = Plasma progesterone

  LH = Luteinizing hormone (urinary)

MED, medical treatment on the day of cycle administered (Rx)

Cx (cervix) MUCUS Amount

  Viscosity (T, thin; M, moderate; k, thick)

  Spinnbarkeit

  White blood cells

  Ferning

  PH

  Cervix score

  Vaginal smear cytology: 1–4, estrogen; 5 and 6, exfoliation; 7, smear cannot be evaluated

PC (postcoital test): HRS, hours postcoital

  No 100X, number of spermatozoa × 100x; % Motil, percentage motility

  Grade, grade of 1–4 (4 being the best forward motility)

Estradiol PG/ML, picograms per ml

Ultrasound No., number of follicles

Follicle # 1 mm and # 2 mm, size in mm of the two largest follicles.

*PATIENT P.G. # 18990:*

— Laparoscopy on February 8, 1980 showed mild endometriosis and anovulation

— Danazol 800 mg daily was prescribed from 20 February 1980 through 20 May 1980

— Conception occurred during the second month of clomiphene and HCG therapy plus husband insemination

— Clomiphene citrate 2 tablets daily from day 5 through day 9 was prescribed

— HCG 10 000 units was administered on day 14 of the cycle

— Note hostile mucus on days 14 and 16 of the cycle

— Intrauterine husband insemination (AIH) was performed on days 14 and 16 of the cycle

— On 26 August 1980 a UCG was strongly positive

— 27 April 1981 the patient was delivered of a baby girl weighing 7 lbs 7 ounces the intrauterine technique (Fig. 20.9). If conception fails to occur after an adequate trial with clomiphene, with or without hCG, we would offer therapy with human menopausal and chorionic gonadotropin.

## LONG-TERM SURVEILLANCE

Inasmuch as endometriosis is a long-term disease complex and inasmuch as 40–50% of infertile patients with endometriosis will never achieve a pregnancy, one must provide long-term follow-up of these patients. Even when endometriosis is presumably cured, there may be recurrences, hence I would prefer to use the term 'arrested endometriosis' rather than 'cure' of the disease. Perhaps patients with recurrent endometriosis, and especially those who have no desire for pregnancy, should be treated with gestagens in the form of injectable medroxyprogesterone acetate. This regimen would be contraindicated in the patient who desired pregnancy because long-term ovulation suppression would be the result of such therapy.

Danazol therapy for six plus months is quite benign. However, no one knows whether this drug can be safely used for many more months or even years in patients with annoying symptoms of recurrent endometriosis who do not desire pregnancy. For example, a patient with catamenial pneumothorax was recently seen. Would it be safe to give such a patient danazol for years?

In a letter, Lieberman (personal communication) discussed a patient with symptomatic endometriosis who had no desire for pregnancy and who was successfully treated with danazol 100 mg daily. He wondered about long-term side-effects. He called my attention to a letter by Fraser & Allen (1979) who reported metabolic changes in a group of patients treated for endometriosis with danazol in doses varying from 400 and 800 mg daily. In all, 19 women were studied over a 6-month period. Total plasma cholesterol in fasting patients rose progressively. Furthermore, in eight patients studied subsequently a dramatic fall in high density lipoprotein cholesterol (HDL) was observed 2 months after therapy was initiated compared with the pretreatment levels. They concluded that patients taking danazol may be at risk of coronary heart disease.

The treatment of mild endometriosis has been shown to be controversial since similar pregnancy rates are described when comparing conservative surgery (Schenken & Malinak 1982) to hormonal modalities (Butler et al 1984) as well as to expectant management. Our approach has gradually shifted to surgical removal at the time of diagnosis. The benefit of surgically removing mild endometriosis is in retarding the progression of the disease and eliminating potential for pain, rather than in increasing the pregnancy rate.

Endometriosis is usually a progressive disease with symptoms increasing in severity. The disease may spread from small implants to involve other pelvic and extrapelvic structures. Hence, constant surveillance of patients with endometriosis is mandatory, especially in those who do not achieve a pregnancy. Repeat medical therapy may be indicated and, furthermore, repeat surgical laparoscopy or laparotomy may be necessary to solve recurrent problems.

## THE INCIDENCE OF ENDOMETRIOSIS IN ISRAEL

A very low incidence of endometriosis has been reported from Israel. For example, in a report by Dor et al (1977) there is no mention of endometriosis. Also, in a recent report from the Kaplan Hospital, Rehovot, Israel, Lancet reported that in a series of 392 major operative procedures, there were only four patients with endometriosis (1.26%). Among a total of 2350 minor surgical operations, there were 40 patients in whom diagnostic laparoscopy was performed. The possible reasons for the low incidence of reported endometriosis from Israel could be the limited use of diagnostic laparoscopy.

Another possibility would be hereditary. Simpson et al (1980) stated that systematic genetic studies in endometriosis have not been conducted. Therefore they studied 123 patients with histologically proven endometriosis. Nine of 153 (5.8%) female sibs over age 18 of patients with histologically proven endometriosis were considered similarly affected; ten of 123 mothers (8.1%) were affected; 19 of 276 (6.9%) of all first-degree relatives were affected. By contrast, only one of 104 (1.0%) female sibs of their husbands and only one of 107 (0.6%) mothers of their husbands were affected. They postulated that polygenetic multifactorial inheritance was probably involved; hence the low incidence of endometriosis in Israel could be hereditary.

## ACKNOWLEDGEMENTS

I wish to acknowledgement the assistance of Dr Isaac Ben-Nun, former Fellow in Reproductive Medicine, who reviewed the extensive literature on endometriosis. I further would like to thank Dr Robert T. Chatterton, Director of the Endocrine Laboratory, Northwestern Memorial Hospital for his critical review of the role of prostaglandins in endometriosis.

## REFERENCES

Acosta A A, Buttram V C Jr, Besch P K, Malinak R L, Franklin R R, Vanderheyden J D 1973 A proposed classification of Adamson G D 1986 Unpublished data endometriosis. Obstet Gynecol 42: 19

Baggish M S, Daniell J F 1989 Death secondary to air embolism associated with Nd-YAG laser surgery and artificial sapphire tips. Am J Obstet Gynecol 161: 877

Bayly H A, Gossack L L 1956 External endometriosis and abnormal uterine bleeding. Am J Obstet Gynecol 72: 147

Biberoglue K O, Behrman S J 1981 Dosage aspects of danazol therapy in endometriosis: short-term and long-term effectiveness. Am J Obstet Gynecol 139: 645

Butler L, Wilson E A, Belisle S, Gibson M, Albrecht B, Schiff I, Stillman R 1984 Collaborative study of pregnancy rates following danazol therapy of stage I endometriosis. Fertil Steril 41: 373

Cheesman K L, Ben-Nun I, Cohen M R, Chatterton R T 1982 Gonadotropin and pregnanediol excretion patterns associated with endometriosos. Presented at the Society for Gynecologic Investigation. Annual Meeting

Cohen M R 1967 Peritoneoscopy vs: culdoscopy, Exhibit, 14 April, American Fertility Society, Washington, DC

Corson S L, Unger M, Kwa D et al 1989 Laparoscopic laser treatment of endometriosis with the Nd : YAG sapphire probe. Am J Obstet Gynecol 169: 718

DeLeon F D, Vijayakumar R, Rao C V, Yussman M 1988 Production of $PGF_{2\alpha}$ and $PGE_{2\alpha}$ by peritoneum involved with and without endometriosis. Int J Fertil 32: 6

Dmowski W P, Cohen M R 1975 Treatment of endometriosis with an antigonadotropin, danazol: a laparoscopic and histologic evaluation. Obstet Gynecol 46: 2

Dmowski W P, Cohen M R 1978 Endometriosis: current concepts in hormonal therapy using a new antigonadotropin (Danazol). Exhibit, American Medical Association, St Louis

Dmowski W P, Scholer H F, Mahesh V B, Greenblatt R B 1971 Danazol: a synthetic steroid derivative with interesting physiologic properties. Fertil Steril 22: 9

Dmowski W P, Rao R, Scommegna A 1980 The luteinized unruptured follicle syndrome and endometriosis. Fertil Steril 33: 30

Dmowski W P, Kapetanakis M, Scommegna A 1982 Variable effects of danazol on endometriosis at four low-dose levels. Obstet Gynecol 59: 408

Dor J, Homburg R, Rabau E 1977 An evaluation of etiologic factors and therapy in 665 infertile couples. Fertil Steril 28: 718

Drake T S, O'Brien W F, Ramwell P W, Metz S A 1981 Peritoneal fluid thromboxane $B_2$ and 6-keto-prostaglandin $F_{1\alpha}$ in endometriosis. Am J Obstet Gynecol 140: 401

Feste J R 1985 Laser laparoscopy a new modality. J Reprod Med 30: 413

Fraser I S, Allen J K 1979 Danazol and cholesterol metabolism. Lancet i:

Goldberg F J, Ramwell P W 1975 Role of prostaglandins in reproduction. Physiol Rev 55: 325

Greenblatt R B, Dmowski W P, Mahesh V B, Scholer H F L 1971 Clinical studies with an antigonadotropin—danazol. Fertil Steril 22: 102

Halban J 1924 Hysteroadenosis metastica (di lymphogene genese der sog: Adenofibromatosis heterotopica). Wien Klin Wochenschr 37: 1025

Hamada Y, Bronson R A, Wright K H, Wallach E E 1977 Ovulation in the perfused rabbit ovary: the influence of prostaglandins and prostaglandin inhibitors. Biol Reprod 17: 58

Hamada Y, Wright K H, Wallach E E 1979 The effects of progesterone and human chorionic gonadotropin on ovulation in the in vitro perfused rabbit ovary. Fertil Steril 32: 335

Henzl M R, Corson S L, Moghissi K, Buttram V C, Berquist C, Jacobson J 1988 for the Nafarelin Study Group. Administration of nasal nafarelin as compared with oral danazol for endometriosis: a multicenter double-blind comparative clinical trial. N Engl J Med 318: 485

Horne H W Jr, Clyman M, Debrovner C et al 1973 The prevention of postoperative pelvic adhesions following conservative operative treatment for human infertility. A final 3-year follow-up report. Int J Fertil 18: 109

Iwanoff M S 1898 Drusiges cystenhaltiges uterus-fibromyom kompliziert durch sarcom und carcinom. Wschr Geburtsh Gunakol 7: 295

Jacobsen V C 1922 Intraperitoneal implantation of endometrial tissue. Arch Surg 5: 281

Jansen R P S, Russel P 1986 Non-pigmented endometriosis: clinical, laparoscopic and pathologic definition. Am J Obstet Gynecol 155: 1154

Keye W R, Hansen L W, Astin M, Paulson A M S 1987 Argon laser therapy of endometriosis: a review of 92 consecutive patients. Fertil Steril 47: 208

Kistner R W 1959 The treatment of endometriosis by inducing pseudopregnancy with ovarian hormones: a report of 58 cases. Fertil Steril 10: 539

Kistner R W 1962 Infertility with endometriosis. A plan of therapy. Fertil Steril 13: 237

Kistner R W, Siegler A M, Behrman S J 1977 Suggested classification for endometriosis: relationship to infertility. Fertil Steril 28: 1008

Litchen E M, Bombard J 1987 Laparoscopic treatment of primary dysmenorrhea with laparoscopic uterine nerve ablation. J Reprod Med 32: 37

Manson A J, Stonner F W, Neumann H C et al 1963 Steroidal heteromolecules: VII. Androstano(2,3-d) isoxazoles and related compounds. J Med Chem 6: 1

Martin D C 1986 Intra-abdominal laser surgery. The Resurge Press, Memphis, USA

Martin D C, Absteen G T, Levinson C J 1986 In: Photopulos G J (ed) Intra-abdominal Surgery. The Resurge Press, Memphis, p 116

Meldrum D R, Chang R J, Lu J, Vale W, Rivier J, Judd H L 1982 'Medical oophorectomy' using a long-acting GnRH agonist—a possible new approach to the treatment of endometriosis. J Clin Endocrinol Metab 54 1081

Meyer R 1903 Eine unbekannte art von adenomyom des uterus, mit einer kritischen besprechung der urnierinhypothese von Recklinghausen. Z Gerburtshilfe Gynaekol 49: 464

Moncada S, Vane J R 1979 Pharmacology and endogenous roles of prostaglandin endoperoxides, thromboxane A$_2$ and prostacyclin. Pharmacol Rev 30: 293

Moore E E, Harger J H, Rock J A, Archer D F 1981 Management of pelvic endometriosis with low-dose danazol. Fertil Steril 36: 15

Murphy A A, Green R, De LaCruz I, Rock J A 1986 Unsuspected endometriosis documented by scanning electron microscopy in visually normal peritoneum. Fertil Steril 46: 522

Nezhat C, Crowley S R 1986 Surgical treatment of endometriosis via laser laparotomy. Feril-Steril 45: 778

Nezhat C, Crowley S, Nezhat F 1989 Videolaseroscopy for the treatment of endometriosis associated with infertility. Fertil Steril 51: 237

Nunley W C Jr, Kitchin J D 1980 Congenital atresia of the uterine cervix with pelvic endometriosis. Arch Surg 115: 757

Paulson J D, Asmar P 1986 Analysis of the first 150 pregnancies after laser laparotomy presented at the Annual ASCEP/GLA meeting, Boston, USA

Ridley J H, Edwards I K 1958 Experimental endometriosis in the human. Am J Obstet Gynecol 76: 783

Sampson J A 1925 Heterotopic or misplaced endometrial tissue. Am J Obstet Gynecol 10: 649

Schenken R S, Asch R H 1980 Surgical induction of endometriosis in the rabbit: effects on fertility and concentrations of peritoneal fluid prostaglandins. Fertil Steril 34: 581

Schenken R S, Malinak L R 1982 Conservative surgery versus expectant management for the infertile patients with mild endometriosis. Fertil Steril 37: 183

Semm K 1976 Pelviskopie und hysteroskipie—Lehrbuch und atlas. Schattauer, Stuttgart

Semm K 1979 Der wandel in der therapie der endometriose. In: Beller F K (ed) Tagungsbericht fortschritte in der gynakologie und geburtshilfe - III. Internationales munsteraner gesprach uber fortschritte in der geburtshilfe und gynakologie. G Braun, Karlsruhe, pp 76–104

Semm K 1981 Three-step therapy for endometriosis in infertility. In: Insler V, Bettendorf G (eds) Advances in diagnosis and treatment of infertility. Elsevier North Holland, New York, pp 271–276

Simpson J L, Elias S, Malinak L R, Buttram V C Jr 1980 Heritable aspects of endometriosis; I. Genetic studies. Am J Obstet Gynecol 137: 327

Sterling-Winthrop Research Institute 1981 A clinical comparison of the effectiveness of four dosage regimens in the treatment of endometriosis

TeLinde R W, Scott R B 1950 Experimental endometriosis. Am J Obstet Gynecol 60: 1147

Vernon M S, Beard J S, Graves K, Wilson E A 1986 Classification of endometriotic implants by morphologic appearance and capacity to synthesize prostaglandin F. Fertil Steril 46: 801

Von Rokitansky C, quoted in Ridley J H 1968 The histogenesis of endometriosis: a review of facts and fancies. Obstet Gynecol Surv 23: 1

Wallach E E, Bronson R, Hamada Y, Wright K H, Stevens V C 1975 Effectiveness of prostaglandin F$_{2\alpha}$ in restoration of HMG-HCG induced ovulation in indomethacin-treated rhesus monkeys. Prostaglandins 10: 129

Weed J C, Arquembourg P C 1980 Endometriosis: can it produce an autoimmune response resulting in infertility: Clin Obstet Gynecol 23: 885

Williams T J, Pratt J H 1977 Endometriosis in 1000 consecutive celiotomies; incidence and management. Am J Obstet Gynecol 129: 245

# 21. Assisted reproductive technologies

*R. Ron-El   A. Golan   A. Herman   H. Nachum   Y. Soffer
E. Caspi*

## INTRODUCTION

Assisted reproductive technology (ART) has become the frontier of both infertility treatment and research. The birth of Louise Brown in 1978, following oocyte fertilized in vitro (Edwards et al 1981), constituted the opening shot after which extensive outbreak occurred and tremendous progress has been made. Nowadays, ART is

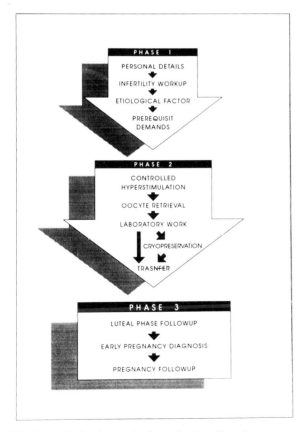

**Fig. 21.1**  Assisted reproductive technology flow chart.

widespread all over the world and has become part of treatment modalities in infertile couples. Therefore, one should be familiar with its basic process, advantages, limitations and complications. The heading ART represents a considerable variety of procedures all comprising the principal step of oocyte collection. With the vast experience gathered up to now there are still many questions with no clear answer. For instance, at what stage of infertility treatment to perform ART, to whom, how many embryos to transfer and where to replace them, how many treatment cycles to perform and many more questions. Beyond practical debates. ART also presents moral and sometimes ethical dilemmas. Society should be alert so that advances in laboratory techniques do not lead to deviant interference in the process of life creation just to satisfy scientific curiousity.

ART can be divided into three main phases (Fig. 21.1). Phase I includes preparations before ART treatment, beginning with an acquaintance meeting in which the couple is questioned on personal details, on previous infertility workup and treatment. At this stage one should decide whether ART should be instituted, be postponed in order to complete workup or other treatment, or the couple rejected. Patients who are referred to ART have to perform certain examinations and their etiological factor should be assessed. At this stage one should also clarify if specific procedures, such as egg or sperm donation or even embryo donation, are needed.

Phase II comprises the core of the ART program which includes controlled ovarian hyperstimulation, oocyte retrieval, laboratory work and transfer of gametes/zygotes (gametes/zygote intrafallopian transfer (GIFT/ZIFT)), pronuclei stage (pronuclear stage tubal transfer (PROST)) or embryos to either the uterine cavity (UET) or to the Fallopian tubes (tubal embryo transfer (TET)).

Phase III includes luteal treatment and follow-up, including ovarian hyperstimulation syndrome (OHSS), early diagnosis of conception and pregnancy followup until delivery.

## Patient selection

ART should be regarded as one of the procedures within infertility workup and treatment modalities which the couple may undergo. Ideally, although not always practical, the same medical personnel should follow the couples during various infertility stages including the ART program. Both patients and physicians have to know that ART is not the ultimate solution to all infertility problems. Moreover, sometimes better results are obtained with other treatments rather than ART. Many patients do not realize that ART is a complex procedure which deserves substantial practical and moral efforts and resources with limited success rate. On the other hand, ART might be the only chance for many couples to conceive. Thus, sometimes it constitutes a critical procedure before fateful descisions such as adoption or gamete donation are undertaken.

The process of patient selection should be well organized and it is recommended to establish a steady policy for referral so that all patients meet the same criteria. Nevertheless, ART is still developing and dynamic changes occur. Therefore, patients rejected in the past may be reconsidered.

### Personal details

Advanced maternal age presents the most common reason for rejecting patients from an ART program. When enough data was gathered (Edwards & Steptoe 1983, Jones 1986, Padilla & Garcia 1989) it was recognized that above age 40 the expectancy of pregnancy was diminished and associated with high abortion rate. Thus 40 years seems a logical upper limit. These findings are still valid, and according to findings of Dicker et al (1991) in 135 patients aged 41 years and more, 16% conceived resulting in a 61% abortion rate

and 3.7% 'take home baby' rate. Improved results among patients aged 40 years or older were reported by Navot et al (1991) following oocyte donation. This indicates that poor oocyte quality constitutes the major cause of age-related infertility. Attention should be given not only to the 'chronological age' but also to the 'biological age' which may be reflected by basal follicle stimulating hormone (FSH) level (Loumaye et al 1990, Toner et al 1991).

The couple, especially the female, should be enquired on general health condition. Cases with chronic illness including subclinical ones should be carefully evaluated in order to examine the influence of ART treatment and pregnancy on life expectancy. It is advised to consult borderline cases in a multidisciplinary forum and the couple should be informed of the hazards. Some couples may seem to be unsuitable to serve as parents (drug addicts, HIV infected, etc.). An extended committee, including social workers, psychologists and public persons, should confront such dilemmas.

### Infertility workup and treatment

Any ART procedure should be preceded by traditional fertility workup (Blackwell 1989) which involves assessment of ovulation, semen analysis, postcoital test, hysterosalpingography and laparoscopy and/or hysteroscopy. More detailed investigations should be carried out according to findings: hormonal profile, ovarian ultrasonography (US) or pituitary imaging in cases with anovulation; sperm penetration assays (SPA) and electron microscopy in cases with impaired sperm analysis; immunological tests in cases with unsatisfactory postcoital tests; hysteroscopy which in many centers still remains a second-line investigation employed when uterine pathology or an anomaly is seen at hysterosalpingography.

Appropriate treatment should be accomplished according to the finding, prior to ART. It is our policy to use menotropins in ovulatory patients with normal pelvic anatomy (Corsan & Kemmann 1991) before referring to ART. Others (Sunde et al 1988, Dodson & Haney 1991) use also intrauterine insemination (IUI) for the same cases. We use IUI only in cases with impaired semen, cervical factor or unsatisfactory postcoital test (Makler et al 1984, Allen et al 1985, Margallioth et al 1988). The presence of intrauterine adhesions deserves surgical correction prior to ART treatment (Golan et al 1992a, Ron-El et al 1992a), whereas other anatomical findings such as myoma, uterine anomaly or endometriotic cyst present a dilemma whether to recommend surgery or perform ART first.

*Etiological factors*

Originally, ART was directed towards patients with tuboperitoneal infertility. In a short period, indications were expanded and included unexplained infertility, male factor and endometriosis. Although ART is not the panacea of infertility (Thatcher & DeCherney 1989), almost every case, regardless of the etiological factor, undergoes ART in due time. This includes polycystic ovary syndrome (PCOS), immunological and uterine causes and advanced age. As preimplantation genetic diagnosis becomes feasible (Handyside et al 1989), it seems that patients belonging to this category will also seek ART treatment. The proportion of patients according to the various etiological factors and results among our last 1000 cycles are presented in Table 21.1.

**Tubal infertility** Only two decades ago reconstructive surgery of the tubes constituted the sole solution for tubal infertility. Today, use of those procedures is becoming less and less common and since the chances of curing infertility by extensive reconstructive surgery are lessening, repeated ART trials are preferred.

Tureck et al (1988) suggested the combination of ART with reconstructive surgery, but this approach was not accepted. Surgery is primarily recommended to young patients, with relatively uncomplicated problems such as periadnexal adhesions or tubal ligation. Thick-walled phimosis or hydrosalpinx and multilocular hydrosalpinx are primary indications for ART (Wiedemann & Hepp 1989). Surgical correction may be offered to borderline cases following unsuccessful ART attempts. Physicians have to remember that cases with tubal infertility can conceive spontaneously during waiting or after ART trail (Ron-El et al 1991a). Ectopic pregnancy which is common after reconstruction of the tube is also more frequent among patients undergoing ART treatment (Herman et al 1990a, Dubuisson et al 1991).

**Unexplained infertility** This cause is second most frequent in ART (Table 21.1) (Lessing et al 1988, Thatcher & DeCherney 1989). Traditionally, unexplained infertility is diagnosed after comprehensive infertility workup, including laparoscopy in the female and SPA or hemizona assay (HZA) (Oehninger et al 1989a) in the male. Although, superovulation with or without insemination yields a considerable success rate, similar to ART, (Crosignani et al 1991) both patients and physicians become 'short breathing' and ART is the next step around the corner. Comparison of patients undergoing ART, with primary and secondary unexplained infertility, demonstrated higher pregnancy rates in the latter group (Lessing et al 1988). Although ART results in patients with unexplained infertility seem to be inferior to those achieved in patients with tubal

**Table 21.1** Distribution of etiological factors and results in 1000 recent IVF-ET cycles in Assaf Harofe Medical Center

| Etiological factor | Cycles | | Embryo transfer | | Clinical pregnancies | |
|---|---|---|---|---|---|---|
| | No. | % | No. | %* | No. | %* |
| Tubal | 382 | 38 | 246 | 64 | 71 | 19 |
| Unexplained | 318 | 32 | 201 | 63 | 42 | 13 |
| Male | 200 | 20 | 80 | 40 | 18 | 9 |
| Endometriosis | 64 | 6 | 39 | 61 | 8 | 13 |
| Other/combined | 36 | 4 | 20 | 56 | 6 | 17 |
| Total | 1000 | 100 | 594 | 60 | 147 | 15 |

* Percentage of total cycles within each etiological factor.

infertility (Table 21.1) (Audibert et al 1989), reasonable results ate still obtained. Moreover, following a considerable period of time, in vitro fertilization (IVF) programs in which quantity and quality of fertilizations can be validated seem to be of importance in order to rule out sperm and/or oocyte factors contributing to infertility. Therefore, it is suggested to use IVF for both treatment and work-up in unexplained cases and to assign this diagnosis only to cases in which normal fertilization took place. When no fertilization occurs in repeated cycles a cross-over gamete donation should be considered.

*Male factor* It was recognized relatively late that cases with male factor may be successfully treated by ART (Cohen et al 1984, Van Uem et al 1985, Hirsch et al 1986). Initial impression of high successes in IVF in this category (Cohen et al 1984) were realized as being too optimistic thereafter. Nevertheless, ART has become a standard step in male infertility treatment with increasing significance. As criteria for patients' allocation to ART programs vary among the centers, the results are not comparable. Although minimal requirements were published (Riedel et al 1989), even cases with extremely severe problems undergo ART several times before accepting the idea of sperm donation. We refuse further ART attempts following two ART treatments without fertilizations of at least four oocytes, each time. In some cases, oocyte donation may be suggested for subsequent trials, in order to ensure that the problem resides with the sperm. Many believe that the new technique of micromanipulation (see 'Laboratory techniques in ART' below) is going to be the answer to this disturbing problem.

*Endometriosis* Following failed surgical and/or medical treatment for endometriosis, ART is the next step in cases with and without tubal obstruction (Chillik et al 1985, Matson & Yovich 1986). Reduced number of oocytes, impaired oocyte quality and implantation inhibitory factor were mentioned for explaining unfavorable results in ART (Wardle et al 1985, Chillik et al 1985, Yovich et al 1985, Yovich et al 1988a). Results of IVF-ET during 1989 in the USA (Medical Research International 1991) demonstrated increased numbers of cycles in cases due to endometriosis, with results similar to other etiological causes.

*Immunological infertility* Immunological infertility relates to antibodies, either in the male or the female, that involve antigens of the sperm (Jones 1987). Various treatments were suggested, including immunosuppression, sperm washing and IUI, artificial donor insemination, antibiotic therapy (Soffer et al 1990) and use of a condom. Again, ART is an inevitable method when other treatments fail to improve the chances of pregnancy. ART results in this category are also favorable (Medical Research International 1991).

*Polycystic ovary syndrome (PCOS)* Although clomiphene citrate (CC) and exogenous menotropins are successfully employed for ovulation induction in the majority of patients with PCOS, cumulative pregnancy rates are lower than 50%. Those patients are prone to develop ovarian hyperstimulation syndrome (OHSS). The more oocytes recovered in patients with PCOS compared with control group of tubal disease, yielded a similar number of embryos (Dor et al 1990). This suggests reduced fertilization capacity of oocytes harvested from PCOS patients. Nevertheless, the pregnancy rate was comparable and a suggestion was even made to direct patients with PCOS with impending OHSS to ART in order to reduce its risk (Lessing et al 1991).

*Ovarian failure* The first successful pregnancy following oocyte donation was reported in 1984 by Lutjen et al. Whereas in the past this procedure was limited to cases with ovarian failure that was either congenital (Turner's syndrome) or acquired (premature menopause), the indications today are widened and include hereditary diseases, advanced age or repeated embryonal loss.

*Miscellaneous factors* Cases with exposure to diethylstillbestrol in embryonic life (DES syndrome), uterine problems such as uterine myoma, intrauterine adhesion or congenital anomaly and advanced age, are among a broad spectrum of categories which do not belong to either of the above groups.

*Prerequisite demands*

Before ART treatment is employed the couple is

asked to perform certain preliminary examinations. According to our policy this includes: immune status for rubella, hepatitis B antigens, immune status for human immunodeficiency virus, cervical cytology (Pap smear), cultures for *Chlamydia trachomatis*, *Mycoplasma hominis* and *Ureaplasma urealyticum*.

Findings among 187 of the patients admitted to ART in our unit (Ron-El et al 1992a) (Table 21.2) demonstrated that in spite of previous IVF treatment only the minority were examined to rubella antibodies and cervical cytology. Moreover, six cases had pathological cervical findings that were treated with laser, conization or extended hysterectomy in one case.

## OVARIAN STIMULATION OF MULTIPLE FOLLICLE DEVELOPMENT

### Introduction

The first conceptions in the IVF-ET program as reported by Steptoe & Edwards between 1976 and 1980 were the product of a spontaneous cycle (Steptoe & Edwards 1976, Edwards et al 1980). These pioneers in ART had previously had bad experience when stimulating the ovaries with human menopausal gonadotropin (hMG) or CC. The lack of conceptions was explained by abnormal follicular steroid production and derangement of the luteal phase. Interestingly, Lopata et al (1978) had the same lack of success in achieving pregnancies with stimulated cycles. Consequently, it was generally considered that successful fertilization in vitro would be limited to spontaneous ovulatory cycles. However, the technical difficulties associated with ovum retrieval in spontaneous cycles continued to encourage others to re-evaluate stimulation for IVF. Trounson et al (1981) showed that induction of multiple follicular development with CC and final maturation of oocytes with human chorionic gonadotropin (hCG) can be used successfully for establishment of pregnancy. In this mode, there was no necessity for frequent sampling of blood or urine to assess the onset of LH release and to aspirate the follicle 26–28 hours afterwards. Oocyte collection could be programmed 35–36 hours after hCG administration when the leading follicle diameter measured by US was 18–20 mm (Hoult et al 1981).

In 1982 the Australian group started to use the combination of CC and hMG devised by McBain (Lopata 1983). In this protocol an individualized approach to ovarian stimulation was adopted, leading to a higher pregnancy rate in comparison to success with CC alone.

At the same period of time the Norfolk group has gained its experience with hMG and FSH combined with hMG (Jones et al 1982). With their increasing experience, they could nicely correlate between different estradiol response patterns and outcome of IVF programs (Jones et al 1983). The wide use of hMG stimulation raised

**Table 21.2** Findings of prerequisite examinations performed in 187 patients prior to ART treatment

| | Documented prior to ART | | Tests performed in our program | | |
| --- | --- | --- | --- | --- | --- |
| | No. | % | Total | Abnormal | |
| | | | | No. | % |
| Rubella antibodies | 84 | 45 | 103 | 11 | 6* |
| Hepatitis B Ag | 19 | 10 | 164 | 8 | 5 |
| HIV antibodies | – | | 187 | 0 | |
| Pap smear | 55 | 29 | 132 | 6 | 3† |
| C. trachomatis | | | 187 | 23 | 14‡ |
| M. hominis | | | 187 | 26 | 14‡ |
| U. urealyticum | | | 187 | 30 | 16‡ |

* Were referred to rubella vaccination before ART.
† This included three cases with cervical intraepithelial neoplasma (CIN) I, one with CIN II, one with CIN III and one with carcinoma Ib.
‡ Were treated until negative cultures were obtained.

the problem of early luteinization and low response, which turned out to be major obstacles in this mode of treatment. 'Medical hypophysectomy' introduced by Fleming et al (1982) using gonadotropin releasing hormone agonist (GnRHa) prior to exogenous ovarian stimulation with hMG was applied in 1984 by Porter et al in IVF programs to induce multifollicular ovulation in 'low responders'. Since then, the combined GnRHa/hMG treatment is used in many IVF units all over the world.

The increasing success of IVF is amongst other things attributable to improved methods of ovarian stimulation. Therefore, it is of major importance to be acquainted with the protocols leading to multiple follicle development and production of multiple embryos without detrimental influence on establishment of clinical pregnancy.

## CC alone

The use of CC as a single agent for multiple follicle development in IVF was first attempted by Lopata et al (1978). Re-evaluation of the use of CC and the addition of hCG to program oocyte collections as described by Trounson et al (1981) led to four clinical pregnancies in 23 women.

The purpose of CC is to override the physiological phenomenon of follicle selection and to induce maturation of several secondary follicles which would probably undergo the process of atresia in natural cycles. The dosage of CC widely used in normally ovulating women undergoing IVF is 100–150 mg daily for 5 days. A smaller dosage or longer period of CC administration did not improve pregnancy rate (Marrs et al 1983). The ideal starting day of CC is considered to be cycle day 5. Commencement of CC on day 3 of the cycle led to low response in a higher percentage (35% vs 3%) when compared to women starting the medication on day 5. Later initiation of CC, on day 7, resulted in a single follicle in 23% of the stimulated cycles. Spontaneous LH surge occurred in 8% and 10% in the groups with days 3 and 7 as the starting day of CC, and in 2% when CC was initiated on day 5 (Marrs et al 1984). The mean number of recovered eggs via laparoscopy was 2.6 in the CC

protocol compared with four to five oocytes per laparoscopy under the CC/hMG stimulation in the same group and at the same time period (Lopata 1983).

The continuous controversy about the detrimental effect of CC on follicular fluid, oocyte, endometrium and luteal phase has been extended from the in vivo treatment to the IVF program. Animal studies indicate a detrimental effect upon maturation and development of mouse oocytes and embryos. Laufer et al (1983) and Ho Yuen et al (1988) have shown the inhibition of progesterone accumulation in cultured human granulosa cells in the presence of CC which can be corrected by hCG administration. However, some authors have seen no difference in fertilization of ovulated ova exposed to CC in comparison to controls (Yoshimura et al 1986). Talbert (1983) suggested that proper assessment of the outcome of CC treatment should be done by life-table analysis. By doing so he found a pregnancy rate per ovulatory cycle of 22%, which remained constant for at least 10 months. This result was not lower than that observed in women who discontinued diaphragm contraception.

The lower pregnancy rate in IVF when using CC alone as stimulation protocol is probably due to the lower mean number of oocytes and, as a consequence, less embryos placed in the uterine cavity. A comparison of the outcome of CC protocol with others in which the same average number of embryos is replaced to the uterus would have been interesting.

Nevertheless, here and there some centers still use the CC protocol in their IVF program mainly because of its low cost.

## CC and hMG combination

McBain, in 1982, devised a scheme in which CC was used in combination with hMG (Lopata 1983). The length of menstrual cycle and the ovarian response were used as guiding parameters. Thus CC, 50 or 100 mg daily, was commenced on days 3–4 in cycles of 24–26 days' duration and on day 5 in cycles of 28–30 days' length. On the last day of CC, hMG was started. In cases where the second degree follicles were 8–12 mm in diameter 225 IU of hMG was given, and when the diameter of these follicles was 12–16 mm the hMG dose was 150 IU per day. The administration of hMG was maintained until at least one follicle reached a diameter of 18 mm.

A concomitant increase of plasma estradiol was documented. hCG was injected 36–48 hours after the last dose of hMG. A decrease in estradiol levels in the presence of growing follicles was an indication to abandon the cycle. Both the addition of hMG and the individual treatment approach contributed to the higher number of retrieved oocytes, more replaced embryos and higher number of pregnancies – 38% per transfer compared with 15% observed in the single-agent protocol (Lopata 1983).

Since then, there have been several studies changing the dosage of CC or hMG and the timing of their administration, but the results remained nearly the same. In a larger series of 147 CC/hMG cycles, 25% were cancelled due to LH surge, poor estradiol patterns, low response or inadequate follicle development (Taymor et al 1985). The mean number of retrieved oocytes was four per laparoscopy, 78% of them fertilized and the pregnancy rate per laparoscopy was 14%.

Since the stimulation protocols of hMG alone and of hMG combined with FSH were introduced at the same time when the combined CC/hMG protocol was in use, the latter has not been widely accepted. Thus, large multicentric comparable studies have not been done concerning the efficacy of CC/hMG protocol. Quigley et al (1988) have shown in a prospective randomized double-blind study no statistical differences between CC/FSH and CC/hMG protocols regarding cancellation, fertilization and conception rates (11% and 15% per aspiration respectively).

Moreover, the controversial effect of CC at the level of the follicle, oocyte and endometrium is of course also relevant for the combined CC/hMG protocol. When comparing the oocytes found in the GnRHa/hMG and the CC/hMG stimulations, the immaturity rate was 18% in the former and 34% in the latter protocol. Aneuploidy was of the same incidence in both groups (Pieters et al 1991). Endometrial glandular volume was significantly reduced after CC/hMG as compared with GnRHa/hMG, despite a similar histopathological dating in both groups.

The endometrial thickness and echogenicity was found to be reduced in cycles stimulated with CC/hMG compared with GnRHa/hMG cycles, although the mean estradiol level on the hCG day was 20% higher in the CC/hMG group than the corresponding estradiol level in the GnRHa/hMG protocol (Rogers et al 1991).

On analysing the data from the IVF Registry in the USA in the years 1989 and 1990 (Medical Research International 1991, 1992), the pregnancy rate with the CC/hMG stimulation was between 18% and 20%, which did not differ significantly from the results of other protocols in that report. However, the CC/hMG protocol is being slowly abandoned. While in 1989 the CC/hMG was used in the USA in 12% of all stimulated cycles, in 1990 it dropped to 2.5%.

## hMG and FSH

In 1982 Jones et al (1982) proposed to use hMG for multiple follicle development. The rationale of this proposition was that FSH and LH are natural substances with well-known physiological mechanisms of action. Jones et al (1982) administered hMG from cycle day 3 to allow for recruitment of multiple follicles before the selection of the dominant follicle. Serum estradiol levels and ultrasonography of the ovaries were assessed daily from day 6 of the cycles.

The administration of hMG was discontinued when a follicle of ≥ 12 mm was visible on the scan and the 'biologic shift' (the presence of 30% pyknotic cells and four out of five of the following characteristics: cervical mucus volume ≥ 0.2 ml, spinbarkeit ≥ 10 cm, clear mucus, 4+ ferning, dilated cervical os) had occurred on the previous or same day of the ultrasonographic examination. Ten thousand units of hCG were administered intramuscularly approximately 50–52 hours after the last dose of hMG. This interval of 50 hours was termed the 'coasting' period. Oocyte recovery took place 35–36 hours after hCG injection. This period of 80–90 hours was suggested as necessary for adequate cytoplasmic oocyte maturation. The coasting period was shortened to 28–30 hours in the following conditions: leading follicle of ≥ 16 mm in diameter, a plateau estradiol level or doubling of the estradiol from the previous-day level, or a triggered endogenous LH surge.

Early on, it was recognized that certain terminal estradiol patterns were associated with particular oocytes at recovery and pregnancy outcomes (Jones et al 1983). Four major patterns emerged, designated as A, B, C and G (Fig. 21.2).

*Pattern A:* Daily estradiol in the serum showed a continuing rise in levels during hMG administration, which continued to rise during the coasting period and after hCG administration.

*Pattern B:* Daily estradiol continued to rise during hMG administration, with a decrease during the coasting period (upon discontinuation of hMG) and rose again following the hCG administration.

*Pattern C:* Estradiol levels decreased during hMG administration and continued to fall after hCG.

*Patterns D and E* were variations of pattern C.

*Pattern G:* Estradiol levels continued to rise

during hMG stimulation and during the coasting period but decreased after hCG administration.

The mean number of retrieved oocytes, transferred embryos and pregnancy rate was the highest in pattern A, followed by patterns G and B. A shorter coasting period of 36 hours in group B led to a higher success rate, approaching that found in group A pattern. Larger experience has led to cancellation of cycles with patterns C, D and E. Cancellation criteria according to the Norfolk group were:

1. Poor estradiol response (estradiol < 100 pg/ml after 5 days of hMG administration).
2. A decrease of estradiol for 2 consecutive days during hMG stimulation period.
3. A greater than 30% decrease of estradiol level on the day after hCG administration. These patients had an endogenous LH rise on a retrospective analysis.
4. The presence of an ovarian cyst with estradiol level > 100 pg/ml on the first day of hMG stimulation.

***The 'combo' – combination protocol.*** The addition of 150 IU of FSH on days 3 and 4 of the cycle to patients who had previously exhibited poor estradiol responses resulted in an increase in the number of oocytes retrieved and improved pregnancy rate (Bernardus et al 1985).

This success of the combination of hMG and FSH on the first 2 days of the stimulation with further hMG administration gave the origin to the 'combo' protocol. The mean number of oocytes recovered per laparoscopy was 3.0 with the combo protocol (228 laparoscopies) and 1.6 with the hMG scheme (453 laparoscopies). Likewise the pregnancy rate was 32% and 24% per transfer respectively. The explanation of these better results with the FSH/hMG combination was in the authors' view due to the utilization of the highest amount of gonadotropin in the early follicular phase, mimicking the normal menstrual cycle by improving the FSH/LH ratio. However, it seems that the different results with the 'combo' protocol were due to the different criteria of hMG discontinuation in the FSH/hMG protocol, e.g. when estradiol reached ≥ 900 pg/ml and not > 600 pg/ml as in the hMG protocol. By elevating

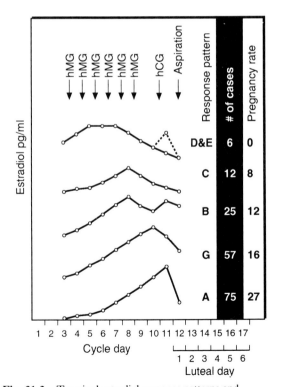

**Fig. 21.2** Terminal estradiol response patterns and associated pregnancy rates. (Reproduced with permission from Jones et al 1983)

the estradiol levels before hMG discontinuation more follicles were sustained, more oocytes were retrieved and so the outcome was improved. With the FSH/hMG combination or FSH protocol, as Jones et al (1985) suggested, a longer stimulation period was possible with less LH and consequently less androgenic interference. However, prospective radomized studies (Scoccia et al 1987) comparing the FSH and hMG protocols, found significantly less cancellation of treated cycles with the FSH protocol but no significant differences regarding pregnancy rate.

Data from the IVF registry in the USA (Medical Research International 1991, 1992) which are shown in Table 21.3 demonstrated no differences in cancellation and clinical pregnancy rates between the hMG and FSH/hMG protocols.

Ovarian stimulation with hMG alone has been shown to be associated with consistent relatively high and reproducible pregnancy rate. However, the cancellation rate with this protocol remains between 20% and 25% (Medical Research International 1991, 1992). The most frequent reasons for cycle cancellation are: spontaneous fall in estradiol before oocyte retrieval, early luteinization (early LH rise), poor response with a single or two follicles or early ovulation.

## GnRH agonist and hMG

Ovulation induction has significantly higher success rate in women with hypothalamo-pituitary failure (group I, WHO Classification) than in women with hypothalamo-pituitary dysfunction (group II) (Lunenfeld & Insler 1978). It was suggested by Fleming et al (1982) to perform temporary pituitary suppression by the GnRHa with subsequent ovarian stimulation by

hMG. Porter et al (1984) chose this combination as an effective way of treatment in low responders in an IVF program. A single dose of GnRHa stimulates the release of gonadotropins and consequently ovarian steroids. Multiple doses of GnRHa cause a reversible blockade of gonadotropic and ovarian function (Sandow et al 1978, Lemay et al 1983).

The action of GnRHa includes the down-regulation of GnRH receptors (Belchetz et al 1978) and the inhibition of postreceptor events (see Ch. 15). The suppression of endogenous gonadotropin secretion, when administering exogenous hMG for superovulation, enhances the efficiency of IVF programs (Porter et al 1984, Wildt et al 1986, MacLachlan et al 1989, Ron-El et al 1991b).

The most frequently used GnRHa in IVF programs are listed in Table 21.4 (see also Ch. 15). The medications are either in the form of solutions for injections, nasal spray, implants or microcapsules (depot preparations) (Sandow 1989). With the nasal spray only 2–5% of the dose is absorbed via the nasal mucosa, in relation to that from the subcutaneous injection site. Nevertheless, nasal spray is an easy self-administration, well-tolerated mode. Doses of 600–900 µg per day led to consistent suppression after 3 weeks of treatment. Subcutaneous buserelin 50 µg 3 times a day, daily single injection of 600 µg buserelin, 0.1 mg Decapeptyl or 1 mg leuprolide are all effective for achieving suppressive state before hMG administration. Likewise, sustained release formulations (Decapeptyl 3.2 mg or Zoladex) with an average duration of 4 or more weeks have also been successfully used in IVF programs. Although very convenient for use, the depot preparations can cause very profound suppression of the gonadotropic function, which in some patients

**Table 21.3** Outcome of IVF and GIFT cycles in hMG and combined hMG/FSH protocols, 1989–90 in the USA

| Stimulation | IVF Cycles (no.) | Cancellation | | Clinical pregnancies per transfer | | Deliveries per retrieval | |
|---|---|---|---|---|---|---|---|
| | | No. | % | No. | % | No. | % |
| hMG | 829 | 188 | 23 | 127 | 20 | 99 | 15 |
| FSH/hMG | 1304 | 393 | 30 | 163 | 18 | 126 | 14 |

Data from IVF-ET Registry (Medical Research International 1991, 1992).

**Table 21.4** GnRH analogs used for IVF

| | Tradename | Company | Half-life | Potency* | Commercially available preparations |
|---|---|---|---|---|---|
| Nonapeptids | | | | | |
| Buserelin (D-Ser (But)$^6$-des Gly$^{10}$-LHRH) | Suprefact | Hoechst | 80 min | 20–40 | Nasal spray, subcutaneous solution |
| Leuprolide (D-Leu$^6$-Pro$^9$-LHRH) | Lupron | Abbott | 1.30 h | 20–30 | Subcutaneous solution |
| Decapeptides | | | | | |
| Triptorelin (D-Trp$^6$-LHRH | Decapeptyl | Salk/Ferring | 7.6 h | 144 | Subcutaneous solution, microcapsules |
| Goserelin (D-Ser (But)$^6$-AzaGly$^{10}$-LHRH) | Zoladex | ICI | 4.5 h | 50–100 | Implant |

* Potency relative to native LHRH.

can lead to difficulties in achieving ovarian stimulation even with high doses of hMG.

## Indications for GnRHa use in IVF

The indications for the use of GnRHa in IVF have not been clearly defined. However, during the last years some consensus about the main indications has been established.

*Premature LH surge.* High LH levels in late follicular phase have been associated with reduced fertilization, lower pregnancy and higher abortion rates (Stanger & Yovich 1985, Howles et al 1986). Moreover, LH surge can be induced by elevated estradiol levels caused by ovarian stimulation (Messinis et al 1986, Glasier et al 1988). LH surge may occur prematurely, before follicles have reached maturation, causing luteinization, disruption of normal follicle and dismaturity of the oocyte. The GnRHa is very effective in suppressing endogenous LH secretion, diminishing frequency of premature LH elevations to < 3% (Caspi et al 1989a, MacLachlan et al 1989, Ron-El et al 1990a).

*Suppression of tonic levels.* GnRHa not only eliminates premature LH surges, but also controls efficiently tonic levels of LH, as in cases with polycystic ovarian disease (PCOD). Considerable disagreement still exists concerning the number and quality of oocytes and outcome of treatment when adding GnRHa to the regimen in PCOD cases undergoing IVF-ET. While Salat-

Baroux et al (1988) observed no differences, irrespective of the type of stimulation, Owen et al (1989) claimed to have a significantly higher fertilization rate when GnRHa was used in PCOD, indicating the oocyte quality is improved by the agonist, probably due to LH suppression (Fleming 1990).

*Poor responders.* A significant proportion of women, ranging from 15% to 30% exhibit an unsatisfactory response to ovarian stimulation, e.g. monofollicular development, low estradiol levels (<300 pg/ml) or estradiol drop after hCG administration (Diedrich et al 1988, Loumaye et al 1990). In many of these repetitive poor responders the use of GnRHa was associated with a significant increase in the number of follicles aspirated, oocytes recovered and fertilized as well as of embryos available for transfer or freezing. This patient population comprised women who failed to respond previously to ovarian stimulation several times and rarely reached oocyte pickup. Nevertheless, patients with occult ovarian failure do not benefit from the analogs and their IVF-ET results remain very low. It is therefore suggested to indentify these women by basal FSH determination (Cameron et al 1988) or with CC challenge test (Loumaye et al 1990) prior to the initiation of treatment.

*Endometriosis.* Since endometriosis is an estrogen-dependent disease, the aim in its treatment is to suppress folliculogenesis. This can be achieved among others with GnRHa. The combined use of GnRHa and hMG in IVF-ET for cases with moderate to severe endometriosis seems to improve significantly the results (Oehninger et al 1989b, Dicker et al 1990). In the severe cases it is advisable to pretreat the patient for 3–6 months by creating the 'pseudo menopause' state and then to directly continue with ovarian stimulation as part of IVF-ET treatment.

*First-line treatment.* Many authors have suggested the use of GnRHa as a first-line treatment in all women undergoing ovarian stimulation for ART (Frydman et al 1988, Caspi et al 1989a, Meldrum et al 1989). It is clear that by using the GnRHa the total cost of IVF-ET treatment is higher due to the cost of the GnRHa medication and the larger hMG amount needed for ovarian stimulation. Nevertheless, the significantly lower cancellation rate, wider possibility to program oocyte recovery and higher number of follicles and oocytes achieved made the combined GnRHa and hMG treatment the most commonly used regimen in IVF programs (Cohen & De Mouzon 1989, Medical Research International 1991, 1992).

## GnRHa protocols

Different protocols have been designed for the administration of GnRHa together with gonadotropins.

*Long protocol (blocking protocol).* This protocol is based on the suppression of ovarian activity (serum estradiol $\leq$ 30 pg/ml) before the initiation of hMG administration. The GnRHa is administered either in the late luteal or early follicular phase. The continued GnRHa effect is presumed to last up to the time of hCG administration. It can be given in its long-acting depot formulation as a single injection or in its short-acting preparation in daily administration. The administration of hMG is started only when the required suppression of the pituitary-gonadal axis has been achieved. The average length of this protocol is 25 days up to the hCG administration day.

*Short protocol (flare-up protocol)* takes advantage of the stimulating phase of the GnRHa. Thus the agonist is given daily from the second or third cycle day and hMG is started at the same time or a day or two after the commencement of the agonist. Both the agonist and hMG are continued up to the hCG day, on average a period of 13–14 days.

*Ultrashort or very short protocol.* This protocol also makes use of the initial stimulation of endogenous gonadotropins caused by the GnRHa in its first phase of administration. Short-acting agonists are given from days 2 to 4, 1 to 7 or 3 to 7 of the cycle, with hMG stimulation starting on the 2nd day of GnRHa administration. On average the length of this treatment is 12–13 days.

*Timing of GnRHa administration.* The importance of rapid and consistent suppression of ovarian activity has given rise to the question: when is the optimal time of GnRHa administration in the long protocol? The administration of GnRHa in early follicular phase causes with its stimulating phase the formation of follicular cysts and a longer stimulating phase. The luteal administration of the agonist was thought not to cause a 'flare up' state and so to prevent cyst formation and to reach a suppressive state in a shorter time period. However, Fraser & Sandow (1985) showed in primates that the initial rise of gonadotropin estradiol and progesterone after midluteal phase GnRHa administration cannot be avoided. The rise was limited to the luteal phase and prevented recruitment of follicles.

In a prospective study (Ron-El et al 1990a) in which two groups of 108 patients each were allocated either to early follicular or midluteal administration of the agonist, a stimulatory phase was evident in both groups. The estradiol peak was 102% higher than the baseline level in the group with early follicular administration (group A) compared with 23% in the group with midluteal initiation (group B) ($P < 0.001$) (Fig. 21.3.).

Fourteen days after the administration of the long-acting GnRHa, which is the standard hMG starting day in the widely used 'long protocol', only 45% of the patients in group A, but 90% in group B ($P < 0.001$) decreased to estradiol levels of $\leq$ 30 pg/ml. The ovarian suppression with the midluteal GnRHa administration is not only more

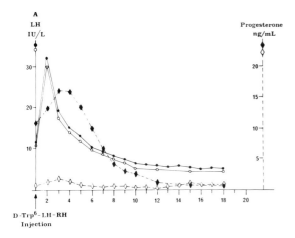

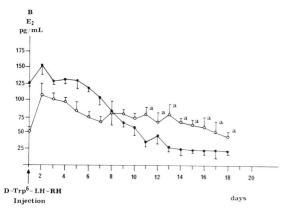

**Fig. 21.3** **a** Daily mean progesterone (group A, ◊; group B, ♦) and LH levels (group A, ○; group B, ●)
**b** Daily mean and SE of estradiol levels in group A (○) and group B (●), after D-Trp[6] injection (a, P <0.01).
Group A, Early follicular phase GnRHa commencement; group B, midluteal phase GnRHa commencement.
(Reproduced with permission from Fertility and Sterility 1990)

prompt but also seems to be more profound. The indirect proof for this suggestion was the higher hMG amounts that were needed in group B compared with group A (45 ± 5 and 41.5 ± 15 ampules respectively, $P = 0.05$). It was clearly expressed also in the different estradiol levels on the hCG administration day, 933 ± 537 pg/ml and 1740 ± 686 pg/ml respectively ($P < 0.001$).

***Outcome of the different GnRHa protocols.***
In large retrospective series more oocytes, more embryos and higher total and viable pregnancy rates were achieved with the long protocol compared with the short one (Cohen & de Mouzon 1989). Among the prospective studies dealing with the comparison of short and long protocols, some of them found no difference in the outcome of both schemes (Foulot et al 1988, Frydman et al 1988). However, these are small series, with 50 cases or less in each group. Contrary to these studies Hedon et al (1988) reported a 38% pregnancy rate per transfer with the long protocol compared to 13% with the short one. Tan et al (1990) reported pregnancy rates of 26% and 16% respectively, and Tarlatzis et al (1992) found a pregnancy rate of 26% and 19% in their series in the short and long protocols respectively. With the long protocol more hMG ampules are needed to stimulate the ovaries, leading to a higher number of oocytes that are recovered and fertilized. It seems that the long protocol offers better results. However, more prospective studies of larger numbers of women are required in order to reach firm conclusions.

The ultrashort protocol originally suggested by Macnamee et al (1989) presumably has the advantages of being a short protocol, with a very low cancellation rate and low estradiol levels in the late follicular phase. This gives the advantage of encouraging the secretory changes in the endometrium facilitating implantation. Relatively low estradiol levels in comparison with the levels found in the long and short protocols, diminish the incidence of ovarian hyperstimulation syndrome. According to Macnamee et al (1989) the pregnancy rate with the ultrashort protocol was 39% per transfer. Our pregnancy rate per transfer was 17% (Ron-El et al 1992b), significantly lower than with other GnRHa protocols. The real validity of the ultrashort protocol will have to be proven by future experience.

***GnRHa protocols and other stimulation regimens.*** The controlled prospective studies dealing with this comparison of GnRHa and non-GnRHa protocols are few. The large retrospective reports mention conflicting results. On analysing the national reports coming from France and the USA in two consecutive years (Table 21.5) in each country, the results are inconsistent and are probably biased by the different number of cycles. Smaller numbers are coming from fewer centers, and thus the results are less universal. While the pregnancy rate is in a wide range in the CC/hMG and hMG protocols (11–22% and 15–28% respectively), the results in the GnRHa/hMG protocol are between 17% and 22%, which may hint on their reliability. However, according to this retrospective data, although the GnRHa/hMG protocol has become the most frequently used, its better outcome is not clearly demonstrated.

Considering the prospective results, Table 21.6 includes studies which were randomly designed and reported in their results all details mentioned in the table. In order to be able to qualify the use of GnRHa as part of stimulation protocol one should know the number of hMG ampules which were used, number of oocytes retrieved and transferred embryos. In our experience, the benefit of the use of GnRHa, if at all, can be achieved only if stimulation was properly carried out. The number of hMG ampules in GnRHa protocol should be significantly higher than in the non-GnRHa protocol (Ron-El et al 1990b). Consequently, more oocytes are obtained, more embryos of high morphological class can be replaced, and so pregnancy chance is higher. In two studies mentioned in Table 21.6 (Antoine et al 1990, Maroulis et al 1991) the number of replaced embryos was similar in the GnRHa and non-GnRHa protocols. In the first study a higher pregnancy rate was achieved with the GnRHa protocol, whereas in the second one (Maroulis et al 1991) the pregnancy rate was higher with the non-GnRHa.

The lower cancellation rate and better possibility of programming oocyte retrieval characterized by the GnRHa, has led to the fact that the GnRHa protocols are the most commonly used today in most of the IVF centers.

Obviously, the costs per cycle with these protocols are high.

### Disadvantages and complications

***Cyst formation.*** Endogenous gonadotropins, secreted soon after GnRHa administration, seem to trigger off primordial follicle growth. The continuous elevated estradiol levels, associated with cyst formation in both early follicular and midluteal GnRHa administration, indicate that the cysts originated from growing follicles that failed to ovulate because of pituitary blockade and abolition of the feedback mechanism (Ron-El et al 1989a, Herman et al 1990b). The cysts were not related to the type of GnRHa formulation nor to the type of protocol (short or long protocol). They were reported as being present in 25% of the cycles (Feldberg et al 1987, Meldrum et al 1988) and in 15% in larger series (Herman et al 1990b, Ron-El et al 1990a). They did not recur in the majority of the repeated cycles, indicating that the phenomenon is not typical to specific patients. The incidence of follicle cyst formation is similar in the early follicular or midluteal GnRHa administration. However, with the midluteal GnRHa initiation the cysts appear earlier and regress more promptly (Herman et al 1990b). The IVF-ET outcome of such cycles was comparable with cycles with no follicular cysts (Ron-El et al 1989a). The management could be either to cancel the cycle, disregard the cyst, aspirate them or to wait until they regress when the long protocol is used. By disregarding them adverse effects like cyst enlargement, disturbed normal follicular development (Feldberg et al 1987) or increased hMG requirement (Tummon et al

**Table 21.5** Outcome of IVF-ET cycles with and without GnRH agonist pre-treatment (retrospective analysis)

| | CC/hMG | | hMG | | GnRHa, | hMG |
|---|---|---|---|---|---|---|
| | Cycles | Preg.* | Cycles | Preg.* | Cycles | Preg.* |
| de Mouzon et al 1988 | | 22 | | 28 | | 22 |
| Cohen & de Mouzon 1989 | | 11 | | 21 | | 17 |
| Medical Research International 1991 | 940 | 18 | 658 | 15 | 2876 | 22 |
| Medical Research International 1992 | 462 | 17 | 171 | 26 | 1992 | 20 |

* Pregnancy rate per embryo transfer.

538   INFERTILITY: MALE AND FEMALE

**Table 21.6**  Results of IVF in GnRHa/hMG (a) and non GnRHa (non a) stimulated cycles (prospective studies)

| | Cycles (no.) | | Cancellation (%) | | hMG ampules (no.) | | Occytes (no.) | | Embryos/transferred (no.) | | Pregnancy (%) | | | |
| | | | | | | | | | | | Cycle | | Transfer | |
| | non a | a | non a | a | non a | a | non a | a | non a | a | non a | a | non a | a |
|---|---|---|---|---|---|---|---|---|---|---|---|---|---|---|
| Antoine 1990 | 90 | 90 | 30 | 14* | 21 | 36* | 7 | 9* | 2.8 | 2.7 | 12 | 21 | 19 | 25 |
| Abdallah 1990 | 102 | 118 | 15 | 8* | 17 | 23* | 6 | 9* | 2.3 | 4.6 | 14 | 28* | 18 | 31* |
| Ron-El 1991 | 151 | 151 | 27 | 3* | 23 | 43* | 6 | 8* | 2.6 | 3.9* | 13 | 26* | 27 | 36 |
| Maroulis 1991 | 99 | 99 | 32 | 12* | 16 | 30* | 6 | 9* | 3.7 | 3.6 | 15 | 14 | 28 | 20 |

* P < 0.05 comparing non a versus a cycles.

1988) were described. Postponement of hMG administration until cyst regression did not affect IVF-ET outcome (Ron-El et al 1989b).

Aspiration of the cyst can be easily performed guided by vaginal ultrasound without any anesthesia. Once the cyst is aspirated, the estradiol level drops quickly and exogenous gonadotropin can be administered. However, aspiration of the cyst 3 weeks after commencement of GnRHa gave no benefit concerning the number of follicles, oocytes, embryos and pregnancy rate (Rizk et al 1990).

***Ovarian hyperstimulation syndrome.*** Ovarian hyperstimulation syndrome (OHSS) is a major serious complication in ovulation induction (see Ch. 16). In our IVF series (Golan et al 1988, Ron-El et al 1991b) the incidence of OHSS was 8.4% and 6.6% respectively when using GnRHa protocol. Half of the cases were classified as severe and the other half as moderate OHSS. The incidence of OHSS in hMG-alone protocols was significantly lower (0.7%, $P < 0.02$) (Ron-El et al 1991b). The reason for this is possibly the significantly higher estradiol level on the hCG administration day (1477 pg/mL versus 836 pg/mL). Asch et al (1991) found that in a patient with > 30 retrieved oocytes the chances of severe OHSS are 23%. In cases where the estradiol level on day of hCG injection was > 6000 pg/mL the chances were 38%. Patients having both these high risk factors had an 80% chance of developing severe OHSS. Witholding hCG supplementation in luteal phase, continuation of GnRHa and cryopreservation of embryos are optional courses of action for prevention (Rizk & Aboulghar 1991). Lately Asch et al (1992) have reported a complete prevention of severe OHSS in 22 high risk cases, in whom 50 gr albumin was administered during the oocyte recovery and immediately afterwards. In our program, in the last 2 years, cycles in which the estradiol level was ≥3000 pg/ml on the hCG day before oocyte retrieval are supplemented with progestational agents and not with hCG in the luteal phase. This has decreased the OHSS incidence to 3% in the GnRHa protocols. The incidence mentioned by Delvigne et al (1991) is 2.5%.

***Inadvertent exposure of concepti to GnRHa.*** With the administration of GnRHa in midluteal phase a possibility of exposure of the conceptus in its early stages to the stimulatory effect of the agonist may occur. Moreover, in cases with deficient luteal phase the stimulus given by flare-up may create a favourable environment for implantation. Ovulation can also be induced by GnRHa in the flare-up phase. A continuous progesterone rise should be interpreted as indicating a pregnancy and can be verified by hCG concentration. The question of the fate of such pregnancies is of great concern. Serafini et al (1988) presumed that pregnancies established under such conditions should be terminated. Since we encountered the pregnancies under inadvertent exposure to GnRHa in couples with longstanding infertility and the only embryo teratogenicity was described in rhesus monkeys in the form of testicular weight reduction when exposed to the agonist for more than 3 months (Sopelak & Hodgen 1987), we did not consider their termination. Supportive therapy of progesterone and estradiol valerate was administered as needed (Herman et al 1992). So far 10 children have been born, one of them with a submucous cleft palate (Golan et al 1990, Ron-El et al 1990c). We had three more pregnancies that terminated in early abortions. Smitz et al (1991) described 13 spontaneous pregnancies in more than 2000 GnRHa cycles, of which three ended in early abortion, three were tubal pregnancies and seven continued uneventfully.

## IVF-ET in the natural cycle

Since the cost of IVF treatment is high, the risk of OHSS, multiple pregnancy rates and luteal phase insufficiency are handicaps of stimulated cycles. Foulot et al (1989) has tried in women with regular menstrual cycles a simplified protocol of IVF without ovarian stimulation. Monitoring of the follicle was done by repetetive estradiol and LH examinations and US scanning. When the follicle arrived at ≥ 18 mm diameter and estradiol exceeded 180 pg/ml, hCG was administered and aspiration of the follicle was performed 34–36 hours later. Cancellation due to spontaneous LH surge was in 36% of the 80 cycles. A pregnancy rate of 22.5% per transfer was obtained, which is favorable for cycles with a single embryo replacement. However, the high cancellation rate and the disadvantage of undergoing the whole IVF-ET procedure relying on a single oocyte-embryo, probably are the causes for the rare use of IVF in spontaneous cycles. Recently Medical Research International (1992) reported only a 5% clinical pregnancy rate in 152 natural cycles.

## OOCYTE RETRIEVAL

Laparoscopy was the primarily used method for oocyte retrieval (Steptoe & Edwards 1970). The three (sometimes four) puncture technique was applied, one for the laparoscope, one for the holding forceps and the third for the aspirating needle. A probe was sometimes also introduced through an additional site in the middle of the lower abdomen.

Aspiration was immediately applied following the puncture of the follicle at a negative pressure of 100–200 mmHg. If the oocyte had not been identified in the first aspirate by the embryologist, the follicle was flushed with a small volume of culture medium and reaspirated. Sometimes the oocyte could have been found in the fluid accumulated in the pouch of Douglas.

Some debate exists in the literature as to the ideal composition of the gas for the pneumoperitoneum. A composition of 5% carbon dioxide, 5% oxygen and 90% nitrogen was suggested as ideal. However, we and many others always used 100% carbon dioxide with no ill effects.

Although the ovarian follicles are directly visualized at laparoscopy, it is an invasive method and not without risk. General anesthesia is necessary, the patient is always left with some abdominal and chest discomfort and usually needs a longer hospitalization. Intraperitonal adhesions, not unusual in IVF patients, are a disadvantage and when severe may even constitute a contraindication.

In the early eighties the Scandinavians were the first to introduce the ultrasound as guidance for oocyte recovery (Lenz et al 1981, Lenz & Lauristen 1982). Three different techniques have been introduced:

- Transvesical retrieval with an abdominal transducer

- Transurethral retrieval also with an abdominal transducer
- Transvaginal retrieval with a vaginal transducer.

In the transvesical approach the urinary bladder is prefilled with 300–500 ml of saline. The needle is firmly inserted into the bladder where its tip is well identified. The tip of the needle is then advanced to the follicle to puncture it. Aspiration is immediately applied and the needle rotated and moved up and down inside the follicle performing an 'intrafollicular curettage' until blood-stained fluid is visible in the silicon tube. The transurethral approach was described by Parsons et al (1985). As with the transvesical approach the ultrasonic transducer is abdominal. The urinary bladder is prefilled and the needle introduced through the urethra, hooked through a side hole of the urinary catheter as it is introduced into the bladder. The needle tip is easily identified as it is almost at a right angle to the ultrasound beam. This technique cannot be applied in patients with ovaries located behind the uterus or high in the pelvis. Although initially promising, this method did not become popular.

Transvaginal approach of aspiration was initially applied with the guide of an abdominal ultrasonic transducer (Delenbach et al 1984), but soon modified to a complete vaginal approach in which a narrow vaginal transducer is introduced into the vagina with a special mount for the aspirating needle. The puncture is carried out through the vaginal fornices with an emptied bladder (Feichtinger & Kemeter 1986). The advantages of this route are the very short puncturing distance, untouched urinary bladder and no skin wounds (Fig. 21.4). Postoperatively, this procedure is associated with less patient discomfort (Russell et al 1987) and is performed as a day case. Regional anesthesia or sedation occasionally supplemented by local analgesia is usually sufficient. Care must be taken when the ovary is behind the uterus and the course of the needle crosses it not to traumatize the endometrium.

An oocyte recovery rate of 70–90% was reported by the Scandinavian groups (Lenz 1984, Wikland & Hamberger 1984). No statistically

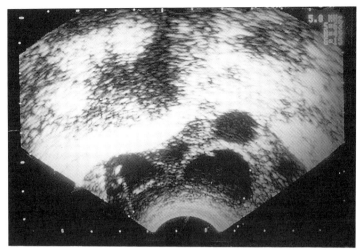

**Fig. 21.4**    Follicles seen on the ultrasound scan during aspiration in the vaginal approach. See the aspiration needle in the left follicle.

significant difference could be found between laparoscopic and ultrasonically guided follicular puncture (Feichtinger & Kemeter 1984, Wikland & Hamberger 1984, Belaish-Allart et al 1985) (Fig. 21.4). In our hands, an oocyte recovery rate of 87% was achieved. The average number of oocytes per successful oocyte retrieval using this approach is $8.9 \pm 6.8$ oocytes.

The possibility of adverse effects of ultrasonic exposure of the preovulatory oocytes had been initially brought up (Demoulin et al 1985), but it is obvious by now that this danger is negligible. Other complications of bleeding or infection connected with the puncture of abdominal structures and vessels were reported, but are extremely rare and probably less frequent than with laparoscopy. Curtis et al (1991) investigated the incidence of bacterial and chlamydial infection in fluid aspirated from the pouch of Douglas in 25 patients undergoing ZIFT. The peritoneal cultures were all negative except one which was positive for *Chlamydia trachomatis*. They reported no occurrence of pelvic infection among their 243 transvaginal ultrasound-guided oocyte recoveries. Prophylactic antibiotic treatment was introduced in various centers, however, there is no consesus as to the type of antibiotic, the timing or the duration of therapy or whether it is required at all (Howe et al 1988, Meldrum 1989). In our last 1000 IVF treatment cycles

869 oocyte retrievals took place, 98% of which were ultrasonically guided via the vagina. The patients were kept for observation for 5–6 hours and then discharged. Two cases showed a significant drop of hemoglobin and tachycardia, probably due to postpuncture bleeding. Both recovered with conservative measures. Pelvic infections of various degrees were noted in four cases, of which a pelvic abscess was palpated and visible by sonography in two. All recovered with antibiotic therapy.

In the most recent global survey (World Collaborative Report 1989), 469 centers participated, with a total number of 76 030 ovum pick ups (OPU). In 91% of the cases ovum retrieval was performed under ultrasonic control. The recent report of the US results of the IVF-ET registry from 180 units reviewed 19 079 treatment cycles of which 16 405 (86%) had oocyte retrievals and 95% of them were performed with ultrasonic control (Medical Research International 1992). Although the vaginal approach for egg collection has become an easy procedure with rare complications, one should remember that the procedure is invasive and not without risks.

## LABORATORY TECHNIQUES IN ART

The laboratory part in the process of IVF-ET is of major importance. In order to obtain embryos of good quality personnel skilled in handling of oocytes and laboratory management are indispensable.

## Laboratory equipment

Three major elements should be under constant rigid quality control in a human IVF laboratory: the microscope, incubation system and culture medium. In this section the minimal acceptable requirements will be briefly discussed.

*The incubator* should be of any standard water-jacketed temperature-controlled variety. The type of gas mixture that is utilized in the majority of the units is 5% carbon dioxide in room air. Some others use a mixture of 90% nitrogen, 5% carbon dioxide and 5% oxygen. Alarm signals should be automatically activated by temperature or gas mixture variations. A high humidity of 98% is also of high importance. Two incubator systems seem to be essential in order to ensure continuous function even when one of them is not working due to a technical problem.

*The microscope* is an important tool in order to achieve a quick and clear visualization of the oocyte and its cytoplasmic configuration. The commonly used microscope is dissecting phase contrast with a magnification power of 5× to 50×. Another light microscope is also necessary for semen evaluation. Other items such as laminar flow hood, heated stages on the microscope and warming trays for the pipettes are advisable measures but not essential.

*Culture media.* Various types of medium have been used so far. Ham's F-10 was the first one that had been used and since then other media such as Earle's, Tyrode's, Heppes and others have also been successfully introduced. The water used in the culture fluid is an important factor and, if coming from a local source, should be 2–5 times distilled and deionized. Many units are using commercially available highly purified water. The medium consists of electrolytes, bicarbonate, lactate and pyruvate. Protein is supplemented to the basic nutrient fluid and is heat inactivated and filtered. Its source can be from patient's serum (Lopata et al 1980) or fetal cord serum (Jones et al 1982). More recently the beneficial effect of purified bovine serum albumin (BSA) was also reported (Ogawa & Marrs 1987).

Insemination culture medium is enriched by 7.5–10% serum, embryo culture medium with 15–20% serum and embryo transfer medium has a high concentration of serum of 50–100% (Leung et al 1984). It has been emphasized that culture medium with a fixed protein concentration of 10% is well accepted for all IVF stages. Moreover, the use of a protein-free medium for up to 24 hours of culture does not harm the zygote-embryo. The osmolarity and pH of the culture medium are very important since the embryo development is strongly related to any variations in these parameters.

Addition of any fluid or cells to the known medium culture is termed co-culture. Human tubal fluid (Quinn et al 1985) or human ampullary cells reduce cleavage abnormalities of the embryo and allow a larger number of embryos to arrive at the blastocyst stage (Bongso et al 1989). Another form of coculture is on monolayers of cells, like Vero cells, which result in increased implantation rate per embryo. The overall pregnancy rate per embryo transfer is not increased (Menezo et al 1992). However, these studies are preliminary and the overall beneficial effect of the coculture technique has still to be demonstrated.

## Oocyte culture technique

The initial step in the IVF culture procedure is to rapidly identify the oocyte in the follicular fluid and to judge the maturational state of the corona–cumulus–oocyte complex. The most common maturity grading of the oocyte was described by Veeck et al (1983) based on the appearance of adjacent formations to the oocyte. A loosely aggregated granulosa, an expanded cumulus and radiant corona indicate a mature oocyte. Compact and tightly aggregated granulosa cells, dense cumulus or absent cumulus and a compact or occasionally absent corona characterize an immature oocyte. The egg itself is usually obscured by the corona cells and often a germinal vescicle can be noted.

Nuclear status at harvest gives a more reliable prediction of oocyte maturity and capacity to fertilize. An oocyte with one polar body (I° polar body) is mature and has a high chance of fertilizing. An oocyte that has no polar body on harvest, but extrudes it 5–15 hours after its collection, has a lower rate of fertilization. A germinal vesicle can be observed in fully immature oocytes. Granular cytoplasm and vacuoles in the cytoplasma are poor prognostic signs (Veeck 1989).

## Sperm preparation

The most common method still in use for sperm preparation is washing in medium 3 times the volume of semen, centrifugation, discarding the supernatant, resuspension of the sperm in the pellet and its layering by medium for an incubation period of 30–60 minutes, (Lopata et al 1976). At this stage the supernatant is carefully collected and normally contains 80–100% motile sperm and a significantly higher percentage of sperm with normal morphology. This well-known technique has the disadvantage of loosing about 90% of the sperm in the pellet. Therefore, other methods are used in cases with oligozoospermia. Among them is the Percoll gradient technique (Gorus & Pipeleers 1981) in which the sperm is layered on an isotonic discontinuous Percoll gradient, centrifuged and collected from the pellet. In this way cell debris, bacteria and malformed sperm are removed. The normal motile sperm are selected according to their specific gravity. Recently, instead of using several Percoll gradients, a mini Percoll gradient of only two different concentrations of Percoll in Ham's F10 has been described (Ord et al 1990). With this technique reduced Percoll gradient volume is used while the ability of sperm filtering is maintained. Van Der Zwalmen et al (1991) have shown that with the Percoll separation technique there was a significant increase in morphologically normal spermatozoa which led also to a higher pregnancy rate as compared with the swim-up technique (33% compared with 21% respectively). These results were confirmed also by other authors and are true for normal and abnormal sperm quality. However, in severe teratozoospermia cases the morphology remains unchanged after Percoll workup. Methods like albumin gradient separation or glass wool separation and storage in *TEST* yolk buffer are less common and still doubtful in their capability to select better sperm. Also the merit of pentoxyphilline is still unclear.

## Sperm quality and minimal requirements

It is well accepted today that correlation exists between fertilizing ability and seminal parameters (Mahadevan & Trounson 1984, Kruger et al 1986). Moreover, there is good evidence that morphologically normal spermatozoa offer the best fertilizing potential (Pousette et al 1986, Hinting et al 1989). Sperm morphology alone evaluated by strict criteria (Kruger et al 1988) appears to be a good predictor of IVF outcome. There is no clear consensus on the threshold values of sperm parameters with regard to fertilizing capacity, yet it is possible to point at the minimal sperm requirements to achieve fertilization. The sperm count of fresh semen should be at least $\geqslant$ 5 million/ml and sperm motility at least 30%. At least 16% normal forms should be present to achieve a normal rate of fertilization. Some oocytes will fertilize with only 5% normal forms of sperm, according to Kruger's strict criteria (Kruger et al 1988, Hinting et al 1989, Ng et al 1989). Triple sperm defect (concentration, motility and morphology) had fertilization rates of less than 8%.

## Preincubation of the oocyte and insemination

A preincubation of the oocyte for 6 hours before insemination was shown by Trounson et al (1982) to improve fertilization rate. Cytogenetic analysis of such oocytes which were fixed after this incubation period showed in some of them break of plasma membrane, exocytosis of granular cortex and vacuolization. Therefore, it is accepted today that insemination of mature oocytes can be performed any time without waiting 6 hours after their collection. In premature oocytes it is worth postponing insemination for 5–10 hours after their recovery to let the extrusion of the first polar body occur.

Insemination includes the addition of

20 000–200 000 motile sperm to a dish of 1 ml of medium where the egg is preincubated. It is noteworthy to mention that in the 1970s $1.0-1.5 \times 10^6$ sperm per ml were employed. Since the reduction of the number of added sperm to the dish, paradoxically the overall fertilization rate has improved. In cases of impaired sperm quality up to 500 000 sperm per dish are added in order to improve the chance of fertilization (Kruger et al 1986). Another method to maximize the sperm/egg exposure is to put microdrops of medium containing motile sperm in the bottom of the dish and to add directly an oocyte to the microdrop, which can then be cultured under paraffin oil (Edwards 1981), or placing several oocytes in the same dish with 1 ml of medium.

The surface characteristics of the spermatozoa and oocyte influence the interaction between the gametes resulting in binding to and penetration of the zona pellucida. Oocyte quality, e.g. maturity, influences the number of sperm bound to the zona. The mean number of sperm bound to mature, immature and atretic oocytes are $51 \pm 50$, $7 \pm 12$ and $10 \pm 18$ respectively (Mahadevan et al 1987). Fertilized mature oocytes have a significantly higher number of sperm bound to the zonae compared to unfertilized oocytes ($81 \pm 53$ compared to $42 \pm 47$ respectively). The sperm motility and the number of motile sperm used to inseminate oocytes were significantly correlated with the number of sperm bound to the zona, whereas sperm morphology and sperm concentration did not correlate (Mahadevan et al 1987).

Secondary insemination is a controversial issue. Many IVF programs perform secondary insemination if fertilization is not seen 18 hours after the first insemination. The oocyte does not fertilize either due to its own immaturity or due to sperm difficulty to penetrate the zona pellucida. In many instances the impression is that secondary insemination has led to fertilization since blastomeres are seen 18 hours after this secondary insemination. Our impression is that this activity in the oocyte is delayed following the first insemination and not related to the second one. According to our data secondary insemination yields only 5–7% of fertilization. This is also the percentage of immature oocytes. Therefore, we perform secondary insemination only in unfertilized oocytes which were immature at the time of their first insemination.

It is interesting that despite the exposure of eggs to supernumerary sperm, the incidence of polyploid fertilization is 2–10%. This incidence is probably related to the functional ability of the polyspermic block of the oocyte rather than to the high number of sperm put in the dish. We have found that polypronuclear fertilization was significantly more frequent in cycles with high fertilization and improved pregnancy rates, which also corroborates the theory of the important role played by the oocyte in the phenomenon of polyspermy (Golan et al 1992b).

## Micromanipulation

Micromanipulation procedures are applied to embryos and gametes in which careful manipulation can be performed with micropipettes under vision via the microscope. The varieties of such procedures are: removal of the zona, dissociation of blastomeres, injection of single or aggregated cells into the oocyte, embryo or blastocyst and pooling out single blastomeres for the purpose of analysis. The main indications for micromanipulation in the human are severe sperm problems such as immotile sperm, severe oligozoospermia or inability to penetrate the oocyte. Cases referred to micromanipulation should be those which failed at least twice to fertilize any of the cohort of recovered eggs when no other technical problems existed in the system. The first human pregnancy after micromanipulation has been reported by Ng et al in 1988.

Several methods of micromanipulation have been described so far:

1. Zona drilling – either mechanical or by local application of a zona solvent like acid Tyrode's or alpha chymotrypsin solution using a microneedle. With the mechanical drilling no pregnancies in the human were achieved (Gordon et al 1988) and with the chemical drilling the meiotic process was affected probably by anaphase II arrest (Ng et al 1989).

2. Partial zona dissection (PZD) – the zona is mechanically torn with a glass needle or cracked by piercing on a glass holding pipette. With these

methods pregnancies were achieved. It should, however, be remembered that in the majority of PZD procedures the oocytes are deposited in a dish with sperm concentrations of $5-10 \times 10^6$/ml which are normally difficult to achieve with severe male factor (Cohen et al 1990a).

3. Subzonal injection (SUZI) – injection of one or several spermatozoa into the perivitelline space. In 771 oocytes Ng et al (1991) injected 7–10 motile sperm and achieved 16% fertilization rate, 2.3% polyspermy, 2.8% parthenogenic activation of the oocyte and 8.6% pregnancies per replaced embryo. All these results were in the group of patients whose sperm density was $< 5.0 \times 10^6$/ml. The fertilization rate of about 15% and pregnancy rate $< 10\%$ per embryo transfer was achieved also by other groups in smaller series. Since fetal wastage in such cases is relatively high, the take home baby rate is 3–5%.

4. Intracytoplasmic injection (ICSI) – the injection of an immotile live spermatozoon directly into the ooplasma. Thirty-one of the 47 oocytes so tested (66%) were fertilized. Of seven patients who underwent embryo replacement, four conceived (Palermo et al 1992). This method is in its first stages and still needs to be elaborated.

It has to be remembered that pregnancy rates with micromanipulation are discouraging. However, pregnancies are achievable in severe male cases and, with larger experience and improvement of the methods, pregnancy rates may increase. The babies born after micromanipulation were normal and had no chromosomal abnormalities.

## Fertilization and embryo development

Human sperm capacitation occurs during a period of 30 minutes which is considered to be a short interval. Only then and following at least another 45 minutes of direct contact with the oocyte sperm is able to penetrate. The presence of a dense or expanded cumulus or its removal before insemination of the oocyte did not change oocyte penetration time (Plachot et al 1986). After gamete contact of 1 hour 84% of the oocytes were fertilized. Insemination time, e.g. time of oocyte exposure to sperm exceeding 4 hours, did not yield more fertilizations. It is for the sake of convenience to leave spermatozoa in contact with eggs overnight and to look for fertilization the next morning, 12–18 hours after sperm were put into the dish. At this stage 2 pronuclei, the female and male ones, are clearly visible. The oocyte is viewed with the aid of the dissecting microscope and the remaining cumulus-corona cells are mechanically stripped off. It is of great importance to view the oocyte in a pronuclear stage. First, to determine whether sperm activity has been good and penetration of the oocyte has occurred. This can be confirmed by the visualization of the second polar body and the two pronuclei. If multiple pronuclei are present, then the diagnosis of polyspermic fertilization can be made. About 40% of the oocytes with polyploidy would begin cleavage and mistakenly can be transferred into the uterus. In rare instances a single pronucleus is visible. This can be either the male or the female one. There has been controversy regarding whether to replace such an oocyte with a single pronucleus once it cleaves. Many authors suggest it should be considered to be an embryo once the second polar body and attached sperm to the zona are visible. The appearance of a single pronucleus when other indications of fertilization exist is probably due to delay in formation of the second pronucleus.

Additional 24 hours of culture will bring the majority of the fertilized eggs into cleavage of two to eight cells. The mean fertilization rate mentioned in the first large series of IVF was >70%. As the indications for IVF-ET have been enlarged and more cases with unexplained and male infertility are treated in IVF programs, the fertilization rate has decreased to 50% or 60% in the majority of centers. The cleavage rate is much higher, 80–95%.

A clear correlation between the morphological appearance of the embryo, its growth rate and the chances to implant have been noticed. Therefore a grading system of morphology is in use to evaluate the embryos, to choose the good ones for replacement and freezing. We use the four grade system which is accepted in many centers: Grade I, equal sized blastomeres and no cytoplasmatic fragments; Grade II, unequal sized blastomeres with or without slight fragmentation aside the polar bodies; Grade III, equal sized blastomeres with some anucleated fragments (> 20%) (Fig. 21.5); Grade IV, unequal sized blastomeres, heavily fragmented (> 50%) and degenerative appearance. We usually do not replace embryos of Grade IV morphology and do not freeze embryos classified as Grades III and IV. The rapidly cleaving embryos, with eight or more blastomeres at 36–48 hours after insemination, are the more likely to establish a pregnancy.

The phenomenon of delayed fertilization can be due to immaturity of the oocytes or impaired sperm quality (Ron-El et al 1991c). In the former etiology, once fertilization took place the chances to achieve embryos with good morphology are almost equal to those observed in oocytes fertilized in time. On the other hand, delayed fertilization due to sperm difficulty in penetrating oocytes usually leads to low fertilization rate, poor embryo morphology and low chances of conceiving.

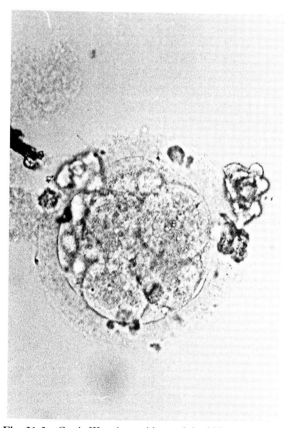

**Fig. 21.5** Grade III embryo with equal sized blastomeres and some anucleated cytoplasmic fragments

## Assisted hatching

Recently implantation enhancement was described following assisted hatching (Cohen et al 1990b). The hypothesis was that an alteration of the zona pellucida by drilling a hole through it, thinning it or altering its stability would promote hatching of embryos which are otherwise unable to escape intact from the zona. In a prospective randomized study Cohen et al (1992) has shown that in cases in which zona thickness was $\geqslant 15$ $\mu$m and was drilled, nine out of ten patients achieved clinical pregnancy in comparison with three out of 13 patients in the control group. Likewise patients aged > 38 years and those with elevated basal FSH levels (> 15 IU/l) showed significantly more pregnancies and ongoing pregnancies when assisted hatching was performed in comparison to the controls (15% compared with 5% and 26% compared with 10% respectively). These results may indicate a possible correlation between age, basal FSH levels and physical or chemical changes in the zona pellucida (Cohen et al 1992).

## Cryopreservation

Embryo cryopreservation is now firmly established in cases with excessive fertilized embryos avoiding the necessity to replace large numbers of embryos with the risk of multiple pregnancy. The additional pregnancies obtained from replacement of cryopreserved embryos has effectively increased the success rate of a cycle of IVF treatment by 1% to 10% (Trounson 1990). Crucial biophysical problems had to be solved in order to achieve viable embryos after the freezing-thawing process. The major problems encountered are formation of intracellular ice during cooling and cell dehydration in response to the increasing concentration of extracellular solutes as water freezes out of the suspending medium. To avoid the formation of intracellular ice, cells must be sufficiently dehydrated by the time they reach the temperature at which intracellular ice nucleation can occur. This may be achieved by proper cooling velocity which is individual to each type of cell depending upon its size and water permeability and cryoprotectants which suppress the injurious effects of the high electrolyte concentrations in the external medium. As cryoprotectants are toxic to the embryo, sucrose solutions are used after thawing of frozen embryos as an osmotic aid in the control of the cryoprotectant removal. Today there are three main embryo freezing protocols:

1. Slow cooling and slow thawing protocol using dimethyl-sulfoxide (DMSO). Embryos are equilibrated in DMSO 0.75 M at room temperature for 10 minutes. The embryo is then cooled at a rate of 2°C/min to −6°C. Seeding is then induced by touching the ampule with cold forceps. The embryo is further cooled at a rate of 0.3°C/min to −80°C and then plunged into liquid nitrogen. Thawing is performed at a rate of 8°C/min to room temperature (Trounson & Mohr 1983).

2. 1,2-Propanediol 1.5 M and sucrose are used as cryoprotectants. The embryo remains for 15 minutes in the medium with the cryoprotectants and then cooled at a rate of 2°C/min to −6°C. Seeding is performed as in the first protocol, and cooling proceeds to −30°C at a rate of 0.3°C/min. The embryo is then plunged into liquid nitrogen. The thawing is very rapidly performed, reaching room temperature at < 1 min (Renaud & Barbinet 1984).

3. Vitrification in which glass rather than ice is formed and problems of ice formation, cooling and thawing rates are significantly diminished. The vitrification requires embryos to be treated with a mixture of DMSO, acetamide, propanediol, and polyethylene glycol at a very high molar concentration. During cooling glass is formed and no ice is present (Rall & Fahy 1985). The ultra-rapid method first described by Trounson & Sjoblam (1988) is a modification of the vitrification method. A high concentration of 2.5 M DMSO and 0.25 M sucrose in buffered saline phosphate is mixed with 10% heat-inactivated patient's serum. The embryos are transferred into the freezing medium and drawn into plastic straws and quickly plunged into liquid nitrogen.

Embryos are suitable for replacement after thawing if the zona is intact or if at least half of the prefreezing number of blastomeres are intact.

Replacement is done preferably in a natural cycle 100 hours after LH peak. However, we had pregnancies also when replacement was performed on days 3 or 5 postovulation. We use ovulatory agents only in anovulatory patients. In a world review by Van Steirteghem & Van den Albeel (1990), 57% of the thawed embryos were suitable for replacement. An implantation rate of 4% of 18 322 embryos and a pregnancy rate of 11% out of 6441 replacements were recorded. The eight-cell embryo is usually preferred for freezing because of its ease in handling and the probability of enough intact blastomeres to be replaced. With the propanediol protocol the two pronuclate stage cryopreservation was promoted. Van Steirteghem et al (1987) found that the best survival with propanediol was in embryos having ≤ two blastomeres, whereas with DMSO it was at the stage of four to eight cells. Pregnancy rate was in favor of the propanediol protocol (23% compared with 15% in the DMSO) but with no significant difference. The results with the ultra-rapid protocol are from small series so far. Survival rate of the embryos was 37.5% and of pronucleated embryos 89%. Four out of 20 patients who underwent embryo transfer conceived (Gordts et al 1990).

A difference in the survival rate of the embryos and pregnancy rate was observed with the ovarian stimulation protocol. Smitz et al (1992b) reported 41% survival of embryos following the GnRHa/hMG protocol compared with 62% with the CC/hMG scheme. The trend in pregnancy rate was also in favor of the CC/hMG protocol. These relatively low results with the long GnRHa protocol were not documented in the short protocols of GnRHa. This observation was also confirmed by others. However, there were some groups who did not observe any difference between both protocols (Macnamee et al 1989, Fugger et al 1991).

Mature unfertilized supernumerary oocytes could have been frozen, especially in countries in which freezing of human embryos is considered unacceptable. However, problems such as non-reversible disassembly of the meiotic spindle during cooling, reduced survival of oocytes after thawing (29%), reduced fertilization rate due to damage to the zona pellucida, increased polyploidy (20–40%) and aneuploidy turned the freezing of oocytes so far into an unacceptable method (Al-Hasani et al 1987, Trounson 1990). Rare pregnancies after freeze-thawing oocytes with later fertilization were described.

## EMBRYO TRANSFER

Although every stage in the IVF-ET process has its own merit, embryo replacement is perhaps the most important of the lot. Two out of three embryo replacements fail to implant and, counting the individual embryos replaced, the proportion of the successfully implanting embryos is even much lower. The successful nidation of an embryo following its replacement is influenced by various factors including the age of the patient, the number and quality of the embryos and the receptivity of the uterus.

The optimal stage of the human embryo for replacement is unknown. Reports exist of pregnancies occurring following replacement of embryos ranging from the pronucleate stage to the blastocyst. Early embryo transfer may decrease the exposure of the developing embryo to many potential risks in the in vitro environment. On the other hand delayed embryo transfer would appear to meet an increased endometrial receptivity. In a randomized prospective study (Caspi et al 1989b) we found no difference in pregnancy rate when we had replaced the embryos 44 or 68 hours after insemination. Sequential replacement (two embryos 24 hours apart) did not change the pregnancy rate. Pregnancy rate obviously increases with the number of embryos replaced. Our results clearly demonstrate that pregnancy rate increases dramatically from 8.1% following the transfer of a single embryo to 25.7% following two, 22.8% following three and 33.5% for four and more embryos. Multiple pregnancy rate rises concomitantly.

The common practice is the replacement of embryos into the uterine cavity through the cervical canal. This transcervical replacement of the embryos must be carried out as quickly and atraumatically as possible. It is believed that the chance of successful implantation increases with the ease and neatness of the replacement. Some investigators considered the appearence of blood on the tip of the catheter as a bad prognostic sign.

We always perform embryo replacement with the patient in the lithotomy position on her own bed. The knee-chest position is suggested by some authors to be used for anteverted uteri. We do not consider such variation of position to be of any significance. The bladder is emptied just prior to the embryo replacement and the procedure is carried out without any anesthesia or analgesia. Following the successful embryo transfer the patient lies on her back for 1 hour and does not get up for an additional 2 hours. Bed rest at home is advised for 48 hours.

No catheter has any preference over the others, as long as the surgeon feels confident and acquainted with it. Gentle catheterization of the cervical canal with a used sterilized catheter is performed to feel the ease and direction. Once a free passage is demonstrated the embryologist loads the embryos into a new catheter and hands it over to the surgeon. Rarely difficulty arises at this stage due to a retroverted uterus or an exaggerated angle between the cervical canal and the uterine cavity. Suprapubic pressure displacing the uterus backwards or alternatively a full bladder may help. If this fails, traction on a volsellum applied to the cervix usually aligns the uterine and cervical axis and facilitates successful embryo replacement.

Although previously reported by some units, we do not perform any cervical dilatation in women with previous difficult embryo transfers. In these women a rigid metal sleeve is successfully used for the replacement with a flexible inner polyethylene catheter.

After the replacement, the catheter flushing is promptly examined under the microscope to ensure that none of the embryos have been left behind.

### Gamete intrafallopian transfer (GIFT)

In an attempt to simplify the IVF-ET process several groups have tried the introduction of gametes directly into the uterine cavity. Few pregnancies were achieved in 1982 (Craft et al 1982). In 1983, Tesarik et al first reported a successful pregnancy occurring following tubal gamete transfer performed at the conclusion of a tubal microsurgical operation. In 1984 Asch et al reported a pregnancy after laparoscopic gamete transfer known as GIFT procedure.

Craft & Brinsden (1989) reported their vast experience in more than a 1000 GIFT cases. They consider GIFT to be the preferred method of treatment if at least one Fallopian tube is functional as shown by hysterosalpingography or laparoscopy.

The oocytes are recovered laparoscopically in the majority of the patients. The recovered oocytes are washed in equilibrated Earl's culture medium. Various numbers of oocytes are transferred to suit different clinical circumstances (even more than ten). Sperm is collected 2 hours before the operation, and 50 000–100 000 sperms are transferred after the preparation by wash, spin and swim up technique. The oocyte/sperm mixture is then instilled 1.5–2.0 cm within the distal end of the Fallopian tube.

Craft & Brinsden (1989) achieved a 33.6% pregnancy rate. They found that the success of the procedure is dependent upon the number and quality of the oocytes transferred and upon the quality of the sperm. The pregnancy rate was 21.4% when up to four oocytes were transferred and almost doubled (40.3%) when four or more were transferred. The multiple pregnancy rate (mostly twins) increased from 17.3% to 32.3% respectively. Treatment by the GIFT technique may have advantages over IVF in terms of relative success for patients with open Fallopian tubes who do not achieve a pregnancy by natural means or by conventional fertility treatment.

In the World Collaborative Report (1989), four to six oocytes were transferred into the tubes in 51% of the GIFT cycles and in another 5% more than six oocytes were replaced.

It is clear that the GIFT technique requires far less extensive oocyte manipulation, and allows for the return of gametes to the Fallopian tubes under the same anesthesia. The potential risks of laparoscopy under general anesthesia were removed from the IVF-ET process but still exist in GIFT. A hysteroscopic GIFT procedure under light sedation has been developed lately (Seracchioli et al 1991). In these cases oocyte retrieval was performed under ultrasonic guidance. The oocytes and sperm were transferred into the tube under $CO_2$ pulsed hysteroscopic visualization. Pregnancy rates were comparable with the laparoscopic GIFT.

## Zygote intrafallopian transfer (ZIFT) or TET (tubal embryo transfer)

The development of few modifications of ART such as ZIFT, PROST and TET has combined the apparent benefits of both worlds, i.e. confirmation of fertilization in vitro and the replacement of the embryo or zygote into the more natural milieu of the Fallopian tube. Oocytes are retrieved as for IVF using the ultrasound technique and embryo or zygote replacements initially performed via the laparoscopic route are now done transcervically.

ZIFT has been proposed for the treatment of unexplained infertility (Devroey et al 1986). Animal studies have shown that the Fallopian tube secretes important substances that coat the embryo and may be important for early development (Kapur & Johnson 1985). Furthermore, natural endotubal transport mechanisms may allow the embryos to enter the uterine cavity at a more synchronized phase of endometrial development (Yovich et al 1988b). Zygote transfer to the tube offers advantages over gamete transfer, as fertilization can be confirmed with selective transfer of the three or four highest quality embryos. However, as oocytes have to be collected in a separate procedure, ZIFT is more time-consuming and expensive. The risks to the patients of two operative procedures must also not be overlooked. Jansen & Anderson (1987) were the first to transcervically catheterize the Fallopian tube with a soft catheter of 0.66 mm diameter documented by vaginal ultrasound. This technique provides the advantage of avoiding an operative procedure under anaesthesia for transfer of gametes or embryos to the tube.

Retrospective studies (Devroey et al 1989, Pool et al 1990, Scholtes et al 1990, Diedrich et al 1991) described a higher rate of pregnancy and implantation with the ZIFT or TET compared with the uterine embryo transfer, namely 29–40% pregnancies per transfer by the ZIFT or TET procedures and 21–28% with the UET. In a prospective randomized study we could not demonstrate any preference in the pregnancy rate in either of the methods (Ron-El et al 1992c).

## LUTEAL PHASE

The importance of the luteal phase was recognized from the very beginning of the ART era when the conception rate following embryo transfer was relatively low (Steptoe et al 1980). In fact, the luteal phase in ART may be subjected to the adverse effect of a variety of factors which include: anesthesia, follicle aspiration, hormonal milieu, mode of ovarian hyperstimulation and luteal support.

It was suggested that endocrinological changes occurring during general anesthesia (Soules et al 1980) may cause impaired function of the corpus luteum. Nevertheless, this phenomenon was not confirmed (Kemeter et al 1981) and the adverse effect of anesthesia on the luteal phase in ART programs is considered to be negligible. Contradictory findings were reported concerning the effect of follicle aspiration on corpus luteum function (Frydman et al 1982, Garcia et al 1981, Kreitmann et al 1981, Kerin et al 1981, Feichtinger et al 1982, Oskowitz et al 1986). Although this issue remains unresolved, it seems that the effect of follicle aspiration on the luteal phase is not crucial. It was found that both ovulation induction with clomiphene citrate (Van Hall & Mastboom 1969, Garcia et al 1977) or menotropins (Olson et al 1983) may cause impaired luteal phase. High estrogens, generally associated with ovarian hyperstimulation, lowered pregnancy rate (Forman et al 1988). Thus, normal postovulatory progesterone levels, found after follicle aspiration, may not be sufficient to contradict the effect of high estrogens. O'Neill et al (1985b) suggested using the ratio between estrogen and progesterone in order to define optimal milieu favoring successful implantation. Nevertheless, randomized prospective studies (Daya 1988, Buvat et al 1988, Kupferminc et al 1990) indicated that there was insufficient data to recommend routine use of luteal support. This was reflected in the world collaborative report (Seppala et al 1984) that pointed out the non-uniform approach to luteal phase supplementa-

tion. Many used progesterone, or its derivatives, others used hCG and some avoided any luteal support. Recently, Yovich et al (1991) found that luteal support may improve ongoing implantation rate, especially in cases with poor embryonic morphology. However, many believe that luteal support is not crucial in cycles treated with clomiphene citrate and/or menotropins.

The introduction of GnRHa to ART has changed the attitude towards luteal support. The luteolytic effect of GnRH and its agonists had been already established before its use in ART (Koyama et al 1978, Casper & Yen 1979, Lemay et al 1979, Asch et al 1981). Smitz et al (1988) showed inadequate corpus luteum function following GnRHa use, when luteal support was omitted. They also showed that serum LH levels remained low until 12 days after cessation of GnRHa administration. Since baseline LH levels are essential for proper function of the corpus luteum (Groff et al 1984), it is obvious that depressed LH levels, during a critical postovulatory period, may cause this phenomenon. Thus, hCG administration (Casper et al 1980) prevented luteolysis when GnRHa was given. Randomized prospective studies demonstrated that while GnRHa is used in ART, luteal supplementation with hCG was associated with higher pregnancy rate compared with nonsupplemented cycles (Smith et al 1987, Belaisch-Allart et al 1990, Herman et al 1990c). Hormonal luteal profile showed that 10 000 IU of hCG administered prior to oocyte retrieval maintains corpus luteum function for an additional 8 days (Smitz et al 1987, Herman et al 1990c). When luteal support was avoided both estradiol and progesterone levels decreased but since progesterone decrease was more pronounced the ratio between them was impaired. If implantation is delayed, endogenous chorionic gonadotropin may be secreted too late for rescuing the corpus luteum. On the other hand, hCG administered 5 days after initial hCG dose effected luteal rescue (Hutchinson-Williams et al 1990). It was found that after GnRHa hCG was superior to progesterone given orally (Buvat et al 1990). On the contrary, Claman et al (1992) did not find any difference between the two regimens although a superior endocrine milieu was associated with hCG. Recently, it was reported (Smitz et al 1992a) that progesterone administered vaginally was associated with a higher pregnancy rate and lower abortion rate compared with intramuscular administration, although plasma progesterone was lower in the former route. More studies are needed to elucidate optimal drug application, route and dosage following various protocols of hyperstimulation. Spontaneous pregnancies that were inadvertently exposed to GnRHa during the luteal phase showed various degrees of impaired corpus luteum function (Smitz et al 1991, Herman et al 1992). Progesterone and estrogen supplementation were given, although the importance of the latter is unknown.

In ART cycles where GnRHa are not used, luteal support is given by most centers despite the fact that it does not seem to be crucial. When GnRHa is administered, luteal support is mandatory in order to oppose the luteolytic effect.

Various assays were suggested for early determination of conception during the luteal phase. This includes: rosette inhibition test (Morton et al 1977); reduced platelet count (O'Neill et al 1985b); pregnancy specific beta-glycoprotein (Sinosich et al 1985); and identification of immunosuppressive factor (Daya & Clark 1988, Bose et al 1989). However, hCG (Kosasa et al 1973) remains the only reliable and practical material whose presence indicates successful implantation. Smitz et al (1988) found that hCG appeared earlier in cycles without GnRHa than in the cycles with the agonist (9.8 ± 1.3 and 11.1 ± 1.3 days after initial hCG administration, respectively), but the significance of this finding is unclear. Quantitative assays of hCG beta subunit may aid in prediction of pregnancy outcome (Yovich et al 1985, Confino et al 1986). However, experience shows that this is true as far as statistics are concerned, whereas in sporadic cases high titers may lead to miscarriage or ectopic gestation and low levels may end with normal live birth. Hormonal follow-up during the first weeks of gestation may help to assess corpus luteum function and the need for supplementary treatment.

In summary, luteal support should not be regarded as an independent process in ART and successful implantation constitutes the final result of various stages that merge together. Moreover, in the framework of the luteal phase, many variables may affect treatment outcome and it is difficult to assess the relative contribution of each one. This includes the real significance of various hormone levels and the interrelationship between them: endometrial receptivity and content of hormonal receptors, proteins and mucupolysacharides, type of luteal support, mode of administration and dosage, and other factors yet unknown. More research and further development may improve implantation rates, thus enabling a reduction of the number of embryos transferred and, consequently, the risk of multiple gestation.

## RESULTS AND OUTCOME

Since ART has become part of treatment modalities suggested to infertile couples in many centers, large national and international registries are now available to analyse the results. The data presented here are based on the:

- Australian and New Zealand National Perinatal Statistics Unit of the Fertility Society of Australia
- The Interim Licensing Authority for IVF of the Medical Research Council and the Royal College of Obstetricians and Gynaecologists (UK)
- FIVNAT, Groupe d'Etude de la Fecondation In Vitro, France
- The IVF-ET Registry (USA) of the Medical Research International and the Society for Assisted Reproductive Technology of the American Fertility Society
- Israel National Registry of IVF Units.

These registries comprise over 40 000 ART babies. Clinical pregnancy and delivery rates in the first four registries in 1988 were found to be quite comparable (Cohen 1991) (Table 21.7). Table 21.8 shows the increasing numbers of retrievals, clinical pregnancies and deliveries in the USA in the years 1985–90 (Medical Research International 1988, 1989, 1990, 1991, 1992). A clinical pregnancy is defined by rising βhCG and the presence of gestational sac within the uterine cavity documented by ultrasound. A live delivery

**Table 21.7**    Clinical pregnancy and delivery rates expressed per puncture in 1988*

|  | Punctures (No.) | Clinical pregnancies/punctures | | Deliveries per puncture | |
|---|---|---|---|---|---|
|  |  | No. | % | No. | % |
| FIVNAT (France) | 13 336 | 2214 | 16.6 | 1587 | 11.9 |
| National Perinatal Statistic Unit (Australia) | 7930 | 1063 | 13.4 | 745 | 9.4 |
| US Registry of IVF-ET (USA) | 13 647 | 2115 | 15.5 | 1638 | 12.0 |
| Interim Licensing Authority for Human IVF (UK) | 8514 | 1354 | 15.9 | 775 | 9.1 |
|  | 43 427 | 6746 | 15.5 | 4745 | 10.9 |

* Reproduced with permission from Cohen 1991.

**Table 21.8**    Outcome by total number of retrievals: US Registry 1986–1990*

|  | Retrievals | Clinical pregnancies † | | Live born deliveries † | |
|---|---|---|---|---|---|
|  |  | No. | % | No. | % |
| A. IVF-ET |  |  |  |  |  |
| 1985 | 2892 | 337 | 12 | 257 | 9 |
| 1986 | 3365 | 485 | 14 | 311 | 9 |
| 1987 | 8725 | 1367 | 16 | 991 | 11 |
| 1988 | 13 647 | 2243 | 16 | 1657 | 12 |
| 1989 | 15 392 | 2811 | 18 | 2104 | 14 |
| 1990 | 16 405 | 3057 | 19 | 2345 | 14 |
| B. GIFT |  |  |  |  |  |
| 1987 | 1968 | 492 | 25 | 362 | 18 |
| 1988 | 3080 | 846 | 25 | 654 | 21 |
| 1989 | 3652 | 1112 | 30 | 848 | 23 |
| 1990 | 3750 | 1093 | 29 | 842 | 22 |

* Data reproduced with permission from Medical Research International 1988–1992.
† Expressed as percentage per retrieval.

is a birth of at least one viable baby. The data show that clinical pregnancies and live born deliveries per retrieval improved with the years, namely from 12% to 19% and from 9% to 14%, respectively. It was also clearly shown that an IVF center which performed 100 cycles and more per year (and there were 30% of such units) achieved a better outcome than the smaller ones. The GIFT procedure had a pregnancy rate and live born delivery rate per retrieval of 29% and 22% respectively (Table 21.8). The results show a better outcome with the GIFT compared with the IVF procedure. The explanation might be due to the higher number of oocytes transferred into the tube compared with the number of embryos transferred into the uterine cavity. Another factor contributing to the better outcome of the GIFT procedure is the fact that the population treated consists mainly of unexplained infertility and mild endometriosis. The former can be treated by superovulation with or without IUI before doing GIFT with a reasonable success rate (Haney et al 1987, Corsan & Kemmann 1991, Dodson et al 1991). A couple with unexplained infertility is accepted to our IVF program only after four to six superovulation cycles with hMG. By doing this preselection the pregnancy rate per cycle in our IVF program in the unexplained infertility group was less than in the tubal factor 13% and 19% respectively (Table 21.1). In the US registry the unexplained group had a 23% pregnancy rate per ET in an IVF program and 33% per GIFT transfer. The tubal group undergoing IVF-ET had a pregnancy rate of 20%. There is a difficulty in analysis of the results, since they are affected by different inclusion criteria.

Pregnancy rate per retrieval is the highest in cases with diseased tubes (Table 21.9). However, when calculated per ET pregnancy rates in all indications are about the same (18–20%). The most influencing parameter on success is the woman's age. Pregnancy decreases with progression of age of the woman. Parallelly, the abortion rate is increasing and the multiple deliveries rate is decreasing. This can be clearly seen in Table 21.10. The break-off point is at 35 years old, and the chances to conceive and to reach term are diminishing dramatically over 40. The number of attempts did not affect the chances of success. The Australian Statistics (National Perinatal Statistics Unit 1990) reported that 42% of the pregnancies were obtained on the first attempt, 24.8% on the second, 14.9% on the third, 7.9% on the fourth and 10.1% on the fifth attempt. The French statistics (FIVNAT 1990) (Cohen 1991)

showed a similar pregnancy rate until the 10th attempt (Table 21.11).

## Outcome of pregnancy

The rate of spontaneous abortion is 20–25% (Table 21.12). In the French register it increases from 18.4% before the age of 25 to 43.7% above 42 years of age, and in the Australian register from 12.3% before 35 to 64.7% after 42. Late abortions were reported in France in 3.1% of the clinical pregnancies.

The rate of ectopic pregnancy is 5.6% which is higher than in the general population. The mechanism of this phenomenom is not yet understood. In a previous report we were able to demonstrate a direct correlation between the occurrence of tubal pregnancy and diseased tubes (Herman et al 1990a). It may be speculated that once the embryos are transferred to the uterine cavity they are passing back and forth into the tubes, and diseased tubes may have difficulties in expelling the embryos back into the uterine cavity,

**Table 21.9**   Rate of clinical pregnancy by indications: US Registry 1988–89*

|  | Retrievals | Pregnancies per retrieval | | Pregnancies per ET |
|---|---|---|---|---|
|  |  | No. | % | (%) |
| Tubal | 5193 | 750 | 14 | 18 |
| Endometriosis | 2988 | 284 | 10 | 18 |
| Male factor | 2660 | 240 | 9 | 18 |
| Unexplained | 1134 | 82 | 7 | 20 |

* Data reproduced with permission from Medical Research International 1991, 1992.

**Table 21.10**   Outcome of IVF and GIFT by woman's age: US Registry 1989–90*

| Age (yr) | Transferred cycles | Clinical pregnancies | | Abortions † | Deliveries ‡ | | Multiple deliveries § |
|---|---|---|---|---|---|---|---|
|  |  | No. | % | (%) | No. | % | (%) |
| A. IVF-ET |  |  |  |  |  |  |  |
| 30–34 | 2718 | 610 | 22 | 19 | 485 | 18 | 6 |
| 35–39 | 2693 | 474 | 18 | 24 | 352 | 13 | 3 |
| ≥ 40 | 947 | 72 | 8 | 35 | 39 | 4 | <1 |
| B. GIFT |  |  |  |  |  |  |  |
| 30–34 | 1315 | 458 | 35 | 15 | 297 | 23 | 10 |
| 35–39 | 1043 | 293 | 28 | 20 | 223 | 21 | 6 |
| ≥ 40 | 348 | 67 | 19 | 42 | 32 | 9 | 1 |

* Data reproduced with permission from Medical Research International (1991, 1992).
† Abortions are expressed as a percentage of clinical pregnancies.
‡ Delivery rate is expressed as a percentage of transfer.
§ Multiple delivery rates are expressed as a percentage of transferred cycles.

**Table 21.11**   Pregnancy rate per puncture for each rank of attempt

| Rank of the attempt | No. of attempts | Pregnancies per puncture | | Cumulative |
|---|---|---|---|---|
| | | No. | % | (%) |
| 1 | 20 761 | 3607 | 17.4 | 17.4 |
| 2 | 11 944 | 1927 | 16.2 | 30.8 |
| 3 | 6762 | 1167 | 17.3 | 42.8 |
| 4 | 3710 | 605 | 16.3 | 52.1 |
| 5 | 2035 | 317 | 15.6 | 59.6 |
| 6 | 1080 | 177 | 16.4 | 66.2 |
| 7 | 583 | 85 | 14.6 | 71.1 |
| 8 | 302 | 48 | 15.9 | 75.8 |
| 9 | 152 | 17 | 11.2 | 78.5 |
| ≥ 10 | 208 | 30 | 14.4 | 81.5 |

Reproduced with permission from Cohen 1991.

**Table 21.12**   Outcome of pregnancies (IVF)

| | Ectopic (%) | Abortion (%) | Stillbirth (%) | Live birth (%) |
|---|---|---|---|---|
| Australia 1988 | 6.3 | 21.1* | 2.6 | 69.5 |
| FIVNAT 1988 | 6.5 † | 20.6 | | 71.5 |
| USA | 5 ‡ | 24 § | | 73.8 § |
| UK 1988 | 4.8 | 21 | | 68 |

Reproduced with permission from Cohen 1991.
* 0.5% abortion for medical reasons.
† 1% ectopic plus intrauterine.
‡ Ectopic pregnancies are expressed as a percentage of all pregnancies.
§ Spontaneous abortion rates and delivery rates expressed as a percentage of clinical pregnancies.

which may explain the significantly higher tubal pregnancy rate (9.1%) in cases with tubal factor etiology. Heterotopic (combined) pregnancies are reported to occur in a much higher incidence than in the normal population. Several authors (Molloy et al 1990, Dor et al 1991, Goldman et al 1992) reported an incidence of around 1% of the clinical pregnancies in ART. Factors such as deep insertion of the uterine transfer catheter and the use of a viscous medium in this process coupled with the multiple embryos replaced may be contributing factors.

The proportion of singleton and multiple deliveries seems to be comparable in the various reports, being 75–77% for singletons, 19–20% for twins and 3–4.5% for triplets or more. In the World Collaborative Report (1989) the multiple pregnancy rate in IVF-ET was 26.5% and 28% for GIFT procedures. In order to reduce multiple pregnancy rate, the Bourn-Hallam group has replaced up to three embryos in the uterine cavity (Steptoe et al 1986). The multiple pregnancy rate among 767 pregnancies was 14%. Twenty-four per cent of them had a vanishing sac. Thus, 11% twins and 1.4% triplets reached delivery. Many countries in Europe are now transferring not more than three oocytes in GIFT, three zygotes in ZIFT and three embryos in TET or in IVF-ET programs. However, since pregnancy rate and multiplicity rate decrease at the age of 35 years we have adopted the individualized transfer, namely transfer of three embryos below 35 years of age and up to four embryos above this age or when previous cycles with three replaced embryos failed to reach pregnancy.

Premature delivery rate (< 37 weeks) was 28% and 36% of the born fetuses weighed < 2500 g (The National Registry for IVF-ET Deliveries 1982–89). The overall prematurity rate is 5–7%. In the Bourn-Hallam group premature deliveries were 25%; 14% in singletons, 59% in twins and 95% in triplets. Thirty-two per cent of the babies had a low birth weight (< 2500 g). Fourteen per cent of singleton babies were small for gestational age compared to 7% of all births in England (Rizk et al 1991).

Mode of delivery (Israel National Registry 1990) was vaginally in 53% and 47% by Cesarian section. Pregnancies were terminated by abdominal delivery in 41% of the singletons, 68% of the twins and 86% of the triplets. The perinatal mortality rate (stillbirths and deaths in first 7 days) per 1000 births was 45 in Australia, 27 in Great Britain and 22 in Israel. The perinatal mortality rate per 1000 births in the total population is between 10 and 15. Multiplicity appears to be the major factor determining the outcome of IVF pregnancies. However, more factors such as higher mean maternal age, e.g. 34.2 years compared with 28 years in the whole population, and concealed problems such as uterine malformations (myomas, congenital and acquired malformations) are heavily influencing the doubled perinatal mortality rate among the ART population.

Major congenital malformations were found in 2.5% of the babies in the Bourn-Hallam series and in the Israel National Registry. The US Registry has found 2.1% of babies with major congenital malformations and the World Collaborative Report had noted 1.5%. In all instances the numbers were not significantly different from the general population of newborns.

The pregnancy rates after replacement of frozen-thawed embryos are 10–12% (Van Steirteghem et al 1990, Medical Research International 1991, 1992). Of the 616 (11%) pregnancies resulting from 5414 replacements of frozen-thawed embryos in the USA, 7.7% were tubal pregnancies and 23% ended with spontaneous abortions. The incidence of congenital malformations among the babies resulting from frozen-thawed embryos was not significantly different compared with the fresh ART babies or the general population newborns.

## FUTURE ASPECTS

Tremendous progress has been made during the last 15 years in the field of ART. Living proof of this advanced technology are the 40 000 babies and children now living among us. People who work in this field have said many times that the achievements have reached the top in ART since pregnancy rate per cycle has reached the natural chance to conceive, a rate of 22% per cycle. However, it seems that there is still a lot left to learn and to do.

Superovulation of the ovaries will probably be performed with GnRH antagonist to prevent stimulation phase disturbances. In-depth studies of embryo culture condition and co-culture are needed. A great deal is still unknown about the implantation of the embryo in the uterus.

Our belief is that male infertility cases will represent a more and more pronounced part of ART. Couples with this problem seek a solution by any means. It may be that results of micromanipulation will improve or some other mode of sperm treatment will be invented.

Regarding cryopreservation, despite the gigantic achievements in this field, we are unable to overcome the poor results in oocyte freezing and the relatively low pregnancy rate after replacement of freeze-thawed embryos. Intensive research in this field will certainly open new horizons.

## REFERENCES

Abdullah H J, Aliuja K K, Leonard T, Morris N N, Honcur J W, Jacobs H S 1990 Comparative trial of luteinizing hormone-releasing hormone analog/human menopausal gonadotrophin and clomiphene citrate/human menopausal gonadotropin in an assisted conception program. Fertil Steril 53: 473

Al-Hasani S, Diedrich K, Van der Ven H, Reinecke A, Hartje M, Krebs D 1987 Cryopreservation of human oocytes. Hum Reprod 2: 695

Allen N C, Herbert C M, Maxson W S, Rogers B J, Diamond M P, Wentz A C 1985 Intrauterine insemination: a critical review. Fertil Steril 44: 569

Antoine J M, Salat-Baroux J, Alvarez S et al 1990 Ovarian stimulation using human menopausal gonadotrophins with or without LHRH analogues in a long protocol for in vitro fertilization: a prospective randomized comparison. Hum Reprod 5: 565

Asch R H, Siler-Khodr T M, Smith C G, Schally A V 1981 Luteolytic effect of D-TRP6-luteinizing hormone-releasing hormone in the rhesus monkey (*Macaca mulatta*). J Clin Endocrinol Metab 52: 565

Asch R H, Ellsworth L R, Balmaceda J P, Wong P C 1984 Pregnancy after translaparoscopic gamete intrafallopian transfer. Lancet ii: 1034

Asch R H, Li H P, Balmaceda J P, Weckstein L N, Stone S C 1991 Severe ovarian hyperstimulation syndrome in assisted reproductive technology: definition and high risk group. Hum Reprod 6: 1395

Asch R H, Ivery G, Stone S C, Balmaced J P, Li H P 1992 Intravenous albumin prevents the development of severe ovarian hyperstimulation syndrome in an ART program. Presented at the 40th Annual Meeting of the Pacific Coast Fertility Society, 8–12 April 1992, Abstract 014

Audibert F, Hedon B, Arnal F et al 1989 Results of IVF attempts in patients with unexplained infertility. Hum Reprod 4: 766

Belaisch-Allart J C, Hazout A, Guillet Rosso F, Glissant M, Testart J, Frydman R 1985 Various techniques for oocyte recovery in an in vitro fertilization and embryo transfer program. J IVF Embryo Trans 2: 99

Belaisch-Allart J C, De Mouzon J, Lapousterle C, Mayer M 1990 The effect of HCG supplementation after combined GnRH agonist/HMG treatment in an IVF programme. Hum Reprod 5: 163

Belchetz P E, Plant T M, Nakai Y, Keogh E J, Knobil E 1978 Hypophyseal response to continuous and intermittent delivery of hypothalonic gonadotropin-releasing hormone. Science 202: 631

Bernardus R E, Jones G S, Acosta A A, Garcia J E, Liu H C, Jones D L 1985 The significance of the ratio in follicle stimulating hormone and luteinizing hormone in induction of multiple follicular growth. Fertil Steril 43: 373

Blackwell R E 1989 The infertility workup and diagnosis J Reprod Med 34 (1 suppl.): 81

Bongso A, Soon-Chye N, Sathananthan H, Lian N P, Rauff S, Ratman S 1989 Improved quality of human embryos when co-cultured with human ampullary cells. Hum Reprod 4: 706

Bose R, Cheng H, Sabbadini E, McCoshen J, Mahadevan M M, Fleetham J 1989 Purified human early pregnancy factor from preimplantation embryo possesses immunosuppressive properties. Am J Obstet Gynecol 160: 954

Buvat J, Marcolin G, Herbaut J C, Dehaene J L, Verbecq P, Fourlinnie J C 1988 A randomized trial of human chorionic gonadotropin support following in vitro fertilization and embryo transfer. Fertil Steril 49: 458

Buvat J, Marcolin G, Guittard C, Herbaut J C, Louvet A L, Dehaene J L 1990 Luteal support after luteinizing hormone-releasing hormone agonist for in vitro fertilization: superiority of human chorionic gonadotropin over oral progesterone. Fertil Steril 53: 490

Cameron I T, O'Shea F C, Rolland J M, Hughes E G, de Kretser D M, Healy D L 1988 Occult ovarian failure: a syndrome of infertility regular menses and elevated follicle-stimulating hormone concentrations. J Clin Endocrinol Metab 67: 1190

Casper R F, Yen S S C 1979 Induction of luteolysis in the human with a long-acting analog of luteinizing hormone-releasing factor. Science 205: 408

Casper R F, Sheehan K L, Yen S S C 1980 Chorionic gonadotropin prevents LRF-agonist-induced luteolysis in the human. Contraception 21: 471

Caspi E, Ron-El R, Golan A et al 1989a Results of in vitro fertilization and embryo transfer by combined long-acting gonadotropin-releasing hormone analog D-Trp$_6$ luteinizing hormone-releasing hormone and gonadotropins. Fertil Steril 51: 95

Caspi E, Ron-El R, Golan A, Herman A, Nachum H 1989b Early, late and sequential embryo transfer in in vitro fertilization program: a preliminary report. Fertil Steril 52: 146

Chillik C F, Acosta A A, Garcia J E et al 1985 The role of in vitro fertilization in infertile patients with endometriosis. Fertil Steril 44: 56

Claman P, Minerva D, Leader A 1992 Luteal phase support in in vitro fertilization using gonadotropin releasing hormone analogue before ovarian stimulation: a prospective randomized study of human chorionic gonadotropin versus intramuscular progesterone. Hum Reprod 7: 487

Cohen J 1991 The efficiency and efficacy of IVF and GIFT. Hum Reprod 6: 613

Cohen J, de Mouzon J 1989 Dossier FIVNAT. Analyse des resultats 1988: Stimulation ovarienne pour PMA. Contracept Fertil Sexual 17: 691

Cohen J, Fehilly C B, Fishel S B et al 1984 Male infertility successfully treated by in vitro fertilisation. Lancet i: 1239

Cohen J, Malter H, Elsner C, Kort H, Massey J, Mayer M P 1990a Immunosuppression supports implantation of zona drilled human embryos. Fertil Steril 53: 662

Cohen J, Elsner C, Kort H et al 1990b Impairment of the hatching process following IVF in the human and improvement of implantation by assisting hatching using micromanipulation. Hum Reprod 5: 7

Cohen J, Alikani M, Trowbridge J, Rosenwaks Z 1992 Implantation enhancement by selective assisted hatching using zona drilling of human embryos with poor prognosis. Hum Reprod 7: 685

Confino E, Demir R H, Friberg J, Gleicher N 1986 The predictive value of hCG β subunit levels in pregnancies achieved by in vitro fertilization and embryo transfer: an international collaborative study. Fertil Steril 45: 526

Corsan G H, Kemmann E 1991 The role of superovulation with menotropins in ovulatory infertility: a review. Fertil Steril 55: 468

Craft I, Brinsden P 1989 Alternative to IVF: the outcome of 1071 first GIFT procedures. Hum Reprod 4 (8 suppl): 29

Craft I, Djahanbakhch O, Mcleod F et al 1982 Human pregnancy following oocyte and sperm transfer to the uterus. Lancet i: 1031

Crosignani P G, Walters D E, Soliani A 1991 The ESHRE multicentre trial on the treatment of unexplained infertility: a preliminary report. Hum Reprod 6: 953

Curtis P, Amso N, Keith E, Bernard A, Shaw R W 1991 Evaluation of the risk of pelvic infection following transvaginal oocyte recovery. Hum Reprod 6: 1294

Daya S 1988 Efficacy of progesterone support in the luteal phase following in-vitro fertilization and embryo transfer: meta-analysis of clinical trials. Hum Reprod 3: 731

Daya S, Clark D A 1988 Indentification of two species of suppressive factor of differing molecular weight released by in vitro fertilized human oocytes. Fertil Steril 49: 360

de Mouzon J, Belaisch-Albert J, Cohen J et al 1988 Dossier FIVNAT, analyze de resultats 1987. Stimulatirus Contracept Fertil Sexual 16: 559

Delenbach P, Nisand I, Moreau L et al 1984 Transvaginal sonographically controlled ovarian follicle puncture for egg retrieval. Lancet i: 1467

Delvigne A, Vandromme J, Barlow P, Lejeune B, Leroy F 1991 Are there predictive criteria of complicated ovarian hyperstimulation in IVF. Hum Reprod 6: 959

Demoulin A, Bologne R, Hustin J, Lambotte R 1985 Is ultrasound monitoring of follicular growth harmless? Ann N Y Acad Sci 442: 146

Devroey P, Braeckmans P, Smitz J et al 1986 Pregnancy after trans-laparoscopic zygote intrafallopian transfer in a patient with sperm antibodies (letter). Lancet i: 1329

Devroey P, Staessen C, Camus M, De Grauwe, Wisanto A, Van Steirteghem A C 1989 Zygote intrafallopian transfer as a successful treatment for unexplained infertility. Fertil Steril 52: 246

Dicker D, Goldman G A, Ashkenazi J, Feldberg D, Voliovitz I, Goldman J A 1990 The value of pretreatment with gonadotrophin releasing hormone (GnRH) analogue in IVF-ET therapy of severe endometriosis. Hum Reprod 5: 418

Dicker D, Goldman J A, Ashkenazi J, Feldberg D, Shelef M, Levy T 1991 Age and pregnancy rates in in vitro fertilization. J IVF Embryo Trans 8: 141

Diedrich K, Van der Ven H, Al-Hasani S, Krebs D 1988 Ovarian stimulation for in vitro fertilization. Hum Reprod 3: 39

Diedrich K, Bauer O, Werner A, Van der Ven H, Al-Hasani S, Krebs D 1991 Transvaginal intratubal embryo transfer: a new treatment of male infertility. Hum Reprod 6: 672

Dodson W C, Haney A F 1991 Controlled ovarian hyperstimulation and intrauterine insemination for treatment of infertility. Fertil Steril 55: 457

Dor J, Shulman A, Levran D, Ben-Raphael Z, Rudak E, Mashiach S 1990 The treatment of patients with polycystic ovarian syndrome by in vitro fertilization and embryo transfer: a comparison of results with those of patients with tubal infertility. Hum Reprod 5: 816

Dor J, Seidman D S, Levran D, Ben-Rafael Z, Ben-Shlomo I, Mashiach S 1991 The incidence of combined intrauterine and extrauterine pregnancy after in vitro fertilization and embryo transfer. Fertil Steril 55: 833

Dubuisson J B, Aubriot F X, Mathieu L, Foulot H, Mandelbrot L, Bouquet de Joliniere J 1991 Risk factors for ectopic pregnancy in 556 pregnancies after in vitro fertilization: implications for preventive management. Fertil Steril 56: 686

Edwards R G 1981 Test tube babies. Nature 293: 253

Edwards R G, Steptoe P C 1983 Current status of in vitro fertilisation and implantation of human embryos. Lancet ii: 1265

Edwards R G, Steptoe P C, Purdy J M 1980 Establishing full-term human pregnancies using cleaving embryos grown in vitro. Br J Obstet Gynaecol 87: 737

Feichtinger W, Kemeter P 1984 Laparoscopic or ultrasonically guided follicle aspiration for in vitro fertilization. J IVF Embryo Transfer 1: 244

Feichtinger W, Kemeter P 1986 Transvaginal sector scan sonography for needle guided transvaginal follicle aspiration and other applications in gynecologic routine and research. Fertil Steril 45: 722

Feichtinger W, Kemeter P, Szalay S, Beck A, Janisch H 1982 Could aspiration of the Graafian follicle cause luteal phase deficiency? Fertil Steril 37: 205

Feldberg D, Ashkenazi J, Dicker D, Yeshaya Y, Goldman G A 1987 Ovarian cyst formation: a complication of gonadotropin releasing hormone analog agonist therapy. Fertil Steril 51: 42

Fleming R 1990 Induction of ovulation with a GnRH analogue and gonadotropins in patients with polycystic ovarian disease. In: Brosens I, Jacobs H S, Runnebaum B (eds) LHRH analogues in gynecology. Parthenon Publishing Cornforth, Lancashire, p 69

Fleming R, Adam A H, Barlow O H, Black W P, Macdaughton M C, Coutts J R 1982 A new systematic treatment for infertile women with abnormal hormone profiles. Br J Obstet Gynaecol 89: 80

Forman R, Fries N, Testart J, Belaisch-Allart J, Hazout A, Frydman R 1988 Evidence for an adverse effect of elevated serum estradiol concentrations on embryo implantation. Fertil Steril 49: 118

Foulot H, Dubuisson B, Ranoux C, Aubriot F X, Poirot C 1988 Etude randomisee entre protocole long de busereline concernanant 100 cycles de Fecondation In Vitro. Contracept Fertil Sexual 16: 628

Foulot H, Ranoux C, Dubuisson J B, Rambaud D, Aubriot F X, Poirot C 1989 In vitro fertilization without ovarian stimulation: a simplified protocol applied in 80 cycles. Fertil Steril 52: 617

Fraser H M, Sandow J 1985 Suppression of follicular maturation by infusion of a luteinizing hormone-releasing hormone agonist starting during the late luteal phase in the stump-tailed macaque monkey. J Clin Endocrinol Metab 60: 579

Frydman R, Testart J, Giacomini P, Imbert M C, Martin E, Nahoul K 1982 Hormonal and histological study of the luteal phase in women following aspiration of the preovulatory follicle. Fertil Steril 38: 312

Frydman R, Parneix I, Belaisch-Allart J 1988 LHRH agonists in IVF: different methods of utilization and comparison with previous ovulation stimulation treatments. Hum Reprod 3: 559

Fugger E F, Bustillo M, Dorfmann A D, Schulman J D 1991 Human preimplantation embryo cryopreservation: selected aspects. Hum Reprod 6: 131

Garcia J, Seegar Jones G, Wentz A C 1977 The use of clomiphene citrate. Fertil Steril 28: 707

Garcia J, Jones G S, Acosta A A, Wright G L 1981 Corpus luteum function after follicle aspiration for oocyte retrieval. Fertil Steril 36: 565

Glasier A F, Thatcher S S, Wickings E J, Hillier S G, Baird D T 1988 Superovulation with exogenous gonadotropin does not inhibit the luteinizing hormone surge. Fertil Steril 49: 81

Golan A, Ron-El R, Herman A, Weinraub Z, Soffer Y, Caspi E 1988 Ovarian hyperstimulation syndrome following D-Trp-6 luteinizing hormone-releasing microcapsules and menotropin for in vitro fertilization. Fertil Steril 50: 912

Golan A, Ron-El R, Herman A, Weinraub Z, Soffer Y, Caspi E 1990 Fetal outcome following inadvertent administration of long-acting D-Trp6 GnRH microcapsules during pregnancy: a case report. Hum Reprod 5: 123

Golan A, Ron-El R, Herman A, Soffer Y, Bukovsky J, Crapi E 1992a Diagnostic hysteroscopy—its value in a IVF-ET unit (in press)

Golan A, Nachum H, Herman A, Ron-El R, Soffer Y, Caspi E 1992b Increased fertilization and pregnancy rate in polypronuclear cycles in IVF-ET. Fertil Steril 57: 137

Goldman G A, Fisch B, Ovadia J, Tadir Y 1992 Heterotopic pregnancy after assisted reproductive technologies. Obstet Gynaecol Surv 47: 217

Gordon J W, Grunfeld L, Garrisia G J, Talansky B E, Richards C, Laufer N 1988 Fertilization of human oocytes by sperm from infertile males after zona pellucida drilling. Fertil Steril 50: 68

Gordts S, Roziers P, Campo R, Noto V 1990 Survival and pregnancy outcome after ultrarapid freezing of human embryos. Fertil Steril 53: 469

Gorus E K, Pipeleers D G 1981 A rapid method for the fractionation of human spermatozoa according to their progressive motility. Fertil Steril 35: 662

Groff T R, Raj H G, Talbert L M, Willis D L 1984 Effects of neutralization of luteinizing hormone on corpus luteum function and cyclicity in Macaca fascicularis. J Clin Endocrinol Metab 59: 1054

Handyside A H, Penketh R J A, Winston R M L, Pattinson J K, Delhanty J D A, Tuddenham E G D 1989 Biopsy of human preimplantation embryos and sexing by DNA amplification. Lancet i: 347

Haney A F, Hughes C L, Whitesides D B, Dodson W C 1987 Treatment independent, treatment-associated and pregnancies after additional therapy in a program of in vitro fertilization and embryo transfer. Fertil Steril 47: 634

Hedon B, Arnal F, Basor E et al 1988 Comparison randomisee protocole long-protocole court dans les stimulation de l'ovaire en association avec un agoniste de la GnRH en vue de fecondation in vitro. Contracept Fertil Sexual 16: 624

Herman A, Ron-El R, Golan A, Weinraub Z, Bukovsky I, Caspi E 1990a The role of tubal pathology and other parameters in ectopic pregnancies occurring in in vitro fertilization and embryo transfer. Fertil Steril 54: 864

Herman A, Ron-El R, Golan A, Nachum H, Soffer Y, Caspi E 1990b Follicle cysts following menstrual versus midluteal administration of gonadotropin releasing hormone analog in IVF. Fertil Steril 53: 854

Herman A, Ron-El R, Golan A, Raziel A, Soffer Y, Caspi E 1990c Pregnancy rate and ovarian hyperstimulation after luteal human chorionic gonadotropin in in vitro fertilization stimulated with gonadotropin-releasing hormone analog and menotropins. Fertil Steril 53: 92

Herman A, Ron-El R, Golan A, Nachum H, Soffer Y, Caspi E 1992 Impaired corpus luteum function and other undesired results of pregnancies associated with inadvertant administration of a long-acting agonist of gonadotropin-releasing hormone. Hum Reprod 7: 465

Hinting A, Comhaire F, Vermulen M, Dhont M, Vermulen A, Vandekerckhove 1989 Value of sperm characteristics and the result of in vitro fertilization for predicting the outcome of assisted reproduction. Int J Androl 13: 59

Hirsch I, Gibbons W E, Lipshultz L I et al 1986 In vitro fertilization in couples with male factor infertility. Fertil Steril 45: 659

Hoult I J, de Crespigny L Ch, O'Herlihy C et al 1981 Ultrasound control of clomiphene human chorionic gonadotropins stimulated cycles for oocyte recovery and in vitro fertilization. Fertil Steril 36: 316

Howe R S, Wheeler C, Mastroianni L Jr, Blasco L, Tureck R 1988 Pelvic infection after transvaginal ultrasound-guided ovum retrieval. Fertil Steril 49: 726

Howles C M, Macnamee M C, Edwards R G, Goswamy R, Steptoe P C 1986 Effect of high tonic levels of luteinizing hormone on outcome of in vitro fertilization. Lancet ii: 521

Ho Yuen B, Mari N, Duleba A J, Moon Y S 1988 Direct effect of clomiphene citrate on the steroidogenic capability of human granulosa cells. Fertil Steril 49: 626

Hutchinson-Williams K A, DeCherney A H, Lavy G, Diamond M P, Naftolin F, Lunenfeld B 1990 Luteal rescue in in vitro fertilization-embryo transfer. Fertil Steril 53: 495

Jansen R P S, Anderson J C 1987 Catheterisation of the fallopian tubes from the vagina. Lancet ii: 309

Jones G S, Acosta A A, Garcia J E, Bernardus R E, Rosenwaks Z 1985 The effect of follicle-stimulating hormone without additional luteinizing hormone on follicular stimulation and oocyte development in normal ovulatory women. Fertil Steril 43: 696

Jones H W J 1986 Introduction. In: Fishel S, Symonds E M (eds) In vitro fertilization. IRL Press, Oxford, p 17

Jones H W J Jr, Jones G S, Andrews M C et al 1982 The program for in vitro fertilization at Norfolk. Fertil Steril 38: 14

Jones H W J Jr, Acosta A A, Andrews M C et al 1983 The importance of the follicular phase to success and failure in in vitro fertilization. Fertil Steril 40: 317

Jones W R 1987 In: Pepperell R J, Hudson B, Wood C (eds) The infertile couple, 2nd edn. Churchill Livingstone, Edinburgh, p 159

Kapur R P, Johnson L 1985 An oviductal fluid glycoprotein associated with ovulated mouse ova and early embryos. Dev Biol 112: 89

Kemeter P, Feichtinger W, Neumark J, Szalay S, Bieglmayer Ch, Janisch H 1981 Influence of laparoscopic follicular aspiration under general anaesthesia on corpus luteum progesterone secretion in normal and clomiphene-stimulated cycles. Br J Obstet Gynaec 89: 948

Kerin J F, Broom T J, Ralph M M et al 1981 Human luteal phase function following oocyte aspiration from the immediately preovular graafian follicle of spontaneous ovular cycles. Br J Obstet Gynaecol 88: 1021

Kosasa T, Levesque L, Goldstein D P et al 1973 Early detection of implantation using a radioimmunoassay specific for human chorionic gonadotrophin. J Clin Endocrinol Metab 36: 622

Koyama T, Ohkura T, Kumasaka T, Saito M 1978 Effect of postovulatory treatment with a luteinizing hormone-releasing hormone analog on the plasma level of progesterone in women. Fertil Steril 30: 549

Kreitmann O, Nixon W E, Hodgen G D 1981 Induced corpus luteum dysfunction after aspiration of the preovulatory follicle in monkeys. Fertil Steril 35: 671

Kruger T F, Menkueld R, Stander F S H et al 1986 Sperm morphology features as a prognostic factor in in vitro fertilization. Fertil Steril 84: 551

Kruger T F, Acosta A A, Simmons K F, Swanson R J, Matta J F, Oehinger S 1988 Predictive value of abnormal sperm morphology in in vitro fertilization. Fertil Steril 49: 112

Kupferminc M J, Lessing J B, Amit A, Yovel I, David M P, Peyser M R 1990 A prospective randomized trial of human chorionic gonadotropin or dydrogesterone support following in vitro fertilization and embryo transfer. Hum Reprod 5: 271

Laufer N, Pratt B M, Decherney A H, Naftolin F, Merino M, Markert C L 1983 The in vivo and in vitro effects of clomiphene citrate on ovulation, fertilization and development of cultured mouse embryos. Am J Obstet Gynecol 147: 633

Lemay A, Labrie F, Ferland L, Raynaud J 1979 Possible luteolytic effects of luteinizing hormone-releasing hormone in normal women. Fertil Steril 31: 29

Lemay A, Faure N, Labrie F, Fazekas A T 1983
Gonadotroph and corpus luteum responses to two
successive intranasal doses of luteininzing hormone-
releasing hormone agonist at different days after the
midcycle luteinizing hormone surge. Fertil Steril 39: 661

Lenz S 1984 Ultrasonically guided aspiration of human
oocytes. Ultrasound A Med Biol 10: 625

Lenz S, Lauritsen J G 1982 Ultrasonically guided
percutaneous aspiration of human follicles under local
anaesthesia: a new method of collecting oocytes for in vitro
fertilization. Fertil Steril 38: 673

Lenz S, Lauritsen J G, Kjellow U 1981 Collection of human
oocytes for in vitro fertilization by ultrasonically guided
follicular puncture. Lancet i: 1163

Lessing J B, Amit A, Barak Y et al 1988 The performance of
primary and secondary unexplained infertility in an in vitro
fertilization-embryo transfer program. Fertil Steril 50: 903

Lessing J B, Amit A, Libal, Yovel I, Kogosowski A,
Peyser M R 1991 Avoidance of cancellation of potential
hyperstimulation cycles by conversion to in vitro
fertilization-embryo transfer. Fertil Steril 56: 75

Leung P C S, Gronow M J, Kellow J N et al 1984 Serum
supplement in human in vitro fertilization and embryo
development. Fertil Steril 41: 36

Lopata A 1983 Concepts in human in vitro fertilization and
embryo transfer. Fertil Steril 40: 289

Lopata A, Patullo M J, Chang A, James B 1976 A method for
collecting motile spermatozoa from human semen. Fertil
Steril 27: 677

Lopata A, Brown J B, Leeton J F, Talbot J Mc, Wood C 1978
In vitro fertilization of preovulatory oocytes and embryo
transfer in infertile patients treated with clomiphene and
human chorionic gonadotropin. Fertil Steril 30: 27

Lopata A, Johnston W H, Hault I H, Spiers A 1980
Pregnancy following intrauterine implantation of an embryo
obtained by in vitro fertilization of a preovulatory egg. Fertil
Steril 33: 117

Loumaye E, Billion J J, Mine J M, Psalti I, Pensis M, Thomas
K 1990 Prediction of individual response to controlled
ovarian hyperstimulation by means of a clomiphene citrate
challenge test. Fertil Steril 53: 295

Lunenfeld B, Insler V 1978 Infertility. Grosse Verlag, Berlin,
p 64

Lutjen P, Trounson A, Leeton J, Findlay J, Wood C, Renou P
1984 The establishment and maintenance of pregnancy
using in vitro fertilization and embryo donation in a patient
with primary ovarian failure. Nature 307: 174

MacLachlan V, Besanko M, O'Shea F et al 1989 A controlled
study of luteinizing hormone-releasing hormone agonist
(Buserelin) for the induction of folliculogenesis before in
vitro fertilization. N Engl J Med 320: 1233

Macnamee M C, Howles C M, Edwards R G, Taylor P J,
Elder K T 1989 Short-term luteinizing hormone-releasing
hormone agonist treatment: prospective trial of a novel
ovarian stimulation regimen for in vitro fertilization. Fertil
Steril 52: 264

Mahadevan M M, Trounson A O 1984 The influence of
seminal characteristics on the success rate of human in vitro
fertilization. Fertil Steril 42: 400

Mahadevan M M, Trounson A O, Wood C, Leeton J F 1987
Effect of oocyt equality and sperm characteristices on the
number of spermatozoa bound to the zona pellucida of
human oocytes inseminated in vitro. J IVF ET 4: 223

Makler A, DeCherney A, Naftolin F 1984 A device for
injecting and retaining a small volume of concentrated

spermatozoa in the uterine cavity and cervical canal. Fertil
Steril 42: 306

Margallioth E J, Sauter E, Bronson R A, Rosenfeld D L,
Scholl G M, Cooper G W 1988 Intrauterine insemination
as treatment for antisperm antibodies in the female. Fertil
Steril 50: 441

Maroulis G B, Emery M, Verkauf B S, Saphier A, Bernhisel
M, Yeko T R 1991 Prospective randomized study of
human menotropin versus a follicular and luteal phase
gonadotropin-releasing hormone analog-human
menotropin stimulation protocols for in vitro fertilization.
Fertil Steril 55: 1157

Marrs R P, Vargyas J M, Gibbons W E, Saito H, Mishell D Jr
1983 A modified technique of human in vitro fertilization
and embryo transfer. Am J Obstet Gynecol 147: 318

Marrs R P, Vargyas J M, Shangold G M, Yee B, 1984 The
effect of time of initiation of clomiphene citrate on
multiple follicle development for human in vitro
fertilization and embryo replacement procedures. Fertil
Steril 41: 682

Matson P L, Yovich J L 1986 The treatment of infertility
associated with endometriosis by in vitro fertilization. Fertil
Steril 46: 432

Medical Research International, The American Fertility
Society Special Interest Group 1988 In vitro
fertilization/embryo transfer in the United States: 1985 and
1986 results from the National IVF-ET Registry. Fertil
Steril 49: 212

Medical Research International Society, The Society for
Assisted Reproductive Technology 1989 In vitro
fertilization/embryo transfer in the United States: 1987
results from the IVF-ET Registry. Fertil Steril 51: 13

Medical Research International Society, The Society for
Assisted Reproductive Technology 1990 In vitro
fertilization/embryo transfer in the United States: 1988
results from the IVF-ET Registry. Fertil Steril 53: 13

Medical Research International Society for Assisted
Reproductive Technology, The American Fertility Society
1991 In vitro fertilization-embryo transfer (IVF-ET) in the
United States: 1989 results from the IVF-ET Registry.
Fertil Steril 55: 14

Medical Research International Society for Assisted
Reproductive Technology, The American Fertility Society
1992 In vitro fertilization-embryo transfer (IVF-ET) in the
United States: 1990 results from the IVF-ET Registry.
Fertil Steril 57: 15

Meldrum D R, Wisot A, Hamilton F, Gutlay A L, Huynh D,
Kempton W 1988 Timing of initiation and dose schedule of
leuprolide influence the time course of ovarian suppression.
Fertil Steril 50: 400

Meldrum D R 1989 Antibiotics for vaginal oocyte aspiration.
J IVF ET 6: 1

Meldrum D R, Wisot A, Hamilton F, Gutlay A L,
Kempton W, Huynh D 1989 Routine pituitary suppression
with leuprolide before ovarian stimulation for oocyte
retrieval. Fertil Steril 51: 455

Menezo Y, Hazout A, Dumont M, Herbaut N, Nicollet B
1992 Coculture of embryos on vero cells and transfer of
blastocysts in humans. Hum Reprod 7(suppl): 101

Messinis I E, Templeton A, Baird D T 1986 Relationships
between the characteristics of endogenous luteinizing
hormone surge and the degree of ovarian hyperstimulation
during superovulation induction in women. Clin
Endocrinol 25: 393

Molloy D, Deambrosis W, Keeping D et al 1990 Multiple

sited (herterotopic) pregnancy after in vitro fertilization and gamete intrafallopian transfer. Fertil Steril 53: 1068

Morton H, Rolfe B, Clunie G J A 1977 An early pregnancy factor detected in human serum by the rosette inhibition test. Lancet i: 394

National Perinatal Statistic Unit 1990 IVF and GIFT pregnancies. Australia and New Zealand 1988. National Perinatal Statistics Unit, Fertility Society of Australia, Sydney

The National Registry for IVF-ET Deliveries 1982–1989 The Israel Fertility Society

Navot D, Bergh P A, Williams M A et al 1991 Poor oocyte quality rather than implantation failure as a cause of age-related decline in female fertility. Lancet 337: 1375

Ng S C, Bongso T A, Ratnam S S et al 1988 Pregnancy after transfer of multiple sperm under the zona. Lancet ii: 790

Ng S C, Bongso T A, Chang S I, Sathananthan H, Ratnam S S 1989 Transfer of human sperm into the perivitelline space of human oocytes after zona-drilling or zona-puncture. Fertil Steril 52: 73

Ng S C, Bongso A, Ratnam S S 1991 Microinjection of human oocytes: a technique for severe oligoasthenoterato zoospermia. Fertil Steril 56: 1117

Oehninger S, Coddington C C, Scott R et al 1989a Hemizona assay: assessment of sperm dysfunction and predictor of in vitro fertilization outcome. Fertil Steril 51: 665

Oehinger S, Acosta A A, Kreiner D, Mausker S J, Jones H W, Rozenwaks Z 1989b In vitro fertilization and embryo transfer in patients with endometriosis: Impact of gonadotropin releasing hormone agonist. Hum Reprod 5: 541

Ogawa T, Marrs R P 1987 The effect of protein supplementation on single cell mouse embryos in vitro. Fertil Steril 47: 156

Olson J L, Rebar R W, Schreiber J R, Vaitukaitis J L 1983 Shortened luteal phase after ovulation induction with human menopausal gonadotropin and human chorionic gonadotropin. Fertil Steril 39: 284

O'Neill C, Ferrier A J, Vaughan J, Sinosich M J, Saunders D M 1985a Causes of implantation failure after in vitro fertilization and embryo transfer. Lancet ii: 615

O'Neill C, Gidley-Baird A A, Pike I L, Porter R N, Sinosich M J, Saunders D M 1985b Maternal blood platelet physiology and luteal-phase endocrinology as a means of monitoring pre- and postimplantation embryo viability following in vitro fertilization. J IVF ET 2: 87

Ord T, Patrizio P, Marello E, Balmaceda J P, Asch R H 1990 Mini-Percoll: a new method of semen preparation for IVF in severe male factor infertility. Hum Reprod 5: 987

Oskowitz S, Seibel M, Smith D, Taymor M L 1986 Luteal phase serum progesterone levels after follicle aspiration with and without clomiphene citrate treatment. Fertil Steril 46: 461

Owen E J, Davies M C, Kingsland C R, Jacobs H S, Mason B A 1989 The use of a short regimen of buserelin, a gonadotropin-releasing hormone agonist and human menopausal gonadotropin in assisted conception cycles. Hum Reprod 4: 749

Padilla S L, Garcia J E 1989 Effect of maternal age and number of in vitro fertilization procedures on pregnancy outcome. Fertil Steril 52: 270

Palermo G, Joris H, Devroey P, Van Steirteghem A C 1992 Pregnancies after intracytoplasmic injection of single spermatozoa in oocytes. Lancet 340: 17

Parsons J, Booker M, Goswamy R et al 1985 Oocyte retrieval for in vitro fertilization by ultrasonically guided needle aspiration via the uretha. Lancet i: 1076

Pieters M H E, Dumoulin J C M, Engelhart C M, Bras M, Evers J L H, Geraedts J P M 1991 Immaturity and aneuploidy in human oocytes after different stimulation protocols. Fertil Steril 56: 306

Plachot M, Junca A M, Mandelbaum J, Cohen J, Salat Baroux J, Lagi C Da 1986 Timing of in-vitro fertilization of cumulus-free and cumulus-enclosed human oocytes. Hum Reprod 1: 237

Pool T B, Ellsworth L R, Garza J R, Martin J E, Miller S S, Atiee S H 1990 Zygote intrafallopian transfer as a treatment for nontubal infertility: a 2-year study. Fertil Steril 54: 482

Porter R N, Smith W, Craft I L, Abdulwahid N A, Jacobs H S, 1984 Induction of ovulation for in vitro fertilisation using buserelin and gonadotropins. Lancet ii: 1284

Pousette A, Akerlof E, Rosenborg L, Fredricsson B 1986 Increase in progressive motility and improved morphology of human spermatozoa following their migration through Percoll gradients. Int J Androl 9: 1

Quigley M M, Collins R L, Blankstein J 1988 Pure follicle stimulating hormone does not enhance follicular recruitment in clomiphene citrate/gonadotropin combinations. Fertil Steril 50: 562

Quinn P, Kerin J F, Warnes G M 1985 Improved pregnancy rate in human in vitro fertilization with the use of a medium based on the composition of human tubal fluid. Fertil Steril 44: 493

Rall W F, Fahy G M 1985 Ice free cryopreservation of mouse embryos at $-196°C$ by vitrification. Nature 313: 573

Renaud J P, Barbinet C 1984 High survival of mouse embryos after rapid freezing and thawing inside plastic straws with 1–2 propanediol as cryoprotectant. J Exp Zool 230: 443

Riedel H H, Hubner F, Ensslen S C, Bieniek K W, Grillo M 1989 Minimal andrological requirements for in vitro fertilization. Hum Reprod 4: 73

Rizk B, Aboulghar M 1991 Modern management of ovarian hyperstimulation syndrome. Hum Reprod 6: 1082

Rizk B, Doyle P, Tan S L et al 1991 Perinatal outcome and congenital malformations in in vitro fertilization babies from the Bourn Hallam group. Hum Reprod 6: 1259

Rizk B, Tan S L, Kingsland C, Steer C, Mason B, Campbell S 1990 Ovarian cyst aspiration and the outcome of in vitro fertilization. Fertil Steril 54: 661

Rogers P A W, Polson D, Murphy C R, Hosie M, Susil B, Leoni M 1991 Correlation of endometrial histology morphometry and ultrasound appearance after different stimulation protocols for in vitro fertilization. Fertil Steril 55: 583

Ron-El R, Herman A, Golan A, Raziel A, Soffer Y, Caspi E 1989a Follicle cyst formation following long acting gonadotropin releasing hormone analog administration. Fertil Steril 52: 1063

Ron-El R, Golan A, Herman A, Raziel A, Nachum H, Caspi E 1989b Flexible menotropins initiation after long acting gonadotropins-releasing hormone analog. Fertil Steril 52: 860

Ron-El R, Herman A, Golan A, Van der Ven H, Caspi E, Diedrich K 1990a The comparison of early follicular and midluteal administration of long acting gonadotropin-releasing hormone agonist. Fertil Steril 54: 233

Ron-El R, Raziel A, Herman A, Golan A, Soffer Y, Caspi E

1990b Ovarian response in repetitive cycles induced by menotrophin alone or combined with gonadotrophin releasing hormone analogue. Hum Reprod 5: 427

Ron-El R, Golan A, Herman A, Raziel A, Soffer Y, Caspi E 1990c Midluteal gonadotropin-releasing hormone analog administration in early pregnancy. Fertil Steril 53: 572

Ron-El R, Herman A, Golan A, Arieli S, Bukovsky I, Caspi E 1991a Spontaneous pregnancies after failed and successful IVF-ET trials. 47th Annual Meeting of the American Fertility Society, abstr 101, p 544

Ron-El R, Herman A, Golan A, Nachum H, Soffer Y, Caspi E 1991b Gonadotropins and combined gonadotropin-releasing hormone agonist-gonadotropins protocols in a randomized prospective study. Fertil Steril 55: 574

Ron-El R, Nachum H, Herman A, Golan A, Caspi E, Soffer Y 1991c Delayed fertilization and poor embryonic development associated with impaired semen quality. Fertil Steril 55: 338

Ron-El R, Bracha Y, Herman A et al 1992a Prerequisite work-up of the couple before in vitro fertilization. Hum Reprod 7: 483

Ron-El R, Herman A, Golan A, Soffer Y, Nachum H, Caspi E 1992b Ultrashort gonadotropin-releasing hormone agonist (GnRH-a) protocol in comparison with the long acting GnRH-a protocol and menotropin alone. Fertil Steril

Ron-El R, Golan A, Herman A et al 1992c Pregnancy rate following tubal and intra uterine embryo transfer. A prospective randomized study. Human Reproduction. Abstracts from the 8th Meeting of the European Society of Human Reproduction and Embryology, abstr 270

Russell J B, DeCherney A H, Hobbins J C 1987 A new tranvaginal probe and biopsy guide for oocyte retrieval. Fertil Steril 47: 350

Salat Baroux J, Alvarez S, Antoine J M 1988 Results of IVF in the treatment of polycystic ovary disease. Hum Reprod 3: 331

Sandow J 1989 Chemistry and metabolism of LHRH and its analogues. In: Shaw R W, Marshall J C (eds) LHRH and its analogues, Butterworth-Heinemann, Oxford, Ch 3, pp 35–48

Sandow J, Von Rechenberg W, Jerabek G, Stoll W 1978 Pituitary gonadotropin inhibition by highly active analog of luteinizing hormone-releasing hormone. Fertil Steril 30: 205

Scholtes M C, Roozenburg B J, Alberda A T, Zeilmaker G H 1990 Transcervical intrafallopian transfer of zygotes. Fertil Steril 54: 283

Scoccia B, Blumenthal P, Wagner C, Prins G, Scommegna A, Maru E L 1987 Comparison of urinary human follicle-stimulating hormone and human menopausal gonadotropins for ovarian stimulation in an in vitro fertilization program. Fertil Steril 48: 446

Seppala M et al 1984 The world collaborative report on in vitro fertilization and embryo replacement: current state of the art in January 1984. Ann NY Acad Sci 558

Seracchioli R, Possati G, Bafaro G et al 1991 Hysteroscopic gamete intra-fallopian transfer: a good alternative, in selected cases, to laparoscopic intra-fallopian transfer. Hum Reprod 6: 1388

Serafini P, Batzofin J, Kerin J, Marrs R 1988 Pregnancy: a risk to initiation of leuprolide acetate during the luteal phase before controlled ovarian hyperstimulation. Fertil Steril 50: 371

Sinosich M J, Grudzinskas J G, Saunders D M 1985 Placental proteins in the diagnosis and evaluation of the 'elusive' early pregnancy. Obstet Gynecol Surv 40: 273

Smith E M, Anthony F W, Gadd S C, Masson G M 1989 Trial of support treatment with human chorionic gonadotropin in the luteal phase after treatment with buserelin and human menopausal gonadotropin in women taking part in an in vitro fertilization programme. Br Med J 298: 1483

Smitz J, Devroey P, Braeckmans P et al 1987 Management of failed cycles in an IVF/GIFT programme with the combination of a GnRH analog and hMG. Hum Reprod 2: 309

Smitz J, Devroey P, Camus M et al 1988 The luteal phase and early pregnancy after combined GnRH-agonist/HMG treatment for superovulation in IVF or GIFT. Hum Reprod 3: 585

Smitz J, Camus M, Devroey P, Bollen N, Tournaye H, Van-Steirteghem A C 1991 The influence of inadvertent intra nasal buserelin administration in early pregnancy. Hum Reprod 6: 290

Smitz J, Devroey P, Faguer B, Bourgain C, Camus M, Van Steirteghem A C 1992a A prospective randomized comparison of intramuscular or intravaginal natural progesterone as a luteal phase and early pregnancy supplement. Hum Reprod 7: 168

Smitz J, Ron-El R, Tarlatzis B C 1992b The use of gonadotrophin releasing hormone agonists for in vitro fertilization and other assisted procreation techniques: experience from three centers. Hum Reprod 7(suppl): 49

Soffer Y, Ron-El R, Golan A, Herman A, Caspi E, Samra Z 1990 Male genital mycoplasmas and Chlamydia trachomatis culture: its relationship with accessory gland function, sperm quality and autoimmunity. Fertil Steril 53: 331

Sopelak V M, Hodgen G D 1987 Infusion of gonadotropin-releasing hormone agonist during pregnancy: maternal and fetal response in primates. Am J Obstet Gynecol 156: 755

Soules M R, Sutton G P, Hammond C B, Haney A F 1980 Endocrine changes at operation under general anesthesia: reproductive hormone fluctuations in young women. Fertil Steril 33: 364

Stanger J D, Yovich J L 1985 Reduced in vitro fertilization of human oocytes from patients with raised basal luteinizing hormone levels during the follicular phase. Br J Obstet Gynecol 92: 385

Steptoe P C, Edwards R G 1970 Laparoscopic recovery of preovulatory human oocytes after priming the ovaries with gonadotropins. Lancet i: 683

Steptoe P C, Edwards R G 1976 Reimplantation of a human embryo with subsequent tubal pregnancy. Lancet i: 880

Steptoe P C, Edwards R G, Purdy J M 1980 Clinical aspects of pregnancies established with cleaving embryos grown in vitro. Br J Obstet Gynaecol 87: 757

Steptoe P C, Edwards R G, Walters D E 1986 Observations on 767 clinical pregnancies and 500 births after human in vitro fertilization. Hum Reprod 1: 89

Sunde A, Kahn J A, Molne K 1988 Intrauterine insemination: a European collaborative report. Hum Reprod 3: 69

Talbert L M 1983 Clomiphene citrate induction of ovulation. Fertil Steril 39: 742

Tan S L, Kingsland C, Campbell S 1990 The use of buserelin in in-vitro fertilization – a comparison between the long and short protocol of administration. Gynecol Endocrinol 4(suppl. 2): abstr 107

Tarlatzis B C, Bontis J, Pados G, Lagos S, Spanos E Mantalenakis S 1992 Ovarian stimulation for assisted procreation with buserelin and gonadotropins: prospective evaluation of short versus long protocol. Hum Reprod (in press)

Taymor M L, Seibel M M, Oskowitz S P, Smith D M, Lee G 1985 In vitro fertilization and embryo transfer: an individualized approach to ovulation induction. J IVF ET 2: 162

Tesarik J, Pilka L, Dvorak M, Travnik P 1983 Oocyte recovery, in vitro insemination and transfer into the oviduct after its microsurgical repair at a single laparotomy. Fertil Steril 39: 472

Thatcher S S, DeCherney A H 1989 A critical assessment of the indications for in vitro fertilization and embryo transfer. Hum Reprod 4(suppl): 11

Toner J P, Philput C B, Jones G S, Muasher S J 1991 Basal follicle-stimulating hormone level is a better predictor of in vitro fertilization performance than age. Fertil Steril 55: 784

Trounson A O 1990 Cryopreservation. Br Med Bull 46: 695

Trounson A O, Mohr L 1983 Human pregnancy following cryopreservation, thawing and transfer of an eight-cell embryo. Nature 305: 707

Trounson A, Sjoblam P 1988 Cleavage and development of human embryos in vitro after ultra rapid freezing and thawing. Fertil Steril 50: 373

Trounson O A, Leeton J E, Wood C, Webb J, Wood J 1981 Pregnancies in human by fertilization in vitro and embryo transfer in the controlled ovulatory cycle. Science 212: 681

Trounson A O, Mohr L R, Wood C, Leeton J 1982 Effect of delayed insemination on in vitro fertilization, culture and transfer of human embryos. J Reprod Fertil 64: 285

Tummon I S, Henig I, Radwanska A, Binor Z, Rawlins R, Dmowski W P 1988 Persistent ovarian cysts following administration of human menopausal and chorionic gonadotropins: an attenuated form of ovarian hyperstimulation syndrome. Fertil Steril 49: 244

Tureck R W, Ben-Rafael Z, Blasco L, Sondheimer S, Mastroianni L 1988 Follicular aspiration and in vitro fertilization associated with pelvic reconstructive surgery. Fertil Steril 50: 447

Van Der Zwalmen P, Bertin-Segal G, Geerts L, Debauche C, Schoysman R 1991 Sperm morphology and IVF pregnancy rate: comparison between Percoll gradient centrifugation and swim-up procedures. Hum Reprod 6: 581

Van Hall E V, Mastboom J L 1969 Luteal phase insufficiency in patients treated with clomiphene. Am J Obstet Gynecol 103: 165

Van Steirteghem A C, Van Den Abbell E, Camus M et al 1987 Cryopreservation of human embryos obtained after gamete intra-fallopian transfer and/or in-vitro fertilization. Hum Reprod 7: 593

Van Steirteghem A C, Van Den Abbeel E 1990 World results of human embryo cryopreservation. In: Mashiach S, Ben-

Rafael Z, Laufer N, Schenker J G (eds) Advances in assisted reproductive technologies. Plenum, New York, pp 601–610

Van Uem J F H M, Acosta A A, Swanson R J et al 1985 Male factor evaluation in in vitro fertilization: Norfolk experience. Fertil Steril 44: 375

Veeck L L 1989 Pregnancy rate and pregnancy outcome associated with laboratory evaluation of spermatozoa, oocytes and pre embryos. In: Mashiach S, Ben Rafael Z, Laufer N, Schenker J G (eds) Advances in assisted reproductive technologies. Plenum, New York, pp 745–765

Veeck L L, Wortham J W, Witmyer J, Sandow B A, Acosta A A, Garcia J E 1983 Maturation and fertilization of morphologically immature human oocytes in a program of in vitro fertilization. Fertil Steril 39: 594

Wardle P G, McLaughlin E A, McDermott A, Mitchell J D, Ray B D, Hull M G R 1985 Endometriosis and ovulatory disorder: reduced fertilisation in vitro compared with tubal and unexplained infertility. Lancet ii: 236

Wiedemann R, Hepp H 1989 Selection of patients for IVF therapy or alternative therapy methods. Hum Reprod 4(suppl): 23

Wikland M, Hamberger L 1984 Ultrasound as a diagnostic and operative tool for in vitro fertilization and embryo replacement (IVF/ER) programs. J IVF ET 1: 213

Wildt L, Diedrich K, Van-der-Ven H, Al-Hasani S, Hubner H, Klasen R 1986 Ovarian hyperstimulation for in vitro fertilization controlled by GnRH agonist administered in combination with human menopausal gonadotropins. Hum Reprod 1: 15

World Collaborative Report 1989 Bilan Modial. 7th World Congress on In Vitro Fertilization and Assisted Procreation, Paris 1991

Yoshimura Y, Hosoi Y, Atlas S J, Wallach E E 1986 Effect of clomiphene citrate on in vitro ovulated ova. Fertil Steril 45: 800

Yovich J L, Stanger J D, Yovich J M, Tuvik A I, Turner S R 1985 Hormonal profiles in the follicular phase, luteal phase and first trimester of pregnancies arising from in vitro fertilization. Br J Obstet Gynaecol 92: 374

Yovich J L, Matson P L, Richardson P A, Hilliard C 1988a Hormonal profiles and embryo quality in women with severe endometriosis treated by in vitro fertilization and embryo transfer. Fertil Steril 50: 308

Yovich J L, Yovich J M, Edirisinghe W R 1988b The relative chance of pregnancy following tubal or uterine transfer procedures. Fertil Steril 49: 858

Yovich J L, Edirisinghe W R, Cummins J M 1991 Evaluation of luteal support therapy in a randomized controlled study within a gamate intrafallopian transfer program. Fertil Steril 55: 131

# Treatment of infertility (male)

# 22. Treatment of disturbed sperm–cervical mucus interaction

## J. Kremer

In couples where the result of the postcoital test (PCT) is poorer than could be expected on the score of the semen qualities, treatment must be performed along one or more of the following lines:

1. Treatment of disturbed sperm deposition
2. Treatment of cervical mucus abnormalities
3. Treatment of immunological infertility in women
4. Treatment of immunological infertility in men

## TREATMENT OF DISTURBED SPERM DEPOSITION

The total number of spermatozoa that will enter the endocervical crypts after coitus is influenced by the following factors:

1. The concentration and motility of the spermatozoa in the ejaculate
2. The physicochemical properties of the cervical mucus
3. The closeness of contact that can be achieved between ectocervical mucus and semen

The dimension of the area of contact achieved between semen and cervical mucus depends on the dimension of the surface area of the ectocervical mucus, the volume of the ejaculate, the depth of the intravaginal penile penetration, and the intensity of coital movements during ejaculation. Coital movements by themselves do not really mix semen and cervical mucus because these two fluids mix poorly. Coital movements do, however, enlarge the area of contact between semen and mucus (Fig. 22.1a). The return of the vaginal walls to their original position after

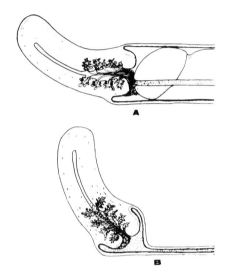

**Fig. 22.1a** Situation during coitus. Coitus movements increase the contact between first part of the ejaculate and the ectocervical mucus. **b** Situation after coitus. A part of the ejaculate is 'trapped' around the vaginal part of the cervix by the vaginal walls. Another part has left the vagina due to lack of space.

withdrawal of the penis then maintains the contact between semen and mucus (Fig. 22.1b). If ejaculation occurs halfway in the vagina without semen and ectocervical mucus coming in contact during and after coitus, the PCT is mostly negative or poor. The content of the vagina is hostile to spermatozoa and they mostly lose their penetrability within half an hour after deposition in the vagina (Kremer 1968).

The pregnancies that occur in virgins after coitus interlabialis are probably due to a long cervical mucus thread beginning in the cervical canal and ending at the opening of the vulva.

Faulty coital technique, severe hypospadias, unnoticed and/or unreported impotence, extreme displacement of the uterus or severe uterine prolapse may be the cause of a poor PCT (Insler et al 1977).

In practice it is surprising how often a poor coital technique is the underlying cause for an unexplained poor result of the PCT. Even thorough inquiries concerning coital techniques do not always reveal the underlying coital disorder.

If there is any doubt as to whether the intromission of the penis during intercourse is sufficiently deep, it is useful to perform a speculum investigation on the wife, in the presence of the husband, in order to show him exactly where he must deposit his semen. The deepest penile penetration into the vagina occurs when the wife lies on her back with her legs flexed on the thighs and her thighs abducted.

This dorsosacral position during coitus is, however, not convenient for women for whom coitus is painful on account of pelvic adhesions, low-lying ovaries, or endometriosis in the pouch of Douglas. In such patients coitus with stretched legs is preferable, in order to avoid dyspareunia. Coitus in this position, however, is not conducive to, and actually prevents deep intravaginal ejaculation from occurring. These women should be advised to have intercourse only in the dorsosacral position during the preovulatory phase of the cycle, restricting this position to the moment of ejaculation. It has never been proved that a horizontal position after coitus prolongs the period of time wherein sperm penetration from the seminal pool into the cervical mucus occurs. It has, however, been a longstanding tradition in the medical world to advise an involuntarily infertile women to lie on her back after coitus for a considerable period of time. On theoretical grounds, however, there is no benefit to be gained in maintaining this uncomfortable position for more than half an hour (Kremer 1968).

A woman who wants to achieve a pregnancy is often worried about the reflux of semen out of the vagina occurring directly after intercourse. She usually imagines that she needs the whole ejaculate in order to get pregnant. Postcoital seminal flux is, however, a normal physiological occurrence. After the penis has been withdrawn, the proximal part of the vagina cannot contain more than about 1 ml of semen (Fig. 22.1b). Under normal circumstances this volume is sufficient to buffer the acid ectocervical mucus for the time needed to allow as many spermatozoa as required for a normal chance of conception to enter the cervical canal.

If the volume of the husband's semen is less than 1 ml (hypospermia), the buffer capacity of the seminal plasma is often not enough to raise the ectocervical mucus pH over 6.3, this being the critical level below which spermatozoa quickly lose their motility. A period of abstinence of 5–6 days' duration is in general sufficient to increase the volume of semen to overcome hypospermia. If after an abstinence period of 6 days hypospermia still exists, a precoital alkalizing vaginal irrigation may raise the pH of the ectocervical mucus enough to permit normal postcoital sperm penetration. An alternative method of treatment is artificial insemination.

Other conditions wherein a physiological reflux of the semen out of the vagina after coitus does not occur (besides hypospermia) are *anejaculation* (mostly psychogenic) and *retrograde ejaculation* (organic or psychogenic). Both disorders result in a negative PCT. In anejaculation orgasmic feelings are absent, despite normal erection and normal intravaginal movements of the penis. Men with retrograde ejaculation experience normal orgasm. Psychotherapy in men with anejaculation is seldom successful. Pregnancy, however, can often be achieved by using artificial insemination with an ejaculate which the patient has obtained with the aid of an electrovibrator (Kremer 1977). The inseminations can be performed by the couple (autoinsemination) or by the doctor. It is important to give clear instructions to the couple. The most common cause of failure is that the man does not press the cup of the vibrator (Fig. 22.2) strongly enough on the glans or that he takes away the cup from the glans as soon as he feels the very early contractions of the ejaculation process (probably due to an unconscious fear of ejaculation). Retrograde ejaculation following retroperitoneal lympadenectomy can often successfully be treated with 25–50 mg imipramine per day (Kelly & Needle 1979). We used this treatment in 12 men; in ten of them antegrade ejaculation was restored during treatment and five

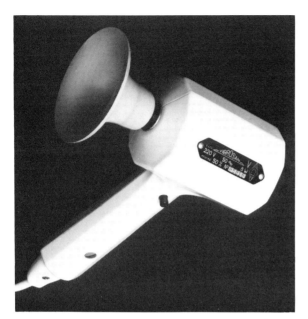

**Fig. 22.2** Electrovibrator to induce the ejaculatory reflex. The rubber cup is placed on the glans penis. The apparatus should be provided with a mechanism to change the vibration frequency.

men impregnated their wives after coitus. Retrograde ejaculation returned after discontinuation of the imipramine treatment (Nijman et al, 1982).

Treatment is difficult if retrograde ejaculation is due to damage of the smooth muscle tissue of the bladder neck and in men with psychogenic retrograde ejaculation. Then, artificial insemination with the retrograde ejaculate is often successful, provided the semen can be collected with a minimum degree of urinary contamination. The best way of collection is masturbation with an empty bladder and thereafter direct voiding of the bladder contents by pressure on the lower abdomen. The first three drops leaving the urethra are suitable for insemination and must be collected in a dry, clean, small bottle. The rest of the ejaculate is contaminated with urine and must be thrown away. The inseminations can be performed by the couple or by the physician (see also Chapter 25). We have performed this method in 12 patients; nine women became pregnant, three of them twice. In one of the men, the (probably psychogenic) retrograde ejaculation resolved spontaneously after the birth of his first child, the pregnancy being achieved by autoinsemination (Kremer, unpublished data).

## TREATMENT OF CERVICAL MUCUS ABNORMALITIES

The treatment of abnormal cervical mucus depends on the cause of this disorder. If the cervical mucus is abundant, thick, yellowish and very cellular during the whole menstrual cycle, then chronic cervicitis may be the cause. In most of the cases the term 'chronic cervicitis' is however, a misnomer, since the poor quality of mucus is usually not due to a chronic inflammatory process (Davajan & Nakamura 1975). The diagnosis cannot be made with a bacteriological culture. Cervical mucus acts as a filter preventing bacteria from entering the uterine cavity and therefore it often contains pathogenic microorganisms. Moderate bacterial or fungal contamination does not affect sperm penetrability of cervical mucus (Insler & Mezkel 1977, Eggert-Kruse et al 1987). The only correct diagnostic method for detecting a chronic cervicitis is a cervical curettage and a histological examination of the material. If this diagnostic method is used the incidence of chronic cervicitis in infertile women proves to be very low. The curettage is also a method of treating chronic cervicitis; it must be combined with a broad-spectrum antibiotic, e.g. doxycycline orally 200 mg per day for 10 days.

Amount, composition and physical properties of the cervical secretions have been proved to be controlled by ovarian steroids (Zondek 1957, Hertzberg et al 1964, Moghissi & Neuhaus 1966, Elstein 1970, Weed & Carrera 1970, Iacobelli et al 1971, Hagenfeldt 1972, Boehr & Moghissi 1973, Masson 1973, Schill & Schumacher 1973, Elstein & Daunter 1973).

An abnormal response of the endocervical epithelium to a normal estrogenic stimulation during the preovulatory period of the cycle is a second cause of abnormal preovulatory cervical mucus. The amount and the properties of the mucus depend on the secretory functions of the epithelial cells. If an abnormally low number of normally secreting epithelial cells are present in the cervical canal or if the secretory capacity of the normal number of secretory epithelial cells in the cervical canal is subnormal, the physicochemical properties of the cervical mucus during the preovulatory phase are normal but the amount of mucus is small (*oligomucorrhea*) and ectocervical mucus for the reception of spermatozoa is often absent. Oligomucorrhea is sometimes combined with a so-called pinhole cervical os. This condition can occur in women exposed to diethylstilbestrol (DES) in utero but the cause is unknown in a majority of the cases. Treatment is not opportune if the result of the PCT is good (Ter Brugge & Kremer 1990).

In cases of dysfunction of the endocervical epithelium the secreted mucus has abnormal properties during the preovulatory period (*dysmucorrhea*). A relatively frequent dysfunction is a too high production of the high viscosity component of the mucus in proportion to the low viscosity component. This results in a normal or large amount of thick but rather clear mucus during the preovulatory phase of the cycle. This material is not a suitable medium for sperm penetration and migration. Estrogen treatment of oligomucorrhea and cervical dysfunction in women with *normal levels of serum estrogens* is not rational and the results are disappointing. If the treatment is started too early in the cycle, ovulation is often delayed and the cycles become irregular. Intrauterine insemination is a more logical approach (see also Chapter 25).

In cases where the oligomucorrhea or the dysmucorrhea is due to the antiestrogenic effect of treatment with clomiphene citrate, the mucus qualities can often be improved if the clomiphene treatment is followed by a high dose of estrogen (Insler & Lunenfeld 1978).

A cause for hostile cervical mucus that is frequently overlooked is an abnormally low pH of the endocervical mucus. Spermatozoa are susceptible to changes in the pH of cervical mucus (Moghissi et al 1964, Moghissi 1966). In normal fertile women the mean pH of the cervical mucus during the periovulatory period is 6.3–7.2 (Kroeks & Kremer 1977). Directly after coitus the pH of the ectocervical and endocervical mucus rises, due to the buffer capacity of the seminal fluid (Kroeks & Kremer 1977, Wolters-Everhardt et al 1980). If the pH of the ectocervical

mucus does not increase beyond the critical value of 6.3, spermatozoa cannot penetrate the mucus because they lose their motility quickly in such an acid environment. If the pH of the endocervical mucus cannot be maintained at a level over 6.3 during a period of at least 24 h, the spermatozoa in the endocervical crypts cannot survive long enough for a normal chance of conception.

If the PCT does not reveal motile spermatozoa during the periovulatory period for at least three cycles and this abnormality is combined with a pH of the endocervical mucus lower than 6.3, as measured with a glass mini-electrode in the cervical canal (Kroeks & Kremer 1977), then precoital alkalizing vaginal irrigation is rational. A suitable irrigation fluid which increases the pH of the preovulatory endocervical mucus within 30 min by 0.5–1.3 and maintains the favourable pH for at least 16 h, is:

| | |
|---|---|
| $Na_2HPO_4 2H_2O$ | 0.144 g |
| $KH_2PO_4$ | 0.025 g |
| NaCl | 0.8 g |
| KCl | 0.02 g |
| $MgSO_4$ | 0.01 g |
| Glucose | 0.2 g |
| Aqua destilata | 100 ml |

The fluid must be kept sterile in order to prevent growth of microorganisms. Approximately half an hour before coitus the fluid must be introduced into the vagina as deep as possible with the woman lying on her back. The horizontal position must be maintained during half an hour. Thereafter the fluid is removed by pressure on the lower abdomen with the patient in an upright position. This removal of fluid prevents dilution of semen in the vagina. Then intercourse occurs and 8–12 h later a PCT is performed. If the treatment was carried out exactly, the pH of the endocervical mucus is generally within the normal range and progressively motile spermatozoa are present. The treatment must be continued for at least six cycles, two to three times per cycle during the preovulatory period. If the complete fertility investigation of husband and wife does not reveal other abnormalities, pregnancy occurs in 50% of the cases (Kremer, unpublished data).

In a relatively large number of cases treatment

of cervical mucus abnormalities does not result in the presence of normal preovulatory cervical mucus and in a good result of the PCT after coitus. Intrauterine insemination is then the method of choice, provided the semen contains a sufficient number of spermatozoa with good forward motility (Te Velde et al 1989). The results are, however, generally no more than 25% pregnancies during a period of one to six insemination cycles.

## TREATMENT OF IMMUNOLOGICAL INFERTILITY IN WOMEN

Until now the significance of antispermatozoal antibodies (ASAs) in the serum of women in respect to their fertility has been doubtful and the results of treatment are unconvincing. In recent years it has been realized that sperm antibodies in cervical mucus may bear a more precise relationship to female infertility (Centaro 1973, Soffer et al 1976, Sudo et al 1977, Cantuaria 1977, Wong 1978, Dor et al 1979, Moghissi et al 1980, Ingerslev 1980, De Almeida et al 1981, Nicotra et al 1982, Cerasaro et al 1982; Chapter 13).

Progressively moving spermatozoa in the semen change their movements into local shaking movements directly after contact with the cervical mucus if agglutinating antisperm antibodies are present in the cervical mucus. This 'shaking phenomenon' can be measured quantitatively with the SCMC test (sperm–cervical mucus contact test) described by Kremer & Jager in 1976. Table 22.1 clearly demonstrates the effect of sperm agglutinins in cervical mucus on in vitro sperm penetration. Sperm immobilizing antibodies in cervical mucus, mentioned by some investigators (Soffer et al 1979, Cantuaria 1977, Wong 1978, Dor et al 1979, Moghissi et al 1980) as a cause of a poor PCT, probably seldom occur (Jager et al 1983). Moreover, these antibodies have no significance for sperm migration in cervical mucus because they need complement to become active. Complement is not present in cervical mucus during the preovulatory period (Schumacher 1980). The significance of antispermatozoal antibodies in the serum in relation to the fertility of women is uncertain, whereas it is known that the presence of antispermatozoal antibodies in cervical mucus strongly reduces female fertility. For this reason, only the treatment of infertile women with sperm agglutinating antibodies in the cervical mucus (resulting in a strongly positive shaking phenomenon in the SCMC test) will be discussed in this chapter.

### Treatment with intrauterine insemination

The five women detailed in Table 22.1 were treated with intrauterine inseminations with 0.2 ml of the first part of a split ejaculate of the husband (Kremer 1979).

Mrs B became pregnant during the fourth

**Table 22.1** Comparison between the results of the SPM test in women with and donors without sperm agglutinins in cervical mucus. The husband of each woman had normospermia

| Couple | Sperm agglutination titer* in cervical mucus | % locally shaking sperm in SCMC test | Penetration in cervical mucus | | | | | |
|--------|-----|-----|-----|-----|-----|-----|-----|-----|
| | | | Of wife | | | Of donor | | |
| | | | Penetration (cm) depth | No. of sperm per LPF | Motility grade† | Penetration (cm) depth | No. of sperm per LPF | Motility grade† |
| A | 64 H-H | 80 | 3 | 0–5 | 1- | 5 | 20–50 | 2+ |
| B | 4069 H-H | >80 | 3 | 0–1 | 1 | 5 | 100–200 | 1+ |
| P | 512 H-H | >90 | 5 | 0–1 | 1 | 5 | 100–200 | 2 |
| S | 128 H-H | 100 | 5 | 0–1 | <1 | 5 | 200 | 2+ |
| Z | 4069 H-H | >80 | 3 | 0–1 | 1 | 5 | 100–200 | 2+ |

In all the women the sperm antibodies in the cervical mucus belonged to the IgA class.
SPM, sperm penetration meter (Kremer 1968); H-H, head to head agglutination
*, The cervical mucus was liquified with bromelin.
†1, Slowly progressive; 2, moderately progressive; 3, quickly progressive.

insemination cycle and did not abort despite a considerable rise of the sperm agglutination titer in the serum (from 64 to 512) during the first trimester of her pregnancy. She delivered a healthy child. After this successful treatment, we performed intrauterine inseminations in another group of six women. As in the first group the sperm antibodies in the cervical mucus in this group belonged to the IgA class and caused head-to-head agglutination. The in vitro and in vivo sperm penetration in cervical mucus was negative or poor and the percentage of shaking spermatozoa in the SCMC test was at least 75. One of the women became pregnant during the insemination cycles. One spontaneous pregnancy occurred in the 11 women during a follow-up period of 3–7 years. Mrs B (Table 22.1) did not achieve a second pregnancy via intrauterine inseminations (nine insemination cycles).

The intrauterine inseminations increased the sperm agglutination titer by at least three titer steps in the serum of the women who already had ASAs in the serum and in the cervical mucus before treatment (booster effect). Intrauterine inseminations did not elicit antispermatozoal antibodies in women where the sperm agglutination titer in serum and in cervical mucus was negative before the treatment (Kremer et al 1978).

## Occlusion therapy

Occlusion therapy (the male partner using a condom for 6–9 months) was apparently first proposed by Franklin & Dukes (1964). It was supposed that if the semen does not come into contact with the tissue of the female genital tract for an extended period of time, the woman's ASA level will subside. The first unprotected intercourse must be timed to occur with the ovulation period, so that fertilization can be expected to happen more quickly than a booster antigenic stimulation. Franklin & Dukes stated that 'antibody titers declined markedly' in a group of women so treated; however, they did not provide any actual titers, as they did not describe any titer for any of their cases in general. Moreover, they only determined the presence of ASAs in serum and not in cervical mucus. A review of the results

of occlusion therapy (Jones 1976) indicates that they compare unfavorably with the outcome in patients with circulating ASAs who remain untreated. A more rational selection of patients for condom therapy on the basis of local immunity demonstrable in the cervical mucus did not lead to better results in a small series of patients (Kremer et al 1978).

## Immunosuppression

Immunosuppression therapy with corticosteroids has been attempted and has led to case reports of decreased ASA titers and the occurrence of pregnancies. We used immunosuppressive therapy in two women with ASAs in the serum and in the cervical mucus. The result of the in vivo and in vitro sperm penetration tests was bad and the shaking phenomenon level in the SCMC test was at least 80%. The period of unvoluntary infertility was of more than 3 years' duration (Mrs Z and Mrs A of Table 22.1). They were treated with 96 mg methylprednisolone daily for 7 days (Kremer et al 1978). No change in the antibody titer in serum and in cervical mucus and no significant influence on the shaking phenomenon in the SCMC test could be demonstrated.

It is possible that a better result would be obtained if the high-dose corticosteroid treatment was given for the 7 days preceding ovulation. This regimen has been used in men with some success (Hendry et al 1981). The occasional severe side-effects and the risks of the high-dose corticosteroid treatment are reason enough to doubt whether it is justifiable to use this treatment for a disorder that is not life-threatening.

## TREATMENT OF IMMUNOLOGICAL INFERTILITY IN MEN

ASAs of the IgA class on the spermatozoa in the ejaculate can cause a severe disturbance in the sperm–cervical mucus interaction (Kremer & Jager 1980). This results in an inhibition of sperm penetration in cervical mucus in vivo and in vitro. The PCT is usually negative or poor despite normal physicochemical properties of the preovulatory cervical mucus and normal concentration and motility of the spermatozoa in the ejaculate (Kremer et al 1978).

Three methods of treatment are described.

## Immunosuppression

The aim of the treatment is to decrease the ASA production. Up until now only corticosteroids are used for this purpose. There are two types of corticosteroid treatment:

1. Intermittent courses of 1 week, each with a very high dosage scheme.
2. One course of 2–3 months with an intermediate dose of corticosteroids.

The largest and best documented series of men treated with intermittent high-dose corticosteroids is that published by Hendry et al (1981). Forty-five men were treated. They used 96 mg methylprednisolone for 7 days during the last week of their wives' menstrual cycles for three alternate cycles; 14 women (31%) became pregnant. There was a positive correlation between the decrease of the ASA titer and the occurrence of pregnancy. Thirty-two per cent of the men had transient side-effects, sometimes rather severe.

We prescribed this treatment to five men. A decrease of the sperm agglutination titer in the seminal plasma and a decrease of the shaking phenomenon in the SCMC test were considered to be relevant for the effect of the treatment. Table 22.2 demonstrates that a one to two titer step decrease of the sperm agglutination titer occurred in three men and a decrease of the shaking phenomenon occurred in four men. One couple achieved a pregnancy. Two of the five men treated complained of Cushing-like side-effects but were able to continue their daily work. Afterwards we treated a group of six men in the same way. No pregnancy occurred and one man got severe pain in his hip joints. Treatment was discontinued and we did not treat another group because of the risks as well as the poor results in terms of pregnancies.

The favourable effect of prednisolone could also not be confirmed by De Almeida et al (1985), and later on not by Haas & Manganiello (1987) as

**Table 22.2**  Results of treatment with 96 mg methylprednisolone for 7 days in five men with ASA

| Time of investigation | Sperm agglutination titer in seminal plasma | | | | | Shaking phenomenon in SCMC+ test | | | | |
|---|---|---|---|---|---|---|---|---|---|---|
| | E | H | J | K | L | E | H | J | K* | L |
| Before treatment | 64 | 16 | 4 | 32 | 8 | 3+ | 3+ | 3+ | 3+ | 3+ |
| 2 weeks after 1st course | 16 | 8 | 4 | 32 | 8 | | | | | |
| 2 weeks after 2nd course | 8 | 4 | <4 | 16 | 4 | | | | | |
| 2 weeks after 3rd course | 16 | 4 | <4 | 32 | 8 | 2+ | 2+ | – | 2+ | 3+ |

* Mr K's wife became pregnant during the first cycle after the 3rd course of her husband's treatment.

well. Both studies were placebo controlled and concerned a 3-month long treatment course. In 1990, however, Hendry et al reported a favorable effect of an intermediate high dose of soluble prednisolone for 9 months, during the first 12 days of the spouse's cycle. This study was also placebo controlled.

## Intrauterine insemination

Intrauterine insemination with the semen of the husband (see Chapter 25) is a logical approach to overcome the disturbed sperm–cervical mucus interaction (Kremer 1979). Until 1 July 1982 we treated 33 infertile couples with a negative or poor PCT and ASAs on the spermatozoa. Eight women achieved a pregnancy (Table 22.3). The husbands of the pregnant women had a sperm concentration of at least 10 million/ml and at least 40% of the spermatozoa had a quick forward motility. The semen qualities were generally poor in the 25 husbands whose wives did not achieve a pregnancy by intrauterine insemination. We have

**Table 22.3**  Result of insemination treatment of infertility due to ASA in the man

| | | |
|---|---|---|
| Women treated by IUI* (no.) | 33 | |
| Women pregnant during an IUI cycle (no.) | 8 | (24%) |
| Women treated with AID after unsuccessful IUI | 12 | |
| Women pregnant during an AID cycle | 9 | (75%) |

*Intrauterine insemination.

therefore restricted intrauterine inseminations to couples where the husband has normospermia in terms of sperm concentration and motility. This could be confirmed by other investigators (Te Velde et al 1989).

## Artificial insemination by donor (AID)

This treatment should be suggested to the couple when the presence of ASAs of the IgA class on the spermatozoa in the ejaculate is combined with severe oligoasthenozoospermia. AID should also be suggested to the couple if treatment with corticosteroids or intrauterine insemination has been unsuccessful. The chance of achieving pregnancy by AID is then high (Table 22.3). It is important for the couples not to have intercourse during the period of insemination because the ASAs in the husband's seminal plasma might get attached to the cervical mucus and inhibit the penetration of donor spermatozoa (Quinlivan & Sullivan 1977).

REFERENCES

Boehr S A, Moghissi K S 1973 Human and bovine cervical mucus. In: Blandau R J, Moghissi K S(eds) The biology of the cervix. University of Chicago Press, Chicago, p 125

Cantuaria A A 1977 Sperm immobilizing antibodies in the serum and cervico-vaginal secretions of infertile and normal women. Br J Obstet Gynaecol 65: 84

Centaro A 1973 The relationship between agglutinating and immobilizing antibodies and sterility. In: Bratanov K, Edwards R G, Vulchanov V H, Dokov V, Somlev B (eds) Immunology of reproduction. Bulgarian Academy of Sciences Press, p 369

Cerasaro M, Nicotra M, Coghi I M, Stampone L, Amodei M, Dondero F 1982 Detection of antispermatozoal isoantibodies in cervical mucus from infertile and fertile women using the Shulman–Hekman capillary test. In: Shulman S, Dondero F, Nicotra M (eds) Immunological factors in human reproduction. Academic, London p 51

Davajan V, Nakamura R M 1975 The cervical factor. In: Behrman S J, Kistner R W (eds) Progress in infertility. Little, Brown and Company, Boston p 19

De Almeida M, Feneux D, Rigaud C, Jouannert P 1985 Steroid therapy for male infertility associated with antisperm antibodies. Results of a small randomized clinical trial. Int J Androl 8: 111

Dor J, Nebel L A, Soffer Y, Maschiach S, Serr D M 1979 Cell mediated and local immunity to spermatozoa in infertility. Int J Fertil 24: 94

Eggert -Kruse W, Gerhard I, Hofmann H, Runnebaum B, Petzholdt D 1987 Influence of microbial colonization on sperm–mucus interaction in vivo and in vitro. Hum Reprod 2: 301

Elstein M 1970 The proteins of cervical mucus and the influence of progestagens. J Obstet Gynaecol Br Cwlth 77: 1443

Elstein M, Daunter B 1973 Trace elements in cervical mucus. In: Elstein M, Moghissi K S, Borth R (eds) Cervical mucus in human reproduction. Scriptor, Copenhagen, p 122

Franklin R R, Dukes C D 1964 Antispermatozoal antibody and unexplained infertility. Am J Obstet Gynecol 89: 6

Haas G G, Manganiello P 1987 A double blind, placebo controlled study of the use of methylprednisolone in infertile men with sperm-associated immunoglobulins. Fertil Steril 47: 295

Hagenfeldt K 1972 Copper and zinc levels in endometrium, cervical mucus and plasma in women using the copper-T device for intrauterine contraception. In: Hasegawa T,

Hayashi M, Ebling F J, Henderson I W (eds) Fertility and sterility. Excerpta Medica, Amsterdam, p 115

Hendry W F, Stedronska J, Parslow J, Hughes L 1981 The results of intermittent high dose steroid therapy for male infertility due to antisperm antibodies. Fertil Steril 36: 4

Hendry W F, Hughes L, Scammell G, Prior J P, Hargreave T B 1990 Comparison of prednisolone and placebo in subfertile men with antibodies to spermatozoa. Lancet 335: 85

Hertzberg M, Joel C A, Katchalsky A 1964 The cyclic variation of sodium choloride content in the mucus of the cervixuteri. Fertil Steril 15: 684

Iacobelli S, Garcea N, Angeloni C 1971 Biochemistry of cervical mucus; a comparative analysis of the secretion from preovulatory, postovulatory and pregnancy periods. Fertil Steril 22: 727

Ingerslev H J 1980 Sperm agglutinating antibodies and sperm penetration of cervical mucus from infertile women with sperm-agglutinating antibodies in serum. Fertil Steril 34: 561

Insler V, Lunenfeld B 1978 Anovulation. In: Keller J P (ed) Contributions to gynecology and obstetrics, vol IV, Female Infertility. Karger, Basel

Insler V, Mezkel A 1977 The effect of bacterial and fungal contamination of the cervical mucus on sperm penetrability. In: Ludwig H, Tauber P (eds) Human fertilization p 96

Insler V, Bernstein D, Glezerman M 1977 Diagnosis and classification of the cervical factor in infertility. In: Insler V, Bettendorf G (eds) The uterine cervix in reproduction. Georg Thieme, Stuttgart p 253

Jager S, Kremer J, Wilde de-Jansen I W 1983 Are sperm immobilizing antibodies in cervical mucus an explanation for a poor post coital test? AJRI 5: 56

Jones W R 1976 Immunological aspects of infertility. In: Scott J S, Jones W R (eds) Immunology of human reproduction. Academic, London, p 374

Kelly M E, Needle M A 1979 Imipramine for aspermia after lymphadenectomy. Urology, 13: 414

Kremer J 1968 The in vitro spermatozoal penetration test in fertility investigations. Thesis, Groningen, The Netherlands, p 73

Kremer J 1977 Infertility: male and female. In: Money J, Musaph H (eds) Handbook of sexology. Excerpta Medica, Amsterdam, p 679

Kremer J 1979 A new technique for intrauterine insemination. Int J Fertil 24: 53

Kremer J, Jager S 1976 The sperm-cervical mucus contact test: a preliminary report. Fertil Steril 27: 335

Kremer J, Jager S 1980 Characteristics of anti-spermatozoal antibodies responsible for the shaking phenomenon with special regard to immunoglobulin class and antigen-reactive sites. Int J Androl 3: 143

Kremer J, Jager S, Kuiken J, Van Slochtern-Draaisma T 1978 Recent advances in diagnosis and treatment of infertility due to antisperm antibodies. In: Cohen J, Hendry W F (eds) Spermatozoa antibodies and infertility. Blackwell Scientific Publications, Oxford, p 117

Kroeks M V A M, Kremer J 1977 The pH in the lower third of the genital tract. In: Insler V, Bettendorf G (eds) The uterine cervix in reproduction. Georg Thieme, Stuttgart, p 109

Masson P L 1973 Carbohydrate component of cervical mucus. In: Elstein M, Moghissi K S, Borth R (eds) Cervical mucus in human reproduction. Scriptor, Copenhagen, p 82

Moghissi K S 1966 Cyclic changes of cervical mucus in normal and progestin treated women. Fertil Steril 17: 663

Moghissi K S, Dabich D, Levine J, Neuhaus O W 1964 Mechanism of sperm migration. Fertil Steril 15: 15

Moghissi K S, Neuhaus O W 1966 Cyclic changes of cervical mucus proteins. Am J Obstet Gynecol 96: 91

Moghissi K S, Sacco A G, Borin K 1980 Immunologic infertility. I. Cervical mucus antibodies and post coital test. Am J Obstet Gynecol 136: 941

Nicotra M, Dondero F, Coghi I M 1982 Follow-up studies in infertile women with antisperm iso-antibodies. In: Shulman S, Dondero F, Nicotra M (eds) Immunological factors in human reproduction. Academic, London p 37

Nijman J M, Jager S, Boer P W, Kremer J, Oldhoff J, Schrafford Koops H 1982 The treatment of ejaculation disorders after retroperitoneal lymphnode dissection. Cancer 50: 2967

Quinlivan W L G, Sullivan H 1978 Spermatozoa antibodies in human seminal plasma as a cause of failed artificial donor insemination. Fertil Steril 28: 1082

Schill W B, Schumacher G F B 1973 Micro radial diffusion in gel methods for the quantitative assessment of soluble proteins in genital secretions. In: Blandau R J, Moghissi K S (eds) The biology of the cervix. University of Chicago Press, Chicago, p 173

Schumacher G F B 1980 Humoral immune factors in the female reproductive tract and their changes during the cycle. In: Dhindsa D S, Schumacher G F B (eds) Immunological aspects of infertility and fertility regulation. Elsevier, North Holland p 93

Soffer Y, Marcus Z H, Bukovsky I, Caspi E 1976 The cervical factor in fertility: diagnosis and treatment. Int J Fertil 21: 89

Sudo N, Shulman S, Stone M L 1977 Antibodies to spermatozoa. IX. Spermagglutination phenomenon in cervical mucus in vitro: a possible cause of infertility. Am J Obstet Gynecol 129: 360

ter Brugge H G, Kremer J 1990 The pin-hole cervical os; a small fertility problem. Eur J Obstet, Gynaecol Reprod Biol 37:247

te Velde E R, Kooy van J H, Waterreus J J H 1989 Intra-uterine insemination of washed husband's spermatozoa: a controlled study. Fertil Steril 51: 182

Weed J C, Carrera A E 1970 Glucose contents in cervical mucus. Fertil Steril 21: 866

Wolters-Everhardt E, Dony J M J, Lemmers W A J G, Doesburg W H, De Pont J J H A M 1986 Buffering capacity of human semen. Fertil Steril 46: 114

Wong W P 1978 Sperm antibodies in the cervical mucus and sera and postcoital tests in infertile women. Eur J Obstet Gynecol Reprod Biol 8: 363

Zondek B 1957 Cervical mucus arborization as an aid in diagnosis. In: Meigs J V, Sturgis S H (eds) Progress in gynecology. Grune and Stratton, New York, p 86

# 23. Medical treatment of male infertility

*W–B Schill    G. Haidl*

## INTRODUCTION

In this chapter the different treatment approaches using pharmacological compounds to improve male fertility will be discussed in detail. The rationale of some of these therapies is based on a logical appreciation of normal physiology e.g. stimulation of testicular function by antiestrogens in an attempt to stimulate pituitary secretion, direct stimulation of the gonads by gonado-tropins, or inhibition of interfering substances. Other therapies may have less valid rationales and are empirically based.

The main problem in the majority of infertility cases is that the cause of reduced fertility is unknown and consequently no specific therapy is available. Hence, basic to the search for effective therapies is the need for a better understanding of the pathophysiology of male infertility. If we know more about the fundamental causes of poor semen formation and function, the development of an effective therapy will become easier.

There is another major problem concerning the objective assessment of the treatment response in the subjects, which is very important for the evaluation of the therapeutic value of a particular form of medical treatment. Several factors contribute to make this a difficult task. The main factor is the great biological variation of the semen parameters that may occur within one individual. Endogenous and exogenous factors like acute illnesses such as viral infections, other specific disease entities, e.g. thyroid dysfunction or hyper-prolactinemia, possible noxious influences to which the patient may be exposed, e.g. heavy smoking, excessive amount of alcohol, work with pesticides or other chemicals or pollutants, side-effects of other drug treatment (e.g. salazosul-fapyridine for the treatment of ulcerative colitis) and particularly emotional and psychological stress, may all influence sperm production and quality.

It is therefore mandatory that the patient selected for treatment should first undergo a careful clinical evaluation including a thorough medical history, physical examination and a complete laboratory workup (Bain & Hafez 1980, Lunenfeld & Glezerman 1981, Hargreave 1983).

Thus, therapy should not be initiated before the above-mentioned exogenous and endogenous factors are excluded, removed or treated appro-priately.

It should be kept in mind that all therapeutic agents stimulating spermatogenesis should be applied for at least 3 months before a significant improvement of sperm count can be expected, due to the fact that spermatogenesis in men takes 74 days from basal stem cells to spermiation and approximately 10–14 days for epididymal passage (Heller & Clermont 1964).

## THEORETICAL BASIS OF TREATMENT

The aim of medical therapy in infertile men is the improvement or normalization of the fertility status of the subfertile individuals in order to increase the chance of a pregnancy within a defined period of time. One leading hypothesis is that by improvement of reduced semen par-ameters (sperm motility, morphology, number) a measurable improvement of the conception chance will be possible. However, in reality, amelioration of semen quality will not always correlate with an increased conception chance, and vice versa. On the other hand, a correlation between sperm penetration in cervical mucus and conception index has been established (Ulstein 1973).

Another important factor is the time required for pregnancy to occur independent of whether or not treatment of the infertile male has been performed. Many pregnancies occur while the patient is on the waiting list to see the doctor. This stresses the great influence of emotional and psychological factors within the interrelationships of a couple. The willingness of the husband to see the andrologist will sometimes help to relax tensions within a disturbed partner relationship of an infertile couple and may result in a spontaneous pregnancy.

Regarding medical therapy of male fertility disturbances one has to distinguish between specific and empirical treatment procedures. Specific treatment is based on a pathophysiological concept and implies accurate patient selection. Predictability of the treatment success is valid. In contrast, empirical treatment involves no patient selection according to specific criteria. Since no selection criteria are given and predictability of results is not assessed, treatment is performed on an empirical basis regardless of whether the mechanism of action of the drug used is hypothetical, partially known, or well established. This is the reason why the response of each patient towards the available pharmacological compounds has to be tested individually.

The different treatment approaches within the specific and empirical forms of therapy are summarized in Table 23.1 according to their mode of action.

### Specific treatment of selected patients

*Replacement therapy* in cases of hormone deficiency is a classical form of specific endocrine treatment with a high rate of predictability concerning restoration and maintenance of fertility. This treatment is employed in congenital (e.g. Kallmann's syndrome, fertile eunuch syndrome) and acquired disorders (tumors, inflammation, trauma).

For hormone substitution generally human gonadotropins are used, but in particular cases also gonadotropin-releasing hormone (GnRH) or its analogs may be applied.

Another therapeutic approach based on a well-defined principle is the *inhibition of an increased prolactin secretion*. To treat hyperprolactinemia bromocriptine is successfully applied (see Chapter 17).

In cases of acute or chronic male genital tract inflammations, a combined *antimicrobial-antiinflammatory treatment* is necessary with antibiotics and antiphlogistics.

If there is evidence of the presence of sperm autoantibodies causing immunological infertility, administration of *immunosuppressive substances*, e.g. corticosteroids or azathioprine, is considered

**Table 23.1**   Specific and empirical forms of medical treatment of male fertility disturbances

1. Specific treatment of selected patients:
    Replacement therapy (hMG/hCG, GnRH)
    Inhibition of prolactin secretion (bromocriptine)
    Antiinflammatory therapy (antibiotics, antiphlogistics)
    Immunosuppressive therapy (glucocorticosteroids, azathioprine)
    Improvement of emission and ejaculation (α-sympathomimetics, anticholinergics)
2. Empirically based therapies:
    Stimulation therapy (with enhancement of physiological hormone levels)
        Antiestrogens (clomiphene, tamoxifen)
        Human gonadotropins (hMG/hCG)
        Androgens (testosterone, mesterolone, testolactone)
    Rebound therapy (testosterone)
    Increased levels of tissue hormones (kallikrein, captopril)
    Improvement of testicular blood microcirculation (pentoxifylline)
    Mast cell block age (ketotifen)
    Immunomodulatory therapy, replacement of zinc deficiency (zinc)
    Antioxidative therapy (vitamin E)
    Improvement of psycho-vegetative functions (psychotropic drugs, spasmolytic agents)

another form of specific therapy (see also Chapters 13 and 22).

Finally, disturbances of semen emission and ejaculation, e.g. retrograde ejaculation after abdominal surgery or in the course of diabetic neuropathy, are specifically treated by *sympathomimetic* or *anticholinergic drugs* in order to increase the sympathetic tone or decrease the parasympathic activity of the bladder neck muscles (Collins 1982).

## Empirically based therapies

The main premise of empirical treatment is that in infertile males with an intact hypothalamic-pituitary-gonadal axis and a normal gonadotropic stimulation of the testes, further enhancement of the spermatogenic function is possible by additional stimulation of the endogenous secretion of gonadotropins, increasing the intratesticular testosterone concentration. This *stimulation therapy* is more or less successfully practised with antiestrogens and human gonadotropins, but is also feasible using GnRH, androgens, and recently also aromatase inhibitors. The stimulation therapy is based on the assumption that there may exist a relative disproportion between the levels of certain hormones and their target cells. An increase of the sex hormone level could therefore lead to improved function of the seminiferous epithelium with a further stimulation of spermatogenesis.

Stimulation therapy is based upon recent knowledge that both follicle stimulating hormone (FSH) and testosterone participate in regulation of spermatogenesis. The target cell of both hormones is the Sertoli cell. However, testosterone seems to be the most important spermatogenic hormone, since for initiation and maintenance of spermatogenesis extremely high intratesticular testosterone concentrations are necessary, being a hundredfold higher than the peripheral plasma testosterone level (Steinberger et al 1974). The role of FSH remains unclear, but it is necessary to complete spermatogenesis. Investigations by Steinberger (1981) demonstrate a significant correlation between testosterone production in vitro, the number of Leydig cells and the number of early spermatids. In contrast, there was no correlation between testosterone production and the number of spermatogonia and spermatocytes. This suggests a relationship between the capacity of the testes to synthesize testosterone and the ability of the germ cells to complete meiotic division. Thus, it seems that testosterone is essential for completion of the meiotic division. This is confirmed by demonstration of a statistically significant direct correlation between the sperm count and in vitro testosterone production. However, according to Steinberger (1981), the modulating influence of other hormones (e.g. FSH, prolactin, estrogen, inhibin, etc.) on spermatogenesis in an in vivo homeostatic state cannot be ruled out.

Another therapeutical principle uses the *rebound phenomenon*, well known since 1950 when Heller and coworkers applied high androgen doses to oligozoospermic men. This treatment leads to a suppression of gonadotropin secretion followed by suppression of spermatogenesis with azoospermia due to an atrophy of the germinal epithelium. After discontinuation of testosterone administration, depressed spermatogenesis recovers, sometimes leading to a substantial improvement of sperm count to higher than pretreatment levels. The reason for this rebound of spermatogenesis is still obscure. However, the biological principle of the rebound phenomenon seems to be a nonspecific reaction.

Another therapeutic approach is based on the principle of *liberation of tissue hormones* from precursor molecules of the kallikrein–kinin system (Geiger 1981) by limited proteolysis through systemic administration of the pancreatic proteinase kallikrein (Fig.23.1). These precursors are high and low molecular weight kininogens found in the blood plasma and different body and tissue fluids. The biologically active substances are kinins released by kallikreins or kininogenases from ubiquitous kininogen. Kinins have been shown to be involved in the proliferation of various tissues (summarized by Haberland et al 1975a, b, 1977, Haberland & Rohen 1973). Clinical and animal studies have also indicated possible interference of the kallikrein–kinin system with the spermatogenic functions of the testis (summarized in Haberland et al 1977, Haberland & Rohen 1981, Schill et al 1989). This

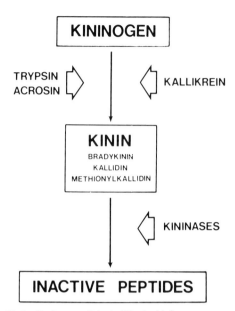

**Fig. 23.1**  Pathways of the kallikrein–kinin system.

concept is also supported by clinical studies aiming at an inhibition of kinin degradation by blocking angiotensin-converting enzyme (ACE) with captopril (Parsch & Schill 1988). ACE is the key regulatory enzyme of the renin–angiotensin system and the kallikrein–kinin system and is the predominant kinin inactivating enzyme found in highest concentrations within the male genital tract, particularly in the prostate and epididymis. Inhibition of ACE activity by captopril treatment leads to a significant increase in the number of spermatozoa. In addition, components of the kallikrein–kinin system apparently participate, in conjunction with other factors, in the stimulation and regulation of sperm motility (Schill et al 1974, 1976, Schill 1982a). The hypothetical mode of action whereby kallikrein and kinins stimulate spermatogenesis and sperm metabolism at the cellular level are (summarized by Schill 1982a): activation of Sertoli cell function, increase of ³H-labelled thymidine incorporation into the DNA of testicular tissue, enhancement of glucose uptake due to an increase in membrane permeability, increase of testicular blood flow, and an acceleration of glucose and fructose transport across the sperm cell membranes enhancing sperm metabolism and sperm motility. In addition, improvement of the secretory activity

of the sex glands and even a small influence on the hormonal balance of the pituitary–gonadal axis has been discussed as possibly leading to an increased intratesticular testosterone level. Locally increased testosterone levels might favor epididymal sperm maturation with an improvement in sperm viability and sperm motility. However, besides the observed small increase of the strictly target-cell-oriented sex hormones, the local action of kinins as biologically active tissue hormones involved in cell proliferation of various tissues must be considered to be primarily responsible for the observed spermatogenic effects.

*Improvement of testicular blood microcirculation* is another empirical therapeutic approach. As suggested by Heite & Koschnicke (1979), amelioration of a possibly disturbed blood circulation in the testes and epididymes may improve the nutritive situation and increase the response of the testes to androgen stimuli. An increase of the testicular circulation and metabolism feasible by influencing the flow properties of erythrocytes with pentoxifylline, a methylxanthine derivative which shows phosphodiesterase inhibitory activity such as caffeine and theophylline. This substance also improves sperm motility in vitro (Aparicio & coworkers 1980a) by increasing the intracellular cAMP level through inhibition of phosphodiesterase activity.

In *inflammatory testicular disorders* the increased occurrence of *mast cells* in close proximity to the seminiferous tubules has been described. This indicates that therapy with the mast cell blocker ketotifen may have positive effects in such cases (Behrendt et al 1981).

Further therapeutic approaches include the administration of *trace elements* and *vitamins*. Zinc, for example, which is found in high concentrations in the testes and accessory sexual glands, is thought to play an important role in human reproduction (Srivastava et al 1983).

The antioxidative effect of *vitamin E* is supposed to protect spermatozoa from damage by peroxidation of endogenous phospholipides and, thus, to improve the motility of spermatozoa (Engel et al 1985)

The use of psychotropic and spasmolytic agents may be considered as a kind of *supportive therapy*. Occasionally, these agents improve the emission phase of the ejaculatory process due to a better voiding of the semen reservoir in the epididymis. In addition, a positive influence on smooth muscle contractions of the vas deferens and the accessory sex glands cannot be excluded. Particularly, this class of agents may be beneficial in patients with disorders at the level of the autonomic nervous system caused by emotional stress (Hornstein 1971, Kockott 1982).

## SELECTION OF PATIENTS

Clinical and laboratory investigations allow the exclusion of patients with irreversible infertility, e.g. chromosomal aberrations or depopulation of the germinal epithelium. Another group of patients must primarily undergo surgery, e.g. varicocele, epididymovasostomy, or rarely implantation of an alloplastic spermatocele (see Chapter 24). A relatively new method is the collection of epididymal spermatozoa by SMART (sperm microaspiration retrieval technique). The rest of the patients will be subjected to some form of medical treatment discussed in this chapter. In addition, in special cases improvement of semen quality by in vitro methods has to be considered for the purpose of instrumental insemination (see Chapter 26). Future research will also determine the role of in vitro fertilization and embryo transfer (IVF-ET) within the treatment schedule of male fertility disturbances (see Chapter 21). Since semen analysis shows only nonspecific indications of different etiopathological diseases, the basis for diagnosis and treatment should also include endocrinological evaluation of the patient. Using radioimmunological methods it is thus possible to classify the patients into one of the following groups:

1. Primary testicular failure with elevated gonadotropin levels, particularly of FSH. Pharmacological treatment in these patients is unsuccessful. In some cases improvement of semen quality may be possible using the split ejaculate technique, swim-up procedures or sperm motility stimulating substances like pancreatic kallikrein, caffeine or pentoxifylline.

2. Secondary testicular failure with gonadotropin deficiency, which comprises 1% of our patients. In this group gonadotropin replacement therapy is successful. Some authors also include patients with relative hypogonadotropic normogonadism, who represent about 5–10% of the oligozoospermic patients and are claimed to have an FSH deficiency (Glezerman & Lunenfeld 1976).

3. Normogonadotropic men with different andrological disturbances such as occlusion, varicocele, retrograde ejaculation, acute and chronic male genital tract infections, other functional disorders of the male accessory sex glands, disturbances of sperm storage and sperm maturation in the epididymis, and idiopathic forms of oligozoospermia. The latter group most probably comprises fertility disturbances of different etiology, however, with a negative medical history, no varicocele, no signs of male genital tract inflammation, and a normal size and consistency of the testes and epididymes. In these patients the results of pharmacological treatment are fair, but rather difficult to predict.

As already mentioned, semen quality is an equivocal selection criterion for treatment. To use it, reproducibility of pathological semen values within a time period of 3–6 months is necessary, suggesting that the observed pathological parameters are not accidental, but represent a pathological condition.

*Azoospermia* necessitates differentiation between occlusion of the efferent duct system, primary or secondary testicular failure, or complete spermatogenic maturation arrest. In *oligozoospermia* FSH determination will allow differentiation between severe tubular failure or other forms of normogonadotropic oligozoospermia. In *asthenozoospermia* a series of possible etiological factors must be excluded (heat, varicocele, inflammation, inherent sperm defects — especially those of the flagella — epididymal dysfunction which can be demonstrated by abnormal staining behavior of the flagella (Haidl et al 1991), drugs, toxins, sperm antibodies, artifacts, epididymal dysfunction, relative androgen deficiency, viscosipathy, dysfunctions of prostate and seminal vesicles). If *teratozoospermia* is diagnosed, exogenous toxins should be excluded. In some men hereditary diseases will be the cause of teratozoospermia, like globozoospermia or decapitated sperm syndrome. Apart from severe acrosomal disturbances, the causes of *polyzoospermia* are still unknown; therefore, further investigations are necessary while empirical therapeutic studies appear less reasonable.

In order to make the selection of patients for treatment more logical and less empirical and to improve the possibility of a more precise localization of the lesion responsible for male infertility, Lunenfeld & Glezerman (1977) have provided algorithmic schemes to classify infertile men into diagnostic groups depending on the etiology and on the location of the disturbance (see Chapter 11). These algorithmic schemes enable assignment of an appropriate management for each diagnostic group, and selection of the most suitable fertility promoting agent for those men classified as susceptible to treatment. An experienced physician will be able to use 'short-cuts', to shift centers of gravity, and to add relevant extensions to the proposed schemes.

## PHARMACOLOGICAL AGENTS, TREATMENT SCHEMES AND RESULTS

For treatment of the different male fertility disorders various pharmacological agents have been suggested. Some of the 'older' compounds in the meantime were found ineffective and showed simply placebo effects. These compounds are vitamins A and D, arginine and triiodothyronine. Recently, however, attention has been drawn to beneficial effects of vitamin E as an antioxidant that may prevent spermatozoa from damage by free oxygen radicals (Engel et al 1985, Aitken & Clarkson 1988, Hofmann 1988). Triiodothyronine will also not work unless thyroid insufficiency can be proven and even then thyroid treatment may not improve spermatogenesis.

In this paragraph only those modes of therapy will be considered that appear rational and that have been subjected to at least some scientific critique. The pharmacological agents will be subdivided into substance classes according to their mode of actions, including sex hormones, tissue homones, xanthine derivatives, antibiotics, antiphlogistics, immunosuppressive agents, peripheral gangliotropic agents and psychotropic drugs. In addition, the available information on some compounds under investigation will be given briefly.

For a comprehensive and critical review of all pharmacological compounds that have been used or suggested for the treatment of male infertility, see also Lunenfeld & Insler (1978), Schill (1979a, 1982 b,d), Bain et al (1982), Bandhauer & Frick (1982), Menchini Fabris et al (1982b), Hargreave (1983) and Haidl & Schill (1991).

## SEX HORMONES AND THEIR INHIBITORS

Sex hormones and their inhibitors are known to interact specifically with receptor sites at the level of the hypothalamus, the pituitary, the testes, and the accessory sex glands. To these groups of substances belong antiestrogens, prolactin inhibitors, GnRH and its analogs, human gonadotropins and androgens.

### Antiestrogens

A large number of compounds with antiestrogenic activity are available (Lunan & Klopper 1975). However, only two major compounds were introduced into clinical medicine with relative success: clomiphene and tamoxifen.

#### Clomiphene

Clomiphene citrate (Fig. 23.2) is a synthetic analog of chlorotrianisene, a nonsteroidal estrogen, which is closely related to stilbestrol. Clomiphene citrate exhibits both antiestrogenic and estrogenic effects. It exists in two forms, *cis* and *trans* isomers, which are both present in commercial preparations. The *cis* compound is much more effective in stimulating ovulation (Greenblatt 1961).

Clomiphene is the best known antiestrogen: it is used with great success in women for induction of ovulation. However, despite its induction of considerable raise in gonadotropin and androgen levels, the use of clomiphene is still controversial in the treatment of oligozoospermia.

First effects on spermatogenesis have been

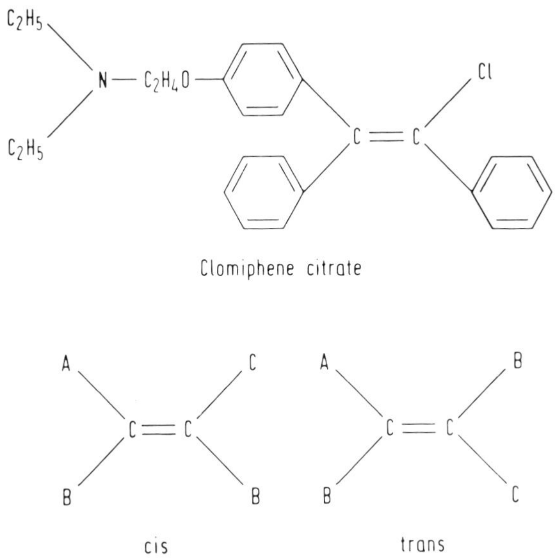

**Fig. 23.2** Structure of the antiestrogen clomiphene citrate and its two isomers. (From Schellen 1982.)

reported by Jungck & coworkers (1964). The dosages applied in the male subjects are between 25 and 400 mg/day. During treatment with high doses of clomiphene (200–400 mg/day) the intrinsic estrogenic activity may cause some adverse effect on the seminiferous tubules by damaging the spermatids (Heller et al 1969). In contrast, lower dosages (25–50 mg/day) show beneficial results on sperm quality by stimulating spermatogenesis. Some reports also claim a beneficial effect on sperm motility. A more favorable effect of therapy was reported when clomiphene citrate was applied in a new regimen (25 mg on alternate days) as compared to a daily dose of 25 mg (25 days on, 5 days off) (Homonnai et al 1988). Using this regimen, a significant improvement in sperm concentration, total sperm count and sperm motility could be achieved. Elimination of clomiphene takes about 5 days; thus cumulative effects have been discussed (Paulson & Wacksman 1976).

***Patients suitable for treatment: idiopathic normogonadotropic oligozoospermia*** Treatment is limited to patients with less than $20 \times 10^6$ spermatozoa/ml, with low or normal FSH and LH levels and a positive response of the pituitary after application of GnRH, clomiphene or tamoxifen (see Chapter 11). Therapy is supposed to be useful only if after antiestrogen application increased FSH, LH and testosterone values are registered. Individuals with increased basal gonadotropin levels and azoospermia are excluded from treatment (Schellen & Beek 1974). Sometimes patients with slightly elevated FSH levels respond positively to an antiestrogen administration (Bartsch & Scheiber 1981). However, the previous concept that therapy is only useful if increased levels of FSH, LH and testosterone are registered after application of antiestrogen must be reconsidered. By means of an antiestrogen test with tamoxifen, Schill & Schillinger (1987) demonstrated that FSH levels remained unchanged in patients who showed a positive reaction to tamoxifen, while a significant increase of FSH was observed in the 'nonresponders'. A direct influence of tamoxifen on spermatogenesis was also discussed by the authors.

***Treatment scheme and results*** There is now general agreement that low-dose clomiphene treatment should be performed with administration of 25–50 mg clomiphene/day for a period of 3–6 months.

Table 23.2 summarizes the results of low-dose clomiphene therapy published in the literature, showing an improvement in sperm count in 50% of 574 treated patients and a conception rate of 14%. Results differ considerably amongst various authors, due to selection of patients, dosage, and duration of treatment. Rönnberg (1980) was able to prove the efficacy of clomiphene in lower doses in a double-blind study. In 30 patients with idiopathic oligozoospermia, Pusch et al (1986a) observed a statistically significant increase in sperm density after low-dose therapy with clomiphene. On the other hand, no therapeutic effect of clomiphene was found by Sokol et al (1988) during a placebo-controlled study in 23 patients with oligozoospermia.

***Side-effects*** In 5–6% of patients clomiphene treatment produces side-effects including vertigo, nausea, gain of body weight, allergic dermatitis, hair loss and visual disturbances (blurring of vision, scintillating scotomas). In case of visual disturbances treatment must be stopped immediately. Most side-effects disappear rapidly after withdrawal of the medication.

**Table 23.2**   Clomiphene treatment in oligozoozpermic men (dosage: 25–50 mg/day) (summarized by Schill 1985)

| Reference | Patients (no.) | Improvement of sperm count | Pregnancies (no.) |
|---|---|---|---|
| Jungck et al 1964 | 29 | 17 | n.m. |
| Mellinger & Thompson 1966 | 13 | 10 | 0 |
| Mroueh et al 1967 | 15 | 1 | 0 |
| Potts 1968 | 20 | 13 | 1 |
| Palti 1970 | 40 | 15 | 3 |
| Halim et al 1973 | 25 | 11 | n.m. |
| Kern & Schirren 1973 | 43 | 21 | n.m. |
| Da Rugna et al 1974 | 33 | 5 | 0 |
| Schellen & Beek 1974 | 101 | 61 | 19 |
| Emperaire et al 1976 | 54 | 16 | 4 |
| Sas et al 1976 | 21 | 15 | 3 |
| Check & Rakoff 1977 | 10 | 5 | 9 |
| Espinasse 1977 | 37 | 16 | 3 |
| Epstein 1977 | 16 | 10 | 5 |
| Paulson 1977 | 57 | 45 | 20 |
| Homonnai et al 1978a | 60 | 28 | 2 |
| Total | 574 | 289(=50%) | 69(=14%) |

n.m., Not mentioned.

In some patients continuous administration of clomiphene may lead to an increase in desmosterol levels (Espinasse 1977) or increase in bromsulftalein retention. Therefore, clomiphene should not be prescribed in cases with a history of serious liver disease.

In all patients undergoing hormonal treatment, testicular and prostatic size should be carefully monitored at regular intervals in order not to overlook tumors whose growth may be stimulated by high testosterone levels.

### Tamoxifen

The antiestrogen tamoxifen has particularly drawn the attention of andrologists for the treatment of idiopathic oligozoospermia, since it exhibits much weaker estrogenic activities than clomiphene and does not increase the concentration of estrogen-sensitive binding proteins in the blood plasma (Comhaire 1982). Grabbe et al (1990) observed a significant increase of sex hormone binding globulin (SHBG) in the seminal plasma of patients who had shown a positive response to tamoxifen therapy as compared to nonresponders. They concluded that apart from its stimulation of the hypothalamus–pituitary gland–Leydig cell system, tamoxifen also has an effect on the Sertoli cells.

Tamoxifen is structurally similar to clomiphene citrate (Fig. 23.3). Whereas clomiphene is a racemic mixture of equal parts of the *cis* and *trans* isomers, tamoxifen, due to its chemical structure, contains only one isomer.

***Patients suitable for treatment: idiopathic normogonadotropic oligozoospermia*** The same selection criteria exist as for clomiphene therapy.

***Treatment scheme and results*** Ten milligrams of tamoxifen is given twice daily for 3–6 months. Tamoxifen was first successfully

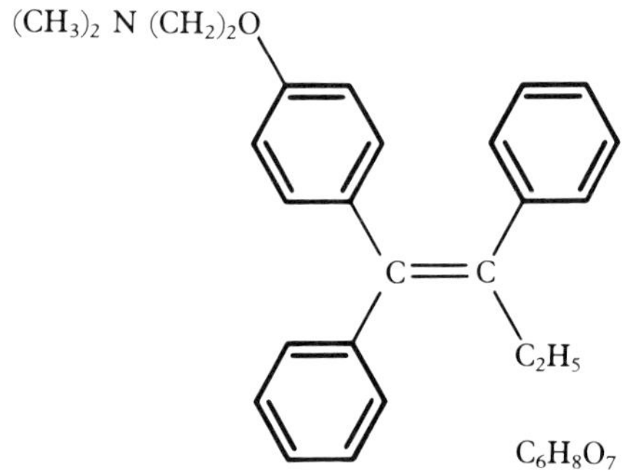

$(CH_3)_2 N (CH_2)_2O$

$C_2H_5$

$C_6H_8O_7$

**Fig. 23.3**   Structure of the antiestrogen tamoxifen, a triphenyl-ethylene derivative.

used by Comhaire (1976) for the treatment of idiopathic oligozoospermia. A statistically significant increase in sperm count was observed. In the mean time several groups have confirmed these results; (Bartsch et al 1979, Ruiz-Velasco et al 1980, Schill & Landthaler 1980, Buvat et al 1981, Traub & Thompson 1981, Schieferstein et al 1987). Török (1985) observed a significant increase in sperm concentration in a group of 20 patients with oligozoospermia who received 20 mg of tamoxifen for 3 months in an open trial; however, in a double-blind study with 54 patients this effect could not be demonstrated. During intake of tamoxifen, testosterone concentrations were found to increase significantly at a constant level between 83% and 100% (Comhaire 1976, Vermeulen & Comhaire 1978, Bartsch & Scheiber 1981). Peripheral estradiol concentration increased parallel to testosterone. Also serum gonadotropin levels increased significantly (Fig. 23.4). The rise in sperm concentration is shown in Fig. 23.5A. The increase is generally apparent 3 months after initiation of therapy. If no increase in sperm count has occurred after 6 months no effect can be expected from further teratment. The best results were seen in patients with sperm concentrations below $20 \times 10^6$ spermatozoa/ml (Vermeulen & Comhaire 1978). Between 55% and 80% of oligozoospermic patients with normal basal FSH levels responded to tamoxifen administration with a two- to three- fold increase in the initially determined basal values. Sperm motility was not affected in the studies performed by Comhaire (1976, 1982). However, Bartsch & Scheiber (1981) and Schill & Landthaler (1981) demonstrated a significant improvement in total motility, but not in progressive motility (Fig. 23.5B). Sperm morphology was not improved. Pregnancy rate was found to be around 38% (Schill & Landthaler 1981). Lewis-Jones et al (1987) observed an improvement in sperm count, motility and progressive motility, which was later confirmed by Schill & Schillinger (1987) (Fig. 23.6).

*Side-effects* During tamoxifen therapy no major side-effects have been observed, particularly no alterations in the number of leukocytes and thrombocytes, in liver parameters, and in

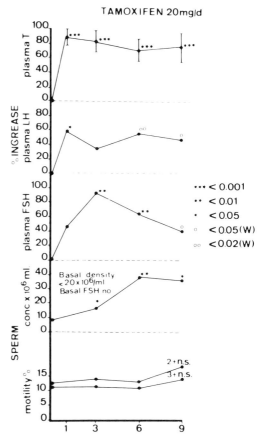

**Fig. 23.4** Influence of tamoxifen treatment on serum concentrations of testosterone, LH and FSH, and on concentration and motility of spermatozoa in patients with oligozoospermia (< 20 million/ml). The abscissa indicates the duration of treatment in months. Motility is subdivided into rapidly progressive (3+) and sluggishly progressive (2+). (For details see Vermeulen and Comhaire 1978.)

serum calcium pool. Some patients reported an increased libido or gain of body weight.

## Prolactin inhibitors

A number of drugs reduce prolactin secretion by the pituitary (for details see Chapter 17). Among them the ergoline derivative bromocriptine (2-Br-α-ergocriptine) was selected because of its strong prolactin-inhibitory action (Flückiger 1972). Bromocriptine is a derivative of lysergic acid, but lacks the hallucinogenic properties of LSD. It does not exhibit vascular and uterotonic effects common to other ergot compounds. Its specificity

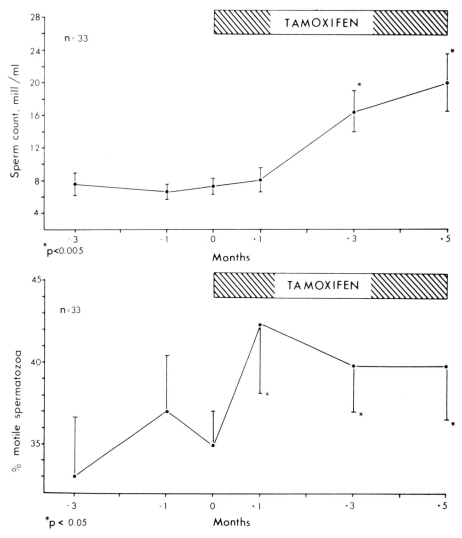

**Fig. 23.5** Tamoxifen treatment (20 mg/day) of 33 patients with idiopathic normogonadotropic oligozoospermia (< 20 × 10⁶/ml) over a period of 5 months. Mean values (± SE) of sperm density (a) and total sperm motility (b) before and during tamoxifen treatment are plotted. (For details see Schill & Landthaler 1981.)

as an agonist of the neurotransmitter dopamine is supported by the strong competitive action with other substances exhibiting high affinity for dopamine receptors. Average daily doses producing maximal prolactin inhibition in humans are 2.5–5 mg, although in some cases dosage increases up to 10 mg or even more may be required (del Pozo 1982).

***Treatment scheme and results*** In cases of prolactinoma with hyperprolactinemia neuro-

surgery may be considered. Persistent pathological prolactin secretion can also be inhibited by daily administration of 2.5–10 mg bromocriptine titrated according to the serum prolactin levels. In case of impotence, this will lead to an improvement in libido and other sexual dysfunctions (del Pozo 1982). If oligozoospermia is caused by hyperprolactinemia, bromocriptine administration will also improve the sperm count (Fig. 23.7).

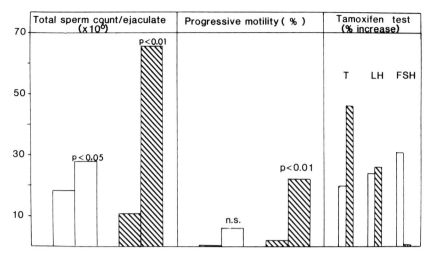

**Fig. 23.6**  Semen parameters before and during tamoxifen therapy (20 mg/day) in 26 oligospermic patients arranged according to men who fathered a child during or shortly after tamoxifen treatment and those who failed to do so. Open bars represent median values of nonfathers ($n = 19$), dashed bars those of fathers ($n = 7$). In addition, the response of testosterone, LH and FSH towards a short-term tamoxifen test (40 mg/day for 1 week) is shown. Increase of serum hormone values compared to basal values in percent is given. n.s.= not significant. (Reproduced with permission from Schill & Schillinger 1987.)

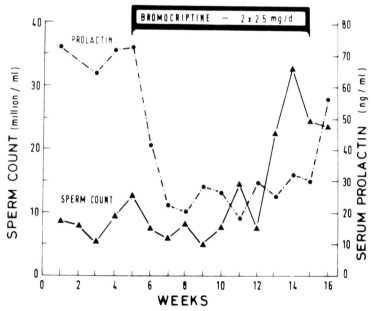

**Fig. 23.7**  The effect of bromocriptine treatment on serum prolactin levels and sperm count. (Reproduced with permission from Segal et al 1976.)

Bromocriptine plays no significant role in the treatment of oligozoospermia in normoprolactinemic men with no other signs of endocrine disturbances. Apart from single reports demonstrating the improvement of fertility by bromocriptine in oligozoospermic patients, most investigators see no relationship between oligozoospermia, prolactin and bromocriptine treatment. In particular, two double-blind trials with bromocriptine and placebo support this concept and showed no difference within the spermiograms of treated patients and controls (Hovatta et al 1979, Pryor & Chaput de Saintonge 1981).

*Side-effects* Vertigo, nausea and emesis may occur initially during bromocriptine intake. However, these side-effects can be overcome by administration of slowly increasing amounts of bromocriptine.

## Gonadotropin-releasing hormone (see also Chapter 15)

Synthesis and release of LH and FSH by the pituitary are regulated by one hypothalamic hormone, which is a polypeptide composed of ten amino acids. This hormone is called LH- and FSH-releasing hormone (LH-RH/FSH-RH) or simply LHRH or gonadotropin-releasing hormone (GnRH) (Schally et al 1973). Some of the amino acids are responsible for the affinity to the receptor, while the remaining ones are responsible for the physiological action of the compound. The compound can be synthesized and can be administered intravenously, intramuscularly or intranasally. Intestinal absorption is poor. The physiological effect is brief due to the short half-life of GnRH (4–9 min). For this reason repeated daily application is required. Efforts were therefore made to obtain a long-lasting vehicle, or GnRH-related compounds with structural modifications and/or substitution of amino acids, able to maintain a longer half-life and/or a higher gonadotropin-releasing potency. These studies have led to the availability of different synthetic GnRH analogs, some showing higher potency and long-lasting effects (Table 23.3), others having the capacity to block the GnRH effect and thus inhibit the pituitary gonadotropic function. As a result of chemical synthesis, GnRH and some analogs have been used therapeutically in men, namely in the treatment of hypogonadotropic hypogonadism (Mortimer et al 1974, Happ et al 1975, Mortimer 1977, Tharandt et al 1977, Vilchez-Martinez et al 1979). GnRH analogs decrease circulating testosterone blood levels and inhibit spermatogenesis

**Table 23.3** Different synthetic GnRH analogs with higher GnRH potency

| Analog | Potency in comparison to GnRH |
| --- | --- |
| D-Ala$^6$-GnRH | 6–7 times |
| D-Leu$^6$-GnRH | 5–9 times |
| D-Phe$^6$-GnRH | 10–13 times |
| D-Trp$^6$-GnRH | 50–100 times |
| D-Ser-(Bu)$^6$-GnRH-EA (HOE 766) | 30–100 times |
| D-Leu$^6$-GnRH-EA | 50–60 times |
| D-Ala$^6$-GnRH-EA | 30 times |

After Schwarzstein & Aparicio 1982

through inhibition of testicular LH and prolactin receptors as well as through a decrease in the number of LH/hCG receptors in the pituitary. These findings suggest application of GnRH analogs for the treatment of androgen-dependent diseases like carcinoma of the prostate and benign hypertrophy of the prostate, and for contraceptive purposes (Labrie et al 1980). When considering treatment of infertile men, GnRH and its analogs are still experimental and may have only limited application in the future.

### GnRH

*Patients suitable for treatment* Pulsatile administration of GnRH should be the treatment of choice in patients with hypothalamic failure (hypogonadotropic hypogonadism) and delayed puberty. Treatment of men with idiopathic normogonadotropic oligozoospermia is another approach, however, controversial results have been obtained so far.

*Treatment scheme and results* In hypogonadotropic hypogonadism prolonged treatment with 500 µg GnRH three times daily led to a restoration of potency and induction of spermatogenesis in some patients (Mortimer et al 1974). Vermeulen (1981) referring to results of Slager who treated ten patients with Kallmann's syndrome and obtained only a deficient spermatogenesis in three patients, questioned this approach. Also Happ et al (1975) and Potashnik et al (1977) reported use of intranasal GnRH (8 × 200 µg/day) in hypogonadotropic hypogonadism with disappointing results. For details about the therapeutic use of GnRH in hypogonadotropic hypogonadism see Schally (1976). GnRH as intranasal spray 6 × 200 μg daily was also shown to be effective in cryptorchidism and thus may be of certain advantage for therapy in children (Bartsch & Frick 1974). However, this form of treatment is still not generally accepted despite published positive results (Happ 1981). The current method of GnRH therapy is pulsatile administration of a 50 ng/kg/pulse by means of a pump (Wagner 1985). Berezin et al (1988) reported to have successfully treated a patient with Kallmann's syndrome: 6 months of therapy resulted in pregnancy and birth of a healthy child. Liu et al (1988) compared pulsatile subcutaneous administration of GnRH and exogenous gonadotropins in the treatment of men with isolated hypogonadotropic hypogonadism. They concluded that pulsatile gonadotropic levels achieved with GnRH are more effective in stimulating testicular growth but not sperm output than are gonadotropic concentrations obtained with hCG/hMG.

In idiopathic oligozoospermia, Zarate & coworkers (1973) reported questionable results of treatment of ten men twice daily by 500 μg GnRH intramuscularly for a period of 6 months. However, there was no clear selection of patients and no criteria for evaluation of therapeutic reasons. At least some patients experienced an increase in sperm output. Later, Schwarzstein et al (1975) successfully treated four men with normogonadotropic oligozoospermia by daily injections of 500–1000 μg synthetic GnRH over a period of 100–135 days. In three of the four men, a significant increase in sperm count was observed. Libido and sexual potency increased in all four subjects. In subsequent studies, long-term (60 days) and short-term (30 days) treatment were compared in 21 men with idiopathic normogonadotropic oligozoospermia using an intramuscular injection of 100–500 μg GnRH daily (Aparicio et al 1976). Short-term treatment was less effective, whereas long-term treatment resulted in an improvement in sperm count and sperm motility in patients with hypospermatogenesis or spermatogenic arrest up to the spermatid stage. Thus in normogonadotropic oligozoospermia GnRH treatment for at least 90 days at an average of 250 μg daily was recom-

mended (Schwarzstein & Aparicio 1982). Fauser et al (1985) could not achieve improvement after 3 months of LHRH therapy in four patients with idiopathic oligozoospermia. Aulitzky et al (1989) administered 4 μg LHRH by means of an infusion pump to 14 patients with oligozoospermia and increased FSH levels. After 6 months of therapy a significant increase in sperm count and reduced FSH levels were observed in eight patients who had previously shown a disturbed LH pulsatility of less than 8 pulses/24 h (normal value: 12 pulses/24 h). Three pregnancies were achieved during this treatment. Decreased FSH levels after pulsatile LHRH therapy were also observed by Wagner (1985) and Gross et al (1986), while the results obtained by Bals-Pratsch et al (1989) were rather disappointing. Further experience with larger groups of patients is required to show a possible efficacy of GnRH therapy in the treatment of subfertile men. Particularly, performance of a double-blind trial is urgently needed.

GnRH analogs are used in the treatment of precocious puberty, prostatic and breast cancer, endometriosis, uterine leiomyoma, polycystic ovarian disease and various other disorders. Due to the downregulation of pituitary and gonadal receptors they are not used for treatment of male fertility disorders (Filicori & Flamigni 1988).

**Side-effects** None have been observed. There was one report of secondary drug failure because of antibody formation in a hypogonadal patient treated for more than 1 year with GnRH (van Loon & Brown 1975). However, due to the rapid disintegration of GnRH in vivo it rarely becomes immunogenic.

### Human gonadotropins

LH and FSH are glycohormones which are required for normal testicular functions: LH stimulates testosterone production by the Leydig cells and FSH stimulates the Sertoli cells in the seminiferous tubules.

For clinical purposes human menopausal gonadotropin (hMG) extracted from postmenopausal urine and human chorionic gonadotropin (hCG) extracted from pregnancy urine are used. Pregnant mare gonadotropin should not be used because of its strong antibody-inducing effect.

After a single dose of hCG (as LH substitute) a prolonged biphasic response of plasma testosterone is observed with a first increment 2–8 h after injection and a second peak 2–3 days after intramuscular injection (Saez & Forest 1979, Nankin et al 1980, Padron et al 1980). The physiological significance of this biphasic phenomenon remains to be established.

***Patients   suitable   for   treatment*** The following are indications for treatment:

1. Hypogonadotropic hypogonadism, which is characterized by clinical hypogonadism, hypospermatogenesis and low serum testosterone levels associated with low serum LH and FSH concentrations. The cause of the disease may be within either the hypothalamus or the pituitary. A differential diagnosis of hypogonadotropic hypogonadism is given in Table 23.4.

2. Idiopathic normogonadotropic oligozoospermia. It is postulated that in some patients a relative FSH deficiency may occur (Glezerman & Lunenfeld 1976, Lunenfeld et al 1979).

3. Oligozoospermia due to histologically confirmed disorders at the spermatid stage (Schwarzstein 1974).

4. Oligoasthenozoospermia and asthenozoospermia caused by a relative androgen deficiency due to a latent Leydig cell insufficiency (Hofmann et al 1975a, Lunenfeld & Glezerman 1981).

5. Cryptorchid children (Bierich et al 1977).

***Treatment   schemes   and   results***
*1. Hypogonadotropic hypogonadism* Gonadotropin treatment in hypogonadotropic hypogonadism is the only replacement therapy that shows a high grade of predictability for restoration of fertility. However, no standardized regimen of treatment is available since experience has shown substantial variations from patient to patient. Nevertheless, general agreement exists that combined application of hMG and hCG gives better results with more predictable testicular maturation (MacLeod et al 1966, Mancini et al 1969).

In hypogonadotropic men with testicular atrophy first hCG is administered for full maturation of Leydig cells, thus increasing testosterone production and estradiol secretion by the testes (Kelch et al 1972, Smith et al 1974). After 4–6 weeks, hMG should be added. Once spermatogenesis is achieved, it can usually be maintained with hCG alone. Liu et al (1988) did not observe any advantage of pulsatile GnRH administration as compared to hCG/hMG therapy. Replacement therapy should be monitored by sporadic testosterone determinations.

The treatment schedule is usually as follows: every 5–7 days 5000 IU hCG are injected intramuscularly to maintain a testosterone level of at least 5 mg/ml. hMG is given by weekly intramuscular injections of 3 × 75 IU FSH. Sometimes, 2 × 75 IU FSH will be sufficient; in other cases, an FSH dose of up to 300 IU FSH daily may be necessary (Glezerman & Lunenfeld 1982). In

**Table 23.4**   Disorders associated with hypogonadotropic hypogonadism

| | |
|---|---|
| Idiopathic hypogonadotropic hypogonadism and related syndromes | Hypothalamic tumors and cysts |
| Kallmann's syndrome | Dysgerminoma |
| 'Fertile eunuch' syndrome | Craniopharyngioma |
| Prader–Willi syndrome | CNS infections |
| Lawrence–Moon–Biedl syndrome | Meningitis (bacterial and fungal) |
| Möbius's syndrome | Encephalitis |
| Idiopathic hypopituitarism (partial and complete) | Miscellaneous |
| Pituitary adenomas | Head trauma |
| Chromophobe adenomas | Sarcoidosis |
| Prolactinomas | Hemochromatosis |
| Cushing's syndrome | Histiocytosis |
| Acromegaly | Pituitary irradiation |
| | Anorexia nervosa |

(After Winters & Troen 1982)

contrast, Sherins & coworkers (1977) showed that induction of spermatogenesis in hypophysectomized males may be possible using only 10–30% of the conventional FSH dosage. This is confirmed by our own experience. Similarly, the hCG doses recommended are probably excessive. At these doses, downregulation of hCG receptors may take place and the efficacy of the treatment may therefore be compromised (Steinberger & Rodriguez-Rigau 1981).

The length of treatment needed to restore spermatogenesis may vary considerably and take between 3 and 12 months and sometimes 2 years or longer. If a pregnancy is achieved, combined gonadotropin medication may be discontinued and followed with hCG alone or with testosterone replacement. If fertility is desired again, long-term therapy with testosterone seems to have no negative effects on the subsequent induction of spermatogenesis with hMG/hCG (Burger et al 1976, Johnsen 1978, Schroffner 1978).

Figure 23.8 illustrates combined gonadotropin therapy in a hypophysectomized man over a period of more than 3 years. During the time of replacement therapy three pregnancies occurred.

Tables 23.5–23.7 summarize the therapeutic results obtained in different centers with

**Table 23.5**  Effect of human gonadotropins on hypophysectomized men

| Reference | Patients (no.) | Instances of complete spermatogenesis |
| --- | --- | --- |
| Gemzell & Kjessler 1964 | 1 | 1 |
| Lytton & Kase 1966* | 1 | 1 |
| Johnson & Christiansen 1968* | 1 | 1 |
| Granville 1970 | 1 | 1 |
| MacLeod 1970 | 2 | 2 |
| Mancini 1970 | 15 | 15 |
| Lunenfeld 1978† | 2 | 2 |
| Schroffner 1978 | 1 | 1 |
| Schill (unpublished) | 2 | 2 |
| Total | 26 | 26(=100%) |

\* Quoted from Rosemberg 1976.
† Quoted from Glezerman et al 1978.

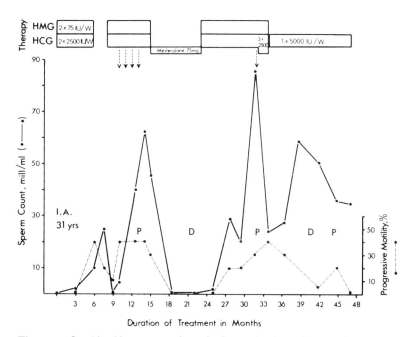

**Fig 23.8**  Combined human gonadotropin therapy in a hypophysectomized man over a period of more than 3 years. Sperm count (10⁶/ml) and progressive sperm motility (%) are plotted. Three pregnancies (P) with spontaneous deliveries (D) were observed. ·→, insemination by cervical cap. (For details see Schill 1979a.)

**Table 23.6**  Effect of human gonadotropins on hypogonadotropic hypogonadism (eunuchoidal men)

| Reference | Patiens (no.) | Instances of complete spermatogenesis |
|---|---|---|
| Davies & Crooke 1965* | 1 | 1 |
| Heller 1965* | 1 | 1 |
| Paulsen 1965* | 2 | 2 |
| Johnsen 1966* | 2 | 2 |
| Martin 1967 | 1 | 1 |
| Crooke et al 1968* | 5 | 3 |
| Paulsen et al 1970 | 5 | 4 |
| Sherins et al 1977 | 9 | 8 |
| Lunenfeld 1978† | 7 | 6 |
| Schill (unpublished) | 5 | 4 |
| Total | 38 | 32(=84%) |

\* Quoted from Rosemberg 1976.
† Quoted from Glezerman et al 1978.

**Table 23.7**  Effect of human gonadotropins on noneunuchoidal azoospermic men

| Reference | Patients (no.) | Instances of complete spermatogenesis |
|---|---|---|
| Pasetto 1965* | 2 | 1 |
| Joel 1966* | 4 | 4 |
| Anton et al 1968 | 2 | — |
| Conti et al 1969* | 13 | 1 |
| Marchesi et al 1969* | 6 | 2 |
| Pomerol and Morer 1969* | 15 | 7 |
| Kjessler 1971† | 38 | 24 |
| Pellegrini et al 1971† | 14 | 4 |
| Rosemberg 1976 | 5 | — |
| Lunenfeld 1978† | 29 | 17 |
| Schill (unpublished) | 4 | 4 |
| Total | 132 | 64(=48%) |

\* Quoted from Rosemberg 1976.
† Quoted from Glezerman et al 1978.

hMG/hCG treatment of hypophysectomized men, eunuchoidal men with hypogonadotropic hypogonadism and noneunuchoidal hypogonadotropic men. The success rate in these hypogonadotropic men in terms of a complete gonadal maturation with recovery of spermatozoa in the ejaculate is between 48% and 100%. All hypophysectomized patients respond to gonadotropin therapy. However, since slow progressive thickening and hyalinization of the tunica propria of the seminiferous tubules has been described (Wong et al 1974), reinitiation of spermatogenesis by gonadotropins after hypophy-sectomy is recommended before the testes are completely hyalinized. In eunuchoidal patients the success rate is 84%, while it is reduced to 48% in postpubertal noneunuchoidal hypogonadotropic men. For further detailed information concerning gonadotropin therapy see Rosemberg (1976), Schill (1979a), Lunenfeld & Glezerman (1981), Isidori (1981) and Winters & Troen (1982).

*2. Idiopathic normogonadotropic oligozoospermia*
In contrast to hypogonadotropic men, the effect of combined gonadotropin therapy in patients with idiopathic normogonadotropic oligozoospermia is inconsistent, predominantly due to the polyetiology of idiopathic oligozoospermia. In addition, no deficiency in gonadotropin secretion is evident in this group of patients (Nankin et al 1977, Winters & Troen 1982). In some patients with low normal testosterone concentrations associated with slightly increased gonadotropin secretion, a primary testicular defect is suggested (de Kretser et al 1972). In another group of patients relative FSH deficiency is presumed (Glezerman & Lunenfeld 1976, Maroulis et al 1977). Lunenfeld et al (1979) recommended use of the GnRH test to select patients with relative FSH deficiency for a more predictable gonadotropin treatment. Other investigators could not confirm this (Bain et al 1978, Schill et al 1982). The known stimulatory effect of gonadotropins on spermatogenesis serves as a rationale for performing gonadotropin therapy in oligozoospermia. During in vitro studies of testicular tissues from subfertile men Okoyama et al (1989) observed a significantly higher DNA synthesis after hMG/hCG therapy compared to patients who had not been treated. However, the response to treatment is unpredictable and the treatment must be considered purely empirical. Knuth et al (1987) did not observe any effect of such a therapy during a double-blind study in 39 patients with oligozoospermia.

For treatment of idiopathic normogonadotropic oligozoospermia the following schedule is recommended: 5000 IU hCG per week together with 1 ampule of hMG (75 IU FSH + 75 IU LH) per day or two ampules hMG three times a week. Duration of treatment is 3 months. In case of a significant response of the individual the treatment may be continued longer, until pregnancy occurs.

Tables 23.8 and 23.9 summarize the results of various studies evaluating the effect of hMG/hCG on hypospermatogenesis with division of the patients into two groups; those with severe (less than $10 \times 10^6$ spermatozoa/ml) and those with moderate ($11-20 \times 10^6$ spermatozoa/ml) oligozoospermia. Moderate oligozoospermia responds more favorably than severe oligozoospermia.

Our own experience with hMG/hCG combination in the treatment of idiopathic normogon-

adotropic oligozoospermia is summarized in Figure 23.9 (Schill et al 1982). A significant increase in sperm count 3 months after initiation of treatment was observed as well as an increase in the percentage of motile spermatozoa 1, 3 and 5 months after the start of gonadotropin medication. Thirty-three per cent of the men (responders) showed a distinct improvement in the semen parameters (Fig. 23.10). Conception chance within the whole patient group was 30%. In the responder group the pregnancy rate was 50%. In contrast, the pregnancy rate of the nonresponder

**Table 23.8**    Effect of human gonadotropins on oligozoospermic men: severe oligozoospermia ($<10 \times 10^6$/ml)

| Authors | Patients (no.) | Improvement to moderate oligozoospermia (11–20 million/ml) | Improvement to > 30 million/ml | Pregnancies (no.) |
|---|---|---|---|---|
| Dörner et al 1960 | 4 | 1 | 1 | n.m. |
| Schoysman 1964 | 4 | 1 | 1 | 1 |
| Pasetto 1965* | 5 | 1 | 3 | — |
| Abelli & Falagario 1966* | 6 | 2 | 1 | — |
| Cittadini & Qwartaravo 1966* | 12 | 5 | 1 | 1 |
| Heeres 1966† | 15 | — | 15 | 4 |
| Lytton & Mroueh 1966 | 9 | 1 | 1 | — |
| Andersson & Perklew 1967† | 34 | — | 6 | — |
| Danezis & Batrinos 1967 | 9 | 2 | 1 | 1 |
| Debiasi & Misurale 1967* | 8 | 1 | 2 | 1 |
| Lunenfeld et al 1967 | 27 | 6 | 8 | 1 |
| Polishuk et al 1967 | 9 | 1 | 3 | 1 |
| Anton et al 1968 | 7 | — | — | — |
| de Kretser et al 1968 | 2 | 1 | — | — |
| Natoli 1968† | 12 | — | 2 | — |
| Da Rugna 1968† | 33 | 30 | 3 | 3 |
| Alvares Rivas 1969† | 17 | 3 | 6 | — |
| Conti et al 1969* | 5 | — | 1 | — |
| Lavieri 1969† | 10 | 7 | — | — |
| Marchesi et al 1969* | 22 | 9 | 3 | 2 |
| Pomerol & Morer 1969* | 20 | 7 | 7 | — |
| Tronchetti et al 1969† | 5 | 1 | 3 | — |
| Troen et al 1970 | 9 | 1 | — | — |
| Landes & Müller 1971 | 4 | — | — | — |
| Pellegrini et al 1971* | 7 | 2 | 4 | 3 |
| Reich & Günther 1973 | 13 | — | 1 | 4 |
| Sherins 1974 | 5 | — | — | — |
| Sina et al 1974 | 25 | 7 | 4 | 6 |
| Schwarzstein 1974 | 3 | 1 | — | 1 |
| Rosemberg 1976 | 4 | 1 | 1 | 1 |
| Niermann (unpublished) | 50 | 5 | — | 1 |
| Schellen & Bruinse 1980 | 30 | 13 | — | 5 |
| Schill et al 1982 | 14 | 3 | — | 2 |
| Total | 439 | 112(=25.5%) | 78(=18%) | 38(=9%) |

n.m., not mentioned
\* Quoted from Rosemberg 1976.
† Quoted from Glezerman et al 1978.

**Table 23.9**  Effect of human gonadotropins on oligozoospermic men: Moderate oligozoospermia ($11-20 \times 10^6$ml)

| Authors | Patients (no.) | Improvement to > 30 million/ml | Pregnancies (no.) |
|---|---|---|---|
| Dörner et al 1960 | 3 | 3 | n.m. |
| Schoysman 1964 | 4 | 2 | — |
| Abelli & Falagario 1966* | 26 | 9 | 6 |
| Cittadini & Quartaravo 1966* | 2 | 2 | — |
| Lytton & Mroueh 1966 | 9 | 6 | 2 |
| Danezis & Batrinos 1967 | 1 | 1 | 1 |
| Debiasi & Misurale 1967* | 7 | 4 | 2 |
| Lunenfeld et al 1967 | 24 | 12 | 4 |
| Mroueh et al 1967 | 2 | 1 | — |
| Polishuk et al 1967 | 5 | 1 | — |
| Makler et al 1968† | 2 | 2 | 1 |
| Troen et al 1970 | 2 | 1 | — |
| Landes & Müller 1971 | 15 | 2 | 5 |
| Reich & Günther 1973 | 18 | 5 | 4 |
| Schwarzstein 1974 | 3 | 3 | 1 |
| Sherins 1974 | 2 | — | — |
| Sina et al 1974 | 13 | 6 | 3 |
| Rosemberg 1976 | 4 | 3 | — |
| Homonnai et al 1978* | 37 | 8 | 3 |
| Niermann (unpublished) | 50 | 5 | 2 |
| Schill et al 1982 | 12 | 4 | — |
| Total | 241 | 80 (=33%) | 34 (=14%) |

n.m., not mentioned.
\* Quoted from Rosemberg 1976.
† Quoted from Glezerman et al 1978.

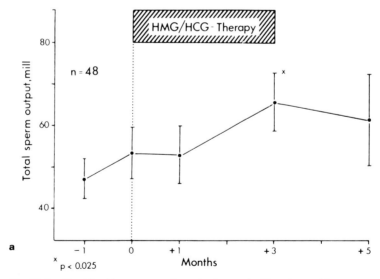

**Fig. 23.9**  Combined human gonadotropin therapy in 48 patients with idiopathic normogonadotropic oligozoospermia ($< 20 \times 10^6$/ml) treated over a period of 3 months with three times weekly 2 ampules hMG (1 ampule $\triangleq$ 75 IU FSH + 75 IU LH) and weekly two times 1 ampule hCG (1 ampule $\triangleq$ 2500 IU LH). Mean values ($\pm$ SE) of the total sperm output (spermatozoa/ejaculate) (**a**) and total sperm motility (**b**) before, during and after therapy are plotted.

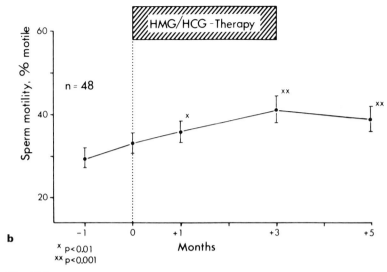

**Fig. 23.9**

group was 19%, being in the range of the spontaneous conception rate. When investigating semen parameters during gonadotropin therapy with respect to fathers ($n = 10$) and nonfathers ($n = 23$), a significant improvement in sperm count and progressive motility could only be observed in the group of fathers (Fig. 23.11).

No abnormalities were seen in the offspring obtained after hMG/hCG therapy in men with idiopathic normogonadotropic oligozoospermia, nor were any reported by other authors.

It should be pointed out that others have treated patients with idiopathic normogonadotropic oligozoospermia using hMG alone

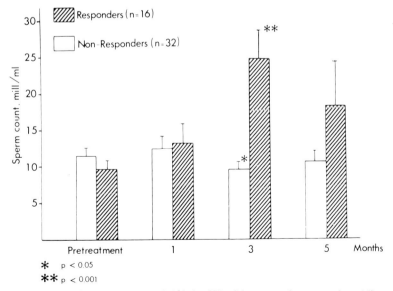

**Fig. 23.10**    Mean sperm count ($10^6$/ml ± SE) of the responders group ($n = 16$) and the nonresponders group ($n = 32$) before, during and after treatment with human gonadotropins in the same patient material as illustrated in Figure 23.9.

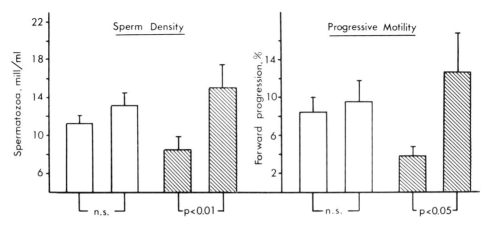

**Fig. 23.11** Combined human gonadotropin therapy in the same patient group as illustrated in Figures 23.9 and 23.10. Among 33 patients who responded to a questionnaire asking for a possible conception, ten pregnancies could be recorded after 1 year of treatment. Sperm count and progressive motility before and 3 months after gonadotropin therapy in the groups of fathers and nonfathers are compared. Open bars represent mean values (± SEM) of non-fathers (*n* = 23), dashed bars those of fathers (*n* = 10). n.s., not significant. (From Schill 1982d.)

and have found strikingly similar results to the combined hMG/hCG treatment with regard to improvement in sperm count and pregnancy rate (Winters & Troen 1982). Therefore, in order to properly evaluate gonadotropin treatment in patients with idiopathic normogonadotropic oligozoospermia, more multicenter double-blind studies are urgently needed.

Gonadotropin therapy should not be applied to oligozoospermic men with elevated FSH levels and to patients in whom the etiology of oligo-zoospermia is outside of the pituitary-gonadal axis (e.g. varicocele).

*3. Oligozoospermia due to disturbed spermatogenesis at the spermatid stage* Schwarzstein (1974) reported successful hMG therapy without hCG in oligozoospermic patients with histologically confirmed disturbed spermatogenesis at the spermatid stage. In 50% of these cases positive results were obtained with significant improvement of sperm count using three weekly injections of one ampule hMG for 30–270 days. The results of Schwarzstein (1974) raised the question as to whether FSH (and LH indirectly) could act selectively at the spermatid stage or whether histological analysis of testicular tissue may help to predict patients with oligozoospermia who can be treated most successfully with hMG alone.

*4. Oligozoospermia and asthenozoospermia due to relative androgen deficiency* Low normal androgen levels were attributed to a latent Leydig cell insufficiency by Hofmann et al 1975a. Relative androgen deficiency may also be diagnosed after positive response of patients with oligozoospermia and asthenozoospermia to hCG treatment (Glezerman & Lunenfeld 1976).

hCG without hMG was used successfully in infertile men with persistently low sperm motility (asthenozoospermia and oligoasthenozoospermia) either using biweekly injections of 10 000 IU hCG (Futterweit & Sobrero 1968), or 2500 IU hCG every 5 days for 75–90 days (Misurale et al 1969), or twice weekly 2500 IU hCG (Dörner et al 1960). Of 30 patients with isolated astheno-zoospermia who had received 5000 IU hCG intramuscularly for 3 months, 16 showed an improvement in total motility from 34% to 40%, and six pregnancies were achieved (Pusch et al 1986b). However, it should be kept in mind that repeated high doses of hCG have been found to result in refractoriness to acute hCG stimulation due to a loss of LH receptor activity and a relative enzymatic defect in testosterone biosynthesis (Cigorraga et al 1978, Saez & Forest 1979).

*5. Cryptorchid children* hCG is successfully used in the treatment of cryptorchidism (Richter et al 1976, Bierich et al 1977). According to modified recommendations of the International Health Foundation, Geneva, hCG is injected intramuscularly once weekly for 5 weeks in different doses according to the patient's age. Thus, within the first year 1 × 500 IU hCG are applied, up to the sixth year 1 × 1000 IU hCG, and above this age 1 × 2000 IU hCG are recommended. If possible descent of the testes should be completed at the end of the second year after birth. If gonadotropin treatment is unsuccessful, a second hCG regimen can be applied 5 weeks later, followed immediately by surgery. Intranasal therapy with GnRH is also possible to induce descent of the testes (Happ 1981). At present, a combined GnRH/hCG treatment is recommended according to the following regimen: 3 × 2 sprays of 0.2 mg GnRH intranasally per day for 4 weeks, followed immediately by 1500 IU hCG per week intramuscularly for another 3 weeks. A success rate between 30% and 70% has been reported.

*Side-effects* Apart from moderate weight increase no adverse effects of hMG therapy in men have been reported. hCG treatment is usually without any side-effect, but with larger doses increased libido and potency are observed and sometimes transient nipple tenderness and gynecomastia can occur. There is no evidence of tubular damage during hCG treatment (Mancini et al 1969, Sherins 1974). Failure of gonadotropin therapy due to the induction of antibodies against hCG was reported (Sokol et al 1980). Since the antibodies could also cross-react with endogenous LH molecules, gonadotropin treatment in eugonadal patients should be performed with care and limited exclusively to men with an urgent wish to father a child.

## Androgens

Testosterone (Fig. 23.12) is the most important androgen secreted by the testes. It reaches the target organs via the bloodstream. If given orally, it is absorbed from the gut, but is so effectively metabolized in the liver that it will never reach the target organs. The metabolizing capacity of the liver, which is age and sex dependent, is only exceeded if the dosage is increased to 200 mg

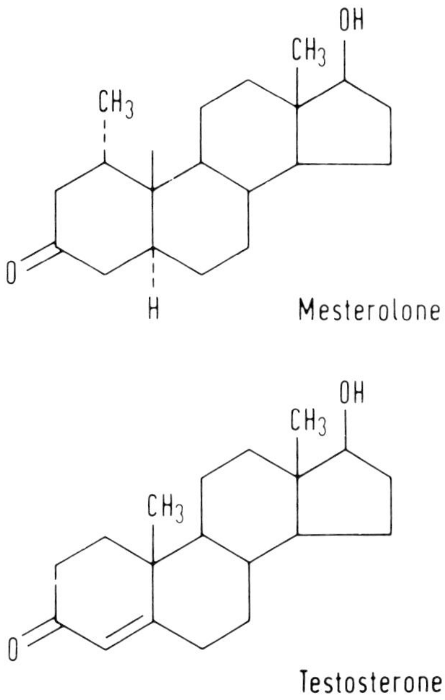

**Fig. 23.12**    Structure of testosterone and mesterolone.

(about 30-fold the amount produced daily by a normal adult). 400–600 mg of free unesterified testosterone must be administered daily in order to effectively replace the endogenous testosterone production (Johnsen et al 1974). However, using this high steroid concentration, which is uneconomical, toxic side-effects cannot be excluded. Therefore, oral administration of testosterone is not generally recommended.

To bypass the liver, the following routes have been suggested: testosterone suppositories (Hamburger 1958), 2 × three times daily; application of testosterone by nasal spray (Danner & Frick 1980); subcutaneous implants of testosterone pellets (Heller & Maddock 1947); and subcutaneous application of silastic capsules (Frick et al 1976). However, apart from suppositories, all other forms of testosterone application have remained experimental.

In a randomized clinical trial of testosterone replacement therapy in hypogonadal men, Conway et al (1988) compared the following applications: 250 mg mixed testosterone esters intramuscularly at 2-weekly intervals, 120 mg testosterone undecanoate by mouth twice daily, and subcutaneous testosterone pellets (6 × 100 mg). The authors concluded that testosterone pellets give the closest approximation to zero order (steady state) delivery conditions for up to 4 months after a single insertion. Furthermore, new formulations like biodegradable injectable microspheres (Asch et al 1986) or more convenient noninvasive modes of application such as transdermal preparations have been developed. Place et al (1990) summarized the results of several testosterone replacement studies in hypogonadal males using a transdermal scrotal route. This provided a circadian rhythm of testosterone and proved to be safe and effective. However, parenteral administration by intramuscular injection is still the method with widespread use. To increase the length of effectiveness of the parenteral route several testosterone esters have been synthesized. The following esters are commonly used: testosterone propionate, testosterone enanthate, and testosterone cypionate (Fig. 23.13). Following the injection of 25–50 mg testosterone propionate, elevated serum testosterone concentrations can be measured for 1–2 days (Nieschlag et al 1976). An increase in the length of effectiveness due to a longer side-chain is found with testosterone enanthate where elevated testosterone serum levels can be observed for 12–14 days in normal men (Nieschlag et al 1976). For long-term replacement therapy of endocrine testicular insufficiency, intramuscular injection of 250 mg testosterone enanthate must be given every 2–3 weeks. Testosterone cypionate and testosterone enanthate can be considered equivalent in terms of clinical effectiveness because of their bioavailability and duration of effectiveness (Schulte-Beerbühl & Nieschlag 1980). Another modification for application of testosterone was successfully developed: esterification of testosterone in position 17 (Fig. 23.13) with undecanoic acid (11 carbon atoms) produces a compound which can be given orally, since it is partially incorporated into chylomicrons in the intestines, absorbed into lymphatic fluid, and reaches the circulation via the ductus thoracicus (Horst et al 1976). Thus, before testosterone may be inactivated by the liver, it reaches the target organs. Maximum concentrations in blood are observed 4 h after oral ingestion, whereas basal levels are reached after 8 h (Nieschlag et al 1975).

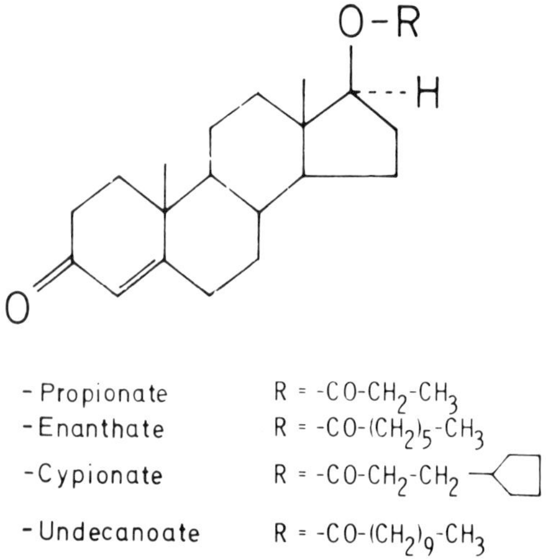

- Propionate    $R = -CO-CH_2-CH_3$
- Enanthate    $R = -CO-(CH_2)_5-CH_3$
- Cypionate    $R = -CO-CH_2-CH_2-$
- Undecanoate    $R = -CO-(CH_2)_9-CH_3$

**Fig. 23.13**   Testosterone esters available for treatment.

In total, however, therapy with testosterone undecanoate is more difficult to control than parenteral application of other testosterone esters, because absorption conditions depend on food intake and may be different (Schürmeyer et al 1983, Schill 1985).

Apart from the use of esterified testosterone, several attempts have been made to chemically modify the steroid molecule in order to delay its metabolism in the liver and thus produce a synthetic androgen which can be used effectively by oral intake. A series of synthetic compounds with androgenic activity were developed; however, all increased the risk of hepatotoxicity with long-term use (17-α-methyltestosterone, fluoxymesterone). Only one substance showed no hepatotoxicity: mesterolone, which can be considered a derivative of the 5-α-reduced testosterone metabolite dihydrotestosterone. Mesterolone (17 β-hydroxy-1-α-methyl-5-α-androstane-3-one) has no double bond between C4 and C5 (Fig. 23.12). Thus, the A-ring in the steroid molecule is saturated and cannot be aromatized to estrogens. Unfortunately, mesterolone is only a partially active androgen and is only weakly active or inactive in target organs requiring the direct effect of testosterone (e.g. muscle) or aromatization to estrogens (e.g. the hypothalamo-pituitary system). This is why mesterolone administration does not affect the pituitary secretion of LH and FSH at doses around 100 mg/day. On the other hand, mesterolone cannot be used for complete substitution in cases of Leydig cell insufficiency (Nieschlag & Freischem 1982).

***Patients suitable for treatment*** These include: men with endocrine testicular insufficiency who require replacement therapy; patients with normogonadotropic and hyper-gonadotropic oligozoospermia in whom high-dose androgen therapy is performed for induction of rebound phenomenon; those with astheno-zoospermia due to relative androgen deficiency; and those with functional disturbances of the epididymis and the accessory sex glands, particu-larly androgen-sensitive insufficiency of the seminal vesicles (low seminal plasma fructose levels), who will be subjected to low-dose androgen therapy. Special indications for androgen administration are idiopathic delayed puberty, excessively tall boys, and androgen insufficiency associated with advanced age.

***Treatment schemes and results***
1. *Replacement therapy* Testosterone replacement therapy is necessary in all types of primary testic-ular failure and in patients with secondary hypo-gonadism on a long-term basis. Replacement therapy should be performed throughout the life of the patient to avoid manifestations of osteo-porosis. Two types of treatment are:

a. Administration of long-acting depot testos-terone preparations: 200–250 mg testosterone enanthate or cypionate intramuscularly every 2–4 weeks. Both esters are clinically equivalent (Nieschlag & Freischem 1982). Therapy is controlled by occasional testosterone determina-tions immediately before the next depot injection. The therapeutic effectiveness is further clinically monitored by observation of physical and mental activity, libido, potency, and somatic signs of virility such as muscular strength, beard growth and male hair pattern. A particularly reliable para-meter to assess the therapeutic efficacy is sexual activity, as shown by Davidson & co-workers (1979) and Seimimies & co-workers (1982).

b. Oral administration of testosterone undecanoate with daily application of 80–160 mg divided into two to three doses. However, there may be great individual variations concerning resorption of testosterone undecanoate by the intestines through the lymphatic fluid via the ductus thoracicus. Satisfactory clinical results have been reported by Franchi & coworkers (1978) and by Della Casa et al (1982). As the effect of testosterone undecanoate on suppression of spermatogenesis is only incomplete, it cannot be used for this purpose (Nieschlag et al 1978, Kloer et al 1980).

2. *Intratesticular testosterone implantation* Theoreticallly, restitution of fertility is possible by implantation of testosterone into the testes (Hohlweg et al 1961, Hohlweg 1981). This approach is supported by the fact that androgen receptors responsible for maintaining spermato-genesis are available within the testes. However, the practicability of such an approach is question-able, since regular intratesticular testosterone applications will not be tolerated by the patient. Nevertheless, limited clinical experience exists in men with severe oligozoospermia after intratesti-cular injections of testosterone crystal suspensions (Laffont & Ezes 1948, Oshima et al 1977, Fahim et al 1979). Three months after intratesticular application of testosterone, a significant improve-ment in sperm count and/or sperm motility was observed in 44% of the men (Fahim et al 1979). Testicular biopsies showed no response in patients with tubular hyalinization and spermatogenic arrest at the stage of the spermato-cytes. In contrast, in cases of moderate tubular disturbances (desquamation and disorganization, or partial spermatogenic arrest) sperm count or sperm motility were improved. However, admin-istration of hCG or of antiestrogens would be a more physiological and easier way to increase intratesticular testosterone levels.

3. *High-dose androgen treatment to induce rebound phenomenon* For this type of treatment, 200–250 mg testosterone enanthate or cypionate intramuscularly twice weekly are recommended in order to suppress gonadotropin secretion and spermatogenesis until azoospermia ensues as illustrated in Figure 23.14. To determine azoospermia numerous semen analyses are neces-sary and a careful control of the patient is mandatory. Duration of treatment is around 5 months. After discontinuation of testosterone administration improvement in semen quality is

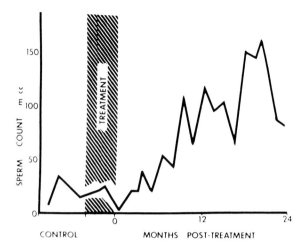

**Fig. 23.14**   The effect of testosterone 'rebound' treatment on sperm count of one patient. (For details see Rowley & Heller 1972.)

short (83% for only 2–3 months, 10% for 4–6 months, 7% for 12 months) and rebound to fertile levels is seen within 3–4 months following cessation of therapy. Improvement of sperm count may occur also at unpredictable intervals after withdrawal of treatment (Charny & Gordon 1978). In some patients rebound activation of spermatogenesis is seen up to 2 years after treatment (Heller et al 1950). Reproducibility of the rebound phenomenon has also been reported (Charny & Gordon 1978).

Table 23.10 summarizes the results of several groups using testosterone rebound therapy. A significant increase in sperm count was observed in 43% of the patients, while the conception rate was 16%. Controlled clinical studies are not available. Wang et al (1983) performed a double-blind crossover trial in 46 patients and demonstrated no

beneficial effect of high-dose testosterone treatment after induction of the rebound phenomenon.

Other authors have seen, in 2–9% of men with oligozoospermia below $20 \times 10^6$ spermatozoa/ml, permanently reduced sperm counts due to damage of the tubular architecture (sclerosis, hyalinization or fibrosis of the tubular wall) (Joel 1960, Tonutti et al 1960, Schirren 1961, Walsh & Amelar 1977). A similar disappointing experience was reported by Glezerman & Lunenfeld (1982).

In conclusion, since a further impairment of the fertility status of an infertile man cannot be excluded and therapy may thus be hazardous for the patient, use of rebound therapy for treatment of male infertility cannot be generally recommended.

*4. Low-dose androgen treatment*   For a long time low-dose androgen treatment was felt to be the only effective empirical therapy in oligozoospermia and asthenozoospermia. Since a direct tubular effect of exogenously administered androgens in therapeutic dosage cannot be completely excluded (Barwin 1982), but is not very probable, the only rationale for low-dose androgen medication of idiopathic oligozoospermia is a direct effect on the activity of the accessory sex glands and the epididymis. Androgen therapy is therefore possible in oligozoospermic and asthenozoospermic men with relative androgen deficiency or functional disturbances of the epididymis and the accessory sex glands (Harvey & Jackson 1957, Hornstein 1966, Schirren 1967, Dondero et al 1976). In case of androgen-sensitive insufficiency of the seminal

**Table 23.10**   Effect of testosterone rebound therapy on oligozoospermic men

| Reference | Patients (no.) | Improvement of sperm count | Pregnancies (no.) |
|---|---|---|---|
| Heckel & McDonald 1952 | 36 | 23 | 5 |
| Getzoff 1955 | 840 | 276 | 56 |
| Joel 1960 | 58 | 14 | 6 |
| Rowley & Heller 1972 | 163 | 110 | 67 |
| Lamensdorf et al 1975 | 145 | 85 | 39 |
| Charny & Gordon 1978 | 225 | 133 | 65 |
| Total | 1467 | 641(=43%) | 238(=16%) |

vesicles, decreased fructose levels would return to the normal range during androgen applications.

For low-dose androgen therapy the synthetic androgen mesterolone in a dose of 75 mg daily or testosterone undecanoate in a dose of 120 mg are recommended. Implantation of polydimethyl-siloxane capsules filled with dry crystalline testosterone, subcutaneously in the submamillary regions (Swyer 1953, Frick 1974, Frick et al 1976) is also possible. Therapeutic doses of the hormone are released for 13 months. Others do not suggest use of testosterone for treatment of male infertility, but do apply hCG in order to stimulate the functions of the epididymis and the accessory sex glands (Glezerman & Lunenfeld 1982).

Most publications report experience with treatment by mesterolone. The results are controver-

sial. Several authors found beneficial effect on sperm count and motility (Schellen & Beek 1972, Hendry et al 1973, Schirren 1973, Giarola 1974, Mauss 1974, Mudemann 1976, Glezerman et al 1978, Barwin 1982). Others could not confirm these results (Somazzi et al 1973, Keogh et al 1976, Jackamann et al 1977, Schill 1982b), and saw no statistical difference compared with placebo (WHO 1989). In a multicenter double-blind study a higher pregnancy rate was observed after doses of 150 mg mesterolone, but this was not statistically significant. Gerris et al (1991) performed a double-blind study in 52 patients with idiopathic oligozoospermia and/or terato-zoospermia. The patients received 150 mg mesterolone per day or placebo for 12 months. A significant increase in motility and in the proportion of normal-shaped spermatozoa was observed in both groups so that the usefulness of high-dose

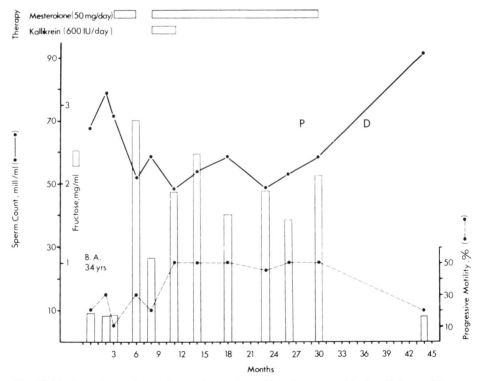

**Fig. 23.15** Low-dose androgen therapy in a patient with androgen-sensitive insufficiency of the seminal vesicles indicated by decreased seminal plasma fructose levels. Sperm count ($10^6$/ml), progressive motility (%) and fructose levels (mg/ml) are plotted. A pregnancy (P) followed by a spontaneous delivery (D) occurred during androgen medication. Normalization of fructose levels was observed after androgen medication which again decreased after withdrawal of therapy. (For details see Schill 1979a.)

mesterolone therapy on idiopathic male infertility was questioned. Nevertheless, this does not exclude positive effects of mesterolone on some individuals. Using testosterone undecanoate in a dose of 120 mg daily in a double-blind controlled trial, Pusch (1989) reported an improvement of semen parameters in patients with oligozoospermia. In contrast, Comhaire (1990) could not observe an effect in a double-blind study of patients with idiopathic oligozoospermia, asthenozoospermia or teratozoospermia who received high-dose therapy with 240 mg testosterone undecanoate.

There is agreement about the stimulatory effect of androgens on the secretory activity of the accessory sex glands. An increase in previously subnormal fructose production (< 1.2 mg/ml) in androgen-sensitive insufficiency of the seminal vesicles was reported (Schirren 1963, Mauss et al 1974, Schill 1976). After normalization of the decreased fructose levels by mesterolone (75 mg daily for 6 months or 75 mg from day 1 to day 16 of the female cycle) pregnancies sometimes occur (Schirren 1966, Schill 1978b, 1979a) as illustrated in Figure 23.15. Very probably the fertility-improving principle is not the increase in fructose concentrations per se, but the increase in another, so far unknown, seminal plasma factor which may be stimulated by androgen administration in the same way as fructose. Moreover, Hofmann (1988) points out that the use of androgens (mesterolone, testosterone undecanoate) is quite reasonable in cases of noninflammatory epididymal disorders and disturbed spermatozoal outlet. Androgens can be given to patients with vegetative dysregulation in addition to roborant measures, e.g. autogenous training.

5. *Special indication for androgen administration* Testosterone can also be used in the treatment of idiopathic delayed puberty to initiate puberty and ameliorate growth retardation (Nieschlag & Freischem 1982). Monthly injections of 250 mg testosterone enanthate for 3 months (Figure 23.16) are administered followed by another course of three injections 3–6 months later. In order to avoid premature epiphyseal closure, testosterone must be administered carefully. Because of this possible undesired effect Richman & Kirsch (1988) recommended low-dose testos

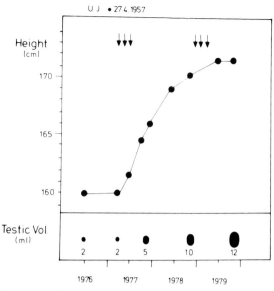

**Fig. 23.16**  Treatment of delayed puberty and growth retardation with testosterone enanthate. Each arrow indicates one injection of 250 mg testosterone enanthate given at monthly intervals. (Reproduced with permission from Nieschlag & Freischem 1982.)

terone therapy with 50 mg testosterone enanthate. They found it effective in the treatment of 15 boys with constitutional delay in growth and development who received this regimen for 1 year on average without compromising the final adult height.

In contrast, premature epiphyseal closure can be achieved in excessively tall boys with high testosterone doses administered at short intervals (Zachmann et al 1976). Treatment should start before the age of 14 and should last for 1 year.

Lastly, testosterone may be administered in advanced age in cases of androgen deficiency (Nieschlag & Freischem 1982).

***Side-effects***  During testosterone replacement therapy the following side-effects may be observed: weight gaining, acne vulgaris, and increase in red blood cell count and hemoglobin. There is no evidence of the induction of prostatic carcinoma by androgens; however, since growth of carcinoma is enhanced, regular examinations of the prostate are recommended during androgen therapy. Lastly, damage of the tubular

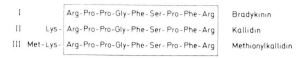

| I | | Arg-Pro-Pro-Gly-Phe-Ser-Pro-Phe-Arg | Bradykinin |
| II | Lys- | Arg-Pro-Pro-Gly-Phe-Ser-Pro-Phe-Arg | Kallidin |
| III | Met-Lys- | Arg-Pro-Pro-Gly-Phe-Ser-Pro-Phe-Arg | Methionylkallidin |

**Fig. 23.17**   Primary structure of kinins.

architecture in severe oligozoospermia cannot be excluded during testosterone rebound therapy.

## TISSUE HORMONE-RELEASING PROTEINASES

Tissue hormones are polypeptides which are liberated enzymatically from precursor molecules within the blood plasma. They belong to a class of biologically active substances that are not produced by specific glands like steroid hormones. The most prominent polypeptides are angiotensins and kinins, the latter including the nonapeptide bradykinin, the decapeptide kallidin and methionylkallidin (Fig. 23.17).

Kinins are involved in enhancing vascular permeability and lowering blood pressure, have pain-producing properties, stimulate smooth muscle contractions, and improve glucose transport through cell membranes (Erdös 1970, Meng & Haberland 1973, Wicklmayr et al 1978). Kinins also contribute to the vascular reactions of the carcinoid syndrome, hereditary angioedema and inflammation, where they are effective mediators. Involvement of the kinin system in cell proliferation of various tissues was shown (Rixon et al 1971, Haberland & Rohen 1973, Haberland et al 1975a, b, 1977). In addition, there is a close interrelation between the kinin system and coagulation and fibrinolysis, the complement system, the prostaglandin system, and the angiotensin–renin system (Erdös 1970, Fujii et al, 1979a, b).

Kinins are liberated from high and low molecular weight kininogens by kininogenases or kallikreins which are present in blood plasma and tissues, particularly in secretory glands (pancreas, submandibular glands, and kidneys) (Dietl et al 1978, Lemon et al 1979, Fink et al 1980). Kinins are biologically active in the nanogram range and have normally short life spans due to the rapid degradation by exopeptidases and endopeptidases, the kininases, which are present in blood plasma, body fluid, and tissue extracts. Two

kininases occur in human serum (kininases I and II) and degrade kinins to inactive polypeptides by cleavage of the C-terminal arginine residue or hydrolysis of the Pro–Phe bond between positions 7 and 8. Kininase II corresponds to the angiotensin-converting enzyme which occurs in highest concentrations within the secretory compartments of the male genital tract.

Liberation of kinins from kininogen is possible by kininogenases (kallikreins) with high substrate specificity, like organ kallikreins, and those with broad substrate specificity, like trypsin, plasmin and acrosin. One excellently characterized organ kallikrein is pancreatic kallikrein (EC 3.4. 2.1. 8), a glycoprotein with a molecular weight of approximately 36 000 daltons, which belongs to the class of serin proteinases. It is isolated from autolysed hog pancreas and shows multiple enzymatic forms due to its varying carbohydrate content (5–12%). Commercially available kallikrein preparations contain two molecular forms (kallikrein A and B) which differ in the composition of the carbohydrate portion, but not in the amino acid composition (232 amino acid residues) and the enzymatic properties (Fritz 1975). There is a close structural homology between hog pancreatic kallikrein and trypsin (Tschesche et al 1979).

Like sex hormones, kinins are natural mediators which, according to a series of experimental and animal studies, seem to be involved in reproductive functions by stimulating the transport of spermatozoa through the female genital tract by means of smooth muscle contractions of the uterus and activation of sperm motility. Kinins also seem to be involved in spermatogenesis by improving total sperm output. Together with the renin–angiotensin system, the kallikrein–kinin system is very probably involved in the paracrine regulation of testicular functions, particularly at the level of the Sertoli cell, where the occurrence of significant amounts of kallikrein has been demonstrated by Saitoh et al (1985).

The physiological significance of the kinin system in reproductive functions is supported by the fact that all components of this system are present in male and female genital secretions: low amounts of kininogen as specific substrate for kininogenases; kininases as the kinin-inactivating enzymes, and kinin-liberating proteinases, the kininogenases (Palm et al 1976, Fink & Schill 1983). As long as these three components are present in the body fluids, generation and inactivation of kinins take place continuously (Schill et al 1988).

As potent kininogenases within the genital tract the following proteinases must be discussed: a tissue kallikrein from the prostate, traces of kallikrein from the blood plasma, leukocytic proteinases, and the sperm-specific proteinase acrosin. The latter occurs in seminal plasma as an inactive enzyme–inhibitor complex. However, within the female genital tract the inhibitor is removed from the spermatozoa, and then acrosin released from disintegrating spermatozoa may activate vital sperm cells via liberation of kinins in the presence of ubiquitously occurring kininogen (Schill et al, 1979). Recently, the occurrence of tissue kallikrein in nanogram amounts could be identified in human seminal plasma (Fink & Schill 1983). Moreover, Miska et al (1991) were able to demonstrate intestinal absorption of orally administered porcine pancreatic kallikrein in 26 healthy volunteers by means of a highly sensitive bioluminescence-enhanced enzyme immunoassay.

Apart from major components of the kinin system, other substances are directly or indirectly involved in kinin generation or degradation: prekallikrein activator, inhibitors of kininases, and inhibitors of kallikreins, such as $\alpha_2$-macroglobulin, $C_1$-inactivator and $\alpha_1$-antitrypsin. Of these, only $\alpha_1$ proteinase inhibitor occurs in human seminal plasma. Since $\alpha_1$-proteinase inhibitor is a progressive type of kallikrein inhibitor, inactivation of kallikrein in the seminal plasma takes only slowly.

From the above data it can be concluded that the kinin system seems to play a certain physiological role within the reproductive tract and that alterations of the homeostasis of this system, e.g. low kininogenase levels, must be considered pathophysiological. This is supported by recent observations by Miska & Schill (1990) who demonstrated that sperm motility can be increased by addition of bradykinin to washed spermatozoa. In contrast, the kinin analogs Des-Arg-Bk and T-kinin from rats were unable to stimulate sperm motility. Therefore, exogenous administration of kininogenases like pancreatic kallikrein is considered a way to overcome a kininogenase deficiency.

***Patients suitable for treatment*** Idiopathic normogonadotrophic oligozoospermia, hypergonadotropic oligozoospermia, idiopathic asthenozoospermia, polyzoospermia, and mild teratozoospermia are all indications for treatment. Furthermore, the positive influence of kallikrein on varicocele orchiopathy before and after surgical or sclerosing therapy is known and supported by several studies (Schill 1983, Schroeder-Finck et al 1986, Micic et al 1990).

***Treatment schemes and results*** Pancreatic kallikrein can be administered either parenterally (40 KU three times weekly) (Fig. 23.18) or orally (600 KU daily) in the form of lacquer-coated tablets in order not to come into contact with the acid environment of the stomach, which would inactivate the enzyme. The treatment period is 3–6 months; in case of a positive response, long-term administration for 6–12 months is possible until conception occurs. At present, pancreatic kallikrein is available only in some countries.

Kallikrein therapy is empirical and there are no parameters available to predict whether it will be successful in a given individual. The best results are obtained in idiopathic forms of oligozoospermia and asthenozoospermia, whereas in spermatogenic arrest or severe tubular failure no effects are seen (for review see Schill 1982a). In some men with polyzoospermia normalization of sperm number is described (Stüttgen 1975); in men with mild teratozoospermia the number of morphologically abnormal spermatozoa is sometimes reduced (Hofmann et al 1975b, Schill 1975a).

Several open clinical trials have demonstrated improvement in total and progressive motility, an increase in the number of spermatozoa, and a slight improvement in the percentage of morphologically normal spermatozoa in about 30–50% of infertile men with idiopathic fertility disturbances. In asthenozoospermia (Fig. 23.19) improvement of fertility is the primary effect (Schill 1975a, Lunglmayr 1976, Schütte & Schirren 1977, Kamidono et al 1981). Sometimes a decrease in sperm count is found, but it stays within the

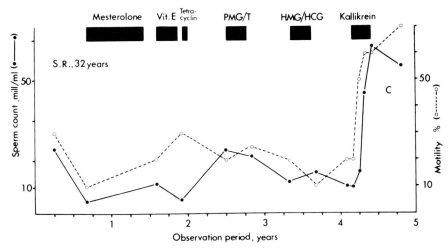

**Fig. 23.18**  Parenteral administration of pancreatic kallikrein (40 KU intramuscularly 3 times weekly) over a period of 3 months in a case of idiopathic.normogonadotropic oligozoospermia. Several agents were administered without any significant improvement of the semen parameters. Kallikrein led to a dramatic improvement of sperm count and sperm motility. A conception (C) occurred 3 months after withdrawal of the medication. (From Schill 1982a.)

normal range and will completely recover after cessation of therapy (Hommonai et al 1978b, Schill et al 1980). In oligozoospermia (Fig. 23.20) the number and/or motility of spermatozoa will be improved (Hofmann et al 1975b, Schill 1975a, 1978a, Schirren 1978, Sato et al 1979, Török 1979). Conception rates within an observation period of 1 year were found to be between 25% and 55%, whereas most pregnancies occurred within the first 5 months after initiation of therapy.

Four double-blind studies were performed in oligozoospermic patients. One study showed a significant increase in sperm count (Fig. 23.21) and sperm motility and a significant improvement ($P < 0.05$) in the conception rates (38%) compared to the placebo (16%) (Schill 1979b). Another double-blind study confirmed improve-

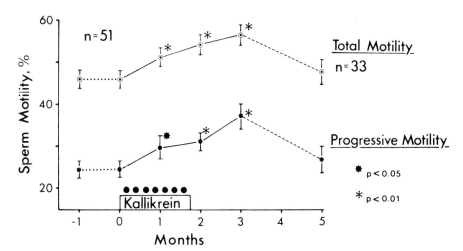

**Fig. 23.19**  Kallikrein therapy in 51 subfertile patients with idiopathic asthenozoospermia. Daily oral administration of 600 IU kallikrein over a period of 7 weeks. Mean values (± SE) of total and progressive sperm motility (%) are plotted. (Reproduced with permission from Kienitz and Schill 1977.)

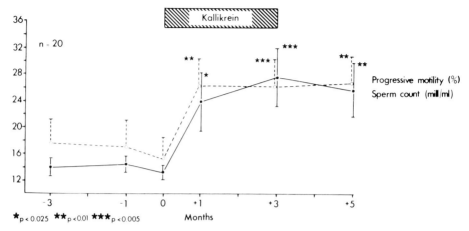

**Fig. 23.20**    Kallikrein treatment (600 KU/day) in 20 patients with idiopathic normogonatropic oligozoospermia ($< 20 \times 10^6$/ml) over a period of 3 months. Mean values ($\pm$ SE) of the sperm count ($10^6$/ml) and the progressive sperm motility (%) are plotted. (From Schill 1982b.)

ment in sperm count (Bedford & Elstein 1981), while the third study reported significantly more conceptions in the kallikrein group, compared to the placebo group (Propping et al 1978). In contrast, Nürnberger & Grassow (1977) were unable to show any effect of systemic kallikrein administration; however, the patient group was too small to draw any final conclusions. Further studies, both randomized and controlled, confirmed a positive effect of kallikrein in patients with oligozoospermia and asthenozoospermia (Berzin et al 1987, Giovenco et al 1987, Saitoh et al 1987).

Micic (1988) observed a pregnancy rate of 32% in patients with genital tract infections who had received combined therapy with kallikrein and antibiotics, while it was only 17% in the group who had been treated with antibiotics alone.

***Side-effects***    Side-effects of kallikrein therapy

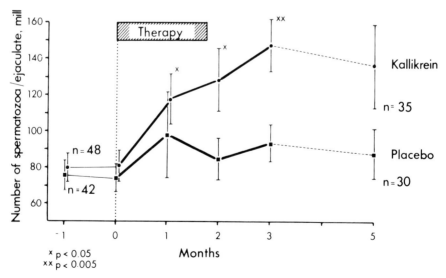

**Fig. 23.21**    Double-blind study in 90 subfertile patients with idiopathic oligozoospermia ($< 40 \times 10^6$/ml) treated over a period of 7 weeks either with placebo or with kallikrein (600 KU/day). Mean values ($\pm$ SE) of the total sperm output ($10^6$/ejaculate) are plotted. (For details see Schill 1979b.)

are rare and include vertigo, diarrhea, allergic eruptions, and exacerbation of chronic male genital tract infections with development of acute prostatitis or epididymitis due to kinin liberation. These may be treated effectively.

As kallikrein is a potent mediator of inflammation, intratesticular inflammations that are otherwise not recognizable in the ejaculate may intensify and lead to reduced sperm quality (Schroeder-Finckh et al 1986). Thus, kallikrein may be used not only therapeutically but also diagnostically with regard to different inflammatory testicular disorders (Hofmann 1981).

## METHYLXANTHINES

Methylxanthine derivatives, such as caffeine and theophylline, are well known for their phosphodiesterase inhibitory activity interfering with the intracellular cAMP level of different cell systems. For example, caffeine is experimentally used to stimulate sperm metabolism and motility of fresh and frozen spermatozoa (Schill 1975b, Barkay et al 1977, Schill et al 1977). Another methylxanthine derivative is pentoxifylline (Fig. 23.22) which has been found suitable for systemic application in infertile men (Aparicio 1979). The substance can be given orally or by infusion intravenously. In clinical medicine, pentoxifylline is widely used for the treatment of vascular diseases, improving circulation and metabolism by influencing the flow properties of erythrocytes (Hess et al 1973). It also seems to improve disturbed microcirculation in the testis and epididymis (Heite & Koschnicke 1979).

***Patients suitable for treatment*** Idiopathic asthenozoospermia, and oligozoospermia due to a reduced testicular blood microcirculation are indications for treatment.

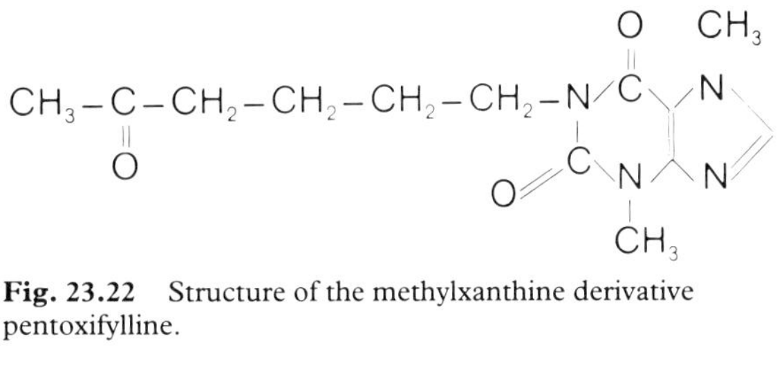

**Fig. 23.22** Structure of the methylxanthine derivative pentoxifylline.

***Treatment schemes and results*** Oral administration of 1.2 g pentoxifylline daily for a period of 3–6 months is used.

In idiopathic asthenozoospermia a significant improvement of the percentage of forwardly progressive spermatozoa was first described by Aparicio & coworkers (1980a,b) in 15 men. This was confirmed by Schill (1982c) in 25 asthenozoospermic patients (Fig. 23.23). Seven (28%) of the patients showed a significant increase in progressive motility. The conception rate was 37%.

In oligozoospermia, Heite & Koschnicke (1979) reported a significant increase in sperm count, sperm motility and sperm morphology in 44 men after 4–9 months' administration of pentoxifylline. Schramm (1981) confirmed these positive effects of pentoxifylline in oligozoospermia. In contrast, Schill (1982c) found no improvement in semen parameters in 40 patients with idiopathic normogonadotropic oligozoospermia ($< 20 \times 10^6$ spermatozoa/ml) after 3 months' treatment with pentoxifylline. There was only a small statistically significant increase in the ejaculate volume and the seminal plasma fructose level during pentoxifylline therapy. The conception rate was 17%, in the range of the spontaneous pregnancy rates. During a 6-month therapy with daily doses of 1200 mg pentoxifylline, Marrama et al (1985) observed a significant improvement in sperm count and motility in 22 men with idiopathic oligoasthenozoospermia.

Yovich et al (1990) described a PROST (pronuclear stage tubal transfer) or TEST (tubal embryo stage transfer) program in which pentoxifylline was added to the semen samples prior to insemination. The study included 57 couples with male factor infertility due to oligozoospermia. Compared to the controls in which pentoxifylline had not been added, a significant improvement in sperm motility and progressive motility and a higher fertilization rate with 17 pregnancies were achieved (30%). Thus, addition of pentoxifylline to semen samples of asthenozoospermic and oligozoospermic men may be of value when methods of assisted reproduction are considered.

***Side-effects*** During pentoxifylline administration side-effects such as vertigo, headache,

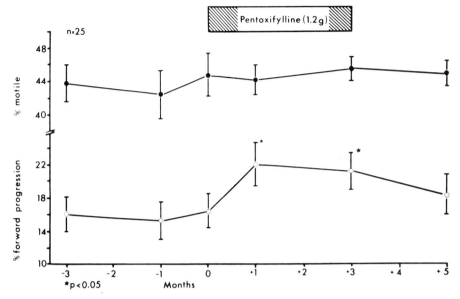

**Fig. 23.23**    Pentoxifylline treatment (1.2 g/day) in 25 subfertile patients with idiopathic asthenozoospermia over a period of 3 months. Mean values (± SE) of the total and progressive sperm motility (%) are plotted. (Reproduced with permission from Schill 1982c.)

nausea, and flatulence may be observed, but are rare. Acute epididymitis was seen in one patient, probably as a result of an improved blood circulation with exacerbation of a silent male genital tract infection.

## ANTIINFLAMMATORY AGENTS

Since acute and chronic male genital tract infections are known to impair male fertility, diagnosis and treatment of inflammatory reactions are an important task in the management of infertility. A review of the literature about diagnosis and success of treatment was given by Nahoum (1982).

***Patients suitable for treatment*** Adequate criteria to select patients for treatment of male genital tract infections remain to be established (Nahoum 1982). Likewise, Comhaire et al (1986) pointed out that features of male accessory gland infection may regress spontaneously and are not influenced by doxycycline treatment. Eggert-Kruse et al (1988) concluded from their studies that microbial colonization is of minor importance for sperm–mucus interaction and that the benefits of antimicrobial therapy in asymptomatic

couples are limited. Pathogenic microorganisms in semen or prostatic-vesicular fluid, abnormalities as shown by rectal examination, altered exfoliative cytology, pyospermia, viscosipathy, agglomeration phenomena, asthenozoospermia, and decreased secretory functions of the accessory sex glands may be indicative of an inflammatory response (Eliason et al 1966, Comhaire et al 1980; see Chapters 7 and 11).

Recently, Sanchez et al (1990) pointed out that mollicutes may cause significant alterations in sperm tails so that antibiotic therapy is recommended in case of mollicute involvement. After treatment with doxycyline or erythromycin a significant improvement in sperm morphology could be observed.

***Treatment schemes and results*** For the treatment of inflammatory reactions two classes of substances are available: antibiotics and antiphlogistics.

*Antibiotics* The selection of an antibiotic for treatment is dependent on the antibiogram. However, in most cases, clinical experience will determine the use of a suitable antibiotic. Tetracyclines are by far the most suitable and are used as first choice for treatment, particularly if

**Table 23.11**  Antimicrobial therapy of male adnexitis

*Non-gonorrhoic adnexitis:*
1. Classic tetracyclines
   — Tetracycline, oxytetracycline daily 1.5–2.0 g
   — Doxycycline daily 200 mg
   — Minocycline daily 200 mg
   — Methacycline daily 600 mg
2. Cotrimoxazole daily 320 mg trimethoprim + 1.6 g sulfamethoxazole
3. Erythromycin daily 1.5–2.0 g
4. Gyrase inhibitors daily 0.8–1 g
also possible:    semisynthetic oral penicillins e.g. ampicillin daily 2–4 g
                  thiamphenicol daily 1.5 g
                  Duration of treatment: 7–28 days
*Gonorrhoic adnexitis:*
   Penicillin G daily $4 \times 10^6$ IU + probenecid daily 1 g
   Duration of treatment: 3 days but according to the clinical situation even longer
*Adnexitis by trichomonas:*
   Metronidazole daily 500 mg for 6 days

culture and sensitivity studies are not yet completed. The duration of therapy is 1–2 weeks in higher dosage followed by 2 weeks in lower dosage. In addition, gyrase inhibitors (ofloxacin, norfloxacin, ciprofloxacin) have been found to be effective (Schill 1986a, Comhaire 1987). If pathogenic germs are the cause of inflammation simultaneous treatment of the female partner is recommended. The achievement of a sufficient concentration of the antibiotic in the secretions of the male accessory sex glands is very important.

Depending on the cause of the male adnexitis, three etiopathological forms may be determined: nongonorrhoic and gonorrhoic adnexitis, and adnexitis caused by *Trichomonas vaginalis*. Table 23.11 summarizes the different chemotherapeutics available for the treatment of male adnexitis. They are used in all cases where pathogenic microorganisms are found or cannot be excluded.

*Antiphlogistics* Antibiotic and antiphlogistic drugs are a common combination utilized in the treatment of chronic bacterial and chronic

**Table 23.12**  Sperm parameters in 22 patients with chronic epididymitis before and after treatment

|  | No.(mill/ml) | Mot.(%) | Mot. 1(%) | nForm(%) |
| --- | --- | --- | --- | --- |
| Before therapy | | | | |
| Mean value | 19.2 | 29.3 | 10.3 | 16.2 |
| SD | 20.5 | 16.0 | 15.7 | 10.6 |
| After therapy | | | | |
| Mean value | 25.3 | 40.5 | 24.8 | 17.5 |
| SD | 24.5 | 16.0 | 18.9 | 10.8 |
| P < | — | 0.025 | 0.005 | — |

|  | Spd(%) | Leuko (mill/ml) | Macro (mill/ml) | Flp (%) | Fl1a (%) |
| --- | --- | --- | --- | --- | --- |
| Before therapy | | | | | |
| Mean value | 7.1 | 2.4 | 2.1 | 70.0 | 52.6 |
| SD | 3.5 | 2.0 | 1.2 | 16.4 | 13.2 |
| After therapy | | | | | |
| Mean value | 5.9 | 0.7 | 0.9 | 58.3 | 32.3 |
| SD | 2.8 | 0.8 | 0.7 | 15.1 | 12.1 |
| P < | — | 0.05 | 0.001 | 0.025 | 0.001 |

No., Concentration of spermatozoa; Mot., global motility; Mot. 1, progressive motility; nForm, portion of normal-shaped spermatozoa (including flagella); Spd, portion of spermatids; Leuco, concentration of leukocytes; Macro, concentration of macrophages; Flp, portion of pathological flagella; Fl1a, flagella with abnormal staining (% of Flp). (From Raidl 1990.)

abacterial nonacute types of prostatitis (Hommonai et al 1975). Treatment should last for a period of at least 2–4 weeks. In inflammatory epididymal diseases where macrophages are involved, nonsteroidal antiphlogistic therapy is recommended in addition to antibiotic treatment in order to prevent local occlusions and the induction of local immunity phenomena (Haidl 1990). After combined antiphlogistic and antibiotic treatment of 22 patients with chronic epididymal infection, a significant increase in sperm motility and progressive motility accompanied by a significant decrease in leukocytes and macrophages as well as of epididymis-related flagellar disturbances was observed (Haidl 1990) (Table 23.12).

The indication for additional antiphlogistic therapy is supported by studies with experimentally induced epididymal *Escherichia coli* infections in rats. After a few days, no pathogens could be identified; however, numerous leukocytes and macrophages were found (Weidner et al 1989). Furthermore, nonsteroidal antiphlogistic therapy is indicated for patients with inflammatory testicular damage. Barkay et al (1984) observed an improvement in sperm count and motility after administration of indomethacin and ketoprofen for 60 days. The antiphlogistic drugs diclofenac, indomethacin and aspirin are used for 3–6 weeks (Barkay et al 1984, Schroeder-Finckh et al 1986).

The available antiphlogistic drugs for treatment of male genital tract inflammations are shown in Table 23.13. Antiinflammatory therapy will improve semen quality and fertility. In the case of chronic noninfectious orchitis, beneficial effects of 30 mg prednisolone daily for a period of 2 weeks followed by a slow reduction of the glucocorti-

**Table 23.13** Antiphlogistic drugs for the therapy of noninfectious male adnexitis

Acetylsalicylic acid daily 3–6 g
Phenylbutazone daily 400–600 mg
Oxyphenylbutazone daily 400–600 mg
Indomethacin daily 100–150 mg
Ibuprofen daily 600–1200 mg
Diclofenac daily 100 mg
Ketoprofen daily 100–150 mg
Naproxene daily 500–750 mg
Glucocorticoids (prednisolone) daily 7–30 mg

coids have been reported (Hofmann & Kuwert 1979).

***Side-effects*** Occasionally diarrhea and nausea are observed; during long-term treatment transient impairment of semen quality cannot be excluded.

## IMMUNOSUPPRESSIVE AGENTS

Treatment of immunological infertility in the male is still experimental (see Chapters 14 and 22). The following possibilities are available:

1. In cases of genital infection causing immunological disorders antibiotic treatment is preferred.
2. In cases of unilateral chronic epididymitis or epididymoorchitis the organ should be removed by surgery (see Chapter 24).
3. Antibodies in seminal plasma can be removed by washing the spermatozoa followed by intrauterine insemination (see Chapter 25).
4. Testosterone rebound therapy with transitory suppression of spermatogenesis leading to a temporary decrease of the antibody titers.
5. Immunosuppressive therapy by low- and high-dose glucocorticoids or azathioprine.

A detailed review of all problems involved in immunological infertility was published by Friberg (1982).

***Patients suitable for treatment*** Treatment of male patients with antispermatozoal antibodies in the seminal fluid (rather than in the serum) is suggested (WHO 1987). Recently, however, assisted reproductive technologies are preferred in these patients.

***Treatment schemes and results*** *Corticosteroids* Low-dose corticosteroid therapy with 10–20 mg prednisolone daily for 3–6 months is questionable. High-dose corticosteriod medication is being experimentally studied; it seems to be more efficient in the treatment of immunological male infertility. Shulman (1976) administered a daily dosage of 96 mg methylprednisolone orally for a period of 7 days. The beneficial effects of high-dose corticosteroid therapy on the spermiogram and the cervical mucus penetration ability of spermatozoa was confirmed by Kremer & coworkers (1978), Hendry & coworkers (1979).

and Fredricsson (1988). Alexander et al (1983) applied 60 mg prednisone for 7–21 days to 24 patients with circulating antisperm antibodies and observed significantly more pregnancies in the treated group as compared to a control group. There were no changes in sperm counts, motility and morphology, but significant reductions in the levels of circulating immobilizing and agglutinating antisperm antibodies were achieved.

Hargreave & Elton (1982) recommend 2 mg betamethasone for 3 days, followed by 1 mg or 0.5 mg for another 2 days. In a small randomized clinical trial de Almeida et al (1985) did not observe any effect of prednisolone therapy (1 mg/kg/day for 9 days over 3 cycles) except for a slight decrease in the titer of seminal antibodies. Hinting et al (1989), too, questioned the effectiveness of steroids in the presence of antispermatozoal antibodies and therefore recommended in vitro fertilization (IVF).

Since the maximum decrease in the serum immunoglobulins is observed 2–3 weeks after initiation of corticosteroid medication, a short-term therapy adapted to the female cycle is recommended. Thus, methylprednisolone is administered during the 15th to 21st day of the female cycle. Three consecutive cycles of treatment are recommended.

*Azathioprine* Initial dosage is 100 mg azathioprine daily for 1–3 months. Depending on the reduction in serum antibody titer, the dosage may be slowly decreased to 50 mg azathioprine daily. Treatment may be continued for months until pregnancy occurs. During therapy, the patient must be carefully monitored with respect to leukocytes, infections, etc.

Azathioprine was once used for the reduction of circulating sperm antibodies until a pregnancy occurred (Krause & Meyhöfer 1973). During the treatment the antibody titer decreased considerably from initially 1 : 1024 to zero. Since this form of therapy is not of vital interest for the patient and may have hazardous side-effects, azathioprine should be administered only in very special cases.

**Side-effects** For corticosteroid therapy side-effects and contraindications are the same as for other forms of corticosteroid medication (diabetes, hypertension, infections, etc.)

Azathioprine should be handled with extreme care, with regular blood monitoring. Side-effects will be those of general immunosuppression.

## DRUGS AFFECTING AUTONOMOUS NERVOUS SYSTEM

Contractions of the smooth muscles of the vas deferens, the accessory sex glands, and the closure of the bladder neck to allow seminal emission into the posterior urethra and antegrade ejaculation, are predominantly regulated by sympathetic innervation. In addition to adrenergic receptors, small numbers of parasympathetic cholinergic receptors are also found in this part of the genital tract (Glezerman et al 1976).

In case of a temporary or permanent deficiency of the sympathetic innervation, either retrograde ejaculation with propulsion of seminal fluid from the posterior urethra into the bladder will occur, or transport of the secretions of the accessory sex glands and the vas deferens will be completely absent. A number of drugs have been used in order to improve the smooth muscle functions of the accessory sex glands, the vas deferens and particularly the bladder neck. The mode of action of these drugs is either to increase the sympathetic activity or to decrease the parasympathetic activity at the bladder neck (Stockamp et al 1974, Kragt & Schellen 1978). A further approach is the increase of the spermatozoal output by drugs affecting the autonomous nervous system. Yamamoto et al (1986) found an increase in sperm output and seminal volume in 16 out of 20 patients after oral administration of an $\alpha_1$-blocker (Bunazosin, 2 mg/day) and a $\beta$-stimulator (procaterol 100 µg/day). The increase in sperm output was referred to relaxation of myoid cells leading to dilatation of stenotic areas of seminiferous tubules.

Most experience in the treatment of retrograde ejaculation has been gained with sympathomimetic medication producing $\alpha$-adrenergic stimulation particularly in patients with bladder neck incompetence resulting from retroperitoneal lymph node dissection (Schill 1986a). Anticholinergic medication shows similar effects due to a decreased parasympathetic activity and a relatively increased sympathetic tone in the bladder neck. However, it is most effective in patients with retrograde ejaculation due to diabetes mellitus.

*Patients suitable for treatment* Retrograde ejaculation or absence of emission or ejaculation due to different causes (see Collins 1982) are indications for treatment.

*Treatment schemes and results* Retrieval of semen from the bladder and subsequent instrumental insemination is described in detail in Chapter 25. Emission of semen and bladder neck closure is possible by α-adrenergic stimulation using sympathomimetic medication. Antegrade ejaculation is achieved by the following chemicals:

1. Alpha-sympathomimetic drugs:
   a. Phenylpropanolamine 1 capsule twice daily (Stewart & Bergant 1974)
   b. Oxedrine 60 mg intravenously (Stockamp et al 1974)
   c. Midodrine $3 \times 5$ mg orally for 10 days (Jonas et al 1979) or $5-15$ mg intravenously. (Schwale et al 1980, Schill 1986b)
   d. Imipramine $25-50$ mg daily (Kelly & Needle 1979, Nijman et al 1981)
2. Anticholinergic drugs:
   Brompheniramine 8 mg twice daily (Andraloro & Dube 1975) or three times daily.

Antegrade ejaculation is easily achieved even by oral medication in patients with minimal sympathetic dysfunction (e.g. diabetic lesions). With more pronounced disturbances (e.g. retroperitoneal lymphadenectomy) parenteral administration is the only possibility to produce antegrade ejaculation. Successful treatment with pregnancies has occasionally been reported (Glezerman et al 1976, Thiagarajah et al 1978, Schill 1990).

*Side-effects* Alpha-sympathomimetic drugs may induce acute hypertension and bradycardia. In case of emergency 10 mg phentolamine will normalize blood pressure and cardiac rhythm.

## PSYCHOTROPIC DRUGS

Knowledge of the use of psychotropic agents for improvement of male fertility is scanty. In contrast, more is known about the fertility—and sexuality-inhibiting effects—of psychopharmacological compounds (Benkert 1980, Przybilla & Schill 1981).

Blair et al (1962) reported a positive influence of the monoamine oxidase inhibitor phenelzine sulphate on sperm production during treatment of schizophrenic patients. Later, Vogel & Braun-Falco (1971) described beneficial effects of the antidepressant amitryptyline (30 mg daily for $4-6$ weeks) on sperm count and ejaculate volume in men with oligozoospermia. It is speculated that amitryptyline would stimulate the voidance of the epididymal sperm reservoir.

Controlled clinical trials are urgently required to properly evaluate the effect of psychotropic drugs on human semen parameters.

In general, psychopharmacological agents, spasmolytics, and tranquilizers could exert an influence via an improvement of the smooth muscle contractions of the epididymis, the vas deferens, and the accessory sex glands. In addition, central nervous effects have to be considered, such as alteration of the brain dopamine turnover or interference with specific dopamine receptors.

Psychotropic drugs like diazepam can occasionally be used as a kind of supporting therapy in infertile patients with disturbances at the level of the vegetative nervous system or due to functional disorders induced by emotional stress (Hornstein 1971). However, it is not possible to give any general recommendations for treatment with this kind of pharmacological agents.

## NEW THERAPEUTICAL APPROACHES

A number of pharmacological compounds are currently under clinical evaluation for their potency to improve the fertility status of certain patients. Most of these investigations are Phase-One studies. It will be important for the future of our patients whether the reported positive results are confirmed and extended by other authors. Particularly necessary, however, is the performance of double-blind studies in order to discriminate between real pharmacological and placebo effects.

Positive effects on sperm count and/or sperm

motility in oligozoospermia are claimed to be exerted by the following compounds:

## Aromatase inhibitors

Teslac ($\Delta^1$-testolactone) is an inhibitor of testosterone aromatization blocking the conversion of testosterone to estradiol and of androstenedione to estrone (Siiteri & Thompson 1975). The application of inhibitors of testosterone aromatization is based on the postulate that estradiol may play a role in regulating human spermatogenesis since it appears to directly inhibit spermatogenesis in the rat (Kalla et al 1980). Estradiol may also indirectly inhibit spermatogenesis by preventing the Leydig cells from maximal production of testosterone in response to LH. Therefore, decrease of estradiol formation might lead to an improvement in both sperm count and fertility in patients with infertility due to oligozoospermia.

During preliminary investigations Teslac therapy caused a fall in serum estradiol and estrone levels of 34% and 41%, respectively, and a rise in serum testosterone and androstenedione of 47% and 70%, respectively, in ten men with idiopathic normogonadotropic oligozoospermia (Vigerski & Glass 1981). Sperm density rose from 10.8 to $19.8 \times 10^6$/ml and total sperm count from 26.8 to $60.6 \times 10^6$/ml. There was no significant change in motility or semen volume. Similar results were reported by Dony et al (1986) who achieved pregnancy in two of nine cases. Likewise, Schill et al (1987) observed a significant increase in sperm count, total sperm output and absolute number of motile and progressively motile spermatozoa in 13 subfertile men after treatment with 1 g testolactone for 3–6 months; the fertility rate was 17%. In contrast, Schütte (1989) did not see any positive effect of testolactone therapy.

New inhibitors with a 1000-fold higher potency are currently being tested and will soon be available for clinical trials (Leschber et al 1989).

## Antiserotonin agents

Animal experiments demonstrated that short- and long-term administration of serotonin (5-hydroxy-tryptamine) to mature rats and mice was followed by tubular and intratubular damage to the testis (Liu & Kinson 1973). The damage resembled ischemic lesions caused by occlusion of the testicular artery. In humans, levels of serotonin and its metabolite 5-hydroxyindole acetic acid (5-HIAA) were found to be elevated in infertile men with oligozoospermia and azoospermia (Segal et al 1975). Thus, serotonin seems to play an etiopathological role in male infertility. It may cause testicular damage or impaired spermatogenesis through constriction of testicular vessels, inhibition of androgen production, or alteration of prostaglandin metabolism.

This prompted studies with treatment of a selected group of infertile patients with high serotonin levels by a serotonin antagonist, cyproheptadine HCl, 4 mg three times daily for two courses of 90 days each. Improvement of sperm count and motility was achieved in 33–55% of the men (Segal 1978).

The mechanism whereby serotonin affects the testis is unclear. However, serotonin antagonists probably act by reducing serotonin uptake, but their effect on the brain serotonin and its antihistaminic properties must also be taken into account.

## Ketotifen

The occurrence of numerous mast cells associated with the boundary tissue of the seminiferous tubules was shown in infertile men in contrast to healthy males (Behrendt et al 1981, Maseki et al 1981). The increase of mast cells is accompanied by a loss of ATPase activity of the specialized fibroblast layer of the boundary tissue as well as by a thickening and/or splitting of the basal lamina underlying the seminiferous epithelium. This finding indicates that there is a correlation between mast cell proliferation and blood–testis barrier dysfunction. Therefore, the effect of ketotifen (an inhibitor of histamine release from mast cells) on the semen parameters of infertile men was investigated. Clinical results indicate particularly beneficial effects on the spermiogram of patients with chronic noninfectious orchitis of different etiology (Hofmann et al 1982). Minor side-effects such as fatigue were reported and attention should be paid to alcohol incompatibility. In 17 patients with normogonadotropic oligozoospermia Schill et al (1986) observed a moderate, but statistically significant, improvement of sperm density after 3 months' therapy with ketotifen. In another group of 22 patients with idiopathic asthenozoospermia a significant increase in sperm count and progressive and total motility was achieved. The usual dosage is 1 mg twice daily for 3–6 months. However, double-blind studies have not been performed so far.

## Nucleotides

Some nucleotides, such as adenosine triphosphate (ATP) are essential for sperm motility providing energy for metabolic processes of the germ cell (Nelson 1975). Other nucleotides (GTP, UTP) are important during sperm formation providing the energy necessary for protein synthesis (Hoskins & Casillas 1975). These important functions of nucleotides initiated studies regarding their usefulness in the therapy of oligoasthenozoospermia. A neonatal calf extract derived from heart/lymph node tissue, rich in amino acids and deoxyribosil nucleotides, was administered to 227 men with oligoasthenozoospermia of various etiology including a placebo group (Menchini-Fabris & Mariani 1982). The patients received 2 ml of the preparation intramuscularly for 20 days followed by a rest period of 10 days. This scheme was repeated over a period of 3 months. The semen analyses showed an effect on sperm count and motility. It is suggested that this preparation exerts its action by providing a substrate for the meiotic process and by providing energy-rich compounds utilized in flagellar movement. The authors observed also an increase of pregnancies in the treated group. Future studies should give information whether the reported positive effects really are the consequence of the treatment.

## Zinc

Since high concentrations of zinc are found in the testes and the accessory sex glands of various animals and man, it was suggested that zinc might play an important role in the reproductive physiology of vertebrates. This is supported by the observation that certain cases of nutritional dwarfism with hypogonadism in man are associated with zinc deficiency and that zinc administration reverses both disorders (Prasad et al 1963). However, little is known about plasma zinc levels in infertile males (Hartoma et al 1977). Treatment of male fertility disorders with zinc can be performed as combination therapy with ketotifen in the indications mentioned above, because zinc deficiency may be detrimental to the maturation and motility of spermatozoa and because zinc is thought to stimulate immunity in a hitherto unknown way (Chvapil 1973, Srivastava et al 1983, Hofmann 1988). Zinc may also be given in cases of strong exfoliation of immature cells of spermatogenesis; the cytoplasm of the exfoliated cells is abundant in zinc which is normally reabsorbed intratesticularly but is lost by exfoliation (Kruczynski & Passia 1986).

Furthermore, zinc is indicated for treatment of secretory dysfunction of the prostate and vesicular glands (Hofmann 1988). It is administered as zinc aspartate 50 mg twice daily for 3–6 months. Netter et al (1981) treated 37 oligozoospermic men with plasma zinc levels within the low normal range by application of 120 mg of zinc sulfate twice daily over a period of 40–50 days. The patients were subdivided into two groups according to the basal plasma testosterone level (group I below 4.8 ng/ml, group II over 4.8 ng/ml). In group I zinc therapy significantly increased plasma levels of zinc and testosterone as well as the sperm count (from $8 \times 10^6$/ml to $20 \times 10^6$/ml). Group II showed only a significant increase in plasma testosterone level and sperm count. Nine pregnancies occurred in group I and none in group II. Kynaston et al (1988) observed a significant improvement in sperm motility in 33 patients with idiopathic asthenozoospermia and/or oligozoospermia after administration of 220 mg zinc sulfate twice daily for 3 months. More studies are necessary to confirm these data. The only available experimental data are animal studies showing depression of spermatogenesis during zinc deprivation (Trentini et al 1968). In contrast, impotence during chronic renal failure is alleviated and plasma testosterone increases under zinc therapy (Antoniou et al 1977, Mahajan et al 1979).

## Captopril

Treatment with captopril was described by Parsch & Schill (1988) as an alternative or additive means of interfering with the kinin system. Captopril inhibits angiotensin converting enzyme (ACE = kininase II) and thereby improves kinin levels within the male genital tract secretion. In a comparison of 50 mg captopril versus placebo ($n = 58$) for 3 months, a significant increase in the number of spermatozoa was observed in patients with oligozoospermia and asthenozoospermia, which may indicate a possible involvement of the angiotensin system within the paracrine regulation of spermatogenesis. Further studies are required to confirm this treatment concept. Contraindications to captopril therapy are inflammatory testicular or adnexal diseases.

## Vitamin E

Treatment of male fertility disorders with the antioxidant vitamin E, as previously performed, is now under discussion again (Engel et al 1985). It is known that spermatozoa may be damaged by peroxidation of endogenous phospholipids, which results in decreased motility. An improved motility of spermatozoa in patients with asthenozoospermia was observed by Engel et al (1985) after oral administration of 300–600 mg vitamin E daily for 6 weeks. Aitken & Clarkson (1988) reported that the damaging influence of centrifugation on the spermatozoal membrane during sperm preparation was reduced by the addition of vitamin E to the culture medium. Furthermore, a significant improvement in sperm–oocyte fusion was observed.

## Vitamin $B_{12}$

Vitamin $B_{12}$ is thought to be effective in the treatment of oligozoospermia (Sandler & Faragher 1984). After administration of Mecobalamin (vitamin $B_{12}$) to mice with experimentally induced oligozoospermia, Oshio et al (1989) observed an increase in sperm count and motility and in the diameter of the seminiferous tubules when compared to a control group.

## CONCLUDING REMARKS

In this chapter, various methods of treatment of different types of male infertility are summarized. Some approaches appear to be rational and based on known mechanisms, others are empirical and may be subjected to scientific critique.

To improve the results of therapy we must strive to better understand the pathophysiology of male infertility. This will, we hope, lead to the development of new therapies rendering the treatment more effective and predictable. At present, there is general agreement that, despite the rather wide spectrum of agents available, the results of andrological therapy are rather poor. Nevertheless, when all available therapeutic approaches are consistently and logically applied, conception rates of 30–40% may be expected (Schill 1982d) and this is over and above the spontaneous conception rate which was determined to be between 10% and 20% (Broer et al 1977, Schill 1979b, Freischem et al 1982).

## REFERENCES

Aitken R J, Clarkson J S 1988 Significance of reactive oxygen species and antioxidants in defining the efficacy of sperm preparation techniques. J Androl 9: 367

Alexander N J, Sampson J H, Fulgham D L 1983 Pregnancy rates in patients treated for antisperm antibodies with prednisone. Int J Fertil 28: 63

Andraloro V A, Dube A 1975 Treatment of retrograde ejaculation with brompheniramine. Urology 5: 520

Anton J P, Gueguen J, Genet P, Patoiseau J Y 1968 Etude de 26 cas d'azoospermies et d'oligoasthenospermies traites par les gonadotrophines humaines extraites durines de femmes menopausées (hMG). Gynecol Obset 67: 509

Antoniou C D, Shalhoub R J, Sudhakar T, Smith J C Jr. 1977 Reversal of uraemic impotence by zinc. Lancet ii: 895

Aparicio N 1979 Therapeutical use of pentoxifylline in disturbed male fertility. Singapore Med J 20 (suppl 1): 43

Aparicio N J, Schwarzstein L, Turner E A, Turner D, Mancini R, Schally A V 1976 Treatment of idiopathic normogonadotropic oligoasthenospermia with synthetic luteinizing hormone–releasing hormone. Fertil Steril 27: 549

Aparicio N J, de Turner E A, Schwarzstein L, Turner D 1980a Effect of the phosphodiesterase inhibitor pentoxifylline on human sperm motility. Andrologia 12: 49

Aparicio N J, Schwarzstein L, de Turner E A 1980b Pentoxifylline (BL 191) by oral administration in the treatment of asthenozoospermia. Andrologia 12: 228

Asch R, Heitmen T O, Gilley R M, Tice T R 1986 Preliminary results on the effects of testosterone microcapsules. In: Zatuchni G I, Goldsmith A, Spieler J M, Sciarra J J (eds) Male contraception: advances and future prospects. Harper and Row, London, pp 347–360

Aulitzky W, Frick J, Hadziselimovic F 1989 Pulsatile L4RH therapy in patients with oligozoospermia and disturbed LH pulsatility. Int J Androl 12: 265

Bain J, Hafez E S E 1980 Diagnosis in andrology. Martinus Nijhoff, The Hague.

Bain J, Moskowitz J P, Clapp J J 1978 LH and FSH response to gonadotropin releasing hormone (GnRH) in normospermic, oligospermic and azoospermic men. Arch Androl 1: 147

Bain J, Schill W B, Schwarzstein L 1982 Treatment of male infertility. Springer, Berlin

Bals-Pratsch M, Knuth U A, Hönigl W, Klein H M, Bergmann M, Nieschlag E 1989 Pulsatile GnRH therapy in oligozoospermic men does not improve seminal parameters despite decreased FSH levels. Clin Endocrinol 30: 549

Bandhauer K, Frick J 1982 Disturbances in male fertility. Springer, Berlin

Barkay J, Zuckerman H, Sklan D, Gordon S 1977 Effect of caffeine on increasing the motility of frozen human sperm. Fertil Steril 28: 175

Barkay J, Harpaz-Kerpel S, Ben-Ezra S, Gordon S, Zuckerman H 1984 The prostaglandin inhibitor effect of antiinflammatory drugs in the therapy of male infertility. Fertil Steril 42: 406

Bartsch G, Frick J 1974 Therapeutic effects of luteinizing hormone releasing hormone (LH-RH) in cryptorchidism. Andrologia 6: 197

Bartsch G, Scheiber K 1981 Tamoxifen treatment in oligospermia. Eur Urol 7: 283

Bartsch G, Scheiber K, Janetschek G 1979 Tamoxifen treatment in oligospermic males. Arch Androl 2 (suppl): (abstr 177)

Barwin B 1982 Mesterolone: a new androgen for the treatment of male infertility. In: Bain J, Schill W-B, Schwarzstein L (eds) Treatment of male infertility. Springer, Berlin, p 117

Bedford N A, Elstein M 1981 The effect of kallikrein on male infertility: a double-blind study. In: Insler V, Bettendorf G (eds) Diagnosis and treatment of infertility. Elsevier/North Holland, New York, p 339

Behrendt H, Hilscher B, Passia D, Hofmann N, Hilscher W 1981 The occurrence of mast cells in human testis. Acta Anat 111: 14

Benkert O 1980 Pharmacotherapy of sexual impotence in the male. In: Ban T A, Freyhan F A (eds) Drug treatment of sexual dysfunction. Karger, Basel, p 158

Berzin M, Bilgeri Y R, Zanzinger A, Wing J, Kalk W J, Mendelsohn D 1987 The effect of kallikrein on spermatozoal ATP and other semen parameters. Andrologia 19: 273

Berezin M, Weissenberg R, Rabinovitch O, Lunenfeld B 1988 Successful GnRH treatment in a patient with Kallmann's syndrome, who previously failed HMG/HCG treatment. Andrologia 20: 285

Bierich J R, Rager K, Ranke M B 1977 Maldescensus Testis, Urban und Schwarzenberg, München

Blair J H, Simpson G M, Kline N S 1962 Monoamine oxidase inhibitor and sperm production. JAMA 181: 192

Broer K H, Winkhaus J, Kaiser R 1977 Parameters of semen analysis in relation to sterility. Fertil Steril 23: 334

Burger H G, de Kretser D M, Hudson B 1976 Effects of preceding androgen therapy on testicular response to human pituitary gonadotropin (HPG) in hypogonadotropic hypogonadism (H.H): a study of two patients. Int J Androl 1 (suppl): 140

Buvat J, Ardaens K, Ganthier A, Buvat-Herbaut M, Lemaire A 1981 Treatment of 80 cases of hypospermia by tamoxifen. Isr J Med Sci 17: 57

Charny Ch W, Gordon J A 1978 Testosterone rebound therapy: A neglected modality. Fertil Steril 29: 64

Check J H, Rakoff A E 1977 Improved fertility in oligospermic males treated with clomiphene citrate. Fertil Steril 28: 746

Chvapil N 1973 New aspects in the biological role of zinc: a stabilizer of macromolecular and biological membranes. Life Sci 13: 1041

Cigorraga S B, Dufau M L, Catt K J 1978 Regulation of luteinizing hormone receptors and steroidogenesis in gonadotropin-desensitized Leydigs cells. J Biol Chem 253: 4297

Collins J P 1982 Retrograde ejaculation. In: Bain J, Schill W B, Schwarzstein L (eds) Treatment of male infertility. Springer, Berlin, p 179

Comhaire F H 1976 Treatment of oligozoospermia with tamoxifen. Int J Fertil 21: 232

Comhaire F H 1982 Tamoxifen. In: Bain J, Schill W-B, Schwarzstein L (eds) Treatment of male infertility. Springer, Berlin, p 45

Comhaire F H 1987 Concentration of Pefloxacine in split ejaculate of patients with chronic male accessory gland infection. J Urol 138: 828

Comhaire F H 1990 Treatment of idiopathic testicular failure with high-dose testosterone undecanoate: a double blind pilot study. Fertil Steril 54: 689

Comhaire F H, Verschraegen G, Vermeulen L 1980 Diagnosis of accessory gland infection and its possible role in male infertility. Int J Androl 3: 32

Comhaire F H, Rowe P J, Farley T M M 1986 The effect of doxycycline in infertile couples with male accessory gland infection: a double-blind prospective study. Int J Androl 9: 91–98

Conway A J, Boylan L M, Howe C, Ross G, Handelsman D J 1988 Randomized clinical trial of testosterone replacement therapy in hypogonadal men. Int J Androl 11: 247

Danezis J M, Batrinos M L 1967 The effect of human postmenopausal gonadotropins on infertile men with severe oligospermia. Fertil Steril 18: 788

Danner C, Frick J 1980 Androgen substitution with testosterone-containing nasal drops. Int J Androl 3: 429

Da Rugna D, Dedes M, Ghossein E 1974 Erfahrungen mit Humangonadotropinen und Clomiphenzitrat bei Fertilitätsstörungen des Mannes. Der informierte Arzt Z für moderne Therapie 2: 470

Davidson J M, Camargo C A, Smith E R 1979 Effect of androgens on sexual behavior in hypogonadal men. J Clin Endocrinol Metab 48: 955

de Almeida M, Feneux D, Rigaud C, Jouannet P 1985 Steroid therapy for male infertility associated with antisperm antibodies. Results of a small randomized clinical trial. Int J Androl 8: 111

de Kretser D M, Taft H P, Brown J B, Evans J H, Hudson B 1986 Endocrine and histological studies on oligospermic men treated with human pituitary and chorionic gonadotrophin. J Endocrinal 40: 107

de Kretser D M, Burger H G, Fortune D et al 1972 Hormonal, histological and chromosomal studies in adult males with testicular disorders. J Clin Endocrinol Metab 35: 392

Della Casa L, Grandi M, Carani C, Sighinolfi R 1982 Effects of oral testosterone undecanoate therapy in andrological pathology. In: Menchini Fabris G F, Pasini W, Martini L (eds) Therapy in andrology. Excerpta Medica, Amsterdam, pp 78–86

del Pozo F 1982 Hyperprolactinemia in male infertility: treatment with bromocriptine. In: Bain J, Schill W B, Schwarzstein L (eds) Treatment of male infertility. Springer, Berlin, p 73

Dietl T, Kruck J, Fritz H 1978 Localization of kallikrein in porcine pancreas and submandibular gland as revealed by the indirect immunofluorescence technique. Hoppe-Seylers Z Physiol Chem 359: 49

Dondero F, Pozza D, Mazzilli F, Isidori A 1976 Response of adnexal glands to testosterone stimulation in the normal adult male. Fertil Steril 27: 806

Dony J M J, Sonals A G H, Rolland R, Fauser B C J M Thomas C M G 1986 Effect of chronic aromatase inhibition by 1-Testolactone on pituitary-gonadal function in oligozoospermic men. Andrologia 18: 69

Dörner G, Moch G, Zabel H 1960 The 'overproduction effect' of the testes after cessation of human chorionic gonadotropin administration in men with oligoasthenozoospermia. Fertil Steril 11: 457

Eggert-Kruse W, Hofmann H, Gerhard I, Bilke A, Runnebaum B, Petzoldt D 1988 Effect of antimicrobial therapy on sperm-mucus interaction. Hum Reprod 3: 861

Eliasson R, Fredrickson B, Johannisson E, Leander G 1966 Biochemical and morphological changes in semen from men with disease in the accessory genital glands. Excerpta Med Int Congr Ser 133: 629

Emperaire J C et al 1976 (cited by Espinasse)

Engel S, Möckel C, Diezel W 1985 Der Einfluß von α-Tokopherolazetat auf die Spermienmotilität. Dermatologische Monatsschrift 171: 800

Erdös E G 1970 Bradykinin, Kallidin and Kallikrein (Handbook of Experimental Pharmacology, vol XXV). Springer, Berlin

Epstcin J A 1977 Clomiphene treatment in oligospermic infertile males. Fertil Steril 28: 741

Espinasse J 1977 Utilisation du citrate de clomiphene isolément ou en association avec les androgènes dans le traitement des hypofertilités masculines idiopathiques. A propos de 74 cas. PhD dissertation, University of Toulouse, France

Fahim M S, Girgis S M, Ibrahim A A, Karaksy A 1979 Local male hormonal therapy in male infertility: A preliminary report. Arch Androl 3: 181

Fauser B C J M, Rolland R, Dony J M J, Corbey R S 1985 Long term, pulsatile, low dose, subcutaneous luteinizing hormone-releasing hormone administration in men with idiopathic oligozoospermia. Failure of therapeutic and hormonal response. Andrologia 17: 143

Filicori M, Flamigni C 1988 GnRH agonists and antagonists. Current clinical status. Drugs 35: 63

Fink E, Schill W-B 1983 Tissue kallikrein in human seminal plasma. In: Fritz H Back N B Dieize E Haberland G L (eds) Kinins III. Plenum, New York, p 1175

Fink E, Geiger R, Witte J, Biedermann S, Seifert J, Fritz H 1980 Biochemical, pharmacological and functional aspects of glandular kallikrein. In: Gross F, Vogel G (eds) Enzymatic release of vasoaction peptides. Raven, New York, p 101

Flückiger E 1972 Drugs and the control of prolactin secretion. In: Boyns A R, Griffith K (eds) Prolactin and carcinogenesis. Alpha Omega Alpha, Cardiff, p 162

Franchi F, Luisi M, Kicovic P M 1978 Long-term study of oral testosterone undecanoate in hypogonadal males. Int J Androl 3: 1

Fredricsson B 1988 Infertility caused by antispermatozoal antibodies in the male. Experience from an intermittent high dose cortisone regimen. Andrologia 20: 238

Freischem C W, Goldmann D B, Hanker J P, Schneider H P G, Nieschlag E 1982 Characteristics of male fertility (German). Dtsch Med Wochenschr 107: 486

Friberg J 1982 Immunological infertility in men. Clinical and therapeutical considerations. In: Bain J, Schill W-B, Schwarzstein L (eds) Treatment of male infertility. Springer, Berlin, p 153

Frick J 1974 Effect of androgens and progestins on spermatogenesis. In: Mancini R E, Martini L (eds) Male infertility and sterility. Academic, London, p 441

Frick J, Bartsch G, Marberger H 1976 Steroidal compounds (injectable and implants) affecting spermatogenesis in men. J Reprod Fertil Suppl 24: 35

Fritz H 1975 The kallikrein-kinin system in reproduction: biochemical aspects. In: Haberland G L, Rohen J W, Schirren C, Huber P (eds) Kininogenases. Kallikrein 2, Schattauer, Stuttgart, p 9

Fujii S, Moriya H, Suzuki T 1979a Kinins II: biochemistry. pathophysiology and clinical aspects. Plenum, New York

Fujii S, Moriya H, Suzuki T 1979b Kinins II: systemic proteases and cellular function. Plenum, New York

Futterweit W, Sobrero A J 1968 Treatment of normogonadotropic oligospermia with large doses of chorionic gonadotropin. Fertil Steril 19: 971

Geiger R 1981 The kallikrein-kinin system. In: Turk V, Vitale Lj (eds) Proteinases and their inhibitors. Mladinska knjiga–Pergamon Press, Ljubljana–Oxford, p 353

Gemzell C, Kjessler B 1964 Treatment of infertility after partial hypophysectomy with human pituitary gonadotrophins. Lancet 644

Gerris J, Comhaire F, Hellemans P, Peeters K, Schoonjans F 1991 Placebo-controlled trial of high-dose mesterolone treatment of idiopathic male infertility. Fertil Steril 55: 603

Getzoff P L 1955 Clinical evaluation of testicular biopsy and the rebound phenomenon. Fertil Steril 6: 465

Giarola A 1974 Effect of mesterolone on the spermatogenesis of infertile patients. In: Mancini R E, Martini L (eds) Male fertility and sterility. Academic, London, p 479

Giovenco P, Amodei M, Barbieri C, Fasani R, Carosi M, Dondero F 1987 Effects of kallikrein on the male reproductive system and its use in the treatment of idiopathic oligozoospermia with impaired motility. Andrologia 19: 238

Glezerman M, Lunenfeld B 1976 Hormontherapie männlicher Fertilitätsstörungen. In: Kaden R, Lübke F, Schirren C (eds) Fortschritte der Fertilitätsforschung III. Grosse, Berlin, p 17

Glezerman M, Lunenfeld B 1982 Treatment of male

infertility. In: Bandhauer K, Frick J (eds) Disturbances in male fertility. Springer, Berlin, p 287

Glezerman M, Lunenfeld B, Potashnik G, Oelsner G, Beer R 1976 Retrograde ejaculation: pathophysiologic aspects and report of two successfully treated cases. Fertil Steril 27: 796

Glezerman M, Lunenfeld B, Insler V 1978 Male infertility. In: Lunenfeld B, Insler V (eds) Infertility. Grosse, Berlin, p 114

Grabbe S, Kövary P M, Traupe H 1990 Mechanism of tamoxifen action: evidence for differential Sertoli cell responsiveness. A D Z, Hamburg, 17–19 November, 1989

Granville G E 1970 Successful gonadotropin therapy of infertility in a hypopituitary man. Arch Intern Med 125: 1041

Greenblatt R B 1961 Induction of ovulation with M R L-41. JAMA 178: 101

Gross K M, Matsumoto A M, Berger R E, Brenner W J 1986 Increased frequency of pulsatile luteinizing hormone-releasing hormone administration selectively decreases follicle stimulating hormone levels in men with idiopathic azoospermia. Fertil Steril 45: 392

Haberland G L, Rohen J W 1973 Kininogenases. Kallikrein 1. Schattauer, Stuttgart

Haberland G L, Rohen J W 1981 Kininogenases. Kallikrein 5. Schattauer, Stuttgart

Haberland G L, Rohen J W, Schirren C, Huber P 1975a Kininogenases. Kallikrein 2. Schattauer, Stuttgart, New York

Haberland G L, Rohen J W, Blümel G, Huber P 1975b Kininogenases. Kallikrein 3. Schattauer, Stuttgart, New York

Haberland G L, Rohen J W, Suzuki T 1977 Kininogenases. Kallikrein 4. Schattauer, Stuttgart, New York

Haidl G 1990 Macrophages in semen are indicative of chronic epididymal infection. Arch Androl 25: 5

Haidl G, Schill W-B 1991 Resorption studies with porcine pancreatic kallikrein in man. Gordon research conference on kallikreins and kinins. Ventura, California

Haidl G, Hofmann N, Weidner W, Weiske W H 1991 Demonstration of epididymis-related motility disturbances by abnormal staining behavior of human sperm tails (German). Fertilität 7: 25

Halim A, Antoniou D, Leedham P W, Blandy J P, Tresidder G C 1973 Investigation and treatment of the infertile male. Proc R Soc Med 66: 373

Hamburger C 1958 Testosterone treatment and 17-ketosteroid excretion. Acta Endocrinol 28: 529

Happ J 1981 Therapie mit Gonadotropin-Releasing-Hormon. Untersuchungen zur Anwendung bei Hypogonadismus, Pubertas tarda und Kryptorchismus. Urban und Schwarzenberg, München

Happ J, Neubauer M, Egri A, Demisch K, Schöffling K, Beyer J 1975 GnRH therapy in males with hypogonadotrophic hypogonadism. Horm Metab Res 7: 526

Hargreave T B 1983 Male infertility. Springer, Berlin

Hargreave T B, Elton R A 1982 Treatment with intermittent high-dose methylprednisolone or intermittent betamethasone for antisperm antibodies: preliminary communication. Fertil Steril 38: 586

Hartoma R, Nahoul K, Netter A 1977 Zinc, plasma androgens and male sterility. Lancet ii: 1125

Harvey C, Jackson M H 1957 Intermittent methyltestosterone therapy in male subfertility. Lancet i: 711

Heckel N J, McDonald J H 1952 The rebound phenomenon of the spermatogenic activity of the human testis following the administration of testosterone propionate. Fertil Steril 3: 49

Heite H-J, Koschnicke H 1979 The influence of pentoxifylline on the spermiogram—a clinical study in patients with reduced fertility (German). Akt Dermatol 5: 247

Heller C G, Clermont Y 1964 Kinetics of the germinal epithelium in man. Recent Prog Horm Res 20: 545

Heller C G, Maddock W O 1947 The clinical uses of testosterone in the male. Vitam Horm 5: 393

Heller C G, Nelson W O, Hill J B et al 1950 Improvement in spermatogenesis following depression of the human testis with testosterone. Fertil Steril 1: 415

Heller C G, Rowley M J, Heller G V 1969 Clomiphene citrate: a correlation of its effect on sperm concentration and morphology, total gonadotropins, ICSH, estrogen and testosterone excretion and testicular cytology in normal men. J Clin Endocrinol Metab 29: 638

Hendry W F, Sommerville F, Hall R R, Pugh R C B 1973 Investigation and treatment of the subfertile male. Br J Urol 45: 684

Hendry W F, Stedronska J, Hughes L, Cameron K M, Pugh R C B 1979 Steroid treatment of male subfertility caused by anti-sperm antibodies. Lancet ii: 498

Hess H, Franke I, Jauch M 1973 Medikamentöse Verbesserung der Fließeigenschaften des Blutes. Fortschr Med 91: 743

Hinting A, Vermeulen L, Comhaire F, Dhont M 1989 Pregnancy after in vitro fertilization and embryo transfer in severe immune male infertility. Andrologia 21: 516

Hofmann N 1981 Kallikrein-test. Andrologia 13: 265

Hofmann N 1988 Wege zur Andrologie. 2. Teil: Klinik der Fertilitätsstörungen des Mannes. Edition TAD, Cuxhaven

Hofmann N, Kuwert E 1979 Die chronische, nicht-Erreger-bedingte Orchitis. Z Hautkr 54: 173

Hofmann N, Becker H, Gall H 1975a Grenzen und Chancen einer Gonadotropintherapie bei Fertilitätsstörungen des Mannes. Therapiewoche 25: 7575

Hofmann N, Schönberger A, Gall H 1975b Investigations on kallikrein treatment of male infertility disturbances (German). Z Hautkr 50: 1003

Hofmann N, Behrendt H, Hilscher B, Passia D, Hilscher W 1982 First results of ketotifen treatment in 'inflammatory' fertility disorders (German). Z Hautkr Geschlechtskr 57: 609

Hohlweg W 1981 Effect of testosterone on the incretory and excretory function of the testis. Endocrinologie 77: 117

Hohlweg W, Dörner G, Kopp P 1961 Über die Wirkung intratestikulärer Testosteronimplantationen auf Sexualverhalten und Fertilität östrogenbehandelter Rattenmännchen. Acta Endocrinol 36: 299

Homonnai T Z, Sasson S, Paz G, Kraicer P F 1975 Improvement of fertility and semen quality in men treated with a combination of anticongestive and antibiotic drugs. Int J Fertil 20: 45

Homonnai T Z, Peled M, Paz G F 1978a Changes in semen quality and fertility in response to endocrine treatment of subfertile men. Gynecol Obstet Invest 9: 244

Homonnai T Z, Shilon M, Paz G F 1978b Evaluation of semen quality following kallikrein treatment. Gynecol Obstet Invest 9: 132

Homonnai T Z, Yavetz H, Yoger L, Rotem R, Paz G F 1988 Clomiphene citrate treatment in oligozoospermia:

comparison between two regimens of low-dose treatment. Fertil Steril 50: 801

Hornstein O 1966 Beitrag zur Langzeitbehandlung schwerer Zustände von Androgenmangel mit 1 α-Methyl-5 α-androstan-17 β-o1-3-on (Mesterolon). Arzneimittel forschung 16: 466

Hornstein O 1971 Behandlung einiger wichtiger Fertilitätsstörungen des Mannes. Hautarzt 22: 373

Horst H J, Höltgi W J, Dennis M, Coert A, Geelen J, Voigt K D 1976 Lymphatic absorption and metabolism of orally administered testosterone undecanoate in man. Klin Wochenschr 54: 875

Hoskins D D, Casillas E R 1975 Function of cyclic nucleotides in mammalian spermatozoa. In: Greep R O, Astwood E B, Hamilton D W, Geiger S R (eds) Endocrinology, handbook of physiology, section 7, vol V. Waverly, Baltimore, p 453

Hovatta D, Koskimies A J, Ranta T, Stenman U H, Seppälä M 1979 Bromocriptine treatment of oligospermia: a double-blind study. Clin Endocrinol 11: 377

Hudemann C Th 1976 Untersuchungen zur Wirkung von Mesterolon auf die Spermaqualität im Doppelblindversuch. In: Kaden R, Lübke F, Schirren C (eds) Fortschritte der Fertilitätsforschung III. Grosse, Berlin, p 81

Isidori A 1981 A modern approach to the gonadotropin treatment in oligospermia. Andrologia 13: 187

Jackaman F R, Ansell J D, Ghanadian R, McLoughlin P V A, Lewis J G, Chisholm G D 1977 The hormone response to a synthetic androgen (mesterolone) in oligospermia. Clin Endocrinol 6: 339

Joel C A 1960 The spermiogenetic rebound phenomenon and its clinical significance. Fertil Steril 11: 384

Johnsen S G 1978 Maintenance of spermatogenesis induced by hMG treatment by means of continuous hCG treatment in hypogonadotrophic men. Acta Endocrinol 89: 763

Johnsen S G, Bennet E P, Jensen V G 1974 Therapeutic effectiveness of oral testosterone. Lancet ii: 1473

Jonas D, Linzbach P, Weber W 1979 The use of Midodrin in the treatment of ejaculation disorders following retroperitoneal lymphadenectomy. Eur Urol 5: 184

Jungck E C, Roy S, Greenblatt R B, Matesh V B 1964 Effect of clomiphene citrate on spermatogenesis in the human. A preliminary report. Fertil Steril 15: 40

Kalla N R, Nisula B C, Menard R, Loriaux D L 1980 The effect of estradiol on testicular testosterone biosynthesis. Endocrinology 106: 35

Kamidono S, Hazama M, Matsumoto O, Tokada K J, Tomioka O, Ishigami J 1981 Kallikrein and male subfertility. Usefulness of high-unit kallikrein tablets. Andrologia 13: 108

Kelch R P, Jenner M R, Weinstein R L, Kaplan S L, Grumbach M M 1972 Estradiol and testosterone secretion by human and canine testis, in males with hypogonadism and in male pseudohermaphrodites with the feminizing testes syndrome. J Clin Invest 51: 824

Kelly M E, Needle M A 1979 Imipramine for aspermia after lymphadenectomy. Urology 13: 414

Keogh E J, Burger H G, de Kretser D M, Hudson B 1976 Nonsurgical management of male infertility. In: Hafez E S E (ed) Human semen and fertility regulation in men. Mosby, St Louis, Miss, p 452

Kern D, Schirren C 1973 Ergebnisse der Behandlung von subfertilen Männern mit Clomiphenzitrat. Andrologie 5: 59

Kienitz T, Schill W B 1977 Oral kallikrein therapy in asthenozoospermia (German). Fortschr Med 95: 2102

Kloer H, Hoogen H, Nieschlag E 1980 Trial of high-dose testosterone undecanoate in treatment of male infertility. Int J Androl 3: 121

Knuth U A, Hönigl W, Bals-Pratsch M, Schleicher G, Nieschlag E 1987 Treatment of severe oligozoospermia with hCG/hMG: a placebo-controlled double-blind trial. J Clin Endocrinol Metab 65: 1081

Kockott G 1982 Sexual dysfunction in the male. In: Bain J, Schill W-B, Schwarzstein L (eds) Treatment of male infertility. Springer, Berlin, p 191

Kragt F, Schellen A 1978 Clinical report about some cases with retrograde ejaculation. Andrologia 10: 380

Krause W, Meyhöfer W 1973 Unterdrückung Spermagglutinierender Autoantikörper im Serum durch Azathioprin (Imurek). Hautarzt 24: 551

Kremer J, Jager S, Kuiken J 1978 Treatment of infertility caused by anti-sperm antibodies. Int J Ferti 23: 270

Kruczynski D, Passia D 1986 The distribution of heavy metals in human ejaculate: a histochemical study. Acta Histochem 79: 187

Kynaston H G, Lewis-Johnes D I, Lynch R V, Desmond A D 1988 Changes in seminal quality following oral zinc therapy. Andrologia 20: 21

Labrie F, Bélanger A, Pelletier G et al 1980 LH-RH agonists: inhibition of testicular functions and possible clinical application. In: Cunningham G R, Schill W-B, Hafez E S E (eds) Regulation of male fertility. Martinus Nijhoff, The Hague, p 65

Laffont A, Ezes H 1948 La testosterone peut-elle avoir une action locale sur la spermatogénèse? Gynécol Obstét 47: 769

Lamensdorf H, Compere D, Begley G 1975 Testosterone rebound therapy in the treatment of male infertility. Fertil Steril 26: 469

Landes E, Müller H 1971 Behandlungsergebnisse bei Oligospermie und HMG (Pergonal 500). Hautarzt 22: 305

Lemon M, Fiedler F, Förg-Brey B, Hirschauer C, Leysath G, Fritz H 1979 The isolation and properties of pig submandibular kallikrein. Biochem J 177: 159

Leschber G, Nishino Y, Neumann F 1989 Influence of an aromatase inhibitor (4-acetoxy-4-androstene-3, 17-dion) on experimentally induced impairment of spermatogenesis in immature rats. Andrologia 21: 529

Lewis-Jones D I, Lynch R V, Machin D C, Desmond A D 1987 Improvement in semen quality in infertile males after treatment with tamoxifen. Andrologia 19: 86

Liu C C, Kinson G A 1973 Testicular gametogenic and endocrine responses to melatonin and serotonin peripherally administered to mature rats. Contraception 7: 153

Liu L, Chaudhari N, Corle D, Sherins R J 1988 Comparison of pulsatile subcutaneous gonadotropin-releasing hormone and exogenous gonadotropins in the treatment of men with isolated hypogonadotropic hypogonadism. Fertil Steril 49: 302

Lunan C B, Klopper A 1975 Antioestrogens: a review. Clin Endocrinol 4: 551

Lunenfeld B, Glezerman M 1977 Versuch eines algorithmischen Ansatzes zur Diagnose männlicher Fertilitätsstörungen. Akta Dermatol 3: 119

Lunenfeld B, Glezerman M 1981 Diagnose und Therapie männlicher Fertilitätsstörungen. Grosse, Berlin

Lunenfeld B, Insler V 1978 Diagnosis and treatment of functional infertility. Grosse, Berlin

Lunenfeld B, Mor A, Mani M 1967 Treatment of male infertility. I. Human gonadotropins. Fertil Steril 18: 581

Lunenfeld B, Olchowsky D, Tadir Y, Glezerman M 1979 Treatment of male infertility with human gonadotropins: Selection of cases, management and results. Andrologia 11: 331

Lunglmayr G 1976 Sperm motility during kallikrein treatment (German). Wien Klin Wochenschr 88: 709

Lytton B, Mroueh A 1966 Treatment of oligospermia with urinary human menopausal gonadotrophin: a preliminary report. Fertil Steril 17: 696

MacLeod J 1970 The effects of urinary gonadotropins following hypophysectomy and in hypogonadotropic eunuchoidism. In: Rosemberg E, Paulsen C A (eds) The human testis. Plenum, New York, p 577

MacLeod J, Pazianos A, Ray B 1966 The restoration of human spermatogenesis and of the reproductive tract with urinary gonadotrophins following hypophysectomy. Fertil Steril 17: 7

Mahajan S, Abassi A, Prasad A, Briggs W, McDonald F 1979 Effect of zinc (Zn) therapy on uremic hypogonadism: a double-blind study. Kidney Int 16: 893

Mancini R E 1970 Effect of urinary FSH and LH on the testicular function in hypogonadal patients. In: Rosemberg E, Paulsen C A (eds) The human testis. Plenum, New York, p 563

Mancini R E, Seiguer A C, Perez L, Loret A P 1969 Effect of gonadotropins on the recovery of spermatogenesis in hypophysectomized patients. J Clin Endocrinol 29: 467

Martin F J R 1967 The stimulation and prolonged maintenance of spermatogenesis by human pituitary gonadotrophins in a patient with hypogonadotrophic hypogonadism. J Endocrinol 38: 431

Maroulis G B, Parlow A F, Marshall J R 1977 Isolated follicle-stimulating hormone deficiency in man. Fertil Steril 28: 818

Marrama P, Baraghini G F, Carani et al 1985 Further studies on the effects of pentoxifylline on sperm count and sperm motility in patients with idiopathic oligo-asthenozoospermia. Andrologia 17: 612

Maseki Y, Miyake K, Mitsuya H, Kitamura H, Yamada K 1981 Mastocytosis occurring in the testes from patients with idiopathic male infertility. Fertil Steril 36: 814

Mauss J 1974 Ergebnisse der Behandlung von Fertilitätsstörungen des Mannes mit Mesterolon oder einem Placebo. Arzneimittelforschung 24: 1338

Mauss J, Börsch G, Török L 1974 Differential diagnosis of low or absent seminal fructose in man. Fertil Steril 25: 411

Mellinger R C, Thompson R J 1966 The effect of clomiphene citrate in male infertility. Fertil Steril 17: 94

Menchini-Fabris G F, Mariani M 1982. Treatment of male infertility with nucleotides. In: Bain J, Schill W B, Schwarzstein L (eds) Treatment of male infertility, Springer, Berlin, p 143

Menchini Fabris G F, Pasini W, Martini L 1982 Therapy in andrology. Excerpta Medica, Amsterdam

Meng K, Haberland G L 1973 Influence of kallikrein on glucose transport in the isolated rat intestine. In: Haberland G L, Rohen J W (eds) Kininogenases. Kallikrein 1. Schattauer, Stuttgart, p 75

Micic S 1988 Kallikrein and antibiotics in the treatment of infertile men with genital tract infections. Andrologia 20: 55

Micic S, Tulic C, Dotlic R 1990 Kallikrein therapy of infertile men with varicocele and impaired sperm motility. Andrologia 22: 179

Miska W, Schill W-B 1990 Enhancement of sperm motility by bradykinin and kinin analogs. Arch Androl 25: 63

Miska W, Schill W-B 1991 Absorption study with porcine pancreatic kallikrein in man. Drug re 41 (II): 1061 (German)

Misurale F, Cagnazzo G, Storace A 1969 Asthenozoospermia and its treatment with HCG. Fertil Steril 20: 650

Mortimer L H 1977 Clinical applications of the gonadotropin releasing hormone. Clin Endocrinol Metab 6: 167

Mortimer L H, McNeilly A S, Fisher R A, Murray M A F, Besser G M 1974 Gonadotropin releasing hormone therapy in hypogonadal males with hypothalamic or pituitary dysfunction. Br Med J 4: 617

Mroueh A, Lytton B, Kase N 1967 Effects of human chorionic gonadotropin and human menopausal gonadotropin (Pergonal) in males with oligospermia. J Clin Endocrinol Metab 27: 53

Nahoum C R C 1982 Inflammation and infection. In: Bain J, Schill W B, Schwarzstein L (eds) Treatment of male infertility. Springer, Berlin, p 5

Nankin H R, Castaneda E, Troen P 1977 Endocrine profiles in oligospermic men. In: Troen P, Nankin H R (eds) The testis in normal and infertile men. Raven, New York, p 529

Nankin H R, Lin T, Murono E, Osterman J, Troen P 1980 Testosterone and 17-OH-progesterone responses in men to 3-hour LH infusions. Acta Endocrinol 95: 110

Nelson L 1975 Spermatozoan motility. In: Greep R O, Astwood E B, Hamilton D W, Geiger S R (eds) Endocrinology: handbook of physiology, section 7, vol V. Waverly, Baltimore, p 421

Netter A, Hartoma R, Nahoul K 1981 Effect of zinc administration on plasma testosterone, dihydrotestorone, and sperm count. Arch Androl 7: 69

Nieschlag E, Freischem C W 1982 Androgen therapy in hypogonadism and infertility. In: Bain J, Schill W B, Schwarzstein L (eds) Treatment of male infertility, Springer, Berlin, p 103

Nieschlag E, Mauss J, Coert A, Kicovic P 1975 Plasma androgen levels in men after oral administration of testosterone or testosterone undecanoate. Acta Endocrinol 79: 366

Nieschlag E, Cüppers H J, Wiegelmann W, Wickings E J 1976 Bioavailability and LH-suppressing effect of different testosterone preparations in normal and hypogonadal men. Horm Res 7: 138

Nieschlag E, Hoogen H, Bölk M, Schuster H, Wickings E J 1978 Clinical trial with testosterone undecanoate for male fertility control. Contraception 18: 607

Nijman J M, Kremer J, Jager S, Schraffordt-Koops H, Boer P W, Oldhoff J 1981 Treatment of ejaculation disorders following retroperitoneal lymphadenectomy. Isr J Med Sci 17: 789

Nürnberger F, Grassow J 1977 Kallikrein therapy in oligozoospermia and asthenozoospermia during a double-blind trial. Hautarzt 28 (suppl II): 308 (German)

Okoyama A, Nonomura N, Nakamura M et al 1989 Effectiveness of hMG-hCG treatment for DNA/RNA syntheses in subfertile human testis in vitro. Arch Androl 22: 167

Oshima H, Negishi T, Yokowa M, Ochi-Ai K 1977 Clinical evaluation of testosterone pellet implantation in the testis as a treatment of male infertility. In: Troen P, Nankin H R (eds) The testis in normal and infertile men. Raven, New York, p 561

Oshio S, Ozaki S, Ohkawa I, Tajima T, Kaneko S, Mohri H 1989 Mecobalamin promotes mouse sperm maturation. Andrologia 21: 167

Padron R S, Wischusen J, Rennie G C, Burger H G, de Kretser D M 1980 Proceedings of the International Congress of Endocrinology, Abstract no 566, p 492. Melbourne, Australia, 10 February

Palm S, Schill W B, Wallner O, Prinzen R, Fritz H 1976 Occurrence of components of the kallikrein-kinin system in humen genital secretions and their possible function in stimulation of sperm motility and migration. In: Sitcuteri F, Back N, Haberland G L (eds) Kinins: pharmacodynamics and biological roles. Plenum, New York, p 271

Palti Z 1970 Clomiphene therapy in defective spermatogenesis. Fertil Steril 21: 838

Parsch E M, Schill W-B 1988 Captopril: a new approach for treatment of male subfertility? Andrologia 20: 537

Paulsen C A, Espeland D H, Michals E L 1970 Effects of HCG, HMG HLH and HGH administration on testicular function. In: Rosemberg E, Paulsen C A (eds) The human testis. Plenum, New York, p 547

Paulson D F 1977 Clomiphene citrate in the management of male hypofertility: predictors for treatment selection. Fertil Steril 28: 1226

Paulson D F, Wacksman J 1976 Clomiphene citrate therapy in the management of male infertility. J Urol 115: 73

Place V A, Atkinson L, Prather D A, Trunnell N, Yates F E (1990) Transdermal testosterone replacement through genital skin. In: Nieschlag E, Behre H M (eds) Testosterone. Action, deficiency. substitution. Springer, Heidelberg, pp 165-181

Polishuk W Z, Palti Z, Laufer A 1967 Treatment of defective spermatogenesis with human gonadotropins. Fertil Steril 18: 127

Potashnik K G, Ben-Adereth N, Lunenfeld B, Rofe C 1977 Assessment of pituitary response to nasal application of synthetic gonadotropin-releasing hormone in men. Fertil Steril 28: 650

Potts J F 1968 A clinical evaluation of two types of therapy for male infertility. Med J Aust 17: 707

Prasad A S, Miale A J, Farid Z, Sandsted H H, Schulert A R 1963 Zinc metabolism in patients with the syndrome of iron deficiency anemia, hepatosplenomegaly, dwarfism and hypogonadism. J Lab Clin Med 61: 537

Propping D, Tauber P F, Plewa G, Katzorke T 1978 Kallikrein treatment of the subfertile male: results of a double-blind cross-over study. Vth European Congress on Fertility and Sterility, October 1978, Venice, Italy (Abstr), p 93

Pryor, J P, Chaput de Saintonge M 1981 Controlled clinical trial of bromocriptine for oligozoospermic men. Isr J Med Sci 17: 773

Przybilla B, Schill W B 1981 Drug side effects on male sexuality. Ther Gegenw 120: 923 (German)

Pusch H H 1989 Oral treatment of oligozoospermia with testosterone undecanoate: results of a double-blind placebo-controlled trial. Andrologia 21: 76

Pusch H H, Haas J, Pürstner P 1986a Results of a low-dose treatment of oligozoospermia with clomiphene citrate. Andrologia 18: 561 (German)

Pusch H H, Purstner P, Haas J 1986b Treatment of asthenozoospermia with HCG. Andrologia 18: 201

Reich P, Günther E 1973 Results of treatment with homologous FSH-preparation by the pituitary gland. Andrologie 5: 339

Richman R A, Kirsch L R 1988 Testosterone treatment in adolescent boys with constitutional delay in growth and development. Engl J Med 319: 1563

Richter W, Pröschold M, Butenandt O, Knorr D 1976 Die Fertilität nach HCG-Behandlung des Maldescensus Testis. Klin Wschr 54: 467

Rixon R H, Whitfield J F, Bayliss J 1971 The stimulation of mitotic activity in the thymus and bone marrow of rats by killikrein. Horm Metab Res 3: 279

Rönnberg L 1980 The effect of clomiphene citrate on different sperm parameters and serum hormone levels in preselected infertile men: a controlled double-blind cross-over study. Int Androl 3: 479

Rosemberg E 1976 Gonadotropin therapy of male infertility. In: Hafez E S E (ed) Human semen and fertility regulation in men. Mosby, St Louis, p 464

Rowley M J, Heller C G 1972 The testosterone rebound phenomenon in the treatment of male infertility. Fertil Steril 23: 498

Ruiz-Velasco V, Domville E, Rosas Arceo J 1980 Treatment of 'idiopathic oligoasthenospermia' with tamoxifen. Preliminary report. J Androl 1: 74

Saez J M, Forest M G 1979 Kinetics of human chorionic gonadotropin-induced steroidogenic response of the human testis. I. Plasma testosterone: implications for human chorionic gonadotropin stimulation test. J Clin Endocrinol Metab 49: 278

Saitoh S, Kumanoto Y, Ohno K, Maruta H, Shimomoto K, Iimura O 1985 Studies of kallikrein–kinin system in human and sexual organ. Jap J Fertil Steril 30: 276

Saitoh S, Kumamoto Y, Shimamoto K, Iimuro O 1987 Kallikrein in the male reproductive system. Arch Androl 19: 133

Sanchez R, Hein R, Concha M, Vigil P, Schill W-B 1990 Mollicutes in male infertility: is antibiotic therapy indicated? Andrologia 22: 355 (German)

Sandler B, Faragher N 1984 Treatment of oligozoospermia with vitamin $B_{12}$. Infertility 7: 133

Sas M, Szöllösi J, Falkay G 1976 Traitement par clomiphene de la subfertilité de l homme. Ther Hung 3: 127

Sato H, Mochimaru F, Kobayashi T, Iizuka R, Kaneko S, Moriwaki C 1979 Kallikrein treatment of male infertility. In: Fujii S, Moriya H, Suzuki T (eds) Kinins II: biochemistry, pathophysiology and clinical aspects. Plenum, New York, p 529

Schally A V 1976 Clinical application of synthetic hypothalamic releasing hormones. In: Ebling F J G, Henderson J W (eds) Biological and clinical aspects of reproduction. Excerpta Medica, Amsterdam, p 238

Schally A V, Arimura A, Kastin A J 1973 Hypothalamic regulatory hormones. Science 179: 341

Schellen A M 1982 Clomiphene citrate in the treatment of male infertility. In: Bain J, Schill W-B, Schwarzstein (eds) Treatment of male infertility. Springer, Berlin-Heidlberg, New York p 34

Schellen A M, Beek J M J 1972 The influence of high doses of mesterolone on the spermiogram. Fertil Steril 23: 712

Schellen A M, Beek J M J 1974 The use of clomiphene treatment for male sterility. Fertil Steril 25: 407

Schellen A M, Bruinse H W 1980 Evaluation of the treatment with gonadotropic hormones in cases of severe and moderate oligozoospermia. Andrologia 12: 174

Schieferstein G, Adam W, Armann J et al 1987 Therapeutic results with tamoxifen in oligozoospermia. II. Hormonal analysis and semen parameters. Andrologia 19: 333 (German)

Schill W B 1975a Influence of kallikrein on sperm count and sperm motility in patients with infertility problems: preliminary results during parenteral and oral application with special reference to asthenozoospermia and oligozoospermia. In: Haberland G L, Rohen J W, Schirren C, Huber P (eds) Kininogenases. Kallikrein 2, Schattauer, Stuttgart, p 129

Schill W B 1975b Caffeine- and kallikrein-induced stimulation of human sperm motility: a comparative study. Andrologia 7: 229

Schill W B 1976 Fructosebestimmung im Spermaplasma. Aussage, differential-diagnostische Bedeutung und praktische Hinweise. Med Klin 71: 1031

Schill W B 1978a Clinical experience with kallikrein in the treatment of oligozoospermia and asthenozoospermia (German). In: Schillen C (ed) Fortschritte der Andrologie, Vol 6 kallikrein in der Andrologie. Grosse, Berlin, p 55

Schill W B 1978b Neuere Aspekte der Hormontherapie männlicher Fertilitätsstörungen. Ther Gegenw 117: 24

Schill W B 1979a Recent progress in pharmacological therapy of male subfertility—a review. Andrologia 11: 77

Schill W B 1979b Treatment of idiopathic oligozoospermia by kallikrein: results of a double-blind study. Arch Androl 2: 163

Schill W B 1982a Kinin-releasing pancreatic proteinase kallikrein. In: Bain J, Schill W B, Schwarzstein L (eds) Treatment of male infertility. Springer. Berlin, p 125

Schill W B 1982b Medical treatment of idiopathic normogonadotropic oligozoospermia. Int J Androl 5 (suppl): 135

Schill W B 1982c Therapy of idiopathic astheno-and oligozoospermia with pentoxifylline. Fortschr Med 100: 696 (German)

Schill W B 1982d Recent advances in medical treatment of male fertility disturbances. Hautarzt 33: 468 (German)

Schill W-B 1983 The effect of pancreatic kallikrein on semen parameters of men with varicocele. In: Fritz et al (eds) Kinins—III Part B. Plenum, New York, pp 1181–1186

Schill W-B 1985 Neue Aspekte der medikamentösen Therapie der männlichen Infertilität. Hautarzt 36(suppl VII): 170

Schill W-B 1986a Established and new approaches in medical treatment of male sterility. Fertilität 2: 7 (German)

Schill W-B 1986b Diagnosis and treatment of ejaculatory sterility. In: Paulson J A, Negro-Villar A, Lucena E, Martini L (eds) Andrology. Male fertility and sterility. Academic, Orlando, pp 599–617

Schill W-B 1990 Pregnancy after brompheniramine treatment of a diabetic with incomplete emission failure. Arch Androl 25: 101

Schill W B, Landthaler M 1980 Tamoxifen treatment of oligozoospermia. Andrologia 12: 546

Schill W B, Landthaler M 1981 Erfahrungen mit dem Antiöstrogen Tamoxifen zur Therapie der Oligozoospermie. Hautarzt 32: 306

Schill W B, Schillinger R 1987 Selection of oligozoospermic men for tamoxifen treatment by an antiestrogen test. Andrologia 19: 266

Schill W B, Braun-Falco O, Haberland G L 1974 The possible role of kinins in sperm motility. Int J Fertil 19: 163

Schill W B, Wallner O, Palm S, Fritz H 1976 Kinin stimulation of spermatozoa motility and migration in cervical mucus. In: Hafez E S E (ed) Human semen and fertility regulation in men. Mosby, St Louis, Miss, p 442

Schill W B, Pritsch W, Preissler G 1977 Effect of kallikrein and caffeine on frozen human semen. Fertil Steril 28: 312

Schill W B, Preissler G, Dittmann B, Müller W P 1979 Effect of pancreatic kallikrein, sperm acrosin and high molecular weight (HMW) kininogen on cervical mucus penetration ability of seminal plasma-free human spermatozoa. In: Fujii S, Moriya H, Suzuki T (eds) Kinins II: systemic proteases and cellular function, Plenum, New York, p 305

Schill W B, Jüngst D, Unterburger P, Braun S 1982 Combined HMG/HCG treatment in subfertile men with idiopathic normogonadotropic oligozoospermia. Int J Androl 5: 467

Schill W-B, Schreider J, Ring J 1986 The use of ketotifen, a mast cell blocker, for treatment of oligo – and asthenozoospermia. Andrologia 18: 570–573

Schill W-B, Korting H C, Schweikert H U 1987 Treatment of oligozoospermia by testolactone. Acta Endocrinol 114(suppl 283): 22

Schill W-B, Miska W, Parsch E M, Fink E 1989 Significance of the kallikrein–kinin system in andrology. In: Fritz F, Schmidt I, Dietze G (eds) The kallikrein–kinin system in health and disease. Limbach Verlag, Braunschweig, pp 171–204

Schill W B, Rjosk H K, Krizic A 1990 Andrological, biochemical and endocrinological investigations in subfertile men during kallikrein treatment. Hautarzt 31: 191 (German)

Schirren C 1963 Relation between fructose content of semen and fertility in man. J Reprod Fertil 5: 347

Schirren C 1966 Die Behandlung der postpuberalen Leydig-Zell-Insuffizienz mit 1 α-Methly-5 α-androstan-17 β-o1-3-on (Mesterolon). Arneimittelforschung 16: 463

Schirren C 1967 The treatment of the postpuberal Leydig cell insufficiency. Excerpta Medica Int Congr Series 133: 808

Schirren C 1973 Therapieprobleme in der Andrologie. Urologe B 13: 1

Schirren C 1978 Clinical results of kallikrein therapy in men with disturbed fertility (Germany). In: Schirren C (ed) Fortschritteder Andrologie. Grosse, Berlin, p 35 (German)

Schirren C 1981 Fertilitätsstörungen des Mannes. Diagnostik, Biochemie des Spermaplasmas, Hormontherapie. Enke, Stuttgart

Schoysman R 1964 Essais preliminaires de traitement des oligospermies moyennes par la gonadotrophine humaine extraite de lurine de femmes menopauses (HMG). Bull Soc R Belge Gynecol Obstet 34: 399

Schramm P 1981 Pentoxifyllin in der andrologischen Therapie. Z Hautkr 56: 1046

Schroeder-Finckh R, Hofmann N, Hartmann R 1986 Kallikrein: a contribution to the pathophysiology of testicular disorders and its implications for therapy. Fertilität 2: 171 (German)

Schroffner W G 1978 Restoration of male fertility five years after total hypophysectomy. Hawaii Med J 37: 331

Schürmeyer T, Wickings E J, Freischem C W, Nieschlag E 1983 Saliva und serum testosterone following oral testosterone undecanoate administration in normal and hypogonadal men. Acta Endocrinol 102: 456-462

Schütte B 1989 Die medikamentöse Behandlung männlicher Fertilitätsstörungen. Medizinische Welt 40: 1252

Schütte B, Schirren C 1977 Therapeutic administration of kallikrein in patients with sperm motility disturbances. Z Hautkr 52: 930 (German)

Schulte-Beerbühl M, Nieschlag E 1980 Comparison of testosterone, DHT, LH and FSH in semen after injection of testosterone enanthate or testosterone cypionate. Fertil Steril 33: 201

Schwale M, Frosch P, Tölle E, Niermann H 1980 Behandlung retrograder Ejakulation und Anorgasmie mit einem Alpha-Sympathomimetikum (Midodrin). Z Hautkr 55: 756

Schwarzstein L 1974 HMG in the treatment of oligozoospermic patients. In: Mancini R E, Martini L (eds) Male fertility and sterility. Academic, London, p 567

Schwarzstein L, Aparicio N 1982 LH-RH and its analogs in the treatment of idiopathic normogonadotropic oligozoospermia. In: Bain J, Schill W B, Schwarzenstein L (eds) Treatment of male infertility. Springer, Berlin, p 55

Schwarzstein L, Aparicio N J, Turner D, Calamera J C, Mancini R, Schally A V 1975 Use of synthetic luteinizing hormone-releasing hormone in the treatment of oligospermic men: a preliminary report. Fertil Steril 26: 331

Seiminies P, Kockott G, Pirke K M, Vogt H J, Schill W B 1982 Effect of testosterone replacement on sexual behavior in hypogonadal men. Arch Sex Behav 11: 345

Segal S 1978 The role of serotonin in male infertility. In: Fabbrini A, Steinberger E (eds) Recent progress in andrology. Academic, London, p 343

Segal S, Sadovsky E, Palti Z, Pfeifer Y, Polishuk W Z 1975 Serotonin and 5-hydroxyindoleacetic acid in fertile and subfertile men. Fertil Steril 26: 314

Segal S, Polishuk W Z, Ben-David M 1976 Hyperprolactinemic male infertility. Fertil Steril 27: 1425

Sherins R J 1974 Clinical aspects of treatment of male infertility with gonadotropins: testicular response of some men given hCG with and without Pergonal. In: Mancini R E, Martini L (eds) Male fertility and sterility. Academic, London, p 545

Sherins R J, Winters S J, Waschlicht H 1977 Studies of the role of hCG and low-dose FSH in initiating spermatogenesis in hypogonadotropic men. In: Proceedings of the 59th Annual Meeting of the Endocrine Society, p 312 (Abstr)

Shulman S 1976 Treatment of immune infertility with methylprednisolone. Lancet ii: 1243

Siiteri P K, Thompson E A 1975 Studies of human placental aromatase. J Steroid Biochem 6: 317

Sina D, Taubert H D, Karschnia R 1974 Human menopausal gonadotrophin in the treatment of infertility in men. Dtsch med Wschr 99: 2639 (German)

Smith K D, Ficher M, Steinberger E 1974 Clinical and laboratory findings during gonadotropin therapy of postpubertal hypogonadotropic hypogonadism. Andrologia 6: 147

Sokol R Z, Steiner B S, Bustillo M, Petersen G, Swerdhoff R S 1988 A controlled comparison of the efficacy of clomiphene citrate in male infertility. Fertil Steril 49: 865

Sokol R Z, Swerdloff R S, McClure R D, Peterson M 1980 Gonadotropin therapy failure secondary to HCG induced antibodies. Proceedings of the International Congress of Endocrinoloy, abstr No 484, p 451, Melbourne, Australia, 10 February

Somazzi S, Goor W, Ott F 1973 Therapieresultate bei Oligospermien. Dermatologica 147: 37

Srivastava A, Chaudhuri A R, Setty B S 1983 Zinc content of maturing spermatozoa in oestrogen treated rats. International J Androl 6: 103

Steinberger E 1981 Regulation of spermatogenesis. Second International Congress on Andrology, Postgraduate Course, Tel Aviv, Israel

Steinberger E, Rodriguez-Rigau L J 1981 Treatment of male infertility. In: Frajese G, Hafez E S E, Conti C, Fabbrini A (eds) Oligozoospermia: recent progress in andrology. Raven, New York, p 407

Steinberger E, Smith K D, Tcholakian R K et al 1974 Steroidogenesis in human testis. In: Mancine R E, Martini L (eds) Male fertility and sterility. Academic, London, p 149

Stewart B, Bergant J 1974 Correction of retrograde ejaculation by sympathomimetic mediation: preliminary report. Fertil Steril 25: 1073

Stockamp K, Schreiter F, Altwein J 1974 Alphaadrenergic drugs in retrograde ejaculation. Fertil Steril 25: 817

Stüttgen G 1975 Kallikrein effects: a short comment. In: Haberland G L, Rohen J W, Schirren C, Huber P (eds) Kininogenases. Kallikrein 2, Schattauer, Stuttgart, p 171

Swyer G J M 1953 Effects of testosterone implants in men with defective spermatogenesis. Br Med J 2: 1080

Tharandt L, Schulte H, Benker G, Hackenberg K, Reinwein D 1977 Treatment of isolated gonadotropin deficiency in men with synthetic LH-RH and a more potent analogue of LH-RH. Neuroendocrinology 24: 195

Thiagarajah S, Vaughan E D, Kitchin J D 1978 Retrograde ejaculation: successful pregnancy following combined sympathomimetic medication and insemination. Fertil Steril 30: 96

Tonutti E, Weller O, Schuchardt E, Heincke E 1960 Die männliche Keimdrüse. Struktur, Funktion, Kinetik. Grundzüge der Andrologie. Thieme, Stuttgart

Török L 1979 Treatment of male subfertility with kallikrein. Münch Med Wochenschr 121: 1047 (German)

Török L 1985 Treatment of oligozoospermia with tamoxifen (open and controlled studies). Andrologia 17: 497

Traub A J, Thompson W 1981 The effect of tamoxifen on spermatogenesis in subfertile men. Andrologia 13: 486

Trentini G P, Ferrari De Gaetani C, Saviano M S 1968 Rapporti dello zinco con laccrescimento e la riproduzione del ratto albino. Boll Soc Ital Biol Sper 45: 602

Troen P, Yanaihara T, Nankin H, Tominaga T, Lever H 1970 Assessment of gonadotropin therapy in infertile men. The human testis. Adv Exp Biol Med 10: 591

Tschesche H, Mair G, Godec G et al 1979 The primary structure of porcine glandular kallikrein. In: Fujii S, Moriya H, Suzuki T (eds) Kinins II: biochemistry, pathophysiology and clinical aspects. Plenum, New York, p 245

Ulstein M 1973 Fertility of donors at heterologous insemination. Acta Obstet Gynecol Scand 52: 97

Van Loon G R, Brown G M 1975 Secondary drug failure occurring during chronic treatment with LH-RH: appearance of an antibody. J Clin Endocrinol Metab 41: 640

Vermeulen A 1981 Hormonal treatment of male infertility. In: Frajese G, Hafez E S E, Conti C, Fabbrin A (eds) Oligozoospermia: recent progress in andrology. Raven, New York, p 413

Vermeulen A, Comhaire F 1978 Hormonal effects of an antiestrogen, tamoxifen, in normal and oligospermic men. Fertil Steril 29: 320

Vigersky R A, Glass A R 1981 Effect of Δ-testolactone on the pituitary-testicular axis in oligospermic men. J Clin Endocrinol Metab 52: 897

Vilchez-Martinez J A, Pedroza E, Arimura A, Schally A V 1979 Paradoxical effects of D-Trp—luteinizing hormone-releasing hormone on the hypothalamic-pituitary-gonadal axis in immature female rats. Fertil Steril 31: 677

Vogel P G, Braun-Falco O 1971 Behandlung von Oligospermien mit Amitryptylin. Münch med Wschr 113: 1028

Wagner TOF 1985 Pulsatile LHRH therapy of the male. TM Verlag, Hameln

Walsh P C, Amerlar R D 1977 Medical management of male infertility. In: Amelar R D, Dubin L, Walsh P C (eds) Male infertility. Saunders, Philadelphia, pp 179

Wang C, Chang C W, Wong K K, Yeung K K 1983 Comparison of the effectiveness of placebo, clomiphene citrate, mesterolone, pentoxifylline, and testosterone rebound therapy for the treatment of idiopathic oligospermia. Fertil Steril 40: 358

Weidner W, Prudlo J, Schiefer H G, Jantos C, Altmannsberger M, Aumüller G 1989 *Escherichia coli*–Epididymitis der Ratte: ein tierexperimentelles Modell der akut-eitrigen und chronisch-obstruktiven Entzündung. Fertilität 5: 151

WHO 1987 Laboratory manual for the examination of human semen and semen–cervical mucus interactions. Cambridge University Press, Cambridge

WHO 1989 Mesterolone and idiopathic male infertility: a double blind study. Int J Androl 12: 254

Wicklmayr M, Dietze G, Günther B et al 1978 Improvement of pathological glucose tolerance by bradykininin diabetic and in surgical patients. Klin Wochenschr 56: 1077 (German)

Winters S J, Troen P 1982 Gonadotropin therapy in male infertility. In: Bain J, Schill W B, Schwarzstein L (eds) Treatment of male infertility. Springer, Berlin, p 85

Wong T W, Strauss F, Warner N E 1974 Testicular biopsy in the study of male infertility. III. Pretesticular causes of infertility. Arch Pathol 89: 1

Yamamoto M, Takaba H, Hashimoto J, Miyake K, Mitsuya H 1986 Successful treatment of oligozoospermic and azoospermic men with $\alpha_1$-blocker and $\beta$-stimulator: new treatment for idiopathic male infertility. Fertil Steril 46: 1162

Yovich J M, Edirisinghe W R, Cummins J M, Yovich J L 1990 Influence of pentoxifylline in severe male accessory gland infection: a double blind prospective study. Int J Androl 9: 91

Zachmann M A, Murset G, Gnehm H E, Prader A 1976 Testosterone treatment of excessively tall boys. J Pediatr 88: 116

Zarate A, Valdez-Vallina F, Gonzales A, Perez-Ubierna L, Ganales E S, Schakly A V 1973 Therapeutic effect of synthetic luteinizing hormone-releasing hormone (LH-RH) in male infertility due to idiopathic azoospermia and oligozoospermia. Fertil Steril 24: 485

# 24. Surgical treatment of male infertility

*R. Schoysman*

Surgical treatment of the male genital tract aims at the diagnosis of infertility (biopsy, vasogram), at correcting obstruction, at improving patency at different levels of the genital tract, and at treating vascular disorders, such as varicocele.

We shall not discuss in this chapter orchidopexy, urethral disorders, testicular autotransplantation or penile implant operations performed for vascular impotence.

Operations performed to create patency of the genital tract after obstruction have definitively entered the field of microsurgery over the past decade. Loupes and conventional surgical equipment have become completely obsolete.

## PRINCIPLES OF MICROSURGICAL TREATMENT OF MALE INFERTILITY

The main purpose of microsurgical therapy of epididymal or deferential block is not only to obtain spermatozoa in the ejaculate; other essentials have to be equally considered by the surgeon:

1. The presence of mature sperm with full motility. This requires a correct knowledge of epididymal function and environment (Orgebin-Crist et al 1981).

2. The presence in the ejaculate of as high a number of spermatozoa as can be expected considering spermatogenesis at the testicular level.

3. Both mature and motile sperm in adequate numbers can be obtained by performing an atraumatic operation, creating minimal tissue reaction and avoiding secondary scarring down of the anastomosis, either partially or completely.

This requires gentle tissue handling, meticulous hemostasis, and the use of adequate microinstruments and sutures.

4. The value of spermatogenesis, relying on testicular biopsy (the normality of hormonal investigation does not give sufficient information in this respect). Since nowadays good correlation has been established between spermatid count in biopsy readings and sperm count in the ejaculate, biopsy will prove most effective in predicting chances of repair as well as in evaluating postoperative results (Silber & Rodriguez-Rigau 1981).

Doubts about the importance of testicular biopsy still persist and the issue remains a permanent subject of controversy, when mere descriptive histology is used. A semiquantitative approach (Van Dop 1979) allows a better correlation between spermatogenesis and sperm output but is very time consuming and not totally satisfying.

The very elaborate quantitative measurements of Paulsen & Steinberger are far too time consuming to be practical. We think that the simple approach mentioned above (Silber & Rodriguez-Rigau 1981) may prove a useful and practical preoperative investigation.

## INSTRUMENTS AND MATERIALS

### The operating microscope

A large variety of optical equipment is available, ranging from simple devices to more sophisticated ones, including zooming foot pedals and all fittings for photographic and video recordings. Indispensable features are stability, a long articulated arm between the column and the optics, and a 200–300 mm lens allowing easy surgery.

Double optics for both the surgeon and the assistant are highly advisable.

## Seating

Some surgeons prefer to be seated during microsurgical operations. In this case a simple saddle chair will do. More complicated models including arm support have proved to be more nuisance than help. Surgeons find a support attached to the operating table mostly adequate.

## Microinstruments

A wide range of instruments are available; they vary in design and quality, according to the firm that manufactures them. This equipment is expensive and completion of a set requires a careful choice. Of equal importance is the care with which they should be handled, especially after the operation while sterilizing and packing them. A specially trained nurse will avoid cleaning them together with more conventional and heavier instruments. It must be realized that clumsy handling can easily damage delicate instruments.

A basic set, strictly for microsurgery of males, would be composed of:

— A vasovasostomy clamp
— A curved and straight microneedleholder
— Jeweler forceps number 3 or 5
— Ophthalmological swabs
— Blunt lacrimal duct needles.

## PROCEDURES TO RESTORE PATENCY OF GENITAL TRACT

### Epididymiolysis

Periepididymal adhesions may have a very different appearance, ranging from a simple loose veil which does not interfere with transit at all to very close coalescence of the scrotal lining, epididymis and testis so as to create an undissectable scar. There are nevertheless cases in which postinflammatory adhesive bands enclose the epididymis tightly, giving rise to well-localized structures. Their progressive liberation along the edge of the free portion of the epididymis is usually quite easy. It is enough to take care not to injure the organ and to perform microcoagulation of the vessels at a distance of more than 1 mm from the epididymal tubules.

## Epididymal cysts

### Diagnosis

The epididymis is frequently the location of congenital cysts, which are mainly situated in the head. Their diagnosis is usually simple since at the upper pole of the testis a round, sometimes resilient or comparatively hard mass is felt. The diameter of these cysts varies and may be several centimeters.

When the scrotum is opened it may be found that the cyst is situated immediately below the serosa; such cysts rarely cause compression of the epididymal tract. The epididymis itself is easily recognized and both inspection and palpation give sufficient proof of the complete independence of the epididymal tract in relation to the cystic mass.

Epididymal cysts, which are sometimes multiple, located in the organ itself, give greater cause for concern. We have found up to six with diameters varying between 2 and 8 mm in the same epididymal head. These cysts cause definite difficulties of transit and their removal may be indispensable for the restoration of normal epididymal function.

### Choice of incision

The incision of the serosa must always be longitudinal, i.e. it must follow the main axis of the epididymis. Its length should be proportional to the size of the cyst to be removed. The incision must never be such as to cause the loss of part of the serous membrane, because this would lead to further stenosis.

The incision must be quite superficial and involve only the serosa. If, as is most frequently the case, part of the cyst is on the same level as the subserosa, the cystic wall proper is recognized and every care must be taken not to pierce it. With the aid of curved round-tipped scissors the serous membrane is gradually separated from the cystic wall and special care must be taken in places where epididymal tubules come into view. It is not rare for the distension of the cyst to have involved epididymal loops which are therefore drawn out and not recognizable to the naked eye. The dissection of the cystic wall must therefore be performed under the microscope so as to recognize these structures in time. The operating field is constantly irrigated and the dissection is carried out under an uninterrupted fine stream of physiological saline. While the plane of cleavage between serous membrane and cystic wall is always easily identified, the same cannot be said for the part of the cyst adhering to the epididymal tubules. In some cases this adherence is very close, and the separation of the epididymal tubules must be carried out with the greatest caution in order not to injure them. The epididymal tissue must on no account be touched or pulled aside, since it is extremely fragile.

Any attempt to create tension of the plane of cleavage should only be made from the side of the already separated wall of cyst. This wall is as a rule completely avascular and it is quite exceptional for vessels to be found on it except at one pole which is usually oriented towards the depth of the epididymal tissue.

The proximity of this small vascular pole is usually noticed because at this point the plane of cleavage comes to an end and in progressing cautiously one finds a few thin vessels. In order to avoid coagulating these in the immediate vicinity of the epididymal loops, it is better to free them for a length of 1 or 2 mm and only then to coagulate them.

Once the cyst has been removed, the dissection area is again irrigated and, according to the extension of the excised structure, one or more clusters of loops or epididymal tubules will be seen. If the extirpation has been carried out correctly, this whole surface is bloodless. The serosa is closed with a few 6/0 nylon stitches, which should simply approximate the two edges of the incision.

If, when the serosa has been incised, the cyst is found to be covered entirely by epididymal tissue, the anatomy of the epididymis should be taken into consideration before beginning the dissection.

The head of the epididymis itself is formed by the efferent tubes; the number of these is variable but as a rule there are about a dozen. Thus, injury to one of them does not lead to severe consequences as far as the outcome of the operation is concerned. On the contrary, beyond the head, all the tubules are joined in one single structure, injury to which implies total loss of patency. Macroscopically, this difference in anatomical structure is found 12–15 mm from the upper end of the epididymis. Consequently, the removal of any cyst beyond this limit must be performed with even greater care than that of lesions situated in the head.

However, not even the epididymal head itself has uniform structure; the tubules are grouped into several lobular structures separated from each other by partitions of loose connective tissue. If the cysts are situated in the head, they must be approached via one of these interlobular planes, the choice of which depends on the localization of the lesion. With the aid of the microscope, the slightly grayish zones separating the whitish-yellow clusters of tubules in which the loops are perfectly visible are easily identified. However cautiously one proceeds, dissecting can only reach a depth of 3 mm from the epididymal surface. Every care must be taken not to compress or injure the epididymal tubules.

If several cysts are located in the same epididymis, even if they are very close together, it is preferable to make a separate incision of the serous membrane for each of them, even if one is tempted to remove two cystic masses by the same surgical approach. In fact, only at the point where the cyst bulges most obviously under the serosa is the likelihood of finding stretched epididymal tubules least. It is impossible to avoid these tubules if the cyst is approached more laterally as would be the case if a single incision of the serosa were used.

### Vasectomy reversal

Vasectomy reversal is today in the USA the most frequent microsurgical andrological operation and will probably also reach this level in Europe in the years to come.

Considering the increasing demand for this contraceptive method linked with the higher frequency of divorce in permissive societies, this evolution is logical. Henceforth the search for improved vasectomy techniques that give the male the best chances for a successful reversal, as well as the search for better reversal techniques, will occupy an important place in clinical research.

There is no doubt that the report of Schmidt et al (1976), advising minimal tissue loss of the vas with his coagulation technique, is an improvement with regard to ligation technique. This technique, combined with care in selecting a straight portion of the vas for vasectomy, gives the patient and the surgeon the highest probability of success if a subsequent reversal is decided on.

Since vasovasostomy technique is so linked with the foregoing vasectomy technique, it is worthwhile illustrating Schmidt's technique (Figs 24.1–24.3).

Two more remarks about the safety of male contraception by vasectomy in those males who may later regret it, concern sperm banking and the age factor.

Sperm banking has been advocated and has already proved useful in a few cases, but there are drawbacks to it. Amongst them is the actual rarity of banks, which would be totally insufficient if this demand were to spread. Furthermore, not all semen samples, though proven fertile, are necessarily of such quality as to allow storage. Finally,

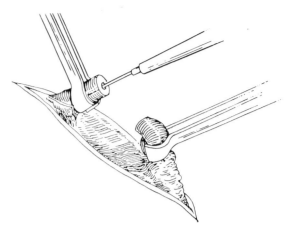

**Fig. 24.2**  After simple section (no vas removed!) testicular extremity is coagulated by inserting an electrode over 5 mm. The coagulating process aims at only destroying the inner part of the vas.

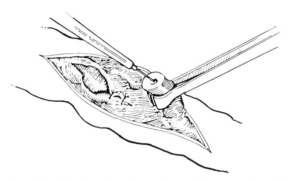

**Fig. 24.3**  Fascia is closed over the testicular extremity and the prostatic end is also coagulated (not mandatory).

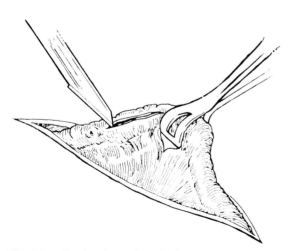

**Fig. 24.1**  Freeing the vas from the fascia.

the duration of storage should not exceed 10 years and the semen must be of very good quality at the start to allow this long freezing period (see also Chapter 25).

When considering the age factor, the experience of those who have the largest series of reversals (Silber 1978a) show that 10 years after vasectomy the chances of performing a successful reversal drop very markedly, almost to zero.

Two main technical procedures have been advocated for reversal operation: the one-layer technique; and the double-layer technique (Silber 1977, 1978a).

*Single-layer technique*

This technique (Fig. 24.4) consists of placing

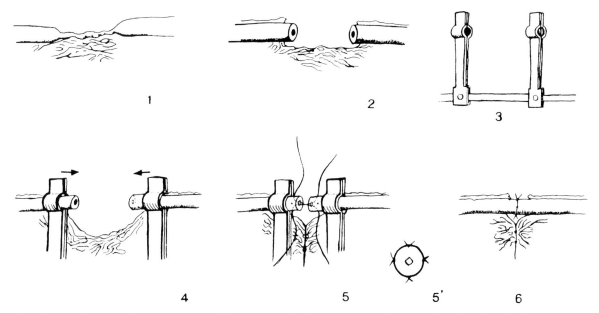

**Fig. 24.4**   1, Status of old vasectomy scar. 2, Preparation of both sections in healthy vas. 3, Double adjustable clamp. 4, Facing both sections. 5, Inserting the stitches (nylon 6/0); 5', cross-section. 6, End result.

from three to six, and sometimes eight, stitches on the circumference of the vas deferens with sutures varying in thickness from 4 to 7/0. Some surgeons involve the mucosa in these stitches, others recommend that they should be confined to the submucous layer. Ideas also differ as to the use of a splint at the level of the suture — this splint comes out higher up in the ductus deferens and should be pulled out a few days later. Some authors even suggest that a catgut should be left in place instead of a splint and be absorbed. Following the work of Smith we performed vasovasostomy at first with the single-layer technique and included the deferential mucosa in the stitches.

The scrotum is incised in the neighbourhood of the vasectomy scar, and it is usually very easy to isolate the ductus deferens for a stretch including some 2 cm of intact duct both distal and proximal to the vasectomy site. Sometimes a granuloma is found in this place. It may be very thick and we have seen some that were 2–3 cm long and had a diameter of 1 cm. Once the occluded area and the healthy stumps on each side have been well laid bare, the vas is sectioned with a scalpel in a single cut so as to have an even edge running perpendicular to the axis of the ductus deferens. This is done on either side of the obliterated stretch, which is usually 2–3 cm in length and is then excised with electric cutting, the few bleeding points being immediately coagulated.

At this stage, one must make sure that the healthy portions of the vas have been found. Downstream this is done by introducing a fine lacrimal probe into the opening of the vas, whereas upstream it is sufficient to compress the epididymal tail slightly in order to see a whitish fluid drip from the section of the vas. Microscopic examination of this fluid should confirm the presence of spermatozoa. In additon, microscopic inspection of the section shows whether the lumen is patent. If the cut has not yet involved the intact portion of the duct, it must be repeated to 2 or 3 mm distance until a patent lumen is found on either side. The two ends are then aligned on a small fixing device with two parallel branches which hold the ductus deferens and can be brought closer together or drawn apart on a sliding rod. Before placing the first stitch, the two ends are brought close together as in the final stage of the operation.

Prolene 6 or 8/0 is used as suture material. The easiest way of placing the stitches is to start from the prostatic segment. At this point the diameter of the vas is in fact smaller than that of the testicular segment. A small counterpressure forceps is introduced into the lumen in order to place a stitch involving both the mucosa and submucous tissue of the vas for 1.5 mm. Care must be taken not to touch the mucous membrane of the opposite side. Once the needle has passed the thickness of the ductus deferens on this side, it is reintroduced from inside the lumen on the side of the testis at a distance of 1 mm and passed out on the outside of the duct at 1.5 mm from the cut edge. This knot is tied immediately and followed by two further stitches on either side of the ductus deferens visible to the surgeon.

Once the anterior side has been sutured, the whole operating field is reversed by turning the fixing device and the opposite side is sutured with three more stitches. The two last stitches may prove somewhat difficult to insert exactly, but by separating the two cut surfaces with the aid of a jeweler's forceps, one can ensure their correct position. Experience has shown that six stitches ensure that the suture holds tight. Older techniques with only three or four stitches had the drawback of allowing fluid to escape from the lumen, thus creating small granulomas which were detrimental to the ultimate prognosis of the operation.

At present, we do not have sufficiently comparable case series to judge the advisability of placing the stitches immediately below the mucous membrane and joining only the muscular wall. This technique, which is recommended by some authors, has the disadvantage that, unless the submucosal stitch is ideally placed, there is the risk of having a fringe of mucous membrane jutting out into the lumen of the vas deferens, which does not allow an ideal anatomical reconstruction.

Some authors describe large series of cases operated according to this technique with up to 80% patency. The percentage of pregnancies is smaller for a number of reasons that cannot be discussed here, but is decidedly larger than after epididymo-deferential anastomosis because, obviously, epididymal maturation has never been impaired.

When the ductus deferens is opened and the lumen on the side of the testis is well visible but sperm is not seen to issue from this end, the tunica vaginalis should be opened and the epididymis carefully examined. In fact, in some cases of vasectomy, increased intraepididymal pressure has caused the rupture of the loops at this level giving rise to secondary obliteration. In certain situations, the problem can then be solved by creating an epididymo-deferential anastomosis; but these possibilities are limited, in view of the distance between the epididymis and the healthy portion of the ductus deferens above the vasectomy.

*Two-layer technique*

This is illustrated in Figure 24.5. The operating field is prepared as described above. Once the two stumps have been freed and their patency has been checked, it is useful to place a silastic sheet under them so as to obtain better visualization of the two ends to be joined. We have already said that the vas deferens is opened by a cut running perpendicular to its axis; thus, as a rule, a straight cut edge is obtained. However, in some cases there is a certain amount of retraction of the central portion of the ductus deferens with the result that the cut edge becomes funnel shaped. This is no great problem for the one-layer vasovasostomy but creates an additional difficulty for the first mucomucosal suture in two-layer vasovasostomy. In order to avoid this difficulty it is useful,

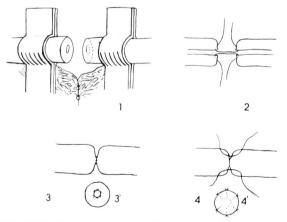

**Fig. 24.5** Vaso-vasostomy: double-layer technique. 1, Preparing both sections. 2, Inserting mucosal stitches (nylon 10/0). 3, Completion of the mucosal layer; 3', cross-section. 4, Muscular suture (nylon 6/0); 4', cross-section.

when sectioning the vas, to hold the resected cicatrical portion firmly and to apply traction in the opposite direction to the periphery of the ductus deferens. By doing this, cut edges are obtained which are practically never funnel shaped and as a rule are even convex. The first stitch, using Prolene 10/0, takes a few muscle fibers as well as the mucosa. The diameters of the two cut edges must be made equal; this is achieved by inserting a jeweler's forceps into the distal portion of the vas deferens and releasing it slightly several times until the two diameters are equal. The mucosa is never seized with a forceps and the stitches are inserted and passed through the mucous membrane by taking advantage of the counterpressure of the forceps introduced into the lumen. The first stitch is tied immediately and is followed by two stitches placed on either side on the part of the vas exposed to the surgeon. This requires constant irrigation, because the semen leaking from the testicular end of the vas impinges upon the visibility of the delicate mucosal edge.

The operation is done under the microscope with a magnification of $16\times$ to $25\times$. It is advisable to use the zoom of the microscope frequently to employ maximum magnification only when inserting the stitches, and then to reduce it for placing and tying the knots. The ductus deferens is then turned by $180°$ and the deep layer is at once made visible. The suture will be the more leakproof the more perfectly identical the stitches are with regard to their insertion and the amount of mucosa they charge. Ths precaution is essential if the presence of fringes of mucosa inside the lumen is to be avoided.

The tissues involved are so thin that as a rule the whole loop of the knots in the deep layer can be seen and not only the part of the thread that has penetrated into the lumen. The other three stitches are then inserted in identical fashion. In some cases of a particularly wide ductus deferens it may be necessary to place up to eight stitches. As a last stage of the operation, the muscularis is joined with six stitches of Prolene 6/0.

*Comment*

Compared to the single-layer technique, two-layer vasovasostomy has the advantage of a tighter suture. This is due to the greater precision of the insertion of the stitches in the mucosa and because irregularities at the level of suture are avoided, which is less easy during single-layer vasovasostomy. We have repeatedly stressed that each stitch should involve the same amount of tissue; obviously this precision will be enhanced by dealing separately with the mucous and the muscular layer.

*Results*

Increasing numbers of statistics are published regularly by population reports and progressively the picture clarifies and allows some general conclusions.

Training and skill of the surgeon is paramount and reversals will have to be restricted to a limited number of operators with suffcent expertise. The double-layer technique gives roughly 10% better results compared to the one-layer technique.

The most impressive series, those by Lee (1981), Schmidt et al (1976) and Silber (1978a), mention 80–90% patency, and Silber obtained a 71% pregnancy rate.

Most authors have a pregnancy rate of about 50%. The better results published by Silber may be linked to his selection on basis of previous testicular biopsies.

Our own experience covers 320 demands for vaso-vasostomies. Patency rate is 85% and pregnancy rate 52%.

**Vasoepididymostomy**

*Epididymal patency: a matter of degree*

Commonly, the presence of even a few spermatozoa in the ejaculate is taken as evidence of a normally patent epididymis. As a consequence, the correct diagnosis of epididymal disease is often overlooked and patients are treated for a long time by stimulation of spermatogenesis (insofar as such stimulation seems possible) without any obvious beneficial results. Despite this, the frequent discrepancy between the good quality of spermatogenesis and the inadequacy of sperm in the ejaculate caught the attention of many investigators working in the field of male infertility (Steinberger, Rodriguez, Schoysman). It must therefore be emphasized that suspicion of epididymal pathology is justified mainly in cases of azoospermia, but also in some forms of oligozoospermia and even asthenozoospermia.

### Pathology of epididymal obstruction

There are many causes of ductal obstruction in the male genital tract. The most frequent are postinfectious. With effective antibiotic treatment, however, the incidence of postinfectious obstructions has progressively diminished and congenital lesions are becoming more significant. A group of small cystic lesions of the epididymal tract are another cause of epididymal obstruction. The ratio of infectious to congenital azoospermia depends on the country where the study is carried out and on the method of patient selection.

Epididymal obstruction is not an all or none phenomenon, all degrees of obstruction being present. This is especially true when the obstruction is secondary to an infective process.

**Congenital causes.** As stated previously, this group is becoming more important and accounts for 2% of all infertile males. There are many different anomalies, but the most frequent is the total absence of the cauda epididymis, the loop of the vas, and the vas deferens itself, although the caput epididymis is left intact. In addition, the seminal vesicles are also commonly absent in this anomaly, leading to an ejaculate of very small volume (usually less than 1 ml). These findings can be explained by considering the embryological development of the epididymis. The caput is of testicular origin and consists of the cones efferentes, whereas the cauda epididymis and vas deferens are derived from the urethra. Thus, even if the vas developed normally, it could have failed to join with the caput. Congenital absence of the vas deferens is relatively frequent, and techniques to construct an artificial spermatocele in such cases generally lead to disappointing results (Schoysman, Wagenknecht, Kelami).

**Management of cases of congenital absence of vas deferens by IVF with epididymal sperm** In 1985, an Australian group (Temple-Smith et al 1985) obtained a pregnancy by aspirating spermatozoa from the isolated caput epididymis and using them to fertilize oocytes in vitro after their echoguided retrieval in the wife. The first breakthrough in this important group of patients was followed by other successes mainly by the group of Asch and Silber in the USA, who obtained nine pregnancies on 33 attempts. Other groups have also published successes and our own experience is gathered in Table 24.1 where five pregnancies have been obtained in 16 attempts (July 1991).

The successes with this approach have led to some astonishing observations: the closer spermatozoa are collected to the rete testis the better is their motility. This is not a uniform observation as seen in Table 24.1, but it is nevertheless frequently observed. It has led to some doubt about the physiological function of the epididymis but more precise biochemical workup of the particular epididymal secretions in these circumstances will explain the, at first view, contradictory behaviour of spermatozoa in these collected samples.

For this particular work the aspiration of sperm must be realized with the help of the operative microscope. It is mandatory that the tubule would be prepared by careful dissection in order to avoid all bleeding and that after its incision with a diamond scalpel the obtained fluid should be aspirated in a tuberculine syringe filled with some culture medium. The sperm is then further handled on a mini-Percoll column and surprisingly good motility can ultimately be obtained. Combining this approach with further use of pentoxyphyllin and eventual subzonal insemination of spermatozoa may significantly improve the results. This extremely interesting new area of approach for situations that in the past were of poor prognosis is raising much enthusiasm both from the IVF teams and from the physiologists of epididymal function.

Although retrograde ejaculation does not actually belong to the group of azoospermic males, a similar approach can be mentioned in these cases. When the usually advocated procedure of collecting sperm in the bladder has failed during several insemination cycles, sperm collection from the vas can also be used in IVF attempt.

Finally, the same approach has been used for

**Table 24.1**  Deferential agenesis

| Site of collection (mm from the rete testis) | | | | | | | Concentration motility | Treatment of sperm | No. of fertilizations | Transfers |
|---|---|---|---|---|---|---|---|---|---|---|
| 30 | 25 | 20 | 15 | 10 | 5 | 0 | | | | |
| SP IM | SP IM | SP MOT | — | — | SP IM | — | $20\times10^6$ 20% MOT S/PL | PTF MINIPERCOL | 7/9 | Pregnancy Miscarriage 9 Weeks |
| — | — | NO SP | SP MOT | SP IM | SP IM | — | $5.0\times10^6$ 5% MOT S/PL | MINIPERCOL | 0/4 | — |
| — | NO SP | — | SP MOT | — | — | — | $30\times10^6$ 10% MOT S/PL | PTF MINIPERCOL | 1/8 | |
| — | — | — | — | SP IM | SP IM | — | | | | |
| — | NO SP | NO SP | NO SP | NO SP | NO SP | — | | | | |
| — | NO SP | — | SP MOT | — | SP MOT | — | $30\times10^6$ 10% MOT S/PL | PTF MINIPERCOL | 7/19 | Pregnancy |
| — | — | SP IM | SP IM | SP MOT | — | — | $20\times10^6$ 9% MOT S/PL | PTF MINIPERCOL | 0/4 | |
| — | NO SP | — | SP MOT | SP MOT | — | — | $5\times10^6$ 5% MOT S/PL | PTF MINIPERCOL | 5/7 | Pregnancy |
| — | SP IM | — | SP IM | SP IM | — | — | | | | |

SP IM, immotile spermatozoa; SP MOT, motile spermatozoa; NO SP, no spermatozoa; 9, sperm collections; 8, with spermatozoa; 6, with motile spermatozoa; 20, embryos/51 oocytes; 3, pregnancies.

failed vasovasostomies or failed vasoepididy- mostomies. Some authors had successes with sperm collected from the caput epididymis after failed vasoepididymostomy but generally in this indication the outcome is much more debatable.

***Postinfectious causes*** In the 1950s, gonor- rhea was the most frequent cause of epididymal obstruction. However, looking at all the series of epididymal lesions, one finds that obstruction has occurred subsequent to a gonorrheal infection in less than 20% of the current cases. Gonorrhea frequently destroys the distal section of the epididymis and spares the caput. The vas deferens may be affected in addition to the epididymis, focally or along its entire length. A surgical repair, in this last instance, is of course impossible. A significant number of patients may suffer from other types of infections, resulting in epididymal obstruction. Any lower urinary tract infection can ascend the ejaculatory duct, enter the vas deferens, and reach the epididymis. This may cause clinical or subclinical epididymitis, and may be associated with varying degrees of prostatitis or seminal vesiculitis which may be clinically inapparent. Genital tuberculosis on the other hand is almost nonexistent in Western Europe. It causes severe destruction of the entire epididymis, including the caput.

Because of the importance of identifying postinfectious causes of epididymal obstruction, we will give a more detailed description of the pathogenesis of this condition.

***Subacute epididymal infection and its sequelae*** Males with this condition are in most cases referred to the infertility clinic because of oligospermia and are completely unaware of any degree of genital infection. Study of the ejaculate itself is unlikely to help in diagnosis because there are usually no signs of infection. Clinical investi- gation shows the epididymis to be soft, tender, and slightly enlarged. This situation can last unchanged for a long time, occasionally 1 or 2 years, and respond dramatically to antibiotics and antiinflammatory drugs.

Once the acute or subacute epididymitis is cured, by treatment or by its own natural course, we have to face different types of sequelae. It is unreasonable to look for a classification of these, because, depending on the level of the epididymis

which was infected, there may be variable degrees of sclerosis. Consequently, the degree to which the epididymal tubules are blocked may vary and only the study of several ejaculates together with a thorough evaluation of the condition of the epididymis would allow a correct diagnosis. The erroneous idea that spermatogenesis stops when the epididymis is blocked still lives on but should be finally laid to rest. If a patient showed both epididymal disease and inhibited spermatogen- esis, it is either due to the fact that he had some degree of orchitis associated with his epididymal infection, or that he already had some disturbance of spermatogenesis before suffering from epididymal complications.

***Final postinfectious status*** The first result of infection is sclerosis, causing a progressive constriction of the tubules, either very high in the head of the epididymis or lower down along the organ. The most severe type of postinfectious sclerosis is generally located halfway down the organ. If the tubules are narrowed and spermato- genesis proceeds unchanged, there will be a progressive engorgement in the tubules above the obliteration site. It is important to point out here that, owing to transit difficulties, complete or incomplete, the testis shows no significant differ- ence as far as the quality of spermatogenesis is concerned. Although one occasionally finds some cases where there seems to be some relationship between the level of the epididymal block and the degree of alteration in the testicular function, detailed studies do not substantiate this hypoth- esis. In 15 carefully selected patients in whom localization of the site of their epididymal blockage was very accurate, we studied spermato- genesis in the obstructed testicle and found that the level of obstruction did not affect its quality.

Dilatation of the epididymal tubules is not uniform. First of all it occurs close to the block and progressively spreads out higher up until occasionally the entire caput epididymis is swollen. Clinically, one can palpate a thickened caput of the epididymis and by visual inspection, the diagnosis is easy: tubules are dilated and have a yellow or buff-colored aspect.

Microscopically, the epididymal duct proximal to the obstruction becomes dilated and tortuous, with early phagocytosis of sperm cell, which collect there in excessive numbers. As spermato-genesis continues, progressive packing of the epididymal ducts occurs. With increasing luminal pressure, rupture of the ducts with extravasation of sperm cells into interstitial tissue eventually occurs, finally leading to the development of spermatic granulomas. If this process takes place close to the organ, one is not aware of it unless careful palpation occasionally reveals some hard nodules; but when it is located just underneath the serosa, brownish blot of variable diameter appears. Ultimately this granuloma is itself invaded by vessels and progressively reabsorbs, but then a new sclerotic area appears, and hence-forth a new block. Inspection of the epididymis shows that such an area of sclerotic granuloma has a bluish aspect and feels rather hard. When such lesions are located very high in the epididymis, although they will have destroyed a certain number of vasa efferentia, sperm can still progress along those vasa that were not involved in the sclerotic process. However, once these types of lesions appear lower down, where the epididymal tubule is single, the chances of their causing a complete block are much higher. The time span necessary to provoke lesions like this is variable. Clear information will only be available if the patient remembers the exact time at which he suffered the acute condition, for instance gonorrhea, which can be presumed to have been the start of this epididymal disease.

## The diagnosis of epididymal obstruction

Most patients with epididymal obstruction present with azoospermia or severe oligo-zoospermia and the differential diagnosis is there-fore between primary testicular disease, such as germinal aplasia or maturation arrest, and a congenital ductal agenesis or acquired obstruc-tion. In primary testicular disorders, physical examination usually reveals testes that are smaller and softer than normal, with normally palpable epididymes and vasa deferentia. Serum follicle stimulating hormone (FSH) is considerably elevated.

Usually, the diagnosis of epididymal occlusion is relatively easy. A firm testis of normal volume is found, while the ejaculate is azoospermic. The

caput epididymis is slightly enlarged, sometimes soft, and rarely painful. The vas deferens is easily palpable. If the caput epididymis is swollen, and more than 2 cm long, epididymal occlusion is the most likely diagnosis.

## Surgical repair of epididymal obstruction

Management of the incomplete epididymal block is an open question. One does not really know what to do. When the infection is very recent and limited to edema, as said before, antibiotics and antiinflammatory drugs can be used, but for the older subtotal obliteration, there is no good medical cure.

As to the complete blocks causing azoospermia, the same types of lesions are present and their management can cause great difficulties. It is out of the question to repair epididymal tubules in situ. Therefore the principle of curing epididymal blocks is to create a bypass or anastomosis between the caput epididymis and the vas deferens.

### Surgical technique by latero-lateral vaso-epididymostomy. The incision is not a scrotal incision but somewhat higher and midway between the scrotum and the inguinal canal. This allows a higher dissection of the vas if necessary. Once the scrotum is opened, the testis is completely exposed and the epididymis carefully inspected. The vas is then retained with a Babcock clamp and the operation begins with its dissection. It is exposed over a length of 12–15 mm, carefully avoiding the vessels. The muscular coat is never completely freed all around from its fascia; only the area that lies opposite the epididymis is completely exposed. During the dissection, an assistant keeps the operative field moist with a drip infusion of 5% glucose with addition of 5000 units of heparin and 200 mg of hydrocortisone. When half a cylinder of the muscular layer is exposed over a length of 12–13 mm, it is incised sharply with an iridec-tomy knife over a length of 10–12 mm. Before the operation continues, patency of the distal vas must be confirmed. It suffices to inject 20–30 ml of 5% glucose solution (because the seminal vesicles contain up to 20 ml, the injection of only

a few millilitres does not prove that the entire genital tract is patent).

The vas is now wrapped in moist swabs and the epididymis is opened. The incision must be made as low as possible in the corpus, for two reasons. First, by leaving part of the caput above the sutures intact the option remains of performing a reanastomosis in case of failure of the first attempt. Secondly, and more important, the low anastomosis allows the sperm to flow through a greater length of the epididymis than does a high anastomosis, permitting better maturation of the spermatozoa. The low anastomosis, if successful, thus produces sperm of better motility. The high anastomosis, although technically easier and giving the patient a better chance of high sperm count, leads to an ejaculate containing mainly immotile spermatozoa. The epididymis is held firmly between the thumb and index finger while a straight deep incision of 12–13 mm is made with a very sharp pointed scalpel. The incision must be 5 mm deep from the start. A mixture of blood and white to yellowish epididymal secretion will immediately ooze out. A drop of this secretion is immediately studied under the microscope by an assistant. Although sometimes motile sperm are found, usually only degenerated spermatozoa are present. However, if no cells at all are found, the incision must be repeated at a higher level until spermatozoa, motile or not, are found in large numbers. The upper angle (distal vas to cephalid portion of the epididymal incision) is the best location to start suturing the vas and epididymis together. For years we have used a straight 6 cm needle with 6/0 tantalum wire but we recently replaced this material with 7/0 or 8/0 nylon. At the side of the vas deferens, the needle takes both the muscular layer and the mucosa. By including the mucosa, the stitches act more or less like a very localized splint. One must not be mistaken about the rationale of the latero-lateral technique and imagine that sperm is likely to flow through an opening 12 or 13 mm in length. Even if tubules let sperm ooze out lower down, in the end the real passage along the vas will only be obtained through the upper angle. Additional stitches uniting the deferential and epididymal incisions lower down generally work as a firm support of the anastomosis (Fig. 24.6).

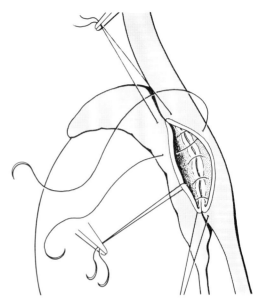

**Fig. 24.6**  Latero-lateral anastomosis between epididymis and vas deferens.

This again stresses the utmost importance of dealing with the upper angle stitch at the level of the vas, it will include both muscular and mucosal layers; in the epididymis one must make sure the needle moves as close as possible to the tubules (generally two or three) whither viable spermatozoa leak. Once this area is secured by three or four mucoepididymal stitches, the anastomosis continues progressively by interrupted sutures every alternate 2 mm on both sides of the epididymal and deferential incisions, taking care to have it watertight over its entire length. At the end of the operation, two more stitches are inserted, one above and the other below the anastomosis to avoid excessive tension.

***Microsurgical termino-terminal vasoepididymostomy.*** The first approach of latero-lateral vasoepididymostomy we have described is now totally abandoned for more precise microsurgical end-to-end termino-terminal anastomosis. This operation was first advocated by Silber (1978b) and consists of a direct anastomosis between an epididymal tubule and the lumen of the vas. The preparation of the operation is similar as in the previous technique. The epididymis being inspected, the location of obstruction is determined and at this level the epididymis is completely divided with straight scissors. The section shows than a large number of leaking tubules and numerous bleeders. We must, however, keep in mind that beyond 10–12 mm of the rete testis the epididymal tubule is a unique one and that, even if many loops are opened at the lower level, only one of them is in continuity with the rete testis. It is important to locate that precise loop, which is easy to do since spermatozoa continue oozing out of it. Once the patent loop has been definitely recognized and its contents checked for the presence of spermatozoa, a 10.0 Prolene stitch is immediately passed outside – inside through its wall and left in place. The vas deferens is then prepared by an eventual high dissection of the cord, in order to avoid all traction, and also divided. The section of the vas brought close to the prepared tubule and first sutured to the serosa of the epididymis by two posterior stitches. A direct anastomosis between the tubule and the mucosa of the vas is then realized either by 3 or 4 Prolene 10.0 stitches. Once this mucosal suture has been realized the circumference of the vas is further sutured to the serosa of the epididymis by either 8.0 or 5.0 Prolene stitches (Fig. 24.7).

The advantages of this operation are obvious. It is a much more precise anastomosis than the latero-lateral one and it is therefore not surprising that the results on the whole are undoubtedly much better. The drawback, however, is twofold. First, the difficulty in locating the patent tubule. It is indeed not always easy to make up one's mind what tubule will be ultimately the patent one. Another difficulty is the fact that that particular tubule may not be centered in the middle of the epididymal section. As a consequence, the anastomosis of the vas to the epididymis will occasionally be difficult. In the original drawing of Silber a fine anastomosis is shown, but this is only so if the epididymal block is located very low. If it is located in the caput epididymis the section of the organ will be very large and clearly difficulties in suturing the vas are to be expected.

***Latero-terminal vasoepididymostomy (Thomas)*** (Fig. 24.8) The latest approach for correcting epididymal blocks avoids the above-said difficulties. It consists of incising the serosa of the epididymis at a level containing dilated tubules, dissecting one of them and preparing a

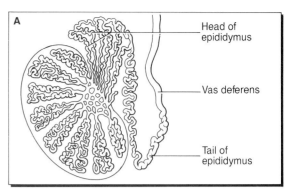

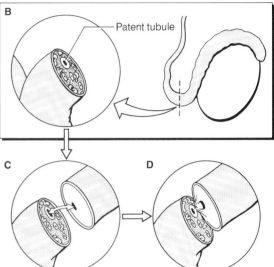

**Fig. 24.7** Original drawing of Silber illustrating termino-terminal anastomosis.

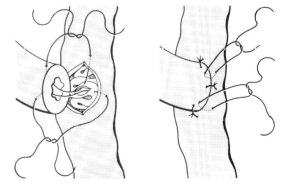

**Fig. 24.8** Original drawing of the latero-terminal anastomosis according to Thomas & Wagenknecht.

longitudinal incision into it. Its content is checked for spermatozoa and, if found positive, the vas is prepared and approximated as for a termino-terminal anastomosis. In the first place we unite by two posterior stitches the serosa of the epididymis and the circumference of the vas. The opening in the tubule is then sutured to the mucosa of the vas by four stitches of 10.0 Prolene.

After the mucosal suture the anastomosis is completed by support stitches between the circumference of the vas deferens and the incision of the epididymal serosa (Fig. 24.7).

## Results of surgery

The results of surgery reported in the literature vary considerably, ranging from very little success up to 30% pregnancy rate. We have performed 320 epididymal-deferential anastomoses with known follow-up in 261 patients. After 1 year patency reaches an average of 51%, but the pregnancy rate is much lower. To our knowledge this figure is 21% at most and could be even lower if all patients lost to follow-up failed to achieve fatherhood. The delay in obtaining pregnancy can take up to 4 years. Even in successful cases, several problems remain unsolved. One of them is the delay in postoperative results. After operation, azoospermia can persist for up to 12 months. Judging whether or not an anastomosis is unsuccessful is thus only possible 1 year following surgery.

Semen samples after anastomosis show a varia-tion in quality that, regardless of total sperm concentration, is certainly related to the level of the epididymis at which the operation was performed. Almost without exception high anastomosis results in very poor motility whereas this criterion of sperm quality is dramatically improved with a lower anastomosis. This again stresses the importance of carefully checking the site of the anastomotic area, starting low and proceeding gradually higher and higher, until finally sperm cells are found in the epididymal fluid.

Since we abandoned the latero-lateral technique in favor of the termino-terminal and the latero-lateral, our experience covers at this time slightly over 1 000 treatments of excretory azoo-spermic males. One must accept, however, that a significant percentage of those patients are in-operable.

In discussing the results of vasovasostomy we have mentioned that many candidates for this surgery had severely diminished spermatogenesis and the same is observed in postinfectious epididymal blocks. Furthermore, 8% of the patients also have deferential blocks. Finally, epididymal damage can be very high causing sclerosis up to the vasa efferentia. In short, 30% of the patients are inoperable. Tables 24.2–24.4 summarize the experience with the three aforesaid operations. The two first groups concern latero-lateral approaches performed either on the lower segment or cauda epididymis or the higher caput

**Table 24.2**    Macrosurgical side-to-side vasoepididymostomy

| Author | Patients (no.) | Sperm No. | Sperm % | Pregnancies No. | Pregnancies % |
|---|---|---|---|---|---|
| Jequier 1985 | 24 | 3 | 12.5 | 1 | 4.2 |
| Hanley 1955 | 71 | 11 | 15.5 | 5 | 7 |
| Dubin & Amelar 1984 | 69 | 14 | 20 | 7 | 10 |
| O'Connor 1953 | 61 | 14 | 20 | 5 | 8 |
| Lee 1981 | 82 | 25 | 30.4 | 11 | 13.4 |
| Wagenknecht et al 1980 | 170 | 48 | 32 | — | |
| Hendry et al 1983 | 83 | 29 | 35 | 9 | 10.8 |
| Kar & Phadke 1975 | 281 | 137 | 48.8 | 40 | 14.2 |
| Schoysman 1982 | 261 | 146 | 56 | | 21 |
| Hendry 1981 | 5 | 3 | 60 | — | |
| Schoysman & Bedford 1993 | 565 | 350 | 62 | | 18 |
| Hagner 1936 | 33 | 21 | 64 | 16 | 48.5 |
| Bayle 1953 | 65 | 43 | 66 | 20 | 30.7 |

**Table 24.3**    Microsurgical tubule-to-tubule vasoepididymostomy

| Author | Year | Patients (no.) | Sperms No | Sperms % | Pregnancies No. | Pregnancies % |
|---|---|---|---|---|---|---|
| McLoughlin | 1982 | 23 | | — | 9 | 39 |
| Wagenknecht | 1985 | 50 | | — | 12 | 23 |
| Dubin & Amelar | 1984 | 46 | 18 | 39 | 6 | 13 |
| Thomas | 1986 | 50 | 33 | 66 | 18 | 41.9 |
| Schoysman | 1990 | 161 | 126 | 78 | 67 | ↗ 41 on total  ↘ 53 on patency |
| Fogdestam et al | 1986 | 41 | 35 | 85.3 | 15 | 36.6 |
| Silber | 1978 | 14 | 12 | 86 | — | |
| Belgrano et al | 1984 | 4 | 4 | 100 | 1 | 25 |

**Table 24.4**    Detailed personal results

| | No. | Patency (%) | Pregnancies (%) of patent cases | Pregnancies (%) of total |
|---|---|---|---|---|
| Low latero-lateral anastomosis | 210 | 62 | 24 | 15 |
| Termino-terminal anastomosis | 78 | 82 | 45 | 38 |
| Latero-terminal anastomosis | 40 | 82 | 50 | 42 |
| Selected 'ideal' group | 43 | 93 | 70 | 65 |

epididymis. The last group (Table 24.4) is a particularly favorable, one in which all aspects of the pathological situation are optimal for surgical repair. In such a group statistics are of course optimalized to the extreme.

*Postoperative management*

Customarily, we first request a semen specimen 2 months after the anastomosis, but the curiosity of the patient often leads to this control sample being supplied earlier. We have seen positive specimens as early as 7 days postoperatively. Nevertheless, a negative sample at 2 months postoperatively is certainly no indication that the operation was a failure. We have had patients whose ejaculate became positive only after a period of 8 months.

CONCLUSIONS

The surgery of male infertility is thankless work but nevertheless allows some hope for success. This surgery should be restricted to a limited number of specialists, in order to give them an opportunity to gain adequate experience. If one performs a single epididymal-deferential anastomosis every other year, good results will never be obtained and the already poor chances of success will be reduced even more.

Summarizing this intricate and confusing field, the following statements should be born in mind:

1. Epididymal pathology is a potentially recognizable factor in up to 21% of male subfertility.

2. Spermatogenesis in the testis remains unaltered whatever the level of the epididymal block.

3. Epididymal patency is a matter of degree. Epididymal pathology can cause both incomplete and complete blocks, leading consequently to oligozoospermia as well as to azoospermia.

4. Not looking at the epididymis while performing testicular biopsy may result in the loss of at least one-half of the value of scrotal exploration.

5. Microsurgical epididymovasostomy is best reserved for azoospermic males. In some cases oligospermic males have been treated but this is so far a very uncertain field for microsurgery. Amongst the variable techniques the latero-terminal one is clearly the most favorable since it offers an up to 50% chance of fertilization in the partner within the year after surgery.

The older latero-lateral anastomosis definitely belongs to the past.

## PROCEDURES TO IMPROVE VASCULAR DISORDERS—VARICOCELE

### A. The problem of varicocele

The problem of varicocele is the perfect illustration of that very peculiar situation where opinions range between overenthusiasm and complete neglect.

Operation of varicocele was never performed on infertile males until Tulloch, in 1928, drew attention to its salutary effects on spermatogenesis. This observation was practically unnoticed but reappeared in 1961 during the infertility congress in Stockholm. Varicocele ligation became the andrological bombshell of the year. However, the problem did not receive the enthusiasm of all urologists or andrologists since it is a fact that a lot of males with varicocele have fathered many children. Nevertheless, the lowered fertility of many oligospermic males justified backing up the idea of varicocele ligation as a possible help, especially since medical therapy proved so disappointing.

In the sixties, a large number of very enthusiastic papers were published about varicocele ligation and its success, but progressively careful studies of pre- and post-operative semen samples led to more doubtful attitudes.

After 20 years of 'pros and cons' we have a better view of the impact of vascular disorder on spermatogenesis and on the possibilities for improving the quality of sperm output.

*Varicocele and semen characteristics*

Varicocele meant a unique chance to link a particular seminological pattern to a clinical condition. One of the problems in andrology is the lack of such correlations, since the testis responds in a fairly similar way to all types of interferences to its function.

MacLeod (1965) described a typical 'stress pattern', in connection with the presence of varicocele. This consisted of an elongation of the nucleus leading to tapering forms, and the presence of many immature cells with markedly decreased motility.

However, it has been recognized that some patients with second or third degree varicocele do not necessarily show the particular seminological pattern in their ejaculates and, on the other hand, that the stress pattern was not systematically associated with clinical varicocele. In our experience, the seminological pattern fits the clinical situation in approximately 20–25% of the patients.

The most logical way to approach the impact of varicocele on fertility was suggested by Stewart Scott, keeping in mind that parameters of seminal values are distributed along a Gauss curve. Undoubtedly for all males having seminal values on the left side of the Gauss curve, varicocele definitely represents a greater danger to their spermatogenesis than for the other ones. This explains why there is a percentage of varicocele among a fertile population practically identical to its incidence in husbands of barren couples.

Classification of clinical varicocele recognizes several groups according to volume and scrotal extent. They are generally localized in the left scrotal area (5–7% are bilateral). Usually three groups are recognized — group 3 being the extreme from where the entire left or bilateral scrotal tissue is filled with dilated veins. Moreover, over the last few years, the occult varicocele has drawn a lot of attention. According to some authors the occult form of varicocele would be just as harmful to testicular function as the very severe degrees, but these statements are controversial.

Although there is no clear-cut relation between the severity of oligospermia and the extent of the vascular disorder, in our material the 'larger the varicocele, the poorer the sperm' seems to be the trend.

Its discovery is possible using the Valsalva manoeuvre with the patient in a standing position, but more adequately by thermography, Doppler effect, or by retrograde phlebography.

Good data are available (Comhaire & Kunnen 1976) about varicocele detection, by thermography and retrograde phlebography. A difference of more than 2° between both testis means an alarm signal, revealing occult varicocele. Retrograde phlebography has shown a variety of vascular anomalies that are interesting to study both to detect venous deficiency or to recognize incomplete surgical ligation (since the venous plexus shows extreme anatomical variations some veins may be overlooked during surgery).

## B. Causal part of varicocele interfering with spermatogenesis

There are several theories attempting to explain the influence of varicocele on testicular function. The most obvious causes are diminished oxygenation of the tissue and increased scrotal temperature. Furthermore, good evidence is available proving that catecholamines and steroids from the suprarenal can reach the testis by the retrograde bloodflow, and so affect both gonads through the extensive cross circulation between them.

Each theory of course has sound arguments. Therefore the most obvious conclusion seems to consider it as a fact that varicocele has a multifactorial deleterious effect on the testes.

## C. Surgical therapy

### Contraindications

Contraindications for surgery are an abnormal karyotype, an elevated level of FSH and occurrence of cryptorchidism in the anamnesis. Although it has been claimed by several authors that the clinical degree of varicocele has no relation to the degree of impairment of spermatogenesis, some authors feel that the very discrete varicoceles and also the subclinical varicoceles

would indeed have very little influence on spermatogenesis. A group of 40 patients with subclinical varicocele detected by retrograde phlebography and corrected either surgically or by immediate embolization has not shown significant improvement of semen parameters (Schoysman 1982). Other contraindications are age over 40 years and of course general poor health.

### Techniques

The two most commonly advised surgical approaches are the Ivanissevitch operation and the Palomo operation. We favour the Ivanissevitch operation since it is the easiest and gives the best approach to the plexus pampiniformis of the spermatic vein.

An inguinal incision of 6 cm is performed in the middle third of the inguinal canal. The aponeurosis is freed and opened over a similar length. Introducing the mid-finger towards the inner inguinal canal easily localizes the transverse muscle that can be elevated with a retractor, exposing the spermatic cord. The latter is then grasped with atraumatic forceps and gently freed from some loose adhesions. Opening of the cord allows spermatic veins to extrude easily and elevation of the plexus pampiniformis allows good recognition of the vas deferens.

The latter is easily separated from the plexus pampiniformis. Arterial vascularization is generally very close to the vas deferens, but damage to it can usually be avoided. The plexus pampiniformis is then transected, divided, and both extremities ligated with catgut 1. Before ligating it is best to inspect the entire area for eventual deeper veins that might have escaped at first view. Both stumps are re-entered into the inguinal canal and the aponeurotic incision is closed with three or four stitches of a nonresorbable material.

The Palomo operation follows the same principle but is performed at a higher level and consists of freeing the spermatic vein retroperitoneally by an incision at the level of the iliac crest. It offers the advantage of being above the plexus pampiniformis and is thus in a better position to ligate the total venous testicular circulation.

Some surgeons prefer an even higher approach at ligating the spermatic vein a few centimeters beneath the renal vein.

Although we do not deny the value of these higher retroperitoneal approaches, the Ivanissevitch approach is simpler, identical for both right and left sides if the varicocele is bilateral, and in our view represents the preferable technique.

## Embolization of the spermatic vein

In recent years embolization of the spermatic vein has been advocated to avoid the complications of surgery and to handle the case on an outpatient basis. Embolization of the spermatic vein is carried on by injection of iso-butyl-2-cyano acrylat (Bucrylat). Catheterization starting in the right femoral vein allows us to bring the catheter into the left spermatic vein under radioscopic control. Actually this technique is similar to retrograde phlebography so that diagnosis and immediate therapy by embolization can be combined. The procedure is simple and very rewarding. After the first publications several devices have been advocated to obliterate the spermatic vein.

## Embolization versus surgery in varicocele therapy

Routinely after varicocele ligation, we perform scrotal exploration of the infertile patient, aiming at evaluation of the epididymis and also allowing for two testicular biopsies, one for routine pathology examination and one for genetic study of the meiosis. The finding of epididymal transit disturbances in at least 20% of all our investigations and meiotic anomalies in 8% proves clearly that infertile patients afflicted with varicocele can have other associated causes of their poor semen quality.

Not recognizing these predominant reasons for asthenoteratospermia will leave the andrologist with an incomplete diagnosis and generate erroneous statistics with regard to the results of varicocele therapy.

In 700 varicocele ligations marked improvement in sperm quality was noted only in 25%, and pregnancies were recorded in 17%. If, however, we excluded from this group all epididymal and genetic causes, the improvement of sperm quality by varicocele ligation is over 40% and the pregnancy rate approaches 30%. Embolization without associated scrotal exploration will thus leave a certain number of pathological conditions unrecognized.

The results of varicocele ligation and pregnancy rate vary significantly from one surgical team to another with discrepancies as large as 5–60%.

Improvement is usually seen within 6–18 months after surgery. Often a moderate to marked increase in sperm count is seen, with marked improvement in motility and decrease of immature forms. Best results usually follow when a preoperative oligospermia has been present but occasionally improvement follows when the man is almost azoospermic (Stewart 1974).

Clear conclusions are still not available since one should also consider the age of the treated patient. Obviously the longer the testis has been exposed to the deleterious influence of the varicocele, the poorer are the chances for recovery of good spermatogenesis.

In our own studies, patients in the age group between 25 and 30 years stand a far better chance than those aged 35–40. Beyond that age it is our opinion that the chances for improvement are practically nil. However, on the other hand, this would be an argument for preventive ligation of varicocele in adolescents. Some andrologists today are convinced that the preventive approach will offer better help to a male population afflicted with varicocele than a therapeutic one when testicular dysfunction has already become obvious.

Such an attitude, however, is also open to criticism since a fairly large number of males in a fertile population do have a varicocele and systematic ligation in adolescents would undoubtedly lead to a great deal of useless operations, that, however benign, do nevertheless present the hazards inherent to all surgical interventions.

BIBLIOGRAPHY

A complete bibliography on the topic of surgery of the male genital tract, including work on testicular biopsy and immunology, is exhaustive and only the most significant publications are listed below.

Bayle H 1953 Traitement chirurgical des oblitérations du canal déférent. 1st World Congress on Fertility and Sterility, New York

Bedford J M, Calvin H, Cooper G W 1973 The maturation of spermatozoa in the human epididymis. J Reprod Fert Suppl 18: 199

Beer A E, Naeves W B 1978 Antigenic status of semen from the viewpoints of the female and the male. Fertil Steril 29: 3

Brown J S, Dubin L, Hotchliss R S 1967 The varicocele as related to fertility. Fertil Steril 18: 46

Comhaire F, Kunnen M 1976 Selective retrograde venography of the internal spermatic vein: a conclusive approach to the diagnosis of varicocele. Andrologia 8: 11

Dubin L, Amelar R D 1970 Varicocele size and results of varicocelectomy in selected subfertile men with varicocele. Fertil Steril 21: 606

Hanley H G 1955 The surgery of male subfertility. Ann R Coll Surg Eng 17: 159

Hanley H G, Hodges R D 1959 The epididymis in male sterility: a preliminary report of microdissection studies. J Urol 82: 508

Hellinga G, Swaen G J V, Van Der Esch E P 1972 Morphological semiquantitative scoring of testicular biopsy in infertility. Andrologie 4: 55

Holstein A F 1969 Morphologische Studien am Nebenhoden des Menschen. Thieme Verlag, Stuttgart

Kelami A, Roloff D, Preu K et al 1976 Alloplastic reservoir on epididymis—an experimental study on minipigs and beagle dogs. Proceedings of the International Congress on Andrology, Barcelona

Klosterhalfen H, Schirren C 1964 Operative Wiederherstellung der Zeugungsfähigkeit des Mannes. Dtsch Med Kschr 47

Kunnen M 1980 Neue Technik zur Embolisation der Vena spermatica interna: intravenoser Gewebekleber. Fortschr Róngenstr 133, 6: 625

Kunnen M, Comhaire F 1983 Extratesticular factors in male infertility. Clin Endocrinol (in press)

Lee H Y 1981 Evaluation of vasovasostomy: macroscopic vs. microscopic anastomosis. J Kor Med Assoc 24: 243

Lunenfeld B, Mör A, Mani M 1976 Treatment of male infertility—I. Human gonadotropins. Fertil Steril 18: 581

Mann T 1974 Secretory function of the prostate, seminal vesicle and other male accessory organs of reproduction. J Reprod Fertil 37: 179

Nankin H R, Troen P 1976 Endocrine profiles in idiopathic oligozoospermic men. In: E S E Hafez (ed) Human semen and fertility regulation in man. Mosby, St Louis, p 370

O'Connor V 1953 Mechanical aspects and surgical management of sterility in men. J A M A

Orgebin-Crist M C, Olson G E, Danzo B J 1981 Factors influencing maturation of spermatozoa in the epididymis. In: Franchimont P, Channing C P (eds) Intragonadal regulation of reproduction. Academic, London, p 39

Sachse H 1965 Morphologie und Funktion des Semenwegsverschlusses. Med Klin 60: 1925

Schmidt S S, Schoysman R, Stewart B H 1976 Surgical approaches to male infertility. In: Hafez E S E (ed) Human semen and fertility regulation in man. Mosby, St Louis, p 299

Schoysman R 1969 La création d'un spermatocèle artificiel dans les agénésies du canal déférent. Andrologie 1: 33

Schoysman R 1969 Surgical treatments in male sterility. Andrologie 31: 33

Schoysman R 1976 Exploration and treatment of obstruction and infections in the seminal duct and accessory genital glands, surgical procedures. Proceedings of the International Congress on Andrology, Barcelona

Schoysman R 1982 Epididymal causes of male infertility: pathogenesis and management. Int Androl Suppl 5: 120

Schoysman R, Bedford J M 1993 The role of the human epididymis in sperm maturation and sperm storage as reflected in the consequences of epididymovasostomy. (in press)

Schoysman R, Drouart J M 1972 Progrès récent dans la chirurgie de al stérilité masculine et féminine. Acta Chir Belg 71: 261

Silber S J 1977 Microscopic vasectomy reversal. Fertil Steril 28: 1191

Silber S J 1978a Vasectomy and vasectomy reversal. Fertil Steril 2: 125

Silber S J 1978b Microscopic vaso-epididymostomy; specific microanastomosis to the epididymal tubule. Fertil Steril 30: 565

Silber S J 1979a Epididymal extravasation following vasectomy as a cause for failure of vasectomy reversal. Fertil Steril 31: 309

Silber S J 1979b Microsurgery. Williams and Wilkins, Baltimore

Silber S J 1982 Recent advances in microsurgery of the male genitalia. Ann Chir Gynaecol 71: 80

Silber S J, Rodriguez-Rigau L J 1981 Quantitative analysis of testicle biopsy: determination of partial obstruction and prediction of sperm count after surgery for obstruction. Fertil Steril 36: 480

Silber S, Balmaceda J, Borreco C, Ord T, Asch R 1988 Pregnancy with sperm aspiration from the proximal head of the epididymis: a new treatment for congenital absence of the vas deferens. Fertil Steril 50(3)

Steinberger E 1951 Hormonal control of mammalian spermatogenesis. Physiol Rev 51: 1

Temple-Smith P D, Southwick G J, Yates, C A, Trounson A O, Kretser D M 1985 Human pregnancy by in vitro fertilization (IVF) using sperm aspirated from the epididymis. J In Vitro Fert Embryo Transf 2: 119

Thomas A J 1987 Vasoepididymostomy. Male infertility. Urol Clin North Am 14(3)

Van Dop P A 1979 Quantitative morphology of the testis of fertile and infertile males. Thesis, Vrije Univesiteit, Amsterdam

Wagenknecht L V 1982 Obstruction in the male reproductive tract. In: Bain J, Schill W B, Schwarztein L (eds) Treatment of male infertility. Springer Verlag, Berlin, p 231

Wagenknecht L V, Weitze K F, Hoppe L P et al 1976 Alloplastic spermatocele for treatment of male infertility. Proceedings of the International Congress on Andrology, Barcelona

Wagenknecht L V, Leidenberger F A, Schutte B et al 1978 Clinical experiences with an alloplastic spermatocele. Andrologia 10: 417

Wagenknecht L V, Klosterhalfen H, Schirren C 1980 Microsurgery in andrologic urology I. Refertilization J Microsurg 1: 370

# 25. Artificial insemination

*M. Glezerman*

## HISTORICAL BACKGROUND OF ARTIFICIAL INSEMINATION

The first reported successful pregnancy following homologous insemination (AIH) was performed by John Hunter at the end of the 18th century. The indication for this procedure was severe hypospadias in the male partner of a barren couple (Shields 1950).

In 1835 Marion Sims performed a procedure which was to be termed later the 'etheral copulation' (McIntosh 1909). Sims obtained semen from the husband of a woman who suffered from a 'hyperesthetic' vagina, most probably vaginism, anesthetized her with ether and injected the semen. Sims, whose name has been immortalized in the postcoital test (PCT), was one of the pioneers in the evaluation of sperm–mucus interaction. In 1886 he carried out intracervical homologous artificial inseminations in six women with negative PCTs. Semen was obtained from the vagina following intercourse. Unfortunately, the only patient who became pregnant eventually aborted.

The first reported human donor insemination (AID) was performed in 1884 by William Pancoast in Philadelphia, Pennsylvania (Hard 1909, Gregoire & Mayer 1965). The indication for the procedure was therapy-resistant azoospermia. When discussing the case with his students, they suggested to solve the problem by a 'hired man'. Eventually, the 'best looking member of the class' provided the semen and the patient was inseminated under anesthesia without her or her husband having been informed about the procedure. The patient conceived and delivered later a healthy male infant.

It was 25 years later that a student of Pancoast, most probably the said 'best looking member of the class' of 1884, published an article reporting about this first successful donor insemination in humans (Hard 1909). Working meanwhile as a general practitioner in Milwaukee, he traveled all the way to New York in order to personally shake the hand of a 25-year-old successful businessman, the 'result' of the experiment of 1884.

Probably without knowing about Dr Pancoast, John Dickinson started to perform AID in women in 1890 with utmost secrecy. Sophia Kleegman shared his office and later became one of the foremost practitioners in the field (Kleegman & Kaufman 1966). The first reported study on a larger number of inseminations comes from the UK and dated back to 1946 (Barton et al). The report included 31 cases of AIH and 15 cases of AID. Since then both AIH and AID have become important tools in the treatment of infertility.

## RATIONALE FOR ARTIFICIAL INSEMINATION

There are a variety of indications for AIH. Yet, this procedure is certainly no panacea. If applied indiscriminately, one may expect a placebo rather than a therapeutic effect and the stress situation associated with AIH may even reduce fertility chances.

AIH is not per se superior to intercousrse if not based on sound indication.

Fertilization of a properly released ovum requires three basic prerequisites: the availability of a sufficient number of motile and morphologically normal sperm cells, the intravaginal deposition of these cells, and ascension of sperm cells into the higher parts of the female genital tract.

While the production of normal semen results solely from normal functioning of the male reproductive system, the second and third prerequisites require adequate interaction between the anatomical and physiological systems of both partners. When any of these three conditions is not fulfilled, fertility may be impaired. When medical, surgical and other treatment schemes have failed, an attempt may be made to employ artificial insemination procedures.

Artificial insemination is not an innocuous procedure and its value must be weighed carefully against possible adverse effects. Whenever AIH is employed, mechanization of the sexual relationship enters into consideration. The process of AIH may not be perceived by the couple as a purely medical procedure, but rather as a corrective measure for performance inability. Consequently, the archaic perception that procreative failure equals failure of sexuality may surface and guilt feelings, subconscious accusation of the partner, and a severe injury to the ego of the 'responsible' partner may ensue. It is not rare to observe previously ovulatory cycles turn anovulatory as soon as treatment with AIH is started and various degrees of impaired sexual response may occur in either partner (Beck 1976). For the male who has to produce an ejaculate on demand at a given time, performance coercion is even more evident and presents the most immediate psychological drawback to AIH. The resulting continuous stress situation for the couple and cumulative month-to-month failures exert a tremendous emotional effect on the marriage in general and the sexual relationship in particular.

Considering this background, the decision for AIH has to be made very carefully.

As we learn more and more about the physiology of reproduction, we become increasingly able to define disturbances along the tract which have to be negotiated by the sperm cells on their journey from the testicle to the fertilization site in the female oviduct. In therapy-resistant spermatogenetic disturbances, or when genetic causes oppose progeny from the male partner, AID may be the solution. Subnormal semen may be treated in vitro for subsequent AIH. Inadequate

sperm–cervical contact due to anatomical abnormalities in either partner may be corrected by artificial placing of the semen. A hostile uterine cervix can be circumvented by intrauterine insemination.

## TECHNIQUE OF ARTIFICIAL INSEMINATION

Artificial insemination may be accomplished by deposition of semen into the vagina, around the cervix, into the cervix, into the uterus or into the oviduct. Special insemination instruments such as cervical caps are available.

These techniques aim at protection of a given sperm sample from the vaginal or cervical environment without attempting to improve its qualities. Fertilization chances of a given sample will improve markedly if quality-promoting factors are added to the protective ones. Many attempts have been made to concentrate spermatozoa prior to insemination using centrifugation (Hanson & Rock 1971), pooling, etc. However, one of the most efficient ways of concentrating sperm cells may be found by observing the natural process of ejaculation: MacLeod & Hotchkiss (1942) observed that the first ejaculatory spurt contains a significantly higher concentration of sperm cells than the following spurts. Harmann (1962) reported that this first portion contains about 90% of all sperm cells destined to leave the male genital tract during a given ejaculation. The first ejaculatory spurt is made up mainly of products from the testes, epididymes, vasa deferentia, and prostate gland. Thus, the first ejaculatory portion contains the highest concentration of sperm cells. The following ejaculatory spurts consist of secretions from the seminal vesicles which act as a buffering agent, as a source of nutrition (due to high fructose content) and a vehicle for spermatozoa. By splitting the ejaculatory spurts into different fractions, one will obtain the highest sperm concentration in the first 'split'. The first ejaculatory split is therefore uniquely suited for AIH if the major seminal problem is reduced sperm concentration. Prior to insemination the different fractions should be examined, since in about 6% of cases sperm concentration is higher in the second ejaculatory spurt, and in 5%

of cases sperm concentration is equally distributed in the different fractions (Amelar et al 1977). This may be due to a disturbance in the sequence of ejaculatory synchronization.

The use of split ejaculates for AIH in cases of subnormal semen may be advantageous also from other points of view. Lindholmer (1973) has postulated suppressive factors in the secretions of the seminal vesicles which may have a deleterious effect on sperm survival.

## Intravaginal insemination

Intravaginal insemination is easily performed by means of a plastic syringe using the whole specimen. This method does not require exposure of the cervix and may be performed by the couple. The female partner is in the supine Trendelenburg position. If the procedure is performed by the couple at their home, the pelvis may be elevated slightly by means of a pillow. The position should be maintained for about 20 min following insemination. Extreme care must be taken not to inject air into the vagina and cervix since this could cause air embolism.

## Pericervical and intracervical insemination

Usually pericervical and intracervical insemination are used concomitantly. The patient is placed in the Trendelenburg position, 0.2–0.5 ml semen is injected slowly into the cervical canal by applying the blunt tip of a plastic syringe to the external os. The rest of the specimen is placed in the anterior vaginal fornix. The patient remains in the supine position for some 20 min.

## 'Cap' insemination

While the small amount of semen deposited intracervically will be stored there for future release to the fertilization site, the major part of the specimen, placed in the vagina will pour out very soon following insemination. Remaining spermatozoa will be inactivated rather quickly by vaginal acidity. Furthermore, all insemination techniques mentioned above require that the patient remains supine for almost half an hour following insemination. This may tie up rooms in a busy practice. The cervical cap technique overcomes these drawbacks (Fig. 25.1).

This cap consists of a plastic hood available in two sizes connected to a flexible plastic tubing which may be closed by a 'roll-on' clamp. Following exposure of the cervix by a speculum and cleaning of the vagina and cervix the cap is placed on the portio vaginalis using a grasping instrument. Vacuum is produced either by a commercially available small hand pump or simply by means of a 10 ml syringe. During this process the application to the cervix is controlled visually. The clamp is then closed and the semen-containing syringe is attached. The clamp is now opened and the semen is injected under vision. The speculum is withdrawn and the patient may leave the table immediately. The cap remains in situ for 8–16 h. The patient is advised to open the clamp upon rising the next morning and to remove the cap by simply pulling on the plastic tubing.

For some patients the production of an ejaculate on demand presents a serious problem. In these cases one should not exert further pressure on the patient, but offer the vacuum cap as an alternative. The instrument is fixed to the uterine cervix by the physician just prior to the time when ovulation is expected. Within the next 16 h the male partner may at his leisure fill the syringe with semen and complete the insemination procedure at a time convenient for him and his wife. Diamond et al (1983) have treated 61 couples with cap-home insemination. The overall pregnancy rate was 53%. Home insemination has been also used successfully in AID programs. The

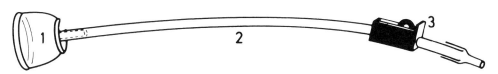

**Fig. 25.1** The vacumn insemination cap (Semm et al 1976). 1, Plastic cap; 2, tubing; 3, roll-on clamp.

husband is instructed in the use of the speculum and the woman is taught to prepare the semen straw for insemination. Portable liquid nitrogen containers were provided for cryopreservation of the semen throughout the insemination period. This approach was used in a randomized study and did not reveal significant differences in pregnancy rates between home and clinical inseminations (Hogerzeil et al 1988). Obviously, this type of collaboration is reserved for highly sophisticated and motivated patients.

### Intrauterine insemination

By means of intrauterine insemination (IUI) the uterine cervix is bypassed and seminal fluid is injected directly into the uterine cavity. This may be done by the use of an infant feeding tube or the plastic tubing of an intracath, attached to the sperm-containing syringe. Specifically designed devices for IUI are commercially available (Makler et al 1984). Intrauterine insemination is not physiological and may pose several problems. First, spermatozoa are introduced into the uterine cavity together with seminal fluid (Asch et al 1977). Secondly, spermatozoa deposited in utero leave the female genital tract rather quickly via the uterine tubes and disappear into the peritoneal cavity, while no supply from the endocervical storage space is available to replace the loss. There is therefore a decreased chance that spermatozoa will be able to meet a short-lived fresh ovum on their way through the oviduct. More frequent inseminations (e.g. daily) compensate only partially for this drawback. Alternatively, ultrasonographic monitoring of follicular growth may be very helpful for more exact timing of impending ovulation, thereby reducing the need for multiple inseminations.

Thirdly, the bactericidal properties of the endocervix are bypassed by IUI. The risk of infections may thus increase. Meticulous cleansing of the vagina and cervix by the use of ample amounts of, for example, lactated Ringer's solution prior to insemination and strict sterile handling of the seminal specimen is of paramount importance. In addition, we advocate prophylactic antibiotic treatment during the insemination period. Doxycycline, 100 mg daily in a single dose, results

in good penetration into the secretions of the female genital tract and is thus suitable for this purpose (Whelton et al 1980).

Fourthly, intrauterine insemination may lead to very painful uterine cramps due to the effect of the prostaglandin content of human semen. (Taylor & Kelly 1974). Most authors advocate therefore to restrict the inseminated volume to 0.3 ml (White & Glass 1976). Prostaglandins are secreted by the seminal vesicles, which contribute to the last ejaculatory spurts. Thus the first ejaculatory portion, consisting mainly of epididymal and prostatic contributions, contains relatively little prostaglandin but a high concentration of spermatozoa. It is thus uniquely suited for intrauterine inseminations and we have exclusively used the first split fraction for this purpose, injecting up to 0.8 ml per insemination without observing any side-effects (Glezerman et al 1984). Alternatively, the so-called 'swim-up technique' may be used to prepare semen in vitro for IUI. Centrifuging sperm cells and replacing the supernatant plasma with a nutrient such as Eagle's solution, Tyrode's solution or HAM F-10 medium will allow motile and optimally configured cells to swim away from the pellet and concentrate in the nutrient solution from where they can be retrieved. This method, as the methods using columns is associated with a high loss of sperm cells and is aimed to replace quantity with quality. Retrieved spermatozoa may be used for IUI.

IUI has become rather popular in recent years for a variety of indications. Results are difficult to compare since many reports fail to list adequately important parameters such as timing and technique of insemination, preparation method for semen, and very often there is no stratification for diagnostic criteria (Allen et al 1985). IUI seems to offer little advantage in cases of male infertility (Allen et al 1985, Ho et al 1989, Moeslein-Rossmeissl & Taubert 1989, Yavetz et al 1990). Immunological infertility is a relative indication for IUI. Bronson et al (1982) have suggested that sperm-specific isoantibodies and autoantibodies may inhibit the binding of human sperm cells to the zona pellucida, and this may be the reason for the relatively low pregnancy rate following IUI for immunological infertility. Allen et al (1985) have summarized results of five studies of IUI-treated immunological infertility. The average pregnancy rate was 22%. The truly logical indication for IUI is related to a situation in which the uterine cervix has to be bypassed because it poses an hostile environment to sperm cells. This is the case after destruction of cervical crypts by conization or if the produced mucus is either too scanty or impenetrable to sperm cells as evidenced by sperm penetration tests (Insler et al 1977). Results of IUI for a cervical factor of infertility have been encouraging (Table 25.1). Bypassing of vagina and uterine cervix may also be indicated in those rare cases where vaginoseminal contact leads to an allergic reaction in the female. Shapiro et al (1981) have reported on IUI in such a case followed by pregnancy.

## TIMING OF INSEMINATION

Before initiating insemination, the fertility status of the female partner must be thoroughly assessed and any abnormalities detected should be treated appropriately. The periovulatory period must be identified as accurately as possible.

The life span of the human ovum is believed to average 6–24 h, while motile human sperm cells have been observed in the cervical mucus for periods up to 205 h following intercourse. Thus (except for IUI), two or three inseminations per cycle on alternative days will usually suffice to 'cover' the periovulatory period and ensure that sufficient sperm cells are available at the fertilization site when the ovum arrives.

Serial scoring of the cervical mucus, i.e. observation of its amount, spinnbarkeit, ferning, and the appearance of the external cervical os has been very useful as an adjunct in scheduling repeated insemination. The use of urinary LH immunoassay for timing apparently offers little benefit over conventional methods of timing such as basal body temperature and cervical mucus assessment (Kossoy et al 1988).

## HOMOLOGOUS INSEMINATION (AIH)

### Indications

Mere substitution of the natural sperm delivery mechanism by mechanical means (e.g. vaginal insemination) does not ameliorate the decreased fertilization capacity of a given semen. Only if artificial insemination can provide additional protective, promotive or corrective features will its use be superior to sexual intercourse for procreative purposes.

### Hypospermia

Hypospermia is defined as a condition in which repeated semen analysis reveals a seminal volume of less than 2 ml. In cases of severe hypospermia, i.e. seminal volume below 1 ml, infertility may be due to failure of the small amount of seminal fluid to make contact with the cervical os and its secretion. In these cases protective AIH may improve the fertilizing ability of the semen sample. One may either use the cap or intrapericervical AIH.

### Oligozoospermia

The term oligozoospermia indicates a condition in which the seminal plasma contains less than the normal concentration of sperm cells per

**Table 25.1** Intrauterine AIH for cervical factor of infertility

| Authors | CS | PCT | SP | Patients (no.) | Pregnancies | |
|---|---|---|---|---|---|---|
| | | | | | No. | % |
| Barwin 1974 | — | Poor | Negative | 18 | 13 | 70 |
| White & Glass 1976 | — | Poor | — | 9 | 5 | 56 |
| Glezerman et al 1984 | Poor | Poor | Negative | 25 | 13 | 52 |
| Yavetz et al 1990 | Poor | Poor | — | 7 | 3 | 43 |
| Total | | | | 59 | 34 | 57.6 |

CS, Cervical score; PCT, postcoital test; SP, sperm penetration test.

milliliter. For practical purposes we consider the lower normal limit of sperm concentration to be $20 \times 10^6$ ml, measured in at least two consecutive examinations. Yet, men with semen samples containing less than this concentration may be perfectly fertile. It seems that sperm concentration per se is not the most important feature of a given semen sample unless markedly decreased and accompanied by reduced motility and reduced percentage of normally configured sperm cells.

In cases of isolated oligozoospermia a rational approach would be to concentrate as many as possible of the available spermatozoa at the external cervical os while avoiding as much as possible direct contact with vaginal secretions and spilling from the vagina. Unfortunately, AIH has not been very successful in patients with oligozoospermia (Allen et al 1985, Ho et al 1989, Yavetz et al 1990).

### Asthenospermia

Progressive motility is crucial for the fertilizing capacity of sperm cells. Reduced motility has been more often associated with infertility than reduced sperm concentration or increased percentage of abnormally configured sperm cells (Glezerman et al 1980). Normally, more than 50% of sperm cells in a given semen sample present with fast progressive motility. Asthenospermia is a condition in which less than 50% of sperm cells move progressively.

Artificial insemination with asthenospermic semen seems to offer no distinct advantage over the natural insemination process. However, various methods have been suggested which aim at in vitro improvement of the motility rate of a given semen sample for subsequent insemination.

In vitro treatment of semen has been employed by many investigators with various results. It appears that methylxanthines and kinins are the most promising agents. These agents are discussed in Chapter 23. In the seventies, some authors reported beneficial results with L-arginine, with prostaglandins, and with acetylcarnitine. Since no further corroboration followed, these treatment modes were abandoned.

### Increased seminal viscosity and delayed seminal liquefication

Increased seminal viscosity may be a possible cause of infertility, particularly when coinciding with decreased motility. In these cases the use of the first ejaculatory spurt for insemination may be of value. Amelar et al (1977) have proposed either forcing the semen specimen through an 18–19 gauge needle several times or mixing the semen with a mucolytic solution. Both methods yield a semen sample with highly reduced viscosity suitable for AIH.

Nonliquefying semen may be treated in vitro by adding a 4% solution of α-amylase in Locke's solution (Bunge & Sherman 1954). Following this procedure the specimen may be used for AIH. Another possibility is the treatment of nonliquefying semen by the proteolytic enzyme α-chymotrypsin (5 mg/ejaculate) as suggested by Schill (1973).

### Factors interfering with sperm–ovum contact.

**1. Male factors** *Anatomical abnormalities* As mentioned earlier, the first reported case of AIH was performed because severe hypospadias impeded semino-vaginal contact. Today surgical correction of such an abnormality would be preferred, but one may still choose to perform intravaginal AIH until a normal urethral orifice is reconstructed. In cases of partially obstructed or absent ductus deferens, attempts have been made to produce artificial spermatoceles made of alloplastic material (Wagenknecht 1976). These artificial spermatoceles are then punctured and the obtained semen is used for AIH. Pregnancies were reported in animals as well as in humans.

*Male impotence and anejaculation* Occasionally couples are referred for AIH because of erective failure or premature ejaculation. Often these couples perceive parenthood as a solution for their sexual difficulties. To respond to the demand of these couples and to perform AIH would be to circumvent the major problem of sexual inadequacy. We feel that AIH is contraindicated until sexual therapy has been tried and proven unsuccessful. Even then, AIH should be instituted only after marriage counseling has been provided.

Some couples may not volunteer or may withhold information about sexual problems while requesting AIH. Repeated negative postcoital tests in the female, concomitant with normal semen analysis and normal sperm penetration tests, may reveal the sperm deposition problem. In cases of organic impotence (paraplegics, diabetic neuropathy) in whom causal treatment has been ineffective, intravaginal AIH is the treatment of choice. This may be performed by the couples themselves following appropriate explanation. AIH performed by the male partner in the home surroundings will be much more convenient for the couple, relieve some of the stress connected with the procedure and provide the male partner with a more active role, relieving him of some of the emotional stress.

Anejaculation may have a variety of causes (endocrine, anatomical, psychogenic). Following evaluation and treatment, some patients may still require artificial procedures to obtain semen for insemination. Electrovibration may be used for this purpose (Glezerman & Lunenfeld 1976).

*Retrograde ejaculation* Retrograde ejaculation has been often mistakenly described as anejaculation, and presents a clear indication for AIH. In this condition, the semen is ejected backwards into the bladder, rather than forward through the urethra. The diagnosis of retrograde ejaculation is made by observing sperm cells in the postcoital urine. In these patients fertility could be achieved by restoration of antegrade ejaculation by sympaticomimetic agents (Virupannavar & Tomera 1982) or through efforts to regain viable and fertile sperm from the urinary bladder after sexual intercourse or masturbation with subsequent artificial insemination. In order to avoid possible damage to the sperm cells by contact with urine, its acidity is neutralized by administering alkalizing agents prior to intercourse. When the urine is received, it is washed with nutrient solutions (Eagle's solution, Ringer's solution, etc.), and centrifuged, and the female partner is inseminated with the sediment using the pericervical or cap technique (Glezerman et al 1976). Scammel et al (1982) have used human serum albumin for suspension of retrieved semen and subsequent successful AIH.

**2. *Female factors*** *Anatomical abnormalities* Occasionally, extreme displacement of the uterus or uterine cervix may necessitate AIH.

*Vaginismus* Intravaginal AIH is very effective in these cases. However, we feel that fertility-promoting therapy in couples in whom a potency problem such as vaginismus exists should be postponed until adequate sexological treatment has been provided.

*The cervical factor of infertility* The uterine cervix and its secretions play an important role in the reproductive process. The main element of this function is the transport and preservation of spermatozoa so that a sufficient number of sperm cells may be sustained long enough to reach the Fallopian tube at a time appropriate for fertilization of the ovum. It is now generally accepted that ill function of the uterine cervix will impede sperm transport and infertility may ensue. The clinical expression of this ill function may be 'relative or absolute dysmucorrhea', i.e. inability of the uterine cervix to produce sufficient amounts of cervical mucus of adequate physical and chemical properties, and 'penetration dysmucorrhea', i.e. cervical mucus hostility to sperm. On the other hand, migration failure may be due to an 'inherent penetration inability' of sperm cells which seem normal on routine seminal analysis (Insler et al 1979). The evaluation of the cervical factor of infertility is discussed elsewhere in this volume (see Chapters 13 and 22). Any of the disturbances mentioned will require the artificial bypassing of the uterine cervix by introducing semen directly into the uterine cavity. Intrauterine insemination has been rather successful in women with a cervical factor of infertility.

*Tubal factors of infertility* Advances in extracorporeal fertilization have provided some hope for those women in whom surgical treatment for tubal factors of infertility is not available or has failed. This issue is discussed elsewhere extensively in this volume (see Chapter 21). Reintroduction of the zygote is based on IUI techniques.

*Sex preselection*

It is estimated that modern methods of separation

of X and Y sperm yield an accuracy rate of 75–80%. Ericsson et al (1980) in reviewing the topic, state that 'it is doubtful if any procedure used within the next decade or ever, will be 100% reliable'. Sex preselection is certainly a very controversial issue, touching on deep ethical, philosophical and sociological problems. Yet in cases where genetic diseases prohibit the generation of one of the sexes, this form of genetic screening may be justified. Methods employed for sex preselection have been reviewed by Ericsson et al (1980). AIH techniques are applied to treated semen.

### Cryopreservation of sperm and subsequent AIH

During the past decade, semen banking has received much public attention because of its potential as fertility insurance for patients prior to therapy negatively affecting fertility, for men whose professional activity may decrease their fertility, and in those contemplating vasectomy. The cryopreserved semen can then be used for intracervical, pericervical or cap artificial insemination. In men with subnormal semen, most notably oligozoospermia, many attempts have been made to freeze semen samples for subsequent pooling and AIH. Subnormal semen sustains further loss of quality during the freezing and thawing process so that this technique may not offer any advantage.

### Contraindications for AIH

Absolute or relative contraindications for AIH are present:

1. Whenever pregnancy is contraindicated for medical or psychological reasons.
2. In cases of incompatibilities (such as the RH factor).
3. If either of the partners carries a hereditary disease.
4. In cases of severe systemic diseases in either of the partners (such as lues, severe forms of diabetes mellitus, malignant diseases, etc.).
5. When cytostatic or immunosuppressive treatment has been applied recently (up to 1 year before attempted AIH).
6. When either partner has received therapeutic X-ray (up to 4 months before attempted AIH).
7. When acute genital infection is present in either partner.

### Results of AIH

The success rate of AIH varies widely with its indication, and ensuing pregnancies are not always easily attributable to the AIH procedure. For example, in eight out of 34 oligospermic patients treated with AIH by Russell (1960), pregnancies occurred when the insemination scheme was discontinued while only two of these 34 patients reported pregnancies during the treatment period. In the same study, ten females with apparent cervical hostility were treated with AIH and three pregnancies ensued. However, two women conceived spontaneously after discontinuation in inseminations. Generally, comparison of data is difficult, since often multifactorial infertility is treated by AIH, equivocal indications are sometimes used, and data are not always completely reported.

Cervical hostility is a logical indication for AIH and has been discussed above. With IUI pregnancy rates averaging 58% have been achieved (Table 25.1). AIH in cases of severe oligozoospermia (less than $10 \times 10^6$ sperm cells/ml), asthenospermia (less than 50% motility) or teratospermia (less than 50% normally configured sperm cells) has rarely produced pregnancy rates in a range which might be considered beyond the rate of chance. We too have not been able to demonstrate the benefit of simple protective AIH in these cases. However, if the quality of semen is improved before insemination, treatment success is considerably higher. We have employed AIH in 21 patients in whom reduced sperm concentration was due to high seminal volume (dilution oligozoospermia). The mean spermatozoal concentration was $12.4 \times 10^6$/ml (SE $4.8 \times 10^6$/ml). In 11 cases the first ejaculatory spurt contained at least twice as many sperm cells per milliliter than the following spurts. These males were advised to perform 'split intercourse' during the periovulatory period. The method consists of a modified coitus interruptus during which only the first ejaculatory spurt is allowed to enter the vagina while the following spurts are ejaculated ante portas. Five of these 11 patients reported difficulties in performing split intercourse and 'split AIH' was applied, using the first ejaculatory spurt. The wives of all 11 men conceived within 7 months. In ten males the first ejaculatory spurt contained less than twice the spermatozoal concentration than the following spurts. Split intercourse or split AIH resulted in five pregnancies in this group. Thus, the total pregnancy rate in these 21 couples was 76.2% following either split intercourse or split AIH (Glezerman et al, 1980).

## ARTIFICIAL DONOR INSEMINATION (AID)

Numerous reports in the scientific literature concerning AID and discussion in the lay press have disseminiated information about this procedure, have contributed to its demystification, and have effected a reserved acceptance by society.

In Denmark and France, AID services have been organized on a national scale. Undoubtedly the demand for AID is steadily increasing. This is also due to decreasing availability of babies for adoption in Western countries.

Yet, notwithstanding the triumphant advance of AIS as evidenced by numbers, the prospect of AID for the individual couple is often perceived as a verdict, a disaster, and may induce a complex spectrum of emotional problems involving both partners. The realization of being irreversibly infertile leads almost invariably to an identity crisis in the male, amplified by guilt feelings toward the female partner. She may often produce guilt feelings for her part toward the husband for not sharing his reproductive failure, and it is not a rare phenomenon for previously ovulatory cycles to turn subsequently anovoluatry (Glezerman, 1981). Hopes nourished for prolonged periods of time, during which exhaustive attempts with treatments have been tried and various doctors have been consulted, must be abandoned, and the long avoided truth must be faced. The couple must come out of this crisis with a new self-definition without the biologic procreative dimen-

sion. The archaic connection between sexuality and procreation must be untied. This identity crisis, involving both partners, must be solved in a psychosocial vacuum without the support of family and friends. The physician who gave the verdict of irreversible infertility bears a heavy responsibility and must provide help to enable the couple to come through the painful process of adaptation to a new form of identity.

It would be unwise to proceed to AID very soon after the husband has been confronted with his infertility. Adjustment of both partners takes time, and both AID and adoption should be discussed extensively leaving the choice to the couple.

There may be questions regarding the legitamacy of a child born after AID, religious and ethical problems may arise, and the couple must be given enough information and time to overcome suspicion as to the other partner's attitude toward the use of donor sperm. Parenthood is as much a psychosocial relationship toward the child and toward society as a biologic one. The myth of 'blood and flesh' must be uprooted.

A state of consciousness must be achieved in which the donor, from the psychological point of view, does not exist. Donor semen should be then regarded as 'material' from an anonymous testis, the donor being actually a 'nonperson'. For this purpose we restrict information given about the donor to an absolute minimum, revealing only ethnnic origin and negativity of familial and personal history of diseases, and possible resemblance to the husband.

### Indications for AID

The most common indication is absolute male sterility, such as in cases of Klinefelter's syndrome, hypergonadotropic hypogonadism, and therapy-resistant azoospermia, teratospermia, or asthenospermia. If the husband's semen remains resistant to therapy that is the next common indication. Inheritable diseases in the husband's line (e.g. Tay-Sachs disease, juvenile diabetes, Huntington's chorea, etc.) are also indications for AID. So are incompatibles, such as those concerning the Rh factor when the female partner is sensitized. Finally, in long-standing infertility with no apparent etiology when the female partner is approaching the end of her reproductive years, AID may be considered as a last measure.

## Fresh versus frozen semen

Most clinicians feel that AID with fresh semen is more succesful than when cryoreserved semen is used. Recent data cast some doubt on this impression. Sherman (1987) states that most of the data on conception rates are not suitable for valid comparisons between fresh and frozen semen. This may be due to different methods of data analysis and variations in investigation protocols of women undergoing AID. A prospective randomized study using life-table analysis produced equal pregnancy rates for frozen and fresh semen used for AID (Iddenden et al, 1985). Other investigators reported similar results (Bordson et al 1986, Hammond et al 1986, Hummel & Talbert 1989, Keel & Webster 1989). On the other hand, Richter et al (1984) have reported that fresh semen is more than three times as likely to induce pregnancies as frozen semen. However, their minimum cut-off point for post-thaw semen was as low as $9\times10^6$ motile sperm cells/insemination. When post-thaw ejaculates with less than $10\times10^6$ motile sperm cells/ml were excluded (Keel & Webster 1989), there was no apparent difference in pregnancy rates between fresh and frozen semen. It seems that a fair comparison between pregnancy rates using fresh and frozen semen should not be based, as it is so often, on sperm characteristics before freezing but on post-thaw parameters. Freezing obviously causes a decrease in post-thaw sperm motility on which fecundity is dependent. If post-thaw semen is used only when conforming to certain minimal criteria, then there should be no significant difference in pregnancy rates between fresh and frozen semen. The problem lies therefore not in the use of cryopreserved semen for insemination but in the technology of freezing and thawing which at this time still reduces qualities of some semen samples. These samples should be discarded to achieve comparable results with fresh semen. Further advances in cryotechnology will hopefully lead to less waste of semen samples.

The use of sperm banks make the AID program much easier and safer. Furthermore, the potential risks associated with the use of fresh semen have lead the CDC (Center for Disease Control) and the AFS (American Fertility Society 1988) to strongly discourage its use for AID. Finally, there are many advantages which will most probably cause the disappearance of AID services using fresh semen:

1. Logistics of donor organization are much easier and cheaper.
2. Matching is easier when there is a large number of different semen specimens to choose from.
3. Frozen semen can be exchanged or transported over a large geographical area, minimizing the likelihood of inbreeding for the offspring of a donor.
4. Couples can be given the opportunity of multiple pregnancies from the same donor.
5. Frozen semen is cheaper, since one ejaculate can be used for several inseminations.
6. Quarantization of semen permits longitudinal observation of prospective donors and significantly reduces risks for transmitting infectious diseases, especially AIDS.

## Selection of donors

Some patients offer a relative as donor to ensure 'blood bondage'. This choice should be definitely discouraged since serious emotional complications may ensue. The principle of the donor being a 'nonperson' will be neutralized, positive or negative identification of either partner with the donor may result, and a theoretical possibility that the donor may one day claim the child, a very archaic fear, can hang like the sword of Damocles above the heads of the couples. It should be only the physician to whom the donor's identity is known. As trivial as this statement sounds, this is one of the basic pillars for AID.

Usually, patients request that the physical characteristics of the donor be matched to those of the husband. The couple should be fully informed that matches of this kind in the human by no means guarantee resemblance and that the child may well inherit physical characteristics of a remote and unknown relative and not resemble either of the parents. However, attempts should be made to choose donors of the same ethnic origin, body proportions and hair and eye color as those of the husband. If feasible, the same blood type as the husband's or at least the wife's should be present.

The donor should be intelligent and fully aware about the use of his semen. The first laboratory step in the evaluation of a potential donor is of course the semen evaluation. At least two consecutive semen analyses should be performed and demonstrate excellent qualities. A thorough physical examination should not reveal any pathologies which might be hereditary, and an extensive familial and personal anamnesis should be negative for hereditary diseases. Intravenous drug users should be rejected. Basic laboratory tests should include complete blood count, blood typing, glucose tolerance test, urinary cultures, and basic bacteriological testing for sexually transmitted diseases. The American Fertility Society (1986) has suggested guidelines for genetic and health screening for sperm donors. Serological tests for syphilis are advisable. There is a growing need to perform repeated tests for gonorrhea in potential and active donors. Jennings et al (1977) demonstrated that *Neisseria gonorrhoeae* contaminating semen collected for AID do not lose viability in vitro in the time which most specimens are used. Garcia et al (1981) have documented the survival of *N. gonorrhoeae* after cryopreservation of semen. Since hepatitis B may be transmitted by infected semen (Berry et al 1987), donors should be screened for HBsAg and HBcAg. The most dangerous infectious agent which might be transmitted by artificial insemination is the human immunodeficiency virus (HIV). Stewart et al have reported in 1985 on transmission of HIV by artificial insemination. Therefore, legislation in many countries requires today screening of donors for HIV. Current practice calls for freezing and quarantization of semen from HIV-negative donors for 6 months. At this time the donor is again screened for HIV. If at this time the donor is found negative for HIV the frozen semen may be released for AID. In different countries specific tests should be performed to detect certain diseases especially common for the given area (e.g. sickle cell anemia for American blacks, enzymatic assays of serum or skin fibroblasts for Tay–Sachs disease in Jews of European origin, etc.).

## Technique of insemination

The technique of insemination with donor's semen is essentially the same as with husband's sperm. A specific problem arises when the couple requires mixing of the husband's sperm with that of the donor. A great advantage of this method is the positive doubt as to which spermatozoa eventually fertilized the ovum. Even in highly sophisticated couples we have often observed the phenomenon that the husband, while being fully aware of his irreversible infertility, discovers later features in his child that are interpreted by him as proof that his semen fertilized the ovum. On the other hand, adding husband's semen to the specimen provided by the donor will dilute it and may even have immobilizing and agglutinating effects (Quinlivan & Sullivan 1977a,b). We feel, nevertheless, that if preliminary tests for immobilization and agglutination in mixed specimen are negative and postcoital tests following insemination with mixed sperm are good, one should perform inseminations with mixed semen. The husband will thus be given a chance to identify himself better with his role as a father. Furthermore, when the husband has to provide semen for each insemination and is thereby actively involved in the therapeutic process, the abstraction of the donor's person is achieved more easily and the AID program is perceived by both partners as treatment for both. For the same purpose, we encourage sexual intercourse following inseminations in couples in whom mixing is not feasible. Excluded from this reasoning are obviously couples in whom the husband's procreation is not advisable (inheritable diseases in the husband, etc.).

## Legal aspects of AID

Artificial insemination using donor semen raises legal questions as to the legitimacy of the child and to the child's rights in relation to the husband

and to the donor, especially as far as inheritance rights and support claims are concerned. The State courts and legislatures have generally ignored these issues, and only sporadically have the legal problems surrounding AID found their way into the courts. In the USA, the statutes of 29 states accept the recipient and husband as the legal parents following delivery of an AID child (Hummel & Talbert 1989). No court has stated that AID is illegal. For the time being, the physician performing AID should be well aware of the fact that husband, wife, child and donor are all in a rather unsatisfactory position with regard to the law. The least one can do is to provide extensive information to the couple and to obtain written consent upon entering the AID program.

Another important legal question is the birth certificate's validity concerning legitimacy. In many countries, birth certificates are documents stating fatherhood. Consequently, the physician who enters the name of the husband on the birth certificate, knowing that the baby was born following AID, may be accused of falsifying records. Amelar et al (1977) reported on an English physician who had been charged with this offence and was consequently jailed for 3 years. In these circumstances it would be wise for the physician who has performed the successful insemination not to attend the birth of the baby and not to sign a birth certificate.

Many legal aspects remain to be solved. It should be one of the goals of conscientious medicine to promote discussion and legislation to provide a sound basis from which help can be offered to desperate childless couples to whom other alternatives are not available.

## Results of AID

The results of artificial insemination using donor semen are excellent. Chances for conception compare favorably even with spontaneous pregnancy rates in fertile couples after discontinuation of contraception (Table 25.2). Using fresh donor semen, more than 70% of treated women will eventually become pregnant, the specific technique playing no significant role. An analysis of the cumulative distribution of 1566 pregnancies according to number of insemination cycles and based on four series with more than 100 pregnancies each reveals that 52% of those women who will eventually be pregnant will do so within the first three treatment cycles, and 78% will conceive within the first six treatment cycles (Table 25.3). In our material, the accumulative pregnancy rate after six treatment cycles was 86.8% (Table 25.4). Of

**Table 25.2** Cumulative conception rate in patients receiving artificial donor insemination (AID) and spontaneous pregnancy rates in women following discontinuation of contraception (observed)

| Cycle (no.) | Women(no.) | | Pregnancies(no.) | | Cumulative pregnancy rate(%) | |
|---|---|---|---|---|---|---|
| | AID | Observed | AID | Observed | AID | Observed |
| 1 | 270 | 611 | 69 | 199 | 30.0 | 32.6 |
| 3 | 201 | 412 | 57 | 103 | 54.7 | 49.4 |
| 3 | 144 | 309 | 34 | 64 | 69.5 | 59.9 |
| 4 | 110 | 245 | 13 | 36 | 75.2 | 65.8 |
| 5 | 97 | 197 | 11 | 33 | 80.0 | 71.5 |
| 6 | 81 | 157 | 15 | 30 | 86.5 | 77.0 |
| 7 | 64 | 118 | 6 | 18 | 89.1 | 80.5 |
| 8 | 53 | 95 | 6 | 13 | 91.7 | 83.2 |
| 9 | 43 | 77 | 4 | 9 | 93.4 | 85.1 |
| 10 | 37 | 63 | 2 | 10 | 94.3 | 87.5 |
| 11 | 31 | 48 | 4 | 3 | 96.0 | 88.3 |
| 12 | 21 | 43 | 2 | — | 96.9 | 88.3 |
| Later | 18 | 38 | 7 | 9 | | |
| Total | | | 230 | 257 | | |

Data on AID from Glezerman (1981); data on spontaneous pregnancy rate following discontinuation of contraception from Tietze (1968).

**Table 25.3**  Accumulative pregnancy rates relative to number of insemination cycles following AID with fresh semen

| Authors | Patients (no.) | 3-month pregnancies | | 6-month pregnancies | |
|---|---|---|---|---|---|
| | | No. | % | No. | % |
| Behrman 1959 | 126 | 74 | 59 | 108 | 86 |
| Haman 1959 | 303 | 203 | 67 | 264 | 87 |
| Whitelaw 1974 | 766 | 271 | 35 | 532 | 70 |
| Glezerman & Potashnik 1988 | 371 | 258 | 70 | 322 | 87 |
| Total | 1566 | 806 | 52 | 1226 | 78 |

**Table 25.4**  Accumulative pregnancy rate in 371 pregnancies following AID. From Glezerman & Potashnik, 1988 (with permission from Blackwell Wissenschafts-Verlag)

| | Treatment Cycle | | | |
|---|---|---|---|---|
| | 3 | 6 | 12 | >12 |
| Pregnancies(no.) | 258 | 64 | 42 | 7 |
| Pregnancy rate(%) | 69.5 | 17.3 | 11.3 | 1.9 |
| Accumulative pregnancy rate(%) | 69.5 | 86.8 | 98.1 | 100 |

all patients who eventually became pregnant 98.1% did so after 12 treatment cycles. The longest treatment period in this series was 32 months. It seems from these data that not very much can be gained if AID is continued for longer than 1 year, and that at this time other treatment modalities should be discussed with the couple (in vitro ferilization, GIFT, etc.). A fair chance for treatment success should thus be based on at least six ovulatory cycles following which the wife should be reevaluated and continuation of the AID program discussed with both partners.

The cumulative distribution of pregnancies relative to the number of insemination cycles using cryopreserved semen, however, was similar to that achieved with fresh semen.

**Factors affecting success of AID**

Variation in methods of recording information make comparison of success rates somewhat difficult. Patients who discontinue treatment within the first 3 months of AID should be considered not to have been exposed to a fair chance of conception and should therefore not be regarded as AID failures. They should, however, enter the calculation of pregnancy rate per cycle of insemination.

*Age*

Dixon & Buttram (1976) noted a decline in pregnancy rates if the patients were older than 30 years, but Corson (1980) could not confirm this observation. Evaluating 371 pregnancies in 440 patients treated by AID, we (Glezerman & Potashnik 1988) did not find a significant difference in pregnancy rates between patients aged 20–34 years and those aged 35–41 years (Table 25.5). This is in contrast to our previous report (Glezerman 1981), the data of which were included in our report of 1988. With the larger number of patients, a previously statistically significant difference became not significant.

In our material there was also no difference in pregnancy rates between women suffering from primary infertility and those suffering from secondary infertility. As duration of infertility increased, pregnancy rates decreased significantly and more treatment cycles per pregnancy were required (Table 25.5).

*Socioeconomic state*

We divided our patients into three groups according to their socioeconomic state. Couples were classified by the partner of the higher socioeconomic state. With a rising socioeconomic class a significant increase in the pregnancy rates was observed. The number of treatment courses per pregnancy did not differ (Table 25.5).

**Table 25.5**    The influence of various factors on pregnancy rates in women treated by artificial donor insemination (with permission from Blackwell Wissenschafts-Verlag.)

| Factor | Patients | | Pregnancy rate | Significance |
|---|---|---|---|---|
| | No. | % | (%) | |
| Age (yr) | | | | NS |
| < 35 | 396 | 90.0 | 89.2 | |
| > 35 | 44 | 10.0 | 80.9 | |
| Infertility | | | | NS |
| Primary | 294 | 66.8 | 86.3% | |
| Secondary | 146 | 33.2 | 91.2% | |
| Duration of infertility | | | | $P < 0.001$ |
| < 3 yr | 176 | 40.0 | 93.8% | |
| 3–6 yr | 192 | 43.6 | 88.0% | |
| >–6 yr | 72 | 16.4 | 76.9% | |
| Socioeconomic | | | | $P < 0.01$ |
| Low | 47 | 11.2 | 76.6% | |
| Middle | 239 | 56.8 | 87.6% | |
| High | 135 | 32.1 | 94.5% | |
| Type of ovulation | | | | $P < 0.03$ |
| Normal | 238 | 54.1 | 91.7% | |
| Abnormal | 202 | 45.9 | 84.1% | |

From Glezerman & Potashnik 1988.

## Ovulatory pattern

The patients were divided into two groups according to ovulatory pattern prior to and at initiation of the pre-AID investigation scheme. Patients who required ovulation induction therapy had significantly lower pregnancy rates than those who did not (Table 25.5). One out of five of our patients ceased to ovulate as soon as the prospect of AID became real.

## Office presentation

Couples were always asked to appear together for AID (Glezerman 1981). Yet, in 35 of 270 cases (13%) the male partner did not accompany his wife to the treatment appointments. In this group, abortion rates were twice as high and pregnancy rates were significantly lower than in patients enjoying the support of their husbands (Table 25.6).

Couples in whom the male partner failed to accompany his wife for AID appointments were interpreted as influenced strongly by resistance of the husband in spite of his formal acceptance of the AID program. The impact of this resistance was astonishingly high.

**Table 25.6**    Influence of husband's resistance on pregnancy rate in AID

| Office presentation | Patients (no.) | Pregnancy (no.) | Pregnancy rate (%) |
|---|---|---|---|
| Group I | 35 | 10 | 28.6 |
| Group II | 235 | 220 | 93.6 |
| Significance | $P < 0.0005$ | | |

Group I, couples in whom the male partner failed to accompany his wife to AID appointments; group II, couples appearing together for AID appointments.

## Mechanical factors of infertility and previous surgery

In women who have undergone pelvic surgery, pregnancy rates following AID are reduced significantly. Reasons for this are obvious.

## Are there adverse effects of AID on pregnancy outcome?

In a study on 440 couples who were treated by AID using fresh semen, we could not find higher rates for ectopic pregnancies, spontaneous abortions and perinatal deaths than those observed in the general population (Glezerman & Potashnik 1988). Schwartz et al (1986) reported on 1345 pregnancies resulting from AID using cryopreserved semen. They reported on an abortion rate of 19%, similar to that observed in the general population. It seems, therefore, that AID does not adversely affect the outcome of pregnancies.

## REFERENCES

Allen N C, Herbert C M III, Maxson W S, Rogers B J, Diamond M P, Wentz A C 1985 Intrauterine insemination: a critical review. Fertil Steril 44: 569

Amelar R D, Dubin L, Walsh P C 1977 Male infertility. Saunders, Philadelphia

American Fertility Society 1986 New guidelines for the use of semen donor insemination. Fertil Steril 46(suppl 2): 97

American Fertility Society 1988 Revised new guidelines for the use of semen-donor insemination. Fertil Steril 49: 211

Asch R H, Balmaceda J, Pauerstein C J 1977 Failure of seminal plasma to enter the uterus and oviducts of the rabbit following artificial insemination. Fertil Steril 28: 671

Barton M, Walker K, Weiser P P 1946 Artificial insemination. Br Med J 1: 40

Barwin B N 1974 Intrauterine insemination of husband's semen. J Reprod Fertil 101

Beck W W 1976 A critical look at the legal, ethical and technical aspects of artificial insemination. Fertil Steril 27: 1

Berry W R, Gottesfeld R L, Alter H J, Vierling J M 1987 Transmission of Hepatitis B virus by artificial insemination. JAMA 257: 1079

Behrman S I 1959 Artificial insemination. Fertil Steril 10: 248

Bordson B L, Ricci E, Dickey R P, Dunaway H, Taylor S N, Curole D N 1986 Comparison of fecundability with fresh and frozen semen in therapeutic donor insemination. Fertil Steril 46: 466

Bronson R A, Cooper G W, Rosenfeld D L 1982 Sperm-specific isoantibodies and autoantibodies inhibit the binding of human sperm to the zona pellucida. Fertil Steril 38: 724

Bunge R G, Sherman J K 1954 Liquefaction of human semen by alpha amylase. Fertil Steril 5: 353

Corson S L 1980 Factors affecting donor artificial insemination success rates. Fertil Steril 33: 415

Diamond M P, Christianson C, Daniell J F, Wentz A C 1983 Pregnancy following use of the cervical cup for home artificial insemination utilizing homologous semen. Fertil Steril 39: 480

Dixon R E, Buttram V C 1976 Artificial insemination using donor semen: a review of 171 cases. Fertil Steril 27: 130

Ericsson R J, Dmowski W P, Broer K H, Gasser G 1980 Separation of X and Y spermatozoa for sex selection. In: Emperaire J C, Audebert A, Hafez E S E (eds) Clinics in andrology vol 1, homologous artificial insemination (AIH). Martinus Nijhoff, The Hague, p 98

Garcia A, Sierra M F, Friberg J 1981 Survival of bacteria after freezing of human semen in liquid nitrogen. Fertil Steril 35: 549

Glezerman M 1981 270 cases of artificial donor insemination. Management and results. Fertil Steril 35: 180

Glezerman M, Lunenfeld B 1976 Zur Therapie der maennlichen Anorgasmie ein Fallbericht. Akta Dermatol 2: 167

Glezerman M, Potashnik G 1988 Artificial donor insemination using fresh donor semen. Andrologia 20: 384

Glezerman M, Lunenfeld B, Potashnik G, Oelsner G, Beer R 1976 Retrograde ejaculation: pathophysiological aspects and report of two successfully treated cases. Fertil Steril 27: 796

Glezerman M, Brook I, Potashnik G, Ben-Aderet N, Insler V 1980 Fertility pattern and reported pregnancies in 33 patients referred to male infertility clinics. In: Proceedings of V ESCO Venice. Edizioni Internazionali Gruppo Editoriale Medico, Rome, p 495

Glezerman M, Bernstein D, Insler V 1984 The cervical factor of infertility and intrauterine insemination. Int J Fertil 29: 16

Gregoire A T, Mayer R C 1965 The impregnators. Fertil Steril 16: 130

Hammond M G, Jordan S, Sloan C S 1986 Factors affecting pregnancy rates in a donor insemination program using frozen semen. Am J Obstet Gynecol 155: 480

Haman S J 1959 Therapeutic donor insemination. Calif Med 90: 130

Hanson F M, Rock J 1971 Artificial insemination with husband's semen. Fertil Steril 122: 162

Hard A D 1909 Artificial impregnation. Med World 27: 253

Hartman C G 1962 Science and the safe period: a compendium of human reproduction. Williams and Wilkins, Baltimore

Ho P-Ch, Poon I M L, Chan S Y W, Wang Ch 1989 Intrauterine insemination is not useful in oligoasthenospermia. Fertil Steril 51: 682

Hogerzeil H V, Hamerlynck J V Th H, Amstel N van, Nagelkerke N J D, Lammes F B 1988 Results of artificial insemination at home by the partner with cryopreserved donor semen: a randomized study. Fertil Steril 49: 1030

Hummel W P, Talbert L M 1989 Current management of a donor insemination program. Fertil Steril 51: 919

Iddenden D A, Sallam J C, Collins W P 1985 A prospective randomized study comparing fresh semen and cryopreserved semen for artificial insemination by donor. Int J Fertil 30: 54

Insler V, Bernstein D, Glezerman M 1977 Diagnosis and classification of the cervical factor of infertility. In: Insler V, Bettendorf G (eds) The uterine cervix in reproduction. Thieme Verlag, Stuttgart p 253

Insler V, Bernstein D, Glezerman M, Misgav N 1979 Correlation of seminal fluid analysis with mucus penetrating ability of spermatozoa. Fertil Steril 32: 316

Jennings R T, Dixon R E, Nettles J B 1977 The risks and prevention of Neisseria gonorrheae transfer in fresh ejaculate donor insemination. Fertil Steril 28: 554

Keel B A, Webster B W 1989 Semen analysis data from fresh and cryopreserved donor ejaculates: comparison of cryoprotectants and pregnancy rates. Fertil Steril 52: 100

Kleegman S J, Kaufman S A 1966 Infertility in women. Oxford, Blackwell Scientific Publications

Kossoy L R, Hill G A, Herbert C M et al 1988 Therapeutic donor insemination. The impact of insemination timing with the aid of a urinary luteinizing hormone immunoassay. Fertil Steril 40: 1026

Lindholmer C 1973 Survival of human spermatozoa in different fractions of split ejaculate. Fertil Steril 24: 521

McIntosh T M 1909 Artificial inpregnation. Med World 27: 196

MacLeod J, Hotchkiss R S 1942 Distribution of spermatozoa and of certain chemical constituents in human ejaculate. J Urol 48: 225

Makler A, DeCherney A, Naftolin F 1984 A device for injecting and retaining a small volume of concentrated spermatozoa in the uterine cavity and cervical canal. Fertil Steril 42: 306

Moeslein-Rossmeissl S, Taubert H-D 1989 Male subfertility and the outcome of intrauterine insemination. Andrologia 21: 519

Quinlivian W L G, Sullivan H 1977a Spermatozoal antibodies in human seminal plasma as a cause for failed artificial donor insemination. Fertil Steril 28: 1028

Quinlivian W L G, Sullivan H 1977b The immunologic effect of husband's semen on donor spermatozoa during mixed insemination. Fertil Steril 28: 448

Richter M A, Haning R V, Shapiro S S 1984 Artificial donor insemination: fresh versus frozen semen; the patient as her own control. Fertil Steril 41: 277

Scammel G E, Stendronska J, Dempsey A 1982 Successful pregnancies using human serum albumin following retrograde ejaculation. Fertil Steril 37: 277

Schill W B 1973 Probleme der homologen und heterologen Insemination aus andrologischer Sicht. In: Braun-Falco O, Petzoldt D (eds) Fortschritte der praktischen Dermatologie und Venerologie. Springer Verlag, Heidelberg, p 187

Schwartz D, Mayaux M J, Guihard-Moscato M L, Czuglik F, Gavid G 1986 Abortion rate in AID and semen characteristics: a study of 1345 pregnancies. Andrologia 18: 292

Semm K, Brandl E, Mettler 1976 Vacuum insemination cap. In: Hafez E S E (ed) Human semen and fertility regulation in men. Mosby, St Louis, p 439

Shapiro S S, Kooistra J B, Schwartz D, Yunginger J W, Haning R W 1981 Induction of pregnancy in a woman with seminal plasma allergy. Fertil Steril 36: 405

Sherman J K 1987 Frozen semen: efficiency in artificial insemination and advantage in testing for aquired immune deficiency syndrome. Fertil Steril 47: 19

Shields F E 1950 Artificial insemination as related to female. Fertil Steril 1: 271

Stewart G J, Tyler J P P, Cunningham A L 1985 Transmission of human T-cell lymphotropic virus type III by artificial insemination by donor. Lancet ii: 581

Taylor P L, Kelly R W 1974 19-OH E Prostaglandins as the major prostaglandin of human semen. Nature 250: 665

Tietze Ch 1968 Fertility after discontinuation of intrauterine and oral contraception. Int J Fertil 13: 385

Virupannavar Ch, Tomera F 1982 An unusual case of retrograde ejaculation and a brief review of management. Fertil Steril 37: 275

Wagenknecht L V 1982 Obstruction in the male reproductive tract. In: Bain J, Schill W-B, Schwarzstein L (eds) Treatment of male infertility. Springer Verlag, Berlin, p 221

Whelton A, Lucas J B, Carter G C et al 1980 Therapeutic implications of doxycycline and cephalothin concentrations in the female genital tract. Obstet Gynecol 55: 28

White R M, Glass R H 1976 Intrauterine insemination with husband's semen. Obstet Gynecol 47: 119

Whitelaw M J 1974 Observations on 1000 consecutive AID patients. 8th World Congress on Fertility and Sterility, Buenos Aires (abstr)

Yavetz H, Mosek A, Yogev L, Paz G, Homonnai T Z 1990 Intrauterine insemination in subfertile couples. Andrologia 22: 29

# Special aspects of infertility

# 26. Polycystic ovarian disease

*Vaclav Insler    Bruno Lunenfeld*

Polycystic ovarian disease (PCOD) has for years been one of the most controversial entities in gynecological endocrinology. There is still a difference of opinion whether the condition should be regarded as a disease (PCOD) or a syndrome (PCOS) consisting of an array of signs and symptoms. Despite the fact that a vast amount of clinical, laboratory and experimental data have been accumulated since the initial report of Stein & Leventhal in 1935, our knowledge of the endocrine mechanism underlying the clinical signs of the disease is still fragmentary, incomplete and often confusing.

## THE EPIDEMIOLOGICAL DIMENSION

The incidence of PCOD varies immensely in different reports, depending on the parameters analysed.

In a series of 12 160 unselected gynecological laparotomies, polycystic ovaries (PCO) were found in 1.4% of cases (Vara & Niemineva 1951). Sommers & Wadman (1956), in 740 consecutive autopsies, including an unspecified number of children and old women, noticed the presence of bilateral polycystic ovaries in 3.5%. In large groups of infertile women a prevalence of PCO ranging between 0.6% and 4.3% was observed (Breteche 1952, McGoogan 1954).

Adams et al (1986) examined by ultrasound 173 women with anovulation or hirsutism and found PCO in 26% of patients with amenorrhea, 87% with oligomenorrhea and 92% of women with hirsutism.

Hull (1987) analysed a consecutive series of women with oligomenorrhea or amenorrhea. Patients with primary damage to the hypothal-amic-pituitary-gonadal axis and with disorders of other endocrine systems were excluded. Women with hirsutism were classified as 'overt presumed PCOD' and patients without hirsutism but having evidence of endogenous estrogen production were designated as 'occult presumed PCOD'. Using epidemiological methods of incidence prediction, he then estimated that the total 'overt' and 'occult' PCOD incidence would be 90% and 37%, in infertile women with oligomenorrhea and amenorrhea respectively.

## CLINICAL SYMPTOMATOLOGY

The classical picture of PCOS (Stein–Leventhal syndrome) is characterized by infertility, menstrual disorders, hirsutism and obesity. However, the incidence of every one of the aforementioned symptoms is inconsistent.

Goldzieher & Green (1962) reviewed 505 cases of *surgically proven* PCO. This series was enlarged to 1079 patients (Goldzieher & diZerega 1985). The symptoms which appeared with highest average incidence were: menstrual disorders (80%), infertility (74%) and hirsutism (69%). However, the range reported by different authors for each symptom was tremendous (Table 26.1). It should also be noted that this review based on 187 reports showed that cyclic menses was observed in 7–28% of women and the mean incidence of finding a corpus luteum at operation was 22%. This indicates that certainly not all women with PCO must present with infertility.

Looking at the above findings from proper perspective implies two conclusions:

1. PCOD can not be considered a well-defined

**Table 26.1** Clinical symptoms in patients with surgically proven PCOD: 1079 cases collected from 187 references

| Symptoms | Cases Surveyed (no.) | Incidence range (%) in reports |
|---|---|---|
| Infertility | 596 | 35–94 |
| Obesity | 600 | 16–49 |
| Hirsutism | 819 | 17–83 |
| Virilization | 431 | 0–28 |
| Amenorrhea | 640 | 15–77 |
| Spontaneous menses | 395 | 7–28 |
| Irregular bleeding | 547 | 6–25 |
| Corpus luteum found at operation | 391 | 0–71 |

Modified from Goldzieher & diZerega 1985

clinical entity. On the contrary, it probably represents a whole array of different disturbances leading to a similar structural change in the ovaries.

2. Since ovarian biopsy or wedge resection are no longer regarded as obligatory procedures, clinical diagnosis of PCOD must remain presumptive in many cases. The sonographic diagnosis proposed by Adams et al (1986) seems to provide an important addition to the existent means. The typical 'necklace' of cystic follicles in the periphery and the dense echogenicity of the ovarian stroma are regarded as the main parameters of sonographic diagnosis of PCO (Fig. 26.1). It should, however, be remembered that the above parameters may not be distinct in all cases or may not be accurately recognized by all sonographers. Many women with clinical and hormonal indicators of PCOD can have apparently normal ovaries on sonographic examination, while others showing a sonographic picture typical for polycystic ovary do not necessarily exhibit the characteristic clinical and laboratory findings.

## MORPHOLOGICAL FEATURES OF PCOD

The typical polycystic ovary has been traditionally described as being grossly enlarged, pearly white, with a thick capsule and numerous subcapsular cysts. The following microscopic features have been thought to be characteristic for the disease:

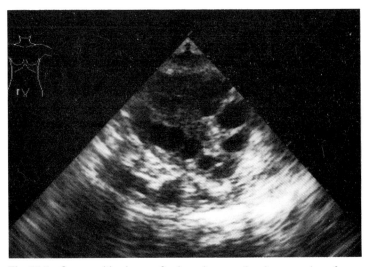

**Fig. 26.1** Sonographic picture of polycystic ovary showing a number of cystic follicles in the periphery and dense echogenicity of the stroma.

— Thickened tunica albuginea
— Hyperthecosis
— Luteinization of theca interna
— Thickening of basement membrane
— Reduction of granulosa cells.

The histological examination usually reveals several typical findings. The ovarian capsule is thick and sometimes fibrotic. Goldzieher & Green (1962) reported that the width of the normal ovarian capsule was approximately 100 µm, compared to 144–595 µm in PCO. Dozens of cystic follicles lined with between one and three layers of granulosa cells and myriads of atretic follicles are found under the thickened capsule. Hyperthecosis may also be apparent. Jones (1962) found that while in the normal ovary the theca layer consisted of 6–14 rows of cells, in PCO it comprised 17–34 layers of cells. Sometimes the theca cells were luteinized. In some cases of PCOS (proven by histology) hyperplasia of the stromal cells in the medulla and/or hilus was observed (Greenblatt 1963).

When reviewing the literature, one is surprised by the large number of deviations from the typical morphological features reported by many authors. First of all PCOD with all its clinical symptoms may appear in women having ovaries of normal size and appearance. Moreover, the existence of unilateral PCO in patients presenting with a clinical course consistent with PCOD has also been documented (Delahunt et al 1975, Vejlsted & Albrechtsen 1976). Smith et al (1965) reported that not all PCO had a thickened tunica albuginea. Other authors questioned the point whether hyperthecosis is one of the inherent morphological features of PCOD or represents a completely separate entity (Givens et al 1971, Aiman et al 1978, Farber et al 1978, 1981). Hofmeister & Byce (1966) analysed the records of 104 patients who underwent bilateral wedge resection or ovarian biopsy. In 91 cases, microscopic examination identified the ovaries as multicystic, polycystic or as containing multiple cystic follicles with evidence of cortical fibrosis. There were, however, 13 patients whose ovaries were diagnosed as polycystic at operation, but this diagnosis was not confirmed microscopically. The authors state in the discussion that 'The director

of the department of pathology designated 34 of 81 of the previously judged positive slides as indicative of definite Stein ovaries...'. It is also noteworthy that only 18 of the latter specimens showed a pronounced hyperplasia of theca interna cells.

Some or all morphological characteristics of PCO may appear in individuals certainly not having the disease. Merrill (1963) observed that in 80% of the ovaries of 2-year-old children and prepubertal and adolescent girls gross cysts could be found, and in 50% luteinization and thecal hyperplasia were present.

## HORMONAL FINDINGS

Three endocrine findings are usually considered to be indicative of PCOD: elevated luteinizing hormone/follicle stimulating hormone (LH/FSH) ratio, abnormally high androgen (androstenedione and/or testosterone) values and persistent relatively high endogenous estrogen production. McArthur and her coworkers, using then available bioassays, reported already in 1958 that LH levels were continuously, albeit moderately, elevated in patients with PCO. Since then most investigators have pointed out that women with PCOD present with exaggerated pulsations or persistently high LH levels (Rebar et al 1976, Hull 1987) (Fig. 26.2). Others reported that these findings are encountered only in some patients (Berger et al 1975, Vejlsted & Albrechtsen 1976 Adams et al 1986).

This discrepancy may stem from the conflict between the nature of LH secretion and the method used for measuring the level of this hormone in the blood. LH is secreted in a pulsatile manner and the difference between the peak and nadir of each pulse may be substantial. Measuring the hormone levels in plasma once daily may obviously produce confusing results depending on the timing of blood sampling in relation to the oscillation of the hormone. Moreover, Laaitikainen et al (1983) showed that in obese women with PCOD the mean levels and pulse amplitudes were lower than in nonobese PCOD patients. Our own study (Insler et al 1991) indicated that in obese PCOD women the mean LH values in 24 consecutive blood samples

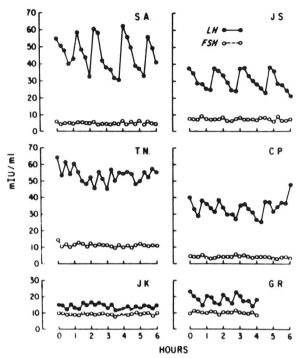

**Fig. 26.2**   LH pulsatility in women with PCOD. (Reproduced with permission from Rebar et al 1976.)

obtained every 20 min over 8 h were lower than in nonobese patients (Fig. 26.3), both before and during pituitary suppression by GnRH analog.

The use of androgen levels as a basis for diagnosis of PCOD creates even more complicated problems. First, the secretion of all steroid hormones is oscillating in pulses of relatively high

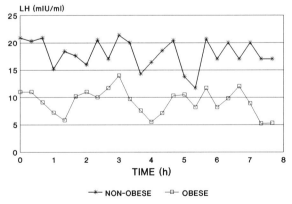

**Fig. 26.3**   LH pulsatility in obese and non-obese women with PCOD.

frequency and is also subject to a circadian rhythm. Secondly, androgens such as testosterone and androstenedione are produced by both the ovary and the adrenal glands, the final blood levels of the former being also increased by peripheral conversion of the latter. Thirdly, the physiological effects of the most potent androgen —testosterone—depend not only on the amount of the hormone produced, but also on how much of it circulates in the blood in its free form and how much is bound to sex hormone binding globulin (SHBG) or to serum albumins. In normal women only 1% of testosterone is free. Since in most PCOD patients SHBG is low, in some hirsute women the amount of free testosterone may be doubled. Extremely high levels of androgens appear almost exclusively in women with functioning ovarian or adrenal tumors.

Persistent endogenous production of estrogens is also of limited diagnostic value in identifying and/or classifying patients with PCOD. First of all, some patients with histologically proven PCOD may ovulate as indicated by biphasic basal body temperature (BBT) curves observed in approximately 15% and corpus luteum found at operation in 22%. The above figures may represent an overestimate, since luteinization of unruptured follicles may be mistaken for ovulation. Many women with oligo- or anovulation show persistent estrogen production although their gonads do not exhibit the characteristic structural changes of PCO. It should also be remembered that the absolute values of estrogens measured in plasma do not identify the source of their secretion. Estrone and estradiol may be produced by the ovary, by the adrenal or by peripheral conversion of androgens. Moreover, even in women with presumably ovulatory cycles, a considerable variability of hormone levels between cycles in the same subject and a ten-fold variability between different individuals has been observed (Johansson et al 1971, Landgren et al 1980).

## PATHOPHYSIOLOGICAL MECHANISMS LEADING TO PCOD

PCOD may result from disturbances of various endocrine systems. It has been reported to appear in patients with Cushing's syndrome, adrenal hyperplasia, hypothyroidism, adrenal or ovarian tumors, and hyperprolactinemia (Axelrod et al 1965, Stevens & Goldzieher 1968, Futterweit & Krieger 1979, Alger et al 1980, Lisse et al 1980, Lobo & Goebelsmann 1980). Some authors found either genetic abnormalities or familial patterns to be connected with the disease (Cooper et al 1968, Parker et al 1980). Within the last few years several new facts have been observed and studied in depth in different fields of neuroendocrinology, molecular biology and reproductive medicine. These studies could help us to rearrange the components of the PCOD puzzle and to obtain a concise logical general picture.

Recently, several reports appeared showing that PCOD may be connected with acanthosis nigricans and insulin resistance (Kahn et al 1976, Burghen et al 1980, Shapiro 1981). This indicates clearly that PCOD may be linked with insulin action and its control. It also became apparent that growth factors (GF) play a role in the ovarian response to gonadotropic stimulation (Adashi et al 1985, 1988). Urdl (1988) studied 33 women

with PCOD and in 18 of them observed decreased human growth hormone (hGH) levels and increased somatomedin-C (Sm-C) values. Pekonen et al (1989) found that patients with PCOD had decreased levels of human insulin-like growth factor-1 binding protein (hIGFBP-1). All these observations indicate definitely that growth hormone and other growth factors as well as their binding proteins may play an important role in the pathophysiology of PCOD. Growth hormone stimulates the systemic release of insulin-like growth factor (IGF-1) from the liver. GH and probably other growth factors binding proteins are also produced by the liver. At this stage it could be speculated that PCOD is connected with higher levels of *free* IGF-1 (Sm-C) and possibly also other growth factors of either intra- or extra-ovarian origin. Since Sm-C increases the ovarian response to gonadotropins, this may explain the excessive production of androgens by the LH-responsive structural ovarian components. Furthermore, it also explains the hyperresponsiveness of the ovarian follicular elements to FSH stimulation. If these stipulations are confirmed, one pathophysiological basis of the PCOD could be explained as follows: the increased levels of *free* IGF-1 result in excessive follicular stimulation on the one hand and in overproduction of androgens leading to follicular atresia on the other (Fig. 26.4). This hypothesis can also clarify the type of response obtained to exogenous stimulation by either human menopausal gonadotropin (hMG) or human follicle stimulating hormone (hFSH) in PCOD patients. Since hIGFBP-1 and the level of free or bound IGF-1 are not affected by GnRH analog, it is also logical that in this group of PCOD patients, the basic ovarian response to hMG or hFSH stimulation is not significantly changed by pituitary downregulation.

Neuroendocrinology has been another area in which a possibility of a new insight into the pathophysiologic mechanisms of PCOD was generated. It is well known that brain tissue contains estrogen receptors. Naftolin et al (1990) showed that estrogen may induce alterations in synaptic density and in postsynaptic membrane structure in the rat arcuate nucleus tissue. As established in animal experiments, estrogen may affect

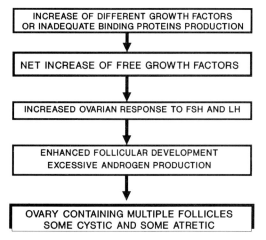

**Fig. 26.4** The excessive levels of free growth factors as a possible pathophysiological mechanism leading to PCOD.

neurogenesis in the fetus (Rasmussen et al 1990), synaptogenesis in the perinatal and adult rat (Matsumoto & Arai 1981) and synaptic remodelling and, consequently, gonadotropin control in adult rodents (Garcia-Segura et al 1986) (Fig. 26.5). Moreover, the brain tissue is capable of converting androgens into estrogens (Naftolin & Brawer 1978) and thus, many if not all the androgen effects which lead to sex differences in the pattern of gonadotropin release are actually elicited by estrogens. Availability of sufficient amounts of estrogen during the intrauterine and perinatal period results in the development of an LHRH delivery system allowing only tonic gonadotropin release (male pattern). If during the 'critical period' of sexual development insufficient amounts of estrogen reach the brain, a female-type synaptology, resulting in a cyclic-LHRH

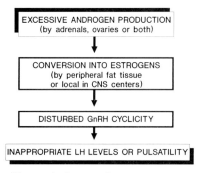

**Fig. 26.5** Changes in the central nervous system possibly leading to PCOD.

delivery system, will develop. Estrogen was shown to be capable of permanently altering the pattern of gonadotropin release not only during the 'critical period' (i.e. perinatal), but also throughout the life of the rat (Finch et al 1984, Naftolin et al 1988).

It could be presumed that a permanent disturbance of CNS function controlling the gonadotropin release pattern might result from the following sequence of events: The ovaries or the adrenal glands may produce apparently normal but relatively excessive amounts of androgens. If this overproduction is chronic and/or if the enzymatic apparatus required for aromatization of androgens into estrogen (in the fat tissue or in the brain) is either too sensitive or quantitatively excessive, constant hyperestrogenism will inevitably follow. Hyperestrogenism may affect the synaptic remodelling and finally produce a synaptology and postsynaptic membrane resembling the male type. In consequence, the brain centers will be unable to generate signals appropriate for the cyclic pattern of gonadotropin release and this will obviously lead to persistent disturbance of ovarian function.

Obesity should also be regarded as a possible basis for the development of PCOD (Nestler et al 1989) (Fig. 26.6). It is well known that fat tissue contains significant amounts of aromatase and may thus efficiently convert androgens into estrogen (Forncy et al 1981). It has also been established that many obese women develop insulin resistance and, consequently, may become hyperinsulinemic. Hyperinsulinemia can result in a whole array of effects. It can lead to excessive ovarian androgen production (Barbieri et al 1988) and to enhanced conversion of testosterone into the more potent $5\alpha$-dihydrotestosterone (DHT). The expression of 5-$\alpha$–reductase activity and the number of DHT receptors may also be increased (Kaufman et al 1981). Rosenfield et al (1990), showed that in some cases of PCOD hyperandrogenism may result from unbalanced production or function of the cytochrome P-450 c 17-alpha. It should also be remembered that ovarian hyperandrogenism may inhibit the liver production of sex hormone binding globulin (SHBG) resulting in a further increase in bioactive androgens.

Compounding the facts discussed above, Insler

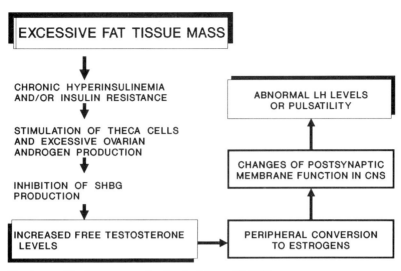

**Fig. 26.6** Obesity as a part of pathophysiology of PCOD.

& Lunenfeld (1991) proposed that the following sequence of events (mechanisms) may lead to the development of polycystic ovarian disease (Fig. 26.7): Increased adrenal function during the pre- or peri-pubertal period may result in elevated androgen production. At least a part of these androgens is changed to estrogens by peripheral conversion in fat or brain tissues. The excessive

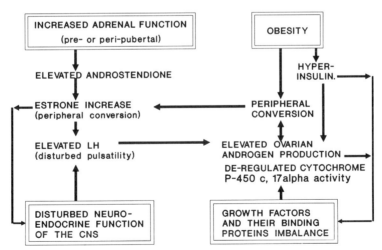

**Fig. 26.7** Possible pathophysiological mechanisms of PCOD. The 'circulus viciosus' finally leading to clinical manifestation of PCOD consists of elevated androgen levels, increased ability of fat and other tissues to convert androgens into oestrogens and, consequently, disturbed LH pulsatility. The generating or triggering factors may originate in the adrenals; the hypothalamus or higher CNS centers; in the ovary itself (deregulated cytochrome P-450 c, 17-alpha); may stem from excess of fat tissue usually combined with hyperinsulinism; or may be the result of a net increase in active growth factors. Each of the above disturbances probably appears early in life much before the clinical signs of the disease are evident. (Reproduced with permission from Insler & Lunenfeld 1991.)

estrogen levels alter the synaptology type and postsynaptic membrane function of the arcuate nucleus and possibly other centers in the brain. This results in a disturbed LH secretion pattern. The abnormal LH secretion may, in turn, stimulate the thecal compartment of the ovary to produce androgens, which on the one hand would increase the estrogen pool due to peripheral conversion, and on the other hand would disturb the follicular development and ripening by local action within the ovary. If this mechanism will act for a sufficient period of time, the vicious circle of disturbed gonadotropin secretion pattern and abnormal ovarian response will be established leading to the typical structural changes of the ovary.

It can also be presumed that a net increase in some growth factors resulting either from increased production or from lack of specific binding protein, may initiate an overproduction of ovarian androgens or estrogens which, in turn, could affect the function of the CNS and initiate the vicious circle leading to PCOD.

The synaptic function and postsynaptic membrane structure could be disturbed during intrauterine life. There is no doubt that the fetal endocrine systems are capable of function and it would be overoptimistic to assume that this function cannot be deranged. For example, gestational diabetes resulting in both enlarged quantity of fetal fat tissue and in hyperinsulinemia could be regarded as a logical candidate for initiating the vicious circle of disturbed CNS function and ovarian response. According to our knowledge, no studies were performed correlating gestational diabetes (i.e. the glucose and insulin levels in pregnant women and neonatal birthweight) with the incidence of PCOD during the fertile period in the offspring in appropriately chosen cohorts. One additional point should be stressed here. Although PCOD may be initiated by each of the four above-mentioned disturbances (increased adrenal function, obesity, relative excess of growth factors or male-type synaptology), in many cases the vicious circle is probably a result of a synergistic action of more than one of them.

On the basis of the ideas presented, it is also logical to presume that the disease may be genetic

in some cases (deranged function of the cytochrome P-450 17-alpha; attenuated adrenal hyperplasia) or may start during intrauterine life (maternal gestational diabetes), but it expresses itself mainly during the peripubertal period. If this is the case, screening of adolescent girls, determination of probable risk factors and elaboration of methods for their detection, as well as devising preventive therapy, would certainly be of enormous value. It should not be overlooked that although infertility is at present perceived as the main disturbance related to PCOD, hyperestrogenism or a wide 'estrogen window' must be regarded as risk factors for the development of uterine or breast cancer in later years. Its role in disturbing lipid metabolism, consequently leading to atherosclerosis and possibly cardiovascular diseases, must also be seriously regarded (Obhrai et al 1990). This makes early detection and preventive therapy even more important. The possible early predisposing factors and late consequences of PCOD are summarized in Figure 26.8.

## MANAGEMENT OF PCOD

### Prevention approach

It seems that in the majority of patients, PCOD begins at the peripubertal period. This is the time when many endocrine systems undergo significant functional changes. The hypothalamus alters its release pattern of GnRH, effecting a profound modification of the frequency and amplitude of FSH and LH pulses. The follicular and stromal

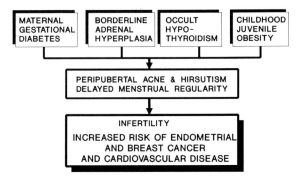

**Fig. 26.8** Predisposing factors and late consequences of PCOD. (Reproduced with permission from Insler & Lunenfeld 1991.)

ovarian compartments change their response to gonadotropin stimulation. The relative levels of different adrenal steroids undergo a pronounced, although graduate, shift. The sensitivity of various target organs to respond to steroids is being modified. These critical changes in the hypothalamic-pituitary-ovarian axis may be adversely influenced by some extraneous factors. Childhood or juvenile obesity may result in excessive extragonadal estrogen production by the fat tissue mast cells. Late-onset adrenogenital syndrome (AGS) is associated with excessive adrenal androgen secretion. This could result in the appearance of hirsutism, acne and seborrhea on the one hand, and in peripheral conversion of androgens into estrone on the other hand. Prolonged stress could produce a similar effect in the presence of normal adrenal glands.

It has been accepted that a peripubertal girl must 'learn to ovulate'. However, the length of this 'learning period' was never accurately established. As usual in medicine, significant individual variations are presumed to be a rule. Would it not be logical to conclude that a girl who is incapable of establishing regular cycles within 6 months after menarche and who develops during that period a slight or moderate hirsutism, has a high chance of eventually creating the circulus viciosus of disturbed LH oscillations, inappropriate ovarian response to gonadotropin stimulation and hyperandrogenism? Would it be surprising if, 10 years later, she would be received in infertility clinic with a diagnosis of PCOD? Accepting this line of thinking, peripubertal obesity and stress must receive proper attention. These girls should also be treated with combined contraceptive pills (preferably containing antiandrogens such as cyproterone acetate) and in that way improve the symptoms of acne, seborrhea and hirsutism and possibly prevent the development of PCO. In order to prove that the above theory is indeed correct, a well-planned properly randomized double-blind study using placebo and contraceptive pills should be carried out. Although expensive, difficult and long, such research could probably help to shed some light on the enigma of PCOD.

It should also be remembered that excessive estrone levels and prolonged unopposed estrogen effects represent significant risk factors for breast and endometrial cancers, cardiovascular diseases and cerebrovascular accidents. Thus, PCOD patients should probably be treated with contraceptive pills during the periods between pregnancies.

## Clinical management protocols

As pointed out in previous sections of this chapter ('Hormonal findings' and 'Clinical symptomatology'), diagnostic parameters of PCOD, i.e. menstrual disorders, infertility, obesity, elevated LH levels or LH/FSH ratio, persistent estrogen production, hyperandrogenism and distinct sonographic picture are not constantly found. Thus, the management must be based mainly on two criteria: the severity of androgenization and fertility intentions of the patient.

Insler & Lunenfeld (1990) proposed a practical management scheme for patients presumed to have PCO. According to anamnesis, primary physical examination and plasma testosterone levels the patients are divided into two groups, each being managed in a different way.

*Group A* is characterized by a sudden onset of hirsutism and menstrual disorders. Very often other signs of virilization such as change in body contour, enlargement of the clitoris and deepening of the voice are also present. The plasma total testosterone levels usually exceed 2 ng/ml (Fig. 26.9). In these patients the tentative diagnosis is functioning ovarian tumor. Since some of these tumors may be malignant, further examination by CT scan and sonography is performed. If the diagnosis is confirmed, an explorative laparotomy should be carried out. The extent and type of the following surgical procedure is determined by the results of microscopic examination of frozen sections of the tumor, other intraabdominal findings, the patient's age and her future fertility goals.

If the presence of an ovarian tumor is ruled out, the patient should be reexamined in order to find the source of elevated testosterone production. In extremely rare instances this may be found in the adrenal glands. When CT and ultrasound do not show any specific anatomical findings within the adrenals or the ovaries, catheterization of

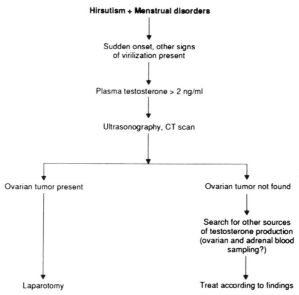

**Fig. 26.9**  Management flowsheet of patients with pronounced hirsutism (or virilization) of sudden onset.

the ovarian and adrenal veins to obtain blood samples for hormonal examinations may be indicated.

*Group B* includes the great majority of cases of hirsutism, menstrual disorders and infertility. In this group the intensity of symptoms progresses slowly and gradually. Signs of virilization are usually absent or very scanty. Plasma total testosterone levels do not exceed 2 ng/ml (Fig. 26.10). Dehydroepiandrosterone sulfate (DHEA-S) is now measured. If found to be elevated, the patient should be examined for the presence of late-onset adrenocortical hyperplasia, Cushing's syndrome or ACTH secreting pituitary tumor.

In women having normal levels of DHEA-S, thyroid function tests are performed. Even slight (subclinical) hypothyroidism may interfere with the normal function of the hypothalamic-pituitary-ovarian axis and result in menstrual disorders, anovulation, possible hyperandrogenism and finally in the development of PCO. Obviously, hypothyroidism, if present, must be taken into consideration when the therapy is planned.

In patients with normal thyroid function tests, a prolactin assay is performed. The presence of moderate hyperprolactinemia does not exclude the possibility of polycystic changes in the ovary, but may influence the type of treatment.

All hyperandrogenized women with a variety of menstrual disorders, but having normal adrenal and thyroid function and prolactin levels, are designated as functional ovarian hyperandrogenism, this term being actually synonymous with PCOD.

The treatment to be instituted depends on the fertility plans of the patient. In women not desiring pregnancy in the immediate future, a whole array of synthetic and natural steroids has been applied. The basic aim of the therapy is to reduce the excessive LH levels and possibly also to exert some beneficial local effect upon the ovary. It seems that contraceptive pills containing different combinations of estrogen and gestagens are the most commonly used. Our group prefers to treat these patients with a combination of cyproterone acetate and ethinyl estradiol. The former has a good effect in diminishing hirsutism and the latter ensures normal cyclic bleeding. In this context the report of Falsetti & Galbignani (1990) is of special interest. They treated 66 PCOD women with a combination of 0.035 mg of ethinyl estradiol and 2 mg of cyproterone acetate over 36 consecutive cycles. At the end of this

**HIRSUTISM/ACNE/MENSTRUAL DISORDERS**

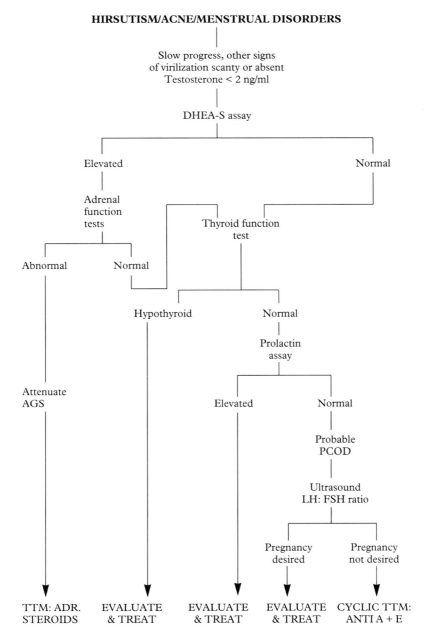

**Fig. 26.10**   Management flowsheet of patients with menstrual disorders and hirsutism.
TTM, treatment; ADR. STEROIDS, corticosteroids; ANTI A, antiandrogen; E, estrogen.

treatment, in addition to improvement of acne and hirsutism, the LH/FSH ratios were normalized, the estrogen androstendione and testosterone values were markedly reduced, and the levels of SHBG increased significantly. Moreover, the ovarian size and the number of cystic follicles diminished considerably. Unfortunately, this report does not provide information on whether the improved hormonal status and ovarian morphology persisted after cessation of therapy.

Patients presumed to suffer from PCOD who desire to conceive as soon as possible are usually offered ovulation-inducing treatment (Fig. 26.11). Again, a number of stimulating agents and protocols have been used.

Clomiphene citrate (CC) is most often applied as a first-line therapy (see also Chapter 18). Raj et al (1977) studied 55 women with PCOD and achieved a pregnancy rate of 55% using CC. Most reports, however, claim that clomiphene treatment results in pregnancy only in approximately 30% of cases. This is also our own experience.

hMG has been for years applied as an ovulation inducer in infertile women who failed to conceive following CC therapy. According to our own experience, patients with PCOD respond well to this therapy, but the pregnancy rates are not higher and hyperstimulation occurs more often than in women having normal ovaries (see also Chapter 16). Similar findings were reported by Wang & Gemzell (1980). Kemmann et al (1981) reported on exceptionally good clinical results obtained with hMG in patients with PCO. The pregnancy rate was 58% and none of the women developed ovarian hyperstimulation. His series was, however, relatively small, comprising only 24 patients. In a review article describing the general principles and overall results of gonadotropin therapy (Insler 1988), it has been pointed out that in small groups of meticulously selected patients the pregnancy rates were usually

higher than in large series treated routinely in busy fertility clinics. In recent years a gonadotropin preparation containing 'pure' FSH without the addition of LH has become available. Since the excessive LH secretion has been considered to be a characteristic feature of PCOD, it seemed that induction of ovulation in these patients by application of 'pure' FSH should be more efficient than the use of hMG containing equal amounts of both FSH and LH. It has been observed that ovaries stimulated with 'pure' FSH secrete a nonsteroidal factor which suppresses the secretion of LH (Schenken & Hodgen 1983). The reduction of LH levels following application of 'pure' FSH was also observed in clinical studies of ovulation-induction cycles (Kamrawa et al 1982, Venturoli et al 1984, Jones et al 1985). Recently, a pharmacodynamic study of Anderson et al (1989) showed that serum levels of LH decreased significantly following a single dose of hFSH. In normal controls the effect (a 24% decrease) was observed within 30 min and in PCOD patients the LH levels decreased by 27% within 18 h. The above observations are supportive of the theoretical advantages of hFSH over hMG in PCOD patients. This has, however, not yet been confirmed by wide scale clinical trials.

Birkhauser et al (1988) treated 30 PCOD women over 68 cycles and achieved a pregnancy rate of 58.6%. The severe hyperstimulation rate was, however, rather high (8.8%), and in almost half of the treatment cycles premature LH surges were noticed. Reviewing recent literature, Traub & McFaul (1989) concluded that the pregnancy rates that have been achieved using 'pure' FSH were not significantly different from those obtained by hMG therapy.

When discussing ovulation-induction therapy by FSH in PCOD patients one more aspect should be mentioned. Some authors proposed to use a 'low-dose' and 'stepwise increase' of FSH (Sagle et al 1991, Shoham et al 1991). The gist of this protocol has been to start the therapy by injecting 75 IU FSH (1 ampule) daily and either to reduce or to increase the daily dose by 37.5 IU after 7–14 days according to the ovarian response assessed by sonography. This treatment resulted in higher ovulation rates, smaller number

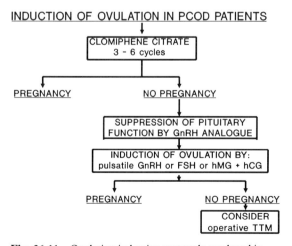

**Fig. 26.11** Ovulation induction protocols employed in PCOD patients desiring pregnancy. TTM, treatment.

of leading follicles and lower cancellation incidence than the 'standard' FSH or hMG therapy. For the sake of synoptic accuracy it should be mentioned that the 'stepwise' increments (by 1.3) of gonadotropin dose was proposed by Townsend & his collegues in 1966, and the 'low' or 'decreasing' dose to be applied according to ovarian response of individual patients was recommended by Lunenfeld in 1963 and elaborated by Insler and Lunenfeld in 1974.

It has been recently reported that several esters of alcohols containing a cyclohexyl ring were potent inhibitors of human placental aromatase and of the rat testicular 17α-hydroxylase/C17, 20-lyase complex (McCague et al 1990). Morita et al (1990) showed that ketoconazole (an imidazole containing antimycotic drug) reduced 17α-hydroxylase and C17, 20-lyase activities in a dose-dependent manner and inhibited testosterone biosynthesis in man. This would indicate that ketoconazole (and possibly other related drugs) could regulate the levels and/or action of cytochrome P-450 connected enzymes. Bar et al (1991) reported on a small series of infertile women with PCOD treated by a combination of ketoconazole/hMG/hCG for induction of ovulation. Previous treatment of the same women with hMG/hCG alone served as control. The combined therapy resulted in lower estradiol levels, development of one to three dominant and less small follicles, lower hyperstimulation and higher pregnancy rates than in the control cycles. If confirmed by larger clinical experiments, the above results may inspire development of a tailored treatment scheme for a subgroup of PCOD women in whom the underlying patho-physiological mechanism involves deregulated function of the cytochrome P-450 enzymes family.

The introduction of potent GnRH analogs capable of eliciting a temporary 'medical hypophysectomy' (Crowley et al 1982, Meldrum et al 1982, Yen 1983, Bettendorf et al 1988) seemed to carry a great promise for an efficient treatment of PCOD (see also Chapter 15). However, the initial hopes proved to be excessively optimistic. The combined therapy consisting of pituitary suppression by GnRH

analog and ovarian stimulation by gonadotropins does not produce higher pregnancy rates, nor does it result in lower hyperstimulation incidence. There is no doubt that this therapy does significantly reduce the frequency of ill-timed LH surges (Insler et al 1988, Schoemaker et al 1988) and/or reduces the excessive LH levels during the follicular phase.

Timely maturation of the oocyte is essential if fertilization and the development of an embryo are to occur. Before ovulation the chromosomes of the oocyte are arrested in the prophase stage of meiosis by an inhibiting factor that is itself inhibited by the action of LH at midcycle. This ensures the release of a mature egg at the appropriate time (Tsafriri & Pomerantz 1986). Premature reactivation of meiosis caused by high basal concentrations of LH may lead to kariotypic abnormalities and death of the embryo or fetus. It has been suggested that a high concentration of LH through the follicular phase allows the developing oocyte to mature prematurely (Homburg et al 1988), producing at ovulation an oocyte that is physiologically aged. These oocytes are unlikely to fertilize or, if conception is achieved, early abortion may result. From work involving women undergoing in vitro fertilization (IVF) several authors have reported that high concentrations of LH in the few days before oocytes are collected were associated with reduced rates of fertilization and conception (Stanger & Yovitch 1985, Howles et al 1986, Punnonen et al 1988). The above results were confirmed by McFaul et al (1989). These authors also demonstrated that if conception is achieved in a cycle in which the oocyte is prematurely exposed to elevated LH, there is a significantly higher probability that an early abortion will result. They pointed out that this situation occurs in patients diagnosed as PCOD, where ovulation rates following ovulation induction are high but pregnancy rates are low. Johnson & Pearce (1990) supported this concept and concluded that pituitary supression by GnRH analog before induction of ovulation (reducing LH levels) reduces the risk of spontaneous abortion in women with PCOD and primary recurrent spontaneous abortion following induction of ovulation. Spontaneous abortion occurred in 11 of 20 women given CC, compared with only two of 20 who had pituitary suppression with buserelin followed by administration of pure FSH.

Of particular interest is also the report by Filicori et al (1990) who achieved a significant improvement of the results of pulsatile GnRH therapy by pretreating PCOD patients with GnRH analog.

At present, the combined pituitary suppression/ovarian stimulation therapy is used in many centers as the main infertility treatment in women with PCOD.

The conclusion of Coutts et al (1990) that combined pituitary suppression/ovarian stimulation therapy is capable of improving pregnancy rates in PCOD patients but is inadequate to permanently cure the underlying disease should, however, not be disregarded.

### In vitro fertilization and embryo transfer (IVF-ET)

Macnamee (1989) in a retrospective study of IVF patients found that approximately 60% of women who showed no ovarian response to prolonged clomiphene and/or hMG stimulation had the typical ultrasound pattern of PCOD. The majority of these patients showed also high basal LH levels during the follicular phase. He concluded that elevated LH levels in the follicular phase may be detrimental to oocyte development. The LH elevation can be successfully suppressed by concomitant application of GnRH analogs. The combined therapy resulted in IVF-ET results similar to those obtained in other groups of patients (21% of clinical pregnancies). Obviously, IVF is not the first-line therapy for PCOD patients who do not present with additional (mechanical or male) infertility factors (see also Chapter 21).

### Ovarian wedge resection

A whole series of surgical procedures, ranging from puncture of cystic follicles by the vaginal route, through wedge resection, to hilus excision and decortication of the ovary was advocated (Lunenfeld et al 1968). The main rationale of operative therapy is most probably just the removal of some of the mass of androgen-producing ovarian tissue (atretic follicles, stroma, hyperplastic theca). This should improve the ovarian reaction to gonadotropin stimulation and, consequently, also correct the hypothalamic-pituitary function with regard to the levels and oscillations of LH secretion. Wedge resection in the majority of cases resulted in a significant reduction of plasma testosterone and estrogen

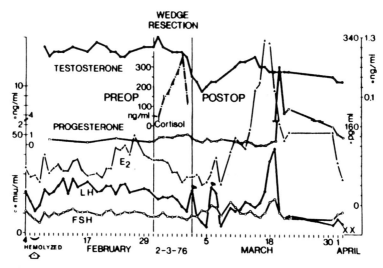

**Fig. 26.12**  Hormonal levels before, during and following wedge resection in a patient with PCOD. (Reproduced with permission from Katz et al 1978.)

**Table 26.2**   The results of ovarian wedge resection in patients with PCOD

| Postoperative findings | Cases evaluated (no.) | Range (%) |
|---|---|---|
| Regular cycles | 447 | 6–95 |
| Pregnancy | 640 | 13–89 |
| Diminished hirsutism | 205 | 0–18 |

Recalculated from Goldzieher & Green 1962

levels (Fig. 26.12). The LH and FSH levels and their ratios returned to normal only in some cases and this result usually appeared later than the effect of surgery on steroids (Judd et al 1976, Katz et al 1978, Mahesh et al 1978, Belisle et al 1981).

The clinical results of wedge resection reported in the literature were summarized by Goldzieher & Green (1962). It seems that the procedure has been much more effective in improving menstrual disorders and infertility than in decreasing hirsutism (Table 26.2). It has also been pointed out that the effects of wedge resection are usually temporary and the signs and symptoms of the disorder return within months following the operation. Moreover, it has been proven that ovarian wedge resection results quite often in formation of periovarian and peritubal adhesions (Butram & Vaquero 1975) which may significantly reduce the future fertility potential of the patient (Adashi et al 1981).

Recently a cauterization electrode for treatment of PCOD has been introduced (Aakvaag & Gjonnaess 1985, Greenblatt & Casper 1987, Amar et al 1990). The procedure is performed under laparoscopic control. The depth of cauterization is limited by the design of the instrument. The results reported so far seem to be promising. The question regarding the span of clinical improvement is still open. It has also not yet been definitely proven whether the operation may be used repeatedly and whether it engenders any damage to the ovaries or their surroundings. When the above questions will be satisfactorily answered, it seems that this procedure will be employed for treatment of infertility in PCOD women, particularly after failure of other ovulation-inducing therapies.

## REFERENCES

Aakvaag A, Gjonnaess H 1985 Hormonal response to electrocautery of the ovary in patients with polycystic ovarian disease. Br J Obstet Gynaecol 92: 1258

Adams J, Polson D W, Franks S 1986 Prevalence of polycystic ovaries in women with anovulation and idiopathic hirsutism. Br Med J 293: 355

Adashi E A, Rock J A, Guzick D, Wentz A C, Jones G, Jones H W 1981 Fertility following bilateral ovarian wedge resection: a critical analysis of 90 consecutive cases of the polycystic ovary syndrome. Fertil Steril 36: 320

Adashi E A, Resnick C E, Svoboda, M E, van Wyk J J 1985 Insulin-like growth factors as intraovarian regulators of granulosa cell growth and function. Endocrinol Rev 6: 400

Adashi E A, Resnick C E, Svoboda M E, van Wyk J J 1988 Somatomedin C enhances induction of LH receptors by FSH in cultured rat granulosa cells. Endocrinology 116: 2369

Aiman J, Edman C D, Worley J R, Vellios F, MacDonald P C 1978 Androgen and estrogen formation in women with ovarian hyperthecosis. Obstet Gynecol 51: 1

Alger M, Vazquez-Matute L, Mason M, Canales E, Zarate A 1980 Polycystic ovarian disease associated with hyperprolactinemia and defective metoclopramide response. Fertil Steril 34: 70

Amar N A, McGarrigle H H G, Honour J, Holownia P, Jacobs H S, Lachelin G C L 1990 Laparoscopic ovarian diathermy in the management of anovulatory infertility in women with polycystic ovaries: endocrine changes and clinical outcome. Fertil Steril 53: 45

Anderson R E, Cragun J M, Chang R J, Stanczyk F Z, Lobo R A 1989 A pharmacodynamic comparison of human urinary follicle-stimulating hormone and human menopausal gonadotropin in normal women and polycystic ovarian syndrome. Fertil Steril 52: 216

Axelrod L R, Goldzieher J W, Ross S D 1965 Concurrent 3beta-hydroxysteroid dehydrogenase deficiency in adrenal and sclerocystic ovary. Acta Endocrinol 48: 392

Bar A, Gal M, Triger A, Samama A, Porat E, Diamant J 1991 The clinical use of ketoconazol as an adjuvant antiandrogen therapy in induction of ovulation by hMG/hCG in women with PCOD. Proceedings of The Congress of Israel Society for the Study of Fertility, Tel-Aviv, p 38

Barbieri R L, Smith S, Ryan K J 1988 The role of hyperinsulinemia in the pathogenesis of ovarian hyperandrogenism. Fertil Steril 50: 197

Belisle S, Lehoux J G, Bernard B, Ainmelk Y 1981 Ovarian hyperthecosis; in vivo and in vitro correlations of the androgen profile. Obstet Gynecol 57: 70

Berger M J, Taymor M L, Patton W C 1975
Gonadotropin levels and secretory patterns in patients with
typical and atypical polycystic ovarian disease. Fertil Steril
26: 619

Bettendorf G, Braendle W, Lichtenberg V, Lindner Ch 1988
Pharmacologic hypogonadotropism-an advantage for
gonadotropin stimulation. Gynecol Endocrinol 2
(suppl 1): 66

Birkhauser M H, Huber P R, Neuenschwander E, Naepflin S
1988 Induktion der follikelreifung mit 'reinem' FSH beim
polyzystichen ovar-syndrom. Geburtshil Frauenheilkd
48: 220

Breteche J 1952 Kystes ovariques et ovaries sclero-cystique
dans la sterilite. Bull Fed Gynecol Obstet Franc 4: 149

Burghen G A, Givens J R, Kitabachi A E 1980 Correlation of
hyperandrogenism with hyperinsulinism in polycystic
ovarian disease. J Clin Endocrinol Metab 50: 113

Butram V C, Vaquero C 1975 Post ovarian wedge resection
adhesive disease. Fertil Steril 26: 874

Cooper H E, Spellacy W N, Prem K A, Cohen W D 1968
Hereditary factors in the Stein–Leventhal Syndrome. Am J
Obstet Gynecol 100: 371

Coutts J R T, Hamilton M P R, Yates R, McNally W,
Finnie S, Fleming R 1990 Primary oligomenorrhea in
women: pathophysiology and the treatment of
associated infertility using combined GnRH-a and
exogenous gonadotrophins. Gynecol Endocrinol 4(suppl
2): 55

Crowley F, Comite W, Vale J, Rivier D L, Loriaux,
Cutler G B 1982 Inhibition of serum androgen levels by
chronic intranasal and subcutaneous administration of a
potent luteinizing hormone-releasing hormone (LH-RH)
agonist in adult men. Fertil Steril 27: 240

Delahunt J W, Clements R V, Ramsay R D, Newton J,
Collins W P, Landon J 1975 The monocystic ovary
syndrome. Br Med J 4: 621

Falsetti L, Galbignani E 1990 Long-term treatment with the
combination ethinylestradiol and cyproterone acetate in
polycystic ovary syndrome. Contraception 42: 611

Farber M, Millan V G, Turksoy R N, Mitchell G W 1978
Diagnostic evaluation of hirsutism in women by selective
bilateral adrenal and ovarian catheterization. Fertil Steril
30: 283

Farber M, Madanes A, O'Brian D S, Millan V G, Turksoy
R N, Rule A H 1981 Asymmetric hyperthecosis ovarii.
Obstet Gynecol 57: 521

Filicori M, Flamigni C, Meriggiola M C et al 1990 The use of
GnRH analogues to enhance susceptibility to pulsatile
GnRH ovulation induction. Gynecol Endocrinol
4(suppl 2): 54

Finch E C, Felicio L S, Mobbs C V, Nelson J F 1984 Ovarian
and steroidal influences on neuroendocrine aging process in
the female rodents. Endocrinol Rev 5: 467

Forncy J P, Milewich L, Chen G T 1981 Aromatization of
androstenedione to estrone by human adipose tissue in
vitro: correlation with adipose tissue mass, age and
endometrial neoplasia. J Clin Endocrinol Metab 53: 192

Futterweit W, Krieger D T 1979 Pituitary tumor associated
with hyperprolactinemia and polycystic ovarian disease.
Fertil Steril 31: 608

Garcia-Segura L M, Baetens D, Naftolin F 1986 Synaptic
remodelling in arcuate nucleus after injection of estradiol
valerate in adult female rats. Brain Res 366: 131

Givens J R, Wiser W L, Coleman S A, Wilroy R S,
Andersen R N, Fish S A 1971 Familial ovarian

hyperthecosis: a study of two families. Am J Obstet Gynecol
110: 959

Goldzieher J W, Green J A 1962 The polycystic ovary.
I. Clinical and histologic features. J Clin Endocrinol Metab
22: 325

Goldzieher J W, diZerega G S 1985 Polycystic ovarian
disease. In: Shearman R P (ed) Clinical reproductive
endocrinology. Churchill Livingstone, Edinburgh, p 406

Greenblatt R B 1963 The hirsute female. Thomas,
Springfield, Ill., p 154

Greenblatt E, Casper R F 1987 Endocrine changes after
laparoscopic ovarian cautery in polycystic ovarian
syndrome. Am J Obstet Gynecol 156: 279

Hofmeister F J, Byce K R 1966 The clinical aspects of the
Stein-Leventhal syndrome. Obstet Gynecol 28: 264

Homburg R, Armar N A, Eshel A, Adams J, Jacobs H S 1988
Influence of serum luteinising hormone concentration on
ovulation, conception and early pregnancy loss in polycystic
ovary syndrome. Br Med J 297: 1024

Howles C M, Macnamee M C 1989 The endocrinology of
superovulation: lessons from assisted conception therapy.
In: Howles C M, Macnamee M C (eds) The endocrinology
of superovulation; the influence of luteinizing hormone.
Excerpta Medica, Amsterdam, p 6

Howles C M, Macnamee M C, Edwards R G, Goswamy R,
Steptoe P C 1986 Effect of high tonic levels of luteinizing
hormone on outcome of in vitro fertilisation. Lancet ii: 521

Hull M G R 1987 Epidemiology of infertility and polycystic
ovarian disease: endocrinological and demographic studies.
Gynecol Endocrinol 1: 235

Insler V 1988 Gonadotropin therapy: new trends and insights.
Int J Fertil 33: 85

Insler V, Lunenfeld B 1974 Application of human
gonadotropins for induction of ovulation. In: Campos da
Paz A, Hasegava T, Notake Y, Hayashi M (eds) Human
reproduction. Igaku Shoin, Tokyo, pp 25–38

Insler V, Lunenfeld B 1990 Polycystic ovarian disease: a
challenge and controversy. Gynecol Endocrinol 4: 51

Insler V, Lunenfeld B 1991 Pathophysiology of polycystic
ovarian disease: new insights. Hum Reprod 6: 1025

Insler V, Potashnik G, Lunenfeld E, Meizner I, Levy J 1988
Ovulation induction with hMG following down regulation
of the pituitary-ovarian axis by LH-RH analogs. Gynecol
Endocrinol 2(suppl 1): 67

Insler V, Barash A, Zadin Z, Lunenfeld B, Barensteri R,
Chen M 1991 The effect of pituitary suppression on follicle
stimulating hormone and luteinizing hormone pulsatility
problems in PCOD. Isr J Obstet Gynecol 2: 157

Johansson E D B, Wide L, Gemzell A 1971 Luteinizing
hormone (LH) and progesterone in plasma and LH and
oestrogens in urine during 42 normal menstrual cycles.
Acta Endocrinol 68: 502

Johnson P, Pearce J M 1990 Recurrent spontaneous abortion
and polycystic ovarian disease: comparison of two
regimens to induce ovulation. Br Med J (Clin Res)
300: 154

Jones G S, Acosta A A, Garcia J E, Bernados R E,
Rosenwaks Z 1985 The effect of follicle-stimulating
hormone without additional luteinizing hormone on
follicular stimulation and oocyte development in normal
ovulatory women. Fertil Steril 43: 696

Jones R V 1962 cited by Lunenfeld et al 1968

Judd H L, Rigg L A, Anderson D C, Yen S S C 1976 The
effect of ovarian wedge resection on circulating
gonadotropin and ovarian steroid levels in patients with

polycystic ovary syndrome. J Clin Endocrinol Metab 43: 347

Kahn C R, Flier J S, Bar R S et al 1976 The syndrome of insulin resistance and acanthosis nigricans. Insulin-receptor disorders in man. New Engl J Med 294: 739

Kamrawa M M, Seibel M M, Berger M J, Thomson I, Taymor M L 1982 Reversal of persistent anovulation in polycystic ovarian disease by administration of chronic low dose follicle-stimulating hormone. Fertil Steril 37: 520

Katz M, Carr P J, Cohen M B, Millar R P 1978 Hormonal effects of wedge resection of polycystic ovaries. Obstet Gynecol 51: 437

Kaufman M, Pinsky L, Feder-Hollander R 1981 Defective upregulation of the androgen receptor in human androgen insensitivity. Nature, 297: 735

Kemmann E, Tavakoli F, Shelden R M, Jones J R 1981 Induction of ovulation with menotropins in women with polycystic ovary syndrome. Am J Obstet Gynecol 141: 58

Laatikainen T, Tulenheimo A, Anderson B, Karkkainen J 1983 Obesity, serum steroid levels, and pulsatile gonadotropin secretion in polycystic ovarian disease. Eur J Obstet Gynecol Reprod Biol 15: 45

Landgren B M, Unden A L, Diczfalusy E 1980 Hormonal profile of the cycle in 68 normally menstruating women. Acta Endocrinol 94: 89

Lisse K, Schurenkamper P, Friedrich W, Rutkowsky J 1980 Diurnal change of serum androstenedione and testosterone and response to hCG and dexamethasone in women with polycystic ovaries, adrenal hyperandrogenism and unexplained hirsutism. Acta Endocrinol 93: 216

Lobo R A, Goebelsmann U 1980 Adult manifestation of congenital adrenal hyperplasia due to incomplete 21-hydroxylase deficiency mimicking polycystic ovarian disease. Am J Obstet Gynecol 138: 720

Lunenfeld B 1963 Treatment of anovulation by human gonadotrophins. Int J Gynecol Obstet 1: 153

Lunenfeld B, Eshkol A, Insler V, Kraiem Z 1968 Metabolic disorders of the ovary. In: Levine R, Luft R (eds) Advances in metabolic disorders Vol 3. Academic, New York, p 153

McArthur J W, Worcester J, Ingersoll F M 1958 cited by Lunenfeld et al 1968

McCague R, Rowlands M G, Barrie S E, Houghton J 1990 Inhibition of enzymes of estrogen and androgen biosynthesis by esters of 4-pyridylacetic acid. J Med Chem 33: 3050

McFaul P B, Traub A I, Thompson W 1989 Premature luteinization and ovulation induction using human menopausal gonadotrophin or pure follicle stimulating hormone in patients with polycystic ovary syndrome. Acta Eur Fertil 20: 157

McGoogan L S 1954 Sterility and ovarian pathology. Obstet Gynecol 3: 254

Macnamee M C 1989 The role of in vitro fertilization in polycystic ovarian disease. In: Cooke I D, Lunenfeld B (eds) Current understanding of polycystic ovarian syndrome. Research and clinical forums, vol 11, no 4. Royal Wells Medical Press, UK, p 89

Mahesh V B, Toledo S P A, Mattar E 1978 Hormone levels following wedge resection in polycystic ovary syndrome. Obstet Gynecol 51: 64

Matsumoto A, Arai Y 1981 Neuronal plasticity in the deafferented hypothalamic arcuate nucleus of adult female rats and its enhancement by treatment with estrogen. J Comp Neurol 197: 197

Meldrum D, Chang R J, Lu J, Vale W, Rivier J, Judd H L 1982 Medical oophorectomy using a long-acting GnRH agonist—a possible new approach to treatment of endometriosis. J Clin Endocrinol Metab 54: 1081

Merrill J A 1963 The morphology of the prepubertal ovary: relationship to the polycystic ovary syndrome. South Med J 56: 225

Morita K, Ono T, Shimakawa H 1990 Inhibition of testosterone biosynthesis in testicular microsomes by various imidazole drugs. Comparative study with ketoconazole. J Pharmacobiodyn 13: 336

Naftolin F, Brawer J R 1978 The effect of estrogens on hypothalamic structure and function. Am J Obstet Gynecol 132: 758

Naftolin F, MacLusky N J, Leranth C, Sakamoto H S, Garcia-Segura L M 1988 The cellular effects of estrogens on neuroendocrine tissues. J Steroid Biochem 30: 195

Naftolin F, Garcia-Segura L M, Keefe D, Leranth C, MacLusky N J, Brawer J R 1990 Estrogen effects on the synaptology and neural membranes of the rat hypothalamic arcuate nucleus. Biol Reprod 41: 21

Nestler J E, Clore J N, Blackard W G 1989 The central role of obesity (hyperinsulinemia) in the pathogenesis of the polycystic ovary syndrome. Am J Obstet Gynecol 161: 1095

Obhrai M, Samra J S, Brown P, Lynch S 1990 Effects of medical oophorectomy on fasting lipids and lipoproteins in women with polycystic ovarian syndrome. Gynecol Endocrinol 4(suppl 2): 72

Parker R, Ming P L, Rajan R, Goodner D M, Reme G 1980 Clinical and cytogenetic studies of patients with polycystic ovarian disease. Am J Obstet Gynecol 137: 656

Pekonen F, Laatikainen T, Buyalos R, Rutanen E M 1989 Decreased 34K insulin-like growth factor binding protein in polycystic ovarian disease. Fertil Steril 51: 972

Punnonen R, Ashorn R, Vilja P, Heinonen P K, Kunjansuu E, Tuohimaa P 1988 Spontaneous luteinizing hormone surge and cleavage of in vitro fertilized embryos. Fertil Steril 49: 479

Raj S G, Thompson I E, Berger M J, Taymor M L 1977 Clinical aspects of the polycystic ovary syndrome. Obstet Gynecol 49: 552

Rasmussen J, Torres-Alleman I, McLusky N J, Naftolin F, Robbins J R 1990 The effect of estradiol on the growth patterns of estrogen receptor positive hypothalamic cell lines. Endocrinology 126: 235

Rebar R, Judd H L, Yen S S C, Rakoff J, Vandenberg J, Naftolin F 1976 Characterization of the inappropriate gonadotropin secretion in polycystic ovary syndrome. J Clin Invest 57: 1320

Rosenfield R L, Barnes R B, Cara J F, Lucky A W 1990 Dysregulation of cytochrome P450c 17alpha as the cause of polycystic ovarian syndrome. Fertil Steril 53: 785

Sagle M A, Hamilton-Fairley D, Kiddy D S, Franks S 1991 A comparative, randomized study on low-dose human menopausal gonadotropin and follicle-stimulating hormone in women with polycystic ovarian syndrome. Fertil Steril 55: 56

Schenken R S, Hodgen G D 1983 Follicle-stimulating hormone induced ovarian stimulation in monkeys: blockade of the luteinizing hormone surge. J Clin Endocrinol Metab 57: 50

Schoemaker J, Hompes P G A, Scheele F, Weissenbruch M M 1988 PCOD: treatment with LHRH analogues. Gynecol Endocrinol 2(suppl): 51

Shapiro A G 1981 Pituitary adenoma, menstrual disturbance, hirsutism and abnormal glucose tolerance. Fertil Steril 35: 226

Shoham Z, Patel A, Jacobs H S 1991 Polycystic ovarian syndrome: safety and effectiveness of stepwise and low-dose administration of purified follicle-stimulating hormone. Fertil Steril 55: 1051

Smith K D, Steinberger E, Perloff W H 1965 Polycystic ovarian disease (PCO). A report of 301 patients. Am J Obstet Gynecol 93: 994

Sommers S C, Wadman P J 1956 Pathogenesis of polycystic ovaries. Am J Obstet Gynecol 72: 160

Stanger J D, Yovitch J L 1985 Reduced in vitro fertilization of human oocytes from patients with raised basal luteinising hormone levels during the follicular phase. Br J Obstet Gynecol 92: 385

Stein I F, Leventhal M L 1935 Amenorrhea associated with bilateral polycystic ovaries. Am J Obstet Gynecol 29: 181

Stevens V C, Goldzieher J V 1968 Urinary excretion of gonadotropins in congenital adrenal hyperplasia. Pediatrics 41: 421

Townsend S L, Brown J B, Johnstone J W, Adey F D, Evans J H, Taft H P 1966 Induction of ovulation. J Obstet Gynaecol Br Cwlth 73: 529

Traub A I, McFaul P B 1989 Injectable gonadotropins in the treatment of PCOS. In: Cooke I D, Lunenfeld B (eds) current understanding of polycystic ovarian syndrome. Research and clinical forums, vol 11, no 4. Royal Wells Medical Press, UK, p 71

Tsafriri A, Pomeranz S H 1986 Oocyte maturation inhibitor. Clin Endocrinol 15: 157

Urdl W 1988 Polycystic ovarian disease: endocrinological parameters with specific reference to growth hormone and somatomedin-C. Arch Gynecol Obstet 243: 13

Vara P, Niemineva K 1951 Small cystic degeneration of ovaries as incidental finding in gynecological laparotomies. Acta Obstet Gynecol Scand 31: 94

Vejlsted H, Albrechtsen R 1976 Biochemical and clinical effects of ovarian wedge resection in the polycystic ovary syndrome. Obstet Gynecol 47: 575

Venturoli S, Paradisi R, Raffaella F, Magrini O, Porcu E, Flamigni C 1984 Comparison between human urinary follicle-stimulating hormone and human menopausal gonadotropin treatment in polycystic ovary. Obstet Gynecol 63: 6

Wang C F, Gemzell C R 1980 The use of human gonadotropins for the induction of ovulation in women with polycystic ovarian disease. Fertil Steril 33: 479

Yen S S C 1983 Clinical application of gonadotropin-releasing hormone analogs. Fertil Steril 39: 257

# 27. Sexually transmitted diseases and their impact on fertility

*E. Lunenfeld    A. H. DeCherney*

Among the many causes of infertility sexually transmitted disease (STD) is one which is well recognized. Many studies such as that from Westrom (1987) have established an association between STD, pelvic inflammatory disease (PID) and Fallopian tube pathology. Acute salpingitis is the most prevalent important complication of some of the sexually transmitted pathogens. Tubal infertility in conjunction with ectopic pregnancy is a recognized sequelae of salpingitis. Salpingitis may be caused by a variety of organisms, the relative importance of which, however, seems to vary in different populations. Mardh et al (1981) in Sweden examined paired sera from 60 consecutive patients with laparoscopically confirmed acute salpingitis and concluded that the acute episode of salpingitis was associated with concurrent chlamydial infection in 58%, gonococcal infection in 8% and concurrent *Mycoplasma hominis* in 12%. In a review of 415 women treated for laparoscopy-verified acute salpingitis and followed up for 9.5 years, Westrom (1980) found that the incidence of tubal obstruction increased significantly after each episode of acute salpingitis, i.e from 12% after one episode to 75% after three episodes. It has been estimated that the annual incidence of PID among women less than 35 years of age in the USA reaches 425 000 cases. About 16% of that group (68 000) will experience involuntary infertility each year. Furthermore, it has been demonstrated by Rosenfeld et al (1983) and others that about 50% of cases with tubal infertility had no history of PID referred to by some authors as silent salpingitis. Distal tubal occlusion associated with hydrosalpingx, intratubal fibrosis and peritoneal adhesions are the major pathological abnormalities in tubal infertility which is associated with sexually transmitted pathogens, especially gonorrhea and chlamydia. Histological examination of those tubes revealed variable findings including dilated lumen, a single layer of uniformly flattened columnar epithelial cells and occasionally lymphocytes which had migrated into the epithelium (Fig. 27.1). Scanning electron microscopy as shown by Patton et al (1989) revealed in these cases mucosal folds which were flattened, attenuated and were devoid of ciliated epithelial cells. The secretory epithelial cells of the Fallopian tubes appeared smooth or contained thickened microvilli with clubbed appendages (Fig. 27.2). Transmission electron microscopy by the same authors revealed degenerative changes within the epithelial cells, extensive vacuole formation within the cells' cytoplasm and decreased numbers of intracellular organelles (Fig. 27.3). The secretory epithelial cells contained fewer secretory granules which were often irregular in size and in shape. At the plasma membrane of the secretory cells the microvilli were fewer in number and the ciliated epithelial cells had fewer cilia. It had also been demonstrated by Patton et al (1989) that ciliary beat frequency is lowered to one-third of the control. In addition to salpingitis, it has been suggested that certain sexually transmitted pathogens such as chlamydia and genital mycoplasma may directly contribute to infertility or reproductive wastage.

In men the most common local complication of sexually transmitted pathogens, especially gonorrhea and chlamydia, is epididymitis. Patients with acute epididymitis tend to present with unilateral testicular pain and swelling and most patients had

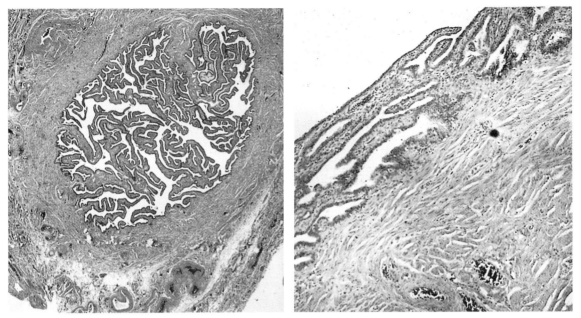

**Fig. 27.1a** (left)   Ampulla from a normal Fallopian tube which is filled with delicate mucosal folds containing epithelium on both surfaces. The lumen is only a potential space (x6). **b** (right) Light micrograph of the lumen of a Fallopian tube ampulla of a patient with 'silent PID' with greatly distended lumen. The epithelium is dramatically thinned (x10). (Reproduced with permission from Patton et al 1989.)

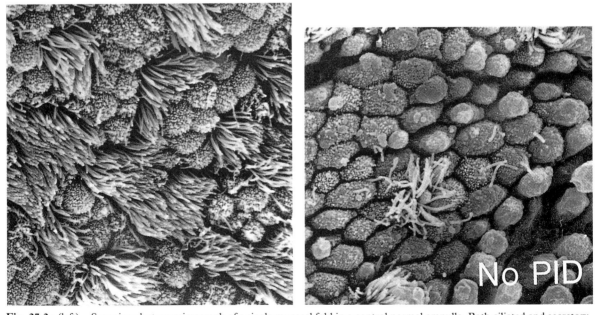

**Fig. 27.2a** (left)   Scanning electron micrograph of a single mucosal fold in a control normal ampulla. Both ciliated and secretory epithelial cells are present and cover the entire surface of the mucosal fold. Note that the normal ciliated cell contains 250–300 cilia per individual cell (x1920). **b** (right) Scanning electron micrograph of an ampula of a patient with 'silent PID'. The secretory epithelial cells appear smooth and flattened. Few microvillous projections are present on their surface. Individual cilia appear thickened and clumped. Widespread deciliation of the mucosal surface is observed (x1920). (Reproduced with permission from Patton et al 1989.)

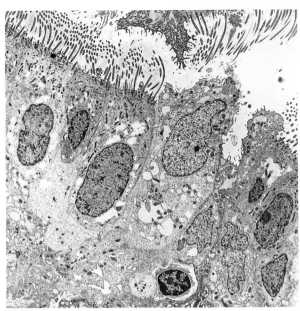

**Fig. 27.3**  Transmission electron micrograph of the endosalpinx from a patient with 'silent salpingitis'. Both ciliated and secretory epithelial cells are present. Extensive vacuolization is noted in the perinuclear region of the secretory cells, and little secretory granule production is observed. The ciliated cells contain few cilia. Beneath the basement membrane, a lymphocyte is observed near a damaged secretory epithelial cell (x1200). (Reproduced with permission from Patton et al 1989).

overt urethritis when they presented. Most cases of acute epididymitis begin in the tail of the epididymis with an acute intraluminal exudate, tubular epithelial damage and subjacent microabscesses. Some cases show predominantly mononuclear and perivascular infiltration. The inflammation in acute epididymitis is not limited to the epididymis and testicular involvement may occur. Wolin (1975) found on testes biopsy during acute epididymitis that 20 of 28 patients had decreased spermatogenesis and nine of 28 had testicular inflammation. Nilsson et al (1968) did aspiration biopsies on testicles in acute epididymitis and found that 16 of 22 showed inflammatory cells. Follow-up biopsy of these testicles after 2–3 years showed that five of nine had reduced or absent spermatogenesis. Berger et al (1979) have found low sperm counts in a high proportion of patients with acute epididymitis. Ludwig & Haselberger (1977) reported on 46 patients with unilateral epididymitis followed for 1 year. They found

initially that 66% were oligozospermic, however only 20% remained so after 1 year. Patients with bilateral epididymitis and bilateral occlusion of the vas deferens or epididymis have virtually a very low potential for fertility. As in women with subclinical or silent salpingitis and tubal damage, in infertile men with no history of epididymitis Gartman (1961) reported histological evidence of the condition which may lead to asymptomatic scarring and decreased fertility. Since sperm transit through the epididymis is known to be necessary for development of normal sperm function, it is possible that acute inflammation and damage to the epididymis could ultimately lead to decreased fertility even in the absence of occlusion of the epididymal tubules. In addition to epididymitis, evidence of previous gonococcal or chlamydial infection has been found in about 10% of prostatitis cases.

The diagnosis of STD in general and STD-associated infertility in particular should be confirmed at least by demonstrating the suggested causative organism, either by microscopy, culture, antigen or techniques based on DNA hybridization. Unfortunately to date obtaining material from internal organs such as Fallopian tubes, endometrium or epididymis still necessitates invasive procedures which are impractical for screening or routine diagnosis. Furthermore, the time interval between the genital infection and the complaint of infertility is often in the magnitude of years. It is therefore sometimes difficult to identify the causative organisms or the sequence of events leading to infertility. The recent development and refinement of serological techniques for identifying previous infection with all their limitations have contributed to establish the relative importance of the different pathogens in infertility. Among the many causes of infertility, those related to STD are difficult to treat but possible to prevent. It is with this in mind that we have reviewed the information on gonorrhea, chlamydia and genital mycoplasma and their possible effect on fertility. The biological background, pathogenesis and clinical data which seem relevant to infertility on each of these pathogens are discussed below.

### Neisseria gonorrhoea

Gonococci are nonmotile and nonspore forming Gram-negative diplococci which usually grow in pairs (diplococci). Neisseria gonorrhoea infect only mucous membrane lined by columnar cuboidal noncornified squamous epithelial cells, most often in the urogenital tract. They are transmitted almost exclusively by sexual contact or perinatally. The initial event in gonococcal infection is the adherence to mucosal cells. The pathogenic part of the gonococci is the fibrillar pili, which have been shown by Pearce & Buchanan (1978) to increase adhesion and invasion to host tissue. The second important documented adherence mechanisms are other gonococcal surface proteins described by Newhall et al (1980) known as protein II. The gonococci adhere selectively to the mucus-secreting nonciliated cells of the Fallopian tube and are gradually enfolded by pseudopodes and engulfed by the host epithelial cells. Gonococci appear to be able to multiply and divide intracellular. Once inside the epithelial cell

gonococci are immune to antibody complement or neutrophil attack. By pinocytosis the gonococci are transported from the mucosal surface to the subepithelial space. Gonococci produce extracellular products that might damage host cells including enzymes but are not considered to be a true protein toxin. Tissue damage appears to be due to two structural components on the gonorrhea cell surface, the peptidoglycan and the lipid A protein on the lypopolysaccharide component. Carney & Taylor-Robinson in 1983 have shown by utilizing human tube organ cultures that as gonococci reach the endosalpinx they become attached to mucosal epithelial cells, penetrate them and cause cell destruction. Although gonococci do not attach to Fallopian tube ciliated cells, diminished beating of cilia was evident hours after infection as observed and described by Gregy et al (1980) and McGee et al (1981). This effect is probably due to membrane blebs containing lipid A which are released from gonococci attached to the nonciliated cells. Progressive mucosal cell damage and submucosal invasion are accompanied by submucosal micro-abscess formation and exudate of purulent material. Leukocytic polymorphonuclear response is replaced later, if untreated, by infiltrates of mononuclear and abnormal round cells.

Clinical gonorrhea has a multiple presentation, including asymptomatic and symptomatic local infection, local complicated infection and systemic dissemination. Ascending genital infection, salpingitis, ectopic pregnancies, epididymitis, infertility and bacteremic dissemination are relatively common and account for most of the serious morbidity due to gonorrhea. In gonococcal salpingitis the usual route of infection is thought to be direct cannalicular spread of the organism from the endocervix along the endometrial surface to the tubal mucosa leading to endosalpingitis. Factors that determine whether the gonococci are localized in the endocervix or gain access to the uterus and tubes are unknown. It has been postulated that the gonococci either migrate into the Fallopian tubes or are carried there with either refluxed menstrual blood or via sperm attachment.

In men the most common local complication of gonococcal urethritis is epididymitis. In 1941

Pelouze reported that with a history of gonococcal urethritis, 10.5% of patients had a history of involuntary infertility. With unilateral and bilateral epididymitis he reported 23% and 42% incidences of infertility respectively.

### Chlamydia trachomatis

Chlamydiae are obligate intracellular bacteria which parasitize the host cell for nutrients and energy. They lack the ability to synthesize high energy compounds, hence they depend on the host cell to supply them with ATP and necessary nutrients. They lack a system for electron transport, have no cytochromes and cannot synthesize ATP and GTP. The growth cycle initially involves attachment and penetration into susceptible host cells. The chlamydiae undergo a complex and unique developmental cycle with two main structures: a small one (300 nm in diameter) named elementary body (EB) which is the infectious particle and a larger (1000 nm in diameter) named reticulate body (RB) which is engaged in intracellular multiplication. The EB is relatively resistant to the extracellular environment but is not metabolically active and is responsible for cell-to-cell and host-to-host transmission. The initial contact of the chlamydial EB with the susceptible host cell may involve a specific receptor site, but no such structures have clearly been identified. Once attached, the EB are rapidly internalized by the host cells. Penetration of chlamydia into the host cell involves an enhanced phagocytic process which is induced by the chlamydiae. The chlamydial particle enters the cell within a phagosome and stays within that phagosome throughout its entire life cycle but phagolysosomal fusion does not occur probably due to an EB surface antigen as suggested by Eissenberg et al (1983). Approximately 8 h after entry into the cell the EB changes into an RB. The RBs are not stable outside the host cell. They are the reproductive and metabolically active form of the chlamydiae. RBs contain three times more RNA than DNA, in contrast to EBs which contain equal amounts of RNA and DNA. The number of ribosomes in the RBs is much higher than in the EBs. The RB cell envelope resembles that of the EB in that it consists of an inner cytoplasmic membrane and an outer membrane that contains a major outer protein (MOMP) similar to that of Gram-negative bacteria. The importance of the MOMP in the infectious process was indicated by Caldwell & Perry (1982), as they were able to neutralize *C. trachomatis* infectivity in vitro with antibodies to MOMP. The MOMP of *C. trachomatis* contains species, subspecies and perhaps type-specific antigenic domains. The RBs take up ATP and required nutrient. They divide by binary fusion for approximately 24 h. About that time some of the RBs become EBs by a condensation process which is not clearly understood, while others continue to divide. During the replication of the RBs there is budding and blabbing of the outer membrane. This entire cycle takes place within the phagosome which undergoes a large increase in size. The mature inclusion contains hundreds to thousands of elementary bodies (EBs) and the entire cytoplasm of the cell may be displaced by the inclusion. Glycogen accumulates within the inclusions reaching levels detectable by iodine stain 30–48 h post infection. At some time between 48 and 72 h post infection lysosomal enzyme activity is noted and the cell ruptures releasing the infectious EBs to start a new cycle. Phagolysosomal fusion does not occur until the death of the cell is imminent. The EBs might be toxic if many particles are ingested by the host cell but chlamydia does not produce an extracellular toxin.

*C. trachomatis* isolates of human origin are classified into 15 serotypes. Types D through K are associated mainly with sexually transmitted infections and types L1, L2 and L3 with lymphogranuloma venereum (LGV), which will not be discussed in this chapter since it is not known to cause infertility. Non-LGV *C. trachomatis* strains have a very limited tissue host range in vivo. They appear to be almost exclusively parasites of squamocolumnar epithelial cells. Because they are obligate intracellular parasites and kill host cells at the end stages of their growth cycle, they must cause some cell damage where they persist.

The disease process and clinical manifestations of chlamydial infections probably represent the combined effect of tissue damage resulting from chlamydial replication as well as inflammatory responses caused by the presence of chlamydiae and necrotic material from the destroyed host cells. There is now evidence that chlamydial diseases result in part from hypersensitivity or are diseases of immunopathology. There must be some sort of protective immune response to the organisms since chlamydial infections tend to follow a fairly self-limited acute course resolving into a low-grade persistent infection which may last for years. These infections may be activated by a variety of stimuli. In animals and other in vitro models chlamydial infections induce lymphokines such as tumor necrosis factor (TNF) in macrophages as shown by Manor & Sarov (1988). Those lymphokines may play a role in controlling the infection and may also contribute to pathological consequences. Lymphokines have been shown by Holtman et al (1990) to have inhibitory effect on chlamydia. Furthermore, *C. trachomatis* is sensitive to alpha, beta and gamma interferons. Shemer & Sarov (1988) have demonstrated that gamma interferon delays the chlamydial developmental cycle so that the RBs persist longer. This may result in persistent inapparent infection and may also play a role in immunopathogenesis. Lymphokines can induce collagen deposition, collagenase production and fibroblast proliferation, and it is possible that they are involved in the development of scarring.

Patton et al (1982, 1983, 1987) in several studies on animal models of chlamydia salpingitis induced by genital serovars have shown that after 1 year following a single infection only a self-limited tubal inflammation with little residual damage was demonstrated. However, repeated tubal infections produced extensive tubal scarring, chronic salpingitis, distal obstruction and moderate to severe peritubal adhesions. From the animal models and from case reports, such as Moller et al (1979), one can conclude that *C. trachomatis* infection causes tubal dysfunction probably by destroying the ciliated and secretory mucosa of the distal Fallopian tube. The similarity of damage seen in the experimental models and in women with tubal infertility which had positive chlamydial serology supports this conclusion. Studies by Aurbiot et al (1984) and Patton et al (1989) have suggested that chlamydia

salpingitis causes not only deciliation but also persistent dyskinesia. Ciliary dyskinesia may be a contributing factor to persistent infertility even after reestablishment of a patent tubal lumen. A common pathological end point of chlamydial infection is scarring of the affected mucus membranes which probably leads to infertility and ectopic pregnancies after acute, overt or silent salpingitis.

*C. trachomatis* is currently acknowledged as being one of the most common sexually transmitted pathogens. The final type of damage to the genital tract by this organism closely resembles that due to *N. gonorrhoeae*. *C. trachomatis* is responsible for a significant proportion of nongonococcal urethritis and acute epididymitis in men. It is found in association with cervicitis, endometritis and salpingitis in women. Mardh et al (1977) isolated *C. trachomatis* directly from the Fallopian tubes of women with acute salpingitis. Subsequently, Henry-Suchet et al (1980, 1987) based on Fallopian tube cultures suggested that *C. trachomatis* is associated with tubal infertility. They found *C. trachomatis* among 30% of patients with infertility due to tubal obstruction using direct Fallopian tubes' and peritoneal cultures, while in only 19% they found positive cervical cultures. Recently Soong et al (1990), using a DNA hybridization technique in endocervical cells, have demonstrated a 49% recovery rate of chlamydial DNA among infertile patients with tubal infertility in comparison to 13.4% and 12% in nontubal infertility and pregnant women respectively. Many studies based on chlamydial serology (Punnonen et al 1979, Jones et al 1982, Conway et al 1984) have all demonstrated a high prevalence rate of antichlamydial antibodies in infertility due to tubal disease. Likewise, an association between serological evidence of chlamydial infection and ectopic pregnancy has been observed by many authors (Gump et al 1983, Svensson et al 1985, Hartford et al 1987). From these data one can conclude that chlamydial salpingitis may have a variety of clinical consequences, ranging from absolute infertility with bilateral oviductal obstruction to relative tubal infertility with ectopic pregnancy. Sweet et al (1983) have demonstrated that *C. trachomatis* can persist in the endometrial cavity following therapy for acute salpingitis despite an apparent clinical cure. Such stubborn chlamydial infection could result in relapse and chronic infection. Furthermore, Cleary & Jones (1985) found positive chlamydial endometrial cultures in 26% of infertile women with serum antichlamydial antibodies. These data are of special interest since modern reproductive medicine offers to many of those infertile patients in vitro fertilization and intrauterine embryo transfer (IVF-ET).

Since the introduction of IVF several studies (Rowland et al 1985, Torode et al 1987, Lunenfeld et al 1989, Osser et al 1990) have emerged, which try to evaluate the role of chlamydia on IVF-ET success rate. Despite the fact that antichlamydial antibodies are present in follicular fluid as shown by Lunenfeld et al (1990), none of the studies have shown any effect of those antibodies on fertilization rates. While Rowland et al (1985) demonstrated that in IVF-ET programs the pregnancy rates among patients who were seropositive chlamydia-specific IgG were halved compared to chlamydia-specific IgG seronegative women. Torode et al (1987) and Osser et al (1990) could not confirm these results. On the other hand, Lunenfeld et al (1989) have demonstrated that the take-home baby rate among patients who conceived in an IVF-ET program is much higher if they are found to be

antichlamydial seronegative (Table 27.1). Further well-designed studies including endometrial biopsies for chlamydial isolation and or chlamydial DNA hybridization are needed to pursue the role of chlamydia on IVF-ET pregnancy outcome.

The relative role of chlamydial genital tract infection in the etiology of male infertility is less clear compared with female infertility. In vitro studies by Wolner-Hanssen & Mardh (1984) have demonstrated that C. trachomatis is able to adhere to human spermatozoa but there is little information on the influence of this microorganism on semen quality. Close et al (1987) demonstrated that positive chlamydial serology was associated with the presence of sperm agglutinating antibodies in serum and suggested that chlamydial genital inflammation may activate an autoimmune response to sperm.

Although Stortz et al (1960) have shown that *Chlamydia psittaci* is involved in bovine abortion, there has been little documentation of the role of chlamydial infection in spontaneous clinical abortions. Quinn et al (1987) have demonstrated an increased prevalence of detectable chlamydial antibody in patients with a history of recurrent abortion compared to normal fertile couples. In our study (Lunenfeld et al 1989) on IVF patients we were impressed with the high prevalence rate of positive chlamydial serology among patients

**Table 27.1** The association between chlamydial-specific IgG and IVF

| | Outcome | Seropositive (%) | Seronegative (%) |
|---|---|---|---|
| Prevalence of chlamydial IgG among 52 women receiving three embryos after IVF-ET (Rowland et al 1985) | Pregnant<br>Not pregnant | 6(30)<br>21(65.6) | 14(70)<br>11(34.4) |
| Prevalence of chlamydial IgG among 159 women undergoing IVF-ET (Torode et al 1987) | Pregnant<br>Not pregnant | 11(52)<br>62(45) | 10(48)<br>76(55) |
| Prevalence of chlamydial IgG by various outcomes of IVF-ET (Lunenfeld et al 1989) | Term pregnancies<br>Spontaneous abortions<br>Ectopic pregnancies<br>Chemical pregnancies<br>Not pregnant | 14(29)<br>15(56)<br>4(66)<br>17(71)<br>52(55) | 35(71)<br>12(44)<br>2(34)<br>7(29)<br>42(45) |
| Prevalence of chlamydial IgG among 121 women undergoing IVF-ET | Pregnant<br>Not pregnant | 23(72)<br>67(75) | 9(28)<br>22(25) |
| Prevalence of chlamydial IgG by various outcomes of IVF-ET (Osser et al 1990) | Term pregnancies<br>Spontaneous abortions<br>Ectopic pregnancies | 15(80)<br>6(66)<br>2(66) | 5(20)<br>3(34)<br>1(34) |

with chemical pregnancies compared to other pregnancy outcome in IVF-ET.

## GENITAL MYCOPLASMAS

The mycoplasma fall somewhere between bacteria and viruses. They differ from bacteria in that they have no cell wall but are surrounded by a triple-layered membrane. They differ from viruses because they contain both DNA and RNA and because they can grow and replicate on cell-free medium. Two species can frequently be isolated from the human genital tract: *Mycoplasma hominis* and *Ureaplasma urealyticum* (T mycoplasmas). Studies on both *M. hominis* and *U. urealyticum* have resulted in the identification of multiple serotypes; at least eight for *M. hominis* and 14 for *U. urealyticum*. Growth of the genital tract mycoplasma in broth medium can be detected by the use of their metabolic activity. *M. hominis* metabolizes arginine to ammonia while *U. urealyticum* metabolizes urea to ammonia.

Fraser & Taylor-Robinson (1977) and Taylor-Robinson et al (1975) have shown in rodents that intraperitoneal or intravenous infection or exposure of murine sperm to mycoplasma species will cause reproductive failure. Many species of mycoplasma stimulate lymphocytes to undergo blast formation. The immunopathological consequences of this stimulation are not known but an inflammatory tissue response with resultant tissue damage is a possibility. Experimental infections of grivet monkeys with *M. hominis* (Moller et al 1978), have shown that the organism spreads from lesions along the cervical and endometrial epithelium via lymphatics and blood vessels to the parametria and then to the Fallopian tube. Biopsy specimens of affected tubes have shown congestion and lymphoid infiltration of the mucosa. Mardh et al (1976) have observed that *M. hominis* caused clubbing, swelling of cilia and slowing of the mucociliary wave activity in tissue cultures of human Fallopian tube epithelium. Ureaplasma have been shown by Stalheim et al (1976, 1977) to cause marked ciliostasis in cultures of bovine oviduct which could be enhanced by the addition of ammonia to the cultures, which suggests means by which these organisms might cause the insult. In contrast (Taylor-Robinson & Carney 1974),

showed that although various strains of mycoplasma were capable of growing in human Fallopian tube organ cultures, they did not produce any demonstrable tissue damage.

*M. hominis* and *U. urealyticum* have been suggested to be associated with PID and infertility. However, mycoplasmas are part of the normal genital tract flora of many sexually active men and women who have no obvious clinical disease or abnormalities. Thus any pathogenic role of the genital mycoplasmas must be evaluated with this epidemiological background in mind. Sweet (1986) recovered from the endometrium of patients with acute PID *M. hominis* and *U. urealyticum* in 39% and 15% respectively. Furthermore, the same investigators demonstrated a coexistence of pathogens in the endometrial cavity of women with acute salpingitis. Of the patients with *N. gonorrhoeae* isolation, *C. trachomatis* was present in 42% and genital mycoplasmas in 58%. For patients with *C. trachomatis* 50% had concomitant *N. gonorrhoeae* and 80% had genital mycoplasmas. These investigators (Sweet et al 1981) noted that *U. urealyticum* was recovered from the Fallopian tubes only from patients with initial or recurrent episodes of PID who had been symptomatic for more than 72 h. This may suggest that ureaplasmas are secondary invaders.

Contradiction exists concerning epidemiological data when trying to associate the prevalence of genital *M. hominis* and *U. urealyticum* and infertility (Table 27.2). The first to postulate that mycoplasmas are etiological factors in infertility were Gnarpe & Friberg in 1972. They cultivated these microorganism in a significantly higher percentage from both unexplained infertile women and men (91% and 85% respectively) compared to fertile pregnant couples (23% and 26% respectively). Upandhyaya et al (1983) in a Welsh study found a highly significant difference in the distribution of ureaplasma between infertile and pregnant women, whereas Gump et al (1984) could find no causal relationship between genital mycoplasma and ureaplasma and either infertility or subsequent pregnancy. Definitive conclusion about the significance of cervical colonization cannot therefore be drawn. Henry-Suchet et al (1980) reported the recovery of *U. urealyticum*

**Table 27.2**  Infertility and *U. urealyticum*

| Author | Sample Size | Source of Culture | Isolation Rates(%) | | *P* |
|---|---|---|---|---|---|
| | | | Infertile women | Fertile women | |
| Idress et al 1978 | 40 | Cervix | 55 | 32 | 0.03 |
| Gnarpe & Friberg 1972 | 55 | Cervix | 92 | 22 | 0.001 |
| Stray-Pederson et al 1978 | 64 | Endometrium | 26–50 | 7–8 | 0.0001 |
| Koren & Spigland 1978 | 59 | Endometrium | 27 | 6 | 0.01 |
| Cassel et al 1983b | 193 | Endometrium | 1 | 0 | NS |
| | | Cervix | 40 | 35 | NS |
| Henry-Suchet et al 1980 | 46 | Peritoneal cavity and/or Fallopian tube | 15 | NS | NS |

Adapted with permission from Sweet 1986.
NS, not significant.

from the peritoneum and/or Fallopian tube from 23% of patients with infertility and tubal obstruction who had mild inflammation and from 10% of patients with infertility and tubal obstruction but no inflammation. On the other hand, Cassel et al (1983b) recovered *U. urealyticum* and *M. hominis* from the endometrial cavity in only a small number of infertile patients undergoing laparoscopy. In that study they noted that *M. hominis* was more frequently recovered from the cervicovaginal specimens of patients undergoing tubal reanastomosis than from other infertility patients. There was no statistically significant difference in *U. urealyticum* recovery from cervicovaginal specimens among the infertile patients and control groups. Moller et al (1985) have demonstrated that antibodies to *M. hominis* occurred three times more often in women with tubal infertility than in other infertile women (36% versus 11%). There is a fairly high correlation between positive vaginal or cervical *M. hominis* and *U. urealyticum* cultures and the presence of these organisms in the male partners. Cassel et al (1983a) categorized a large group of infertile patients according to their infertility diagnosis and found a significant increase in the frequency of cervically isolated ureaplasma among the male factor group compared to the other infertility diagnosis.

In men there is substantial evidence for documenting the capacity of *U. urealyticum* to cause acute nongonococcal urethritis, however evidence for residual disease after clearance of the acute episode is scanty. The same is also true for

ureaplasma chronic prostatitis. As far as we know ureaplasma-induced epididymitis has not been reported. Ureaplasma are frequently a part of the urethral flora of males and are known to infect and attach to spermatozoa, as shown by Fowlkers et al (1975a) using electron microscopy. However, Taylor-Robinson (1986) has shown that in 33 men with ureaplasma and six with *M. hominis* in their semen none had these organisms isolated from their vas deferens, supporting the concept that sperm are infected with genital mycoplasmas as they pass through the urethra during ejaculation. Witkin & Toth (1983) have found antisperm antibodies in semen of ureaplasma carriers more often than in men who were culture negative. Thus the presence of these organisms might induce autoimmune infertility. As with cervicovaginal colonization with genital mycoplasma and female infertility, contradictory results exist concerning the effect of ureaplasma on semen parameters. While some authors (Fowlkers et al 1975b, O'Leary & Frick 1975, Toth et al 1978) have shown that in some cases ureaplasmas can affect semen parameters, others (Cintron et al 1981, Upandhyaya et al 1984) have been unable to correlate the presence of ureaplasmas with any alteration in semen characteristics. Furthermore, Cintron et al (1981) and Eggert-Kruse et al (1987) found that the presence of genital mycoplasma in the cervical mucus or in the semen fails to inhibit sperm penetration through the cervical mucus. Recently Talkington et al (1991) have investigated the in vitro effect of three serotypes of *U. urealyticum* (4, 1 and 11) on spermatozoal motility and on penetration of polyacrylamide gels. Their results indicated that at least in the in vitro system these three ureaplasma serotypes had no detrimental effects on spermatozoal motility or penetration ability. In 1985 Busolo & Zanchetta reported that exposure of test sperm samples to *M. hominis* resulted in a diminished hamster ovum penetration rate. The same was also true for *U. urealyticum* serotype 4, while serotype 1 gave penetration rates similar to controls. Preincubation of sperm with the supernatant from ureaplasma cultures decreased the penetration rate. This effect could be reversed by heating the supernatant before sperm exposure.

Since the data concerning the association between genital mycoplasmas and infertility have been controversial, attempts at treatment were being undertaken in order to improve fertility. Toth et al (1983) using doxycycline successfully eradicated ureaplasmas from 129 infertile couples. The 3-year conception rate was 60%, compared with only 5% for 32% of infertile couples in whom ureaplasmas could not be eliminated. Busolo et al (1984) reported that conception had occurred in five of 19 treated patients in whom ureaplasma was eradicated, in contrast to nonconception among 29 couples in whom ureaplasma persisted after treatment. In contrast, Upandhyaya et al (1983) reported that pregnancy rates were the same whether or not ureaplasmas were eradicated. Harrison et al (1975) assigned infertile couples to doxycycline, placebo and nontreatment groups with about equal numbers of culture-positive and culture-negative individuals in each group. During a 6-month period there was no significant difference in the pregnancy rate among the three groups. Hinton et al (1979) on the other hand performed a randomized double-blind crossover study and found a significant increase in pregnancies after treatment with doxycycline. Unfortunately the contradictory results concerning genital mycoplasmas, antibiotic therapy and fertility results only add to the yet unsolved enigma of genital mycoplasma and infertility. Foulon et al (1986) found ureaplasmas more often in endocervical specimens from women with a history of spontaneous abortion, especially recurrent spontaneous abortion, compared to a control group of women. Munday et al (1984) and Harrison (1986) have found no relation between lower genital tract colonization with ureaplasma and fetal loss.

## CONCLUSIONS

When considering the female partner there is no question about the role of *N. gonorrhoeae* and *C. trachomatis* in causing either acute or silent salpingitis and consequently tubal damage, ectopic pregnancies and infertility. The role of genital tract mycoplasma in female infertility remains unclear. As for the male partner the role of genital tract infection by sexually transmitted pathogens in the etiology of male infertility except for obstruction of the male epididymis or vas deference is less clear. It is interesting to note that although most authors agree that the presence of serum chlamydial antibodies or the presence of genital mycoplasma does not usually affect semen characteristics, both were suggested as being associated with the presence of sperm agglutinating antibodies in serum.

As we have already stated at the beginning of this chapter, prevention of STD is the most effective way of preventing damage which results in reduced natural fertility potential. Due to the life-threatening consequences of AIDS public awareness to the prevention of STD has recently increased. Furthermore, screening programs and very motivated health personnel are needed for early detection of sexually transmitted reservoirs. Once detected, vigorous and appropriate treatment and follow up for all sexually involved partners is necessary in order to reduce possible damage. Once damage has occurred it is important to properly diagnose it and to be aware that it is STD related. This understanding is important, since in some instances the sexually transmitted pathogens are still present in the genital tract and might cause further damage which will reduce fertility potential, as implied for *C. trachomatis* by Moss & Steptoe in 1983. Studies using modern techniques such as polymerase chain reaction (PCR) for the detection of sexually transmitted pathogens and refining the diagnosis of genital mycoplasma by serotyping these microorganisms might increase our understanding of the role of

STD on fertility potential and might enable us to try specific therapy to increase the chances of an

STD-associated infertile couple conceiving and bringing home a healthy baby.

## REFERENCES

Aurbiot J B, Dubuisson A, Eyquem A, Schwartz J, Vacher-Lavenu M C 1984 Etude de l'activite ciliare des cellules de la trompe de fallope (a propos de sequelles de salpingite). J Gynecol Obstet Biol Reprod 13: 617

Berger R E, Alexander E R, Haruish J P et al 1979 Etiology, manifestation and therapy of acute epididymitis: prospective study of 50 cases. J Urol 121: 750

Busolo F, Zanchetta R 1985 The effect of *Mycoplasma hominis* and *Ureaplasma urealyticum* on hamster egg in vitro penetration by human spermatozoa. Fertil Steril 43: 110

Busolo F, Zancheta R, Lanzone E, Cusinato R, 1984 Microbial flora in semen of asymptomatic infertile men. Andrologia 16: 269

Caldwell H D, Perry L J 1982 Neutralization of *Chlamydia trachomatis* with antibodies to the major outer membrane protein. Infect Immunol 38: 745

Carney F F, Taylor-Robinson D 1983 Growth and effect of *Neisseria gonorrhoeae* in organ cultures. Br J Venereol Dis 49: 435

Cassel G H, Brown M B, Young J B 1983a Incidence of genital mycoplasmas in women at the time of diagnostic laparoscopy. Yale J Biol Med 56: 557

Cassel G H, Young J B, Brown M B et al 1983b Microbiologic study of infertile women at the time of diagnostic laparoscopy. N Engl J Med 308: 502

Cintron R D, Wortham J W E, Acosta A 1981 The association of semen factors with the recovery of *Ureaplasma urealyticum*. Fertil Steril 36: 648

Cleary R E, Jones R B 1985 Recovery of *Chlamydia trachomatis* from the endometrium in infertile women with serum antichlamydial antibodies. Fertil Steril 44: 233

Close C E, Wand S P, Roberts P L, Berger R E 1987 The relationship of infection with *Chlamydia trachomatis* to the parameters of male fertility and sperm autoimmunity. Fertil Steril 48: 880

Conway D, Glazener C M A, Caul E O et al 1984 Chlamydial serology in fertile and infertile women. Lancet i: 191

Eggert-Kruse W, Gerhard I, Hofmann H, Runnebaum B, Petzoldt D 1987 Influence of microbial colonization on sperm–mucus interaction in in vivo and in vitro. Humm Reprod 2: 301

Eissenberg L G, Wyrick P B, David C H, Rumpp J W 1983 *Chlamydia psittaci* elementary body envelopes: ingestion and inhibition of phagolysosome fusion. Infect Immunol 40: 741

Fowler J E 1984 Genital tract infection and male infertility. In: Gracia C R, Mastroianni L Jr, Amella R D, Dubin L (eds) Current therapy of infertility 1984–1985. Decker, Philadelphia, pp 173–179

Fowlkers D M, Dooher G B, O'Leary W M 1975a Evidence by scanning electron microscopy for an association between spermatozoa and T-mycoplasma in men of infertile marriage. Fertil Steril 26: 1203

Fowlkers D M, MacLeod J, O'Leary W M 1975b T-mycoplasmas and human infertility: correlation of infection with alterations in seminal parameters. Fertil Steril 26: 1212

Fraser L R, Taylor-Robinson D 1977 The effect of

*Mycoplasma pulmonis* on fertilization and preimplantation development in vitro of mouse eggs. Fertil Steril 28: 488

Foulon W 1986 Epidemiology and pathogenesis of *Ureaplasma urealyticum* in spontaneous abortion and early premature labor. Pediatr Infect Dis 5: S353

Gartman E 1961 Epididymis: a reappraisal. Am J Surg 101: 736

Gnarpe H, Friberg J 1972 Mycoplasma and human reproductive failure. Am J Obstet Gynecol 114: 727

Gregy C R, Mebly M A, McGee Z A 1980 Gonococcal lipopolysacharide A toxin for human fallopian tube muccosa. Am J Obstet Gynecol 138: 981

Gump D W, Gibson M, Ashikaga T 1983 Evidence of prior pelvic inflammatory disease and its relationship to *Chlamydia trachomatis* antibody and intrauterine contraceptive device use in infertile women. Am J Obstet Gynecol 146: 153

Gump D W, Gibson M, Ashikaga T 1984 Lack of association between genital mycoplasma and infertility. N Engl J Med 310: 937

Harrison H R 1986 Cervical colonization with *Ureaplasma urealyticum* and pregnancy outcome: prospective studies Pediatr Infect Dis 5: S266

Harrison R F, Blades M, deLouvois J, Hurley R 1975 Doxyline treatment and human infertility. Lancet i: 605

Hartford S L, Silva P D, diZerega G S, Yonekura M L 1987 Serologic evidence of prior chlamydial infection in patients with tubal ectopic pregnancy and contralateral tubal disease. Fertil Steril 47: 118

Henry-Suchet J, Loffredo V, Serfaty D 1980 *Chlamydia trachomatis* and *mycoplasma* research by laparoscopy in cases of pelvic inflammatory disease and in cases of tubal obstruction. Am J Obstet Gynecol 138: 1022

Henry-Suchet J, Ultzmann C, DeBrux J, Ardoin P, Catalan F 1987 Microbiologic study of chronic inflammation associated with tubal factor infertility: role of *Chlamydia trachomatis*. Fertil Steril 47: 274

Hinton R A, Egdell L M, Andrews B E, Clarke S K R, Richmond S J 1979 A double blind cross over study of the effect of doxycicline on mycoplasma infection and infertility. Br J Obstet Gynaecol 86: 379

Holtmann H, Shemer-Avni Y, Wessel K, Sarov I, Wallach D 1990 Inhibition of growth of *Chlamydia trachomatis* by Tumor Necrosis Factor is accompanied by increased prostoglandin synthesis. Infect Immunol 58: 1017

Idress W M, Patton W C, Taymor M L 1978 On the etiologic role of *Ureaplasma urealyticum* infection in infertility. Fertil Steril 30: 293

Jones R B, Ardery B R, Hui S L, Cleary R E 1982 Correlation between serum antichlamydial antibodies and tubal factor as cause of infertility. Fertil Steril 38: 553

Koren Z, Spigland I 1978 Irrigation technique for detection of mycoplasma intrauterine infection in infertile patients. Obstet Gynecol 52: 588

Ludwig V G, Haselberger J 1977 Epididymitis und fertilität: behandlungsergebnisse bei akuter anspezifischer epididymitis. Fortschr Med 05: 397

Lunenfeld E, Shapiro B S, Sarov B, Sarov I, Insler V,

Decherney A H 1989 The association between chlamydial specific IgG and IgA antibodies and pregnancy outcome in an in vitro fertilization program. J In Vitro Fert Embryo Trans 6: 222

Lunenfeld E, Sarov B, Sarov I et al 1990 Chlamydial IgG and IgA in serum and follicular fluid among patients undergoing in vitro fertilisation. Eur J Obstet Gynecol Reprod Biol 37: 163

McGee Z A et al 1981 Pathogenic mechanism of Neisseria gonorrhoeae: observations on damage to human fallopian tubes in organ culture by gonococci of colony type 1 or type 4. J Infect Dis 143: 413

Manor E, Sarov I 1988 Inhibition of Chlamydia trachomatis replication in HEp-2 cells by human monocyte-derived macrophages. Infect Immunol 56: 3280

Mardh P A, Westrom L, von Mecklenburg C et al 1976 Studies on ciliated epithelia on the human genital tract. Br J Vener Dis 52: 52

Mardh P A, Ripa T, Svensson L, Westrom L 1977 Chlamydia trachomatis infection in patients with acute salpingitis. N Engl J Med 296: 1377

Mardh P A, Lind I, Svensson L, Westorm I, Moller B R 1981 Antibodies to Chlamydia trachomatis, Mycoplasma hominis and Neisseria gonorrhoeae in serum from patients with acute salpingitis. Br J Vener Dis 57: 125

Moller B R, Freundt E A, Black F T, Fredriksen P 1978 Experimental infection of the genital tract of female grivet monkeys by Mycoplasma hominis. Infect Immunol 20: 248

Moller B R, Westrom L, Ahrons S et al 1979 Chlamydia trachomatis infection of the fallopian tubes. Histological findings in two patients. Br J Vener Dis 55: 422

Moller B R, Taylor-Robinson D, Furr P M, Toft B, Allen J 1985 Serological evidence that chlamydiae and mycoplasmas are involved in infertility in women. J Reprod Fertil 73: 237

Moss T R, Steptoe P C 1984 Chlamydia trachomatis: importance in in vitro fertilisation. J R Soc Med 77: 70

Munday P E, Porter R, Falder P F et al 1984 Spontaneous abortion—an infectious etiology? Br J Obstet Gynecol 91: 1177

Nahoum C R D 1982 Inflamation and infection. In: Bain J, Schill W B, Schwarzstein L (eds) Treatment of male infertility. Springer-Verlag, Berlin, pp 5–32

Newhall W J, Sawyer W D, Heak R A 1980 Cross-linking analysis of the outer membrane proteins of Neisseria gonorrhoeae. Infect Immunol 28: 785

Nilsson S, Obrant K O, Persson P S 1968 Changes in the testis parenchyma caused by acute non specific epididymitis. Fertil Steril 19: 748

O' Leary W M, Frick J 1975 The correlation of human male infertility with the presence of mycoplasma T strains. Andrologia 7: 309

Osser S, Persson K, Wramsby H, Liedholm P 1990 Does previous Chlamydia trachomatis infection influence the pregnancy rate of in vitro fertilization and embryo replacement? Am J Obstet Gynecol 162: 40

Patton D L, Halbert S A, Wang S P 1982 Experimental salpingitis in rabbits provoked by Chlamydia trachomatis. Fertil Steril 37: 691

Patton D L, Halbert S A, Kuo C O, Wang S P, Holmes K K 1983 Host response to primary Chlamydia trachomatis infection of the fallopian tube in pig tailed monkeys. Fertil Steril 40: 829

Patton D L, Kuo C C, Wang S P, Halbert S A 1987 Distal tubal obstruction induced by repeated Chlamydia trachomatis salpingeal infections in pig tailed macaques. J Infect Dis 55: 1292

Patton D L, Moore D E, Spadoni L R, Soules M R, Halbert S A, Wang S P 1989 A comparison of the fallopian tube's response to overt and silent salpingitis. Obstet Gynecol 73: 622

Pearce W A, Buchanan T M 1978 Attachment role of gonococcal pili: optimum conditions and quantitation of adherance of isolated pili to human cells in vitro. J Clin Invest 61: 931

Pelouze P S 1941 Epididymitis in gonorrhea in the male and female. Saunders, Philadelphia

Punnonen R, Terho P, Nikkanen V, Meurman D 1979 Chlamydial serology in infertile women by immunofluorescence. Fertil Steril 31: 656

Quinn P A, Petric M, Barkin M et al 1987 Prevalence of antibody to Chlamydia trachomatis in spontaneous abortion and infertility. Am J Obstet Gynecol 156: 291

Rosenfeld D L, Seidman S M, Bronson R A, Scholl G M 1983 Unsuspected chronic pelvic inflammatory disease in the infertile female. Fertil Steril 39: 44

Rowland G F, Forsey T, Moss T R, Steptoe P C, Hewitt J, Darougar S 1985 Failure of in vitro fertilization and embryo replacement following infection with Chlamydia trachomatis. J In Vitro Fertil Embryo Transfer 2: 151

Shemer Y, Sarov I 1988 Inhibition of growth of Chlamydia trachomatis by human gamma interferon. Infect Immunol 48: 592

Soong Y K, Kao S M, Lee C J, Lee P S, Pao C C 1990 Endocervical chlamydial deoxyribonucleic acid in infertile women. Fertil Steril 54: 815

Stalheim O H U, Proctor S J, Gallagher J E 1976 Growth and effects of ureaplasmas (T-Mycoplasmas) in bovine oviductul cultures. Infect Immunol 13: 915

Stalheim O H U, Gallagher J E 1977 Ureaplasmal epithelial lesions related to ammonia. Infect Immunol 15: 995

Storz J, McKercher D, Horwath J A et al 1960 The isolation of a viral agent from an episodic bovine abortion. Am Vet Med Assoc J 137: 509

Stray-Pederson B, Eng J, Reikvam T M 1978 Uterine T-mycoplasma colonization in reproductive failure. Am J Obstet Gynecol 130: 307

Svensson L, Mardh P A, Ahlgren M, Nordenskjold F 1985 Ectopic pregnancy and antibodies to Chlamydia trachomatis. Fertil Steril 44: 313

Sweet R L 1986 Colonization of the endometrium and fallopian tubes with Ureaplasma urealyticum. Pediatr Infect Dis 5: S214

Sweet R L, Draper D L, Hadley W K 1981 Etiology of acute salpingitis: influence of episode number and duration of symptoms. Obstet Gynecol 58: 62

Sweet R L, Robbie M O, Schachter J 1983 Failure of beta-lactam antibiotics to eradicate Chlamydia trachomatis from the endometrium of patients with acute salpingitis despite prompt clinical response. JAMA 250: 2641

Talkington D F, Davis J K, Canupp K C et al 1991 The effects of three serotypes of Ureaplasma urealyticum on spermatozoal motility and penetration in vitro. Fertil Steril 55: 170

Taylor-Robinson D 1986 Evaluation of the role of Ureaplasma urealyticum in infertility. Pediatr Infect Dis 5: S262

Taylor-Robinson D, Carney F E 1974 Growth and effect of mycoplasmas in fallopian tube organ cultures. Br J Vener Dis 50: 212

Taylor-Robinson D, Rassner C, Furr P M, Humber D P, Barness R D 1975 Fetal wastage as a consequence of *Mycoplasma pulmonis* infection in mice. J Reprod Fertil 42: 483

Torode H W, Wheeler P A, Saunders D M, McPetrie R A, Medcalf S C, Ackerman V P, 1987 The role of chlamydial antibodies in an in vitro fertilization program Fertil Steril 48: 987

Toth A, Swenson C E, O'Leary W M 1978 Light microscopy as an aid in predicting ureaplasma infection in human semen. Fertil Steril 30: 586

Toth A, Lesser M L, Brooks C, Labriola D 1983 Subsequent pregnancies among 161 couples treated for T-mycoplasma genital tract infection. N Engl J Med 308: 505

Upandhyaya M, Hibbard B M, Walker S M 1983 The role of mycoplasmas in reproduction. Fertil Steril 39: 814

Upandhyaya M, Hibbard B M, Walker S M 1984 The effect of *Ureaplasma urealyticum* on semen characteristics. Fertil Steril 41: 304

Westrom L 1980 Incidence, prevalence and trends of acute pelvic inflammatory disease and its consequences in industrialized countries. Am J Obstet Gynecol 138: 880

Westrom L 1987 Pelvic inflammatory disease: bacteriology and sequelae. Contraception 36: 111

Witkin S S, Toth A 1983 Relationship between genital tract infections, sperm antibodies in seminal fluid and infertility. Fertil Steril 40: 805

Wolin L H 1975 On the etiology of epididymitis. J Urol 105: 531

Wolner-Hanssen P, Mardh P A 1984 In vitro tests of the adherence of *Chlamydia trachomatis* to human spermatozoa. Fertil Steril 42: 102

# 28. Psychosomatic aspects of infertility

## M. Stauber   C. Brucker

Fertility is an existential necessity, and as such has assumed overwhelming importance to men and women in all times. Existence depended upon fertility of land and livestock, as well as upon human procreation. With time, social habits and religion influenced human perception of fertility or infertility.

Recently, the human outlook on fertility has been modified by the affluence of modern industrial nations; the intrinsic value of fertility is now relatively lessened. Additionally, modern conceptive and contraceptive methods have caused a segregation of sexuality and fertility — further devaluing fertility as a single factor in modern life.

While several decades ago there were relatively few couples who voluntarily wished no children, this phenomenon is now fairly common in some parts of the world. This is supported by the work of Johnson et al (1987), who found a significant increase in voluntary childlessness in the last 15 years — from 3.2% to 11% in the UK (Table 28.1).

It may be concluded that the modern couple does not have to define its existence by its offspring, at any cost.

Modern infertility studies should address themselves to the couple in a balanced fashion — and not to the woman as the central symbol, as overemphasized during the World Congress in Marrakesh (1989). The same studies should stress the psychosomatic aspects of the desire for procreation, which is too often lacking in recent fertility meetings.

## MOTIVATION OF THE DESIRE FOR A CHILD

The question as to the motivation for childbirth applies most intensively to couples who wish for children with no result. The answers to the question 'Why a child?' reflect the intense desire of these patients for a child — this desire may eclipse all other thoughts and aims.

As a rule, the desire for one's own child has no rational foundation. In our own experience, compliance with social standards plays a minor role, althogh it should be noted that parenthood is judged positively throughout society. Infertile patients may have difficulty in explaining the need for children. We received a letter from a patient stating 'to have children is a basic need just like hunger, sleep, and avoidance of pain'. A successful 30-year-old librarian noted 'I cannot

**Table 28.1** Involuntarily or voluntarily childless?

| Year of birth | m | Childless (%) | Voluntarily childless (%) | Involuntarily childless (%) | Result |
|---|---|---|---|---|---|
| 1935 | 533 | 7.7 | 3.2 | 4.5 | Significant increase in |
| 1950 | 617 | 14.3 | 11.0 | 3.3 | voluntary childlessness |

From Johnson et al 1987.

find rational reasons for my wish to have children. There is no plausible reason for it, it is just based on some feeling...'. Here, the wish for children is expressed as a basic need, to which an outsider might have difficulty relating. This often 'irrationally' unproportional wish for children becomes once again more understandable, if the formerly mentioned existential necessity of fertility is brought to mind.

Sigmund Freud has defined the wish for a child as an absolute criterion of female behavior. The girl recognizes the reality of not having a penis, envying the boy, and subsequently wishes for a child as a penile substitute. The child-wish is actually the admission of her own female gender. Therese Benedek points out that the monthly cycle of the female is a permanent reminder of procreation from a biological point of view. The female's behavior changes throughout the monthly cycle, a possible reflection of biological-hormonal forces. She describes behavior in the first phase of the cycle as being rather active, while throughout the second phase of the cycle, an introverted attitude is assumed, much as is typical for the time of pregnancy.

The more one thinks about the motivation behind procreation, the more the wish for a child appears to be deeply anchored within the basic character and basic biological function of the female. Primarily, therefore, one is tempted to define the wish for children as 'normal' and 'healthy'. An unfulfilled wish for children may lead to a respectively 'disproportionate ("unhealthy") wish' for children; an inappropriate reaction. External as well as internal motives are especially obvious. In such cases, one can find that a role is prospectively ascribed to the wished-for child. Drug-addicted females expect 'to make everything better' in their lives with their expected child, and with depressive patients one can sense some 'Messiah Expectancy' in their wish for procreation.

Until now, there have been few investigations concerning the male wish for procreation (Frick-Bruder & Schuett 1991). Münkel (1982) conducted a thorough investigation and showed that men wishing for children mostly have positive, sympathetic memories about their own childhood, that they have an ongoing good

**Table 28.2** Frustrated wish for children (after unsuccessful therapy): psychological inquiry ($n = 72$)

As compared to a control group, frustrated wish for children often leads to:
1. Increased functional problems,
2. Negative social resonance,
3. Depressed mood,
4. Conflicts of disturbed individual life perspective ('the biggest problem that has ever been encountered'),
5. Coping problems (partnership, isolation tendencies),
6. Defence efforts with negation and projection.

relationship with their parents, and that they show positive perspectives for the future in their descriptions. It was thus concluded that the wish for procreation in males is seen more in the context of satisfying experiences—as opposed to the male without the wish for procreation—and as opposed to the basic biological need as in the female.

## RESULTS FROM FOLLOW-UP STUDIES

Coping with an ultimately frustrated desire for children by couples is accompanied by great difficulties in many cases (Table 28.2). Schultz-Ruthenberg & Stauber (1980) noted that women from infertile marriages exhibited tendencies to narrowed self-awareness as compared to women who did not experience difficulties in their wish for procreation. An increase in psychosomatic symptoms in this group was found, such as abdominal pain, dysmenorrhea and disturbance of sexual function. Men from marriages with a frustrated wish for children also showed greater difficulties in coping and more functional sexual disturbances as compared to a control group.

On the other hand, fulfilment of the wish for children in couples that have been treated earlier (Becker 1980) does not necessarily resolve all problems. Evaluating 655 patients' histories, a far greater incidence of pregnancy-related complaints was found, which were interpreted primarily as psychosomatic. In addition, a higher abortion rate and a higher preterm delivery rate were noted, although the psychological component of these complications is difficult to analyse. (Table 28.3).

In a non-representative retrospective question-naire (15 years after unsuccessful infertility

**Table 28.3**  Finally fulfilled wish for children: $n = 655$ couples from the infertility clinic

As compared to a control group, pregnancy, delivery and postpartum period in former infertility patients were characterized by:
1. Five times higher frequency of hyperemesis gravidarum
2. Double rate of pregnancy-related complaints
3. Double abortion rate
4. Higher frequency of gestational hypertension, proteinuria and oedema
5. Double rate of vaginal surgical deliveries
6. Triple rate of caesarean sections
7. Lower frequency of breast feeding and shorter duration

Becker 1980

treatment) we noted that in some couples, former treatment for infertility was considered by them to be a wrong step in their lives (Stauber 1988). In individual cases, patients actually considered treatment to be negligent because the psychosomatic aspects of unvoluntary childlessness were not reviewed.

## PSYCHOSOMATIC COUNSELLING

Psychosomatic aspects of infertility have been included—to a certain extent—in the counselling of infertile couples in recent years. This has been accomplished in part by psychologists and psychotherapists, in the secondary care set-up, usually for special cases only. It is of greater importance that gynecologists and andrologists themselves become more sensitive towards their male and/or female patients and offer integrated, primary psychosomatic counselling.

The psychosomatic view towards therapy of infertile couples is necessary for the following reasons:

1. The unfulfilled wish for children often represents a major life crisis for the couple, causing:
  a. disturbed life perspectives
  b. strong suffering
  c. coping with renunciation
  d. negative social resonance
  e. depressed mood.
2. Sterility/infertility may have its causes (alone or combined with other causes) in a psychopathology. Examples include symptomatic sexual disturbances, endocrinopathy, and male subfertility.

3. Psychosomatic support is indicated when high-pressure psychological situations are incurred, such as in vitro fertilization (IVF), insemination or donor insemination.

Trying to estimate the pressure created by the unfulfilled wish for children can bring the physician to a better understanding of the couple, and improve the physician–patient relationship. Longstanding experience with infertile couples allows us to draw the simplified scheme shown in Table 28.4.

A special problem is the late desire for children, which has become more frequent since the advent of IVF. It concerns primarily women between the ages of 40 and 50. The high pressure these women exert upon the physician is readily apparent, even at the first interview. The patient signals the physician that she is willing that he 'do with me as you will, if only my wish for children can be fulfilled'. Risk taking without reasonable limitations is also apparent. The patient – physician relationship is strongly hampered, and an open discussion about background and motivation is avoided or remains superficial. Psychosomatic interventions are seen in a

**Table 28.4**  Wish for children

'Healthy' wish for children:
— Pressure moderately strong
— Hesitant concerning invasive medical procedures
— Renunciation appears possible
— Frustrated wish for children is socially tolerable
— Balanced relationship between physician and patient is well possible.

'Strong' wish for children:
— Pressure very strong
— Urge for invasive medical procedures
— Renunciation appears hardly possible
— Life-perspective is obviously disturbed (negative social resonance/reactive depression)
— Balanced relationship between physician and patient is more difficult.

'Overemphasized' wish for children:
— Massive pressure ('attacks of hunger for children'), search for specialists)
— Only invasive methods are accepted (risk-taking without limitation!)
— Frequent activities ('going through many doctors')
— Search for a relationship between physician and patient which stands for an 'ominous alliance' (patient's position: 'a child at any cost'/physician's position: 'the only success is a child').

negative light by the patient, since they 'want a child, not a psychotherapist'. Women with a very late wish for children often show unstable partner relationships. Often, the formerly successful professional woman, now going through a preclimacteric crisis, can be found repeatedly among these patients. The very late wish for a child (in common language a 'frost flower') may represent ones' own unfulfilled wishes, such as protection from inner feelings of emptiness or depressive feelings and other individual impulses (Table 28.5).

The comparison between risk and benefit that the physician must make before any medical intervention, should discourage the application of modern reproductive technology — such as IVF — with the very late wish for children. At times, the patient will seek out a physician who will be willing to grant any treatment. We see this alliance as a negative one, as the psychological level is neglected completely between the physician who is willing to undertake anything possible with medical technology, and the patient, who wishes a child at any cost. In this situation, a chance to work on the patient's basic problems, and to put her life into perspective, is lost.

## SPONTANEOUS PREGNANCIES DURING INFERTILITY TREATMENT

Analysis of therapeutic results in the Berlin-Charlottenburg University Hospital Infertility Clinic is most validly made from pre-IVF results. An extensive correlation between therapeutic success and previous therapeutic measures was found (Stauber 1988). Cumulative results showed that the highest pregnancy rate was achieved

independently of active therapeutic measures; often, pregnancies occurred in the interim before a scheduled invasive procedure. A higher pregnancy rate was noted after diagnostic procedures such as laparoscopy, possibly reflecting the conscious knowledge that 'everything is alright'. Finally, many pregnancies were tallied during therapy pauses, vacations and unilateral psychotherapeutic measures. Seeing that there are centers where invasive procedures are applied without clear-cut indications or criteria, this evidence is of great importance. The University of Melbourne Center for Reproductive Medicine also reported that couples on the IVF waiting list registered a pregnancy rate similar to those undergoing IVF at the same center. Permitting some time to pass, to allow for a possible spontaneous pregnancy to occur, has some psychological benefit as well as achieving the couples' aim. It may be concluded that invasive treatment should be administered only for clear-cut indications, and in every case, the risk–benefit comparison should be made.

Infertility solely or partially caused by psychological reasons, which is often also called functional, psychogenic or psychosomatic, can be described in the widest sense as depicted in Table 28.6.

The graphic presentation of an attempt to make a retrospective determination of functional infertility is presented in Figure 28.1. Five hundred and sixty-six of 2000 thoroughly investigated couples in two combined studies conducted at the Women's Hospital of the Free University Berlin-Charlottenburg (28.3%) were found to suffer from functional sterility. In other terms, up to one-fourth of all infertile couples have some psychological component to attribute their infertility. Distribution of all causes of infertility

**Table 28.5**  The very late wish for children: women aged 40–50 years

| | |
|---|---|
| Actualized by: | Overproportional trust in the modern reproductive technologies (e.g. IVF) |
| Appearance: | Extreme pressure |
| | Search for invasive procedures |
| | Risk-taking without limits |
| | Primary refusal of psychosomatic intervention |
| Psychodynamics: | Wish for children as an attempt to solve own conflicts |
| Therapeutic intervention: | Clarify 'shine solution' |

**Table 28.6**  'Psychogenic sterility' (in the widest sense)

Phenomenology:
— Asymptomatic ('idiopathic')
— Symptomatic, e.g. amenorrhoea, anovulation, sexual disturbances, impaired semen quality
Pathogenesis:
— Via hormonal system or neurovegetative tract
Aetiology:
— Psychological conflict, e.g. unconscious denial of pregnancy, problem of sexual identity

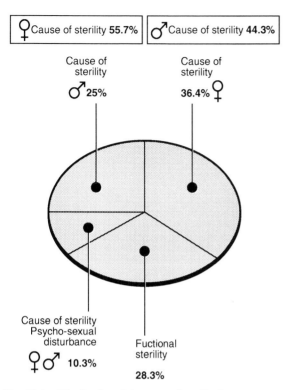

Fig. 28.1   Distribution of the cause of sterility between female and male: retrospetive overview of $n = 1994$ couples with the admitting diagnosis of sterility.

**Table 28.7**   Functional sexual disturbances in sterile couples (primary sexual disturbances)

1. 'Virgin marriages'
2. Isolated disturbances within the female (e.g. vaginismus, dyspareunia without organic findings)
3. Isolated disturbances within the male (e.g. impotentia coeundi)
4. Infrequent sexual intercourse and avoidance of conception optimum

naires in the infertile group. We also found that the partner relationship was significantly more often pathological in psychological childlessness, typically exhibiting a clinging, symbiotic pattern. Both partners viewed themselves as being unattractive to their surroundings, neglected and unpopular. Both partners also considered themselves — on the average — more depressive than the control group.

Data concerning psychosomatic andrology are especially impressive (Daiger 1988, Stauber 1988). Low quality semen was found to be positively correlated with work-related stress and stress within the family as well as with increased psychosomatic symptoms. Table 28.8 represents an overview of that investigation as well as its conclusions.

We conclude that a more sophisticated individual diagnosis is of importance in andrology. Attention must be paid to indicators of psychological components of infertility, which occasionally consist of changing spermatogram parameters.

## CONCLUSIONS

A number of practical suggestions concerning the treatment of infertile couples can be deduced from the aforementioned results. The holistic

between the two sexes shows a female cause in 55.7% and a male cause in 44.3%.

Primary sexual disturbances are frequently encountered in infertile couples, at a rate of up to 10%, therefore including the partner in a counselling session is especially important in order not to miss any 'partner pathology'. Frequently encountered sexual disturbances are listed in Table 28.7. Infrequent intercourse and subconscious avoidance of the optimum conception time is seen often, a point not to be missed by the physician with a holistic approach. Additionally, during treatment, secondary sexual disturbances can be noted which are often induced by the mechanistic approach of many physicians (too many inseminations per cycle, timed intercourse, etc.).

Psychosomatic disturbances and complaints should bring to mind (more frequently) the diagnosis of psychologically caused infertility. Compared to a control group, a significant rise in somatic symptomatology was elicited by question-

**Table 28.8**   Results concerning psychosomatic andrology $n = 1454$ primary spermatograms and questionnaires, compare Stauber 1988 and Daiger 1988)

Reduced semen quality correlates positively with:
1. Work-related stress
2. Family-related stress
3. Psychosomatic complaints
Conclusions:
— Follow-up of indicators (e.g. great differences in spermatogram parameters)!
— More sophisticated individual diagnostics in andrology

view of the infertile couple should start with consideration of psychological interrelationships within both partners, as well as with various organic causes of childlessness. Furthermore, the overemphasized wish for children should be discussed at the onset of treatment. Finally, an individualized treatment plan is mandatory during the first part of infertility treatment. Within the often time-consuming treatment plan for infertility, a stepwise confrontation, clarification and interpretation of the psychosomatic interrelationships is warranted. Primary and secondary sexual disturbances, which can be seen as a result of the 'mechanistic' therapeutic procedures, should be diagnosed and clarified early. Discussing adoption options and necessary treatment pauses is helpful. The physician in charge should be prepared to accept that the possible best solution in any specific case may be renunciation of the potential child, and be able to confront the couple with an honest appraisal of the facts. Termination or 'abandoning' infertility treatment should always include a contact offer for later problems, or queries which may arise at a later time. Discussing the option of entering an encounter group of infertile couples has provided good support. Exchange of experiences, as well as allowing for necessary emotional letdown, are positive tools provided by support groups, which should be led by properly schooled physicians or psychotherapists.

Table 28.9 provides a model of fertility counselling for both partners, in which psychosomatic aspects are routinely integrated. Grouped by history, diagnostics and therapy, the primary organic therapeutic steps of the female and of the male are shown. In parallel, the psychosomatic treatment measures are conducted, which may be linked to conventional therapy directly in the physician's office or gynecology department.

## NEW REPRODUCTIVE TECHNOLOGIES

New reproductive technologies, and especially IVF, have opened up a new dimension in medicine. For the first time, it is possible to watch and perhaps even manipulate the very origin of a human being within the laboratory. Perspectives are thereby opened which can create discomfort within most of us. Fear of abusing these methods and subsequent questions of limitations of methods must be dealt with. Reference should be made to new literature which has dealt with the questions of the new reproductive technologies (Morse & van Hall, 1987, Baram et al 1988, Brody 1989, Bydlowski & Dayan-Lintzer 1988, van Hall 1988a,b, Dennerstein & Morse 1988, Shaw et al 1988, Newman 1989, Reading 1989).

During the 18th Congress for Psychosomatic Obstetrics and Gynecology in Dusseldorf in 1989, we conducted an inquiry among psychosomatically oriented gynecologists about IVF; 95% were in favor of professional as well as legal limitations for modern reproductive medicine.

**Table 28.9** Fertility clinic for both partners: 'Model for integrated psychosomatics'

|  | History | Diagnostics | Therapy |
|---|---|---|---|
| Female | Duration of wish for children, primary/secondary sterility, illnesses, previous treatments, cycle | Genital findings, basal temperature curve, cervical factor, hormones, genetics, ultrasound, extended laparoscopy | Treatment of inflammation, determination of ovulation, insemination, adoption?, microsurgery, IVF |
| Male and Female | Suffering by unfulfilled wish for children, partner relationship (stable?), motivation for wish for children, sexual life | Psychosomatic symptoms, personality structure, partner interaction, psychosomatic interventions, ('here and now') | Psychological guidance (e.g. at IVF), encounter groups, treatment pauses, psychotherapy, contact offer (be careful of fixated wish for children) |
| Male | Diseases of the genital tract, previous treatments, surgeries, risk factors (cigarettes, prescriptions) | Genital findings, spermatogram (stress?), hormones, SH, immunology, testicular biopsy | Treatment of inflammation, hormone therapy, surgery, adoption?, preservation of semen for insemination |

IVF has resolved fertility problems for some groups of patients, but has created new pathologies for another group of patients (Table 28.10). Extrauterine pregnancy, spontaneous abortion and premature delivery are more common in IVF patients, and the incidence of multifetal pregnancy, and caesarean delivery are increased. Multifetal pregnancies have drawn attention as a potential complication, since they can endanger both mother and fetus. Hepp (1991) has pointed out the various risks, to both mother and child. The mother is at risk from hyperstimulation, hyperemesis, spontaneous abortion, EPH-gestosis, bleeding, polyhydramnios, premature rupture of membranes, and anemia. For the child, the risks of preterm birth, intrauterine growth retardation, fetal presentation pathologies, prolapse of the cord, twin-to-twin transfusion syndrome, intrapartum death or permanent damage are increased. The physician indicating IVF should be prepared to answer the question whether the risk to benefit ratio had been adequately estimated. The same physician should not fail to take into account possible psychological problems encountered in IVF by both partners, as presented by Kentenich et al (1989, 1991) (Table 28.11).

**Table 28.10** Medical risks of IVF after successful conception

— High abortion rate (about 25%)
— High rate of extrauterine pregnancies (about 4%)
— High rate of pregnancy-related complications (e.g. bleedings, premature labour)
— High incidence of premature birth (approx. 20%) (danger of developmental disturbances of the newborn)
— High incidence of caesarean sections (approx. 40%)
— High incidence of multifetal pregnancies (approx. 15%) (possibly with vital problems for mother and child)

**Table 28.11** IVF: psychological problems

1. During stimulation:
   fear, feeling of insufficiency, tension, regulation of sexual needs
2. During the time in the reproduction laboratory:
   fear of gamete mix-up, fear of gamete damage
3. After embryo transfer:
   fear of implantation impairment (?), fear of complications, such as abortion, extrauterine pregnancy, multifetal pregnancy

Stauber 1985, Kentenich 1989.

The finding that a high percentage of the couples did not wish to reveal to their child later that he/she had been conceived by IVF was of special interest. This problem of conscious secrecy is well known from the area of heterologous inseminations, and the question arises whether one should not discuss this 'life lie' with such a couple. From a psychoanalytical point of view, identity conflicts are to be expected for the child, if the parents' conscious and unconscious communications are not congruent. Openness in a parent–child relationship is an all-important condition for the successful emotional development of the child. The Berlin group at Charlottenburg conducts a psychosomatic support program, and results of long term follow-up will undoubtedly bring forth conclusions concerning IVF children and the interaction between them and their parents.

The patient–physician relationship should be carefully nurtured, but at the same time continuously monitored for the appearance of any imbalance in the consideration of the risk-benefit ratio. The physician who judges the success of his sterility treatment only by the obtainment of a child—without considering if an underlying crisis has not been resolved (or perhaps even enhanced) —will be willing to take unlimited risks to succeed. The matching patient wishes a child at any cost, and shows unlimited risk taking. This 'ominous alliance' is to be condemned. Our conscience can be deftly tucked away by the day-to-day routine of infertility treatments, and the 'higher tech' these treatments become, the narrower our sense of limitation becomes.

Modern indications for IVF now include unexplained infertility, whereas originally the primary indication for IVF was tubal dysfunction. The rationale for expanding the indications includes the argument 'We need a more effective treatment for infertility'. This easily leads to viewing the patient's wish as the only valid one to consider, and from there, acceptance of oocyte donation, semen donation, surrogate mothers and even commercial embryos is facilitated. IVF as an elective procedure, with appropriate commercial remuneration, might be next in this futuristic scenario, and there are some groups who would see no problem with this development, and there are those who already practise it. Relaxation of conscience will bring the next step in embryo research. The argument that 'We want to advance our knowledge for genetically healthy children and to cure cancer' easily dissolves any inner resistance that one might still have. We feel that specific limitations should be applied to modern reproductive technologies, and a consensus reached with regard to:

- Embryo research
- Embryo manipulation
- Homologous versus heterologous fertilization
- Semen, oocyte, and embryo donations
- Surrogate mothers
- Embryo reduction in utero.

Finding a consensus will not be easy, considering the fact that well-known and responsible physicians hold quite different views on the possibilities of embryo research, the ethics of such research, and even on the beginning of life itself. Nevertheless, it is imperative to reach a consensus, which should have a wide, interdisciplinary base. If concrete answers are impossible, then at least concrete attitudes and clear guidelines should be laid down. Good judgement and farsightedness are necessary, and every new step should be planned.

The psychosomatic aspect of infertility treatments, while not being the backbone of therapeutic importance, still has utmost validity. Balancing the wish for children—in the context of all other life wishes—with a realistic situation in the context of infertility, will set the stage for a constructive patient–physician relationship. Supporting the couple, and supplying them with coping strategies throughout such a trying period of their life, will invariably enhance their peace of mind, and may even be the major factor in success.

## REFERENCES

Baram D E, Tourtelot E, Muechler K E, Huang 1988 Psychosocial adjustment following unsuccessful in vitro fertilization. J Psychosom Obstet Gynecol 9: 181

Becker R 1980 Schwangerschaftsverlauf, Geburt und postpartale Entwicklung bei Sterilitätspatientinnen mit schließlich erfülltem Kinderwunsch. Inauguraldissertation. Freie Universität, Berlin

Brody E B 1989 Human rights aspects of traffic in human fetuses: an international perspective. In: van Hall E, Everaerd W (eds) The free woman. Parthenon Publishing, Carnforth, Lancashire

Bydlowski M, Dayan-Lintzer M 1988 A psycho-medical approach to infertility: suffering from sterility. J Psychosom Obstet Gynecol 9: 139

Daiger M E 1988 Untersuchungen zur sterilen Partnerschaft unter besonderer Berücksichtigung andrologischer psychosomatischer Befunde. Inauguraldissertation. Freie Universität, Berlin

Dennerstein L, Morse C 1988 A review of psychological and social aspects of in vitro fertilisation. J Psychosom Obstet Gynecol 9: 159

Frick-Bruder V, Schütt E 1991 Zur Psychologie des männlichen und weiblichen Kinderwunsches. In: Stauber M, Conrad F, Haselbacher G (eds) Psychosomatische Gynäkologie und Geburtshilfe. Springer, Berlin

Hepp H 1991 Klinik, Ethik und Recht der operativen Reproduktionsmedizin. In: Stauber M, Conrad F, Haselbacher G (eds) Psychosomatische Gynäkologie und Geburtshilfe. Springer, Berlin

Johnson G D, Roberts R, Brown E et al 1987 Infertile or childless by choice? A multipractice survey of women aged 35 and 50. Br Med J 294: 98

Kentenich H 1989 Ergebnisse aus einer Nachuntersuchung von IvF-Paaren. Vortrag auf dem 9. Internationalen Kongreß für psychosomatische Geburtshilfe und Gynäkologie, Amsterdam

Kentenich H, Wilcke M, Fuhrmann S, Stief G, Blankau A, Schmiady H 1991 Ergebnisse einer Nachuntersuchung von IvF-Paaren und deren Kindern. In: Stauber M, Conrad F, Haselbacher G (eds) Psychosomatische Gynäkologie und Geburtshilfe. Springer, Berlin

Morse C, van Hall E 1987 Psychosocial aspects of infertility: a review of current concepts. J Psychosom Obstet Gynecol 6: 157

Münkel W 1982 Bevölkerungsrückgang als Folge veränderten generativen Handelns des Mannes. Explikation anhand Theorien. Inauguraldissertation. Freie Universität, Berlin

Newman L F 1989 Reproduction and technology. In: van Hall E, Everaerd W (eds) The free woman. Parthenon Publishing Group, Carnforth, Lancashire p 523–528

Reading A E 1989 Psychological and social aspects of the new reproductive technologies. In: van Hall E, Everaerd W (eds) The free woman. Parthenon Publishing Group, Carnforth, Lancashire

Schultz-Ruthenberg C, Stauber M 1980 Zur Verarbeitung des frustranen Kinderwunsches (unveröff. Ergebnisse)

Shaw P, Johnston M, Shaw R 1988 Counselling needs, emotional and relationship problems in couples awaiting IVF. J Psychosom Obstet Gynecol 9: 171

Stauber M 1985 Psychosomatisches Modell für die extrakorporale Fertilisation. In: Fervers-Schorre B, Poettgen H, Stauber M (eds) Psychosomatische Probleme in der Gynäkologie und Geburtshilfe, S 39–51. Springer, Berlin

Stauber M 1988 Psychosomatik der sterilen Ehe 2. Aufl Grosse, Berlin

Stauber M 1991 Kinderwunschbehandlung aus

psychosomatischer Sicht-Ergebnisse und
Schlußfolgerungen. In: Stauber M, Conrad F, Haselbacher
G (eds) Psychosomatische Gynäkologie und Geburtshilfe.
Springer, Berlin

van Hall E 1988a Infertility. J Psychosom Obstet Gynecol
9: 155
van Hall E 1988b Manipulation of human reproduction.
Commentary. J Psychosom Obstet Gynecol 9: 207

# 29. Medical conditions leading to infertility

*Yair Liel    Ilana Harman-Boehm    Jonathan E. Arbelle*
*Seymour M. Glick*

## INTRODUCTION

Serious medical illnesses of many kinds are associated with infertility as a result of many factors. The present chapter deals with a selected group of illnesses which either are most commonly associated with problems in fertility, which are of special interest to the general physician, or have been foci of recent advances in our knowledge. The chapter is by no means intended to deal with all the diseases that may affect fertility, but only to touch upon several specific areas of interest.

## NUTRITIONAL STATES

### Undernutrition and exercise

*Female*

Anorexia nervosa will not be reviewed in detail since the patient suffering from this disease is not likely to present to the gynecologist with a chief complaint of infertility. A consideration of the endocrine defects of anorexia nervosa, however, may help us to answer the more relevant question: does being thin affect fertility? Anorexia nervosa is accompanied by amenorrhea associated with low levels of luteinizing hormone (LH), follicle stimulating hormone (FSH), estrogen, nocturnal and daytime prolactin (Fichter & Pirke 1984), androgens, and often a delayed or blunted LH response to a single bolus of GnRH (Palmer et al 1975, Hurd et al 1977, Drossman et al 1979, Isaacs et al 1980, Schwabe et al 1981), and regression to an immature or early pubertal circadian pattern of pulsatile LH secretion, i.e. sleep entrained episodic LH release (Boyar et al 1974, Kapen et al 1981). Repeated pulses (Drossman et

al 1979), and in some instances a single dose (Katz et al 1977), of GnRH can evoke an appropriate increase in LH, FSH and estrogen, and may induce ovulation (Drossman et al 1979). As weight returns towards normal the mature pattern of LH secretion reappears, and menses resume, (McArthur et al 1976). These observations, and the fact that growth hormone responses to clonidine stimulation were blunted in adolescent girls with early anorexia nervosa (Nussbaum et al 1990), suggest a functional defect at the hypothalamic level involving GnRH secretion, rather than a defect at the pituitary or ovary (Boyar et al 1974).

Indeed, Van de Wiele has emphasized the presence in both anorexia nervosa and involuntary starvation of similar disturbances of hypothalamic function including: altered thyroid-stimulating hormone (TSH) response to thyrotropin-releasing hormone (TRH); partial diabetes insipidus; abnormalities of temperature regulation; and abnormalities of gonadotropin secretion (Van de Wiele 1977). Quantitatively less pronounced, but qualitatively similar, defects in hypothalamic function have also been reported in mildly overweight patients with secondary amenorrhea associated with simple weight loss (Vigersky et al 1977), in college women participating in competitive athletics (Feicht et al 1978), in long distance runners (Dale et al 1979) as well as in participants in other strenuous sports such as rowing, cycling and swimming (Sanborn et al 1982) and in students at professional ballet schools (Frisch et al 1980). Young women with regular menstrual cycles develop menstrual disturbances after only a few weeks of exercise (Bullen et al 1985). An open population study in Holland also supports a relationship between thinness and menstrual disturbance (Vandenbroucke & Valkenburg 1981).

Fishman, in a cogent editorial (Fishman 1980), discussed the relation of fatness to ovulation, specifically the concept that there is a critical weight, in particular, the fat : lean body composition (Frisch & Revelle 1971, Frisch 1980), which must be attained to initiate the menarche and to maintain ovulatory cycles, presumably by generating the appropriate physiological signal for mature gonadotropin releasing hormone (GnRH) secretion (Fishman 1980).

The known effects of adipose tissue on estrogen economy could account for a dependency of normal ovulation on a critical mass of fat. A possible direct regulatory effect of adipose tissue on sex hormone binding globulin (SHBG) levels (Plymate et al 1981) and the capacity of adipose tissue to aromatize androstenedione to estrogen (Siiteri & MacDonald 1973) would alter the supply of estrogen, while the effectiveness of circulating estrogen could be modified by conversion of estradiol to 2-hydroxy estrone (Fishman et al 1975, Fishman 1980). Thus, a reduction in body fat as seen in anorexia nervosa (Jeuniewic et al 1978), simple weight loss (Vigersky et al 1977), athletes (Feicht et al 1978, Dale et al 1979, Smith 1980) or ballerinas (Frisch et al 1980) could alter estrogen balance, causing the mature hypothalamus to regress to the prepuberal functional (anovulatory) state.

There are, however, several observations which do not support this concept:

1. Between 25% and 50% of patients with anorexia nervosa develop amenorrhea before substantial weight loss (Beck & Brochner-Mortensen 1954, Warne et al 1973, Schwabe et al 1981).

2. Amenorrhea and abnormalities of GnRH response may persist despite an approach to ideal weight (Isaacs et al 1980).

3. Ballet dancers who interrupt training because of illness or injury may resume menses before significant weight gain (Frisch 1980, Abraham et al 1982).

4. Although, compared to the control group, female long distance runners were thinner, had a smaller proportion of body fat and a higher incidence of amenorrhea, the athletic women with menstrual disturbances weighed no less than athletes with regular menses.

5. When compared to a group of patients with cystic fibrosis, and matched for body weight and menstrual age, 100% of the anorexia nervosa patients and only 33% of the patients with cystic fibrosis had had amenorrhea, suggesting that body weight is not the only factor for amenorrhea in patients with anorexia (Weltman et al 1990).

Although these exceptions to the critical weight concept could be ascribed to limitations of the methods for measuring body weight or body fat, other possibilities exist. Adipose tissue may not be homogeneous. The capacity of adipose tissue to aromatize androstenedione increases as the mass of adipose tissue increases, but the capability of enhanced aromatization may be found in women of any build, suggesting the presence of a subpopulation of adipose cells (Forney et al 1981). A small increase in the quantity of this subpopulation, consequent to a decrease in caloric expenditure, while too small to discern, might none the less significantly affect estrogen balance. A change in energy utilization could alter aromatization activity even before a change in body composition occurred or could, perhaps, affect nonadipose sites of estrogen production (Rizkallah et al 1975).

Insufficient attention has been given to variables not directly related to fat content which may affect hypothalamic function, e.g. stress, exercise and thyroid function. Although the emotional influences are different in the young woman with advanced anorexia nervosa and her equally thin athletic counterpart, the aversions to food seen in athletes can mimic anorexia nervosa (Smith 1980) and few would deny that participation in competitive sports or professional ballet is stressful. While the medical and endocrine adjustments to physical training have been reviewed (Björntorp 1976), the effect of exercise on the pituitary-gonadal axis in the undernourished has not been assessed. Both fasting (Portnoy et al 1974) and anorexia nervosa (Moshang et al 1975) are associated with a reduced serum T3 level. The altered relationship between circulating and intra-cellular T3 (Larsen et al 1981) might modify the flux of T3 to the hypothalamus and affect GnRH secretion (see also section on 'Thyroid disease'). Acute exercise increases plasma growth hormone, testosterone, adrenocorticotropic hormone and androgens (Hale et al 1983, Mathur et al 1986). Plasma catecholamines have also been found to be elevated during exercise, more so in amenor-rheic runners than in eumenorrheic runners, and it has been suggested that periodic marked eleva-tions in norepinephrine levels during maximal exercise may interfere with pulsatile LH release and thereby play a role in the occurrence of menstrual dysfunction in women runners (Chin et al 1987). In addition, augmentation of prolactin concentration and responsiveness by exercise, even in the absence of weight loss or underweight, could account for the menstrual dysfunction developing during physical training (Boyden et al 1982). Yet another theory proposes that a suprahypothalamic abnormality could cause both disturbances in hypothalamic function as well as multiple behavioral disorders. Impaired secre-tion of central nervous system neuropeptides such as neuropeptide Y, corticotrophin-releasing-hor-mone, and β-endorphin might account for multiple effects including amenorrhea as well as increased physical activity, reduced sexual interest and pathological feeding behavior (Kaye et al 1989, Seifer & Collins 1990). Suh and associates have found that activation of the ACTH-adrenal axis and inhibition of the GnRH pulse generator are associated with functional hypothalamic amenorrhea in nonathletic women (Suh et al 1988), and increased glucocorticoid levels and β-endorphins have been found to be higher in amenorrheic athletes than in eumenorrheic athletes, or nonathletic women (Ding et al 1988, Hohtari et al 1988). Alternatively the increased plasma concentrations of β-endorphins found after exercise may have an inhibitory effect on the hypothalamic-pituitary axis thereby leading to amenorrhea (De Cree 1989).

In summary, although the mechanism remains uncertain, young women 10–30% below ideal weight may develop a functional hypothalamic hypogonadal state resulting in amenorrhea (Jeuniewic et al 1978, Isaacs et al 1980).

### Male

Whether being thin can affect male fertility is not known. Just as there may be a critical weight to initiate the menarche, the initial growth spurt in boys appears to be associated with a weight of approximately 55 kg (Frisch et al 1971). Anorexia nervosa occurs in men (Hay & Leonard 1979), and in athletes, food aversion simulating anorexia nervosa, has been described (Smith 1980). Men like women who engage in strenuous sport such as marathon running may develop hypothalamic dysfunction (MacConnie et al 1986) manifested by lower amplitudes and frequency of sponta-neous LH pulses and a lower LH response to GnRH than nonrunners. Testosterone levels have not consistently been found to be low, and may depend on the duration of training. In these situa-tions reduced serum testosterone levels are difficult to interpret since psychosocial stress, even without weight loss, may depress testos-terone levels (Kreuz et al 1972, Doering et al 1975).

Animals subjected to severe caloric restriction develop gonadotropin deficiency (Rogers 1958). Some investigators have shown that adult men suffering from protein-caloric malnutrition demonstrate elevated gonadotropins and subnormal responses to human chorionic gonadotropin (hCG), findings consistent with testicular damage (Smith et al 1975), and others have found that a decrease in caloric intake and a subsequent weight loss cause initially a loss of libido, and with continued weight loss, a reduc-tion of prostatic fluid and then lessened longevity and motility of sperm (Frisch 1988).

### Fad diets

Fad diets have become popular in recent years, especially vegetarian diets. The abrupt switch to a vegetarian diet in an otherwise healthy woman frequently causes oligomenorrhea and anovula-tion. The mechanism is unclear, though there is evidence that vegetarians have a higher fecal output with increased fecal estrogen excretion compared with nonvegetarians. It has been suggested that the increased fecal bulk and reduced glucuronidase activity among vegetarians interrupt the enterohepatic circulation of estrogen, thereby reducing the overall impact of secreted estrogens. An alternative explanation is that the switch to a vegetarian diet is accompanied by a rapid reduction in total caloric intake and consequent amenorrhea (Reid & Van Vught 1987).

## Overnutrition

### Female

Obesity may seriously compromise reproductive potential in women. Inadequate luteal phase (Sherman & Korenman 1974), dysfunctional bleeding, polycystic ovary syndrome (Yen 1980) and amenorrhea are mentioned among the gynecological complications of obesity (Rogers & Mitchell 1952, Glass et al 1978, Hartz et al 1979). The amenorrhea in very fat women is generally reversible with weight loss (Glass et al 1981), but menstrual cyclicity may cease during rapid weight loss in the mildly obese (Vigersky et al 1977). In the polycystic ovary syndrome weight loss has been shown to bring about a reduction in estrone levels, a return of normal gonadotropin secretion and resumption of normal menses (Harlass et al 1984). The complicated changes in sex steroid metabolism and pituitary gonadal function observed in obesity have been reviewed (Glass et al 1981) but remain difficult to unravel.

Although the ovaries of obese women show increased capsular hyalinization, atypical follicles and atresia, FSH and LH levels are not consistent with primary ovarian failure. Indeed FSH levels are often low (Dignam et al 1969, Fisher et al 1974, Kopelman et al 1980), and when elevated levels of LH are seen, as in the polycystic ovary syndrome (PCO), this can be ascribed to the increased estrogen levels (Yen 1980) rather than to ovarian failure.

Hypothalamic-pituitary status, as assessed by response to GnRH (Kopelman et al 1980), pulsatile gonadotropin release (Newmark et al 1979) and positive feedback response to estradiol (Glass et al 1981) is generally intact. However, others have observed diminished gonadotropin secretion (Dignam et al 1969), absence of the midcycle surge of LH or FSH, and clomiphene response varying from normal to poor (Dignam et al 1969, Glass et al 1978, 1981).

Excess androgen production by the adrenal (Fehér & Halmy 1975), or by the adrenal and the ovary (Yen 1980) may be associated with amenorrhea and with hirsutism (Hartz et al 1979), but hirsutism is not invariably seen despite high levels of free androgen (Housseinian et al 1976). Further factors contributing to the hyperandrogenism are: (a) a metabolic shift to the more highly potent 5-$\alpha$ steroids as indicated by the increased ratio of androsterone to etiocholanolone (Scuro et al 1977); and (b) a decrease in SHBG levels (Housseinian et al 1976, Kopelman et al 1980, Plymate et al 1981). With weight loss, both the hyperandrogenic state (Glass et al 1978) and the amenorrhea can reverse (Rogers & Mitchell 1952, Newmark et al 1979, Glass et al 1981), as can hirsutism and acanthosis nigricans, when present (Pasquali et al 1989).

The excess of androgen, in turn, results in increased estrogen as a consequence of conversion, presumably by adipose tissue, (Schindler et al 1972, Nimrod & Ryan 1975) to estrone and estradiol (Siiteri et al 1973, Edman & MacDonald 1978, MacDonald et al 1978). The effectiveness of circulating estrogen is further enhanced by decreased production of the weaker estrogens, estriol and 2-hydroxyestrone from their precursors (Fishman et al 1975). This peripherally generated, noncycling, excess estrogen may play a role in the pathogenesis of the PCO syndrome (Yen 1980) and dysfunctional bleeding.

Attention has been drawn recently to the triad: insulin resistance, hyperandrogenism and acanthosis nigricans. Controversy exists as to whether hyperandrogenism causes insulin resistance, as supported by findings of decreased basal insulin levels after suppression of androgen levels by spironolactone, or whether increased insulin levels stimulate androgen production from the ovary (see also Chapter 26). Possibly the obesity associated hyperinsulinism, and not the obesity per se cause the hyperandrogenism and menstrual disorders in this situation (Reid & Van Vught 1987).

Finally, even when estrogen and androgen balance are not disturbed and ovulation takes place, fertility may be impaired by reduced progesterone levels and an inadequate luteal phase (Sherman & Korenman 1974).

## Male

As a consequence of excess fat, we would anticipate the following abnormalities in the obese man: increased estrogen production, elevated estrogen levels, a rise in SHBG, some degree of FSH suppression, variable LH levels, and clinical evidence of hypogonadism, including oligospermia. What, in fact, is observed? With few exceptions (Barbato & Landau 1974, Glass et al 1977, Amatruda et al 1978), increased levels of estradiol and estrone (Kley et al 1979, Schneider et al 1979) and increased rates of production of estrogen proportional to body weight (Schneider et al 1979) have been confirmed. The presumed mechanism is enhanced peripheral conversion of androgen to estrogen (Siiteri et al 1973, Schneider et al 1979, Glass et al 1981) by fat tissue (Schindler et al 1972, Nimrod & Ryan 1975, Perel & Killinger 1979), or by a subpopulation of fat cells (Forney et al 1981). In the morbidly obese (Barbato & Landau 1974, Amatruda et al 1978, Kley et al 1979, Schneider et al 1979), particularly in those men more than 200% over ideal body weight (IBW), testosterone levels are subnormal, and inversely related to weight (Glass et al 1981).

However, except for mechanical limitation, sexual performance and libido are generally unimpaired (Glass et al 1977) and there is no substantial evidence of hypoandrogenism, gynecomastia or testicular atrophy (Glass et al 1977, Amatruda et al 1978, Kley et al 1979, Schneider et al 1979), although some decrease in facial hair may be seen.

The absence of feminization, despite an increase in estrogen and a decrease in testosterone, can be explained, in part, by the unexpected decrease in SHBG in obese men (Glass et al 1977, Amatruda et al 1978, Kley et al 1979, Schneider et al 1979). Even a small decrease in SHBG produces a dramatic increase in the percentage of free testosterone (Dunn et al 1981), thereby maintaining a normal quantity of the physiologically active moiety, free testosterone. Sex steroid-mediated alterations in

binding affinity for testosterone may also be involved (Burke & Anderson 1972). Furthermore, since a decrease in SHBG has only a limited effect on the percentage of bound estradiol, a reduction in SHBG has a net androgenic effect; free testosterone increases out of proportion to free estrogen. However, in the occasional enormously obese man (200% over IBW) free as well as total testosterone is reduced more than 2 SD below normal (Amatruda et al 1978). Since in these men basal LH and FSH levels are not elevated and GnRH response is not enhanced (Glass et al 1981), a defect at the hypothalamic-pituitary level must be present. In most obese men, basal levels of FSH and LH are normal (Kley et al 1979, Schneider et al 1979, Glass et al 1981), and there is a substantial response to dynamic testing with clomiphene, GnRH or hCG (Schneider et al 1979). Whether dynamic responses are 'truly' normal has been questioned (Glass et al 1981). A reduced level of testosterone and of FSH, and a decreased FSH response to GnRH may be seen during even a short-term fast in obese men (Klibanski et al 1981). While the defense of normal free testosterone levels may adequately explain the absence of hypogonadism or feminization despite elevated estrogen levels, it seems likely that obesity somehow impairs the biological effectiveness of estrogen (Schneider et al 1979). The presence of normal, rather than consistently elevated, levels of thyroxine binding globulin (TBG) in obese men (Burman et al 1979, Moreira-Andres et al 1980) supports this suggestion. In summary, with the major qualification that semen analysis data are lacking (Glass et al 1981), it appears that fat men, unless too corpulent to copulate, are acceptable reproductive partners. The clinical significance of the apparent hypogonadotrophic hypogonadism in the occasional massively obese man is uncertain.

## DRUGS

An encyclopedic review of every pharmacological substance or physical agent known to adversely affect sexual performance or pituitary-gonadal function is beyond the scope of this chapter, nor do we intend to cover chemicals such as dibromochloropropane (Potashnik et al 1978, Glass et al 1979) affecting specific groups of workers. This information is available elsewhere (Jackson 1970, Patanelli 1975) and has been succinctly summarized (Anonymous 1987).

Instead we shall discuss:

1. Sedatives, antidepressants, and histamine $H_2$-receptor blockers, since these drugs may be of particular relevance in the highly stressed subfertile couple
2. Opiates, cannabis and alcohol, since these are used extensively as 'entertainment'
3. Antihypertensives
4. Ketoconazole, a systemic fungicide which affects steroid hormones biosynthesis.

The effects of chemotherapy and radiation are dealt with under 'Oncological chemotherapy and radiation' below.

### Sedatives and antidepressants

Erectile impotence may be seen with imipramine, and may resolve with dose reduction (Greenberg 1965). Delayed ejaculation and failure of ejaculation have been reported in patients using chlordiazepoxide (Hughes 1964), amitryptiline (Hollister 1978, Nininger 1978), thioridazine (Singh 1961) and monoamine oxidase inhibitors, which have in fact been used to treat premature ejaculation (Bennett 1961). In addition to these erectile disorders, probably due to disturbances of sympathetic and parasympathetic control, as recently reviewed (Schiavi 1981), reduced sperm counts and diminished semen volume have been noted in a third of patients on antipsychotic drugs (Blair & Simpson 1966). These findings could in part be due to elevated prolactin levels occurring during the use of antipsychotic drugs, as has been demonstrated after concomitant therapy of metoclopramide and sulpiride (Garcia Diez & Gonzalez Buitrago 1982). The newer antipsychotic agent fluvoxamine, a serotonin reuptake inhibitor, has been shown not to affect basal or stimulated levels of LH, FSH or prolactin (Kletzky 1983).

These reports of drug-induced sexual dysfunction and semen abnormalities are not altogether convincing. Many of the observations quoted represent case reports of five of fewer psychiatric

patients (Greenberg 1965, Nininger 1978, Kletzky et al 1979). The interpretation is further clouded by evidence of hypothalamic-pituitary dysfunction in patients with endogenous depression, before drug therapy (Carroll et al 1980). Depression per se could, of course, be the cause of sexual inadequacy.

### Ketoconazole

Ketoconazole is a broad-spectrum antifungal agent which has been used increasingly frequently in recent years for the treatment of superficial and systemic fungal infections. Ketoconazole inhibits steroid synthesis by inhibition of cytochrome P-450-dependent enzyme systems (Loose et al 1983). As a result, several endocrine abnormalities may occur. In females menstrual irregularities may occur in up to 10% of treated patients. In males decreased libido and potency as well as gynecomastia have been reported. In high doses transient azoospermia has been reported. Low doses of ketoconazole can cause a transient drop in plasma concentrations of free testosterone and 17-β estradiol (De Coster et al 1985).

### Sulphasalazine

Sulphasalazine is a drug commonly used for the treatment of inflammatory bowel disease. In animal studies it has not been found to cause infertility, but in humans 40% or more of semen samples from treated patients showed abnormalities: 39.6% showed oligospermia, 41.7% showed an increased number of abnormal forms and 91.7% showed impaired motility (Riley et al 1987). The adverse effect of the drug on male fertility is attributed to the sulfapyridine component of the drug rather than the 5-aminosalicylic acid moiety which is the active antiinflammatory component (O'Morain et al 1984). The mechanisms underlying the toxic effects of the drug might include an antifolate action which influences the rapidly dividing spermatogenic cells, and an antiprostaglandin effect which impairs sperm motility (Steen 1984). Changing therapy to 5-aminosalicylic acid enemas (Chatzinoff et al 1988) or an enteric-coated preparation mesalazine (Riley et al 1987) leads to reversal of the sperm abnormalities.

## Histamine H₂-receptor blocking agents

The histamine $H_2$ antagonists, cimetidine, ranitidine, famotidine and nizaditine are frequently employed for a prolonged period of time in the management of peptic disease (Feldman & Burton 1990). Cimetidine, the most extensively studied member of its class, has the most profound influences on the endocrine system. Unfortunately, although an effective drug, it has antiandrogenic actions which may be manifested by hyperprolactinemia, sexual dysfunction (Biron 1979, Peden et al 1979b), gynecomastia (Hall 1976, Delle Fave et al 1977), and reduced sperm count (Van Thiel et al 1979). Impotence, loss of libido and gynecomastia occur more often in men receiving prolonged therapy with high doses of cimetidine (Knigge et al 1980).

A group of presumably fertile men, given cimetidine, 1200 mg/day for 9 weeks, developed significantly reduced sperm counts and impaired LH-FSH responses to LHRH. Although in these men prolactin levels remained normal (Van Thiel et al 1979), others (Delle Fave et al 1977, Peden et al 1979a) have observed hyperprolactinemia. However, since hyperprolactinemia is not invariably induced by cimetidine, other causes must be considered (Spiegel et al 1978). Peden also found slight increases in basal gonadotropin levels in the presence of normal testosterone levels, suggestive of a degree of androgen resistance, in three men. Cimetidine has been shown to have androgen antagonistic properties caused by the inhibition of binding of dihydrotestosterone to androgen receptors, as shown in studies of cytoplasmic receptor binding and nuclear uptake of DMT by rat prostate slices (Winters et al 1979). This effect of cimetidine, which is also a cause of impotence and loss of libido (Peden et al 1981, Kingge et al 1983), has not been shown with other $H_2$-blockers (Brogden et al 1982, Price & Brogden 1988, Langtry et al 1989). Cimetidine also uniquely raises serum estradiol levels by inhibition of the metabolism of estradiol (Galbraith & Michnovicz 1989). Indeed cimetidine-induced impotence has been shown to disappear within 1 month of changing to ranitidine (Jensen et al 1983). Ranitidine also increases serum prolactin but to a lesser extent than does cimetidine (Nelis & Van de Meene 1980). None the less, ranitidine causes gynecomastia in men and breast swelling, tenderness and galactorrhea in women. These effects are not shared by the other $H_2$-receptor antagonists such as famotidine or nizatidine (Van Thiel et al 1987, Feldman & Burtan 1990).

## Narcotics

Male heroin addicts, while on heroin or during methadone detoxification, have an increased frequency of impotence and ejaculatory problems (Mintz et al 1974). Most (85%) opiate-dependent women have major menstrual disturbances; 25% have galactorrhea, and 90% are infertile (Bai et al 1974). These findings are due presumably to anovulation associated with hypothalamic suppression, since gonadotropin levels are not elevated, and other evidence of hypothalamic dysfunction may be present (Bai et al 1974).

While in the heroin addict it may be difficult to separate the CNS effects of opiates from the influences of stress, malnutrition and infection, a significant dose-related depression of plasma testosterone levels and sperm count is seen in otherwise healthy marihuana users (Kolodny et al 1974a). These men respond to hCG or to the cessation of drug abuse with a prompt rise in testosterone; their FSH and LH levels are normal or low and they are normoprolactinemic; observations compatible with hypothalamic-pituitary suppression (Kolodny et al 1974a). Comparable studies relating marihuana use to ovarian dysfunction are not available.

## Antihypertensive agents

Physicians familiar with the therapy of hypertension are aware that orgasmic difficulties, erectile disturbances and loss of libido may be the price paid for the drug control of hypertension. A review (Anonymous 1987) of drugs that cause sexual inadequacy lists the following antihypertensive drugs: reserpine, clonidine, guanethidine, hydralazine, phenoxybenzamine, methyldopa, the β-adrenergic receptor blocking drugs, propranolol and metoprolol, as well as the thiazide diuretics and spironolactone. The newer antihypertensives calcium-channel blockers and ACE (angiotensin converting enzyme) inhibitors do not appear to cause these adverse effects. Chronic moderate to high dose spironolactone therapy frequently results in gynecomastia, decreased libido and impotence (Clark 1965, Spark & Melby 1968), and is of particular interest because of its complex effects, some of which, such as gynecomastia, are dose dependent (de Gasparo et al 1989).

Although spironolactone does inhibit testosterone production by reducing the level of microsomal cytochrome P-450 in testes and thereby reducing 17-hydroxylase activity (Loriaux et al 1976), this effect does not explain fully the estrogenic effect, since this is demonstrable in animals on fixed doses of testosterone (Steelman et al 1969, Rasmussen et al 1972). Nor does this effect account for the antiestrogenic action of spironolactone (Levy et al 1980). A unifying concept for the effects of spironolactone on sex steroids is based on the observation that spironolactone competitively binds both to estrogen receptors and to dihydrotestosterone receptors in cytosol (Levy et al 1980). Differences in ambient levels of endogenous estrogen and testosterone, and possible differences in testicular versus mammary receptor systems (Levy et al 1980) for example, could determine the net effect of spironolactone. Thus, in men spironolactone would act upon breast as an estrogen agonist as well as by an enhanced conversion of testosterone to estradiol (Rose et al 1977). This in turn, in concert with decreased testosterone production (Loriaux et al 1976), would account for the observed decreased testosterone to estrogen ratio (Rose et al 1977) which magnifies the feminizing effect of spironolactone.

In women, because of the high (relative to male) endogenous estrogen levels, spironolactone would act as an estrogen antagonist (Levy et al 1980). This could explain the observed menstrual disturbance.

Although many of the currently used antihypertensive drugs can affect sexual function (Anonymous 1987), the problem should be seen in proper perspective. Patients with malignant hypertension will not complain of infertility, while patients being treated to minimize the long-term complications of mild to moderate hypertension could switch therapy to a calcium-channel blocker or ACE inhibitor, reduce the dose or interrupt their therapy under medical supervision for the few months needed to permit conception.

## Alcohol

Certainly, from the standpoint of the physician treating infertility, alcohol is the most important Leydig cell toxin (Lipsett 1980, Van Thiel et al 1983a), its effects having been likened to 'chemical' castration (Cicero 1981). One of the commonest causes of male impotence is acute or excessive ethanol ingestion (Masters & Johnson 1970), with most hard-core alcoholics suffering from sexual inadequacy (Van Thiel & Lester 1979). As many as 80% of these men are sterile (Van Thiel et al 1974a,b), their testes showing seminiferous tubule atrophy, loss of sperm cells and abnormal sperm (Morrione 1944, Bennett et al 1950) with thickening, hyalinization and sclerosis of the lamina propria (Haider et al 1985). Alcohol and its oxidation metabolite, acetaldehyde, which is an even more potent toxin (Cicero & Bell 1980, Cicero et al 1980), damage the Leydig cell in several ways. At the membrane level alcohol causes a decrease in gonadotropin receptors at least in vitro (Bhalla et al 1979) and a loss of $Ca^{++}$ ATPase activity (Haider et al 1985). Acetaldehyde causes membrane damage which exposes testicular antigens which in turn provoke the formation of autoantibodies to Leydig cells that maintain the damage even after the cessation of alcohol ingestion (Van Thiel & Gavaler 1986). Intracellularly, the oxidation of alcohol causes a decrease of $3\beta$ and $17\beta$-hydroxysteroid dehydrogenase activity (Johnston et al 1981) and a decrease in the NAD/NADH ratio of the Leydig cell cytosol (Van Thiel et al 1986), thus decreasing steroidogenesis and testosterone biosynthesis. Alcohol, and its metabolite acetaldehyde, also limit the production of testosterone by their inhibitory effect on the mitochondria of the Leydig cell where cholesterol is converted to pregnenolone (Van Thiel et al 1986). In addition, as a result of decreased $\Delta^5\beta$-dehydrogenase conversion of pregnenolone to progesterone

(Gordon et al 1980), and perhaps as a result of impairment of the conversion of androstenedione to testosterone (Cicero & Bell 1980), the intracellular production of testosterone is inhibited (Ellingboe & Varanelli 1979, Cicero et al 1980). Alcohol-induced inhibition of vitamin A metabolism (Van Thiel et al 1974a) may also play a role.

In addition to these disturbances at the level of the testes alcohol has a direct toxic effect on the pituitary and hypothalamus (Gavaler et al 1983), since the testicular atrophy and the reduced testosterone values are not followed by an increase in gonadotropins (Gordon et al 1976, Van Thiel et al 1978a, Cicero 1981). Although the acute ingestion of alcohol may produce a surge in LH (Mendelson et al 1977, 1978a,b), possibly related to the reported alcohol-induced sexual arousal (LaFerla et al 1978), LH levels subsequently fall to low or inappropriately 'normal' levels (Van Thiel et al 1978a).

The central defect is most likely hypothalamic rather than pituitary since:

1. There is no FSH/LH response to clomiphene (Van Thiel et al 1974b)
2. Normal LH responsiveness to GnRH is generally demonstrated (Baker et al 1976, Cicero et al 1978a,b, Cicero 1981)
3. GnRH remains effective even in the presence of alcohol blockade of the LH rise following castration (Baker et al 1976, Cicero et al 1978a,b).

However, since not all patients respond to LHRH (Van Thiel et al 1978a), direct inhibition of the pituitary may be involved at times. Abnormalities of the circadian patterns of prolactin secretion have been noted in alcoholism, providing further evidence of hypothalamic-pituitary dysfunction (Tarquini et al 1977).

Despite the many mechanisms by which alcohol inhibits sexual and testicular function there appears to be no linear correlation between the abnormalities of the sperm and the amount and duration of alcohol consumption (Kucheria et al 1985), though a dose dependency is seen with chronic consumption (Mendelson & Mello 1974, Gordon et al 1976, Mendelson et al 1978a). It should be noted that a defect in testosterone production does not require years of

alcoholism and cirrhosis; reduced testosterone levels are seen within a month of daily ethanol ingestion in normal men (Gordon et al 1976). The toxic effects of alcohol on sexual function and fertility are reversible if testicular atrophy has not yet occurred and if responses to LHRH or clomiphene are normal (Gavaler et al 1983, Kucheria et al 1985).

Compounding the insult of hypoandrogenism, chronic alcoholics often have evidence of hyperestrogenism as well, i.e. a female escutcheon, palmar erythema and gynecomastia (Van Thiel & Lester 1979). Excellent reviews of alcohol-gonadal and hepatic interrelations have been published (Mendelson & Mello 1979, Van Thiel et al 1979a, Lipsett 1980, Cicero 1981, Gavaler et al 1983, Van Thiel et al 1986, Mello et al 1989). There is a consensus that alcohol per se even in the absence of the associated liver disease is responsible for the sexual dysfunction and the decreased fertility in acute and chronic alcohol abuse (Ylikahri et al 1974, Gordon et al 1976, Mendelson et al 1978a, Cicero 1981, Van Thiel et al 1986), although coexistent liver disease may play a role (Summerskil et al 1960). It is primarily the direct toxic effect of alcohol rather than the derivative disorder of estrogen metabolism consequent to liver disease which causes testicular atrophy and demasculinization. (Engel 1944, Galvão-Teles et al 1973, Mendelson et al 1974, Mendelson et al 1978a, Gavaler et al 1983). However, sexual dysfunction is seen with nonalcoholic liver disease (Van Thiel & Lester 1979, Van Thiel et al 1986) and the role of the liver connot be dismissed. The effects of chronic alcoholism on the hepatic metabolism of testosterone are not clear. There are reports of enhanced $5\alpha$-reductase activity resulting in accelerated degradation of testosterone with acute or short-term ethanol exposure (Gordon et al 1976, 1979c, Rubin et al 1976), but the same authors have also reported no change or a decrease in $5\alpha$-reductase activity (Gordon 1979a,c) with chronic exposure. This is an important observation, since a generalized reduction in the activity of this enzyme could diminish the supply of dihydrotestosterone to the peripheral tissues, thus aggravating the hypoandrogenism. In addition, it is accepted that alcohol increases the capacity of the liver to aromatize testosterone to estradiol (Gordon et al 1975, 1979b). This results in increased estrogen levels and could explain the observed signs of hyperestrogenism. Furthermore, a direct stimulating effect of alcohol and its metabolite acetaldehyde on adrenocortical steroid production has been described (Cobb et al 1979). The increase in androgenic precursors could, by conversion to estrone (Gordon et al 1975) also contribute to a hyperestrogenic state. However, Van Thiel & Lester (1979) in their review of gonadal function in alcoholic men cite numerous reports of normal estradiol and even free estradiol levels in alcoholics with liver disease. Thus, estrogen levels per se do not satisfactorily account for the feminization of alcoholics. Since estrogen receptors are highly specific for estrogen, it seems unlikely that a shift in the ratio of estrogen to testosterone, as such, can explain the hyperestrogenism (Gorski & Gannon 1976, Van Thiel & Lester 1979a). There is evidence, however, that hepatic estrogen receptor activity is modulated by testosterone (Lester et al 1979), a fall in testosterone enhancing receptor activity. It has been tentatively proposed that feminization in the presence of low testosterone levels and normal or only moderately elevated estrogen levels could be ascribed to this mechanism.

Surprisingly, despite the extensive documentation of the damaging effects of alcohol on male gonadal functions, there is little information on the adverse effect of alcohol on ovulation and virtually no data on the reversibility of alcohol-induced gonadal dysfunction. Menstrual abnormalities and, in rats, decreased progesterone levels and atrophy of the ovaries and of estrogen responsive tissues, have been described (Van Thiel et al 1978b, Van Thiel & Lester 1979a). In an animal model Mello et al (1989) found a negative correlation between daily alcohol dose and prolactin levels but in human female social drinkers persistent hyperprolactinemia was found (Mello et al 1989). Amenorrhea, anovulation luteal phase dysfunction and ovarian pathology may occur in alcohol-dependent women (Mello et al 1989). Wilsnack et al (1984) in a survey of 917 women found that dysmenorrhea, heavy menstrual flow and premenstrual discomfort increased with drinking level and were particularly strongly associated with consumption of six or more drinks a day at least once a week. The major disturbances of fetal growth and development associated with maternal alcoholism are beyond the scope of this chapter.

In summary, steady ethanol intake in men, and most probably in women also, can even in the absence of liver disease, seriously impair sexual adequacy and fertility. While reversibility with cessation of drinking seems likely, documentation of this sequence is lacking. The outlook in any case is no better than that of the underlying alcoholism.

## ONCOLOGICAL CHEMOTHERAPY AND RADIATION

Can a young adult who has been treated for a malignancy with chemotherapy or radiation or both, anticipate normal fertility and healthy offspring? With the rising number of long-term survivors after treatment of malignancies such as Hodgkin's disease (De Vita et al 1972, George et al 1979, Kaplan 1980) or choriocarcinoma (Lewis 1976), this question must be faced frequently by physicians concerned with infertility.

Although there are many retrospective reports of gonadal dysfunction associated with cancer therapy, it is difficult to compare one report with another. There are differences in the specific disease or disease stage, in the ages of the patients, in the drug regimens, and in the duration of follow-up. Neither the possible effect of any ancillary therapy used nor the role of the associated stress, infection or weight loss on the hypothalamic-gonadal axis have received adequate attention in these patients. Despite these reservations about the quality of the data, tentative guidelines can be drawn, which may be helpful to the physician dealing with this group of patients.

Although amenorrhea after radiation (Ray et al 1970, Shalet et al 1976, Thomas et al 1976) or after chemotherapy (Chapman et al 1979a) is common and may be prolonged and associated with menopausal symptoms and elevated gonadotropins (Schilsky et al 1980), recovery of normal fertility is not precluded. Resumption of menses, subsequent pregnancy, and the delivery of a normal child after 3–5 years of amenorrhea has been documented (Horning et al 1981). There is also a report of a 24-year-old woman who conceived and delivered a normal child despite 2 years of temporary amenorrhea followed by 4 years of irregular menses (Baker et al 1972). Age at the time of therapy (radiation and/or chemotherapy) is a critical variable in predicting a return of regular menses and the probability of a pregnancy (Horning et al 1981). At the age of 20, chemotherapy or radiation is associated with a probability of approximately 0.8 for maintaining regular menses, while combined modality therapy reduces the probability to approximately 0.4. By age 30, the probability of regular menses is markedly reduced in all groups (Horning et al 1981). In the same study, the interval after completion of therapy, the stage of disease, the number of cycles of chemotherapy, and the dose of radiation (with midline oophoropexy) were not significant factors predicting regular menses. Combination chemotherapy for Hodgkin's disease has also been shown to cause amenorrhea more commonly in patients over the age of 30 (Whitehead et al 1983), though patients below 30 should also be advised that they are at risk for premature menopause.

Adjuvant chemotherapy for breast cancer with cylophosphamide, methotrexate and fluorouracil (CMF) has been shown to cause permanent amenorrhea in 80% of treated patients. Younger patients under age 35 were more likely to retain or regain menses while on or following CMF therapy (Padmanabhan et al 1987, Beex et al 1988) confirmed these trends and in addition found a positive correlation between the age of the CMF treated patient and the progesterone receptor (PgR) status of the tumor. Ovarian suppression occurred predominantly in PgR-positive patients and permanent amenorrhea was associated with significantly longer relapse-free and overall survival times. In 1939 Jacox reported that a single dose of 500 rad to the ovaries resulted in 6–18 months of amenorrhea in young women, but permanent sterility in women over 40. When treatment requires radiation of the pelvic region, midline oophoropexy reduces the dose of radiation delivered to the ovaries to about 500 rads over 4 weeks (Baker et al 1972).

Although it would be reasonable to suspect that the dosage of chemotherapy would also be a significant variable, this has not been established. There are reports describing a relationship (Morganfeld et al 1972, Dnistrian et al 1983), and denying one (Sherman 1973, Horning et al 1981).

Uncertainty also exists about the role of duration of therapy; Shaw, citing Warne, among others, in a review of cyclophosphamide therapy (of nonmalignant disease) concluded that ovarian failure was related to duration of therapy rather than to age at the time of therapy (Shaw 1979).

The double insult of chemotherapy plus radiation was more damaging to gonadal function than either therapy alone, the difference being especially prominent in younger women. Only 20% of women receiving both modalities of therapy resumed regular menses (Horning et al 1981).

The morphological changes in the ovaries consequent to cancer therapy include a decreased number of oocytes (Warne et al 1973), fibrosis, arrest and destruction of follicles (Miller et al 1971, Sobrinho et al 1971, Shaw 1979). However, ovarian function may return despite a discouraging ovarian biopsy. A 24-year-old woman, who developed ovarian failure after cyclophosphamide therapy for nonmalignant disease, subsequently resumed menses despite a 1 × 0.3 cm ovarian biopsy showing only four ova and no primordial follicles (Warne et al 1973).

Shamberger has evaluated high-dose methotrexate therapy and has found no immediate ovarian toxicity (Shamberger et al 1981). Thus, at least in young women treated intensively for malignancy, a hopeless attitude with regard to fertility is not justified, even if menopausal symptoms are present for as long as 3–4 years. Replacement therapy should be considered to relieve symptoms in amenorrheic women; and hypothyroidism secondary to cervical radiation should be excluded in women with menstrual disturbances (Schimpff et al 1980). In addition the outcome of pregnancy is apparently good. In a report of 24 infants born to women treated for Hodgkin's disease, there were two premature births and one low-birthweight infant, but no increased incidence of abortions or fetal abnormalities (Horning et al 1981). Additionally, described in the literature are 1389 liveborn children to more than 844 cancer patients or survivors. Of these children 53, (4%) suffered from birth defects, a number comparable to that in the general population. Only two were born with true genetic disorders, one with trisomy 18 syndrome and one with Marfan's syndrome (Sherins & Mulvihill 1989). Increased rates of premature delivery and low birth rates have been documented in women having received cancer treatment (Mulvihill et al 1987), but may be limited to those who received abdominal irradiation and who were incapable of carrying the pregnancy to term due to uterine fibrosis and vascular insufficiency. The authors caution, however, that more sensitive means of detection of genetic disorders are warranted before definitive conclusions can be drawn.

In men, it is clear that chemotherapy with alkylating agents (Schilsky et al 1980), doxorubicin (DeCunha et al 1979), cytarabine (Lendon et al 1978), vinblastine (Vilar 1974) and especially procarbazine (Sieber et al 1978) damages the germinal epithelium of the testes. Morphological studies reveal germinal cell aplasia, atrophic tubules lined by Sertoli cells only, occasional spermatids or precursors, and normal appearing Leydig cells, (Schilsky et al 1980, Charak et al 1990), although they too may be functionally abnormal (Booth et al 1987). Although seminiferous tubule damage is the most prominent abnormality and results in testicular atrophy, oligoazoospermia and elevated FSH levels, the reduced libido, elevated LH levels (Charak et al 1990) and the LH hyperresponse to GnRH in the presence of normal or diminished testosterone levels indicate a degree of Leydig cell failure as well (Mecklenburg & Sherins 1974, Chapman et al 1979b, Waxman et al 1982, Whitehead et al 1982). The functional Leydig cell dysfunction contrasts with the intact morphology by light microscopy.

In pubertal boys, gynecomastia may be the first clinical evidence of Leyding cell dysfunction; estradiol levels are normal for age while testosterone levels are in the lower range (Sherins et al 1978). The damage appears to be progressive and dose related but without an established threshold either for the dose or for the period of therapy.

Recovery is unpredictable and may be related to the total dose received, type and combination of drugs, and length of post-therapy period (Schilsky et al 1980, Anselmo et al 1990, Charak et al 1990). Chemotherapeutic regimens for Hodgkin's lymphoma such as MOPP containing an alkylating agent have a greater gonadal toxicity than regimens such as ABVD without alkylating agents: full recovery of spermatogenesis was observed in 67% of ABVD patients as compared to 25% of MOPP-treated patients (Vivani et al 1985, Anselmo et al 1990). Once puberty has been completed, age at the time of therapy does not appear to determine the extent of gonadal damage or the probability of recovery in men of reproductive age. There is evidence that the prepubertal testes are less sensitive to damage by cyclophosphamide (Pennisi et al 1975). However, given a large enough dose of this drug, the prepubertal germinal epithelum is also injured (Rapola et al 1973, Etteldorf et al 1976, Lentz et al 1977). In a study of 14 boys, only one of whom was sexually mature at the onset of combined therapy with prednisone, vincristine, methotrexate and 6-mercaptopurine for acute lymphoblastic leukemia, normal sexual development was unimpeded. Gonadal function, as assessed by virilization, gonadotropins, testosterone levels, semen analysis and fertility (one patient) was maintained (Blatt et al 1981).

Elevation of prolactin and of TSH (hypothyroidism) have also been reported in men treated by combination chemotherapy for Hodgkin's disease (Chapman et al 1971) and must be excluded in men developing sexual dysfunction.

Patients facing combination chemotherapy for nonseminomatous testicular cancer can expect azoospermia with a 50% chance of recovery after 2–3 years (Nijman et al 1987). Approximately 75% of men with this disease have impaired sperm count before chemotherapy (Reed et al 1986). A worrying preliminary report of semen abnormalities in a third of patients with Hodgkin's disease has not been confirmed (Chapman et al 1971). In addition, approximately 40% of patients suffer from ejaculatory and sexual impairment after retroperitoneal lymph node dissection (Newton et al 1988). Surgical procedures are being modified in an attempt to preserve potency (Walsh et al 1983, Lange et al 1984, Walsh & Mostwin 1984, Garnick & Richie 1986), including sparing of the hypogastric arteries in radical prostatectomies and nerve-sparing procedures on men undergoing retroperitoneal lymph node dissection. Recently the technique of electroejaculation has been used in the event of ejaculatory failure following retroperitoneal lymph node dissection (Bennett et al 1987).

Since the likelihood of impaired spermatogenesis is very high after chemotherapy and since recovery is variable, unpredictable and may require even 4–5 years (Cheviakoff et al 1973, Buchanan et al 1975, Schilsky et al 1980), sperm banking must be seriously considered in young men anticipating chemotherapy. Encouraging conception rates of 50%–60% with preserved semen have been achieved (Sherman 1973, Ansbacher 1978, Curie-Cohen et al 1979, Scammell et al 1985). At the very least, the subject of sperm banking should be discussed with men of reproductive age facing chemotherapy.

## SELECTED DISEASES

### Thyroid disease

Hypothyroidism and hyperthyroidism are so easily treated that systematic long-term studies of their effects on fertility are all but impossible. These conditions are usually diagnosed and treated independently of their effects on reproductive function. Most fertility workups routinely include thyroid function tests, and while thyroid hormone continues to be dispensed freely in cases of both male and female subfertility, little objective evidence exists supporting such a practice in any but clear-cut cases of thyroidal hypofunction.

Thyroid hormones have major effects on reproductive tissues and processes in both men and women. These effects have been critically reviewed in recent textbooks (Ingbar & Braverman 1986, Yen & Jaffe 1986) and little new evidence has been published since to change their summaries significantly. Thyroid hormones affect the metabolism of every substance and the rate of every chemical reaction in the body, and it should therefore not be surprising that the complex processes of reproduction might be affected at a variety of sites by disturbances of thyroid function. In many of these situations so many changes are observed that it is not possible to designate which effects are primary and which are secondary.

Thyroid hormones increase the plasma concentration of SHBG several-fold (Ruder et al 1971, Tulchinsky & Chopra 1973), resulting in increased total plasma sex steroid hormone concentrations, with smaller changes in the free, or unbound, levels, and reduced metabolic clearance rate for these hormones (Gordon et al 1969, Ruder et al 1971). Estrogen clearance falls less than does that of testosterone (Chopra 1975), contributing to a disturbance of estrogen/testosterone balance. Enzymatic conversion of androgens, chiefly androstenedione, to estrogens, is increased by thyroid hormones (Southren et al 1974) as is the 2-hydroxylation of estrogens (Fishman et al 1965). The net effect is an elevation of plasma estradiol and estrone. LH levels are also elevated in states of hyperthyroidism (Chopra 1975), but it is not clear whether this is the result of a direct effect of thyroid hormone on the hypothalamic-pituitary axis or a consequence of the changes in SHBG, steroidal hormones and their metabolites. Hyperthyroid men have increased responsiveness to GnRH tests which revert to normal on treatment (Rodmark et al 1988).

In the view of the multiple effects of thyroid hormones on reproductive hormones it is not surprising that hyperthyroidism is associated with a variety of clinical disturbances in menstrual function. Hyperthyroidism in prepubertal girls brings on menarche slightly earlier than in a control population (Saxena et al 1964). Most commonly seen abnormalities are oligomenorrhea, reduced menstrual flow, amenorrhea and anovulation. However, many women retain normal menstrual patterns and others even have menometrorrhagia, more typical of hypothyroidism. In a study of 15 thyrotoxic women, Akande (1975) noted that all had elevated plasma LH, FSH and estrogen levels, but that midcycle gonadotropin peak levels were usually present only in menstruating patients.

No reliable data are available, and none are

likely to become available, on the precise frequency and degree of fertility problems in women with hyperthyroidism. From the coincidence of thyrotoxicosis and pregnancy, it is clear that pregnancy occurs with considerable frequency even in women with definite thyrotoxicosis. In all likelihood mild to moderate thyrotoxicosis does not adversely affect fertility (Burrow 1981). It is, however, obvious that the high incidence of anovulation and other menstrual disorders in thyrotoxicosis must mean reduced fertility. It is generally believed, though not conclusively proven, that the incidence of first trimester abortions is higher in untreated hyperthyroidism. The subsequent management of the pregnant thyrotoxic patient is now relatively standardized, and good maternal and fetal outcomes are the norm. It is important to be aware that the placental passage of thyroid stimulating immunoglobulin to the fetus can result in transitory thyrotoxicosis even in well-controlled patients with Graves' disease.

Hyperthyroidism is much less common in men than in women, and its effects on male human fertility have hardly been studied. The effects of excess estrogen (Chopra & Tulchinsky 1974) in hyperthyroid man are most clearly noted by the signs of gynecomastia, sipider angiomas, smooth skin and decreased libido (Becker et al 1968) which are readily reversible by appropriate therapy of the thyrotoxicosis. Testicular size and consistency are usually normal, but few data are available on testicular histology.

Disorders of the menstrual cycle, usually menometrorrhagia, but occasionally even amenorrhea, are common in hypothyroidism and many of the cycles seem to be anovulatory (Goldsmith et al 1952, Akande 1975). Often the midcycle gonadotropin surge is absent and progesterone levels remain low throughout the cycle (Akande 1975). Estrogen levels are relatively low and constant (Akande 1975). The reported hormonal changes are opposite to those seen in hyperthyroidism and reflect a reduction in SHBG, an increase in estradiol metabolic clearance, an increased production of estriol at the expense of estrone, and enhancement of conversion of androstenedione to testosterone (Fishman et al 1965, Gordon et al 1969). Obviously the

high frequency of anovulation seriously reduces the fertility of hypothyroid women. Thus in cases of persistent anovulation following failure of empirical ovulation-inducing therapy, thyroid function should be evaluated in order to rule out mild hypothyroidism as a major or contributing cause of infertility. (See also Chapters 9 and 26). A recent series of 210 women enrolled in an infertility clinic and screened for subclinical hypothyroidism by the measurement of serum TSH revealed a slightly increased (11.3%) incidence of subclinical hypothyroidism in dysovulatory women (Strickland et al 1990). Patients with longstanding primary hypothyroidism may sometimes present with elevated serum prolactin levels, galactorrhea and amenorrhea with pituitary computerized tomographic scans which demonstrate 'pituitary tumors' (Grubb et al 1987). All the abnormalities including the 'pseudo tumor' disappear after thyroxine administration.

With respect to the results of pregnancy in hypothyroid women, a collective review of the literature by Potter (1980) suggests high rates of abortions, stillbirths and congenital anomalies in untreated hypothyroid women. But many of the cases came from small series, poorly studied, and with tests of thyroid function inadequate by present day standards. A series of 11 cases of hypothyroid pregnant women found one stillborn infant in a patient with pre-eclampsia, and a second infant with Down's syndrome and an ostium primum defect (Montoro et al 1981). The very nature of the study, dealing largely with patients presenting to the obstetrician, excluded those patients who may have had first trimester losses, reported to be extraordinarily high (Burrow 1977). Data in rats (Stempak 1962, Varma et al 1978) indicate reduced fertility and litter size in hypothyroidism. Prospective epidemiological studies to decide on the effects of hypothyroidism in humans on the various indices under question are, of course, impossible and the question will remain open.

It is important to emphasize that hypothyroid women on replacement therapy should not discontinue or reduce the dose in the event of pregnancy, as they are commonly erroneously advised.

In men primary hypothyroidism is relatively

uncommon and not widely studied. It is likely that severe myxedema is associated with abnormal spermatogenesis and Leydig cell atrophy (Taymor & Selenkow 1958, De La Balze et al 1962, Griboff 1962), but that mild hypothyroidism is not. A recent study of eight men with primary hypothyroidism revealed a variety of serious abnormalities of gonadal function (Wortsman et al 1987), but short-term withdrawal of replacement thyroid hormone in hypothyroid men resulted only in slight seminal anomalies, not enough to affect fertility (Corrales-Hernandez et al 1990).

## Diabetes mellitus

While most of the standard textbooks of obstetrics usually make general comments about the impaired fertility of diabetic women, objective modern data are sparse. Many of the older data relate to poorly controlled, malnourished women in whom amenorrhea would be expected to be relatively common. Most of the modern literature relates to the management of pregnancy in the diabetic woman and to problems of sexual dysfunction but not to fertility problems. Although amenorrhea, late menarche, oligomenorrhea (Burkat et al 1989), low pregnancy rate, and early menopause have all been reported in diabetic women, the etiology of these disorders is unclear. Low basal prolactin (Djursing et al 1982) and a blunted prolactin response to metoclopramide (Prelevic et al 1987) suggest a role for increased hypothalamic dopaminergic activity in menstrual dysfunction in diabetic women. In addition, functional hypothalamic-pituitary amenorrhea has also been described (Djursing 1987). The premature menopause associated with type I diabetes has been attributed to associated autoimmune disease and the production of antibodies against ovarian steroid-producing cells (Alper & Garner 1985). Recently a gonadotropic function has been attributed to insulin (Poretsky & Kalin 1987), which has been found in follicular fluid, a function which is supported by the observation that decreased beta-cell function is associated with an increased incidence of amenorrhea (Prelevic et al 1989) and delayed menarche (Burkat et al 1989) in type I diabetes but not in type II diabetics. Conversely, hyperinsulinemia is

associated with hyperandrogenism and the classical profile of PCOD (Prelevic et al 1989). Poretsky & Kalin (1987) in their review of the subject, suggest that insulin alone or in concert with FSH and LH is necessary for steroidogenesis in the ovary (see also Chapter 6). Lack of insulin causes ovarian hypofunction, and insulin excess increases steroidogenesis causing hyperandrogenism. Prolonged exposure of the ovary to excess insulin may cause morphological changes such as hyperthecosis and polycystic changes. The effects of insulin on the ovary are mediated by the insulin receptor and possibly through the IGF-I receptor. The postulated mechanisms by which insulin affects ovarian steroidogenesis include direct action on steroidogenic enzymes, modulation of FSH or LH receptor number or function or a nonspecific effect on cell viability. Low LH levels, LH/FSH ratio and decreased testosterone levels found in insulinopenic type I amenorrheic diabetics but not in amenorrheic diabetics with residual beta-cell function also suggest a role for insulin on hypothalamic-pituitary function in type I diabetics (Prelevic et al 1989).

Despite all the above a significant number of diabetic women become pregnant and a significant number of pregnant women develop gestational diabetes during their pregnancy. The outcome of diabetic pregnancy has improved significantly since the clear demonstration that tight metabolic control can dramatically reduce the frequency of the complications of pregnancy in the diabetic (Pederson 1954, Freinkel 1980, Gabbe 1980). The success in metabolic control of the pregnant diabetic has been aided by the use of hemoglobin Alc measurements as an index of control, multiple insulin injections, insulin infusion pumps and of home-glucose monitoring aids, and by the detailed and sophisticated tools available for evaluation of fetal maturation and distress. Perinatal survival has been increased also by improved neonatal intensive care. It has been demonstrated that good diabetic control early in pregnancy is associated with a decreased incidence of congenital anomalies (Miller et al 1981, Fuhrmann et al 1983) and this had suggested that perhaps efforts need to be expanded to achieve normal maternal metabolism even before conception (Freinkel 1981) in order to assure a good fetal outcome. However, the National Institute of Child Health and Human Development Diabetes in Early Pregnancy study (Mills et al 1988) did not demonstrate the expected decrease in fetal malformations associated with tight blood glucose control, finding 4.9% in the diabetics versus 2.1% in controls with the same level of glycemia and HbAlc. Nevertheless, the study did find a 50% lower malformation rate in patients brought under tight control early in pregnancy as opposed to patients enrolled in the study after organogenesis. Thus it would appear prudent to recommend tight metabolic control to diabetic women planning pregnancy.

Diabetic women have been reported to have a much higher incidence of failure to achieve orgasm than do normal women (Kolodny 1971). Ellenberg (1977) on the other hand denies any disturbance in sexual function in diabetic women, a surprising finding in view of the high incidence of neuropathy. More recently, Schreiner-Engel et al (1987) found that women with type I diabetes suffered no more sexual difficulties than controls, while type II diabetic women had significantly more sexual dysfunctions such as lubrication problems, dyspareunia, problems reaching orgasm, as well as sexual dissatisfaction, than controls. Impaired neurovascular processes which regulate genital vasocongestion cause the lubrication deficiency in a manner analogous to erectile impairment in men. The reasons for the differential effects of the different types of diabetes on sexual function are not entirely clear, but are probably related to the age of onset of the disease and the impact of the disease on perception of self-image and sexual role.

Diabetic men have several well-recognized problems which impair their fertility but are unrelated to actual gonadal function. The existence, extent and importance of gonadal damage or dysfunction are less clearly established.

Impotence, which is extraordinarily frequent in diabetic men, is probably related to neuropathy as well as to vascular insufficiency (Goldstein et al 1983), and occurs in one out of four diabetics aged 30–35 and in 75% of those in the 60–65 years age group (Rubin & Babbot 1958). The overall incidence is 40–60% (Rubin & Babbot

1958, Ellenberg 1971). While some would implicate hormonal disorders as contributing factors (Schöffling et al 1963), the great majority of diabetologists consider the problem to be unrelated to hormonal imbalance (Ellenberg 1971, Kolodny et al 1974b) and not to respond to hormonal therapy. Psychogenic factors, as well as drug-induced impotence, are common in the diabetic population, and multiple etiologies often exist in the same patient. Nocturnal penile tumescence, penile/brachial pressure determinations, Doppler ultrasound, the papaverine test and invasive techniques aid in determining the etiology of impotence in the diabetic (Zorgniotti & Liza 1988). Papaverine injections, mechanical aids as well as silicone rubber penile prostheses may be considered as in other cases of otherwise untreatable impotence.

Another less common cause of infertility in diabetic men is retrograde ejaculation, caused by diabetic neuropathy (Greene et al 1963, Ellenberg & Weber 1966, Kolodny et al 1974b). This problem is not always brought to the attention of the physician to whom the couple turn for help in fertility problems and is particularly likely to be overlooked when the problem is only partial. Pregnancy may be induced by collecting a post-ejaculation specimen of urine, washing and concentrating of the semen, and subsequent artificial insemination (Walters & Kaufman 1959) (see also Chapters 12 and 25).

The evaluation of the hypothalamic-pituitary testicular axis in diabetic men has been carried out by numerous investigators, but the results have been singularly unimpressive in demonstrating a clear pathological pattern and have shown no correlation with reported sexual dysfunction. Testosterone levels have been reported as normal in diabetics (Greene et al 1963, Ellenberg 1971) and in diabetics treated with insulin or diet, but low in those treated with sulfonylureas (Greene et al 1963, Ellenberg 1971, Shahwan et al 1978). Jensen et al (1979) also found largely normal levels but with occasional high or low values. Fushimi et al (1989) found lower free testosterone levels in poorly controlled diabetics compared to well-controlled men and those in turn had significantly lower levels than age-matched controls suggesting gonadal dysfunction in diabetes. Lemaire examined the basal levels of serum testosterone, free testosterone, androstenedione, dihydrotestosterone, SHBG and estradiol, as well as a variety of other hormones, and found all the basal levels to be normal (Lemaire et al 1981). SHBG was reported by Wright et al (1976) to be slightly low. In response to the injection of GnRH, LH has been reported to be normal (Rastogi et al 1974, Jensen et al 1979) or blunted (Wright et al 1976, Distiller et al 1975, Shahwan et al 1978) and FSH to be normal (Wright et al 1976), blunted (Distiller et al 1975) or occasionally increased (Wright et al 1976, Shahwan et al 1978, Jensen et al 1979). It is clear from reviewing the data in the literature that with the exception of the occasional FSH hyperresponsiveness, which may indeed be explained on the basis of gonadal insufficiency, no consistent abnormality can be demonstrated in diabetic men, whether potent or not.

There are limited data also with respect to semen quality in diabetics. Ejaculate volume has been reported to be normal (Barták et al 1975) or low (Rubin 1962, Schöffling 1971), and sperm counts normal or high (Barták et al 1975, Klebanow & Macleod 1960), or low in as many as a third of the patients (Schöffling 1971). Impaired sperm motility as well as an increase in abnormal forms has been observed by several investigators (Rubin 1962, Schöffling 1971, Barták et al 1975). There are also reports of abnormalities on testicular biopsy with decreased spermatogenesis and partial maturation arrest (Schöffling 1971) in diabetic men. These data are in accord also with animal models of diabetes, such as that induced by streptozotocin in rats (Paz & Homonnai 1979a) in which severe impairment of fertility and spermatogenesis have been observed. In the animal studies in particular (Paz & Homonnai 1979a, b) but also in some of the human studies, the diabetes was severe and often under poor control. In the animal studies of Paz & Homonnai (1979b) the investigators could not duplicate the abnormalities by severe inanition and could correct them fully by treatment with both insulin and chorionic gonadotropin but not by either alone, nor by insulin plus testosterone. It is not clear to what extent these conclusions are valid for human diabetes. Available data do not permit firm conclusions as to consistent abnormalities in spermatogenesis in reasonably well-controlled diabetics. Probably most such subjects have only minor abnormalities, if any at all.

## Acquired immunodeficiency syndrome (AIDS)

A great deal of the recent medical literature has been devoted to AIDS and its complications including the maternal–fetal transfer of the disease, but very few studies or reports have dealt with the question of the effects of AIDS on fertility. De Paepe & Waxman (1989) reported the histological features of the testes of 57 AIDS patients and found a lower degree of spermatogenesis, prominent thickening of the basement membrane and interstitial fibrosis when compared to heterosexual controls without AIDS. The cause of the testicular atrophy has not been determined but several factors may act in concert to cause the damage: malnutrition, testicular infection, chemotherapy, zinc deficiency and antisperm antibodies. Supporting evidence for this last cause has been provided by Nunez et al (1987) who found higher titers of antisperm antibodies in a patient with AIDS than in heterosexual males without AIDS. As the AIDS epidemic continues we can expect more insight into this aspect of the disease.

## Chronic renal failure

An impaired reproductive capacity, often heralded by a decreased libido and erectile dysfunction, is a well-recognized consequence of renal failure (Elstein et al 1969, Bailey 1977, Massry et al 1980). A recent study indicates that patients who became ill before adulthood were less likely to have married or have had children (Schover et al 1990). The issues related to the reproductive capacity in chronic renal failure have been comprehensively reviewed (Handelsman 1985).

Disturbances in homeostasis at all levels of the hypothalamic-gonadal axis have been identified. In addition, decreased renal degradation of hormones is an important mechanism in these patients and results in a normal, or increased, LH peak in response to GnRH and an extended half-life. (Schalch et al 1975, Holdsworth et al 1977).

Low testosterone levels, not explained by a decrease in SHBG, and an abnormally decreased response to hCG, indicate primary hypogonadism (Chen et al 1970). Testicular size diminishes and semen volume, sperm density and sperm motility are all decreased (Freeman et al 1968, Schmitt 1968, Elstei et al 1969, Chen et al 1970, Lim & Fang 1975). Histological changes consisting of reduced numbers of Leydig cells, hyalinization of the tubular basement membranes, and paucity of spermatogonia (Schmitt et al 1968, Bailey 1977, Holdsworth et al 1977) may also occur in children and adolescents with chronic renal failure (Burke et al 1989).

Since gonadotropins, as evidenced by testosterone levels, are disproportionately low in these men, there must be a disturbance at the hypothalamic-pituitary level as well (Lim & Fang 1975). A paradoxical positive correlation between serum testosterone and LH levels has been observed (Lim et al 1978). Moreover, an exaggerated FSH response to clomiphene (Lim & Fang 1975) observed in the majority of the patients, and the normal peak response of LH to GnRH, indicate a defect at the hypothalamic rather than the pituitary level. A similarly diminished feedback response to low plasma testosterone despite a normal response to clomiphene has been observed in nonuremic men with hypogonadotropic hypogonadism associated with hyposmia, and in the Prader–Willi syndrome (Hamilton et al 1973). It is interesting that this presumed hypothalamic disturbance in chronic renal failure disappears following renal transplantation, but is not altered during hemodialysis, suggesting that a nondialysable factor may be involved (Lim et al 1978).

Hyperprolactinemia is observed in more than 50% of men and women with chronic renal failure. The significance of hyperprolactinemia in the pathogenesis of the sexual and reproductive dysfunction in uremic patients is illustrated by the observation of an increase in basal LH and resumed menses in some patients following suppression of prolactin secretion by bromocriptine (Gómez et al 1980). Hyperprolactinemia develops as a result of both decreased renal degradation and increased pituitary production of prolactin (Emmanouel et al 1980). Prolactin secretion may be further increased by concurrent use of drugs stimulating prolactin secretion. Abnormal prolactin responses to stimulatory (TRH, chlorpromazine) and inhibitory (L-dopa, bromocriptine) agents suggest relative lactotroph insensitivity to dopamine and a defect in the regulation of prolactin secretion (Ramirez et al 1977, Gómez et al 1980); however, specific details are lacking.

In women, menstrual abnormalities appear as the serum creatinine rises above 2–3 mg/dl (Rice 1973). Persistently low progesterone levels, flat basal body temperature curves, lack of positive feedback response to exogenous estrogen and absence of pulsatile release of gonadotropins indicate a hypothalamically mediated anovulatory state (Lim et al 1978, Perez et al 1978). In addition, an ovarian defect is suggested by a failure of estrogen and progesterone levels to rise from low or low normal, despite significant increase in gonadotropins following administration of clomiphene (Lim et al 1978, Swamy et al 1979).

Sexual desire often improves within 1–2 months following initiation of hemodialysis (Lindsay et al 1967, Bailey 1977). A favorable effect of hemodialysis on male fertility has not been definitely established (Elstein et al 1969, Finkelstein et al 1976, DeKretser 1979). In women menses may return, but ovulation is uncommon and successful pregnancies are rare (Goodwin et al 1968, Ackrill et al 1975), but some have occurred and were managed in women on chronic ambulatory peritoneal dialysis (CAPD) (Redrow et al 1988). On the other hand cycles with menorrhagia may require oral contraceptive therapy and in extreme cases, hysterectomy (Rice 1973, Perez et al 1978).

Following successful renal transplantation, LH levels increase initially until testosterone levels reach normal, and finally stabilize at a level lower than pretransplantation (Lim et al 1975, Holdsworth et al 1978, Lim et al 1978, Schover et al 1990). In many men sexual dysfunction improves, but 20–43% remain impotent (Penn et al 1980, Schover et al 1990). Obviously, section of the spermatic cord during transplantation will result in infertility and removal of the internal iliac arteries, usually during a second transplantation, could result in impotence due to vascular insufficiency of the corpora cavernosa (Burns et al 1979). Restoration of reproductive potential depends upon the degree of seminiferous tubule damage present at the time of transplantation. A recent study indicates that while recovery of spermatogenesis is substantial, its final level falls short of that in normal individuals (Netto et al 1980). A persistently increased FSH level represents a poor prognostic sign for future fertility (Holdsworth et al 1978).

In a review of 697 renal transplant patients in whom fecundity was possible in 376 cases, 50 men and 37 women were fertile (Penn et al 1980). There was a negligible risk to the offspring of male transplant patients. Pregnancy after renal transplantation has recently been reviewed (Gaudier et al 1988). Pregnancies of female transplant patients are associated with potential hazards both to mother and offspring. In a review of 40 pregnancies in renal transplant patients the incidence of spontaneous abortions, stillbirths, and ruptured ectopic pregnancies was similar to that in a normal pregnant population. However, 26% of the pregnancies were artificially terminated because of a deterioration in maternal renal function, hypertension, ureteral or ilial loop compression, or emotional instability (Rudolph et al 1979). A risk of about 30% exists for preeclampsia (Rudolph et al 1979, Penn et al 1980). Prematurity is reported in 20–45% of all live births (Rudolph et al 1979, Penn et al 1980) and is the result of compromised maternal renal function and in utero exposure to corticosteroid medication. Neonatal complications occur in 25% of live births and include respiratory distress, adrenocortical insufficiency and septicemia (Penn et al 1980).

The reduced life expectancy of many patients should be a consideration in fertility counselling.

## Systemic lupus erythematosus (SLE)

SLE is the prototype of autoimmune disorders. The disease affects primarily women in the reproductive age and is characterized by the production of pathological clones of antibodies directed against self antigens. Multiple organs are involved in a vasculitic process in which the kidney is frequently affected, resulting in renal failure. Reproduction is often impaired (Ramsey-Goldman 1988, Dombroski 1989).

In periods of remission or mild disease activity fertility is not affected (Bulmash 1978, MacCarthy & Pollak 1981) and a long disease-free period prior to conception is associated with a favorable outcome of pregnancy (Devoe & Taylor 1979). However, spontaneous abortion, fetal wastage and stillbirth are frequent (30%) (Devoe & Taylor 1979, Hayslett & Lynn 1980, Lieb 1981). Fetal wastage approaches 50% in pregnancies associated with proteinuria of more than 300 mg/24 h or creatinine clearance of less than 100 ml/min (Hayslett & Lynn 1980, Lieb 1981). This increased fetal loss, and the enhanced perinatal risk due to intrauterine growth retardation and immaturity, can be ascribed to placental insufficiency consequent to placental lupus vasculitis (Grennan et al 1978). The presence of lupus anticoagulant has been implicated with increased fetal death and spontaneous abortions, even in the absence of other clinical signs of SLE (Hayslett & Reece 1985). Newborns of affected mothers carry an overall risk of 1:60 for neonatal SLE, but neonatal SLE is even more frequently associated with maternal anti-Ro (SSA) antibodies and in that case carries a 1:20 risk for congenital heart block (Ramsey-Goldman et al 1986). Medications (high-dose glucocorticoids and immunosuppressive drugs) employed during pregnancy may further worsen this perinatal risk (Barrett 1981).

An adverse influence on SLE during pregnancy and postpartum, although uncertain and controversial, has not been excluded (Cecere & Persellin 1981, Mintz et al 1986, Meehan & Dorsey 1987) and has been ascribed to a stimulatory effect of estrogen on the immunological disorder (Hayslett & Reece 1985). However, it seems that improved management of the disease and avoidance of conception at the time of active disease can minimize the frequency of both renal and nonrenal complications and that many 'therapeutic' abortions done in the past may have had little, if any, beneficial effect on the course of the disease (Devoe & Taylor 1979, Danovitch 1981).

In men, aside from an association between SLE and Kleinfelter's syndrome (Fane et al 1980), we are unaware of any direct effect of lupus on male fertility. Despite the myriad immunological abnormalities recognized in SLE, there are no reports of abnormality due to antisperm antibodies or immune-mediated damage of the testes or the ejaculatory tract in men suffering from lupus.

## Familial Mediterranean fever (FMF; recurrent polyserositis)

FMF is an inherited disorder of unknown etiology characterized by recurrent episodes of one or more of the symptoms including fever, peritonitis, pleuritis, arthritis or skin lesions. Jews of North African origin, Arabs, Turks and Armenians are among the most affected populations. Amyloidosis is seen as a late complication in some patients. Colchicine is currently used extensively to reduce the rate and intensity of the attacks and prevent amyloidosis (Zemer et al 1980).

Untreated men probably have normal fertility, but among colchicine-treated patients infertility, due to azoospermia or impaired sperm penetration, may reach 20% (Ehrenfeld et al 1986).

Infertility has been reported in up to 30% of untreated women suffering of the disease (Ismajovich et al 1973), and is due mainly to ovulatory dysfunction (Ismajovich et al 1973, Ehrenfeld et al 1987). Peritoneal adhesions were not more prevalent in those patients than in the general population women examined for infertility (Ehrenfeld et al 1987). The possibility of adverse sperm–ovum interaction due to increased neutrophil chemotaxis has been suggested (Ehrenfeld et al 1987). An increased rate (25–30%) of pregnancies terminated in miscarriage (Ehrenfeld et al 1987).

Colchicine does not seem to have any significant beneficial effect on fecundity. Nor are there adverse effects on the outcome of pregnancy in women suffering from FMF which could be ascribed to the treatment (Zemer et al 1980, Pras et al 1984, Ehrenfeld et al 1987). Discontinuation of treatment once pregnancy is contemplated or achieved is not recommended.

## Cystic fibrosis

Cystic fibrosis is an autosomal recessive disease characterized by abnormally thick secretions affecting primarily mucous glands. The clinical manifestations are the result of obstruction of organ passages and present mainly as chronic pulmonary disease and pancreatic insufficiency (DiSant'Agnese & Davis 1976). Although earlier reports described a dismal 98% incidence of azoospermia (Denning et al 1968, Kaplan et al 1968), the severity of the disease is variable, and men with normal semen and with progeny have been reported (Taussig et al 1972, Frydman 1979).

Initial studies stressed abnormalities of seminal composition (Denning et al 1968, Kaplan et al 1968), but it is clear now that the sterility should be attributed to structural defects in the ejaculatory tract. There is obstruction or absence of the epididymis (appreciated on physical examination) as well as of the seminal vesicles and the vas deferens (Kaplan et al 1968, DiSant'Agnese & Davis 1979). Whether these abnormalities represent further primary expression of a double genetic defect, or should be ascribed to degeneration and atrophy consequent to secretory obstruction of the vas deferens, is uncertain (DiSant'Agnese 1968). The appearance of these mesonephric structural abnormalities at an early developmental stage suggests that they are primary abnormalities and not secondary to obstruction (Zondek & Zondek 1980). The possibility that some of the older reports on epididymal abnormalities in cystic fibrosis may in fact be related to the Young's syndrome should be considered (Handelsman et al 1984)(see below).

Recently, successful pregnancies have been achieved by in vitro fertilization (IVF) with sperm from the epididymis and vas deferens of men with congenital absence of the vas deferens (Silber et al 1990)(see also Chapter 24). Since testicular biopsies reveal active spermatogenesis and only mild changes (Denning et al 1968, Kaplan et al 1968) we would suggest that men with mild as well as with controlled disease might be considered as candidates for either similar attempts for in vitro fertilization or for surgical reconstruction of the seminal transport system.

Although less severely affected, only 20% of female patients are fertile (Frydman 1979). The infertility is due to the abnormal composition and viscosity of the cervical mucus. A successful attempt to bypass this defect by direct intrauterine insemination (IUI) has been reported (Kredentser et al 1986).

Although it is reasonable to anticipate disturbances of the hypothalamic-pituitary-ovarian axis in severely ill women with cystic fibrosis, this has not been reported.

The pseudopregnancy of oral contraception may aggravate the course of the disease by enhancing hyperplasia and hypersecretion of the goblet cells (Frydman 1979, LeRoy et al 1980). However, pregnancy does *not* seem to impose an additional hazard on the patient (Frydman 1979, Neri & Ovadia 1980), although there are reports of increased fetal loss (Denning et al 1968, DiSant'Agnese & Davis 1979).

Clearly the reduced life expectancy of the woman with cystic fibrosis will be a serious consideration in family planning (Frydman 1979). Since the infertility is a mechanical problem, the infertile, but otherwise mildly ill woman, if highly motivated to be pregnant, should be considered for IUI (Kredentser et al 1986) or IVF.

## Young's syndrome

This relatively newly recognized entity overlaps both cystic fibrosis and the immotile cilia syndrome (Hendry et al 1978, Umeki 1988), manifesting itself by sinopulmonary infections due to abnormal mucociliary clearance (Pavia et al 1980). It is also characterized by obstructive azoospermia. Young's syndrome has been ascribed as a common cause of sinopulmonary infection and azoospermia (Handelsman et al 1984). Respiratory function is only mildly affected. Hormonal indices and libido are preserved. The epididymides are enlarged or cystic, with abundant spermatozoa on puncture of the epididymal head, but no sperm is present in the middle region of the epididymis or below. The vas deferens is normal, unlike some cases of cystic fibrosis. Spermatogenesis, evaluated by testicular

histology, is usually normal, although dilated seminiferous tubules have been observed in some cases. Unlike congenital absence of the vas deferens and following vasectomy, sperm antibodies are absent. Other causes for chronic sinopulmonary infections are readily excluded by the normal levels of serum α 1-antitrypsin, normal sweat test and normal electron microscopic features of the cilia on bronchial mucosal biopsy (Handelsman et al 1984). Attempts at IVF with sperm obtained from the epididymis or vas deferens should be considered (Silber et al 1990). We are not aware of reports of this syndrome in women.

## Immotile cilia syndrome

Kartagener's syndrome, or the immotile cilia syndrome, is an autosomal recessive disorder manifest as various combinations of sinusitis, bronchiectasis and visceral transposition (Greenstone et al 1988). Male infertility due to impaired sperm motility is common (Afzelius & Eliasson 1983) and it is estimated that one in 5000 men referred to fertility clinics suffer from this syndrome (Eliasson et al 1977). A similar syndrome, including chronic sinopulmonary infections, infertility and situs inversus has been described in English Springer Spaniel dogs (Edwards et al 1989).

In men, testicular biopsies reveal only minimal changes, and both seminal fluid volume and sperm density are normal. In spite of findings in one patient which revealed a shortened sperm survival time (less than 24 h) and abnormal sperm heads, routine microscopic examination is usually unremarkable (Arge 1960; see also Chapters 11 and 12) Electron microscopic studies of the sperm tail and of cilia from various epithelial surfaces have demonstrated an ultrastructural defect. The most characteristic abnormality is a deletion of the dynein arms which form temporary bridges between adjacent microtubules in a process which generates ciliary movement (Afzelius 1976, Sturgess et al 1979). As a consequence of the defect, both ciliary transport and sperm motility are compromised (Eliasson et al 1977) resulting in respiratory tract infections and infertility. Nevertheless, there is at least one report of so-called mosaicism in which infertility due to ultrastructurally and functionally abnormal spermatic cilia occurred without concurrent respiratory tract involvement (Walt et al 1983). Recently, fertilization of ova by microinjection of a single immotile spermatozoon into the perivitelline space has been reported. However, no pregnancy resulted from embryo transfer (Bongso et al 1989).

Transport of the ovum is partially dependent on an organized movement of tubal cilia (Guha & Anand 1979). The functional abnormalities of ciliary motion in the Fallopian tubes may consist of immotility or erratic movement. A temporal similarity between the ciliary ultrastructural and functional abnormalities in the respiratory tract and in the Fallopian tubes has been reported (McComb et al 1986). The extent of female reproductive capacity seems to be only partially compromised in some reports (Greenstone et al 1988). However, in another report, pregnancy occurred in only two out of 12 women who attempted to become pregnant (Afzelius & Eliasson 1983).

## Sarcoidosis

A thorough review of the endocrine aspects of sarcoidosis was published in 1968 (Winnacker et al 1968), and few developments of significance have appeared since. Sarcoidosis can impair reproductive capacity by direct involvement of the genital organs or by hypothalamic-pituitary infiltration. Although the diagnosis may be suspected in the presence of typical pulmonary lesions, cutaneous abnormalties, a positive gallium scan (Nosal et al 1979) and elevated angiotensin-converting enzyme levels (Nosal et al 1979, Shultz et al 1979, Rohatgi et al 1981), final proof requires tissue examination.

In men, granulomas have been noted as incidental findings in the prostate and seminal vesicles, and clinically significant involvement of the epididymis, testes, spermatic cord, scrotum and penis have also been described (Winnacker et al 1968). A unilateral painless or painful induration of the epididymis, persisting despite resolution of the disease elsewhere, is the commonest form of male genital sarcoidosis (Winnacker et al

1967, Hefffernan & Blenkinsopp 1978). The disease may present as an acute corticosteroid-responsive epididymitis (Winnacker et al 1967).

Testicular involvement is, in most instances, microscopic and not associated with hypogonadism, but tumorous enlargement of the testes has been reported (Krauss 1958). Biopsy is essential since sarcoid may coexist with testicular neoplasm (Geller et al 1977).

There are scattered reports of genital sarcoidosis in women involving the uterus, cervix, vagina and Fallopian tubes, and associated with menometrorrhagia (Winnacker et al 1968) and infertility (Winslow & Funkhouser 1968). Although in the anergic patient without evidence of tuberculosis sarcoidosis of the Fallopian tubes might be suspected on salpingography, endometrial biopsy or surgical exploration is required to exclude tuberculosis (Campbell et al 1964).

The patient well enough to present with a complaint of infertility, impotence or amenorrhea, is unlikely to have prominent systemic manifestations of sarcoidosis or major intracranial disease, i.e. meningitis, hydrocephalus, hemiplegia, or disturbance of thirst or thermoregulation (Waxman & Sher 1979). Although clinically significant CNS involvement is rare, sarcoid granulomas may be observed at autopsy, and hypothalamic-pituitary infiltrates may be associated with hypogonadism (Waxman et al 1979). Hypogonadism, when present, may be a result of hyperprolactinemia, itself a consequence of hypothalamic involvement (Turkington & Macindoe 1972), or a result of destructive lesions of the anterior pituitary or the hypothalamus. Even in the absence of pulmonary sarcoid or characteristic skin lesions, the combination of diabetes insipidus and anterior pituitary deficits should raise the possibility of sarcoid. It should be noted that anterior pituitary deficits are more often due to hypothalamic disease than to pituitary infiltration. The pituitary usually shows a normal response to stimulation with hypothalamic releasing hormones (Stuart et al 1978), and autopsy studies demonstrate the greatest involvement in the hypothalamus, the brain stem, and the posterior lobe of the pituitary (Winnacker et al 1968, Turkington et al 1972,

Waxman et al 1979). Even when visual field defects are also present, suggesting pituitary destruction with suprasellar involvement, the field defects are usually due to direct infiltration of the optic nerve.

Standard radiography of the sella is generally normal (Winnacker et al 1968), and calcification in the absence of infection is not seen (Israel et al 1961, Scadding 1961). However, enhancing lesions of the pituitary have been recognized by computerized axial tomography (CT) and removed by transsphenoidal hypophysectomy (Decker et al 1979). Reports of the use of gallium scans have not included patients with hypothalamic-pituitary involvement (Nosal et al 1979).

Spinal fluid examination reveals a lymphocytic pleocytosis, occasionally a low sugar, and almost always an elevation, occasionally marked, of spinal fluid protein (Shealy et al 1961, Winnacker et al 1968), although a normal CSF has also been reported (Silverstein et al 1965).

Although spontaneous improvement has been documented (Hook 1954), it is our opinion that in view of the serious potential complications of CNS sarcoid, any evidence of CNS involvement warrants corticosteroid therapy. The systemic symptoms, neurological signs (especially of short duration), and disturbance of thirst may improve but the endocrine deficit usually persists, requiring replacement therapy (Shealy et al 1961, Winnacker et al 1968, Stuart et al 1978).

In summary, the fertility of the patient with sarcoid is threatened by direct genital involvement, and more frequently by granulomatous inflammation of the hypothalamus. Because of the inaccessibility of the hypothalamus, it may be necessary to start corticosteroid therapy on the basis of clinical and radiological findings compatible with hypothalamic-pituitary disease and biopsy proof of extracranial sarcoidosis.

## Liver disease

Impairment of endocrine homeostasis in alcoholic men with liver cirrhosis has been recognized for centuries. Major progress in elucidation of the pathogenesis of these abnormalities has occurred only in the last two decades. A conceptual breakthrough which has greatly facilitated our understanding of the complexities of the disease process was the differentiation between hypogonadism and feminization (Van Thiel et al 1985). Manifestations of the former include testicular atrophy, reduced fertility, libido and potency, reduced beard growth and reduced free and total plasma testosterone. Feminization is manifested by gynecomastia, female escutcheon, palmar erythema, spider angiomas and increased level of estrogen-responsive proteins of pituitary and hepatic origin. A further critical differentation is that between the effects of alcohol per se as separate from liver disease. The data resulting from these more precise definitions and observations are far from complete but clear trends are appearing.

For an even clearer understanding of the pathophysiology of observed changes it is essential for studies to control the data with respect to the nature and the severity of the liver pathology, the degree of portal-systemic shunting, the age of the patient and the ingestion of drugs which might have their own intrinsic effects. Few studies thus far meet these criteria.

Patients with hypogonadism and feminization associated with alcoholic liver disease generally have low plasma total testosterone and dihydrotestosterone levels, and a reduced production rate of testosterone. Plasma free testosterone is reduced both because of lower production rate as well as because of the increased level of SHBG, which binds over 99% of circulating testosterone. Plasma estradiol is not consistently altered, but its weak precursors, estrone and estriol, are elevated in the plasma.

Alcoholism per se seems to be the major factor in the observed hypogonadism, with direct effects on gonadal function. This view is supported by a large number of data from many investigators over several decades (Van Thiel 1989). The absence of obvious hypogonadism in patients with postnecrotic cirrhosis (Van Thiel et al 1980), in spite of fairly advanced liver disease, and similar data from rat cirrhosis induced by carbon tetrachloride (Van Thiel et al 1980), suggest that liver disease per se may have a lesser influence on gonadal function than does alcohol. A direct comparison of 21 patients with alcoholic liver disease revealed that liver disease alone was associated with lowered testosterone and androstenedione levels and raised estradiol and dehydroepiandrosterone levels, and with sexual dysfunction. But alcoholism amplified abnormalities quite significantly (Bannister et al 1987).

In contrast to hypogonadism in which alcohol probably plays a larger role than does liver disease itself, feminization seems related more to the liver disease per se, of whatever etiology (Van Thiel 1989). Whereas hypogonadism appears relatively early in the alcohol abuser, feminization generally occurs only after several years when liver damage is extensive (Gavaler & Van Thiel 1988). The precise causes of the feminization are not clear, but they are probably multiple. Hepatic damage results in a reduced hepatic clearance of estrogens as well as of weak androgens such as androstenedione and dehydroepiandrosterone, which may be converted to estrogens. Portal-systemic shunts result in estrogens bypassing the liver and acting at peripheral sites. A variety of other factors have also been proposed (Van Thiel 1989).

Some but not all of the changes observed in alcoholic cirrhosis may be reversible. Abstinence from alcohol resulted in some improvement in sexual function (Van Thiel et al 1983b), but testosterone administration sufficient to raise serum levels significantly did not improve sexual dysfunction (Gluud et al 1988).

In women with liver disease superfeminization is not observed. It has indeed been suggested that cirrhotic women lose some of their feminine characteristics and tend to be asexual (Gavaler & Van Thiel 1988). Few detailed endocrine studies have been reported in nonalcoholic women with liver disease.

Two recent comprehensive reviews of pregnancy in women with liver disease (Steven 1981, Varma 1987) highlight the rarity of pregnancy in untreated chronic progressive liver disease of whatever etiology. Amenorrhea and anovulation are common. When pregnancy does occur, its fate is a function of the severity of the liver disease. Fetal wastage is high, but many pregnancies have been brought to a successful conclusion. It is not clear to what extent pregnancy is a threat to the life of the mother over and above the prognosis of the basic disease itself, but the management of such pregnancies requires very careful cooperation between several medical disciplines.

## Hemochromatosis

Hemochromatosis is an iron-storage disorder which can involve many organ systems. A genetic predisposition can cause increased intestinal absorption of iron. The more common acquired presentation often develops in patients with transfusion-dependent thalassemia major or sideroblastic anemia.

While pituitary iron overload is probably the major cause of arrested growth and abnormal sexual maturation (Kuo et al 1968, Kletzky et al 1979, Meyer et al 1990), direct gonadal involvement may occur (Bezwada et al 1977, Vogt et al 1987). Involvement of the liver and the pancreas can contribute to hormonal disturbances and infertility when significant organ failure occurs.

A recent study indicates that initiation of chelation therapy with desferoxamine before the age of puberty in children with transfusion-dependent thalassemia major improves LH response to GnRH and can help attain normal growth and sexual maturation (Bronspiegel-Weintrob et al 1990). However, studies in adult patients demonstrated only partial recovery of the pituitary function following desferoxamine treatment for 18 months (Vannasaeng et al 1991). No clear-cut teratogenic effects of desferoxamine have been reported. Nevertheless, during pregnancy a reduction of the dose of desferoxamine to the minimum needed is recommended.

Excessive placental transport of iron from affected mother to fetus (Knisely et al 1989, Baynes et al 1991) probably affects the overall outcome of pregnancies, since it can cause fetal hemochromatosis, stillbirth and severe liver damage in the newborn (Silver et al 1987).

## Hepatolenticular degeneration (Wilson's disease)

Wilson's disease is an hereditary abnormality in hepatic copper excretion resulting in excessive accumulation of copper in various organs, especially in the liver and basal ganglia in the brain.

While fertility is apparently preserved in the asymptomatic phase (Scheinberg & Sternlieb 1975, Marecek & Graf 1976), it is severely compromised by the time symptoms appear (Scheinberg & Sternlieb 1975, Walshe 1977). In four patients an extensive endocrine profile revealed normal thyroid function and adrenal function. Pituitary function was normal except for somewhat blunted response of LH and FSH to GnRH. Serum estradiol was invariably low, testosterone was high and androstendione was mildly elevated (Kaushansky et al 1987). While the authors suggest interference with follicular aromatase activity, a disturbance in gonadotropin secretion cannot be excluded. The introduction of penicillamine treatment improved fertility rates significantly, and despite sporadic reports on connective tissue abnormalities in some newborns (Endres 1981), in most instances penicillamine does not pose an undue risk to the fetus (Scheinberg & Sternlieb 1975, Walshe 1977), and it may be continued, at the lowest effective dose, throughout pregnancy.

Pregnancy does not have any consistent effect on the course of Wilson's disease and exacerbations have usually been the result of cessation of penicillamine treatment (Walshe 1977).

A review of the literature since 1966 revealed no data on male fertility in Wilson's disease.

## SUMMARY

The present selection of diverse diseases with an impact on fertility illustrates the spectrum of effects and mechanisms involved in the interaction of disease and fertility. When one considers the complexity of the processes of spermatogenesis, oogenesis, ovulation, ejaculation, transport, fertilization, implantation, gestation and delivery, it should not be surprising to find effects of systemic disease on fertility. The list of diseases discussed is by no means exhaustive, as almost any serious disease can affect fertility, but serves to illustrate the approach to these problems.

## REFERENCES

Abraham S F, Beumont P J, Fraser I S, Llewellyn-Jones D 1982 Body weight, exercise and menstrual status among ballet dancers in training. Br J Obstet Gynecol 89: 507
Ackrill P, Goodwin F G, Marsh F P, Stratton D, Wagman H 1975 Successful pregnancy in patient on regular dialysis. Br Med J 2: 172
Afzelius B A 1976 A human syndrome caused by immobile cilia. Science 193: 317
Afzelius B A, Eliasson R 1983 Male and female infertility problems in the immotile-cilia syndrome. Eur J Resp Dis 127(suppl) 144
Akande E O 1975 Plasma concentration of gonadotrophins, oestrogen and progesterone in hypothyroid women. Br J Obstet Gynaecol 82: 552
Alper M M, Garner P R 1985 Premature ovarian failure: its relationship to autoimmune disease. Obstet Gynecol 66: 27
Amatruda J M, Harman S M, Pourmotabbed G, Lockwood D H 1978 Depressed plasma testosterone and fractional binding of testosterone in obese males. J Clin Endocrinol Metab 47: 268
Anonymous 1987 Drugs that cause sexual dysfunction. Med Lett Drugs Ther 29: 65
Ansbacher R 1978 Artificial insemination with frozen spermatozoa. Fertil Steril 29: 375
Anselmo A P, Cartoni C, Bellantuono P, Maurizi-Enrici R, Aboulkair N, Ermini M 1990 Risk of infertility in patients treated with ABVD vs MOPP vs ABVD/MOPP. Haematologica 75: 155
Arge E 1960 Transposition of viscera and sterility in men. Lancet i: 412

Bai J, Greenwald E, Caterini H, Kaminetzky H A 1974 Drug-related menstrual aberrations. Obstet Gynecol 44: 713
Bailey G L 1977 The sick kidney and sex. N Engl J Med 296: 1288
Baker H, Berger H G, DeKretser D M et al 1976 A study of the endocrine manifestations of hepatic cirrhosis. Q J Med 45: 145
Baker J W, Morgan R L, Peckham M J, Smithers D W 1972 Preservation of ovarian function in patients requiring radiotherapy to para-aortic and pelvic Hodgkin's Disease. Lancet i: 1307
Bannister P, Oakes J, Sheridan P, Losowsky M S 1987 Sex hormone changes in chronic liver disease. Q J Med 63: 305
Barbato A C, Landau R L 1974 Testosterone deficiency of morbid obesity. Clin Res 22: 647A
Barrett C T 1981 Neonatal outcome of maternal systemic lupus erythematosus. In: Fime L G (Moderator) Systemic lupus erythematosus in pregnancy. Ann Intern Med 94: 667
Barták V, Josífko M, Horácková M 1975 Juvenile diabetes and human sperm quality. Int J Fertil 20: 30
Baynes R D, Meyer T E, Bothwell T H, Lamparelli R D 1991 Maternal and fetal iron measurements in a hemochromatotic pregnancy. Am J Hematol 36: 48
Beck J C, Brochner-Mortensen K 1954 Observations on the prognosis in anorexia nervosa. Acta Med Scand 149: 409
Becker K L, Winnaker J L, Matthews M J, Higgins G A J 1968 Gynecomastia and hyperthyroidism: an endocrine and histologic investigation. J Clin Endocrinol Metab 28: 277

Beex L V, Mackenzie M A, Raemakers J M, Smals A G, Benraad T J, Kloppenborg P W 1988 Adjuvant chemotherapy in premenopausal patients with primary breast cancer; relation to drug induced amenorrhea, age and progesterone receptor status of the tumor. Eur J Cancer Clin Oncol 24: 719

Bennett C J, Seager S W J, McGuire E J 1987 Electroejaculation for recovery of semen after retroperitoneal lymph node dissection. J Urol 137: 513

Bennett D 1961 Treatment of ejaculation praecox with monoamine-oxidase inhibitors. Lancet ii: 1309

Bennett H S, Baggenstgors A H, Butt H R 1950 The testes, breast and prostate in men who die of cirrhosis of liver. Am J Clin Pathol 20: 814

Bezwada W R, Bothwell T H, van de Walt L A, Kronheim S, Pimstone B L 1977 An investigation into gonadal dysfunction in patients with idiopathic haemochromatosis. Clin Endocrinol 6: 377

Bhalla V K, Chen C J H, Gnanaprakasam M S 1979 Effects of in vivo administration of human chorionic gonadotropin and ethanol on the process of testicular receptor depletion and replenishment. Life Sci 24: 1315

Biron P 1979 Diminished libido and cimetidine therapy. Can Med Assoc J 121: 404

Björntorp P 1976 Exercise in the treatment of obesity. Clin Endocrinol Metab 5: 431

Blair J H, Simpson G M 1966 Effect of antipsychotic drugs on reproductive functions. Dis Nerv Syst 28: 645

Blatt J, Poplack D G, Sherins R J 1981 Testicular function in boys after chemotherapy for acute lymphoblastic leukemia. N Engl J Med 304: 1121

Bongso T A, Sathananthan A H, Wong P C et al 1989 Human fertilization by microinjection of immotile spermatozoa. Hum Reprod 4: 175

Booth J D, Merriam G R, Clark R V, Loriaux D L, Sherins R J 1987 Evidence for Leydig cell dysfunction in infertile men with a selective increase in plasma follicle stimulating hormone. J Clin Endocrinol Metab 64: 1194

Boyar R M, Katz J, Finkelstein J W et al 1974 Anorexia nervosa: immaturity of the 24-hour luteinizing hormone secretory pattern. N Engl J Med 291: 861

Boyden T W, Pamenter R W, Grosso O, Stanforth P, Rotkis T, Wilmore J H 1982 Prolactin responses, menstrual cycles and body composition of women runners. J Clin Endocrinol Metab 54: 711

Brogden R N, Carmine A A, Heel R C, Speight T M, Avery G S 1982 Ranitidine: a review of its pharmacology and therapeutic use in peptic ulcer disease and other allied diseases. Drugs 24: 267

Bronspiegel-Weintrob N, Olivieri N F, Tyler B, Andrews D F, Freedman M H, Holland F J 1990 Effects of age at the start of iron chelation therapy on gonadal function in β-thalassemia major. N Engl J Med 323: 713

Buchanan J D, Fairley K I, Barrie J U 1975 Return of spermatogenesis after stopping cyclophosphamide therapy. Lancet ii: 156

Bullen B A, Skrinar G S, Beitens I Z, von Mering G, Turnbull B A, McArthur J W 1985 Induction of menstrual disorders by strenuous excercise in untrained women. N Engl J Med 312: 1349

Bulmash J M 1978 Systemic lupus erythematosus and pregnancy. Obstet Gynecol Annu 7: 153

Burkat W, Fischer-Guntenhoner E, Standl E, Schneider H P 1989 Menarche, menstrual cycle and fertility in diabetic patients. Geburstshilfe Frauenheilkd 49: 149

Burke B A, Lindgren B, Wic M, Holley K, Manivel C 1989 Testicular germ cell loss in children with renal failure. Pediatr Pathol 9: 433

Burke C W, Anderson D C 1972 Sex hormone binding globulin is an estrogen amplifier. Nature 240: 38

Burman K D, Diamond R C, Harvey G S et al 1979 Glucose modulation of alterations in serum iodothyronin concentration metabolism induced by fasting. Metabolism 28: 291

Burns J R, Houttuin J G, Hawatmeh I S, Sullivan T R 1979 Vascular-induced erectile impotence in renal transplant recipients. J Urol 121: 721

Burrow G N 1977 Thyroid and parathyroid function in pregnancy. In: Fuchs F, Klopper A (eds) Endocrinology of pregnancy. Harper and Row, Hagerstown, M D, p 257

Burrow G N 1989 Thyroid disease in pregnancy. In: Burrow G N, Oppenheimer J H, Volpé R (eds) Thyroid function and disease. W B Saunders, Philadelphia, pp 292–323

Campbell J S, Nigam S, Hurtig A, Sahasrabndhe M R, Marino I 1964 Mineral oil granulomas of uterus and parametrium and granulomatous salpingitis with Schaumann bodies and oxalate deposits. Fertil Steril 15: 278

Carroll B J, Greden J F, Feinberg M 1980 Neuroendocrine disturbances and the diagnosis and etiology of endogenous depression. Lancet i: 321

Cecere F A, Persellin R H 1981 The interaction of pregnancy and the rheumatic diseases. Clin Rheum Dis 7: 747

Chapman R M, Sutcliffe J B, Rees L, Malpas J S 1971 Prospective study: the effects of Hodgkin's disease and prednisone on male gonadal function. Proc Am Soc Clin Oncol 20: 321A

Chapman R M, Sutcliffe S B, Malpas J S 1979a Cytotoxic induced ovarian failure in women with Hodgkin's disease: 1. Hormone function. J A M A 242: 1877

Chapman R M, Sutcliffe J B, Rees L H, Edwards C R W, Malpas J S 1979b Cyclical combination chemotherapy and gonadal function. Retrospective study in males. 1: 265

Charak B S, Gupta R, Mandreker P et al 1990 Testicular dysfunction after cyclophosphamide-vincristine-procarbazine-prednisolone chemotherapy for advanced Hodgkin's disease. A long-term followup study. Cancer 65: 1903

Chatzinoff M, Guarino J M, Corson S L, Batzer F R, Freidman L 1988 Sulfasalazine-induced abnormal sperm penetration assay reversed on changing 5-aminosalacylic acid enemas. Dig Dis Sci 33: 108

Chen C J, Vidt D G, Zorm E M, Hallberg M C, Wieland R G 1970 Pituitary-Leydig cell function in uremic males. J Clin Endocrinol Metab 31: 14

Cheviakoff S, Calamera J C, Morgenfeld M, Mancini R E 1973 Recovery of spermatogenesis in patients with lymphoma after treatment with chlorambucil. J Reprod Fertil 33: 155

Chin N W, Chang F E, Dodds W G, Kim M H, Malarkey W B 1987 Acute effects of exercise on plasma catecholamines in sedentary and athletic women with normal and abnormal menses. Am J Obstet Gynecol 157: 938

Chopra I J 1975 Gonadal steroids and gonadotropins in hyperthyroidism. Med Clin North Am 59: 1109

Chopra I J, Tulchinsky D 1974 Status of estrogen–androgen balance in hyperthyroid men with Graves' disease. J Clin Endocrinol Metab 38: 269

Cicero T J 1981 Neuroendocrinological effects of alcohol. Annual Rev Med 32: 123

Cicero T J, Bell R D 1980 Effects of ethanol and acetaldehyde in the biosynthesis of testosterone in the rodent testes. Biochem Biophys Res Commun 94: 814

Cicero T J, Bell R D, Meyer E R, Badger T M 1980 Ethanol and acetaldehyde directly inhibit testicular steroidogenesis. J Pharmacol Exp Ther 213: 228

Cicero T J, Bernstein D, Badger T M 1978a Effects of acute alcohol administration on reproductive endocrinology in the male rat. Alcohol Clin Exp Res 2: 249

Cicero T J, Meyer E R, Bell R D 1978b Effects of ethanol on hypothalamic-pituitary-luteinizing hormone axis and testicular steroidogenesis. J Pharmac Exp Ther 208: 210

Clark E 1965 Spironolactone therapy and gynecomastia. J A M A 193: 163

Cobb C F, Van Thiel D H, Ennis M F, Gavaler J S, Lester R 1979 Pseudo-Cushings in alcoholics: a mechanism. Cin Res 27: 448A

Corrales-Hernandez J J, Miralles-Garcia J M, Garcia Diez L C 1990 Primary hypothyroidism and human spermatogenesis. Arch Androl 25: 21

Curie-Cohen M, Luttell L, Shapiro S 1979 Current practice of artificial insemination by donor in the United States. N Engl J Med 300: 585

Dale E, Gerlach D M, Wilhite A L 1979 Menstrual dysfunction in distance runners. Am J Obstet Gynecol 54: 47

Danovitch G M 1981 Effect of pregnancy on renal function in systemic lupus erythematosus. In: Fime G L (ed) Moderator. Systemic lupus erythematosus in pregnancy. Ann Intern Med 94: 667

De Coster R, Caer S I, Haelterman C, Debroye M 1985 Effect of a single administration of ketoconazole on total and physiologically free plasma testosterone and 17-beta oestradiol levels in healthy male volunteers. Eur J Clin Pharmacol 29: 489

De Cree C 1989 Endogenous opioid peptides in the control of the normal menstrual cycle and their possible role in athletic menstrual irregularities. Obstet Gynecol Surv 44: 720

de Gasparo M, Whitebread S E P G, Jeunemaitre X, Corvol P, Menard J 1989 Antialdosterones: incidence and prevention of sexual side effects. J Steroid Biochem 32: 223

De La Balze F A, Arrilloga F, Mancini R E, Janches M, Davidson O W, Gurtman A I 1962 Male hypogonadism in hypothyroidism: a study of six cases. J Clin Endocrinol Metab 2: 212

De Paepe M E, Waxman M 1989 Testicular atrophy in AIDS: a study of 57 autopsy cases. Hum Pathol 20: 210

De Vita V T J, Canellos G P, Moxley J M 1972 A decade of combination chemotherapy of advanced Hodgkin's Disease. 30: 1495

Decker R E, Mardayat M, Marc J, Rosool A 1979 Neurosarcoidosis with computerized tomography visualization and transphenoidal excision of a supra and intrasellar granuloma. J Neurosurg 50: 814

DeCunha M F, Meistrich M L, Reid H L, Powell M L 1979 Effect of chemotherapy on human sperm production. Proc Am Assoc Cancer Res 20: 100A

DeKretser D M 1979 The effect of systemic disease on the dysfunction of the testis. Clin Endocrinol Metab 8: 487

Delle Fave G F, Tramburrano G, De Magistris L et al 1977 Gynecomastia with cimetidine. Lancet i: 1319

Denning C R, Sommers S C, Quigley H J 1968 Infertility in male patients with cystic fibrosis. Pediatrics 41: 7

Devoe L D, Taylor R L 1979 Systemic lupus erythematosus in pregnancy. Am J Obstet Gynecol 135: 473

Dignam W J, Parlow A F, Daane T A 1969 Serum FSH and LH measurements in the evaluation of menstrual disorders. Am J Obstet Gynecol 105: 679

Ding J H, Sheckter C B, Soules M R, Bremner W J 1988 High serum cortisol levels in exercise associated amenorrhea. Ann Intern Med 108: 530

DiSant'Agnese P A 1968 Fertility and young adults with cystic fibrosis. N Engl J Med 279: 103

DiSant'Agnese P A, Davis P B 1976 Research in cystic fibrosis (three parts). N Engl J Med 295: 481, 534, 597

DiSant'Agnese P A, Davis P B 1979 Cystic fibrosis in adults. 75 cases and a review of 232 cases in the literature. Am J Med 66: 121

Distiller L A, Sagel J, Morley J E, Jaffe B I, Seftel H C 1975 Pituitary responsiveness to luteinizing hormone releasing hormone in insulin dependent diabetes mellitus. Diabetes 24: 378

Djursing H 1987 Hypothalamic-pituitary-gonadal function in insulin treated diabetic women with and without amenorrhea. Danish Med Bull 34: 139

Djursing H, Nyholm H C, Hagen C, Mølsted-Pedersen L 1982 Depressed prolactin levels in diabetic women with anovulation. Acta Obstet Gynecol Scand 61: 403

Dnistrian A M, Schwartz M K, Fracchia A A, Kaufman R J, Currie V G 1983 Endocrine consequences of CMF adjuvant therapy in premenopausal and postmenopausal breast cancer patients. Cancer 51: 803

Doering C H, Brodie H K H, Kraemer H L, Moss R H, Becker H B, Hamburg D 1975 Negative affect and plasma testosterone: a longitudinal human study. Psychosom Med 37: 484

Dombroski R A 1989 Autoimmune disease in pregnancy. Med Clin North Am 73: 605

Drossman D A, Ontjes D A, Heizer W D 1979 Anorexia nervosa. Gastroenterology 77: 1115

Dunn J F, Nisula B C, Rodbard D 1981 Transport of steroid hormones: binding of 21 endogenous steroids to both testosterone-binding globulin and corticosteroid-binding globulin in human plasma. J Clin Endocrinol Metab 53: 58

Edman C D, MacDonald P L 1978 Effect of obesity on conversion of plasma androstenedione to estrone in ovulatory and anovulatory young women. Am J Obstet Gynecol 130: 456

Edwards D F, Kennedy J R, Patton C S, Toal R L, Daniel G B, Lothrop C D 1989 Familial immotile-cilia syndrome in English springer spaniel dogs. Am J Med Genet 33: 290

Ehrenfeld M, Levy M, Margalioth E J, Eliakim M 1986 The effects of long-term colchicin therapy on male fertility in patients with familial Mediterranean fever. Andrology 18: 420

Ehrenfeld M, Brezezinski A, Levy M, Eliakim M 1987 Fertility and obstetric history in patients with familial Mediterranean fever on long-term colchicin therapy. Br J Obstet Gynecol 94: 1186

Eliasson R, Mossberg B, Camner P, Afzelius B A 1977 The immobile cilia syndrome. A congenital abnormality as an etiologic factor in chronic airway infections and male sterility. N Engl J Med 297: 1

Ellenberg M 1971 Impotence in diabetes: the neurologic factor. Ann Intern Med 75: 213

Ellenberg M 1977 Sexual aspects of the female diabetic. Mount Sinai J Med 44: 495

Ellenberg M, Weber H 1966 Retrograde ejaculation in diabetic neuropathy. Ann Intern Med 65: 1237

Ellingboe J, Varanelli C C 1979 Ethanol inhibits testosterone biosynthesis by direct action in Leydig cells. Res Commun Chem Pathol Pharmacol 24: 87

Elstein M, Smith E K M, Curtis J R 1969 Reproductive potential of patients treated by maintenance hemodialysis. Br Med J 2: 734

Emmanouel D S, Lindheimer M D, Katz A 1 1980 Pathogenesis of endocrine abnormalities in uremia. Endocr Reviews 1: 28

Endres W 1981 D-penicillamine in pregnancy- to ban or not to ban? Klin Wochenschr 59: 535

Engel P 1944 A study of inactivation of ovarian hormones by the liver. Endocrinology 35: 70

Etteldorf J N, West C D, Pitcock J A, Williams D C 1976 Gonadal function, testicular histology and meiosis following cyclophosphamide therapy in patients with nephrotic syndrome. J Pediatr 88: 206

Fane A G, Izsak M, Saiphoo C 1980 Systemic lupus erythematosus and Kleinfelter's syndrome. Arthritis Rheum 23: 124

Fehér T, Halmy L 1975 Dehydroepiandrosterone and dehydroepiandrosterone sulfate dynamics in obesity. Can J Biochem 53: 215

Feicht L B, Johnson T S, Martin B J, Sparkes K E, Wagner W W J 1978 Secondary amenorrhea in athletes. Lancet ii: 1145

Feldman M, Burton M E 1990 Histamin H2-receptor antagonists. Standard therapy for acid-peptic diseases. N Engl J Med 323: 1672, 1749

Fichter M M, Pirke K M 1984 Hypothalamic pituitary function in starving healthy subjects. In: Pirke K M, Ploog D (eds) Psychobiology of anorexia nervosa. Springer, Berlin, p 124

Finkelstein F O, Finkelstein S H, Steele T E 1976 Assessment of marital relationship of hemodialysis patients. Am J Med Sci 271: 21

Fisher E R, Gregorio R, Stephan T, Nolan S, Danowski T 1974 Ovarian changes in women with morbid obesity. Obstet Gynecol 44: 839

Fishman J 1980 Fatness, puberty and ovulation. N Engl J Med 303: 42

Fishman J, Boyar R M, Liellman L 1975 Influence of body weight in estradiol metabolism in young women. Metabolism 41: 989

Fishman J, Hellman L, Zumoff B, Gallagher T F 1965 Effect of thyroid on hydroxylation of estrogen in man. J Clin Endocrinol Metab 25: 365

Forney J P, Milewich L, Chen G T et al 1981 Aromatization of androstenedione to estrone by human adipose tissue in vitro. Correlation with adipose tissue mass, age and endometrial neoplasia. Journal of Clinical Endocrinology and Metabolism 53: 192–199.

Freeman R M, Lawton R L, Fearing M O 1968 Gynecomastia: an endocrine complication of hemodialysis. Ann Inter Med 69: 67

Freinkel N 1980 Of pregnancy and progeny. Diabetes 29: 1023

Freinkel N 1981 Pregnant thoughts about metabolic control and diabetes. N Engl J Med 304: 1357

Frisch R E 1980 Pubertal adipose tissue: is it necessary for normal sexual maturation? Evidence from the rat and human female. Fed Proc 39: 2395

Frisch R E 1988 Fatness and fertility. Sci Am 258: 88

Frisch R E, Revelle R 1971 Height and weight at menarche and a hypothesis of menarche. Arch Dis Childhood 46: 695

Frisch R E, Wyshak G, Vincent L 1980 Delayed menarche and amenorrhea in ballet dancers. N Engl J Med 303: 17

Frydman M I 1979 Epidemiology of cystic fibrosis: a review. J Chronic Dis 32: 211

Fuhrmann K, Reiher H, Semmler K, Fischer F, Fischer M, Glockner E 1983 Prevention of congenital malformations in infants of insulin-dependent diabetic mothers. Diabetes Care 6: 219

Fushimi H, Horie H, Inoue T et al 1989 Low testosterone levels in diabetic men and animals: a possible role in testicular impotence. Diabetes Res Clin Pract 6: 297

Gabbe S G 1980 Medical complications of management of diabetes in pregnancy: six decades of experiences. In: Pitkin R M, Zlatuik F S (eds) Year book of obstetrics and gynecology. Year Book, Chicago, pp 37–49

Galbraith R A, Michnovicz J J 1989 The effects of cimetidine on the oxidative metabolism of estradiol. N Engl J Med 321: 269

Galvão-Teles A, Burke G W, Anderson D C 1973 Biologically active androgens and oestradiol in men with chronic liver disease. Lancet i: 173

Garcia Diez L C, Gonzalez Buitrago J M 1982 Semen characteristics and serum and seminal plasma hormones in drug induced hyperprolactinemia. Arch Androl 9: 311

Garnick M B, Richie J P 1986 Toward more rational management for stage I testis cancer: watch out for 'watch and wait'. J Clin Oncol 4: 1021

Gaudier F L, Santiago-Delphin E, Rivera J, Gonzales Z 1988 Pregnancy after renal transplantation. Surg Gynecol Obstet 167: 533

Gavaler J S, Van Thiel D H 1988 Gonadal dysfunction and inadequate sexual performance in alcoholic cirrhotic men. Gastroenterology 95: 1680

Gavaler J S, Urso T, Van Thiel D H 1983 Ethanol: its adverse effects upon the hypothalamic-pituitary-gonadal axis. Subst Alcohol Actions Misuse 4: 97

Geller R A, Kuremsky D A, Copeland J S, Stept R 1977 Sarcoidosis and testicular neoplasm: an unusual association. J Urol 118: 487

George S L, Aur R J, Mauer A M, Simone J V 1979 A reappraisal of the results of stopping therapy in childhood leukemia. N Engl J Med 300: 269

Glass A R, Swerdloff R S, Bray G A, Dahms W T, Atkinson R L 1977 Low serum testosterone and sex hormone binding globulin in massively obese men. J Clin Endocrinol Metab 45: 1211

Glass A R, Dahms W T, Abraham G, Atkinson R L, Bray G A, Swerdloff R S 1978 Secondary amenorrhea in obesity: etiologic role of weight-related androgen excess. Fertil Steril 30: 243

Glass R I, Lyness R N, Mengle D C, Powell K E, Kahn E 1979 Sperm count depression in pesticide applicators exposed to dibromochloropropane. Am J Epidemiol 109: 346

Glass A R, Burman K D, Dahms W T, Boehm T M 1981 Endocrine function in human obesity. Metabolism 30: 89

Gluud C, Wantzin P, Eriksen J 1988 No effect of oral

testosterone treatment in sexual dysfunction in alcoholic cirrhotic men. Gastroenterology 95: 1582

Goldsmith R E, Sturgis S H, Lerman J, Stanbury J B 1952 The menstrual pattern in thyroid disease. J Clin Endocrinol Metab 12: 846

Goldstein I, Siroky M, Krane R 1983 Impotence in diabetes mellitus. In: Krane R, Siroky M, Goldstein I (eds) Male sexual dysfunction. Little Brown, Boston, pp 77–86

Gómez F, De LaCueva R, Wauters J P, Lemarchand-Béraud T 1980 Endocrine abnormalities in patients undergoing long-term hemodialysis. Am J M 68: 522

Goodwin N J, Valenti C, Hall J E, Friedman E A 1968 Effects of uremia and chronic hemodialysis on the reproductive cycle. Am J Obstet Gynecol 100: 528

Gordon G G, Southren A L, Tochimoto S, Rand J J, Olivo J 1969 Effect of hyperthyroidism and hypothyroidism on the metabolism of testosterone and androstenedione in man. J Clin Endocrinol Metab 29: 164

Gordon G G, Olivo J, Rafii F, Southren A L 1975 Conversion of androgens to estrogens in cirrhosis of the liver. J Clin Endocrinol Metab 40: 1018

Gordon G G, Altman K, Southren A L, Rubin E, Lieber C S 1979 Effect of alcohol (ethanol) administration on sex hormone metabolism in normal men. N Engl J Med 295: 793

Gordon G G, Southren A L, Vittek J, Lieber C S 1979a The effect of alcohol ingestion on hepatic aromatic activity and plasma steroid hormone in the rat. Metabolism 28: 20

Gordon G G, Southren A L, Lieber C S 1979b Hypogonadism and feminization in the male: a triple effect of alcohol. Alcohol Clin Exp Res 3: 210

Gordon G G, Vittek J, Ho R, Rosenthal W S, Southren A L, Lieber C S 1979c The effect of chronic alcohol use in hepatic 5-alpha ring reductase in the baboon and man. Gastroenterology 77: 110

Gordon G G, Vittek J, Southren A L, Munnangi P, Lieber C S 1980 Effect of chronic alcohol ingestion on the biosynthesis of steroids in rat testicular homogenate in vitro. Endocrinology 106: 1880

Gorski J, Gannon F 1976 Current models of steroid hormone action: a critique. Annu Rev Physiol 38: 425

Greenberg H R 1965 Erectile impotence during the course of Tofranil therapy. Am J Psychiatry 121: 1021

Greene L F, Kelalis P P, Weeks R E 1963 Retrograde ejaculation of semen due to diabetic neuropathy. Fertil Steril 14: 617

Greenstone M, Rutman A, Dewar A, Mackay I, Cole P J 1988 Primary ciliary dyskinesia: cytological and clinical features. Q J Med 67: 405

Grennan D M, McCormick J N, Wojtacha D, Carty M, Behan W 1978 Immunologic studies of the placenta in systemic lupus erythematosus. Ann Rheum Dis 37: 129

Griboff S 1962 Semen analysis in myxedema. Fertil Steril 13: 436

Grubb M R, Chakeres D, Malarkey W B 1987 Patients with primary hypothyroidism presenting as prolactinomas. Am J Med 83: 765

Guha S K, Anand S 1979 Gamete transport mechanisms. In: Talwar G P (ed) Recent advances in reproduction and regulation of fertility. Elsevier North Holland, Amsterdam, p 211

Haider S G, Hofman N, Passia D 1985 Morphological and enzyme histochemical observations on alcohol-induced disturbances in testes of two patients. Andrologia 17: 532

Hale R W, Kossa T, Kreiger J, Pepper S 1983 A marathon: the immediate effect on female runners' luteinizing hormone, follicle-stimulating hormone, prolactin, testosterone and cortisol levels. Am J Obstet Gynecol 146: 550

Hall W H 1976 Breast changes in males on cimetidin. N Eng J Med 295: 841

Hamilton C R, Henken R L, Weir G, Gordon W, Kliman B 1973 Olfactory status and response to clomiphene in male gonadotrophin deficiency. Ann Intern Med 78: 47

Handelsman D J 1985 Hypothalamic-pituitary gonadal dysfunction in renal failure and renal transplantation. Endocr Rev 6: 151

Handelsman D J, Boylan L M, Turtle J R 1984 Young's syndrome. Obstructive azoospermia and chronic sinopulmonary infections. N Engl J Med 310: 3

Harlass F E, Plymate S R, Fariss B L, Belts R P 1984 Weight loss is associated with correction of gonadotropin and sex steroid abnormalities in the obese anovulatory female. Fertil Steril 42: 649

Hartz A J, Barboriak P N, Wong A, Katayama K P, Rimm A A 1979 The association of obesity with infertility and related menstrual abnormalities in women. Int J Obesity 3: 57

Hay G G, Leonard J C 1979 Anorexia nervosa in males. Lancet ii: 574

Hayslett J P, Lynn R L 1980 Effect of pregnancy in patient with lupus nephropathy. Kidney Int 18: 207

Hayslett J P, Reece E A 1985 Systemic lupus erythematosus in pregnancy. Clin Perinatol 12: 539

Heffernan J L, Blenkinsopp W K 1978 Epididymal sarcoidosis, Br J Urol 50: 211

Hendry W F, Knight R K, Whifield H N et al 1978 Obstructive azoospermia: respiratory function tests, electron microscopy and the results of surgery. Br J Urol 50: 598

Hohtari H, Elovainio R, Salminen K, Laatikainen T 1988 Plasma corticotropin-releasing hormone, corticotropin, and endorphins at rest and during exercise in eumenorrheic and amenorrheic athletes. Fertil Steril 50: 233

Holdsworth S K, Atkins R C, de Krester D M 1977 The pituitary-testicular axis in men with chronic renal failure. N Engl J Med 296: 1245

Holdsworth S R, DeKrester D M, Atkins R C 1978 A comparison of hemodialysis and transplantation in reversing the uremic disturbances of male reproductive function. Clin Nephrol 10: 146

Hollister L E 1978 Tri-cyclic anti-depressants. N Engl J Med 299: 1106

Hook O 1954 Sarcoidosis with involvement of nervous system: Report of 9 cases. Arch Neur 71: 554

Horning S J, Hoppe R T, Kaplan H S, Rosenberg S A 1981 Female reproductive potential after treatment in Hodgkin's disease. N Engl J Med 304: 1377

Housseinian A M, Kim M H, Rosenfeld R L 1976 Obesity and oligomenorrhea are associated with hyperandrogenism independent of hirsutism. J Clin Endocrinol Metab 42: 765

Hughes J M 1964 Failure to ejaculate with chlordiazepoxide. Am J Psychiatry 121: 610

Hurd H P, Palumbro P J, Gharib H 1977 Hypothalamic-endocrine dysfunction in anorexia nervosa. Mayo Clinic Proc 52: 711

Ingbar S M, Braverman L E 1986 The thyroid. J B Lippincott, Philadelphia, pp 920–930, 1194–1199

Isaacs A J, Leslie R D G, Gomez J, Baylis R 1980 The effect

of weight gain on gonadotropins and prolactin in anorexia nervosa. Acta Endocrinol 94: 145

Ismajovich B, Zemer D, Revach M, Serr D, Sohar E 1973 The causes of infertility in females with familial Mediterranean fever. Fertil Steril 24: 844

Israel H L, Sones M, Roy R L, Stein G N 1961 The occurrence of intrathoracic calcification in sarcoidosis. Am Rev Respir Dis 84: 1

Jackson H 1970 Antispermatogenic agents. Bri Med Bull 26: 79

Jensen R T, Collen M J, Pandol S J et al 1983 Cimetidine-induced impotence and breast changes in patients with gastric hypersecretory states. N Engl J Med 308: 883

Jensen S B, Hagen C, Frland A, Pedersen P B 1979 Sexual function and pituitary axis in insulin treated diabetic men. Acta Med Scand 624(suppl): 65

Jeuniewic N, Brown G M, Garfinkel P E, Moldofsky H 1978 Hypothalamic function as related to body weight and body fat in anorexia nervosa. Psychosom Med 40: 187

Johnston D E, Chiao N B, Gavaler J S, Van Thiel D H 1981 Inhibition of testosterone synthesis by ethanol and acetaldehyde. Biochem Pharmacol 30: 1827

Kapen S, Sternthal E, Braverman L 1981 Case report A pubertal 24-hour luteinizing hormone (L H) secretory pattern following weight loss in the absence of anorexia nervosa. Psychosom Med 43: 177

Kaplan E, Shwachman H, Perlumuter A, Rule A, Khaw K T, Holsclow D S 1968 Reproductive failure in cystic fibrosis. N Engl J Med 279: 65

Kaplan H S 1980 Hodgkin's disease. In: (ed) Harvard University Press, Cambridge, Mass, pp 434, 474

Katz J L, Boyar R M, Roffwarg H, Hellman L, Weiner H 1977 LHRH responsiveness in anorexia nervosa: intactness despite prepubertal circadian L H pattern. Psychosom Med 39: 241

Kaushansky A, Frydman M, Kaufman H, Homburg R 1987 Endocrine studies of the ovulatory disturbances in Wilson's disease (hepatobiliary degeneration). Fertil Steril 47: 230

Kaye W H, Berrettini W H, Gwirtsman H E et al 1989 Contribution of CNS neuropeptide (NPY, CRH, and beta-endorphin) alterations to psychophysiological abnormalities in anorexia nervosa. Psychopharmacol Bull 25: 433

Klebanow D, Macleod J 1960 Semen quality and certain disturbances of reproduction in diabetic men. Fertil Steril 11: 255

Kletzky O A 1983 Curr Ther Res 33: 394

Kletzky O A, Costin G, Marrs R P, Berenstein G, March C M, Mishell D R J 1979 Gonadotropin insufficiency in patients with thalassemia major. J Clin Endocrinol Metab 48: 901

Kley H K, Solbach H G, Mckinnan J C, Krüskemper H L 1979 Testosterone decrease and estrogen increase in male patients with obesity. Acta Endocrinol 91: 553

Klibanski A, Beitins I Z, Badger T, Little R, McArthur J W 1981 Reproductive function during fasting in men. J Clin Endocrinol Metab 53: 258

Knigge U, Wollesen F, Christiansen P M 1980 Histamine H2 receptors and parathyroid hormone secretion. Lancet ii: 212

Knigge U, Dejgaard A, Wollesen F, Ingerslev O, Bennett P, Christiansen P M 1983 The acute and long term effect of H2-receptor antagonists cimetidine and ranitidine on the pituitary-gonadal axis in men. Clin Endocrinol (Oxf) 18: 307

Knisely A S, Grady R W, Kramer E E, Jones R L 1989 Cytoferrin, maternofetal iron transport, and neonatal hemochromatosis. Am J Clin Pathol 92: 755

Kolodny R C 1971 Sexual dysfunction in diabetic females. Diabetes 20: 557

Kolodny R C, Masters W H, Kolodner R M, Toro G 1974a Depression of plasma testosterone levels after chronic intensive marihuana use. N Engl J Med 290: 872

Kolodny R C, Rahn C B, Goldstein H H et al 1974b Sexual dysfunction in diabetic men. Diabetes 23: 306

Kopelman P G, Pilkinton T R, White N, Jeffcoate S L 1980 Abnormal sex steroid secretion and binding in massively obese women. Clin Endocrinol (Oxf) 12: 363

Krauss L 1958 Genital sarcoidosis: case report and review of the literature. J Urol 80: 367

Kredentser J V, Pokrant C, McCoshen J A 1986 Intrauterine insemination for infertility due to cystic fibrosis. Fertility and Sterility 45: 425-426

Kreuz L E, Rose R M, Jennings J R 1972 Suppression of plasma testosterone levels and psychosocial stress. A longitudinal study of young men in officer candidate school. Arch Gen Psychiatry 26: 479

Kucheria K, Saxena R, Mohan D 1985 Semen analysis in alcohol dependence syndrome. Andrologia 17: 558

Kuo B, Zaino E, Roginsky M S 1968 Endocrine function in thalassemia major. J Clin Endocrinol Metab 28: 805

LaFerla J J, Anderson D L, Schalch D S 1978 Psychoendocrine response to sexual arousal in human males. Psychosom Med 40: 166

Lange P H, Narayan P, Fraley E E 1984 Fertility issues following therapy for testicular cancer. Semin Urol II 4: 264

Langtry H D, Grant S M, Goa K L 1989 Famotidine: an updated review of its pharmacodynamic and pharmacokinetic properties and therapeutic use in peptic ulcer disease. Drugs 36: 521

Larsen P R, Silva J E, Kaplan M M 1981 Relationships between circulating and intracellular thyroid hormone: physiological and clinical implications. Endocr Rev 2: 87

Lemaire A, Burat J, Racadot A, Buval-Herbaut M, Fossati P 1981 Comparative study of pituitary testicular axis in two populations of diabetic men (with or without erectile impotence). Isr J Med Sci 12: 740 (abstr)

Lendon M, Hann I M, Palmer M K, Shalet S M, Morris-Jones P H 1978 Testicular histology after combination chemotherapy in childhood for acute lymphoblastic leukemia. Lancet ii: 439

Lentz R D, Bergstein J, Steffes M W et al 1977 Post-pubertal evaluation of gonadal function following cyclophosphamide therapy before and during puberty. J Pediatr 91: 385

LeRoy W M, Dearborn D G, Tucker A S 1980 Cystic fibrosis. In: Fishman A P (ed) Pulmonary diseases and disorders. McGraw-Hill, New York, p 600

Lester R, Eagon P K, Van Thiel D H 1979 Feminization of the alcoholic: the estrogen/testosterone ratio (E/T). Gastroenterology 76: 415

Levy J, Burshell A, Marbach M, Afflalo L, Glick S M 1980 Interaction of spironolactone with estradiol receptors in cytosol. J Endocrinol 84: 371

Lieb S M 1981 The effect of systemic lupus erythematosus on fetal survival. In Fime L G (moderator) Systemic lupus erythematosus. Ann Intern Med 94: 667

Lim V S, Fang V S 1975 Gonadal dysfunction in uremic men. A study of hypothalamus-pituitary-testicular axis before and after renal transplantation. Am J Med 58: 655

Lim V S, Kathpalia S C, Henriquez C 1978 Endocrine abnormalities associated with chronic renal failure. Med Clin North Am 62: 1341

Lindsay R M, Briggs J O, Luke R G, Boyle I T, Kennedy A C 1967 Gynecomastia in chronic renal failure. Br Med J 4: 779

Lipsett M B 1980 Physiology and pathology of the Leydig cell. N Engl J Med 303: 682

Loose D S, Kan P B, Hirst M A, Marcus R A, Feldman D 1983 Ketoconazole blocks adrenal steroidogenesis by inhibiting cytochrome P450-dependent enzymes. J Clin Invest 71: 1495

Loriaux D L, Menard R, Taylor A, Pita J, Santen R 1976 Spironolactone and endocrine dysfunction. Ann Intern Med 85: 630

McArthur J W, O'Loughlin K M, Beitins I Z, Johnson L, Hourihan Y, Alonso C 1976 Endocrine studies during refeeding of young women with nutritional amenorrhea and infertility. Mayo Clin Proc 51: 607

MacCarthy E P, Pollak V E 1981 Maternal renal disease. Effect on the fetus. Clin Perinatol 8: 307

McComb P, Langley L, Villalon M, Verdugo P 1986 The oviductal cilia and Kartagener's syndrome. Fertil Steril 46: 412

MacConnie S E, Barkan A, Lampnan R M, Schork M A, Beitins I Z 1986 Decreased hypothalamic gonadotropin releasing hormone in male marathon runners. N Engl J Med 315: 411

MacDonald P C, Edman C D, Hemsell D L, Porter J C, Siiteri P K 1978 Effect of obesity on conversion of plasma androstenedione to estrone in postmenopausal women with and without endometrial cancer. Am J Obstet Gynecol 130: 448

Marecek Z, Graf M 1976 Pregnancy in penicillamine-treated patients with Wilson's disease (letter). N Engl J Med 295: 841

Massry S G, Goldstein D A, Procci W R, Kletzky O A 1980 On the pathogenesis of sexual dysfunction of the uremic male. Proc Eur Dialysis Transplant Assoc 17: 139

Masters W H, Johnson V E 1970 Human sexual inadequacy. Little Brown, Boston

Mathur R S, Neff M R, Landgrebe S C et al 1986 Time related changes in the plasma concentrations of prolactin, gonadotropins, sex hormone binding globulin, and certain steroid hormones in female runners after a long distance race. Fertil Steril 46: 1067

Mecklenburg R S, Sherins R J 1974 Gonadotropin response to luteinizing-hormone releasing hormone in men with germinal aplasia. J Clin Endocrinol Metab 38: 1005

Meehan R T, Dorsey J K 1987 Pregnancy among patients with systemic lupus erythematosus receiving immunosuppressive therapy. J Rheumatol 14: 252

Mello N K, Mendelson J H, Teoh S K 1989 Neuroendocrine consequences of alcohol abuse in women. Ann N Y Acad Sci 562: 211

Mendelson J M, Mello N K 1974 Alcohol, aggression and androgens. Proc Assoc Res Nervous Mental Dis 225

Mendelson J H, Mello N K 1979 Biological concomitants of alcoholism. N Engl J Med 301: 912

Mendelson J H, Mello N K, Ellingboe J 1977 Effects of acute alcohol intake on pituitary gonadal hormones in normal human males. J Pharmacol Exp Ther 202: 676

Mendelson J M, Mello N K, Elligboe J 1978a Effects of alcohol on human males. In: Lipton M A, Dimascio A,

Killam K F (eds) Psychopharmacology: a generation of progress. Raven, New York, p 1677

Mendelson J M, Ellingboe J, Mello N K, Kuehnli J 1978b Effects of alcohol on plasma testosterone and luteinizing hormone levels. Alcohol Clin Exp Res 2: 255

Meyer W R, Hutchison-Williams K A, Jones E E, DeCherney A H 1990 Secondary hypogonadism in hemochomatosis. Fertil Steril 54: 740

Miller E, Hare J W, Cloherty J P et al 1981 Elevated maternal hemoglobin Alc in early pregnancy and major congenital anomalies in infants of diabetic mothers. N Engl J Med 304: 1331

Miller J J, Williams G F, Leissring J L 1971 Multiple late complications in therapy with cyclophosphamide, including ovarian destruction. Am J Med 50: 530

Mills J L, Knopp R H, Simpson J L Janovic-Peterson L, Metzger B E, Holmes L B, Aarons J H et al and the National institute of Child Health and Human Development Diabetes in Early Pregnancy Study 1988 Lack of relation of increased malformation rates in infants of diabetic mothers to glycemic control during organogenesis. N Engl J Med 318: 671

Mintz G, Niz J, Gutierrez G, Garcia-Alonso A, Krachmer S 1986 Prospective study of pregnancy in systemic lupus erythematosus. Results of a multidisciplinary approach. J Rheumatol 13: 732

Mintz J, O'Hare K O, Brien P, Goldschmidt J 1974 Sexual problems of heroin addicts. Arch Gen Psychiatry 31: 700

Montoro M, Collea J V, Frasier S D, Mestman J H 1981 Successful outcome of pregnancy in women with hypothyroidism. Ann Intern Med 94: 31

Moreira-Andres M N, Black E G, Ramsden D B, Hoffenberg R 1980 The effect of caloric restriction in serum thyroid hormone binding proteins and free hormone in obese patients. Clinical Endocrinol 12: 249

Morganfeld M L, Goldberg V, Parisier H, Bugnard S L, Bur G E 1972 Ovarian lesions due to cytostatic agents during the treatment of Hodgkin's diseasse. Surg Gynecol Obstet 134: 826

Morrione T G 1944 Effects of estrogen on testes in hepatic insufficiency. Arch Pathol 37: 39

Moshang T J, Parks J S, Baker L et al 1975 Low serum triiodothyronine in patients with anorexia nervosa. J Clin Endocrinol Metab 40: 470

Mulvihill J J, McKeen E A, Rosner F, Zarrabi M H 1987 Pregnancy outcome in cancer patients: experience in a large cooperative group. Cancer 60: 1143

Nelis G F, Van de Meene J G 1980 Comparative effect of cimetidine and ranitidine on prolactin secretion. Postgrad Med J 56: 478

Neri A, Ovadia Y 1980 Fertility problems associated with cystic fibrosis. Int J Gynaecol Obstet 18: 438

Netto N R J, Pecoraro G, Sabbaga E, Mcnczes G, de Góes M 1980 Spermatogenesis before and after renal transplant. Int J Fertil 25: 131

Newmark S R, Rossini A A, Naftolin F I, Todd R, Rose L I, Cahill G F 1979 Gonadotropin profiles in fed and fasted obese women. Am J Obstet Gynecol 133: 75

Newton R A, Boyack T, Agarwal A et al 1988 The effect of cancer on semen quality and cryopreservation of sperm. In: Mulvihill J J, Sherins R J (eds) Reproductive consequences of cancer and cancer therapy. Raven, New York

Nijman J M, Schraffordt-Koops H, Kremer J, Willemse P H, Sleijfer D T, Oldhoff J 1987 Gonadal function after surgery and chemotherapy in men with stage II and III nonseminomatous testicular tumors. J Clin Oncol 5: 651

Nimrod A, Ryan K J 1975 Aromatization of androgens by human abdominal and breast fat tissue. J Clin Endocrinol Metab 40: 367

Nininger J E 1978 Inhibition of ejaculation by amitryptiline. Am J Psychiat 135: 750

Nosal A, Schleissner L A, Mishkin F S, 1979 Angiotensin-converting enzyme and gallium scan in non-invasive evaluation of sarcoidosis. Ann Intern Med 90: 328

Nunez R M, Raad J, Nunez C A 1987 Antibodies against spermatozoids in homosexuals, AIDS and infertile men. Allergol Immunopathol (Madr) 15: 215

Nussbaum M P, Blethen S L, Chasalow F I, Jacobson M S, Shenker I R, Feldman J 1990 Blunted growth hormone responses to clonidine in adolescent girls with early anorexia nervosa. Evidence for an early hypothalamic defect. J Adolesc Health Care 11: 145

O'Morain C, Dore C J, Levi A J 1984 Sulphasalazine and impaired fertility. Gut 25: 1078

Padmanabhan N, Wang D Y, Moore J W, Rubens R D 1987 Ovarian function and adjuvant chemotherapy for early breast cancer. Eur J Cancer Clin Oncol 23: 745

Palmer R L, Crisp A B, Mackinnon P C B, Franklin M, Bonnar J, Wheeler N 1975 Pituitary sensitivity to 50 µg LH/FSH-RH in subjects with anorexia nervosa in acute and recovery stages. Br Med J 1: 179

Pasquali R, Antenucci D, Casimirri F et al 1989 Clinical and hormonal characteristics of obese amenorrheic hyperandrogenic women before and after weight loss. J Clin Endocrinol Metab 68: 173

Patanelli D J 1975 Suppression of fertility in the male. In: Hamilton D W, Greep R O (eds) Handbook of physiology. Williams and Wilkins, Baltimore, p 245

Pavia D, Agnew J W, Batman J R M, Knight R K, Hendry W F, Clark S W 1980 Lung mucociliary clearance in patients with Young's syndrome. Chest 80(suppl): 892

Paz G, Homonnai Z T 1979a Development of diabetic infertility induced by streptozotocin in the male rat. Int J Androl 2: 182

Paz G, Homonnai Z T 1979b Involvement of insulin and testosterone in the reproduction of streptozotocin diabetic rats. Int J Androl 2: 353

Peden N R, Cargill J M, Browning M C, Sanders J H, Wormsley K G 1979a Male sexual dysfunction during treatment with cimetidine. Br Med J 1: 659

Peden N R, Boyd E J, Browning M C, Saunders J H, Wormsley K J 1981 Effects of two histamine H2-receptor blocking drugs on basal levels of gonadotrophins, prolactin, testosterone and oestradiol-17β during treatment of duodenal ulcer in male patients. Acta Endocrinol (Copenh) 96: 564

Pederson J 1954 Foetal mortality in diabetics in relation to management during the latter part of pregnancy. Acta Endocrinol 15: 282

Penn I, Makowski E L, Harris P 1980 Parenthood following renal transplantation. Kidney Int 18: 221

Pennisi A J, Grnshkin L M, Lieberman E 1975 Gonadal function in children with nephrosis treated with cyclophosphamide. Am J Dis Child 129: 315

Perel E, Killinger D W 1979 The interconversion and aromatization of androgens in human adipose tissue. J Steroid Biochem 10: 623

Perez R J, Lipner H, Abdulla N, Cicotto S, Abrams M 1978

Menstrual dysfunction of patients undergoing chronic hemodialysis. Obstet Gynecol 51: 552

Plymate S R, Fariss B L, Bassett M L, Matej L 1981 Obesity and its role in polycystic ovary syndrome. J Clin Endocrinol Metab 52: 1246

Poretsky L, Kalin M F 1987 The gonadotrophic function of insulin. Endocr Rev 8: 132

Portnoy L I, O'Brian J T, Bush J et al 1974 The effect of starvation on the concentration and binding of thyroxine and triiodothyronine in serum and the response to TRH. J Clin Endocrinol Metab 39: 191

Potashnik G, Ben-Aderet N, Israeli R, Yanai-Inbar I, Sober I 1978 Suppressive effect of 1, 2-dibromo-3-chlorphopane on human spermatogenesis. Fertil Steril 30: 444

Potter J D 1980 Hypothyroidism and reproductive failure. Surg Gynecol Obstet 150: 251

Pras M, Gafni J, Jacob E T, Cabili S, Zener D, Sohar E 1984 Recent advances in familial Mediterranean fever. Adv Nephrol 13: 261

Prelevic G M, Wurzburger M I, Peric L A 1987 Blunted prolactin response to metoclopramide in insulin-dependent diabetic patients with secondary amenorrhea. Arch Gynecol Obstet 241: 145

Prelevic G M, Wurzburger M I, Peric L A 1989 The effect of residual beta cell activity on menstruation and the reproductive hormone profile of insulin-dependent diabetics. Arch Gynecol Obstet 244: 207

Price A H, Brogden R N 1988 Nizatidine: a preliminary review of its pharmocodynamic and pharmacokinetic properties, and its therapeutic use in peptic ulcer disease. Drugs 36: 521

Ramirez G, O'Neill W M J, Bloomer H A, Jubiz W 1977 Abnormalities in the regulation of prolactin in patients with chronic renal failure. J Clin Endocrinol Metab 45: 658

Ramsey-Goldman R 1988 Pregnancy in systemic lupus erythematosus. Rheumat Dis Clin North Am 14

Ramsey-Goldman R, Hom D, Deng J S et al 1986 Anti-SS-A antibodies and fetal outcome in maternal systemic lupus erythematosus. Arthritis Rheum 29: 1269

Rasmussen G H, Chen A, Reynolds G F, Patanelli D J, Patchitt A A, Arth G E 1972 Antiandrogens, 2', 3', α-tetrahydrofuran 2'-spiro-17 (2'-α-methylene-4-androsten-3-ones). J Med Chem 15: 1165

Rastogi G K, Chakraborti J, Sinha M K 1974 Serum gonadotrophin (LH and FSH) and their response to synthetic LHRH in diabetic men with and without impotence. Horm Metab Res 6: 335

Ray G R, Trueblood H W, Enright L P, Kaplan H S, Nelson T S 1970 Oophoropexy: a means of preserving ovarian function following pelvic megavoltage radiotherapy for Hodgkin's disease. Radiology 96: 175

Redrow M, Cherem L, Elliott J et al 1988 Dialysis in the management of pregnant patients with renal insufficiency. Medicine (Baltimore) 67: 199

Reed E, Sanger W G, Armitage J O 1986 Results of semen cryopreservation in young men with testicular carcinoma and lymphoma. J Clin Oncol 4: 537

Reid R L, Van Vught D A 1987 Weight related changes in reproductive function. Fertil Steril 48: 905

Rice G G 1973 Hypermenorrhea in the young hemodialysis patient. Am J Obstet Gynecol 116: 539

Riley S A, Lecarpentier J, Mani V, Goodman M J, Mandal B K, Turnberg L A 1987 Sulphasalazine induced seminal abnormalities in ulcerative colitis: results of mesalazine substitution. Gut 28: 1008

Rizkallah T M, Tovell H M M, Kelly W G 1975 Production of estrone and fractional conversion and circulating androstenedione to estrone in women with endometrial carcinoma. J Clin Endocrinol Metab 40: 1045

Rodmark S, Berg A, Kallner G 1988 Hypothalamic-pituitary-testicular axis in patients with hyperthyroidism. Horm Res 29: 185

Rogers J 1958 Menstruation and systemic disease. N Engl J Med 259: 674

Rogers J, Mitchell G W 1952 The relation of obesity to menstrual disturbances. N Engl J Med 247: 53

Rohatgi P K, Ryan J W 1981 Value of serial measurements of serum angiotensin converting enzyme in the management of sarcoidosis. Am J Med 70: 44

Rose L I, Underwood R H, Newmark S R, Kisch E S, Williams G H 1977 Pathophysiology of spironolactone-induced gynecomastia. Ann Intern Med 87: 398

Rubin A 1962 Studies in human reproduction: IV diabetes mellitus and seminal deficiency. Am J Obstet Gynecol 83: 200

Rubin A, Babbot D 1958 Impotence and diabetes mellitus. J A M A 168: 498

Rubin E, Lieber C S, Altman K, Gordon G O, Southern A L 1976 Prolonged ethanol consumption increases testosterone metabolism in the liver. Science 191: 563

Ruder H, Corrol P, Mahoudeau J A, Ross G T, Lipsett M B 1971 Effects of induced hyperthyroidism on steroid metabolism in man. J Clin Endocrinol Metab 33: 382

Rudolph J E, Schweizer R T, Bartus S A 1979 Pregnancy in renal transplant patients. Transplantation 27: 26

Sanborn C F, Martin B J, Wagner W W J 1982 Is athletic amenorrhea specific to runners? Am J Obstet Gynecol 143: 859

Saxena K M, Crawford J D, Talbot N B 1964 Childhood thyrotoxicosis: a long-term prospective. Br Med J 2: 1153

Scadding J G 1961 Calcification in sarcoidosis. Tubercle 42: 121

Scammell G E, White N, Stedronske J, Hendry W F, Edmonds D K, Jeffcoate S L 1985 Cryopreservation of semen in men with testicular tumor or Hodgkin's disease: results of artificial insemination of their partners. Lancet ii: 31

Schalch D S, Gonzalez-Barcena D, Kastin A J et al 1975 Plasma gonadotropins after administration of LH-releasing hormone in patients with renal or hepatic failure. J Clin Endocrinol Metab 41: 921

Scheinberg I H, Sternlieb I 1975 Pregnancy in penicillamine-treated patients with Wilson's disease. N Engl J Med 293: 1300

Schiavi R C 1981 Male erectile disorders. Annu Rev Med 32: 509

Schilsky R L, Lewis B J, Sherins R J, Young R C 1980 Gonadal dysfunction in patients receiving chemotherapy for cancer. Ann Intern Med 93: 109

Schimpff S C, Diggs C H, Wiswell J C, Salvatore P C, Wiernik P H 1980 Radiation related thyroid dysfunction: implications for treatment of Hodgkin's disease. Ann Intern Med 92: 91

Schindler A E, Ebert N, Friedrich E 1972 Conversion of androstenedione to estrone by human fat tissue. J Clin Endocrinol Metab 35: 627

Schmitt G W, Shehadeh I, Sawin C T 1968 Transient gynecomastia in chronic renal failure during chronic intermittent hemodialysis. Ann Intern Med 69: 73

Schneider G, Kirschner M A, Berkowitz R, Ertel N H 1979 Increased estrogen production in obese men. J Clin Endocrinol Metab 48: 633

Schöffling K 1971 Diabetes mellitus and male gonadal function. In: Rodriquez R R, Vallance-Owen J (eds) Proceeding of the Congress of the International Diabetes Federation. Excerpta Medica, Buenos Aires, p 36

Schöffling K, Federlin K, Ditschuneit H, Pfeiffer E F 1963 Disorders of sexual function in male diabetics. Diabetes 12: 519

Schover L R, Novick A C, Steinmuller D R, Goormastic M 1990 Sexuality, fertility, and renal transplantation: a survey of survivors. J Sex Marital Ther 16: 3

Schreiner-Engel P, Schiavi R C, Smith H 1987 The differential impact of diabetes type on female sexuality. J Psychosom Res 31: 23

Schwabe A D, Lippe B M, Chang R J, Pops M A, Yager J 1981 Anorexia nervosa. Ann Intern Med 94: 371

Scuro L A, Bosella O, Cigolini M, Ros A, Pelloso M 1977 Urinary excretion of androsterone and etiocholanalone in obese women: correlation with the cellularity of adipose tissue. J Steroid Biochem 8: 1269

Seifer D B, Collins R 1990 Current concepts of beta endorphin physiology in female reproductive dysfunction. Fertil Steril 54: 757

Shahwan M M, Spathis G S, Fry D E, Wood P J, Marks V 1978 Differences in pituitary and testicular function between diabetic patients on insulin and oral antidiabetic agents. Diabetologia 15: 13

Shalet S M, Beardwell C G, Morris-Jones P H, Pearson D, Orrell D M 1976 Ovarian failure following abdominal irradiation in childhood. Br J Cancer 33: 655

Shamberger R C, Rosenberg S A, Seipp C A, Sherins R J 1981 Effects of high-dose methotrexate and vincristine on ovarian and testicular function in patients undergoing postoperative adjuvant treatment of osteosarcoma. Cancer Treat Rep 65: 739

Shaw P W 1979 Ovary. In: Federman D D (ed) Clinics in endocrinology and metabolism. W B Saunders, London, p 511

Shealy C N, Kahana L, Engel F L, McPherson H T 1961 Hypothalamic-pituitary sarcoidosis: a report on four patients, one with prolonged remission of diabetic insipidus following steroid therapy. Am J Med 30: 46

Sherins R J, Mulvihill J J 1989 Adverse effects of treatment: gonadal dysfunction. In: De Vita V T, Hellman S, Rosenberg S A (eds) Cancer principles & practice of oncology. J B Lippincott, Philadelphia, pp 2170–2180

Sherins R J, Olweny C L M, Ziegler J L 1978 Gynecomastia and gonadal dysfunction in adolescent boys treated with combination chemotherapy for Hodgkin's disease. N Engl J Med 299: 12

Sherman B M, Korenman S G 1974 Measurement of serum LH, FSH, estradiol and progesterone in disorders of the human menstrual cycle: the inadequate luteal phase. J Clin Endocrinol Metab 39: 145

Sherman J R 1973 Synopsis of the use of frozen human semen since 1964. State of the art of human semen banking. Fertil Steril 24: 397

Shultz T, Miller W L, Bedrosian W M 1979 Clinical application of measurement of angiotensin converting enzyme levels. J A M A 242: 439

Sieber S M, Correa P, Dalgard D W, Adamson R H 1978 Carcinogenic and other adverse effects of procarbazine in non-human primates. Cancer Res 38: 2125

Siiteri P K, MacDonald P L 1973 Role of extraglandular estrogen in human endocrinology. In: Greep R O, Astwood E B (eds) Handbook of physiology. American Physiological Society, p 615

Silber J S, Ord T, Balmaceda J, Patrizio P, Asch R H 1990 Congenital absence of the vas deferens. The fertilization capacity of human epididymal sperm. N Engl J Med 323: 1788

Silver M M, Beverly L S, Valberg L S, Cutz E, Philips M J, Shaheed W A 1987 Perinatal hemochromatosis. Clinical, morphologic, and quantitative iron studies. Am J Pathol 128: 538

Silverstein A, Feuer M M, Siltzbach L E 1965 Neurologic sarcoidisis: study of 18 cases. Arch Neurol 12: 1

Singh H 1961 A case of inhibition of ejaculation as a side effect of Melleril. Am J Psychiatry 117: 1041

Smith N J 1980 Excessive weight loss and food aversion in athletes simulating anorexia nervosa. Pediatrics 66: 139

Smith S R, Chhetri M K, Johanson A J, Radfar N, Migeon C J 1975 The pituitary gonadal axis in men with protein calorie malnutrition. J Clin Endocrinol Metab 41: 60

Sobrinho L G, Levine R A, Deconte R L 1971 Amenorrhea in patients with Hodgkin's disease treated with anti neoplastic agents. Am J Obstet Gynecol 109: 135

Southren A C, Olivo J, Gordon G G, Vittels J, Brener J, Rafii F 1974 The conversion of androgens to estrogens in hyperthyroidism. J Clin Endocrinol Metab 38: 207

Spark R F, Melby J C 1968 Aldosteronism in hypertension. The spironolacton response test. Ann Intern Med 69: 685

Spiegel A M, Lopatin R, Peikin S 1978 Serum prolactin in patients receiving chronic oral cimetidine. Lancet i: 881

Steelman S L, Brooks J B, Morgan E P, Patanelli D J 1969 Anti androgen activity of spironolactone. Steroids 14: 449

Steen O P 1984 Side-effects of salazopyrin on male fertility. Eur J Obstet Gynecol Reprod Biol 18: 361

Stempak J G 1962 Maternal hypothyroidism and its effects on fetal development. Endocrinology 70: 443

Steven M M 1981 Pregnancy and liver disease. Gut 22: 592

Strickland D M, Whitted W A, Wians F H J 1990 Screening infertile women for subclinical hypothyroidism. Am J Obstet Gynecol 163: 262

Stuart C A, Neelon F A, Lebowitz H E 1978 Hypothalamic insufficiency: the cause of hypopituitarism in sarcoid. Ann Intern Med 88: 589

Sturgess J M, Chao J, Wong J, Aspin N, Turne J A P 1979 Cilia with defective radial spokes. A cause of human respiratory disease. N Engl J Med 300: 53

Suh B Y, Liu J H, Berga S L, Quigley M E, Laughlin G A, Yen S S 1988 Hypercortisolism in patients with functional hypothalamic amenorrhea. J Clin Endocrinol Metab 66: 733

Summerskil W H J, Davidson C S, Dible J H et al 1960 Cirrhosis of the liver: a study of alcoholic and non-alcoholic patients in Boston and London. N Engl J Med 262: 1

Swamy A P, Woolf P D, Cestero R V M 1979 Hypothalamic-pituitary-ovarian axis in uremic women. J Lab Clin Med 93: 1066

Tarquini H, Gheri R, Anichini P, Neri B, Buricci L 1977 Circadian study of immunoreactive prolactin in patients with cirrhosis of the liver. 73: 116

Taussig L M, Lobeck C C, DiSant'Agnese P A, Ackerman D R, Kattwinkei J 1972 Fertility in males with cystic fibrosis. N Engl J Med 287: 586.

Taymor M L, Selenkow H A 1958 Clinical experiences with L-triiodothyronine in male infertility. Fertil Steril 9: 560

Thomas P R M, Winstanly D, Peckam M J, Austin D E, Murray M A F, Jacobs H S 1976 Reproductive and endocrine function in patients with Hodgkin disease: effect of oophoropexy and irradiation. Br J Cancer 33: 226

Tulchinsky D, Chopra I J 1973 Competitive ligand binding assay for measurement of sex hormone binding globulin. J Clin Endocrinol Metab 37: 873

Turkington R W, Macindoe J H 1972 Hyperprolactinemia in sarcoidosis. Ann Intern Med 76: 545

Umeki S 1988 Primary mucociliary transport failure. Respiration 54: 220

Van de Wiele R L 1977 Anorexia nervosa and the hypothalamus. Hospital Practice 12(Dec): 45

Van Thiel D H 1989 Disorders of the hypothalamic-pituitary-gonadal adrenal thyroidal axes in patients with liver disease. In: Zakim D, Boyer T D (eds) Hepatology. W B Saunders, Philadelphia, pp 513–530

Van Thiel D H, Lester R 1979 The effect of chronic alcohol abuse on sexual function. Clin Endocrinol Metab 8: 499

Van Thiel D H, Gavaler J S 1986 Hypothalamic-pituitary-gonadal function in liver disease with particular attention to the endocrine effects of chronic alcohol abuse. Prog Liver Dis 8: 273

Van Thiel D H, Gavaler J, Lester R 1974a Ethanol inhibition of Vitamin A metabolism in the testes: possible mechanism for sterility in alcoholics. Sciences 186: 941

Van Thiel D H, Lester R, Sherins R J 1974b Hypogonadism in alcoholic liver disease: evidence for a double defect. 67: 1188

Van Thiel D H, Lester R, Vaitukaitis J 1978a Evidence for a defect in pituitary secretion of luteinizing hormone in chronic alcoholic men. J Clin Endocrinol Metab 47: 499

Van Thiel D H, Gavaler J S, Lester R, Sherins R J 1978b Alcohol induced ovarian failure in the rat. J Clin Invest 61: 624

Van Thiel D H, Gavaler J S, Smith W I J, Paul G 1979 Hypothalamic-pituitary-gonadal dysfunction in men using cimetidine. N Engl J Med 300: 1012

Van Thiel D H, Gavaler J S, Herman G B, Lester R, Smith W I J, Gay V L 1980 An evaluation of the respective roles of liver disease and malnutrition in the pathogenesis of the hypogonadism seen in alcoholic rats. Gastroenterology 79: 533

Van Thiel D H, Gavaler J S, Cobb C F, Sanfucci L, Graham T O 1983a Ethanol, a leydig cell toxin: evidence obtained in vivo and in vitro. Pharmacol Biochem Behav 18(suppl 1): 317

Van Thiel D H, Gaveler J S, Sanghvi A 1983b Recovery of sexual function in abstinent alcoholic men. Gastroenterology 84: 677

Van Thiel D H, Gavaler J S, Schade R R 1985 Liver disease and the hypothalamic-pituitary-gonadal axis. Semin Liver Dis 5: 35

Van Thiel D H, Gavaler J S, Heyl A, Susen B 1987 An evaluation of the antiandrogen effects associated with H2 antagonist therapy. Scand J Gastroenterol Suppl 136: 24

Vandenbroucke J P, Valkenburg H A 1981 Thinness, delayed menarche and irregular cycles. N Engl J Med 305: 229

Vannasaeng S, Fucharoen S, Pootrakul P, Ploybut S, Yansukon P 1991 Pituitary function in thalassemic patients and the effect of chelation therapy. Acta Endocrinol 124: 23

Varma R R 1987 Course and prognosis of pregnancy in women with liver disease. Semin Liver Dis 7: 59

Varma S K, Murray R, Stanbury J B 1978 Effect of maternal hypothyroidism and triiodothyronine on the fetus and newborn in rats. Endocrinology 102: 24

Vigersky R A, Andersen A E, Thompson R H, Loriaux D L 1977 Hypothalamic dysfunction in secondary amenorrhea associated with simple weight loss. N Engl J Med 297: 1141

Vilar O 1974 Effect of cytostatic drugs on human testicular function. In: Mancini R E, Martini L (eds) Male fertility and sterility. Academic, New York, pp 423–440

Vivani S, Santoro A, Ragri G, Bonfante V, Bestch O, Bonadonna G 1985 Gonadal toxicity after combination chemotherapy for Hodgkin's disease: comparative results of MOPP vs. ABVD. Eur J Cancer Clin Oncol 21: 601

Vogt H J, Weidenbach T, Marquart K H, Vogel G E 1987 Idiopathic hemochromatosis in a 45-year-old infertile man. Andrologia 19: 532

Walsh P C, Mostwin J L 1984 Radical prostatectomy and cystoprostatectomy with preservation of potency: results using a new nerve sparing technique. Br J Urol 56: 694

Walsh P C, Lepor H, Eggleston J C 1983 Radical prostatectomy with preservation of sexual function: anatomical and pathological considerations. Prostate 4: 473

Walshe J M 1977 Pregnancy in Wilson's disease. Q J Med 46: 73

Walt H, Campana A, Balerna M et al 1983 Mosaicism of dynein in spermatozoa and cilia and fibrous sheath aberrations in an infertile man. Andrologia 15: 295

Walters D, Kaufman M S 1959 Sterility due to retrograde ejaculation of semen: report of pregnancy achieved by autoinsemination. Am J Obstet Gynecol 78: 274

Warne G L, Fairley K F, Hobbs J B, Martin F I R 1973 Cyclophosphamide-induced ovarian failure. N Engl J Med 289: 1159

Waxman J S, Sher J M 1979 The spectrum of central nervous system sarcoidosis. A clinical and pathologic study. Mount Sinai J Med 46: 309

Waxman J H, Terry Y A, Wrigley P F M et al 1982 Gonadal function in Hodgkin's disease: long-term followup of chemotherapy. Br Med J 285: 1612

Weltman E A, Stern R C, Doershuk C F, Moir R N, Palmer K, Jaffe A C 1990 Weight and menstrual function in patients with eating disorders and cystic fibrosis. Pediatrics 85: 282

Whitehead E, Shalet S M, Blackledge G, Todd I, Crowther R D, Beardwell C G 1982 The effects of Hodgkin's disease and combination chemotherapy on gonadal function in the adult male. Cancer 49: 418

Whitehead E, Shalet S M, Blackledge G, Todd I, Growther R D, Beardwell C G 1983 The effect of combination chemotherapy on ovarian function in women treated for Hodgkin's disease. Cancer 52: 988

Wilsnack S C, Klassen A D, Wilsnack R W 1984 Drinking and reproductive dysfunction among women in 1981 national survey. Alcohol Clin Exp Res 8: 451

Winnacker J L, Becker K L, Katz S, Matthews M J 1967 Recurrent epididymitis in sarcoidosis: report of a patient treated with corticosteroids. Ann Intern Med 66: 743

Winnacker J L, Becker K L, Katz S 1968 Endocrine aspects of sarcoidosis †(two parts). N Engl J Med 278: 427, 483

Winslow R C, Funckhouser J W 1968 Sarcoidosis of the female reproductive organs. Report of a case. Obstet Gynecol 32: 285

Winters S J, Banks J L, Loriaux D L 1979 The histamine H2-antagonist cimetidine as an antiandrogen. Gastroenterology 76: 504

Wortsman J, Rosner W, Dufau M L 1987 Abnormal testicular function in men with primary hypothyroidism. Am J Med 82: 207

Wright A D, London D R, Holder G, Williams J W, Rudd B T 1976 Luteinizing release hormone tests in impotent diabetic males. Diabetes 25: 925

Yen S S C 1980 The polycystic ovary syndrome. Clin Endocrinol 12: 177

Yen S S, Jaffe R B 1986 Reproductive endocrinology. W B Saunders, Philadelphia

Ylikahri R, Huttunen M, Harkonen M, Adlercreutz H 1974 Hangover and testosterone. Br Med J 2: 445

Zemer D, Pras M, Sohar E, Modan M, Cabili S, Gafni J 1980 Colchicin in the prevention and treatment of the amyloidosis of familial Mediterranean fever. N Engl J Med 314: 1001

Zondek L H, Zondek T 1980 Normal and abnormal development of the epididymis of the fetus and infant. Eur J Pediatr 134: 39

Zorgniotti A W, Liza E 1988 Vascular disease as a cause of impotence. Clin Diabetes 137

# 30.  The ethical aspects of infertility and assisted reproduction

*Howard W. Jones Jr*

## TENETS OF ETHICAL EVALUATION

An ethical verdict is reached by the solution of a calculus which involves four principal variables: (1) the human person; (2) the family; (3) the community; and (4) society. Whatever enhances the moral status and dignity of each of these can be considered morally acceptable. Whatever is degrading is morally unacceptable. Generally, there is some tension among these entities so that a solution of the moral calculus requires some compromise of the interest of one or more of these principal variables.

The situation is further complicated by several modifying considerations: (1) experience; (2) cultural background; (3) the law; and (4) religious authority.

The solution of the ethical calculus is very complex. If, however, it is agreed that the mentioned variables and modifiers, and perhaps others, must each be considered, it follows that an ethical judgment by its very nature is not immutable nor universal — what is ethically acceptable in one setting or in one era may not necessarily be acceptable in another setting or era. A moral dilemma often results from attempts to accommodate divergent judgments. Serious mischief is apt to arise if an attempt is made to impose forcibly on others a moral judgment, however derived.

## ETHICAL EVALUATION OF INFERTILITY

To solve the ethical calculus for infertility requires certain modification of the principal variables. Thus, the human person becomes the human couple, although each partner has a unique interest. Furthermore, there is a special variable, the potential child. Note that the doctor or other health provider (an immoral term, as it is degrading) has little claim to a value in the solution of the calculus, except as a partner or as a member of the family, community or society, where the interest may be in conflict with that of the couple.

## THE ETHICS OF INFERTILITY

The following discussion is an attempt to apply the tenets of ethics as briefly outlined to the various facets of infertility by asking a series of questions. Because of space, the questions cannot be exhaustive. Thus, for example, surrogacy will be excluded.

### Who should treat the infertile couple?

As the solution of the problem of infertility of a couple will enhance the moral status of that couple, the objective of overcoming the infertility certainly takes precedence over almost all other considerations in this particular situation. Of the three recognized subspecialties of obstetrics and gynecology — fetal/maternal medicine, oncology and reproductive medicine — poor diagnosis and therapy of the first two subspecialties may be manifest by the obvious and alarming endpoint of death, but with infertility, poor diagnosis and therapy may be quite unrecognized by the couple or others. This means that there is a special moral burden on those who would undertake to advise and treat the infertile couple. Obviously, where access to care is limited, available help must be utilized. Where options exist as in large metropolitan areas, those who accept patients with infertility have a moral imperative to carry the investigation and any therapy only to the limit of their competence and availability of support services, and above all, to do no harm before sending the patient to the next level of specialization. This view is guaranteed to be contentious as impeccable data do not exist to support the just stated attitude. However, anecdotal experience would suggest that infertility, even in highly developed areas, is often not well cared for with failure to achieve pregnancy, delay in applying appropriate therapy, and worse yet, the application of inappropriate therapy, especially surgical, which greatly compromises ultimate success.

## What is the ethical management of the infertile couple?

In this era of reproductive freedom and autonomy, the health care provider has only limited options to question the request for therapy of infertility. This is not true everywhere in the world. The one-child-per-family goal in China, and the tax and other disincentives for increasing numbers of children in Singapore are but examples. Nevertheless, health care providers should realize that they are treating not infertility, but a couple—two individuals, with infertility. This couple suffers special pressures—family and societal — and may have anxieties borne of unfulfilled dreams and guilt from previous reproductive misfortunes.

Furthermore, reproductive freedom does not relieve the provider from counselling the couple about such reproductive alternatives as barrenness, or adoption, and, if necessary, the use of extraconjugal gametes or preembryos. Warnock is particularly insistent on counselling (Department of Health & Social Security 1984) and insists that the counselling be done by other than the physician in charge, presumably to prevent a conflict of interest.

## What diagnostic and therapeutic options should be offered to the infertile couple?

There seems to be no expressed public concern of an ethical nature about diagnosis and treatment options for infertile couples, up to the use of techniques of assisted reproduction, that is, of in vitro fertilization (IVF) and allied technologies. The lack of expressed public concern again puts a special moral imperative on those utilizing standard investigative and therapeutic alternatives. It is not the function of this chapter to set forth minimal standards for an initial infertility investigation, but studies of the cervix, uterus, tubes, ovaries and peritoneum are required for the female, and standard studies for the male. High ethical standards require that the physician carry out these investigations in an orderly sequence uninfluenced by the level of the fee for the service rendered. The insurance industry carries a special burden in this regard. Provision is often made to cover only a limited number of diagnostic procedures, curiously enough, often only *surgical*. It can be considered ethically highly problematical for the initial workup to be only minimal, plus a laparoscopy prior to sending the patient to a higher level of experience.

Thus, the couple with infertility is in a medically vulnerable situation and health providers at all levels bear a heavy responsibility to see that the couple receives impeccable investigation and therapy with conventional methodology, or with assisted reproductive technology, depending on which is appropriate. In general, conventional methodology should be first, but there are circumstances where assisted reproductive technology represents the first and best option for the couple. An example might be in a couple where the woman is approaching 40, and where moderate endometriosis explains the difficulty. This couple would surely benefit by proceeding directly to assisted reproductive technology, rather than spending the time with medical or surgical management at an advanced reproductive age. It is in the best interest of the couple to see that optimum therapy be applied to the particular situation of the couple, and not that the couple receive therapy, which happens to be more convenient or is the only therapy at hand.

It would be tedious to pursue in further detail the ethics of the diagnosis and treatment of infertility short of the application of assisted reproductive technology. Suffice it to summarize that the ethics of assisted reproductive technology has had wide public discussion, while the ethics of standard investigative and conventional therapy has received little ethical attention. As repeatedly mentioned, it is for this reason that those who first see the infertile couple bear a heavy moral responsibility for the application of proper and contemporary techniques.

## Is the use of IVF morally acceptable?

There has probably been no medical procedure which has been examined so carefully from a moral point of view as IVF. There is a general consensus that there is no moral problem intrinsic in the use of this process in the sample case, i.e. with the gametes of husband and wife. Leroy Walters (1987) summarized some 85 reports of various official and unofficial bodies of 20 countries which have studied this question. Among these 85 reports, there were 15 which were over 50 pages in length and, without exception, IVF was found to be acceptable by these committees representing various countries: Australia (six), UK (two), USA (two), France (one), Netherlands (one), Spain (one), West Germany (one) and Canada (one).

The only major document (although less than 50 pages in length) which held that IVF and other allied technologies were ethically suspect was the 'Instruction on the Respect for Human Life in its Origin and on the Dignity Procreation' (Donum Vitae), issued in 1987 by the Congregation for the Doctrine of the Faith of the Vatican. The instruction rejected IVF on the grounds that it involved a separation between 'the goods and meanings of marriage', that is, the unitive and procreative. The separation of these two dimensions meant, according to Donum Vitae, that procreation was 'deprived of its proper perfection', and was therefore 'not in conformity with the dignity of the person'. In other words, the child must be conceived through an act of love, and specifically, through sexual intercourse. The Ethics Committee of The American Fertility Society replied to Donum Vitae in a special supplement in the February 1988 issue of *Fertility and Sterility* published as part of Volume 49. The Ethics Committee found that the conclusion reached by Donum Vitae was quite problematical,

but it agreed with the 'instruction' that 'the one conceived must be the fruit of his parents' love'. The Committee could not understand how the conclusion was drawn in Donum Vitae that this love must in all circumstances mean sexual intercourse. In the opinion of the The American Fertility Ethics Committee, what happens to 'the goods and meaning of marriage' involves the total relationship and not necessarily the individual act. The Committee furthermore questioned that an act 'deprived of its proper perfection' was necessarily morally wrong. The Committee pointed out that human actions are often not ideal, and in that sense, are 'deprived of their proper perfection'. Such actions, however, are not necessarily morally wrong.

Donum Vitae has undoubtedly had its influence on the decision of individual couples to utilize the strategy of IVF; however, in a global sense, it seems unlikely that its influence has been substantial. For example, at the in vitro program in Norfolk, the percentage of Catholic patients seeking assistance corresponds with the percentage of Catholic couples in the USA.

Donum Vitae, on strict reading, would seem to categorize all techniques of artificial reproduction as illicit, including gamete intrafallopian transfer (GIFT). However, individual clergymen within the Catholic tradition have publicly stated that individuals utilizing IVF, GIFT, and indeed, other methods of artificial reproduction, should not be considered to have sinned.

## Are GIFT and other methods of artificial reproduction using conjugal gametes ethically acceptable?

The ethical pros and cons of GIFT and other methods of artificial reproduction are really not too different from those which are applied to IVF. Where these more recent techniques have been considered by ethics committees, their evaluation has been based largely on indications and efficacy. Generally, the evaluation boils down to meeting three minimal standards:

1.  Have the patient and her partner been investigated according to recent standards of investigation as, for instance, those promulgated by the

American Fertility Society for the investigation of infertile couples?

2. Does the patient have a condition which requires the use of some technique of assisted reproduction and, therefore, does not have a condition amenable to less invasive techniques?

3. Does the facility have a gamete laboratory and personnel meeting minimal standards for an IVF program as, for example, those standards promulgated by the American Fertility Society?

The importance of the criteria just mentioned is to guard against the excessive use of techniques of assisted reproduction without adequate investigation and with assurance that simpler techniques are used prior to resorting to the more complicated methodology of assisted reproduction. The importance of the third consideration is to provide for flexibility and therapy during an assisted reproductive technology procedure, wherein it would be found that, for whatever reason, the original technique was not applicable to the anticipated situation.

### Is it ethical to use extraconjugal gametes?

The use of extraconjugal gametes is highly controversial. If religious authority be accepted and if religious authority opposes the use of extraconjugal gametes, they will not be used in this circumstance. It needs to be mentioned that if a couple is prepared to use extraconjugal gametes and the medical advisor is opposed to their use, it is incumbent upon the adviser to recognize the autonomy of the couple and to indicate where further advice can be obtained.

Several theoretical reasons have been advanced for discouraging the use of extraconjugal gametes. It is said that their use violates the marriage covenant wherein exclusive vows are exchanged. Furthermore, it is held that the use of one extraconjugal gamete blurs the child's genealogy. While these objections are substantial, it is probably fair to say that it would be difficult to support these positions by sophisticated experience. On the contrary, experience would suggest, at least in the short term, that children introduced into a family by the use of extraconjugal sperm or extraconjugal eggs, as the case may be, have a very

satisfactory track record. Unfortunately, follow-up of children resulting from the use of extraconjugal sperm which has been in practice for several decades are conspicuous by their absence, and probably for obvious reasons. If practical considerations could be somehow or other overcome, such a study would be of immeasurable value.

If one is prepared to use either donated sperm or donated eggs, there are several clinical circumstances where they might be applicable. First and foremost, and in use for many years, has been the use of donor sperm where there is intractable infertility in the husband, which even now cannot be overcome by IVF. On the other hand, in the situations where there is a premature menopause, or in the case of either male or female when the couple does not wish to risk an undesirable gene, extraconjugal gametes have proven to be a very worthwhile procedure.

In the event that donor gametes are to be used, it seems clear that several guidelines should be invoked. In order to prevent the commercialization of the procedure, compensation to the donors for eggs or sperm should be avoided. This does not mean that reimbursement for expenses, time, risk and inconvenience associated with the donation should not be recognized. There is very little risk to the donation of sperm, but there is risk to the donation of eggs, and donors must be informed about these matters.

The question of anonymity of donors is complex and there has been a certain movement to make all information available to children so conceived. However, it is difficult to believe that there is reason to transmit this information except for assurances on an anonymous basis about inheritable traits, so far as that can be given. Protection of the donor for an act which must be viewed as very charitable has a high priority. Some political jurisdictions have legislation which protects donors, mostly of sperm, by laws enacted before donor eggs were possible, protecting them from responsibility in the event of congenital anomalies or claims for economic support. On balance, evaluating the claim of all participants, it seems reasonable that anonymity is a desirable goal. This is not to say that in very special circumstances, donation by a family member might not be considered, but the pros and cons need to be thoroughly discussed by all concerned.

It is generally considered proper in donor programs to be sure that the donor has been suitably screened for undesirable genetic traits and that appropriate tests have been done to eliminate infections, particularly such infection as AIDS. While there are indeed laudable goals, it is interesting that no genetic screening is required for couples who wish to be married in the ordinary course of events.

## Are there any ethical objections to the use of cryopreservation?

Cryopreservation, like the use of extraconjugal gametes, can be very controversial, especially if there is opposition by religious authority. It is interesting that many moral theologians have been concerned only about the loss of preembryos during the cryopreservation process, pointing out that if cryopreservation were 100% efficient, i.e. that all preembryos frozen would, when thawed, survive, that cryopreservation could not be considered ethically objectionable because it, in fact, preserves individual human life. At the practical level, cryopreservation has proven to be extraordinarily useful in improving pregnancy rates with assisted reproduction, and in avoiding the complication associated with multiple pregnancies. Thus, it is possible to harvest and fertilize any number of eggs and limit the transfer to three or less, or any given number, in order to prevent the obstetrical and social complication of multiple births. At the same time, it is possible to cryopreserve very early in development fertilizing or fertilized eggs, which can be utilized at some time in the future to achieve the reproductive goals of prospective parents. In a recent study in Norfolk for example, among patients who had eggs cryopreserved over a 4-year period, the average pregnancy rate was increased by some 9%. This is a major

accomplishment. It needs to be emphasized, however, that long-term risks cannot be fully assessed at the present time. It seems that there is no increase in fetal anomalies from cryopreserved prezygotes or preembryos, but obviously the assessment of long-term risks cannot be ascertained.

It also needs to be emphasized that there are several issues related to the disposition of unused cryopreserved preembryos which are of extreme importance. Various catastrophies can happen, such as the death of prospective parents or the disability of one of the prospective parents, separation, divorce, abandonment and so forth. In order to try to prevent unpleasant litigation in regard to these matters, it seems important that in programs utilizing cryopreservation, an agreement with the prospective parents should be arranged prior to the cryopreservation, providing for the ultimate utilization of the cryopreserved material in the event that any one of a number of untoward events might occur.

It is far too early to know whether such contracts will prevent all litigation; in a litigious society, it seems unlikely. Nevertheless, these risks are real and prospective parents and programs utilizing cryopreservation should be alerted to these concerns. Those in responsibility should feel a moral obligation to mitigate potential problems in this area.

## SUMMARY

Ethical evaluation is not an exact discipline. It is unlikely that there can be general agreement on an absolute. Thus, there is no absolute moral right and no absolute moral wrong. To impose one's moral imperative unwillingly on another is nothing less than tyranny, from which man has struggled from eternity. In working with infertile couples, the goal is to enhance the moral status and dignity of the human couple and any potential offspring.

REFERENCES

Department of Health and Social Security 1984 In: Warnock M (ed) Report of the Committee of Inquiry into Human Fertilisation and Embryology. Her Majesty's Stationery Office, London, pp 27, 63

Walters L 1987 Biomedical ethics: a multinational view. In: Hastings Center Report June (suppl)

# Index